COMPACT AMERICAN

MEDICAL DICTIONARY

A Concise and

Up-to-Date

Guide to

Medical Terms

HOUGHTON MIFFLIN COMPANY
BOSTON · NEW YORK

Editorial and Production Staff

EDITORIAL STAFF

**Vice President, Director of Lexical Publishing,
Production, and Manufacturing Services**
Margery S. Berube

Executive Editor
Joseph P. Pickett

Senior Editor
Rosemary E. Previte,
Project Director

Contributing Editors
Ann Marie Menting
Lois J. Principe
Marion Severynse

PRODUCTION STAFF

Managing Editor
Christopher Leonesio

Production Supervisor
Elizabeth J. Rubè

Book Design
Joyce C. Weston

**Senior Art and Production
Coordinator**
Margaret Anne Miles

Illustrations
Laurel Cook Lhowe

Library of Congress Cataloging-in-Publication Data

Compact American medical dictionary.
     p.   cm.
   ISBN 0-395-88409-8 (flexi)
   1. Medicine—Dictionaries.
 R121.C665   1998
 610′.3—dc21
                                     98-20456
                                       CIP

ABCDEFG-WCT-998
Manufactured in the United States of America

Contents

Preface

The Compact American Medical Dictionary is designed for general readers, students, and professionals in fields such as medicine, nursing, allied health, insurance, and medical office management — in short, for anyone who needs clear, concise information about the language of medicine and health. The definitions have been written so that they are easy to understand, without including excessive detail or compromising their technical precision. *The Compact American Medical Dictionary* is a user-friendly reference on modern medicine for the home or office, providing updated, vitally important data useful for studying, communicating, and planning personal health strategies.

Guide to the Dictionary

GUIDEWORDS

Guidewords are printed at the top left and top right corners of every two-page spread:

arch of aorta
arthropathy

SYLLABICATION

An entry and its inflected and derived forms are syllabicated with boldface centered dots:

u·ra·ni·um (yōō-rā′nē-əm) *n.*

In compound entries composed of two or more words, individual words within the compound may not be syllabicated if they are entered separately in the Dictionary with syllabication or if they are common English words that can be found in any general dictionary:

digital sub·trac·tion angiography (səb-trăk′shən) *n.*
graft-versus-host disease *n.*

Pronunciations are also syllabicated, but the syllabication of the phonetic form does not necessarily match the syllabication of the graphic form of the entry word. The former follows phonological rules, while the latter represents the typesetting practice of breaking words at the ends of lines of text.

PRONUNCIATION

Pronunciations are immediately after the boldface entry word. Variant pronunciations are given wherever necessary. When there is more than one pronunciation, all are acceptable, even though some may be used more frequently than others. A full pronunciation key is given on page vi.

Schwa. The symbol ə — called a *schwa* — is used to represent a vowel that receives the weakest level of stress within a word and that usually has a different quality than it would if stressed, as in the third syllable of **biology** (bī-ŏl′ə-jē).

Stress. There are three relative degrees of stress or loudness with which the syllables of a word are spoken. A syllable with primary, or strongest, stress is indicated by a boldface mark (′); one with secondary, or weaker, stress has a lighter mark (′); and one with the weakest stress has no mark.

PART-OF-SPEECH LABELS

The following italicized part-of-speech labels appear after the pronunciation:

adj.	adjective
adv.	adverb
n.	noun
v.	verb

And this label indicates inflected forms:

pl.   plural

Entries that are abbreviations, such as *CDC* and *DDI*, are labeled *abbr.*

INFLECTED FORMS

An inflected form differs from the main entry form by the addition of a suffix or by a change in the base form to indicate grammatical features such as number, person, mood, or tense. The following inflected forms are given in the main entries in this Dictionary: (1) principal parts of all verbs, (2) comparative and superlative degrees of adjectives and adverbs formed by inflection, and (3) irregular plurals of nouns.

Inflected forms follow the part-of-speech label and are syllabicated, set in boldface type, and given a pronunciation when necessary. When more than one inflected form is given, the forms are separated by commas. Inflected forms are usually cut back to the last syllable of the original entry word plus the inflected ending. Irregular inflections are written out to the extent that clarity requires. When inflected forms are cut back, the shortened forms are preceded by boldface hyphens:

a·nes·the·tize (ənĕs′thĭ-tīz′) *v.* **-tized, -tiz·ing, -tiz·es.**

Principal parts of verbs. The principal parts of verbs are entered in this order: *past tense, past participle, present participle,* and *third person singular present tense.* When the past tense and past participle are identical, one form represents both:

di·vide (dĭ-vīd′) *v.* **-vid·ed, -vid·ing, -vides.**

Degrees in adjectives and adverbs. Adjectives and adverbs forming the comparative and superlative degrees by addition of *-er* and *-est* to unchanged entry words show these suffixes after their respective part-of-speech labels:

sick (sĭk) *adj.* **sick·er, sick·est.**

Irregular adjectives and adverbs are those whose forms change upon addition of *-er* and *-est.* These forms follow the general rules of style and presentation for all inflections.

Plurals of nouns. Plurals of nouns other than those formed by the addition of *-s* or *-es* are labeled *pl.*

louse (lous) *n., pl.* **lice** (līs).

When a noun has both regular and irregular plural forms, the most common form is shown first:

a·me·ba or **a·moe·ba** (ə-mē′bə) *n., pl.* **-bas** or **-bae** (-bē).

A noun that is plural both in form and in meaning is labeled *pl.n.:*

abdominal reflexes *pl.n.* Contractions of the muscles of the abdominal wall upon stimulation of the skin or upon the tapping of neighboring bony structures.

CROSS-REFERENCES

When two terms are synonymous, a full definition appears at the primary term. The secondary terms are defined by the primary term, set in secondary boldface letters and followed, if necessary, by the number indicating the sense of the main entry at which a full definition can be found. For instance, **lockjaw** is a cross-reference entry referring the reader to sense **1** of **tetanus:**

lock·jaw (lŏk′jô′) *n.* **1.** See **tetanus** (sense 1). **2.** See **trismus.**

At sense **1** of **tetanus,** the full definition is given:

tet·a·nus (tĕt′n-əs) *n.* **1.** An acute, often fatal disease characterized by spasmodic contraction of voluntary muscles, especially those of the neck and jaw, and caused by the neurotoxin of *Clostridium tetani,* which typically infects the body through a deep wound.

If, however, a secondary term falls adjacent to the primary term, it is not given separate entry.

VARIANTS

All variants in this Dictionary are set in boldface type with the word *or* between the main entry term and its variant:

ba·be·si·o·sis (bə-bē′zē-ō′sĭs) or **bab·e·si·a·sis** (băb′ĭ-zī′ə-sĭs) *n.*

UNDEFINED FORMS

At the end of many entries additional boldface words appear without definitions—words that are formed either from the entry word by the addition of suffixes or that are closely related to the entry word. These forms can include the entry word itself with a different part of speech. These *run-on entries* are related to the entry word but may have different grammatical functions as indicated by their part-of-speech labels. Pronunciations are included as required. At the main entry **anesthetize,** the undefined run-on is:

a·nes·the·tize (ə-nĕs′thĭ-tīz′) *v.* **-tized, -tiz·ing, -tiz·es.** To induce anesthesia in. — **an· es′the·ti·za′tion** (-tĭ-zā shən) *n.*

When different run-on forms have the same grammatical function and meaning, they are separated by a comma and share a single part-of-speech label. For example, at **lipogenesis,** these adjectives have the same function and meaning:

lip·o·gen·e·sis (lĭp′ə-jĕn′ĭ-sĭs) *n.* **1.** Production of fat, either fatty degeneration or fatty infiltration. Also called *adipogenesis.* **2.** The normal deposition of fat or the conversion of carbohydrate or protein to fat. — **lip′o·gen′ic** (-jĕn′ĭk), **li·pog′e·nous** (lĭ-pŏj′ə-nəs) *adj.*

Pronunciation Key

The pronunciation symbols used in this Dictionary are listed in the column headed **Symbols.** In the column headed **Examples** a word or words illustrates how the symbol is pronounced. The letters that correspond in sound to the symbols are in boldface type.

Symbols	Examples
ă	pat
ā	pay
âr	care
ä	father
b	bib
ch	church
d	deed, milled
ě	pet
ē	bee
f	fife, phase, rough
g	gag
h	hat

Symbols	Examples
ĭ	pit
ī	pie, by
j	judge
k	kick, cat, pique
l	lid, needle (nēd′l)*
m	mum
n	no, sudden (sŭd′n)*
ng	thing
ŏ	pot
ō	toe
ô	caught, paw, for
oi	noise
ŏŏ	took
ōō	boot
ou	out
p	pop
r	roar
s	sauce
sh	ship, dish
t	tight, stopped
th	thin
th	this
ŭ	cut

Symbols	Examples
ûr	urge, term, firm, heard
v	valve
w	with
y	yes
z	zebra, xylem
zh	vision, pleasure, garage
ə	about, item, edible, gallop, circus
ər	butter

Foreign

œ	*French* feu, *German* schön
ü	*French* tu, *German* über
KH	*German* ich, *Scottish* loch
N	*French* bon

Stress

Primary (′)   **global** (glō′bəl)
Secondary (′)   **globalize** (glō′bə-līz′)

* In English the consonants *l* and *n* often constitute complete syllables by themselves.

A

Ab *abbr.* antibody

a·bar·og·no·sis (ă-băr′ŏg-nō′sĭs) *n.* Loss of the ability to sense weight.

a·ba·sia (ə-bā′zhə) *n.* Inability to walk due to impaired muscular coordination. — **a·ba′sic, a·bat′ic** *adj.*

abasia-astasia *n.* See astasia-abasia.

abasia trep·i·dans (trĕp′ĭ-dănz′) *n.* Abasia due to trembling of the legs.

Ab·bé operation (ăb′ē) *n.* The transfer of a flap of the full thickness of the middle portion of the lower lip into the upper lip.

Ab·bott's method (ăb′əts) *n.* A method of treating scoliosis by applying a series of plaster jackets after partial correction of the curvature by external force.

ab·do·men (ăb′də-mən, ăb-dō′mən) *n.* The part of the body that lies between the chest and the pelvis and encloses the stomach, intestines, liver, spleen, and pancreas. — **ab·dom′i·nal** (ăb-dŏm′-ə-nəl) *adj.* — **ab·dom′i·nal·ly** *adv.*

abdominal cavity *n.* The space bounded by the abdominal walls, diaphragm, and pelvis and containing the major organs of digestion, the spleen, the kidneys, and the adrenal glands.

abdominal external oblique muscle *n.* An abdominal muscle whose action diminishes the capacity of the abdomen and draws the chest downward.

abdominal guarding *n.* A spasm of the abdominal wall muscles to protect inflamed abdominal viscera from pressure; it usually results from inflammation of the peritoneal surface as in appendicitis, diverticulitis, or generalized peritonitis, and is detectable on palpation.

abdominal hernia *n.* A hernia protruding through or into any part of the abdominal wall.

abdominal hysterectomy *n.* A hysterectomy made through an incision in the abdominal wall.

abdominal hysterotomy *n.* Hysterotomy performed through the abdominal wall.

abdominal internal oblique muscle *n.* An abdominal muscle whose action diminishes the capacity of the abdomen and bends the chest forward.

abdominal pregnancy *n.* An ectopic pregnancy developing in the peritoneal cavity, usually secondary to an early rupture of a tubal pregnancy.

abdominal reflexes *pl.n.* Contractions of the muscles of the abdominal wall upon stimulation of the skin or upon the tapping of neighboring bony structures.

abdominal region *n.* Any of the topographical subdivisions of the abdomen, including the right or left hypochondriac, the right or left lateral, the right or left inguinal, and the epigastric, umbilical, or pubic regions.

abdominal respiration *n.* Breathing that occurs primarily by the action of the diaphragm.

abdominal section *n.* See celiotomy.

ab·dom·i·no·cen·te·sis (ăb-dŏm′ə-nō-sĕn-tē′sĭs) *n.* Surgical puncture of the abdomen by a needle to withdraw fluid; abdominal paracentesis.

ab·dom·i·no·cy·e·sis (ăb-dŏm′ə-nō-sī-ē′sĭs) *n.* **1.** See abdominal pregnancy. **2.** See secondary abdominal pregnancy.

ab·dom·i·no·hys·ter·ec·to·my (ăb-dŏm′ə-nō-hĭs′tə-rĕk′tə-mē) *n.* See abdominal hysterectomy.

ab·dom·i·no·hys·ter·ot·o·my (ăb-dŏm′ə-nō-hĭs′tə-rŏt′ə-mē) *n.* See abdominal hysterotomy.

ab·dom·i·no·plas·ty (ăb-dŏm′ə-nō-plăs′tē) *n.* An operation performed on the abdominal wall for cosmetic purposes.

ab·dom·i·nos·co·py (ăb-dŏm′ə-nŏs′kə-pē) *n.* Internal examination of the abdomen through the use of an endoscope; peritoneoscopy.

ab·duce (ăb-dōōs′, -dyōōs′) *v.* **-duced, -duc·ing, -duc·es.** To abduct.

ab·du·cent nerve (ăb-dōō′sənt, -dyōō′-) *n.* The cranial motor nerve supplying the lateral rectus muscle of the eyes.

abducent *adj.* Abducting; drawing away.

ab·duct (ăb-dŭkt′) *v.* **-duct·ed, -duct·ing, -ducts.** To draw away from the midline of the body or from an adjacent part or limb. — **ab·duc′tion** *n.*

ab·duc·tor (ăb-dŭk′tər) *n.* A muscle that draws a body part, such as a finger, arm, or toe, away from the midline of the body or of an extremity.

A·bell-Ken·dall method (ā′bəl-kĕn′dl) *n.* A standard method for estimating serum cholesterol without interference from bilirubin, protein, and hemoglobin.

ab·er·rant (ă-bĕr′ənt, ăb′ər-) *adj.* **1.** Deviating from the usual course, as certain ducts, vessels, or nerves. **2.** Deviating from the normal; untrue to type. **3.** Out of place; ectopic. — **ab·er′ran·cy** *n.*

ab·er·ra·tion (ăb′ə-rā′shən) *n.* **1.** A deviation from the proper or expected course. **2.** A departure from the normal or typical. **3.** A psychological disorder or an abnormal alteration in one's mental state. **4.** A defect of focus caused by a physical defect in an optical element, as in a lens. **5.** A deviation in the normal genetic structure or number of chromosomes in an organism.

a·be·ta·lip·o·pro·tein·e·mi·a (ā-bā′tə-lĭp′ō-prō′tē-nē′mē-ə, -tē-ə-nē′-) *n.* An inherited disorder characterized by the absence of low-density lipoproteins in the plasma, the presence of acanthocytes in the blood, retinal pigmentary degeneration, malabsorption of fats, and neuromuscular abnormalities.

a·bi·o·sis (ā'bī-ō'sĭs) *n.* **1.** Absence of life. **2.** See **abiotrophy.** — a'bi·ot'ic (-ŏt'ĭk) *adj.* — a·bi·ot'-ic·al·ly *adv.*

a·bi·ot·ro·phy (ā'bī-ŏt'rə-fē, ăb'ē-) *n.* **1.** Premature loss of vitality or degeneration of cells or tissues, especially when due to genetic causes. **2.** A hereditary degenerative disease.

ab·ir·ri·tant (ăb-ĭr'ĭ-tənt) *adj.* Relieving irritation; soothing. — *n.* An agent having this property.

ab·ir·ri·ta·tion (ăb-ĭr'ĭ-tā'shən) *n.* The diminution or abolition of a reflex or other irritability in a body part.

abl *n.* An oncogene found in the Abelson strain of mouse leukemia virus and involved in the Philadelphia chromosome translocation in chronic granulocytic leukemia.

ab·late (ă-blāt') *v.* **-lat·ed, -lat·ing, -lates.** To remove or destroy the function of.

ab·la·tion (ă-blā'shən) *n.* Removal of a body part or the destruction of its function, as by a surgery, disease, or noxious substance.

a·ble·phar·i·a (ā'blĕ-fâr'ē-ə) *n.* Congenital absence of the eyelids.

a·blep·si·a (ə-blĕp'sē-ə) or **a·blep·sy** (ə-blĕp'sē) *n.* Lack of sight; blindness.

ab·nor·mal·i·ty (ăb'nôr-măl'ĭ-tē) *n.* **-ties.** An anomaly, deformity, malformation, or difference from the normal.

ABO hemolytic disease of the newborn *n.* See **erythroblastosis fetalis.**

a·bort (ə-bôrt') *v.* **a·bort·ed, a·bort·ing, a·borts.** **1.** To expel or cause to expel an embryo or fetus before it is viable. **2.** To arrest a disease in its earliest stages. **3.** To arrest in growth or development; to cause to remain rudimentary.

a·bor·tion (ə-bôr'shən) *n.* **1.** The expulsion of an embryo or fetus before it is viable. **2.** A miscarriage. **3.** An aborted organism. **4.** Cessation of normal growth, especially of an organ or other body part, before full development or maturation. **5.** The arrest of an action or process before its normal completion.

a·bor·tion·ist (ə-bôr'shə-nĭst) *n.* One who performs abortions, especially criminal abortions.

a·bor·tive (ə-bôr'tĭv) *adj.* **1.** Not reaching completion, as of a disease subsiding before it has finished its course. **2.** Partially or imperfectly developed; rudimentary. **3.** Abortifacient. — a·bor'tive·ly *adv.* — a·bor'tive·ness *n.*

abortive transduction *n.* Transduction in which the genetic fragment from the donor bacterium is not integrated in the genome of the recipient bacterium.

a·bor·tus (ə-bôr'təs) *n.* The product or products of an abortion.

abortus Bang ring test *n.* An agglutination test on the mixed milk of many cows, usually of entire herds, for the detection of bovine brucellosis.

ABO system *n.* A classification system for human blood that identifies four major blood types based on the presence or absence of two antigens,

A and B, on red blood cells. The four types (A, B, AB, and O, in which O designates blood that lacks both antigens) are important in determining the compatability of blood for transfusion.

a·bra·chi·a (ə-brā'kē-ə) *n.* Congenital absence of the arms.

a·bra·chi·o·ce·pha·li·a (ə-brā'kē-ō-sə-fā'lē-ə) or **a·bra·chi·o·ceph·a·ly** (ə-brā'kē-ō-sĕf'ə-lē) *n.* Congenital absence of the arms and head.

a·brade (ə-brād') *v.* **a·brad·ed, a·brad·ing, a·brades. 1.** To wear away by mechanical action. **2.** To scrape away the surface layer from a part.

abraded wound *n.* A wound caused by abrasion.

a·bra·sion (ə-brā'zhən) *n.* **1.** A scraping away of a portion of a surface. **2.** The wearing down or rubbing away or removal of the superficial layers of skin or mucous membrane in a limited area. **3.** The pathological wearing away of tooth substance by mechanical means; grinding.

a·bra·sive (ə-brā'sĭv, -zĭv) *adj.* Causing abrasion. — *n.* A material used to produce abrasion.

ab·re·act (ăb'rē-ăkt') *v.* **-act·ed, -act·ing, -acts.** To release (repressed emotions) by acting out, as in words, behavior, or the imagination, the situation causing the conflict. — ab're·ac'tion *n.*

ab·rup·ti·o pla·cen·tae (ə-brŭp'shē-ō' plə-sĕn'-tē') *n.* Premature detachment of a normally situated placenta.

ab·scess (ăb'sĕs') *n.* **1.** A collection of pus surrounded by an inflamed area appearing in localized infections and formed by tissue destruction. **2.** A cavity formed by liquefactive necrosis within solid tissue. — *v.* **-scessed, -scess·ing, -scess·es.** To form an abscess.

ab·scis·sion (ăb-sĭzh'ən) *n.* The act of cutting off or away.

ab·sco·pal (ăb-skō'pəl, -skŏp'əl) *adj.* Of or relating to the remote effect that irradiation of tissue has on nonirradiated tissue.

abscopal effect *n.* A reaction produced following irradiation but occurring outside the zone of actual radiation absorption.

ab·sence (ăb'səns) *n.* See **petit mal.**

absence seizure *n.* A brief and sudden loss of consciousness, a symptom of petit mal epilepsy.

abs feb. *abbr. Latin.* absente febre (when fever is absent)

ab·so·lute accommodation (ăb'sə-lōōt', ăb'sə-lōōt') *n.* Accommodation of one eye independent of the other eye.

absolute glaucoma *n.* The final stage of blindness in glaucoma.

absolute leukocytosis *n.* An increase in the total number of white blood cells in the blood.

absolute zero *n.* The temperature at which substances possess no thermal energy, equal to $-273.15°C$, $-459.67°F$, or 0 Kelvin.

ab·sorb (əb-sôrb', -zôrb') *v.* **-sorbed, -sorb·ing, -sorbs. 1.** To take in by absorption. **2.** To reduce the intensity of transmitted light.

absorbable suture *n.* A suture used in surgery composed of a material that can be digested by body tissues.

absorbed dose *n.* The quantity of radiation energy, expressed in rads, administered or absorbed per unit mass of target.

ab·sorb·ent (ə-sôr′bənt, -zôr′-) *adj.* Capable of absorption; able to absorb. — *n.* A substance that is capable of absorption.

ab·sorp·tion (ə-sôrp′shən, -zôrp′-) *n.* The taking in or incorporation of something, such as a gas, a liquid, light, or heat.

ab·sti·nence (ăb′stə-nəns) *n.* The act or practice of refraining from indulgence in an appetite, as for certain foods, drink, alcoholic beverages, drugs, or sex. — **ab′sti·nent** *adj.*

ab·strac·tion (ăb-străk′shən, əb-) *n.* **1.** Distillation or separation of the volatile constituents of a substance. **2.** Exclusive mental concentration; absent-mindedness. **3.** The selection of a certain aspect of a concept from the whole.

abstract thinking *n.* Thinking characterized by the ability to use concepts and to make and understand generalizations, as of the properties or patterns shared by a variety of items or events.

a·bu·li·a or **a·bou·li·a** (ə-bōō′lē-ə, ə-byōō′-) *n.* Loss or impairment of the ability to make decisions or act independently. — **a·bu′lic** (-lĭk) *adj.*

abu·lic (ă- bū′lĭk) *adj.* Of, relating to, or suffering from abulia.

a·buse (ə-byōōz′) *v.* **a·bused, a·bus·ing, a·bus·es. 1.** To use wrongly or improperly; misuse. **2.** To hurt or injure physically by maltreatment; ill-use. — *n.* (ə-byōōs′). **1.** Improper use or handling, as of a drug; misuse. **2.** Physical maltreatment, as of a spouse or child. — **a·bus′er** *n.*

ac *abbr. Latin.* ante cibum (before a meal)

a·cal·cu·li·a (ā′kăl-kyōō′lē-ə) *n.* A form of aphasia characterized by the inability to perform mathematical calculations.

a·camp·si·a (ə-kămp′sē-ə, ā-kămp′-) *n.* Stiffening or rigidity of a joint.

a·can·tha (ə-kăn′thə) *n., pl.* **-thae** (-thē). A sharp spiny point or structure, such as the spinous process of a vertebra.

a·can·tha·me·bi·a·sis (ə-kăn′thə-mē-bī′ə-sĭs) *n.* Infection with amebas of the genus *Acanthamoeba* that may result in a necrotizing dermal or tissue infection or in a fulminating and usually fatal meningoencephalitis.

A·can·tha·moe·ba (ə-kăn′thə-mē′bə) *n.* A genus of free-living amebas found in soil, sewage, and water.

a·can·thes·the·sia (ə-kăn′thĕs-thē′zhə) *n.* An abnormal sensation as of a pinprick.

a·can·tho·ceph·a·li·a·sis (ə-kăn′thə-sĕf′ə-lī′ə-sĭs) *n.* Infection with a type of parasitic worm.

a·can·tho·cyte (ə-kăn′thə-sīt′) *n.* A red blood cell characterized by multiple spiny cytoplasmic projections and found in acanthocytosis.

a·can·tho·cy·to·sis (ə-kăn′thə-sī-tō′sĭs) *n.* A rare condition in which the majority of the red blood cells are acanthocytes.

ac·an·tho·ma (ăk′ən-thō′mə) *n., pl.* **-mas** or **-ma·ta** (-mə-tə). A tumor composed of epidermal squamous cells.

ac·an·tho·sis (ăk′ăn-thō′sĭs) *n., pl.* **-ses** (-sēz′). An increase in the thickness of the prickle cell layer of the epidermis; hyperacanthosis. — **ac′an·thot′ic** (-thŏt′ĭk) *adj.*

acanthosis ni·gri·cans (nī′grĭ-kănz′, nĭg′rĭ-) *n.* An eruption of velvety wartlike growths accompanied by hyperpigmentation in the skin of the axillae, neck, anogenital area, and groin, occurring in a benign form in children, but associated with internal malignancy or reticulosis in adults.

a·can·thro·cy·to·sis (ə-kăn′thrə-sī-tō′sĭs) *n.* See **acanthocytosis.**

a·cap·ni·a (ā-kăp′nē-ə) *n.* A condition marked by the presence of less than the normal amount of carbon dioxide in the blood and tissues.

a·car·di·a (ā-kär′dē-ə) *n.* Congenital absence of the heart, sometimes occurring in the smaller parasitic member of conjoined twins when its partner monopolizes the placental blood supply.

ac·a·ri·a·sis (ăk′ə-rī′ə-sĭs) *n., pl.* **-ses** (-sēz′). A disease, usually of the skin, caused by infestation with mites.

ac·a·rid (ăk′ə-rĭd) *n.* An arachnid of the order Acarina, which includes the mites and ticks.

ac·a·ri·di·a·sis (ə-kăr′ĭ-dī′ə-sĭs, ăk′ər-ĭ-) *n., pl.* **-ses** (-sēz′). See **acariasis.**

ac·a·ri·no·sis (ăk′ər-ə-nō′sĭs, ə-kăr′ə-) *n., pl.* **-ses** (-sēz′). See **acariasis.**

ac·a·ro·der·ma·ti·tis (ăk′ə-rō-dûr′mə-tī′tĭs) *n.* A skin inflammation or eruption produced by an acarid.

ac·a·ro·pho·bi·a (ăk′ə-rə-fō′bē-ə) *n.* **1.** An abnormal fear of mites, small insects, or worms. **2.** An abnormal fear of small particles, or of itching.

a·car·y·ote (ā-kăr′ē-ōt′, ə-kăr′-) *n.* See **akaryocyte.**

a·cat·a·la·se·mi·a (ā-kăt′ə-lā-sē′mē-ə) *n.* Hereditary deficiency of catalase in the blood, often manifested by recurrent infection or ulceration of the gums and related oral structures.

a·cat·a·la·si·a (ā-kăt′ə-lā′zē-ə, -zhə) *n.* See **acatalasemia.**

a·cat·a·ma·the·si·a (ā-kăt′ə-mə-thē′zē-ə, -zhə) *n.* Loss of the faculty of understanding.

a·cat·a·pha·si·a (ā-kăt′ə-fā′zē-ə, -zhə) *n.* Loss of the power to formulate a statement correctly.

ac·a·thex·i·a (ăk′ə-thĕk′sē-ə) *n.* Abnormal loss of bodily secretions. — **ac′a·thec′tic** (-thĕk′tĭk) *adj.*

ac·a·thex·is (ăk′ə-thĕk′sĭs) *n.* A mental disorder in which certain objects or ideas fail to elicit an emotional response in the individual.

ac·cel·er·ant (ăk-sĕl′ər-ənt) *n.* Accelerator.

ac·cel·er·a·tor (ăk-sĕl′ə-rā′tər) *n.* **1.** One that increases rapidity of action or function. **2.** A nerve, muscle, or substance that quickens movement or response. **3.** A catalyst.

accelerator nerve *n.* Any of the slender unmyelinated nerves establishing the sympathetic innervation of the heart.

ac·ces·so·ry (ăk-sĕs′ə-rē) *adj.* **1.** Having a secondary, supplementary, or subordinate function. **2.** Of, relating to, or being a body part that is anatomically auxiliary or supernumerary.

accessory gland *n.* A small mass of glandular tissue detached from, but lying near, another gland of similar structure.

accessory ligament *n.* A ligament around a joint that supports or supplements another.

accessory nerve *n.* A nerve that arises by two sets of roots: the cranial set, arising from the side of the medulla, and the spinal set, arising from the first five cervical segments of the spinal cord. Both roots unite to form the accessory nerve trunk, which divides into two branches: the internal, supplying the muscles of the pharynx, larynx, and soft palate; and the external, supplying the sternocleidomastoid and trapezius muscles.

ac·cli·ma·tion (ăk′lə-mā′shən) *n.* **1.** The process of becoming adjusted to a new environment.

ac·com·mo·date (ə-kŏm′ə-dāt′) *v.* **-dat·ed, -dat·ing, -dates.** To become adjusted, as the eye to focusing on objects at a distance.

ac·com·mo·da·tion (ə-kŏm′ə-dā′shən) *n.* **1.** The act or state of adjustment or adaptation. **2.** The automatic adjustment in the focal length of the lens of the eye to permit retinal focus of images of objects at varying distances.

accommodation reflex *n.* The coordinated changes that occur in the eye when viewing a near object, including pupil constriction, eye convergence, and increased lens convexity.

ac·com·mo·da·tive (ə-kŏm′ə-dā′tĭv) *adj.* Of or relating to accommodation.

ac·cor·di·on graft (ə-kôr′dē-ən) *n.* A skin graft in which multiple slits have been made so that it can be stretched to cover a large area.

ac·cre·men·ti·tion (ăk′rə-mən-tĭsh′ən) *n.* **1.** Reproduction by budding or germination. **2.** See **accretion** (sense 2).

ac·cre·tion (ə-krē′shən) *n.* **1.** Growth or increase in size by gradual external addition, fusion, or inclusion. **2.** Foreign material, such as plaque or calculus, collecting on the surface of a tooth or in a cavity. **3.** The growing together or adherence of body parts that are normally separate.

ac·cre·tion·ar·y growth (ə-krē′shə-nĕr′ē) *n.* Growth resulting from an increase of intercellular material.

ACE inhibitor (ās) *n.* Any of a class of drugs that reduce peripheral arterial resistance and are used in the treatment of hypertension and heart failure.

A cell *n.* See **alpha cell**.

a·cel·lu·lar (ā-sĕl′yə-lər) *adj.* **1.** Containing no cells; not made of cells. **2.** Devoid of cells; noncellular. **3.** Of or relating to unicellular organisms that do not become multicellular and are complete within a single cell unit.

acellular pertussis vaccine *n.* A diphtheria, tetanus, pertussis vaccine containing two or more antigens but no whole cells.

a·ces·the·si·a (ā-sĕs′nĭs-thē′zē-ə, -zhə, ā-sĕn′-ĭs-) *n.* Absence of the sensation of physical existence and well-being or of the consciousness of normal bodily functioning.

a·ceph·a·lo·bra·chi·a (ā-sĕf′ə-lō-brā′kē-ə, ə-sĕf′-) *n.* See abrachiocephalia.

a·ceph·a·lo·car·di·a (ā-sĕf′ə-lō-kär′dē-ə, ə-sĕf′-) *n.* Congenital absence of the head and heart in the parasitic member of conjoined twins.

a·ceph·a·lo·chei·ri·a or **a·ceph·a·lo·chi·ri·a** (ā-sĕf′ə-lō-kī′rē-ə, ə-sĕf′-) *n.* Congenital absence of the head and hands.

a·ceph·a·lo·cyst (ā-sĕf′ə-lō-sĭst, ə-sĕf′-) *n.* A hydatid with no daughter cyst; a sterile hydatid.

a·ceph·a·lo·gas·te·ri·a (ā-sĕf′ə-lō-gă-stĕr′ē-ə, ə-sĕf′-) *n.* Congenital absence of the head, chest, and abdomen in the parasitic member of conjoined twins.

a·ceph·a·lo·po·di·a (ā-sĕf′ə-lō-pō′dē-ə, ə-sĕf′-) *n.* Congenital absence of the head and feet.

a·ceph·a·lor·rha·chi·a (ā-sĕf′ə-lō-rā′kē-ə, ə-sĕf′-) *n.* Congenital absence of the head and spine.

a·ceph·a·lo·sto·mi·a (ā-sĕf′ə-lō-stō′mē-ə, ə-sĕf′-) *n.* Congenital absence of most of the head, with the presence of a mouthlike opening.

a·ceph·a·lo·tho·ra·ci·a (ā-sĕf′ə-lō-thə-rā′sē-ə, ə-sĕf′-) *n.* Congenital absence of the head and chest.

a·ceph·a·ly (ā-sĕf′ə-lē, ə-sĕf′-) or **a·ce·pha·li·a** (ā′sə-fā′lē-ə, ăs′ə-) or **a·ceph·a·lism** (ā-sĕf′ə-lĭz′-əm, ə-sĕf′-) *n.* Congenital absence of the head. — **a·ceph′a·lous** (-ləs) *adj.*

a·cer·vu·lus (ə-sûr′vyə-ləs) *n.,* pl. **-li** (-lī′). See **brain sand**.

ac·e·tab·u·lec·to·my (ăs′ĭ-tăb′yə-lĕk′tə-mē) *n.* Excision of the acetabulum.

ac·e·tab·u·lo·plas·ty (ăs′ĭ-tăb′yə-lō-plăs′-tē) *n.* Surgical repair of the acetabulum.

ac·e·tab·u·lum (ăs′ĭ-tăb′yə-ləm) *n.,* pl. **-la** (-lə). The cup-shaped cavity at the base of the hipbone into which the ball-shaped head of the femur fits. — **ac′e·tab′u·lar** *adj.*

ac·et·al·de·hyde (ăs′ĭ-tăl′də-hīd′) *n.* A colorless, flammable liquid formed during ethanol metabolism and used to manufacture acetic acid and drugs.

a·cet·a·min·o·phen (ə-sē′tə-mĭn′ə-fən, ăs′ə-) *n.* A crystalline compound used in chemical synthesis and in medicine to relieve pain and reduce fevers.

a·ce·tic acid (ə-sē′tĭk) *n.* A clear, colorless organic acid with a distinctive pungent odor, the chief component of vinegar, also used as a solvent.

ac·e·to·a·ce·tic acid (ăs′ĭ-tō-ə-sē′tĭk, ə-sē′tō-) *n.* A ketone body that is formed in excessive amounts and excreted in the urine of individuals suffering from starvation or diabetes.

ac·e·tone (ăs′ĭ-tōn′) *n.* **1.** A colorless, volatile, extremely flammable liquid ketone widely used as an organic solvent. **2.** An organic compound produced in excessive amounts in diabetic acidosis. — **ac′e·ton′ic** (-tŏn′ĭk) *adj.*

acetone body *n.* See **ketone body**.

ac·e·ton·e·mia (ăs′ĭ-tō-nē′mē-ə) *n.* The presence of ketone bodies in relatively large amounts in the blood.

ac·e·ton·u·ri·a (ăs′ĭ-tōn-yōōr′ē-ə) *n.* The excretion in the urine of excessive amounts of acetone, an indication of incomplete oxidation of large amounts of fat, and common in diabetic acidosis.

ac·e·to·phe·net·i·din (ăs'ĭ-tō-fə-nĕt'ĭ-dĭn, ə-sē'-tō-) *n.* A white powder or crystalline solid derived from coal tar and used in medicine to reduce fever and relieve pain.

a·ce·tyl·cho·line (ə-sēt'l-kō'lēn') *n.* A white crystalline derivative of choline that is released at the ends of nerve fibers in the somatic and parasympathetic nervous systems and is involved in the transmission of nerve impulses in the body.

acetyl coenzyme A *n.* **1.** An organic compound in which an acetyl group is attached to coenzyme A. **2.** A compound that functions as a coenzyme in many biological acetylation reactions and is formed as an intermediate in the oxidation of carbohydrates, fats, and proteins.

ache (āk) *n.* A dull persistent pain. — **ache** *v.*

a·chei·li·a or **a·chi·li·a** (ə-kī'lē-ə) *n.* Congenital absence of the lips. — **a·chei'lous** *adj.*

a·chei·ri·a or **a·chi·ri·a** (ə-kī'rē-ə) *n.* **1.** Congenital absence of the hands. **2.** A condition sometimes occurring in hysteria in which there is a loss of the sense of possession of one or both hands. — **a·chei'rous** *adj.*

a·chei·rop·o·dy or **a·chi·rop·o·dy** (ə-kī-rŏp'ə-dē) *n.* Congenital absence of the hands and the feet.

a·chieve·ment age (ə-chēv'mənt) *n.* The level of an individual's educational accomplishment as measured by standardized tests and expressed as the age in years of an average child for whom the total score would be an average score.

achievement quotient *n.* The ratio of actual performance to expected performance or to the norm achieved by individuals of a particular age, usually on a standardized test.

Achilles jerk *n.* See **Achilles reflex.**

Achilles reflex *n.* A reflex bending of the foot resulting from contraction of the calf muscles when the Achilles tendon is sharply struck.

Achilles tendon *n.* The large tendon connecting the heel bone to the calf muscle of the leg.

Achilles tendon reflex *n.* See **Achilles reflex.**

a·chil·lo·bur·si·tis (ə-kĭl'ō-bər-sī'tĭs) *n.* Inflammation of a bursa beneath the Achilles tendon.

ach·il·lor·rha·phy (ăk'ĭl-ôr'ə-fē) *n.* Suture of the Achilles tendon.

a·chil·lo·te·not·o·my (ə-kĭl'ō-tĕ-nŏt'ə-mē) *n.* See achillotomy.

ach·il·lot·o·my (ăk'ĭl-ŏt'ə-mē) *n.* Surgical division of the Achilles tendon.

a·chlor·hy·dri·a (ā'klôr-hī'drē-ə) *n.* Absence of hydrochloric acid from the gastric juice. — **a'·chlor·hy'dric** *adj.*

a·cho·li·a (ā-kō'lē-ə) *n.* Suppression or absence of secretion of bile. — **a·chol'ic** (ā-kŏl'ĭk) *adj.*

a·cho·lu·ri·a (ā'-kō-lŏor'ē-ə, -lyŏor'-, ăk'ə-) *n.* Absence of bile pigments from the urine in some forms of jaundice. — **a'cho·lu'ric** *adj.*

a·chon·dro·pla·sia (ā-kŏn'drō-plā'zhə, -zhē-ə, ə-kŏn'-) or **a·chon·dro·plas·ty** (ā-kŏn'drō-plăs'-tē, ə-kŏn'-) *n.* Improper development of cartilage at the ends of the long bones, resulting in a form

of congenital dwarfism. — **a·chon'dro·plas'tic** (-plăs'tĭk) *adj.*

achondroplastic dwarfism *n.* A congenital dwarfism resulting from a failure of cartilage to normally develop into bone, especially cartilage on the ends of long bones.

ach·ro·ma·si·a (ăk'rō-mā'zē-ə, -zhə) *n.* **1.** Pallor associated with the hippocratic facies of extremely severe and chronic illness. **2.** See **achromia** (sense 2).

ach·ro·mat·ic vision (ăk'rə-măt'ĭk) *n.* See **achromatopsia.**

a·chro·ma·tol·y·sis (ā-krō'-mə-tŏl'ĭ-sĭs, ə-krō'-) *n., pl.* **-ses** (-sēz'). Dissolution of the achromatin of a cell or of its nucleus.

a·chro·ma·top·si·a (ə-krō'mə-tŏp'sē-ə) or **a·chro·ma·top·sy** (ə-krō'mə-tŏp'sē) *n.* A severe congenital deficiency in color perception, often associated with nystagmus and reduced visual acuity.

a·chro·ma·to·sis (ə-krō'mə-tō'sĭs) *n., pl.* **-ses** (-sēz'). See **achromia** (sense 2).

a·chro·ma·tu·ri·a (ə-krō'mə-tyŏor'ē-ə) *n.* Passage of colorless or very pale urine.

a·chro·mi·a (ā-krō'mē-ə, ə-krō'-) *n.* **1.** Congenital or acquired deficiency of natural pigmentation. **2.** Lack of capacity to accept stains in cells or tissue.

a·chy·li·a (ā-kī'lē-ə, ə-kī'-) *n.* **1.** Absence of gastric juice or other digestive secretions. **2.** Absence of chyle. — **a·chy'lous** *adj.*

ac·id (ăs'ĭd) *n.* **1.** Any of a large class of sourtasting substances whose aqueous solutions are capable of turning blue litmus indicators red, of reacting with and dissolving certain metals to form salts, and of reacting with bases or alkalis to form salts. **2.** A substance having a sour taste.

acid-ash diet *n.* A diet consisting largely of meat or fish, eggs, and cereals with a minimal quantity of milk, fruit, and vegetables, that when catabolized leaves an acid residue to be excreted in the urine.

acid cell *n.* See **parietal cell.**

ac·i·de·mi·a (ăs'ĭ-dē'mē-ə) *n.* An increase in the hydrogen ion concentration of the blood or a fall below normal in its pH.

a·cid·i·fy (ə-sĭd'ə-fī') *v.* **-fied, -fy·ing, -fies.** To make or become acid.

acid indigestion *n.* **1.** Indigestion resulting from an excess of hydrochloric acid in the stomach. **2.** Heartburn.

a·cid·i·ty (ə-sĭd'ĭ-tē) *n.* The state, quality, or degree of being acid.

ac·i·doph·i·lus milk (ăs'ĭ-dŏf'ə-ləs) *n.* Milk fermented by bacterial cultures that thrive in dilute acid, often used to alter the bacterial flora of the gastrointestinal tract in the treatment of certain digestive disorders.

ac·i·do·sis (ăs'ĭ-dō'sĭs) *n., pl.* **-ses** (-sēz'). An abnormal increase in the acidity of body fluids, caused either by accumulation of acids or by depletion of bicarbonates. — **ac'i·dot'ic** (-dŏt'ĭk) *adj.*

acid-reflux test *n.* A test to detect esophageal reflux by monitoring esophageal pH, performed either basally or after acid is instilled into the stomach.

ac·i·du·ria (ăs′ĭ-dŏŏr′ē-ə, -dyŏŏr′-) *n.* **1.** Excretion of a specific acid in an abnormal amount. **2.** Excretion of an abnormal amount of any specified acid.

ac·i·du·ric (ăs′ĭ-dŏŏr′ĭk, -dyŏŏr′-) *adj.* Of or relating to bacteria that tolerate an acid environment.

acinar cell *n.* A secreting cell lining an acinus, especially one of the cells of the pancreas that furnish pancreatic juice.

acinar cell tumor *n.* A solid, cystic tumor of the pancreas, occurring in young women.

ac·i·ni·tis (ăs′ə-nī′tĭs) *n.* Inflammation of an acinus.

ac·i·no·tu·bu·lar gland (ăs′ə-nō-tŏŏ′byə-lər, tyŏŏ′-) *n.* See **tubuloacinar gland.**

acinous cell *n.* See **acinar cell.**

acinous gland *n.* A gland in which the secretory unit has a grapelike shape and a very small lumen.

ac·i·nus (ăs′ə-nəs) *n., pl.* **-ni** (-nī′). One of the minute grape-shaped secretory portions of an acinous gland. — **a·cin′ic** (ə-sĭn′ĭk), **ac′i·nose′** (-nōs′), **ac′i·nous** *adj.*

ac·mes·the·si·a (ăk′mĕs-thē′zē-ə, -zhə) *n.* **1.** Sensitivity to pinprick. **2.** A sensation of a sharp point on the skin.

ac·ne (ăk′nē) *n.* An inflammatory disease of the sebaceous glands and hair follicles of the skin that is marked by the eruption of pimples or pustules, especially on the face. — **ac′ned** *adj.*

ac·ne·gen·ic (ăk′nē-jĕn′ĭk) *adj.* Causing or exacerbating lesions of acne.

acne punc·ta·ta (pŭngk-tā′tə) *n.* A condition resembling chloracne in that central blackheads are present in all the lesions.

acne pus·tu·lo·sa (pŭs′tyə-lō′sə) *n.* Acne vulgaris in which pustular lesions predominate.

acne vul·gar·is (vŭl-gâr′ĭs) *n.* An inflammatory eruption affecting the face, upper back, and chest, consisting of blackheads, cysts, papules, and pustules, and occurring primarily during puberty and adolescence.

ac·o·nite (ăk′ə-nīt′) *n.* The dried poisonous root of various herbs of the genus *Aconitum* containing aconitine.

ac·o·re·a (ăk′ə-rē′ə) *n.* Congenital absence of the pupil.

a·cous·ma·tam·ne·sia (ə-kŏŏs′mə-tăm-nē′zhə, -kŏŏz′-) *n.* Loss of memory for sounds.

a·cous·tic (ə-kŏŏ′stĭk) or **a·cous·ti·cal** (-stĭ-kəl) *adj.* Of or relating to sound, the sense of hearing, or the perception of sound.

acoustic aphasia *n.* See **auditory aphasia.**

acoustic meatus *n.* **1.** The passage leading inward through the temporal bone, from the auricle to the tympanic membrane; external acoustic meatus. **2.** A canal running through the temporal bone, giving passage to the facial and vestibulocochlear nerves and to the labyrinthine artery and veins; internal acoustic meatus.

acoustic nerve *n.* See **vestibulocochlear nerve.**

a·cous·tics (ə-kŏŏ′stĭks) *n.* The scientific study of sound, especially of its generation, transmission, and reception.

ac·quired (ə-kwīrd′) *adj.* **1.** Of or relating to a disease, condition, or characteristic that is not congenital but develops after birth. **2.** Developed in response to an antigen, as resistance to a disease by vaccination or previous infection.

acquired antibody *n.* An antibody produced by an immune response, in contrast to one occurring naturally in an individual.

acquired character *n.* A nonhereditary change of function or structure in a plant or animal made in response to the environment.

acquired drive *n.* See **secondary drive.**

acquired immune deficiency syndrome *n.* AIDS.

acquired immunity *n.* Immunity obtained either from the development of antibodies in response to exposure to an antigen, as from vaccination or an attack of an infectious disease, or from the transmission of antibodies, as from mother to fetus through the placenta or the injection of antiserum.

acquired immunodeficiency syndrome *n.* AIDS.

ac·qui·si·tion (ăk′wĭ-zĭsh′ən) *n.* The empirical demonstration in psychology of an increase in the strength of the conditioned response in successive trials in which the conditioned and unconditioned stimuli are paired.

ac·ral (ăk′rəl) *adj.* Of, relating to, or affecting peripheral parts, such as limbs, fingers, or ears.

a·cra·ni·a (ā-krā′nē-ə, ə-krā′-) *n.* Congenital absence of all or a part of the skull. — **a·cra′ni·al** *adj.*

a·crit·i·cal (ā-krĭt′ĭ-kəl, ə-krĭt′-) *adj.* **1.** Not critical; not marked by crisis. **2.** Indeterminate, especially concerning prognosis.

ac·ro·ag·no·sis (ăk′rō-ăg-nō′sĭs) *n.* Absence of sensory perception of the limbs.

ac·ro·an·es·the·sia (ăk′rō-ăn′ĭs-thē′zhə) *n.* Loss of sensation in one or more of the extremities.

ac·ro·a·tax·i·a (ăk′rō-ə-tăk′sē-ə) *n.* Ataxia affecting the hands, fingers, feet, and toes.

ac·ro·blast (ăk′rə-blăst′) *n.* A component of the developing spermatid, composed of numerous Golgi elements and containing the proacrosomal granules.

ac·ro·brach·y·ceph·a·ly (ăk′rə-brăk′ĭ-sĕf′ə-lē) *n.* A condition in which there is premature closure of the coronal suture, resulting in an abnormally short anteroposterior diameter of the skull.

ac·ro·cen·tric (ăk′rō-sĕn′trĭk) *adj.* Having the centromere located near one end of the chromosome so that one chromosomal arm is long and the other is short. — **ac′ro·cen′tric** *n.*

acrocentric chromosome *n.* A chromosome with the centromere located very close to one end so that one arm is very short.

ac·ro·ceph·a·lo·syn·dac·ty·ly (ăk′rə-sĕf′ə-lō-sĭn-dăk′tə-lē) or **ac·ro·ceph·a·lo·syn·dac·tyl·i·a** (-sĭn′-dăk-tĭl′ē-ə) or **ac·ro·ceph·a·lo·syn·dac·tyl·ism** (-sĭn-dăk′tə-lĭz′əm) *n.* Any of various congenital syndromes characterized by a peaked head due to

premature closure of the skull sutures and a fusion or webbing of the fingers or toes.

ac·ro·ceph·a·ly (ăk′rə-sĕf′ə-lē) or **ac·ro·ce·pha·li·a** (ăk′rō-sə-fā′lē-ə) n. See **oxycephaly**. — **ac′ro·ce·phal′ic** (-sə-făl′ĭk), **ac′ro·ceph′a·lous** (-sĕf′ə-ləs) adj.

ac·ro·chor·don (ăk′rə-kôr′dŏn′) n. See **skin tag**.

ac·ro·cy·a·no·sis (ăk′rō-sī′ə-nō′sĭs) n. A circulatory disorder in which the hands, and less commonly the feet, are persistently cold, blue, and sweaty. — **ac′ro·cy′a·not′ic** adj.

ac·ro·der·ma·ti·tis (ăk′rō-dûr′mə-tī′tĭs) n. Inflammation of the skin of the extremities.

acrodermatitis en·ter·o·path·i·ca (ĕn′tə-rō-păth′ĭ-kə) n. A genetic defect resulting in the malabsorption of zinc, beginning as a skin eruption on an extremity or around a body orifice, followed by hair loss and diarrhea or other gastrointestinal disturbances.

ac·ro·der·ma·to·sis (ăk′rō-dûr′mə-tō′sĭs) n. Any of several cutaneous diseases affecting the distal portions of the extremities.

ac·ro·dyn·ia (ăk′rō-dĭn′ē-ə) n. **1.** A syndrome in children and infants caused by mercury poisoning, characterized by erythema of the extremities, chest, and nose, polyneuritis, and gastrointestinal disorders. **2.** A syndrome associated with ingestion of mercury by adults, characterized by anorexia, photophobia, sweating, and tachycardia.

ac·ro·dys·os·to·sis (ăk′rō-dĭs′ŏs-tō′sĭs) n. A disorder marked by abnormally small hands and feet, facial changes, and mental retardation.

ac·ro·es·the·sia (ăk′rō-ĕs-thē′zhə) n. **1.** Extreme hyperesthesia. **2.** Hyperesthesia of one or more of the extremities.

ac·rog·no·sis (ăk′rəg-nō′sĭs) n. Sensory perception of the limbs.

ac·ro·ker·a·to·sis (ăk′rō-kĕr′ə-tō′sĭs) n. Overgrowth of the horny layer of the skin, characterized usually by nodular configurations on the backs of the fingers and toes.

ac·ro·meg·a·ly (ăk′rō-mĕg′ə-lē) n. A disorder marked by progressive enlargement of the head, face, hands, feet, and chest due to excessive secretion of growth hormone by the anterior lobe of the pituitary gland. — **ac′ro·me·gal′ic** (-mĭ-găl′ĭk) adj. & n.

ac·ro·me·lal·gi·a (ăk′rō-mə-lăl′jē-ə, -jə) n. A form of erythromelalgia characterized by redness, pain, and swelling of the fingers and toes, headache, and vomiting.

acromial process n. See **acromion**.

a·cro·mi·on (ə-krō′mē-ŏn′, -ən) n. The outer end of the scapula to which the collarbone is attached. — **a·cro′mi·al** adj.

a·crom·pha·lus (ə-krŏm′fə-ləs) n. Abnormal projection of the umbilicus.

ac·ro·my·o·to·ni·a (ăk′rō-mī′ō-tō′nē-ə) or **ac·ro·my·ot·o·nus** (-mī-ŏt′n-əs) n. Myotonia affecting

only the extremities, resulting in spasmodic deformity of the hand or foot.

ac·ro·par·es·the·sia (ăk′rō-păr′ĭs-thē′zhə) n. Numbness, tingling, or other abnormal sensations in one or more of the extremities.

a·crop·a·thy (ə-krŏp′ə-thē) n. Hereditary clubbing of the fingers and toes without an associated progressive disease.

ac·ro·pho·bi·a (ăk′rə-fō′bē-ə) n. An abnormal fear of heights.

ac·ro·scle·ro·der·ma (ăk′rō-sklĕr′ə-dûr′mə) n. See **acrosclerosis**.

ac·ro·scle·ro·sis (ăk′rō-sklə-rō′sĭs) n. A form of progressive systemic sclerosis occurring with Raynaud's phenomenon, marked by stiffness of the skin of the fingers, atrophy of the soft tissue of the hands and feet, and osteoporosis of the distal phalanges.

acrosomal cap n. A caplike structure at the anterior end of a spermatozoon that produces enzymes that aid in egg penetration.

ac·ro·some (ăk′rə-sōm′) n. See **acrosomal cap**. — **ac′ro·so′mal** (-sō′məl) adj.

ac·ro·tism (ăk′rə-tĭz′əm) n. Absent or imperceptible pulse. — **a·crot′ic** (ə-krŏt′ĭk) adj.

ACTH (ā′sē′tē-āch′) n. Adrenocorticotropic hormone; a hormone produced by the anterior lobe of the pituitary gland that stimulates the secretion of cortisone and other hormones by the adrenal cortex.

ac·tin (ăk′tĭn) n. One of the protein components found in muscle into which actomyosin can be split and which acts with myosin in contraction.

actin filament n. One of the contractile elements in skeletal, cardiac, and smooth muscle fibers.

ac·tin·ic (ăk′tĭn) adj. Of or relating to the chemically active rays of the electromagnetic spectrum. — **ac·tin′i·cal·ly** adv.

actinic dermatitis n. Dermatitis caused by exposure to actinic radiation, such as sunlight, ultraviolet light, or x-rays.

actinic keratosis n. A warty lesion, often premalignant, occurring on the sun-exposed skin of the face or hands, especially of light-skinned persons.

ac·ti·nide (ăk′tə-nī′) n. Any of a series of chemically similar radioactive elements with atomic numbers ranging from 89 (actinium) through 103 (lawrencium).

ac·tin·i·um (ăk-tĭn′ē-əm) n. A radioactive element with atomic number 89 and found in uranium ores.

ac·ti·no·der·ma·ti·tis (ăk′tə-nō-dûr′mə-tī′tĭs) n. **1.** Inflammation of the skin produced by exposure to sunlight. **2.** Adverse reaction of skin to radiation therapy.

Ac·ti·no·my·ces (ăk′tə-nō-mī′sēz′) n. A genus of nonmotile, asporogenous, anaerobic to facultatively anaerobic bacteria pathogenic to humans.

ac·ti·no·my·cete (ăk′tə-nō-mī′sēt′, -mī-sēt′) n. Any of various filamentous or rod-shaped, often pathogenic microorganisms of the genus *Streptomyces (Actinomyces)*. — **ac′ti·no·my′ce·tous** adj.

ac·ti·no·my·cin (ăk′tə-nō-mī′sĭn) n. Any of a large

group of red, often toxic, polypeptide antibiotics isolated from soil bacteria of several species of *Streptomyces* that are active against gram-positive bacteria and fungi.

ac·ti·no·my·co·ma (ăk'tə-nō-mī-kō'mə) *n.* A swelling caused by an infection with an actinomycete.

ac·ti·no·my·co·sis (ăk'tə-nō-mī-kō'sĭs) *n.* An inflammatory disease of cattle, hogs, and sometimes humans, caused by actinomycetes and characterized by lumpy tumors of the mouth, neck, chest, and abdomen. — **ac'ti·no·my·cot'ic** (-kŏt'ĭk) *adj.*

ac·ti·no·ther·a·py (ăk'tə-nō-thĕr'ə-pē) *n.* The therapeutic use of ultraviolet light.

ac·tion (ăk'shən) *n.* **1.** The state or process of acting or doing. **2.** A deed. **3.** A change that occurs in the body or in a bodily organ as a result of its functioning. **4.** Exertion of a physical or chemical force or power.

action current *n.* An electrical current generated in a cell such as a neuron or muscle cell during the action potential.

action potential *n.* The change in membrane potential occurring in nerve, muscle, or other excitable tissue when excitation occurs.

ac·ti·va·tor (ăk'tə-vā'tər) *n.* **1.** An agent that renders another substance active or accelerates a process or reaction. **2.** The fragment produced by chemical cleavage of a proactivator that induces the enzymatic activity of another substance.

ac·tive anaphylaxis (ăk'tĭv) *n.* The anaphylactic response produced following inoculation with an antigen to which a person has been sensitized.

active immunity *n.* Immunity resulting from the development of antibodies in response to the presence of an antigen, as from vaccination.

active repressor *n.* A repressor that binds directly with an operator gene to block it and its structural genes from synthesizing enzymes; it is a homeostatic mechanism for the regulation of inducible enzyme systems.

active splint *n.* See **dynamic splint.**

active transport *n.* The passage of ions or molecules across a cell membrane against an electrochemical or concentration gradient or against the normal direction of diffusion.

ac·tiv·i·ty (ăk-tĭv'ĭ-tē) *n.* **1.** The state of being active. **2.** A physiological process. **3.** The presence of neurogenic electrical energy in electroencephalography. **4.** The intensity of a radioactive source. **5.** The ability to take part in a chemical reaction.

ac·to·my·o·sin (ăk'tə-mī'ə-sĭn) *n.* A protein complex that is the essential contractile substance of muscle, composed of myosin and actin.

ac·tu·al cautery (ăk'chōō-əl) *n.* An agent or process, such as electrocautery or a hot iron, that cauterizes tissue using heat and not a chemical means.

a·cu·i·ty (ə-kyōō'ĭ-tē) *n.* Sharpness, clearness, and distinctness of perception or vision.

ac·u·pres·sure (ak'yə-prĕsh'ər) *n.* See **shiatsu.**

ac·u·punc·ture (ăk'yōō-pŭngk'chər) *n.* A procedure in which specific body areas associated with peripheral nerves are pierced with fine needles to produce surgical anesthesia, relieve pain, and promote therapy.

a·cute (ə-kyōōt') *adj.* **1.** Of or relating to a disease or a condition having a rapid onset and following a short but severe course. **2.** Of or relating to a patient afflicted with such a disease.

acute abdomen *n.* A serious condition within the abdomen characterized by sudden onset, pain, tenderness, and muscular rigidity and usually requiring emergency surgery.

acute adrenocortical insufficiency *n.* A severe phase or attack of a chronic adrenocortical disorder such as Addison's disease, characterized by insufficient amounts of the hormones secreted by the cortex of the adrenal glands and resulting in nausea, vomiting, low blood pressure, and life-threatening imbalances in electrolytes.

acute alcoholism *n.* See **alcoholism** (sense 3).

acute anterior poliomyelitis *n.* An acute infectious inflammation of the anterior cornua of the spinal cord caused by the poliomyelitis virus and marked by fever, pains, and gastroenteric disturbances followed by flaccid paralysis and eventual atrophy of one or more muscular groups.

acute ascending paralysis *n.* Paralysis having a rapid course, beginning in the legs and progressively involving the trunk, arms, and neck.

acute brain disorder *n.* An organic brain syndrome caused by temporary, reversible impairment of brain functioning and characterized by mood changes that range from mild disorientation to delirium; can include more serious personality and behavior disturbances.

acute compression triad *n.* The rising venous pressure, falling arterial pressure, and decreased heart sounds of pericardial tamponade.

acute contagious conjunctivitis *n.* An acute, very contagious form of conjunctivitis caused by the hemophilic bacterium *Hemophilus aegyptius* and characterized by inflammation of the eyelids and eyeballs and a mucopurulent discharge.

acute idiopathic polyneuritis *n.* A neurologic syndrome, usually following infection with certain viruses, marked by paresthesia of the limbs and by muscular weakness or a flaccid paralysis.

acute infectious nonbacterial gastroenteritis *n.* See **epidemic nonbacterial gastroenteritis.**

acute inflammation *n.* Inflammation having a rapid onset and coming to a crisis relatively quickly, with a clear and distinct termination.

acute malaria *n.* Any of various forms of malaria that may be intermittent or remittent, consisting of a chill with a fever and its general symptoms and terminating in a sweating stage.

acute neuropsychologic disorder *n.* See **acute brain disorder.**

acute pulmonary alveolitis *n.* Acute inflammation of the pulmonary alveoli resulting in necrosis and hemorrhage into the lungs.

acute rhinitis *n.* See **cold.**

acute situational reaction *n.* See **stress reaction.**

acute tuberculosis *n.* A rapidly fatal disease in which tubercle bacilli are disseminated by the blood, resulting in the formation of miliary tubercles in various organs and tissues and symptoms of profound toxemia.

a·cy·a·not·ic (ā-sī′ə-nŏt′ĭk) *adj.* Characterized by the absence of cyanosis.

a·cy·clo·vir (ā-sī′klō-vĭr, -klə-) *n.* A synthetic purine nucleoside analog derived from guanine and used topically in the treatment of herpes simplex infections, especially of the genitals.

a·cys·ti·a (ā-sĭs′tē-ə, ə-sĭs′-) *n.* Congenital absence of the urinary bladder.

a·dac·ty·ly (ā-dăk′tə-lē) or **a·dac·tyl·i·a** (ā′dăk-tĭl′ē-ə, ə-dăk-) or **a·dac·tyl·ism** (ā-dăk′tə-lĭz′əm) *n.* Congenital absence of fingers or toes. — **a·dac′ty·lous** *adj.*

Ad·am's apple (ăd′əmz) *n.* The slight projection at the front of the throat formed by the largest cartilage of the larynx, usually more prominent in men than in women.

Ad·ams–Stokes syndrome (ăd′əmz-) *n.* An occasional temporary stoppage or extreme slowing of the pulse as a result of heart block, causing dizziness, fainting, and sometimes convulsions.

ad·ap·ta·tion (ăd′ăp-tā′shən) *n.* **1.** The acquisition of modifications in an organism that enable it to adjust to life in a new environment. **2.** An advantageous change in the function or constitution of an organ or tissue to meet new physiological conditions. **3.** Adjustment of the pupil and retina to varying degrees of illumination. **4.** A property of certain receptors through which they become less responsive or cease to respond to repeated or continued stimuli of constant intensity. **5.** The dynamic process in which the behavior and physiological mechanisms of an individual continually change to adjust to variations in living conditions.

a·dap·tive hypertrophy (ə-dăp′tĭv) *n.* Hypertrophic enlargement in response to a condition, such as the thickening of the walls of a hollow organ when there is obstruction to outflow.

ADD *abbr.* attention deficit disorder

ad·dict (ə-dĭkt′) *v.* **-dict·ed, -dict·ing, -dicts.** To become or cause to become compulsively and physiologically dependent on a habit-forming substance. — *n.* (ăd′ĭkt). One who is addicted, as to narcotics. — **ad·dic′tive** *adj.*

ad·dic·tion (ə-dĭk′shən) *n.* Habitual psychological and physiological dependence on a substance or practice beyond one's voluntary control.

Ad·dis count (ăd′ĭs) *n.* The number of red blood cells, white blood cells, and casts in a twelve-hour urine specimen, used to follow the progress of kidney disease.

ad·di·so·ni·an crisis (ăd′ĭ-sō′nē-ən) *n.* See **acute adrenocortical insufficiency.**

Addison's disease *n.* A disease caused by partial or total failure of adrenocortical function, characterized by a bronzelike pigmentation of the skin and mucous membranes, anemia, weakness, nausea, and low blood pressure.

ad·di·tive effect (ăd′ĭ-tĭv) *n.* An effect in which two substances or actions used together produce a total effect equaling the sum of the individual effects.

ad·duct (ə-dŭkt′, ă-dŭkt′) *v.* **-duct·ed, -duct·ing, -ducts.** To draw inward toward the median axis of the body or toward an adjacent part or limb. — **ad·duc′tion** *n.* — **ad·duc′tive** *adj.*

ad·duc·tor (ə-dŭk′tər) *n.* A muscle that draws a body part, such as a finger, an arm, or a toe, inward toward the median axis of the body or of an extremity.

ad·e·nec·to·my (ăd′n-ĕk′tə-mē) *n.* Surgical excision of a gland.

ad·e·nec·to·pi·a (ăd′n-ĕk-tō′pē-ə) *n.* Presence of a gland elsewhere than in its normal anatomical position.

ad·e·nine (ăd′n-ēn′, -ĭn) *n.* A purine base that is a constituent of DNA and RNA and an important energy transport and storage component in cellular metabolism.

adenine nucleotide *n.* See **AMP.**

ad·e·ni·tis (ăd′n-ī′tĭs) *n.* Inflammation of a lymph node or gland.

ad·e·ni·za·tion (ăd′n-ĭ-zā′shən) *n.* Conversion into a glandlike structure.

ad·e·no·ac·an·tho·ma (ăd′n-ō-ăk′ən-thō′mə) *n.* A malignant neoplasm consisting chiefly of usually well differentiated glandular epithelium with foci of metaplasia to squamous neoplastic cells.

ad·e·no·blast (ăd′n-ō-blăst′) *n.* A proliferating embryonic cell with the potential to form glandular parenchyma.

ad·e·no·car·ci·no·ma (ăd′n-ō-kär′sə-nō′mə) *n.* A malignant tumor originating in the epithelial cells of glandular tissue and forming glandular structures.

ad·e·no·fi·bro·ma (ăd′n-ō-fī-brō′mə) *n.* A benign neoplasm composed of glandular and fibrous tissues.

ad·e·nog·e·nous (ăd′n-ŏj′ə-nəs) *adj.* Originating in glandular tissue.

ad·e·no·hy·poph·y·sis (ăd′n-ō-hī-pŏf′ĭ-sĭs) *n.* The anterior glandular lobe of the pituitary gland, consisting of distal, intermediate, and infundibular parts, and secreting many hormones, including ACTH, prolactin, and somatotropin. — **ad′e·no·hy·poph′y·si′al** (-pŏf′ĭ-sē′əl) *adj.*

ad·e·noid (ăd′n-oid′) *n.* **1.** A lymphoid tissue growth located at the back of the nose in the upper part of the throat that when swollen may obstruct normal breathing and make speech difficult. **2. adenoids.** Hypertrophy of the pharyngeal tonsil resulting from chronic inflammation. — *adj.* Of, relating to, or resembling lymphatic glands or lymphatic tissue. — **ad′e·noi′dal** (ăd′n-oid′l) *adj.*

ad·e·noid·ec·to·my (ăd′n-oi-dĕk′tə-mē) *n.* Surgical removal of adenoid growths in the nasopharynx.

ad·e·noid·i·tis (ăd′n-oi-dī′tĭs) *n.* Inflammation of the adenoids.

adenoid tissue *n.* See **lymphatic tissue**.

ad·e·no·li·po·ma (ăd′n-ō-lĭ-pō′mə, -lī-) *n.* A benign neoplasm composed of glandular and adipose tissues.

ad·e·no·lym·pho·ma (ăd′n-ō-lĭm-fō′mə) *n.* A benign glandular tumor usually arising in the parotid gland and composed of two rows of eosinophilic epithelial cells with a lymphoid stroma.

ad·e·no·ma (ăd′n-ō′mə) *n., pl.* **-mas** or **-ma·ta** (-mə-tə). A benign epithelial tumor having a glandular origin and structure. — **ad′e·nom′a·toid** (ăd′n-ŏm′ə-toid′) *adj.*

ad·e·no·ma·to·sis (ăd′n-ō′mə-tō′sĭs) *n.* Development of multiple glandular overgrowths.

adenomatous polyp *n.* A polyp that consists of benign neoplastic tissue derived from glandular epithelium.

ad·e·no·mere (ăd′n-ō-mēr′) *n.* A structural unit in the parenchyma of a developing gland.

ad·e·no·my·o·ma (ăd′n-ō-mī-ō′mə) *n.* A benign tumor of smooth muscle having glandular elements, occurring most frequently in the uterus and in the uterine ligaments.

ad·e·no·pa·thy (ăd′n-ŏp′ə-thē) *n.* Swelling or abnormal enlargement of the lymph nodes.

ad·e·no·phar·yn·gi·tis (ăd′n-ō-făr′ĭn-jī′tĭs) *n.* Inflammation of the adenoids and the pharyngeal lymphoid tissue.

ad·e·no·sar·co·ma (ăd′n-ō-sär-kō′mə) *n.* A malignant tumor arising in mesodermal tissue or glandular epithelium or both.

a·den·o·sine (ə-děn′ə-sēn′) *n.* A nucleoside that is a structural component of nucleic acids and the major molecular component of ADP, AMP, and ATP.

adenosine 3′,5′-cyclic phosphate *n.* See **cyclic AMP**.

adenosine di·phos·phate (dī-fŏs′fāt′) *n.* ADP.

adenosine mon·o·phos·phate (mŏn′ō-fŏs′fāt′) *n.* **1.** AMP. **2.** Cyclic AMP.

adenosine phosphate *n.* AMP.

adenosine tri·phos·phate (trī-fŏs′fāt′) *n.* ATP.

ad·e·no·sis (ăd′n-ō′sĭs) *n., pl.* **-ses** (-sēz′). A disease of a gland, especially one marked by the abnormal formation or enlargement of glandular tissue.

ad·e·not·o·my (ăd′n-ŏt′ə-mē) *n.* Surgical incision of a gland.

ad·e·no·ton·sil·lec·to·my (ăd′n-ō-tŏn′sə-lĕk′tə-mē) *n.* Surgical removal of the tonsils and adenoids.

ad·e·no·vi·rus (ăd′n-ō-vī′rəs) *n.* Any of certain DNA-containing viruses that can infect humans.

ad·e·quate stimulus (ăd′ĭ-kwĭt) *n.* A stimulus to which a particular receptor responds effectively and that gives rise to a characteristic sensation.

ad·her·ence (ăd-hîr′əns, -hěr′-) *n.* **1.** The process or condition of adhering; adhesion. **2.** The extent to which a patient continues an agreed-upon mode of treatment under limited supervision when faced with conflicting demands.

ad·he·sion (ăd-hē′zhən) *n.* **1.** The act or state of sticking together. **2.** A condition in which body tissues that are normally separate grow together. **3.** A fibrous band of scar tissue that binds together normally separate anatomical structures. **4.** The union of opposing surfaces of a wound, especially in healing.

ad·he·si·ot·o·my (ăd-hē′zē-ŏt′ə-mē) *n.* Surgical division or separation of adhesions.

ad·he·sive (ăd-hē′sĭv, -zĭv) *adj.* **1.** Tending to stick things together. **2.** Of, relating to, or having the characteristics of an adhesion. — *n.* A substance that sticks to a surface or causes adherence between surfaces. — **ad·he′sive·ly** *adv.* — **ad·he′sive·ness** *n.*

adhesive absorbent dressing *n.* A sterile dressing consisting of a plain absorbent gauze or compress affixed to a film of fabric coated on one side with a pressure-sensitive adhesive.

adhesive bandage *n.* A dressing of absorbent gauze affixed to plastic or fabric coated with a pressure-sensitive adhesive.

adhesive pericarditis *n.* Pericarditis with adhesions between the two pericardial layers, between the pericardium and heart, or between the pericardium and neighboring structures.

adhib. *abbr. Latin.* adhibendus (to be administered)

a·di·a·do·cho·ki·ne·sis (ə-dī′ə-dō′kō-kĭ-nē′sĭs, -kī-, ăd′ē-ăd′ə-kō-) *n.* Inability to perform rapid alternating movements.

a·di·a·pho·ri·a (ə-dī′ə-fôr′ē-ə) *n.* Failure to respond to a stimulus after a series of previously applied stimuli.

Adie syndrome *n.* See **Holmes-Adie syndrome**.

ad·i·po·cyte (ăd′ə-pō-sīt′) *n.* See **fat cell**.

ad·i·po·gen·e·sis (ăd′ə-pō-jĕn′ĭ-sĭs) *n.* See **lipogenesis** (sense 1). — **ad′i·po·gen′ic**, **ad′i·pog′e·nous** (-pŏj′ə-nəs) *adj.*

ad·i·po·ki·net·ic hormone (ăd′ə-pō-kĭ-nĕt′ĭk, -kī-) *n.* Adipokinin.

ad·i·po·ki·nin (ăd′ə-pō-kī′nĭn) *n.* An anterior pituitary hormone that mobilizes fat from adipose tissue.

ad·i·po·ne·cro·sis (ăd′ə-pō-nə-krō′sĭs, -nĕ-) *n.* Necrosis of fat, as occurs in hemorrhagic pancreatitis.

ad·i·pose (ăd′ə-pōs′) *adj.* Of, relating to, or composed of animal fat; fatty. — *n.* The fat found in adipose tissue. — **ad′i·pose′ness**, **ad′i·pos′i·ty** (-pŏs′ĭ-tē) *n.*

adipose degeneration *n.* See **fatty degeneration**.

adipose tissue *n.* A connective tissue consisting chiefly of fat cells surrounded by reticular fibers and arranged in lobular groups or along the course of one of the smaller blood vessels.

ad·i·po·sis (ăd′ə-pō′sĭs) *n.* Excessive accumulation of fat in the body.

ad·i·po·su·ri·a (ăd′ə-pō-sŏŏr′ē-ə) *n.* See **lipuria**.

ad·just (ə-jŭst′) *v.* **-just·ed**, **-just·ing**, **-justs**. **1.** To bring into proper relationship. **2.** To treat disorders of the spine by correcting slight dislocations between vertebrae using chiropractic techniques.

ad·just·ment disorder (ə-jŭst′mənt) *n.* Any of a class of disorders that result from a person's failure to adapt to identifiable stresses in the environment such as divorce, natural disaster, or retirement, characterized by an impaired ability to function socially or occupationally.

ad·ju·vant (ăj′ə-vənt) *n.* **1.** A pharmacological agent added to a drug, predictably affecting the action of the drug's active ingredient. **2.** An immunological vehicle for enhancing antigenicity, such as a water-in-oil emulsion in which antigen solution is emulsified in mineral oil.

ad lib. *abbr. Latin.* ad libitum (freely, as desired)

admov. *abbr. Latin.* admove (apply)

ad·o·les·cence (ăd′l-ĕs′əns) *n.* The period of physical and psychological development from the onset of puberty to complete growth and maturity.

ad·o·les·cent (ăd′l-ĕs′ənt) *adj.* Of, relating to, or undergoing adolescence. — *n.* A young person who has undergone puberty but who has not reached full maturity; a teenager.

adolescent medicine *n.* The branch of medicine concerned with the treatment of youth between 13 and 21 years of age.

a·dop·tive immunotherapy (ə-dŏp′tĭv) *n.* The passive transfer of immunity from an immune donor through inoculation with sensitized white blood cells, transfer factor, immune RNA, or antibodies in serum or gamma globulin.

ADP (ā′dē′pē′) *n.* Adenosine diphosphate; an ester of adenosine that is converted to ATP for the storage of energy.

ad·re·nal (ə-drē′nəl) *adj.* **1.** At, near, or on the kidneys. **2.** Of or relating to the adrenal glands or their secretions. — *n.* An adrenal gland or tissue.

adrenal cortex *n.* The outer part of the adrenal gland, consisting of the zona glomerulosa, the zona fasciculata, and the zona reticularis and yielding various steroid hormones.

ad·re·nal·ec·to·my (ə-drē′nə-lĕk′tə-mē) *n.* Surgical excision of one or both adrenal glands.

adrenal gland *n.* Either of two small, dissimilarly shaped endocrine glands, one located above each kidney, consisting of the cortex and the medulla, which secretes epinephrine.

a·dren·a·lin (ə-drĕn′ə-lĭn) See **epinephrine** (sense 1).

ad·re·nal·i·tis (ə-drē′nə-lī′tĭs) *n.* Inflammation of one or both of the adrenal glands.

adrenal medulla *n.* Medulla of the adrenal gland.

ad·re·na·lop·a·thy (ə-drē′nə-lŏp′ə-thē) or **ad·re·nop·a·thy** (ăd′rə-nŏp′ə-thē) *n.* Disease of the adrenal glands.

ad·re·ner·gic (ăd′rə-nûr′jĭk) *adj.* **1.** Of or relating to nerve cells or fibers of the autonomic nervous system that release the neurotransmitter norepinephrine. **2.** Of or relating to drugs that mimic the effects of the sympathetic nervous system. — **ad′re·ner′gi·cal·ly** *adv.*

adrenergic amine *n.* See **sympathomimetic amine.**

adrenergic blockade *n.* Selective inhibition by a drug of the responses of effector cells to adrenergic sympathetic nerve impulses and to epinephrine and related amines.

adrenergic blocking agent *n.* A compound that selectively blocks or inhibits responses to sympathetic adrenergic nerve impulses and to epinephrine and other adrenergic amines.

adrenergic fiber *n.* Any of the fibers that transmit impulses to other nerve cells, smooth muscle, or gland cells by norepinephrine.

adrenergic neuronal blocking agent *n.* A drug that blocks sympathetic nerve impulses but does not inhibit the responses of adrenergic receptors to epinephrine and other adrenergic amines.

adrenergic receptor *n.* Any of several reactive components of effector tissues most of which are innervated by adrenergic postganglionic fibers of the sympathetic nervous system and are activated by norepinephrine, epinephrine, and various adrenergic drugs. They are classified as alpha or beta type receptors.

ad·re·no·cor·ti·cal hormone (ə-drē′nō-kôr′tĭ-kəl) *n.* Any of the various hormones secreted by the adrenal cortex, especially cortisol, aldosterone, and corticosterone.

adrenocortical insufficiency *n.* Loss or diminution of adrenocortical function.

ad·re·no·cor·ti·co·trop·ic hormone (ə-drē′nō-kôr′tĭ-kō-trŏp′ĭk, -trō′pĭk) or **ad·re·no·cor·ti·co·troph·ic hormone** (-trŏf′ĭk, -trō′fĭk) *n.* ACTH.

ad·re·no·cor·ti·co·trop·in (ə-drē′nō-kôr′tĭ-kō-trŏp′ĭn, -trō′pĭn) or *n.* or **ad·re·no·cor·ti·co·troph·in** (-trŏf′ĭn, -trō′fĭn) See **ACTH.**

a·dre·no·gen·i·tal syndrome (ə-drē′nō-jĕn′ĭ-tl) *n.* A group of disorders caused by adrenocortical hyperplasia or malignant tumors, resulting in abnormal secretion of adrenocortical hormones.

ad·re·no·lyt·ic (ə-drē′nə-lĭt′ĭk) *adj.* Inhibiting or preventing the action of epinephrine, norepinephrine, and related sympathomimetics. — **ad·re′no·lyt′ic** *n.*

ad·re·no·meg·a·ly (ə-drē′nō-mĕg′ə-lē) *n.* Enlargement of the adrenal glands.

ad·re·no·mi·met·ic amine (ə-drē′nō-mĭ-mĕt′ĭk, -mī-) *n.* See **sympathomimetic amine.**

ad·re·no·re·cep·tor (ə-drē′nō-rĭ-sĕp′tər) *n.* See **adrenergic receptor.**

ad·re·no·tox·in (ə-drē′nō-tŏk′sĭn) *n.* A substance toxic to the adrenal glands.

ad·re·no·trop·in (ə-drē′nō-trōp′ĭn, -trō′pĭn) *n.* See **ACTH.**

A·dri·a·my·cin (ā′drē-ə-mī′sən) A trademark used for an antibiotic containing doxorubicin and used as an antineoplastic agent.

ad sat. *abbr. Latin.* ad saturatum (to saturation)

Ad·son's test (ăd′sənz) *n.* A test for thoracic outlet syndrome in which the patient is seated and, with the neck head extended and turned to the side of the lesion, breathes deeply; a diminution or total loss of radial pulse on the affected side is indicative of the syndrome.

ad·sorb (ăd-sôrb′, -zôrb′) *v.* **-sorbed, -sorb·ing, -sorbs.** To take up by adsorption.

ad·sor·bent (ăd-sôr′bənt, -zôr′-) *adj.* Capable of adsorption. —*n.* **1.** An adsorptive substance. **2.** A pharmacological substance capable of attaching other substances to its surface without any chemical action. **3.** An antigen or antibody used in immune adsorption.

ad·sorp·tion (ăd-sôrp′shən, -zôrp′-) *n.* The property of a solid or liquid to attract and hold to its surface a gas, liquid, solute, or suspension. —**ad·sorp′tive** (-tĭv) *adj.*

adst. feb. *abbr. Latin.* adstante febre (when fever is present)

a·dult (ə-dŭlt′, ăd′ŭlt) *n.* **1.** One who has attained maturity or legal age. **2.** A fully grown, mature organism. —*adj.* Fully developed and mature. —**a·dult′hood** *n.* —**a·dult′ness** *n.*

a·dul·ter·ant (ə-dŭl′tər-ənt) *n.* An additive causing an undesirable effect; impurity.

adult-onset diabetes *n.* Non-insulin-dependent diabetes.

adult T-cell lymphoma *n.* An acute or subacute disease associated with a human T-cell virus and characterized by enlargement of the liver and spleen, skin lesions, and hypercalcemia.

ad us. ext. *abbr. Latin.* ad usum externum (for external use)

adv. *abbr. Latin.* adversum (against)

ad·vanced life sup·port *n.* Emergency medical care for sustaining life, including defibrillation, airway management, and drugs and medications.

ad·vance·ment (ăd-văns′mənt) *n.* A surgical procedure in which a tendinous insertion or a skin flap is severed from its attachment and sutured to a further point on the body.

advancement flap *n.* See **sliding flap.**

ad·ven·ti·tia (ăd′vĕn-tĭsh′ə, -vən-) *n.* The outermost membranous covering of an organ or structure, especially the outer coat of an artery.

adventitial cell *n.* See **pericyte.**

ad·ven·ti·tious (ăd′vĕn-tĭsh′əs, -vən-) *adj.* **1.** Arising from an external source or occurring in an unusual place or manner; extrinsic. **2.** Occurring accidentally or spontaneously, not caused by heredity. **3.** Of or relating to the adventitia of a structure. —**ad′ven·ti′tious·ly** *adv.*

ad·verse reaction (ăd-vûrs′, ăd′vûrs′) *n.* A result of drug therapy that is neither intended nor expected in normal use and that causes significant, sometimes life-threatening conditions.

ad·y·na·mi·a (ăd′ə-nā′mē-ə) *n.* Loss of strength or vigor, usually because of disease.

ae- For words beginning with *ae-* that are not found here, see under *e-*.

A–E amputation *n.* Amputation of a limb from above the elbow.

aer·a·tion (âr′ā′shən) *n.* **1.** Exposure to air. **2.** Saturation of a fluid with air or a gas. **3.** The exchange of carbon dioxide and oxygen in the lungs.

aer·o·al·ler·gen (âr′ō-ăl′ər-jən) *n.* Any of various airborne substances, such as pollen or spores, that can cause an allergic response.

aer·obe (âr′ōb′) *n.* An organism, such as a bacterium, requiring oxygen to live.

aer·o·bic (â-rō′bĭk) *adj.* **1.** Living or occurring only in the presence of oxygen, as certain microorganisms. **2.** Of or relating to aerobes. **3.** Relating to or used in aerobics.

aer·o·bi·cize (â-rō′bĭ-sīz′) *v.* **-cized, -ciz·ing, -ciz·es.** To perform vigorous exercise as part of a program to improve physical fitness.

aerobic respiration *n.* Respiration in which molecular oxygen is consumed and carbon dioxide and water are produced.

aer·o·bics (â-rō′bĭks) *n.* **1.** A system of physical conditioning designed to enhance circulatory and respiratory efficiency that involves vigorous, sustained exercise, thereby improving the body's use of oxygen. **2.** A program of physical fitness that involves such exercise.

aer·o·bi·o·sis (âr′ō-bī-ō′sĭs) *n.* Life sustained by an organism in the presence of air or oxygen. —**aer′o·bi·ot′ic** (-ŏt′ĭk) *adj.*

aer·o·cele (âr′ō-sēl′) *n.* A cavity or pouch filled with air or gas, especially one connected to the trachea or larynx.

aer·o·col·pos (âr′ō-kŏl′pəs) *n.* Distention of the vagina with air or gas.

aer·o·em·phy·se·ma (âr′ō-ĕm′fĭ-sē′mə, -zē′-) *n.* **1.** See **decompression sickness. 2.** A form of chronic pulmonary emphysema resulting from rapid decompression, as may occur in an inadequately pressurized aircraft.

aer·o·gen·e·sis (âr′ō-jĕn′ĭ-sĭs) *n.* The formation of gas. —**aer′o·gen′ic** *adj.*

aer·o·med·i·cine (âr′ō-mĕd′ĭ-sĭn) *n.* The medical study and treatment of physiological and psychological disorders associated with atmospheric or space flight.

aer·op·a·thy (â-rŏp′ə-thē) *n.* A pathological condition induced by a change in the atmospheric pressure.

aer·o·pha·gia (âr′ə-fā′jə) or **aer·oph·a·gy** (-ŏf′ə-jē) *n.* The excessive swallowing of air or gas.

aer·o·pi·e·so·ther·a·py (âr′ō-pī-ē′sō-thĕr′ə-pē) *n.* The treatment of disease using compressed or rarified air.

aer·o·si·nus·i·tis (âr′ō-sī′nə-sī′tĭs) *n.* Inflammation of the paranasal sinuses caused by a difference between the pressure within the sinus cavities and the ambient pressure.

aer·o·sol (âr′ə-sôl′, -sŏl′) *n.* **1.** A gaseous suspension of fine solid or liquid particles. **2.** A substance, such as a pharmaceutical, packaged under pressure with a gaseous propellant for release as a spray of fine particles.

aer·o·ti·tis me·di·a (âr′ə-tī′tĭs mē′dē-ə) *n.* An acute or chronic traumatic inflammation of the middle ear caused by differences between the pressure in the tympanic cavity and the ambient pressure.

aes·cu·la·pi·an (ĕs′kyə-lā′pē-ən) *adj.* Relating to the art of medicine; medical.

aes·the·sia or **es·the·sia** (ĕs-thē′zhə) *n.* The ability to feel or perceive.

aes·the·si·o·gen·e·sis or **es·the·si·o·gen·e·sis** (ĕs-thē'zē-ō-jĕn'ĭ-sĭs) *n.* The production of sensation, especially of nervous erethism.

aes·the·si·o·neu·ro·sis or **es·the·si·o·neu·ro·sis** (ĕs-thē'zē-ō-nŏŏ-rō'sĭs, -nyŏŏ-) *n.* Any sensory neurosis.

aes·the·si·o·phys·i·ol·o·gy or **es·the·si·o·phys·i·ol·o·gy** (ĕs-thē'zē-ō-fĭz'ē-ŏl'ə-jē) *n.* The physiology of sensation and the sense organs.

aes·thet·ic or **es·thet·ic** (ĕs-thĕt'ĭk) *adj.* **1.** Relating to the sensations. **2.** Relating to esthetics.

a·feb·rile (ā-fĕb'rəl, ā-fē'brəl) *adj.* Being without fever; apyretic.

af·fect (ə-fĕkt') *v.* **-fect·ed, -fect·ing, -fects. 1.** To have an influence on or affect a change in. **2.** To attack or infect, as a disease. — *n.* (ăf'ĕkt'). **1.** A feeling or emotion as distinguished from cognition, thought, or action. **2.** A strong feeling having active consequences.

af·fec·tion (ə-fĕk'shən) *n.* **1.** A tender feeling toward another; fondness. **2.** A bodily condition; disease.

af·fec·tive (ə-fĕk'tĭv) *adj.* **1.** Concerned with or arousing feelings or emotions; emotional. **2.** Influenced by or resulting from the emotions, as of a psychological disorder.

affective disorder *n.* Any of a group of disorders characterized by a prolonged, pervasive disturbance of mood together with a full or partial manic or depressive response that is not caused by a separate physical or mental disorder.

affective psychosis *n.* Psychosis characterized chiefly by emotional disturbance.

af·fer·ent (ăf'ər-ənt) *adj.* Carrying inward to a central organ or section, as of nerves.

afferent nerve *n.* A nerve conveying impulses from the periphery to the central nervous system.

af·fin·i·ty (ə-fĭn'ĭ-tē) *n.* **1.** An attraction or force between particles that causes them to combine. **2.** The attraction between an antigen and an antibody. **3.** The selective staining of a tissue by a dye, or the selective uptake of a dye, chemical, or other substance by a tissue.

af·flux (ăf'lŭks') *n.* A flow to or toward an area, especially of blood or other fluid toward a body part.

a·fi·brin·o·ge·ne·mi·a (ā'fī-brĭn'ə-jə-nē'mē-ə, ā-fī'brə-nō-) *n.* The absence of fibrinogen in the blood plasma.

af·la·tox·i·co·sis (ăf'lə-tŏk'sĭ-kō'sĭs) *n.* Poisoning caused by the consumption of substances or foods contaminated with aflatoxin.

af·la·tox·in (ăf'lə-tŏk'sĭn) *n.* Any of a group of toxic compounds produced by certain molds that contaminate stored food supplies such as animal feed and peanuts.

Af·ri·can sleeping sickness (ăf'rĭ-kən) *n.* African trypanosomiasis.

African trypanosomiasis *n.* Either of two types of an often fatal, endemic infectious disease of humans and animals in tropical Africa: Gambian trypanosomiasis or Rhodesian trypanosomiasis.

af·ter·birth (ăf'tər-bûrth') *n.* The placenta and fe-

tal membranes expelled from the uterus following childbirth.

af·ter·care (ăf'tər-kâr') *n.* Care given to convalescent patients after release from a hospital.

af·ter·hear·ing (ăf'tər-hēr'ĭng) *n.* See **aftersound.**

af·ter·im·age (ăf'tər-ĭm'ĭj) *n.* A visual image that persists after the visual stimulus causing it has ceased to act.

af·ter·im·pres·sion (ăf'tər-ĭm-prĕsh'ən) *n.* See **aftersensation.**

af·ter·pains (ăf'tər-pānz') *pl.n.* Cramps or pains following childbirth, caused by contractions of the uterus.

af·ter·per·cep·tion (ăf'tər-pər-sĕp'shən) *n.* Perception of a sensation after the stimulus that produced it has ceased to act.

af·ter·sen·sa·tion (ăf'tər-sĕn-sā'shən) *n.* A sensory impression, such as an afterimage or aftertaste, that persists after the stimulus has ceased to act.

af·ter·sound (ăf'tər-sound') *n.* The sensation of hearing a sound after the cause of the sound has ceased.

af·ter·taste (ăf'tər-tāst') *n.* A taste persisting in the mouth after the substance that caused it is no longer present.

a·func·tion·al occlusion (ā-fŭngk'shə-nəl) *n.* A malocclusion that does not permit normal biting and chewing function of the teeth.

a·ga·lac·ti·a (ā-gə-lăk'tē-ə, -shē-ə, ăg'ə-) *n.* Absence of or faulty secretion of milk following childbirth. — *a'ga·lac'tous* (-təs) *adj.*

a·ga·lac·tor·rhea (ā'gə-lăk'tə-rē'ə) *n.* Cessation of the flow of milk.

a·gal·ac·to·sis (ā-găl'ək-tō'sĭs, ə-găl'-) *n.* See **agalactia.**

a·gam·ma·glob·u·lin·e·mi·a (ā-găm'ə-glŏb'yə-lə-nē'mē-ə) *n.* Congenital or acquired absence of, or extremely low levels of, gamma globulins in the blood.

a·gan·gli·o·no·sis (ā-găng'glē-ə-nō'sĭs) *n.* **1.** Absence of ganglion cells. **2.** Congenital absence of the myenteric plexus ganglion cells.

a·gar (ä'gär', ä'gär') or **a·gar-a·gar** (ä'gär-ä'gär', ä'gär-ä'-) *n.* **1.** A gelatinous material derived from certain marine algae, used as a base for bacterial culture media and as a stabilizer and thickener in many food products. **2.** A culture medium containing this material.

age (āj) *n.* The length of time that one has existed; duration of life. — *v.* **1.** To become old. **2.** To manifest traits associated with old age.

a·gen·e·sis (ā-jĕn'ĭ-sĭs) *n.* Absence or incomplete development of an organ or body part.

a·gen·i·tal·ism (ā-jĕn'ĭ-tl-ĭz'əm) *n.* Congenital absence of genitals.

a·gent (ā'jənt) *n.* A force or substance, such as a chemical, that causes a change.

Agent Orange *n.* A herbicide containing trace amounts of the toxic contaminant dioxin.

a·geu·si·a (ə-gyŏŏ'zē-ə, -zhə, -jŏŏ'-) *n.* Loss of the sense of taste.

ag·glu·ti·nant (ə-glŏŏt'n-ənt) *n.* A substance that holds parts together or causes agglutination.

ag·glu·ti·nate (ə-glo͞ot′n-āt′) *v.* **-nat·ed, -nat·ing, -nates. 1.** To clump together; undergo agglutination. **2.** To cause substances, such as red blood cells or bacteria, to clump together. — *n.* See **agglutination** (sense 3).

ag·glu·ti·na·tion (ə-glo͞ot′n-ā′shən) *n.* **1.** The act or process of agglutinating. **2.** The clumping together of red blood cells or bacteria, usually in response to a particular antibody. **3.** A clumped mass of material formed by agglutination. **4.** Adhesion of the surfaces of a wound in healing.

agglutination test *n.* Any of various tests in which blood serum causes agglutination of bacteria or blood cells of a foreign type, used to identify pathogens and blood types.

ag·glu·ti·nin (ə-glo͞ot′n-ĭn) *n.* **1.** A substance, such as an antibody, that is capable of causing agglutination of a particular antigen, especially red blood cells or bacteria. **2.** A substance, other than a specific agglutinating antibody, that causes organic particles to agglutinate.

ag·glu·tin·o·gen (ăg′lo͞o-tĭn′ə-jən, ə-glo͞o′tn-) *n.* An antigen that stimulates the production of a particular agglutinin, such as an antibody. — **ag′glu·tin′o·gen′ic** (ăg′lo͞o-tĭn′ə-gĕn′ĭk, ə-glo͞o′tn-) *adj.*

ag·glu·to·gen (ə-glo͞o′tə-jən) *n.* See **agglutinogen.** — **ag·glu′to·gen′ic** (-jĕn′ĭk) *adj.*

ag·gre·ga·tion (ăg′rĭ-gā′shən) *n.* A massing together or clustering of independent but similar units, such as particles, parts, or bodies.

ag·gres·sion (ə-grĕsh′ən) *n.* Hostile or destructive behavior or actions.

ag·gres·sive (ə-grĕs′ĭv) *adj.* **1.** Inclined to behave in a hostile fashion. **2.** Tending to spread quickly, as of a tumor; fast-growing.

aggressive infantile fibromatosis *n.* A childhood disorder characterized by firm subcutaneous nodules that grow rapidly in any part of the body but do not metastasize.

ag·ing (ā′jĭng) *n.* **1.** The process of growing old or maturing. **2.** The gradual changes in the structure of a mature organism that occur normally over time and that eventually increase the probability of death.

ag·i·ta (ăj′ĭ-tə) *n.* Acid indigestion.

ag·i·tat·ed depression (ăj′ĭ-tā′tĭd) *n.* A form of depression characterized by restlessness and nervous activity.

a·glos·so·sto·mi·a (ā-glŏs′ə-stō′mē-ə, ə-glŏs′-) *n.* Congenital absence of a tongue and a mouth opening.

ag·lu·ti·tion (ăg′lo͞o-tĭsh′ən) *n.* See **dysphagia.**

a·gly·co·su·ri·a (ā-glī′kə-so͞or′ē-ə, -sho͞or′-, ə-glī′-) *n.* Absence of sugar in the urine. — **a·gly′co·su′ric** *adj.*

ag·nail (ăg′nāl′) *n.* **1.** A hangnail. **2.** A painful sore or swelling around a fingernail or toenail.

ag·na·thi·a (ăg-nā′thē-ə) *n.* Congenital absence or partial absence of the lower jaw. — **ag′na·thous** (ăg′nə-thəs) *adj.*

ag·no·sia (ăg-nō′zhə) *n.* Loss of the ability to interpret sensory stimuli, such as sounds or images.

ag·om·pho·sis (ăg′ŏm-fō′sĭs) or **ag·om·phi·a·sis** (-fī′ə-sĭs) *n.* See **anodontia.**

ag·o·nist (ăg′ə-nĭst) *n.* **1.** A contracting muscle that is resisted or counteracted by an antagonistic muscle. **2.** A substance that can combine with a cell receptor to produce a reaction typical for that substance.

ag·o·ra·pho·bi·a (ăg′ər-ə-fō′bē-ə) *n.* An abnormal fear of open or public places. — **ag′o·ra·pho′bic** *adj.*

a·gram·ma·tism (ā-grăm′ə-tĭz′əm, ə-grăm′-) *n.* A form of aphasia characterized by the inability to produce a grammatical or intelligible sentence.

a·gran·u·lo·cyte (ā-grăn′yə-lō-sīt′, ə-grăn′-) *n.* A nongranular white blood cell.

a·gran·u·lo·cy·to·sis (ā-grăn′yə-lō-sī-tō′sĭs, ə-grăn′-) *n.* An acute disease characterized by high fever, lesions of the mucous membranes and skin, and a sharp drop in circulating granular white blood cells.

a·graph·i·a (ā-grăf′ē-ə) *n.* A form of aphasia characterized by loss of the ability to write. — **a·graph′ic** *adj.*

ag·ri·a (ăg′rē-ə) *n.* An extensive pustular eruption.

a·gue (ā′gyo͞o) *n.* **1.** A febrile condition, especially associated with malaria, characterized by alternating periods of chills, fever, and sweating. **2.** A chill or fit of shivering.

a·gy·ri·a (ə-jī′rē-ə) *n.* Congenital malformation or absence of convolutions in the cerebral cortex.

AI *abbr.* artificial insemination

AID *abbr.* artificial insemination donor

AIDS (ādz) *n.* A severe immunological disorder caused by HIV, transmitted primarily through venereal routes or by exposure to contaminated blood or blood products, resulting in a defect in cell-mediated immune response manifested by increased susceptibility to opportunistic infections and to certain rare cancers.

AIDS-related complex *n.* A combination of symptoms, including fever, lymphadenopathy, blood abnormalities, and susceptibility to opportunistic infections that is a precursor to AIDS in some individuals infected with HIV.

AIDS-related virus *n.* See **HIV.**

ail·ment (āl′mənt) *n.* A physical or mental disorder, especially a mild illness.

ai·lu·ro·pho·bi·a (ī-lo͞or′ə-fō′bē-ə, ā-lo͞or′-) *n.* An abnormal fear of or aversion to cats.

air (âr) *n.* **1.** A colorless, odorless, tasteless, gaseous mixture, mainly nitrogen (approximately 78 percent) and oxygen (approximately 21 percent) with lesser amounts of argon, carbon dioxide, hydrogen, neon, helium, and other gases. **2.** This mixture, with varying amounts of moisture and particulate matter, enveloping Earth; the atmosphere.

air–bone gap *n.* The difference between the threshold for hearing acuity by bone conduction and by air conduction.

air cell *n.* **1.** A terminal dilation of the bronchiole where gas exchange is thought to occur. **2.** Spaces that contain air in the bones of the skull.

air-conditioner lung *n*. Extrinsic allergic alveolitis caused by forced air contaminated by thermophilic actinomycetes and other organisms.

air conduction *n*. The atmospheric transmission of sound to the inner ear through the external auditory canal and via structures of the middle ear.

air embolism *n*. Bubbles of air in the heart or vascular system that create an obstruction and are usually the result of surgery or trauma.

air·plane splint (âr'plān') *n*. A splint that holds the arm in abduction at about shoulder level with the forearm midway in flexion.

air sac *n*. A tiny, thin-walled, capillary-rich sac in the lungs where the exchange of oxygen and carbon dioxide takes place.

airsickness *n*. A form of motion sickness caused by air flight and characterized by nausea, vomiting, and dizziness.

air splint *n*. A hollow tubular inflatable splint.

air·way (âr'wā') *n*. **1.** Any of various parts of the respiratory tract through which air passes during breathing. **2.** A device used to gain an unobstructed route to convey air into and out of the lungs during general anesthesia or when the respiratory passage is blocked.

a·kar·y·o·cyte (ā-kăr'ē-ə-sīt', ə-kăr'-) *n*. A cell having no nucleus.

a·kar·y·ote (ā-kăr'ē-ōt', ə-kăr'-) *n*. See **akaryocyte.**

ak·a·this·i·a or **ac·a·this·i·a** (ăk'ə-thĭz'ē-ə) *n*. **1.** Motor restlessness characterized by muscular quivering and the inability to sit still, often a result of chronic ingestion of neuroleptic drugs. **2.** Intense anxiety at the thought of sitting down; inability to sit down.

a·ker·a·to·sis (ə-kĕr'ə-tō'sĭs) *n*. Deficiency or absence of horny tissue such as nails.

Å·ker·lund deformity (ĕk'ər-lōōnd', ô'kər-) *n*. A deformity of the duodenal cap as seen in a radiograph of a duodenal ulcer, consisting of an indentation of the cap in addition to the ulcerated area.

a·ki·ne·sia (ā'kĭ-nē'zhə, -kī-) or **a·ki·ne·sis** (-sĭs) *n*. A slowness or loss of normal motor function resulting in impaired muscle movement. — **a·ki·ne'sic** (-zĭk, -sĭk), **a·ki·net'ic** (-nĕt'ĭk) *adj*.

a·kin·es·the·sia (ā-kĭn'ĭs-thē'zhə, kĭ'nĭs-) *n*. Loss of the ability to perceive movement.

akinetic mutism *n*. A syndrome characterized by the inability to speak, loss of voluntary movement, and apparent loss of emotional feeling. It is related to lesions of the upper brain stem.

a·la (ā'lə) *n., pl.* **a·lae** (ā'lē). A winglike or expanded structure or part, such as the external ear.

Ala *abbr.* alanine

ALA (ā'ĕl-ā') *n*. Delta-aminolevulinic acid; an intermediate in the biosynthesis of hematin formed from glycine and succinyl-coenzyme A.

a·lac·ri·ma (ā-lăk'rə-mə) *n*. Hereditary or congenital deficiency or absence of tear secretion.

a·la·li·a (ə-lā'lē-ə) *n*. Impairment or loss of the ability to talk.

al·a·nine (ăl'ə-nēn') *n*. A crystalline amino acid that is a constituent of several proteins.

a·larm reaction (ə-lärm') *n*. The initial stage in the body's response to stressful stimuli, characterized by adaptive physiological changes, such as increased hormonal activity and increased heart rate.

al·ba (ăl'bə) *n*. See **white matter.**

al·bi·cans (ăl'bĭ-kănz') *n., pl.* **al·bi·can·ti·a** (ăl'bĭ-kăn'tē-ə). The white fibrous scar tissue in an ovary that results after the involution and regression of the corpus luteum.

al·bi·du·ri·a (ăl'bĭ-dōōr'ē-ə, -dyōōr'-) or **al·bi·nu·ri·a** (-nōōr'ē-ə, -nyōōr'-) *n*. The passing of pale or white urine having a low specific gravity.

al·bi·nism (ăl'bə-nĭz'əm) *n*. **1.** Congenital absence of normal pigmentation or coloration in the eyes or in the skin, hair, and eyes. **2.** The condition of being an albino. — **al'bi·not'ic** (-nŏt'ĭk) *adj*.

al·bi·no (ăl-bī'nō) *n., pl.* **-nos.** A person or an animal lacking normal pigmentation, resulting in abnormally pale or white skin and hair and pink or blue eyes with a deep-red pupil.

Al·bright's disease (ôl'brīts) *n*. Fibrous dysplasia involving multiple bones and characterized by irregular brown spots on the skin, endocrine dysfunction, and precocious puberty, especially in girls.

al·bu·men (ăl-byōō'mən) *n*. **1.** The white of an egg, which consists mainly of albumin dissolved in water. **2.** Albumin.

al·bu·min (ăl-byōō'mĭn) *n*. A class of simple, water-soluble proteins that can be coagulated by heat and are found in egg white, blood serum, milk, and many other animal and plant juices and tissues. — **al·bu'mi·nous** *adj*.

albumin-globulin ratio *n*. The ratio of albumin to globulin in the serum or in the urine in kidney disease.

al·bu·mi·noid (ăl-byōō'mə-noid') *n*. **1.** A fibrous protein. **2.** See **scleroprotein.** — *adj*. Composed of or resembling albumin.

al·bu·mi·nu·ri·a (ăl-byōō'mə-nōōr'ē-ə, -nyōōr-) *n*. The presence of protein, usually albumin but at times globulin, in the urine, indicating either dysfunction or disease. — **al·bu'mi·nu'ric** (-nōōr'ĭk, -nyōōr'-) *adj*.

al·bu·ter·ol (ăl-byōō'tə-rôl', -rōl') *n*. A crystalline powder readily soluble in most organic solvents whose sulfate form is used as a bronchodilator in the treatment of asthma.

al·co·hol (ăl'kə-hôl') *n*. **1.** Any of a series of hydroxyl compounds, the simplest of which are derived from saturated hydrocarbons, including ethanol and methanol. **2.** A colorless, volatile, flammable liquid synthesized or obtained by fermentation of sugars and starches and widely used, either pure or denatured, as a solvent and in drugs. **3.** Intoxicating liquor containing alcohol.

alcohol amnestic syndrome *n*. An amnestic syndrome resulting from alcoholism and vitamin deficiency whose complications may include peripheral neuropathy and cerebellar ataxia.

al·co·hol·ic (ăl'kə-hô'lĭk) *adj*. **1.** Related to or resulting from alcohol. **2.** Suffering from alcoholism. — *n.* One who drinks alcoholic substances habitually and to excess or who suffers from alcoholism.

alcoholic cirrhosis *n.* Cirrhosis that frequently develops in chronic alcoholism, characterized at an early stage by enlargement of the liver due to fatty change with mild fibrosis and later by Laënnec's cirrhosis with contraction of the liver.

alcoholic psychosis *n.* Any of various psychoses that result from alcoholism and involve organic brain damage.

al·co·hol·ism (ăl′kə-hô-lĭz′əm) *n.* **1.** The compulsive consumption of and psychophysiological dependence on alcoholic beverages. **2.** A chronic, progressive, pathological condition, mainly affecting the nervous and digestive systems, caused by the excessive and habitual consumption of alcohol. **3.** Temporary mental disturbance and muscular incoordination caused by excessive consumption of alcohol.

al·de·hyde (ăl′də-hīd′) *n.* **1.** Any of a class of highly reactive organic compounds obtained by oxidation of primary alcohols, characterized by the common group CHO, and used in the manufacture of organic acids. **2.** See **acetaldehyde**.

al·dose (ăl′dōs′, -dōz′) *n.* Any of a class of monosaccharide sugars containing an aldehyde group.

al·dos·ter·one (ăl-dŏs′tə-rōn′) *n.* A steroid hormone secreted by the adrenal cortex that regulates the salt and water balance in the body.

al·dos·ter·on·ism (ăl-dŏs′tə-rō-nĭz′əm, ăl′dō-stĕr′ə-) *n.* A disorder marked by excessive secretion of the hormone aldosterone, which can cause weakness, cardiac irregularities, and abnormally high blood pressure.

A·lep·po boil (ə-lĕp′ō) *n.* The lesion occurring in cutaneous leishmaniasis.

a·leu·ke·mi·a (ā′lōo-kē′mē-ə, ăl′ōo-) *n.* **1.** An absence of white blood cells in the blood. Usually used in reference to certain varieties of leukemic disease. **2.** The leukemic changes in bone marrow associated with a subnormal number of white blood cells in the blood. — a·**leu′ke′mic** *adj.*

aleukemic leukemia *n.* Leukemia characterized by a normal or low number of white blood cells in the blood despite leukemic changes in tissues.

a·leu·ki·a (ā-lōo′kē-ə, ə-lōo′-) *n.* An absence or extreme reduction in the number of white blood cells in the blood.

a·leu·ko·cy·to·sis (ā-lōo′kō-sī-tō′sĭs) *n.* An absence or severe reduction in the number of white blood cells in the blood or in a lesion. — a·**leu′ko·cyt′ic** (-sĭt′ĭk) *adj.*

a·lex·i·a (ə-lĕk′sē-ə) *n.* Loss of the ability to comprehend the meaning of written or printed words and sentences, usually caused by brain lesions. — a·**lex′ic** *adj.*

a·lex·i·thy·mi·a (ə-lĕk′sə-thī′mē-ə) *n.* Inability to describe emotions in a verbal manner.

al·gae (ăl′jē) *pl.n.* Any of various chiefly aquatic, eukaryotic, photosynthetic organisms, ranging in size from single-celled forms to the giant kelp. — **al′gal** (ăl′gəl) *adj.*

al·ge·sic (ăl-jē′zĭk, -sĭk) *adj.* **1.** Relating to hypersensitivity to pain. **2.** Relating to or causing pain; painful.

al·ge·si·om·e·ter (ăl-jē′zē-ŏm′ĭ-tər) or **al·ge·sim·e·ter** (ăl′jĭ-sĭm′ĭ-tər) *n.* An instrument for measuring sensitivity to a painful stimulus.

al·ges·the·sia (ăl′jĕs-thē′zhə) *n.* The ability to sense pain.

al·ges·the·sis (ăl′jĕs-thē′sĭs) *n.* The perception of pain.

al·gid stage (ăl′jĭd) *n.* The stage of collapse in cholera.

al·go·lag·ni·a (ăl′gō-lăg′nē-ə) *n.* Sexual gratification derived from inflicting or experiencing pain.

al·gom·e·ter (ăl-gŏm′ĭ-tər) *n.* See **algesiometer**.

al·go·phil·i·a (ăl′gə-fĭl′ē-ə) *n.* Abnormal pleasure in receiving or inflicting pain.

al·go·pho·bi·a (ăl′gə-fō′bē-ə) *n.* An abnormal fear of pain.

al·gor mor·tis (ăl′gər môr′tĭs) *n.* The cooling of the body that follows death.

al·ien·a·tion (āl′yə-nā′shən, ā′lē-ə-) *n.* A state of estrangement between the self and the objective world or between parts of one's personality.

a·li·e·ni·a (ā′lī-ē′nē-ə) *n.* Absence of the spleen.

al·ien·ist (āl′yə-nĭst, ā′lē-ə-) *n.* A physician who has been accepted by a court of law as an expert on the mental competence of principals or witnesses appearing before it.

al·i·ment (ăl′ə-mənt) *n.* **1.** Something that nourishes; food. **2.** Something that supports or sustains. — *v.* -**ment·ed**, -**ment·ing**, -**ments**. To supply with sustenance, such as food.

al·i·men·ta·ry (ăl′ə-mĕn′tə-rē, -trē) *adj.* **1.** Concerned with food, nutrition, or digestion. **2.** Providing nourishment.

alimentary canal *n.* The mucous membrane-lined tube of the digestive system that extends from the mouth to the anus and through which food passes, digestion takes place, and wastes are eliminated; it includes the pharynx, esophagus, stomach, and intestines.

alimentary glycosuria *n.* Glycosuria developing after the ingestion of a moderate amount of sugar or starch.

alimentary lipemia *n.* Transient lipemia occurring after the ingestion of foods with a large content of fat.

alimentary pentosuria *n.* The urinary excretion of arabinose and xylose as the result of the excessive ingestion of fruits containing these pentoses.

alimentary system *n.* See **digestive system**.

alimentary tract *n.* See **alimentary canal**.

al·i·men·ta·tion (ăl′ə-mĕn-tā′shən) *n.* **1.** The act or process of giving or receiving nourishment. **2.** Support; sustenance.

al·ka·li (ăl′kə-lī′) *n., pl.* -**lis**. **1.** A carbonate or hydroxide of an alkali metal, the aqueous solution of which is basic. **2.** Any of various soluble mineral salts found in natural water and arid soils.

alkali denaturation test *n.* A test for a type of hemoglobin that is not denatured by alkali to alkaline hematin.

alkali metal *n.* Any of a group of soft, white, low-density, low-melting, highly reactive metallic elements, including lithium, sodium, potassium, rubidium, cesium, and francium.

al·ka·line (ăl′kə-lĭn, -līn′) *adj.* **1.** Of, relating to or containing an alkali. **2.** Having a pH greater than 7.

alkaline-ash diet *n.* A diet consisting mainly of fruits, vegetables, and milk with minimal amounts of meat, fish, eggs, cheese, and cereals, that when catabolized leaves an alkaline residue to be excreted in the urine.

alkaline-earth metal *n.* Any of a group of metallic elements including calcium, strontium, magnesium, barium, beryllium, and radium.

alkaline phosphatase *n.* A phosphatase with an optimum functioning at pH 8.6; it is present throughout the body.

al·ka·lin·i·ty (ăl′kə-lĭn′ĭ-tē) *n.* The alkali concentration or alkaline quality of an alkali-containing substance.

alkali reserve *n.* The sum total of the basic ions of the blood and other body fluids that act as buffers and maintain the normal pH of the blood.

al·ka·loid (ăl′kə-loid′) *n.* Any of various organic compounds, such as nicotine, quinine, cocaine, and morphine, that normally have basic chemical properties and usually contain at least one nitrogen atom in a heterocyclic ring.

al·ka·lo·sis (ăl′kə-lō′sĭs) *n.* Abnormally high alkalinity of the blood and body fluids. — **al′ka·lot′ic** (-lŏt′ĭk) *adj.*

al·kap·to·nu·ri·a or **al·cap·to·nu·ri·a** (ăl-kăp′tə-nŏŏr′ē-ə, -nyŏŏr′-) *n.* An inherited disorder that affects phenylalanine and tyrosine metabolism and leads to the excretion of homogentisic acid in the urine.

al·lan·ti·a·sis (ăl′ən-tī′ə-sĭs) *n.* Poisoning due to the ingestion of sausages, usually those containing the toxins of *Clostridium botulinum.*

al·lan·to·in (ə-lăn′tō-ĭn) *n.* **1.** A substance present in allantoic fluid, amniotic fluid, and fetal urine. **2.** A white, crystalline oxidation product of uric acid that is the metabolic end product of vertebrate purine metabolism and is used medicinally to promote tissue growth.

al·lan·to·i·nu·ri·a (ə-lăn′tō-ə-nŏŏr′ē-ə, -nyŏŏr′-) *n.* The excretion of allantoin in the urine.

al·lan·to·is (ə-lăn′tō-ĭs) *n., pl.* **al·lan·to·i·des** (ăl′ən-tō′ĭ-dēz′). A membranous sac developing from the posterior part of the alimentary canal in the embryos of mammals, birds, and reptiles, and important in the formation of the umbilical cord and placenta in mammals. — **al′lan·to′ic** (ăl′ən-tō′ĭk) *adj.*

al·lele (ə-lēl′) *n.* One member of a pair or series of genes that occupies a specific position on a specific chromosome. — **al·le′lic** (ə-lē′lĭk, ə-lĕl′ĭk) *adj.*

allelic gene *n.* Allele.

al·le·lo·morph (ə-lē′lə-môrf′, ə-lĕl′ə-) *n.* See allele.

Al·len's law (ăl′ənz) *n.* The principle that, in contrast to a normal physiology, the more carbohydrate taken by a diabetic, the less carbohydrate is utilized.

Al·len test (ăl′ən) *n.* A test to determine occlusion of the radial or ulnar artery.

al·ler·gen (ăl′ər-jən) *n.* **1.** A substance, such as pollen, that causes an allergy. **2.** See antigen. — **al′ler·gen′ic** (-jĕn′ĭk) *adj.*

allergenic extract or **allergic extract** *n.* An extract of allergenic components prepared from various sources and used to test for an allergy or to produce desensitization to an allergen.

al·ler·gic (ə-lûr′jĭk) *adj.* **1.** Of, characterized by, or caused by an allergy. **2.** Having an allergy to a substance.

allergic reaction *n.* A local or generalized reaction of an organism to internal or external contact with a specific allergen to which the organism has been previously sensitized.

allergic rhinitis *n.* Rhinitis associated with hay fever.

allergic sa·lute (sə-lōōt′) *n.* A wiping or rubbing of the nose with a transverse or upward movement of the hand.

al·ler·gist (ăl′ər-jĭst) *n.* A physician specializing in the diagnosis and treatment of allergies.

al·ler·gy (ăl′ər-jē) *n.* An abnormally high acquired sensitivity to certain substances, such as drugs, pollens, foods, or microorganisms, that may include symptoms such as sneezing, itching, and skin rashes.

al·les·the·sia (ăl′ĕs-thē′zhə) *n.* A condition in which a sensation or stimulus is perceived at a point on the body that is remote from the point that was stimulated.

al·li·ga·tor forceps (ăl′ĭ-gā′tər) *n.* Long forceps with a small hinged jaw on the end.

alligator skin *n.* See ichthyosis.

al·lo·an·ti·bod·y (ăl′ō-ăn′tĭ-bŏd′ē) *n.* See isoantibody.

al·lo·an·ti·gen (ăl′ō-ăn′tĭ-jən) *n.* See isoantigen.

al·lo·bar·bi·tal (ăl′ō-bär′bĭ-tôl′, -tăl′) *n.* A white, crystalline powder used as a sedative and hypnotic.

al·lo·chei·ri·a (ăl′ō-kī′rē-ə) *n.* See allesthesia.

al·lo·cor·tex (ăl′ō-kôr′tĕks′) *n.* Any of the regions of the cerebral cortex that have fewer cell layers than the isocortex, especially the olfactory cortex and the hippocampus.

al·lo·er·o·tism (ăl′ō-ĕr′ə-tĭz′əm) or **al·lo·e·rot·i·cism** (ăl′ō-ĭ-rŏt′ĭ-sĭz′əm) *n.* Sexual attraction toward another person. — **al′lo·e·rot′ic** (-ĭ-rŏt′ĭk) *adj.*

al·lo·ge·ne·ic (ăl′ō-jə-nē′ĭk) or **al·lo·gen·ic** (-jĕn′ĭk) *adj.* **1.** Relating to a different species or race. **2.** Being genetically different although belonging to or obtained from the same species, as in tissue grafts.

allogeneic graft *n.* See allograft.

allogeneic homograft *n.* See allograft.

al·lo·graft (ăl′ə-grăft′) *n.* A graft of tissue obtained from a donor genetically different from, though of the same species as the recipient.

al·lo·ker·a·to·plas·ty (ăl′ō-kĕr′ə-tō-plăs′tē) *n.* The replacement of opaque corneal tissue with a transparent prosthesis usually made of acrylic.

al·lop·a·thy (ə-lŏp′ə-thē) *n.* A method of treating disease with remedies that produce effects antagonistic to those caused by the disease itself. — **al′lo·path′ic** (ăl′ə-păth′ĭk) *adj.*

al·lo·plast (ăl′ə-plăst′) *n.* **1.** A graft of an inert metal or plastic material. **2.** An inert foreign body used for transplantation into tissues.

al·lo·plas·ty (ăl′ə-plăs′tē) *n.* **1.** The repair of defects by allotransplantation. **2.** A surgical operation in which a synthetic material, such as stainless steel, replaces a body part or tissue.

al·lo·ploi·dy (al- ō-ploy′dē) *n.* An individual or cell having two or more sets of chromosomes derived from two different species. — **alloploid** *adj.*

al·lo·pol·y·ploid (ăl′ə-pŏl′ē-ploid′) *adj.* Having three or more complete sets of chromosomes derived from different species. — *n.* An organism with three or more complete sets of chromosomes derived from different species. — **al′lo·pol′y·ploi′dy** *n.*

al·lo·rhyth·mi·a (ăl′ō-rĭth′mē-ə) *n.* An irregularity in the rhythm of the heartbeat or pulse that recurs in a regular fashion. — **al′lo·rhyth′mic** (-mĭk) *adj.*

al·lo·some (ăl′ə-sōm′) *n.* A chromosome that differs from an ordinary autosome in form, size, or behavior; a sex chromosome.

al·lo·trans·plant (ăl′ō-trăns′plănt′) *v.* -plant·ed, -plant·ing, -plants. To transfer an organ or body tissue between two genetically different individuals belonging to the same species. — *n.* An organ or tissue transferred between genetically different individuals of the same species.

al·lo·trans·plan·ta·tion (ăl′ō-trăns′plăn-tā′shən) *n.* The transfer of an organ or tissue between two genetically different individuals of the same species.

al·lo·type (ăl′ə-tīp′) *n.* Any of the genetically determined antigenic differences within a given class of immunoglobulin that occur among members of the same species. — **al′lo·typ′ic** (-tĭp′ĭk) *adj.*

al·lox·u·re·mi·a (ăl′ŏks-yŏŏ-rē′mē-ə) *n.* The presence of purine bases in the blood.

al·lox·u·ri·a (ăl′ŏks-yŏŏr′ē-ə) *n.* The presence of purine bases in the urine.

Al·mei·da′s disease (äl-mā′dəz) *n.* See **paracoccidioidomycosis.**

al·oe (ăl′ō) *n.* **1.** Any of various chiefly African plants of the genus *Aloe,* having rosettes of succulent, often spiny-margined leaves and long stalks bearing yellow, orange, or red tubular flowers. **2.** Aloe vera. **3.** aloes. A laxative drug obtained from the processed juice of a certain species of aloe.

aloe vera (vĕr′ə, vîr′ə) *n.* **1.** A species of aloe (*Aloe vera*) native to the Mediterranean region. **2.** The thick juice or gel obtained from the leaves of this plant, used in cosmetic and pharmaceutical products for its soothing and healing properties.

a·lo·gi·a (ə-lō′jē-ə) *n.* The inability to speak because of mental deficiency, mental confusion, or aphasia.

al·o·in (ăl′ō-ĭn) *n.* A bitter yellow compound obtained from the aloe and used as a laxative.

al·o·pe·cia (ăl′ə-pē′shə, -shē-ə) *n.* The complete or partial loss of hair from the head, face, or other parts of the body; baldness. — **al′o·pe′cic** (-pē′-sĭk) *adj.*

al·pha (ăl′fə) *n.* **1.** The first one in a series; the beginning. **2.** The first position from a designated carbon atom in an organic molecule at which an atom or radical group may be substituted. — *adj.* **1.** Of or characterizing the atom or radical group that is closest to the functional group of atoms in an organic molecule, such as an alpha-amino acid. **2.** Of or relating to one of two or more closely related substances, as in stereoisomers. **3.** Relating to or characterizing a type of polypeptide chain present in immunoglobins.

alpha-adrenergic blocking agent *n.* See **alpha-blocker.**

alpha-adrenergic receptor *n.* Any of various cell membrane receptors that can bind with norepinephrine and related substances that activate or block the actions of the cells containing such receptors; these cells initiate physiological responses such as vasoconstriction and pupil dilation.

alpha-amino acid *n.* Any of the 20 or so amino acids that has the amino and carboxyl groups attached to the same carbon atom, usually has an L-configuration, and is the chemical constituent of a protein.

alpha angle *n.* **1.** The angle between the visual and the optic axes as they cross at the nodal point of the eye. **2.** The angle between the visual line and the major axis of the corneal ellipse.

al·pha-block·er (ăl′fə-blŏk′ər) *n.* A drug that opposes the excitatory effects of norepinephrine released from sympathetic nerve endings at alpha receptors and causes vasodilation and a decrease in blood pressure.

alpha cell *n.* **1.** Any of the cells on the periphery of the islets of Langerhans. **2.** Any of certain granule-containing cells in the anterior lobe of the pituitary gland.

alpha-fetoprotein *n.* An antigen produced in the liver of a fetus that can appear in certain diseases of adults, such as liver cancer, and whose level in amniotic fluid can be used in the detection of certain fetal abnormalities .

al·pha-fu·co·si·dase (ăl′fə-fyōō-kō′sĭ-dās′, -dāz′) *n.* An enzyme that catalyzes the metabolism of fucose and fucose-containing compounds.

alpha globulin *n.* A type of globulin in blood plasma that exhibits great colloidal mobility in electrically charged neutral or alkaline solutions.

alpha helix *n.* The helical form, turned in a right-handed direction, of many proteins.

alpha-hemolytic streptococci *pl.n.* Streptococci

that partially lyse red blood cells cultured on a blood agar medium.

al·pha·hy·drox·y acid (ăl′fə-hī-drŏk′sē) *n.* Any of various fruit acids with the capacity to trap moisture in the skin and initiate formation of collagen.

alpha-lipoprotein *n.* See **high-density lipoprotein.**

alpha ray *n.* A stream of alpha particles or a single high-speed alpha particle.

alpha-receptor *n.* See **alpha-adrenergic receptor.**

alpha rhythm *n.* A pattern of smooth, regular electrical oscillations, as recorded by an electroencephalograph, that occur in the human brain when a person is awake and relaxed.

alpha-tocopherol *n.* A substance obtained from wheat germ oil or by synthesis that biologically exhibits high vitamin E activity.

alpha wave *n.* See **alpha rhythm.**

al·pra·zo·lam (ăl-prā′zə-lăm′) *n.* A benzodiazepine tranquilizer used in the management of anxiety disorders.

al·pros·ta·dil (ăl-prŏs′tə-dĭl) *n.* A vasodilator used to temporarily keep the arterial canal open in newborns with congenital heart defects.

Al·ström's syndrome (ăl′strəm, äl′strœmz) *n.* An inherited syndrome marked by retinal degeneration with nystagmus and loss of central vision, nerve deafness, and diabetes. It is associated with childhood obesity.

ALT (ā′ĕl-tē′) *n.* Alanine aminotransferase; an enzyme found in serum and body tissues that catalyzes the transfer of amino acid groups from L-alanine to 2-ketoglutarate or the reverse, thus allowing nitrogen to be excreted or incorporated into other compounds.

al·ter ego (ôl′tər) *n.* Another side of oneself; a second self.

al·ter·nate cover test (ôl′-tər-nĭt, äl′-) *n.* A test for detecting phoria or strabismus.

alternating pulse *n.* A pulse pattern that occurs at regular intervals but alternates between weak and strong beats; usually indicates myocardial disease.

alternating tremor *n.* A form of hyperkinesia characterized by regular, symmetrical, to-and-fro movements produced by patterned, alternating contraction of muscles and their antagonists.

al·ter·na·tion (ôl′tər-nā′shən, äl′-) *n.* Successive change from one thing or state to another and back again.

alternation of generations *n.* The regular alternation of forms or of mode of reproduction in the life cycle of an organism, such as the alternation between diploid and haploid phases.

alternation of heart *n.* See **mechanical alternation.**

alt. hor. *abbr. Latin.* alternis horis (every other hour)

al·ti·tude sickness (ăl′tĭ-tōōd′, -tyōōd′) *n.* A collection of symptoms, including shortness of breath, headache, nausea, and nosebleed, brought on by decreased oxygen in the atmosphere, such as that encountered at high altitudes.

al·um (ăl′əm) *n.* Any of various double sulfates of a

trivalent metal such as aluminum or iron and a univalent metal such as potassium or sodium that are used as topical astringents and styptics.

a·lu·mi·no·sis (ə-lōō′mə-nō′sĭs) *n.* A form of pneumonoconiosis caused by exposure to alum-bearing dust.

a·lu·mi·num (ə-lōō′mə-nəm) *n.* A silvery-white, ductile metallic element with atomic number 13 and used in light, corrosion-resistant alloys.

al·ve·o·lar (ăl-vē′ə-lər) *adj.* Relating to an alveolus.

alveolar abscess *n.* An abscess in the alveolar ridge of the jaw.

alveolar-arterial oxygen difference *n.* The difference or gradient between the partial pressure of oxygen in the alveolar spaces and the arterial blood.

alveolar dead space *n.* The difference between physiological dead space and anatomical dead space, representing that part of the physiological dead space resulting from ventilation of relatively underperfused or nonperfused alveoli.

alveolar duct *n.* **1.** The part of the respiratory passages beyond the respiratory bronchioles, from which the alveolar sacs and alveoli arise. **2.** The smallest of the intralobular ducts in the mammary gland, into which the secretory alveoli open.

alveolar gland *n.* A gland having a saclike secretory unit and an obvious lumen.

alveolar sac *n.* See **air sac.**

alveolar ventilation *n.* The volume of gas expired from the alveoli to the outside of the body per minute.

al·ve·o·li·tis (ăl′vē-ə-lī′tĭs) *n.* **1.** Inflammation of alveoli. **2.** Inflammation of a tooth socket.

al·ve·o·lus (ăl-vē′ə-ləs) *n., pl.* **-li** (-lī′). A small angular cavity or pit, such as a tooth socket or an air sac.

a·lym·phi·a (ā-lĭm′fē-ə, ə-lĭm′-) *n.* Absence or deficiency of lymph.

a·lym·pho·cy·to·sis (ā-lĭm′fō-sī-tō′sĭs, ə-lĭm′-) *n.* Total or nearly total absence of lymphocytes.

a·lym·pho·pla·si·a (ā-lĭm′fō-plā′zē-ə, -zhə, ə-lĭm′-) *n.* Aplasia or hypoplasia of lymphoid tissue.

Alz·hei·mer's dementia (älts′hī-mərz, ălts′-, ôlts′-) *n.* Alzheimer's disease. No longer in technical use.

Alzheimer's disease *n.* A degenerative disease of the brain, characterized by clumps of neurofibrils and microscopic lesions in the brain and by confusion, disorientation, memory failure, and speech disturbances, and resulting in progressive loss of mental capacity.

a·mal·gam (ə-măl′gəm) *n.* Any of various alloys of mercury with other metals used for filling teeth.

amalgam tattoo *n.* A bluish-black or gray lesion of the oral mucous membrane caused by accidental implantation of silver amalgam into the tissue.

Am·a·ni·ta (ăm′ə-nī′tə, -nē′-) *n.* A genus of mushrooms, many members of which are highly poisonous.

a·man·ta·dine (ə-măn′tə-dēn′) *n.* An antiviral drug also used in the treatment of Parkinson's disease.

am·a·rine (ăm′ə-rĭn, -rīn′) *n.* Any of various bitter substances derived from plants, especially from the oil of bitter almond.

a·mas·ti·a (ā-măs′tē-ə, ə-măs′-) *n.* Congenital absence of one or both breasts.

am·au·ro·sis (ăm′ô-rō′sĭs) *n.* Blindness, especially without apparent change in the eye, as from a cortical lesion. — **am′au·rot′ic** (-rŏt′ĭk) *adj.*

amaurosis con·gen·i·ta of Le·ber (kən-jĕn′ĭ-tə əv lā′bər) *n.* A cone-rod abiotrophy that causes blindness or severely reduces vision at birth.

amaurosis fu·gax (fōō′găks′, fyōō′-) *n.* A temporary blindness that may result from transient ischemia caused by an insufficiency of the carotid artery or exposure to centrifugal force.

am·ba·geu·si·a (ăm′bə-gyōō′zē-ə, -zhə, -jōō′-) *n.* Loss of taste on both sides of the tongue.

am·bi·dex·ter·i·ty (ăm′bĭ-dĕk-stĕr′ĭ-tē) or **am′bi·dex′trism** (-dĕk′strĭz′əm) *n.* The state or quality of being ambidextrous.

am·bi·dex·trous (ăm′bĭ-dĕk′strəs) *adj.* Able to use both hands with equal facility.

am·bi·ent (ăm′bē-ənt) *adj.* Surrounding; encircling.

am·bi·sex·u·al (ăm′bĭ-sĕk′shōō-əl) *adj.* Sexually attracted to either sex indiscriminately. — *n.* An ambisexual person or organism. — **am′bi·sex′u·al′i·ty** (-ăl′ĭ-tē) *n.*

am·biv·a·lence (ăm-bĭv′ə-ləns) *n.* The coexistence of opposing attitudes or feelings, such as love and hate, toward a person, an object, or an idea. — **am·biv′a·lent** *adj.*

am·bi·ver·sion (ăm′bĭ-vûr′zhən, -shən) *n.* A personality trait including the qualities of both introversion and extroversion.

am·bly·a·phi·a (ăm′blē-ā′fē-ə) *n.* Reduced sensitivity or dullness of the sense of touch.

am·bly·o·pi·a (ăm′blē-ō′pē-ə) *n.* Dimness of vision, especially when occurring in one eye without apparent physical defect or disease. — **am′bly·o′pic** (-ō′pĭk, -ŏp′ĭk) *adj.*

am·bly·o·scope (ăm′blē-ə-skōp′) *n.* A reflecting stereoscope used for measuring or training binocular vision and for stimulating vision in an amblyopic eye.

Am·bu bag (ăm′bōō) A trademark used for a self-reinflating bag used with positive pressure respiration during resuscitation.

am·bu·lance (ăm′byə-ləns) *n.* A specially equipped vehicle used to transport the sick or injured.

am·bu·lant (ăm′byə-lənt) *adj.* Moving or walking about.

am·bu·la·to·ry (ăm′byə-lə-tôr′ē) *adj.* **1.** Of, relating to, or adapted for walking. **2.** Capable of walking; not bedridden. **3.** Moving about.

ambulatory surgery *n.* Surgery performed on a person who is admitted to and discharged from a hospital on the same day.

a·me·ba (ə-mē′bə) or **amoeba** *n.,* *pl.* **-bas** or **-bae** (-bē). A protozoan of the genus *Amoeba* and of related genera, occurring in soil and water and parasitic in animals.

am·e·bi·a·sis (ăm′ə-bī′ə-sĭs) or **amoebiasis** *n.* An infection or disease caused by pathogenic amebas, especially *Entamoeba histolytica.*

a·me·bic (ə-mē′bĭk) or **amoebic** *adj.* Relating to, resembling, or caused by amebas.

amebic abscess *n.* An abscess in the liver or other organ, containing amebas and usually following amebic dysentery.

amebic colitis *n.* Inflammation of the colon in amebiasis.

amebic dysentery *n.* Severe intestinal infection of humans caused by the ameba *Entamoeba histolytica* and resulting in diarrhea, cramping, fever, and ulceration of the colon.

a·me·bi·cide (ə-mē′bĭ-sīd′) *n.* Any of various agents that destroy amebas. — **a·me′bi·cid′al** (-cīd′l) *adj.*

a·me·bo·cyte (ə-mē′bə-sīt′) or **amoebocyte** *n.* **1.** An ameboid cell, such as a white blood cell. **2.** A blood cell in an in vitro tissue culture.

a·me·boid (ə-mē′boid′) or **amoeboid** *adj.* **1.** Of or resembling an ameba, especially in changeability of form and means of locomotion. **2.** Having an irregular or asymmetric outline with peripheral projections, as a group of cultured cells.

ameboid cell *n.* A cell, such as a white blood cell, that is able to change its form and move about like an ameba.

a·me·bu·la (ə-mē′byə-lə) *n.,* *pl.* **-las** or **-lae** (-lē′). **1.** Any of the young amebas of species of *Entamoeba* and their immediate progeny that emerge from the cyst in the human gut before localizing in the large intestine. **2.** The ameboid spores of protozoa and other organisms.

a·me·bu·ri·a (ăm′ə-byōōr′ē-ə) *n.* The presence of amebas in the urine.

a·mel·i·a (ə-mēl′ē-ə, ə-mē′lē-ə) *n.* Congenital absence of one or more limbs.

am·e·lo·blast (ăm′ə-lō-blăst′) *n.* One of the cells that is part of the inner layer of the enamel organ of a developing tooth and is involved in enamel formation.

am·e·lo·blas·tic fibroma (ăm′ə-lō-blăs′tĭk) *n.* A benign odontogenic mixed tumor marked by proliferation of both the epithelium and mesenchyme of the tooth bud without the production of hard tissue.

ameloblastic layer *n.* The internal layer of the enamel organ.

am·e·lo·gen·e·sis (ăm′ə-lō-jĕn′ĭ-sĭs) *n.* The formation and development of dental enamel.

a·men·or·rhe·a or **a·men·or·rhoe·a** (ā-mĕn′ə-rē′ə) *n.* Abnormal suppression or absence of menstruation. — **a·men′or·rhe′al** *adj.* — **a·men′or·rhe′ic** *adj.*

amenorrhea-galactorrhea syndrome *n.* Lactation and amenorrhea resulting from endocrinological causes or from a pituitary tumor.

a·ment (ā′mĕnt′, ā′mənt) *n.* A person whose intellectual capacity remains undeveloped.

a·men·tia (ā-měn′shə, -shē-ə, ə-měn′-) *n.* Insufficient mental development or functioning. — a·men′tial *adj.*

am·er·i·ci·um (ăm′ə-rĭsh′ē-əm) *n.* A white metallic synthetic element of the actinide series with atomic number 95. Its longest-lived isotopes are used as radiation sources in research.

Ames test (āmz) *n.* A test in which strains of *Salmonella* that are unable to synthesize histidine are introduced into a test substance lacking in histidine. If the strains regain the ability to synthesize histidine, the substance is considered mutagenic and thus carcinogenic.

a·me·tri·a (ə-mē′trē-ə) *n.* Congenital absence of the uterus.

am·e·trom·e·ter (ăm′ĭ-trŏm′ĭ-tər) *n.* An instrument for measuring the degree of ametropia.

am·e·tro·pi·a (ăm′ĭ-trō′pē-ə) *n.* An eye abnormality, such as nearsightedness, farsightedness, or astigmatism, resulting from faulty refractive ability of the eye. — am′e·trop′ic (-trŏp′ĭk, -trō′pĭk) *adj.*

a·mim·i·a (ā-mĭm′ē-ə, ə-mĭm′-) *n.* Loss of the ability to imitate or to communicate by gestures or signs.

a·mine (ə-mēn′, ăm′ēn) *n.* Any of a group of organic compounds of nitrogen that may be considered ammonia derivatives in which one or more hydrogen atoms have been replaced by one or more hydrocarbon radicals.

a·mi·no (ə-mē′nō, ăm′ə-nō′) *adj.* Relating to an amine or other chemical compound containing an NH_2 group combined with a nonacid organic radical.

amino acid *n.* Any of various organic acids containing both an amino group and a carboxyl group, especially any of the 20 or more compounds that link together to form proteins.

a·mi·no·ac·i·de·mi·a (ə-mē′nō-ăs′ĭ-dē′mē-ə, ăm′-ə-nō-) *n.* An excess of specific amino acids in the blood.

a·mi·no·ac·i·du·ri·a (ə-mē′nō-ăs′ĭ-dŏor′ē-ə, -dyŏor′-, ăm′ə-nō-) *n.* A disorder of protein metabolism in which excessive amounts of amino acids are excreted in the urine.

a·mi·no·ben·zo·ic acid (ə-mē′nō-běn-zō′ĭk, ăm′-ə-nō-) *n.* Any of three benzoic acid derivatives, especially the yellowish para form, which is part of the vitamin B complex.

a·mi·no·gly·co·side (ə-mē′nō-glī′kə-sīd′, ăm′ə-nō-) *n.* Any of a group of bactericidal antibiotics derived from species of *Streptomyces* or *Micromonosporum* that are effective against aerobic gram-negative bacilli and *Mycobacterium tuberculosis*.

am·i·nu·ri·a (ăm′ə-nŏor′ē-ə, -nyŏor′-) *n.* Excretion of an excessive amount of amines in the urine.

am·i·to·sis (ăm′ĭ-tō′sĭs, ā′mĭ-) *n.* Direct division of the nucleus and cell without the changes in the nucleus that usually occur during cell reproduction. — am′i·tot′ic (-tŏt′ĭk) *adj.*

am·i·trip·tyl·ine (ăm′ĭ-trĭp′tə-lēn′) *n.* An antidepressant drug.

am·mo·ne·mi·a (ăm′ə-nē′mē-ə) or **am·mo·ni·e·mi·a** (ə-mō′nē-ē′mē-ə) *n.* The presence of excessive amounts of ammonia or its compounds in the blood.

am·mo·nia (ə-mōn′yə) *n.* A colorless, pungent gas used to manufacture a wide variety of nitrogen-containing organic and inorganic chemicals.

am·mo·ni·u·ri·a (ə-mō′nē-yŏor′ē-ə) *n.* The presence of an excessive amount of ammonia in the urine.

am·ne·sia (ăm-nē′zhə) *n.* Loss or impairment of memory.

am·ne·si·ac (ăm-nē′zē-ăk′, -zhē-ăk′) *n.* One who is afflicted with amnesia.

am·nes·tic syndrome (ăm-něs′tĭk) *n.* An organic brain syndrome marked by short-term memory disturbance.

am·ni·o·cen·te·sis (ăm′nē-ō-sĕn-tē′sĭs) *n., pl.* **-ses** (-sēz′). A procedure in which a small sample of amniotic fluid is drawn out of the uterus through a needle inserted in the abdomen and is then analyzed to detect genetic abnormalities in the fetus or to determine the sex of the fetus.

am·ni·o·gen·e·sis (ăm′nē-ō-jĕn′ĭ-sĭs) *n.* Formation of the amnion.

am·ni·og·ra·phy (ăm′nē-ŏg′rə-fē) *n.* Radiographic examination of the uterine cavity and fetus following injection of a radiopaque substance into the amnion.

am·ni·o·ma (ăm′nē-ō′mə) *n.* A broad flat tumor of the skin caused by the adhesion of the amnion before birth.

am·ni·on (ăm′nē-ən, -ŏn′) *n.* **-ni·ons** or **-ni·a** (-nē-ə). The thin, tough, membranous sac filled with a serous fluid in which the embryo or fetus is enclosed and suspended in the uterus. — am′ni·ot′-ic (-ŏt′ĭk), am′ni·on′ic (-ŏn′ĭk) *adj.*

am·ni·o·ni·tis (ăm′nē-ə-nī′tĭs) *n.* Inflammation of the amnion.

am·ni·or·rhe·a (ăm′nē-ə-rē′ə) *n.* The escape of amniotic fluid from the amnion.

am·ni·or·rhex·is (ăm′nē-ə-rĕk′sĭs) *n.* Rupture of the amnion.

am·ni·o·scope (ăm′nē-ə-skōp′) *n.* An endoscope that allows the fetus and amniotic fluid to be observed directly through the intact amniotic sac.

am·ni·os·co·py (ăm′nē-ŏs′kə-pē) *n.* Examination of the amniotic cavity and fetus using an optical instrument that is inserted directly into the amniotic cavity.

amniotic cavity *n.* The fluid-filled cavity surrounding the developing embryo.

amniotic fluid *n.* The fluid within the amnion that surrounds the fetus and protects it from injury.

amniotic sac *n.* See **amnion**.

am·ni·o·tome (ăm′nē-ə-tōm′) *n.* An instrument for puncturing the fetal membranes.

am·ni·ot·o·my (ăm′nē-ŏt′ə-mē) *n.* Surgical rupture of the fetal membranes to induce or expedite labor.

am·o·bar·bi·tal (ăm′ō-bär′bĭ-tăl′, -tôl′) *n.* A barbiturate that is used as a sedative and a hypnotic.

A-mode (ā'mōd') *n.* A one-dimensional representation of a reflected sound wave in a diagnostic ultrasound.

a·moe·ba (ə-mē'bə) *n., pl.* **-bas** or **-bae** (-bē). **1.** A genus of protozoa of the class Sarcodina or Rhizopoda. **2.** Any of several genera of protozoa that are parasitic in humans.

a·morph (ā'môrf') *n.* A mutant gene that has no phenotypic effect.

a·mor·phous (ə-môr'fəs) *adj.* **1.** Lacking definite form; shapeless. **2.** Lacking organization.

A·moss' sign (ā'məs) *n.* An indication of painful flexion of the spine in which it is necessary to support a sitting position by extending the arms behind the torso and placing its weight on the hands.

a·mox·i·cil·lin (ə-mŏk'sĭ-sĭl'ĭn) *n.* A semisynthetic derivative of ampicillin that is effective against a broad range of gram-negative and gram-positive bacteria.

AMP (ā'ĕm-pē') *n.* Adenosine monophosphate; a mononucleotide found in animal cells and reversibly convertible to ADP and ATP.

am·phet·a·mine (ăm-fĕt'ə-mēn', -mĭn) *n.* **1.** A colorless, volatile liquid used primarily as a central nervous system stimulant. **2.** A derivative of amphetamine used as a central nervous system stimulant in the treatment of conditions such as narcolepsy and depression.

am·phi·ar·thro·sis (ăm'fē-är-thrō'sĭs) *n.* See **movable joint** (sense 2). — **am'phi·ar·thro'di·al** (-thrō'dē-əl) *adj.*

am·phi·as·ter (ăm'fē-ăs'tər) *n.* A double-star figure present in the cell during mitosis, formed just before the division of the nucleus.

am·phi·mix·is (ăm'fə-mĭk'sĭs) *n.* The union of the sperm and egg in sexual reproduction.

amphoric resonance *n.* The sound obtained by percussing over a pulmonary cavity when the patient's mouth is open, similar to that produced by blowing across the mouth of an empty bottle.

am·pho·ter·i·cin B (ăm'fə-tĕr'ĭ-sĭn) *n.* An antibiotic derived from strains of the actinomycete *Streptomyces nodosus* and used in treating systemic fungal infections.

am·pi·cil·lin (ăm'pĭ-sĭl'ĭn) *n.* A semisynthetic of penicillin that is effective against gram-negative and gram-positive bacteria and is used in treating gonorrhea and infections of the intestinal, urinary, and respiratory tracts.

am·pli·fi·ca·tion (ăm'plə-fĭ-kā'shən) *n.* **1.** The process of increasing the magnitude of a single variable quantity, such as the magnitude of voltage. **2.** The result of such a process. **3.** A process by which extra copies of a gene or DNA sequence are formed.

am·pli·fi·er host (ăm'plə-fī'ər) *n.* A host in which infectious agents multiply to high concentrations, providing an important source of infection for vectors in vector-borne diseases.

am·pli·tude of accommodation (ăm'plĭ-tōod' əv,

-tyōod') *n.* The difference in refractivity of the eye at rest and when fully accommodated.

am·poule or **am·pule** or **am·pul** (ăm'pōōl, -pyōol) *n.* A hermetically sealed vial, usually made of glass, that contains a sterile medicinal solution or a powder to be made into a solution for subcutaneous, intramuscular, or intravenous injection.

am·pul·la (ăm-pōōl'ə, -pŭl'ə) *n., pl.* **-pul·lae** (-pōōl'ē, -pŭl'ē). A small dilated portion of a canal or duct, as in the semicircular canal of the ear. — **am·pul'lar** *adj.*

am·pul·li·tis (ăm'pə-lī'tĭəs) *n.* Inflammation of an ampulla, especially of the dilated extremity of the vas deferens.

am·pu·tate (ăm'pyōo-tāt') *v.* **-tat·ed, -tat·ing, -tates.** To cut off a part of the body, especially by surgery.

am·pu·ta·tion (ăm'pyōo-tā'shən) *n.* **1.** Surgical removal of all or part of a limb, an organ, or a projecting part or process of the body. **2.** Traumatic or spontaneous loss of a limb, organ, or part.

am·pu·tee (ăm'pyōo-tē') *n.* A person who has had one or more limbs removed by amputation.

am·ri·none lactate (ăm'rə-nōn') *n.* An inotropic agent that dilates blood vessels, used in treatment of congestive heart failure.

Am·ster·dam syndrome (ăm'stər-dăm') *n.* See **de Lange's syndrome.**

a·mu·si·a (ə-myōo'zē-ə, -zhə) *n.* Loss or impairment of the ability to produce or comprehend music or musical tones.

a·my·e·li·a (ā'mī-ē'lē-ə, ăm'ī-) *n.* Congenital absence of the spinal cord. — **a'my·el'ic** (-ĕl'ĭk, -ē'lĭk) *adj.*

a·my·e·li·na·tion (ā-mī'ə-lə-nā'shən, ə-mī'-) *n.* Congenital absence of the myelin sheath on a nerve. — **a·my'e·li·nat'ed** (-nā'tĭd) *adj.*

a·myg·da·la (ə-mĭg'də-lə) *n., pl.* **-lae** (-lē). **1.** An almond-shaped mass of gray matter in the front part of the temporal lobe of the cerebrum. **2.** The cerebellar tonsil. **3.** Any of the lymphatic tonsils.

a·myg·da·lin (ə-mĭg'də-lĭn) *n.* A glycoside commonly found in seeds and other plant parts of many members of the rose family, such as kernels of the apricot, peach, and bitter almond, which breaks down into hydroeyanic acid, benzaldehyde, and glucose.

a·myg·da·lo·side (ə-mĭg'də-lə-sīd') *n.* See **amygdalin.**

am·y·lase (ăm'ə-lās', -lāz') *n.* Any of a group of enzymes present in saliva and pancreatic juice that catalyze the hydrolysis of starch to sugar.

amylase-creatinine clearance ratio *n.* A ratio determined by measuring amylase and creatinine in serum and urine, used as a test in the diagnosis of acute pancreatitis.

am·y·la·su·ri·a (ăm'ə-lā-sōōr'ē-ə, -syōōr'-) *n.* The presence of an excess of amylase in the urine.

amyl nitrite *n.* A volatile yellow liquid used as a vasodilator and as an antidote in cyanide poisoning.

am·y·lo·gen·e·sis (ăm'ə-lō-jĕn'ĭ-sĭs) *n.* The biosynthesis of starch. — **am'y·lo·gen'ic** *adj.*

am·y·loid (ăm'ə-loid') *n.* A hard, waxy deposit

consisting of protein and polysaccharides resulting from the degeneration of tissue.

amyloid degeneration n. The degeneration of a tissue or an organ characterized by the infiltration of amyloid between cells and fibers.

amyloid nephrosis n. The nephrotic syndrome due to deposition of amyloid in the kidney.

am·y·loid·o·sis (ăm'ə-loi-dō'sĭs) n. A disorder marked by the deposition of amyloid in various organs and tissues of the body that may be associated with a chronic disease such as rheumatoid arthritis, tuberculosis, or multiple myeloma.

am·y·lol·y·sis (ăm'ə-lŏl'ĭ-sĭs) n. The conversion of starch to sugars by the action of enzymes or acids. — **am'y·lo·lyt'ic** (-lō-lĭt'ĭk) adj.

am·y·lop·sin (ăm'ə-lŏp'sĭn) n. The starch-digesting amylase produced by the pancreas.

am·y·lor·rhe·a (ăm'ə-lō-rē'ə) n. The presence of undigested starch in the stool.

am·y·lose (ăm'ə-lōs', -lōz') n. **1.** The inner portion of a starch granule, consisting of relatively soluble polysaccharides. **2.** A polysaccharide, such as starch or cellulose.

am·y·lo·su·ri·a (ăm'ə-lō-sŏŏr'ē-ə, -shŏŏr'-) n. The presence of amylose in the urine.

am·y·lum (ăm'ə-ləm) n. See **starch** (sense 1).

am·y·lu·ri·a (ăm'ə-lŏŏr'ē-ə) n. See **amylosuria**.

a·my·o·es·the·sia (ā-mī'ō-ĕs-thē'zhə, ə-mī'-) or **a·my·o·es·the·sis** (-thē'sĭs) n. Inability to sense motion, weight, and balance.

a·my·o·pla·si·a (ā-mī'ō-plā'zē-ə, -zhə, ə-mī'-) n. The lack of muscle formation.

a·my·o·sta·si·a (ā-mī'ō-stā'zē-ə, -zhə, ə-mī'-) n. A muscular tremor causing difficulty in standing or in coordination. — **a·my'o·stat'ic** (-stăt'ĭk) adj.

a·my·os·the·ni·a (ā-mī'əs-thē'nē-ə, ə-mī'-) n. Weakness of the muscles. — **a·my'os·then'ic** (-thĕn'ĭk) adj.

a·my·o·tax·y (ā-mī'ə-tăk'sē, ə-mī'-) or **a·my·o·tax·ia** (ā-mī'ə-tăk'sē-ə, ə-mī'-) n. Muscular ataxia or incoordination due to difficulties in controlling voluntary movements.

a·my·o·to·ni·a (ā'mī-ə-tō'nē-ə) n. See **myatonia**.

amyotonia con·gen·i·ta (kən-jĕn'ĭ-tə) n. Any of several congenital diseases of children that are marked by general muscle hypotonia.

a·my·o·troph·ic lateral sclerosis (ā-mī'ə-trŏf'ĭk, -trō'fĭk) n. A disease of the motor tracts of the lateral columns and anterior horns of the spinal cord, causing progressive muscular atrophy, increased reflexes, fibrillary twitching, and spastic irritability of muscles.

a·my·ot·ro·phy (ā'mī-ŏt'rə-fē, ăm'ī-) n. Muscular wasting or atrophy.

a·myx·or·rhe·a (ā-mĭk'sə-rē'ə, -mĭk'-) n. Absence of mucus secretion.

an·a·bi·o·sis (ăn'ə-bī-ō'sĭs) n. A restoring to life from a deathlike condition; resuscitation.

an·a·bi·ot·ic (ăn'ə-bī-ŏt'ĭk) adj. Of, relating to, or being restorative; resuscitative. — n. A powerful stimulant; a revivifying remedy.

anabolic steroid n. A group of synthetic hormones that promote the storage of protein and the growth of tissue, sometimes used by athletes to increase muscle size and strength.

a·nab·o·lism (ə-năb'ə-lĭz'əm) n. The phase of metabolism in which simple substances are synthesized into the complex materials of living tissue. — **an'a·bol'ic** (ăn'ə-bŏl'ĭk) adj.

a·nab·o·lite (ə-năb'ə-līt') n. A substance formed as a result of anabolism.

an·a·cid·i·ty (ăn'ə-sĭd'ĭ-tē) n. Absence of acidity, especially the absence of hydrochloric acid in the gastric juices.

an·a·cli·sis (ăn'ə-klī'sĭs, -năk'lĭ-) n. Psychological dependence on others.

an·a·clit·ic (ăn'ə-klĭt'ĭk) adj. Having a physical and emotional dependence on another person, especially relating to the dependence of an infant on a mother or surrogate mother.

anaclitic depression n. The impairment of an infant's physical, social, and intellectual development following separation from its mother or primary caregiver.

an·a·crot·ic pulse (ăn'ə-krŏt'ĭk) n. A slow-rising pulse tracing with a notch in the ascending portion.

a·nac·ro·tism (ə-năk'rə-tĭz'əm) n. The condition in which one or more notches or waves occur on the ascending limb of an arterial pulse tracing.

an·a·cu·sis or **an·a·ku·sis** (ăn'ə-kōō'sĭs) n. Complete deafness.

an·a·di·cro·tism (ăn'ə-dī'krə-tĭz'əm) n. See **anacrotism**.

an·ad·re·nal·ism (ăn'ə-drē'nə-lĭz'əm) n. Complete absence or failure of adrenal function.

an·aer·obe (ăn'ə-rōb', ăn-âr'ōb') n. An organism, such as a bacterium, that can live in the absence of atmospheric oxygen.

an·aer·o·bic (ăn'ə-rō'bĭk, -âr-ō'bĭk) adj. **1.** Of, relating to, or being an anaerobe. **2.** Living without oxygen.

anaerobic respiration n. Respiration in which molecular oxygen is not consumed.

an·aer·o·bi·o·sis (ăn'ə-rō'bī-ō'sĭs, ăn'â-rō'-) n. Life sustained by an organism in the absence of oxygen.

an·a·gen (ăn'ə-jĕn') n. The growth phase of the hair cycle during which new hair is formed.

a·nal (ā'nəl) adj. **1.** Of, relating to, or near the anus. **2.** Of or relating to the second stage of psychosexual development in psychoanalytic theory, during which gratification is derived from sensations associated with the anus. **3.** Relating to or being personality traits that originated during toilet training and are distinguished as anal-expulsive or anal-retentive.

anal atresia n. Congenital absence of an anal opening due to the presence of a membranous septum or to complete absence of the anal canal.

an·al·bu·mi·ne·mi·a (ăn'ăl-byōō'mə-nē'mē-ə) n. The absence of albumin from blood serum.

anal canal n. The terminal portion of the alimentary canal, extending from the pelvic diaphragm to the anal orifice.

an·a·lep·tic (ăn'ə-lĕp'tĭk) adj. Restorative or stimulating, as a drug or medication. —*n*. A medication used as a central nervous system stimulant.

analeptic enema *n*. An enema of lukewarm water with a small amount of table salt.

anal fissure *n*. A crack or slit in the mucous membrane of the anus.

anal fistula *n*. A fistula opening at or near the anus, usually into the rectum above the internal sphincter.

an·al·ge·si·a (ăn'əl-jē'zē-ə, -zhə) *n*. A deadening or absence of the sense of pain without loss of consciousness.

analgesia al·ger·a (ăl'jər-ə) *n*. Spontaneous pain in a part of the body that is not sensitive to painful stimuli.

analgesia do·lo·ro·sa (dō'lə-rō'sə) *n*. See **analgesia algera.**

an·al·ge·sic (ăn'əl-jē'zĭk, -sĭk) *n*. A medication capable of reducing or eliminating pain. —*adj*. Characterized by analgesia.

a·nal·i·ty (ā-năl'ĭ-tē) *n*. The psychological state derived from and characteristic of the anal period of psychosexual development.

an·a·logue or **an·a·log** (ăn'ə-lôg') *n*. **1.** An organ or structure that is similar in function to one in another species but is of dissimilar evolutionary origin. **2.** A structural derivative of a parent chemical compound that often differs from it by a single element.

anal orifice *n*. See **anus.**

anal phase *n*. In psychoanalytic theory, the stage of psychosexual development occurring early in life, usually around the second year, when a child's activities, interests, and concerns are centered around the expulsion and retention of feces.

anal sphincter *n*. Either of the two sphincter muscles of the anus. See under **external** and **internal sphincter muscle of anus.**

a·nal·y·sis (ə-năl'ĭ-sĭs) *n*., *pl*. **-ses** (-sēz'). **1.** The separation of a whole into its constituent parts for individual study. **2.** The separation of a substance into its constituent elements to determine either their nature or their proportions. **3.** The stated findings of such a separation or determination. **4.** Psychoanalysis.

an·a·lyst (ăn'ə-lĭst) *n*. **1.** One that analyzes. **2.** A licensed practitioner of psychoanalysis.

an·a·lyt·ic (ăn'ə-lĭt'ĭk) or **an·a·lyt·i·cal** (-ĭ-kəl) *adj*. **1.** Of or relating to analysis or analytics. **2.** Expert in or using analysis, especially one who thinks in an logical manner. **3.** Psychoanalytic.

an·a·lyz·er or **an·a·ly·zor** (ăn'ə-lī'zər) *n*. **1.** An analyst. **2.** The neural basis of a conditioned reflex, including the sensory side of the reflex arc and its central connections. **3.** Any of various instruments used for performing an analysis.

an·am·ne·sis (ăn'ăm-nē'sĭs) *n*., *pl*. **-ses** (-sēz). **1.** A recalling to memory; recollection. **2.** The complete case history of a patient.

an·am·nes·tic reaction (ăn'ăm-nĕs'tĭk) *n*. Augmented production of an antibody due to previous stimulation by the same antigen.

an·a·phase (ăn'ə-fāz') *n*. The stage of mitosis and meiosis in which the chromosomes move from the equatorial plate toward opposite ends of the nuclear spindle.

an·a·phi·a (ăn-ā'fē-ə) *n*. Total or partial absence of the sense of touch. —**an·ap'tic** (-ăp'tĭk) *adj*.

an·a·pho·ri·a (ăn'ə-fôr'ē-ə) *n*. A tendency of the eyes, when resting, to turn upward.

an·aph·ro·dis·i·a (ăn-ăf'rə-dĭz'ē-ə, -dĭzh'ə) *n*. A decline or absence of sexual desire.

an·a·phy·lac·tic antibody (ăn'ə-fə-lăk'tĭk) *n*. See **cytotropic antibody.**

anaphylactic shock *n*. A sudden, severe, sometimes fatal allergic reaction characterized by a sharp drop in blood pressure, urticaria, and breathing difficulties that is caused by the injection of a foreign substance, such as a drug or bee venom, into the body after a preliminary or sensitizing injection.

an·a·phy·lac·to·gen (ăn'ə-fə-lăk'tə-jən) *n*. A substance capable of producing anaphylaxis in an individual. —**an'a·phy·lac'to·gen'ic** (-jĕn'ĭk) *adj*.

an·a·phy·lac·toid shock (ăn'ə-fə-lăk'toid') *n*. A reaction similar to anaphylactic shock but not requiring the incubation period characteristic of induced sensitivity and unrelated to antibody-antigen reactions.

an·a·phyl·a·tox·in or **anaphylotoxin** (ăn'ə-fĭl'ə-tŏk'sĭn) *n*. A substance that may cause the release of histamine and other compounds that cause hypersensitivity, thus triggering some or all of the symptoms of anaphylaxis.

an·a·phy·lax·is (ăn'ə-fə-lăk'sĭs) *n*., *pl*. **-lax·es** (-lăk'sēz). **1.** Hypersensitivity especially in animals to a substance, such as foreign protein or a drug, that is induced by a preliminary exposure to the substance and that usually produces a contraction of smooth muscle and a dilation of blood vessels. **2.** See **anaphylactic shock.** —**an'a·phy·lac'tic** (-lăk'tĭk) *adj*.

an·a·pla·sia (ăn'ə-plā'zhə) *n*. Reversion of cells to an immature or a less differentiated form, as occurs in most malignant tumors.

an·a·plas·tic cell (ăn'ə-plăs'tĭk) *n*. **1.** A cell that has reverted to an embryonal state. **2.** An undifferentiated cell, characteristic of a malignant neoplasm.

an·a·rith·mia (ăn'ə-rĭth'mē-ə, -rĭth'-) *n*. An inability to count or use numbers because of a lesion in the central lobe of the brain.

an·ar·thri·a (ăn-ăr'thrē-ə) *n*. Loss of the motor ability that enables speech.

an·a·sar·ca (ăn'ə-sär'kə) *n*. An accumulation of serous fluid in various tissues and body cavities. —**an'a·sar'cous** (-sär'kəs) *adj*.

a·nas·to·mose (ə-năs'tə-mōz', -mōs') *v*. **-mosed, -mos·es, -mos·ing. 1.** To join by anastomosis. **2.** To be connected by anastomosis, as blood vessels.

a·nas·to·mo·sis (ə-năs'tə-mō'sĭs) *n*., *pl*. **-ses** (-sēz). **1.** The direct or indirect connection of separate parts of a branching system to form a network, especially among blood vessels. **2.** The surgical connection of separate or severed tubular hollow organs to form a continuous channel, as between two parts of the intestine. **3.** An opening created by surgery, trauma, or disease between two or more normally separate spaces or organs. — **a·nas'to·mot'ic** (-mŏt'ĭk) *adj.*

anastomotic ulcer *n.* An ulcer of the jejunum occurring after gastroenterostomy.

an·a·tom·i·cal (ăn'ə-tŏm'ĭ-kəl) or **an·a·tom·ic** (-tŏm'ĭk) *adj.* **1.** Concerned with anatomy. **2.** Concerned with dissection. **3.** Related to the structure of an organism.

a·nat·o·mist (ə-năt'ə-mĭst) *n.* An expert in or a student of anatomy.

a·nat·o·mize (ə-năt'ə-mīz') *v.* **-mized, -miz·ing, -miz·es.** To dissect an animal or other organism to study the structure and relation of the parts.

a·nat·o·my (ə-năt'ə-mē) *n.* **1.** The morphological structure of a plant or an animal or of any of its parts. **2.** The science of the shape and structure of organisms and their parts. **3.** Dissection of an animal to study the structure, position, and interrelation of its various parts. **4.** A skeleton. **5.** The human body.

an·a·tri·cro·tism (ăn'ə-trī'krə-tĭz'əm, -trĭk'rə-) *n.* A pulse anomaly manifested by a triple beat on the ascending limb of a sphygmographic tracing. — **an'a·tri·crot'ic** (-trī-krŏt'ĭk) *adj.*

an·a·tro·pi·a (ăn'ə-trō'pē-ə) *n.* See **anaphoria.**

an·chor·age (ăng'kər-ĭj) *n.* **1.** The surgical fixation of loose or prolapsed abdominal or pelvic organs. **2.** The part to which something is secured or stabilized.

an·chor splint (ăng'kər) *n.* A splint used for a fracture of the jaw, with wires around the teeth and a rod to hold it in place.

an·co·ni·tis (ăng'kə-nī'tĭs) *n.* An inflammation of the elbow joint.

an·crod (ăn'krŏd) *n.* A proteinase obtained from the venom of the pit viper, used in the treatment of chronic peripheral vascular disease.

An·cy·los·to·ma (ăn'sə-lŏs'tə-mə, ăng'kə-) *n.* A genus of hookworms that includes several species parasitic in the intestines of humans and other mammals.

an·cy·lo·sto·mi·a·sis (ăn'sə-lō-stō-mī'ə-sĭs, ăng'-kə-lō-) *n.* A disease caused by infestation with the hookworm *Ancylostoma duodenale,* characterized by gastrointestinal pain, diarrhea, and progressive anemia.

An·der·son splint (ăn'dər-sən) *n.* A skeletal traction splint having pins inserted into the proximal and distal ends of a fracture; reduction is obtained by an external plate attached to the pins.

an·dro·blas·to·ma (ăn'drō-blă-stō'mə) *n.* A testicular tumor that histologically resembles a fetal testis and contains cells that may produce estrogen.

an·dro·gen (ăn'drə-jən) *n.* A steroid hormone, such as testosterone or androsterone, that controls the development and maintenance of masculine characteristics. — **an'dro·gen'ic** (-jěn'ĭk) *adj.*

androgenic hormone *n.* See **androgen.**

an·drog·e·nize (ăn-drŏj'ə-nīz') *v.* **-nized, -niz·ing, -niz·es.** To treat with male hormones, usually in large doses.

an·drog·y·nism (ăn-drŏj'ə-nĭz'əm) *n.* Female pseudohermaphroditism.

an·drog·y·ny (ăn-drŏj'ə-nē) *n.* **1.** Female pseudohermaphroditism. **2.** The condition of having both masculine and feminine characteristics, as in appearance, attitude, or behavior. — **an·drog'y·nous** (-nəs) *adj.*

an·droid (ăn'droid') *adj.* Possessing human features and form.

an·dro·pho·bi·a (ăn'drə-fō'bē-ə) *n.* An abnormal fear or dislike of men.

an·dros·ter·one (ăn-drŏs'tə-rōn') *n.* A steroid hormone excreted in urine that reinforces masculine characteristics.

a·ne·mi·a (ə-nē'mē-ə) *n.* A pathological deficiency in the oxygen-carrying component of the blood, measured in unit volume concentrations of hemoglobin, red blood cell volume, or red blood cell number. — **a·ne'mic** *adj.*

a·ne·mic anoxia (ə-nē'mĭk) *n.* See **anemic hypoxia.**

anemic hypoxia *n.* Hypoxia resulting from a decreased concentration of functional hemoglobin or a reduced number of erythrocytes.

anemic murmur *n.* A nonvalvular murmur heard on auscultation of the heart and large blood vessels in cases of profound anemia.

an·e·mo·pho·bi·a (ăn'ə-mō-fō'bē-ə, ə-nē'mə-) *n.* An abnormal fear of the wind or drafts.

an·en·ceph·a·ly (ăn'ən-sěf'ə-lē) *n.* Congenital absence of most of the brain and spinal cord. — **an' en·ce·phal'ic** (-sə-făl'ĭk), **an'en·ceph'a·lous** (-sěf'-ə-ləs) *adj.*

a·neph·ric (ā-něf'rĭk, ə-něf'-) *n.* Lacking kidneys.

an·er·gy (ăn'ər-jē) *n.* Absence of sensitivity to substances that would normally elicit an antigenic response. — **an·er'gic** (ă-nûr'jĭk, ăn'ər-) *adj.*

an·e·ryth·ro·pla·si·a (ăn'ĭ-rĭth'rə-plā'zē-ə, -zhə) *n.* A condition in which there is no formation of red blood cells. — **an·e·ryth·ro·plas·tic** (-plăs'-tĭk) *adj.*

an·es·the·sia (ăn'ĭs-thē'zhə) *n.* **1.** Total or partial loss of sensation, especially tactile sensibility, induced by disease, injury, acupuncture, or an anesthetic. **2.** Local or general insensibility to pain with or without the loss of consciousness, induced by an anesthetic.

anesthesia do·lo·ro·sa (dō'lə-rō'sə) *n.* Severe spontaneous pain in an anesthetic zone.

anesthesia record *n.* A written account of drugs administered, procedures undertaken, and cardiovascular responses observed during the course of surgical or obstetrical anesthesia.

an·es·the·si·ol·o·gist (ăn'ĭs-thē'zē-ŏl'ə-jĭst) *n.* A physician specializing in anesthesiology and related areas.

an·es·the·si·ol·o·gy (ăn'ĭs-thē'zē-ŏl'ə-jē) *n.* The medical specialty concerned with the pharmacological, physiological, and clinical basis of anesthesia, including pain management.

an·es·thet·ic (ăn'ĭs-thět'ĭk) *n.* An agent that reversibly depresses neuronal function, producing total or partial loss of sensation. —*adj.* **1.** Characterized by the loss of sensation. **2.** Capable producing loss of sensation. **3.** Associated with or due to the state of anesthesia. —**an'es·thet'i·cal·ly** *adv.*

anesthetic cocktail *n.* A mixture of various drugs, such as painkillers, muscle relaxants, and consciousness-dulling volatile gases, prepared especially for a given procedure and patient.

anesthetic depth *n.* The degree to which the central nervous system is depressed by a general anesthetic agent, depending on the potency and concentration of the anesthetic.

anesthetic ether *n.* Any of various ethers, especially diethyl ether, having anesthetic properties.

anesthetic gas *n.* A gaseous compound capable of producing general anesthesia upon inhalation.

a·nes·the·tist (ə-nĕs'thĭ-tĭst) *n.* A person trained to administer anesthetics.

a·nes·the·tize (ə-nĕs'thĭ-tīz') *v.* **-tized, -tiz·ing, -tiz·es.** To induce anesthesia in. —**an·es'the·ti·za'tion** (-tĭ-zā'shən) *n.*

an·eu·ploid (ăn'yōō-ploid') *n.* A cell or an organism characterized by aneuploidy.

an·eu·ploi·dy (ăn'yə-ploi'dē) *n.* The state of having a chromosome number that is not a multiple of the haploid number.

an·eu·rysm or **an·eu·rism** (ăn'yə-rĭz'əm) *n.* A localized, pathological, blood-filled dilation of a blood vessel caused by disease or weakening of the vessel wall. —**an'eu·rys'mal** (-məl), **an'eu·ris·mat'ic** (-măt'ĭk) *adj.*

aneurysmal bruit *n.* A blowing murmur heard over an aneurysm.

an·eu·rys·mec·to·my (ăn'yə-rĭz-mĕk'tə-mē) *n.* Excision of an aneurysm.

aneurysm of Char·cot (shär-kō') *n.* A small round nodular aneurysm of a small artery or arteriole of the cerebral cortex or basal ganglia, occurring more frequently in hypertensive persons.

an·eu·rys·mo·gram (ăn'yə-rĭz'mə-grăm') *n.* Demonstration of an aneurysm, usually by means of x-rays and a contrast medium.

an·eu·rys·mo·plas·ty (ăn'yə-rĭz'mə-plăs'tē) *n.* **1.** Treatment of an aneurysm by opening the sac and suturing its walls to reconstruct the artery. **2.** See **aneurysmorrhaphy.**

an·eu·rys·mor·rha·phy (ăn'yə-rĭz-môr'ə-fē) *n.* Suture of the sac of an aneurysm.

an·eu·rys·mot·o·my (ăn'yə-rĭz-mŏt'ə-mē) *n.* Incision into the sac of an aneurysm.

an·gi·ec·to·my (ăn'jē-ĕk'tə-mē) *n.* Excision of a section of a blood vessel.

an·gi·i·tis (ăn'jē-ī'tĭs) *n.* See **vasculitis.**

an·gi·na (ăn-jī'nə, ăn'jə-) *n.* **1.** A severe constricting pain, especially angina pectoris. **2.** A sore throat. —**an·gi'nal** *adj.* —**an'gi·nose'** (-jə-nōs') *adj.*

angina pec·to·ris (pĕk'tər-ĭs) *n.* Severe constricting pain in the chest, often radiating from the precordium to the left shoulder and down the arm, caused by insufficient blood supply to the heart muscle that is usually the result of coronary disease.

an·gi·o·blast (ăn'jē-ə-blăst') *n.* **1.** A cell taking part in blood vessel formation. **2.** The primordial mesenchymal tissue from which embryonic blood cells and vascular endothelium are differentiated.

an·gi·o·car·di·og·ra·phy (ăn'jē-ō-kär'dē-ŏg'rə-fē) *n.* Examination of the heart and associated blood vessels using x-rays following the injection of a radiopaque substance. —**an'gi·o·car'di·o·graph'ic** (-ə-grăf'ĭk) *adj.*

an·gi·o·car·di·o·ki·net·ic (ăn'jē-ō-kär'dē-ō-kĭ-nĕt'ĭk) or **an·gi·o·car·di·o·ci·net·ic** (-sə-nĕt'-ĭk) *n.* Causing dilation or contraction in the heart and the blood vessels.

an·gi·o·car·di·op·a·thy (ăn'jē-ō-kär'dē-ŏp'-ə-thē) *n.* A disease affecting the heart and the blood vessels.

an·gi·o·car·di·tis (ăn'jē-ō-kär-dī'tĭs) *n.* Inflammation of the heart and the blood vessels.

an·gi·o·e·de·ma (ăn'jē-ō-ī-dē'mə) *n.* See **angioneurotic edema.**

an·gi·o·fi·bro·sis (ăn'jē-ō-fī-brō'sĭs) *n.* Fibrosis of the walls of blood vessels.

an·gi·o·gen·e·sis (ăn'jē-ō-jĕn'ĭ-sĭs) *n.* The formation of new blood vessels.

an·gi·o·gram (ăn'jē-ə-grăm') *n.* An x-ray of one or more blood vessels produced by angiography and used in diagnosing pathological conditions of the cardiovascular system.

an·gi·og·ra·phy (ăn'jē-ŏg'rə-fē) *n.* Examination of the blood vessels using x-rays following the injection of a radiopaque substance. —**an'gi·o·graph'ic** (-ə-grăf'ĭk) *adj.*

an·gi·o·he·mo·phil·i·a (ăn'jē-ō-hē'mə-fĭl'ē-ə, -fēl'yə) *n.* See **von Willebrand's disease.**

angioid streak *n.* Any of the breaks in the basal layer of the choroid of the eye occurring in a variety of systemic disorders affecting elastic tissue.

an·gi·o·ker·a·to·ma (ăn'jē-ō-kĕr'ə-tō'mə) *n.* An intradermal hemangioma covered by a wartlike thickening of the horny layer of the epidermis.

an·gi·o·ki·ne·sis (ăn'jē-ō-kə-nē'sĭs) *n.* See **vasomotion.**

an·gi·o·ki·net·ic (ăn'jē-ō-kə-nĕt'ĭk, kī-) *n.* See **vasomotor.**

an·gi·o·li·po·ma (ăn'jē-ō-lĭ-pō'mə, -lī-) *n.* A benign tumor composed chiefly of fat cells and containing an unusually large number of vascular channels.

an·gi·o·lith (ăn'jē-ə-lĭth') *n.* A calcareous deposit in a blood vessel wall. —**an'gi·o·lith'ic** *adj.*

an·gi·o·ma (ăn'jē-ō'mə) *n., pl.* **-mas** or **-ma·ta** (-mə-tə). A tumor composed chiefly of lymphatic vessels or blood vessels.

an·gi·o·my·o·li·po·ma (ăn'jē-ō-mī'ō-lĭ-pō'mə) *n.* A benign tumor composed of adipose tissue, muscle cells, and vascular structures.

an·gi·o·my·o·sar·co·ma (ăn'jē-ō-mī'ō-sär-kō'-mə) *n.* A myosarcoma that has an unusually large number of proliferated, frequently dilated, vascular channels.

an·gi·o·neu·rec·to·my (ăn′jē-ō-nŏō-rĕk′tə-mē, -nyŏō-) *n*. Surgical excision of the vessels and nerves of a part.

an·gi·o·neu·rot·ic edema (ăn′jē-ō-nŏō-rŏt′ĭk, -nyŏō-) *n*. Periodically recurring episodes of non-inflammatory swelling of the skin, mucous membranes, viscera, and brain, occasionally accompanied by arthralgia, purpura, or fever.

an·gi·op·a·thy (ăn′jē-op′ə-thē) *n*. Any of several diseases of the blood or lymph vessels.

an·gi·o·pha·co·ma·to·sis or **an·gi·o·pha·ko·ma·to·sis** (ăn′jē-ō-fə-kō′mə-tō′sĭs, -făk′ō-) *n*. **1.** See **Lindau's disease. 2.** See **Sturge-Weber syndrome.**

an·gi·o·plas·ty (ăn′jē-ə-plăs′tē) *n*. **1.** Surgical reconstruction of a blood vessel. **2.** Balloon angioplasty.

an·gi·o·poi·e·sis (ăn′jē-ō-poi-ē′sĭs) *n*. The formation of blood vessels or lymphatic vessels. — **an′-gi·o·poi·et′ic** (-ĕt′ĭk) *adj.*

an·gi·o·pres·sure (ăn′jē-ō-prĕsh′ər) *n*. The application of pressure on a blood vessel to arrest bleeding.

an·gi·or·rha·phy (ăn′jē-ôr′ə-fē) *n*. Suture repair of a vessel, especially a blood vessel.

an·gi·o·sar·co·ma (ăn′jē-ō-sär-kō′mə) *n*. A rare malignant tumor occurring most often in the breast and skin and believed to originate from the endothelial cells of blood vessels.

an·gi·os·co·py (ăn′jē-ŏs′kə-pē) *n*. Visualization of the passage of intravenously injected substances through the capillaries.

an·gi·o·spasm (ăn′jē-ō-spăz′əm) *n*. See **vasospasm.** — **an′gi·o·spas′tic** (-spăs′tĭk) *adj.*

an·gi·o·ste·no·sis (ăn′jē-ō-stə-nō′sĭs) *n*. The narrowing of one or more blood vessels.

an·gi·os·tro·phy (ăn′jē-ŏs′trə-fē) *n*. The twisting of the cut end of a blood vessel to arrest bleeding.

an·gi·o·te·lec·ta·sis (ăn′jē-ō-tĕ-lĕk′tə-sĭs) or **an·gi·o·tel·ec·ta·si·a** (-tĕl′ĭk-tā′zē-ə, -zhə) *n*. Dilation of the terminal arterioles, venules, or capillaries.

an·gi·o·ten·sin (ăn′jē-ō-tĕn′sĭn) *n*. Any of a group of peptides with vasoconstrictive activity that act to control arterial pressure.

angiotensin I *n*. A decapeptide that is the precursor to angiotensin II but is itself physiologically inactive.

angiotensin II *n*. An octapeptide that is a potent vasopressor agent as well as a powerful stimulus for the production and release of aldosterone from the adrenal cortex.

angiotensin III *n*. A heptapeptide derivative of angiotensin II, having some of the same effects of its precursor.

angiotensin amide *n*. A peptide analogue to angiotensin II that is used as a vasopressor agent in the treatment of certain types of shock and circulatory collapse.

an·gi·o·ten·si·nase (ăn′jē-ō-tĕn′sə-nās′, -nāz′) *n*. **1.** A peptidase in tissues and plasma that degrades angiotensin II. **2.** Any of several enzymes in the blood that hydrolyze angiotensin.

angiotensin-converting enzyme *n*. A proteolytic enzyme that catalyzes the removal of dipeptides from a variety of compounds, as from angiotensin I as it is converted to angiotensin II. See **ACE inhibitor.**

angiotensin-converting enzyme inhibitor *n*. See **ACE inhibitor.**

an·gi·o·ten·sin·o·ge·nase (ăn′jē-ō-tĕn-sĭn′ə-jə-nās′, -nāz′) *n*. See **renin.**

an·gi·ot·o·my (ăn′jē-ŏt′ə-mē) *n*. Incision into a blood vessel.

an·gi·o·tribe (ăn′jē-ə-trīb′) *n*. A strong forceps used to arrest hemorrhage by crushing the end of a blood vessel and the surrounding tissue.

an·gi·o·trip·sy (ăn′jē-ə-trĭp′sē) *n*. Use of an angiotribe to arrest hemorrhage.

an·gle (ăng′gəl) *n*. The figure or space formed by the junction of two lines or planes.

angst (ängkst) *n*. A feeling of anxiety or apprehension often accompanied by depression.

angular cheilitis *n*. Inflammation and radiating fissures from the commissures of the mouth, secondary to predisposing factors such as nutritional deficiencies, atopic dermatitis, or *Candida albicans* infection.

angular stomatitis *n*. Inflammation at the corners of the mouth, usually associated with a wrinkled or fissured epithelium.

an·gu·la·tion (ăng′gyə-lā′shən) *n*. The formation of an abnormal angle or bend in an organ. — **an′gu·late′** (-lāt′) *v*.

an·he·do·ni·a (ăn′hē-dō′nē-ə) *n*. Absence of pleasure from the performance of acts that would normally be pleasurable.

an·hi·dro·sis (ăn′hĭ-drō′sĭs) *n*. Absence of sweating.

an·hi·drot·ic (ăn′hĭ-drŏt′ĭk) *adj*. Relating to or characterized by anhidrosis. — *n*. An agent that reduces, prevents, or stops sweating.

a·ni·linc·tion (ā′nə-lĭngk′shən) or **a·ni·linc·tus** (-lĭngk′təs) *n*. Sexual stimulation by licking or kissing the anus.

a·ni·lin·gus (ā′nə-lĭng′gəs) *n*. Anilinction.

a·nil·i·ty (ə-nĭl′ĭ-tē) *n*. See **dotage.**

an·i·ma (ăn′ə-mə) *n*. **1.** The inner self of an individual; the soul. **2.** In Jungian psychology, the unconscious or true inner self of an individual, as opposed to the persona, or outer aspect of the personality. **3.** In Jungian psychology, the feminine inner personality as present in the unconscious of the male.

an·i·mal (ăn′ə-məl) *n*. **1.** A multicellular organism with membranous cell walls of the kingdom Animalia, differing from plants in certain typical characteristics such as capacity for locomotion, nonphotosynthetic metabolism, pronounced response to stimuli, restricted growth, and fixed bodily structure. **2.** An animal organism other than a human, especially a mammal. **3.** A human considered with respect to his or her physical, as opposed to spiritual, nature. — *adj*. **1.** Relating to, characteristic of, or derived from an animal or animals. **2.** Relating to the physical as distinct from the spiritual nature of humans.

animal pole *n.* The point in an ovum where the nucleus is located and from which the polar bodies are extruded during maturation.

animal starch *n.* See **glycogen**.

an·i·ma·tion (ăn′ə-mā′shən) *n.* **1.** The state of being alive. **2.** Liveliness; high spirits.

an·i·mus (ăn′ə-məs) *n.* **1.** An animating or energizing spirit. **2.** Intention to do something; disposition. **3.** A spirit of active hostility; ill will. **4.** In Jungian psychology, the masculine inner personality as present in the unconscious of the female.

an·i·on (ăn′ī′ən) *n.* A negatively charged ion.

an·i·rid·i·a (ăn′ī-rĭd′ē-ə, ăn′ə-) *n.* Congenital absence of all but the root of the iris.

An·i·sa·kis (ăn′ī-sā′kĭs) *n.* A genus of nematodes that includes many common parasites of marine fish-eating birds and marine mammals.

an·i·sei·ko·ni·a (ăn-ī′sī-kō′nē-ə) *n.* A condition in which the shape and size of the ocular image differ in each eye.

an·i·so·ac·com·mo·da·tion (ăn-ī′sō-ə-kŏm′ə-dā′shən) *n.* Variation between the two eyes in accommodation capacity.

an·i·so·co·ri·a (ăn-ī′sō-kôr′ē-ə) *n.* Unequal size of the pupils.

an·i·sog·a·my (ăn′ī-sŏg′ə-mē) *n.* A union between two gametes that differ in size or form. — **an′i·so·gam′ic** (-sə-găm′ĭk) *adj.*

an·i·so·kar·y·o·sis (ăn-ī′sō-kăr′ē-ō′sĭs) *n.* Variation in the size of the nuclei of cells.

an·i·so·mas·ti·a (ăn-ī′sō-măs′tē-ə) *n.* Asymmetry of the breasts.

an·i·so·me·li·a (ăn-ī′sō-mē′lē-ə) *n.* Inequality between paired limbs.

an·i·so·me·tro·pi·a (ăn-ī′sə-mĭ-trō′pē-ə) *n.* A condition in which the refractive power of one eye differs from that of the other. — **an·i′so·me·trop′ic** (-trŏp′ĭk, -trō′pĭk) *adj.*

an·i·so·pi·e·sis (ăn-ī′sō-pī-ē′sĭs) *n.* Unequal arterial blood pressure on the two sides of the body.

an·i·so·trop·ic (ăn-ī′sə-trŏp′ĭk, -trō′pĭk) *adj.* **1.** Not isotropic. **2.** Having physical properties that differ according to the direction of measurement. — **an·i′so·trop′i·cal·ly** *adv.* — **an′i·sot′ro·pism** (-sŏt′rə-pĭz′əm), **an′i·sot′ro·py** (-sŏt′rə-pē) *n.*

an·i·so·tro·pine meth·yl·bro·mide (ăn-ī′sə-trō′pēn′ mĕth′əl-brō′mīd′) *n.* An anticholinergic agent and intestinal antispasmodic.

an·kle (ăng′kəl) *n.* **1.** The joint between the leg and foot in which the tibia and fibula above articulate with the talus below. **2.** The region of the ankle joint. **3.** The anklebone.

anklebone *n.* See **talus** (sense 1).

ankle joint *n.* A hinge joint between the tibia and the fibula above and the talus below.

ankle reflex *n.* See **Achilles reflex**.

an·ky·lo·proc·ti·a (ăng′kə-lō-prŏk′shē-ə) *n.* Imperforation or stricture of the anus.

an·ky·los·ing spondylitis (ăng′kə-lō′sĭng, -lō′-zĭng) *n.* Arthritis of the spine, resembling rheumatoid arthritis and leading to fusion of the vertebrae.

an·ky·lo·sis (ăng′kə-lō′sĭs) *n.* The stiffening or immobility of a joint resulting from disease, trauma, surgery, or abnormal bone fusion. — **an′ky·lot′ic** (-lŏt′ĭk) *adj.*

an·la·ge or **An·la·ge** (än′lä-gə) *n., pl.* **-ges** or **-gen** (-gən). **1.** The initial clustering of embryonic cells from which a part or an organ develops; primordium. **2.** A genetic predisposition to a given trait or personality characteristic.

an·neal·ing lamp (ə-nē′lĭng) *n.* An alcohol lamp with a soot-free flame used to prepare gold foil for use in dental fillings.

an·nu·lar (ăn′yə-lər) *adj.* Shaped like or forming a ring.

annular scotoma *n.* A circular scotoma surrounding the center of the field of vision.

an·nu·lo·plas·ty (ăn′yə-lə-plăs′tē) *n.* Surgical reconstruction of an incompetent cardiac valve.

an·nu·lor·rha·phy (ăn′yə-lôr′ə-fē) *n.* The closure of a hernial ring by suture.

an·nu·lus or **an·u·lus** (ăn′yə-ləs) *n., pl.* **-lus·es** or **-li** (-lī′). A circular or ring-shaped structure.

an·o·don·ti·a (ăn′ō-dŏn′shē-ə, -shə) *n.* Congenital absence of teeth.

an·o·dyne (ăn′ə-dīn′) *n.* An agent capable of relieving pain.

a·nom·a·lous complex (ə-nŏm′ə-ləs) *n.* An electrocardiographic reading that differs significantly from the normal reading for that physiological type.

a·nom·a·ly (ə-nŏm′ə-lē) *n.* A deviation from the average or norm.

an·o·nych·i·a (ăn′ə-nĭk′ē-ə) or **an·o·ny·cho·sis** (ăn′ə-nĭ-kō′sĭs) *n.* Congenital absence of nails.

A·noph·e·les (ə-nŏf′ə-lēz′) *n.* A genus of mosquitoes containing over 90 species, many of which are vectors of malaria.

an·oph·thal·mi·a (ăn′ŏf-thăl′mē-ə, -ŏp-) *n.* Complete absence of tissues of the eyes.

a·no·plas·ty (ā′nə-plăs′tē) *n.* Reconstructive surgery on the anus.

an·or·chi·a (ă-nôr′kē-ə) or **an·or·chism** (ă-nôr′kĭz′əm) *n.* Congenital absence of the testes.

an·o·rec·tic (ăn′ə-rĕk′tĭk) or **an·o·ret·ic** (-rĕt′ĭk) *adj.* **1.** Marked by loss of appetite. **2.** Suppressing or causing loss of appetite. **3.** Of or affected with anorexia nervosa. — *n.* **1.** An agent that causes loss of appetite. **2.** One who is affected with anorexia nervosa.

an·o·rex·i·a (ăn′ə-rĕk′sē-ə) *n.* Loss of appetite, especially as a result of disease.

anorexia nerv·o·sa (nûr-vō′sə) *n.* A psychophysiological disorder usually occurring in teenage women, characterized by fear of becoming obese, a distorted self-image, a persistent aversion to food, and severe weight loss. It is often accompanied by self-induced vomiting, amenorrhea, and other physiological changes.

an·o·rex·i·ant (ăn′ə-rĕk′sē-ənt) *n.* A drug, process, or event that leads to anorexia.

an·o·rex·ic (ăn′ə-rĕk′sĭk) *adj.* Relating to or suffering from anorexia nervosa. — **an′o·rex′ic** *n.*

an·or·gas·my (ăn′ôr-găz′mē) or **an·or·gas·mi·a** (-găz′mē-ə) *n.* Failure to experience an orgasm.

an·or·thog·ra·phy (ăn'ôr-thŏg'rə-fē) *n.* See **agraphia.**

a·no·scope (ā'nə-skōp') *n.* A short speculum for examining the anal canal and lower rectum.

a·no·sig·moid·os·co·py (ā'nō-sĭg'moi-dŏs'kə-pē) *n.* Endoscopy of the anus, rectum, and sigmoid colon.

an·os·mi·a (ăn-ŏz'mē-ə) *n.* Loss of the sense of smell. — **an·os'mic** *adj.*

an·o·ti·a (ă-nō'shē-ə, -shə) *n.* Congenital absence of one or both ears.

an·ov·u·lant (ăn'ŏv'yə-lənt) *n.* A drug that suppresses ovulation.

an·o·vu·lar menstruation (ăn-ō'vyə-lər, -ŏv'yə-) *n.* Menstrual bleeding without the discharge of an ovum.

an·o·vu·la·tion (ăn-ō'vyə-lā'shən, -ŏv'yə-) *n.* Suspension or cessation of ovulation.

an·ox·e·mi·a (ăn'ŏk-sē'mē-ə) *n.* An absence of oxygen in arterial blood.

an·ox·i·a (ăn-ŏk'sē-ə, ə-nŏk'-) *n.* The absence or reduced supply of oxygen in inspired gases, arterial blood, or tissues. — **an·ox'ic** *adj.*

anoxic anoxia *n.* See **hypoxic hypoxia.**

An·rep phenomenon (ăn'rĕp, än'rĕp) *n.* Homeometric autoregulation of the heart in which cardiac performance improves as aortic pressure increases.

an·sa (ăn'sə) *n., pl.* **-sae** (-sē). An anatomical structure shaped like a loop or an arc.

ant·ac·id (ănt-ăs'ĭd) or **an·ti·ac·id** (ăn'tē-ăs'ĭd, ăn'tī-) *adj.* Counteracting or neutralizing acidity, especially of the stomach. — *n.* A substance, such as sodium bicarbonate, that neutralizes acid.

an·tag·o·nism (ăn-tăg'ə-nĭz'əm) *n.* Mutual opposition in action between structures, agents, diseases, or physiological processes.

an·tag·o·nist (ăn-tăg'ə-nĭst) *n.* Something, such as a muscle or physiological process, that neutralizes or impedes the action or effect of another.

an·tag·o·nis·tic muscles (ăn-tăg'ə-nĭs'tĭk) *pl.n.* Muscles having opposite functions, the contraction of one neutralizing the contraction of the other.

ant·al·gic gait (ănt-ăl'jĭk) *n.* A limp in which the stance phase of the gait is shortened on the injured side to alleviate the pain experienced when bearing weight on that side.

an·te·ce·dent (ăn'tĭ-sēd'nt) *n.* A precursor.

an·te·flex·ion (ăn'tē-flĕk'shən) *n.* A sharp forward curve or angulation, especially in the uterus at the junction of the corpus and cervix.

an·te·grade urography (ăn'tĭ-grăd') *n.* X-ray examination of the urinary tract using percutaneous injection of a contrast agent into the renal calices or pelvis, or into the urinary bladder.

an·te·ri·or (ăn-tîr'ē-ər) *adj.* **1.** Of or relating to the front surface of the body, especially of the position of one structure relative to another; ventral. **2.** Near the head or rostral end of certain embryos. — *n.* The front surface of the body.

anterior chamber of eye *n.* The space between the cornea and the iris, filled with the aqueous humor and communicating through the pupil with the posterior chamber.

anterior column of spinal cord *n.* The ventral ridge of gray matter in each half of the spinal cord, containing the motor neurons innervating the muscles of the trunk, neck, and extremities.

anterior focal point *n.* The point where light rays starting parallel from the retina are focused.

anterior horn *n.* **1.** The front section of the lateral ventricle of the brain. **2.** The front or ventral gray column of the spinal cord in cross section.

anterior lobe of hypophysis *n.* See **adenohypophysis.**

anterior pituitary gonadotropin *n.* Any of several polypeptide or protein hormones secreted by the anterior lobe of the pituitary gland.

anterior staphyloma *n.* A bulging near the anterior pole of the eyeball.

an·ter·o·fa·cial dysplasia (ăn'tə-rō-fā'shəl) *n.* The abnormal growth in an anteroposterior direction of the face or cranium.

an·ter·o·grade amnesia (ăn'tə-rō-grăd') *n.* A condition in which events that occurred after the onset of amnesia cannot be recalled and new memories cannot be formed.

ante·ver·sion (ăn'tē-vûr'zhən, -shən) *n.* A turning forward as a whole without bending. — **an'te·vert'ed** (ăn'tē-vûr'tĭd) *adj.*

ant·hel·min·tic (ănt'hĕl-mĭn'tĭk, ăn'thĕl-) or **ant·hel·min·thic** (-thĭk) *n.* An agent that destroys or causes the expulsion of parasitic intestinal worms. — *adj.* Acting to expel or destroy parasitic intestinal worms.

an·thra·co·sil·i·co·sis (ăn'thrə-kō-sĭl'ĭ-kō'sĭs) *n.* Accumulation of carbon and silica in the lungs from inhaled coal dust.

an·thra·co·sis (ăn'thrə-kō'sĭs) *n.* Accumulation of carbon in the lungs from inhaled smoke or coal dust.

an·thrax (ăn'thrăks') *n.* **1.** An infectious, usually fatal disease of warm-blooded animals that is characterized by ulcerative skin lesions, can be transmitted to humans, and is caused by the bacterium *Bacillus anthracis.* **2.** *pl.* **-thra·ces** (-thrə-sēz'). A lesion caused by anthrax.

an·thro·poid (ăn'thrə-poid') *adj.* **1.** Resembling humans in structure and form. **2.** Of or belonging to the family of great apes including the gorilla, chimpanzee, and orangutan. — *n.* An ape of the family that includes the gorilla, chimpanzee, and orangutan.

an·thro·pol·o·gy (ăn'thrə-pŏl'ə-jē) *n.* The scientific study of the origin, the behavior, and the physical, social, and cultural development of humans. — **an'thro·pol'o·gist** *n.*

an·thro·po·mor·phism (ăn'thrə-pə-môr'fĭz'əm) *n.* The attribution of human motivation, characteristics, or behavior to nonhuman organisms or inanimate objects. — **an'thro·po·mor'phic** *adj.* — **an'thro·po·mor'phi·cal·ly** *adv.*

an·ti·ag·glu·ti·nin (ăn'tē-ə-glōōt'n-ĭn, ăn'tī-) *n.* A specific antibody that inhibits or destroys the action of an agglutinin.

an·ti·an·a·phy·lax·is (ăn′tē-ăn′ə-fə-lăk′sĭs, ăn′-tĭ-) *n.* See **desensitization** (sense 1).

an·ti·an·ti·body or **an·ti·an·ti·bod·y** (ăn′tē-ăn′tĭ-bŏd′ē, ăn′tĭ-) *n.* An antibody that is specifically directed against another antibody.

an·ti·an·ti·tox·in (ăn′tē-ăn′tē-tŏk′sĭn, ăn′tĭ-) *n.* An anti-antibody that is directed against an antitoxin and counteracts its effects.

an·ti·anx·i·e·ty agent (ăn′tē-ăng-zī′ĭ-tē, ăn′tĭ-) *n.* Any of a group of drugs used to treat anxiety without causing excessive sedation.

an·ti·bac·te·ri·al (ăn′tē-băk-tîr′ē-əl, ăn′tĭ-) *adj.* Destroying or inhibiting the growth of bacteria. — **an′ti·bac·te′ri·al·ly** *adv.*

anti-basement membrane antibody *n.* An autoantibody to a renal glomerular basement membrane antigen.

an·ti·bi·o·sis (ăn′tē-bī-ō′sĭs, ăn′tĭ-) *n.* **1.** An association between two or more organisms that is detrimental to at least one of them. **2.** The antagonistic association between an organism and the metabolic substances produced by another.

an·ti·bi·ot·ic (ăn′tĭ-bī-ŏt′ĭk, ăn′tĭ-) *n.* A substance, such as penicillin or streptomycin, produced by or derived from certain fungi, bacteria, and other organisms, that can destroy or inhibit the growth of other microorganisms. — *adj.* **1.** Of or relating to antibiotics. **2.** Of or relating to antibiosis.

antibiotic enterocolitis *n.* Enterocolitis caused by oral administration of broad-spectrum antibiotics.

an·ti·bod·y (ăn′tĭ-bŏd′ē) *n.* **1.** A protein substance produced in the blood or tissues in response to a specific antigen, such as a bacterium or a toxin, that destroys or weakens bacteria and neutralizes organic poisons, thus forming the basis of immunity. **2.** An immunoglobulin present in the blood serum or body fluids as a result of antigenic stimulus and interacting only with the antigen that induced it or with an antigen closely related to it.

antibody excess *n.* In a precipitation test, the presence of antibody in an amount greater than that required to combine with all antigen present.

an·ti·cho·lin·er·gic (ăn′tē-kō′lə-nûr′jĭk, ăn′tĭ-) *n.* An agent that is antagonistic to the action of parasympathetic or other cholinergic nerve fibers. — **an′ti·cho′lin·er′gic** *adj.*

an·ti·cho·lin·es·ter·ase (ăn′tē-kō′lə-nĕs′tə-rās′, -rāz′, ăn′tĭ-) *n.* A substance that inhibits the activity of cholinesterases.

an·ti·co·ag·u·lant (ăn′tē-kō-ăg′yə-lənt, ăn′tĭ-) *n.* A substance that delays or prevents the clotting of blood. — *adj.* Acting as an anticoagulant.

an·ti·co·don (ăn′tē-kō′dŏn, ăn′tĭ-) *n.* A sequence of three adjacent nucleotides in transfer RNA designating a specific amino acid that binds to a corresponding codon in messenger RNA during protein synthesis.

an·ti·com·ple·ment (ăn′tē-kŏm′plə-mənt, ăn′tĭ-) *n.* A substance that neutralizes the action of a complement by combining with it and preventing its union with the antibody.

an·ti·con·vul·sant (ăn′tē-kən-vŭl′sənt, ăn′tĭ-) *n.*

A drug that prevents or relieves convulsions. — **an′ti·con·vul′sive** (-sĭv) *adj.*

an·ti·de·pres·sant (ăn′tē-dĭ-prĕs′ənt, ăn′tĭ-) *n.* A drug used to prevent or relieve mental depression. — **an′ti·de·pres′sive** (-prĕs′ĭv) *adj.*

an·ti·di·ar·rhe·al (ăn′tē-dī′ə-rē′əl, an′tĭ-) *n.* A substance used to prevent or treat diarrhea.

an·ti·di·u·re·sis (ăn′tē-dī′ə-rē′sĭs, ăn′tĭ-) *n.* The reduction of urinary volume.

an·ti·di·u·ret·ic (ăn′tē-dī′ə-rĕt′ĭk, ăn′tĭ-) *n.* An agent that reduces the output of urine.

antidiuretic hormone *n.* See **vasopressin**.

an·ti·dote (ăn′tĭ-dōt′) *n.* A remedy or other agent used to neutralize or counteract the effects of a poison. — **an′ti·dot′al** (ăn′tĭ-dōt′l) *adj.* — **an′ti·dot′al·ly** *adv.*

an·ti·e·met·ic (ăn′tē-ĭ-mĕt′ĭk, ăn′tĭ-) *adj.* Preventing or arresting vomiting. — *n.* An agent that prevents or arrests vomiting.

an·ti·en·zyme (ăn′tē-ĕn′zīm′, ăn′tĭ-) *n.* An agent or principle, especially an inhibitory enzyme or an antibody to an enzyme, that retards, inhibits, or destroys the activity of an enzyme. — **an′ti·en′zy·mat′ic** (-zī-măt′ĭk, -zī-), **an′ti·en·zy′mic** (-zī′mĭk) *adj.*

an·ti·es·tro·gen (ăn′tē-ĕs′trə-jən, ăn′tĭ-) *n.* A substance capable of preventing full expression of the biological effects of an estrogen.

an·ti·feb·rile (ăn′tē-fĕb′rəl, -fē′brəl, -brīl′, ăn′tĭ-) *n.* See **antipyretic**.

an·ti·fer·til·i·ty (ăn′tē-fər-tĭl′ĭ-tē, ăn′tĭ-) *adj.* Capable of reducing or eliminating fertility.

an·ti·fi·bri·nol·y·sin (ăn′tē-fī′brə-nŏl′ĭ-sĭn, ăn′tĭ-) *n.* See **antiplasmin**.

an·ti·fun·gal (ăn′tē-fŭng′gəl, ăn′tĭ-) *adj.* Destroying or inhibiting the growth of fungi.

an·ti·gen (ăn′tĭ-jən) *n.* Any of various substances, including toxins, bacteria, foreign blood cells, and the cells of transplanted organs, that when introduced into the body stimulate the production of antibodies. — **an′ti·gen′ic** (-jĕn′ĭk) *adj.*

antigen-antibody reaction *n.* The binding of an antibody with an antigen of the type that stimulated the formation of the antibody, resulting in agglutination, precipitation, complement fixation, greater susceptibility to ingestion and destruction by phagocytes, or neutralization of an exotoxin.

an·ti·gen·e·mi·a (ăn′tə-jə-nē′mē-ə) *n.* The presence of an antigen in circulating blood.

antigen excess *n.* In a precipitation test, the presence of uncombined antigen above that required to combine with all of the antibody.

antigenic determinant *n.* The portion of an antigen with which an antibody or lymphocyte reacts; epitope.

an·ti·ge·nic·i·ty (ăn′tĭ-jə-nĭs′ĭ-tē) *n.* **1.** The capacity to induce an immune response. **2.** The degree to which a substance induces an immune response.

antigen-presenting cell *n.* A cell, originating in the bone marrow and subsequently found as a dendritic cell in various locations, believed to facilitate the immune response.

an·ti·glob·u·lin test (ăn′tē-glŏb′yə-lĭn, ăn′tī-) *n.* See **Coombs test.**

an·ti-HB_c (ăn′tē-āch′bē-sē′, ăn′tī-) *n.* The antibody to the hepatitis B core antigen.

an·ti-HB_s (ăn′tē-āch′bē-ĕs′, ăn′tī-) *n.* The antibody to the hepatitis B surface antigen.

an·ti-HB_e (ăn′tē-āch′bē-ē′, ăn′tī-) *n.* The antibody to the hepatitis B e antigen.

an·ti·he·mag·glu·ti·nin (ăn′tē-hē′mə-gloot′n-ĭn, ăn′tī-) *n.* A substance that inhibits or prevents the effects of hemagglutinin.

an·ti·he·mol·y·sin (ăn′tē-hī-mŏl′ĭ-sĭn, -hē′mə-lī′-, ăn′tī-) *n.* A substance that inhibits or prevents the effects of hemolysin.

an·ti·he·mo·phil·ic factor (ăn′tē-hē′mə-fĭl′ĭk, ăn′tī-) *n.* See **factor VIII.**

antihemophilic globulin *n.* **1.** See **factor VIII. 2.** See **human antihemophilic factor.**

antihemophilic globulin A *n.* See **factor VIII.**

antihemophilic globulin B *n.* See **factor IX.**

antihemophilic human plasma *n.* Normal human plasma in which the labile antihemophilic globulin component has been preserved, used for the temporary relief of dysfunction of the hemostatic mechanism in hemophilia.

an·ti·hem·or·rhag·ic (ăn′tē-hĕm′ə-răj′ĭk, ăn′tī-) *adj.* Arresting or reducing hemorrhage.

an·ti·his·ta·mine (ăn′tē-hĭs′tə-mēn′, -mĭn) *n.* Any of several drugs used to counteract the physiological effects of histamine. — **an′ti·his′ta·mine′** *adj.*

an·ti·his·ta·min·ic (ăn′tē-hĭs′tə-mĭn′ĭk) *adj.* Tending to neutralize or antagonize the action of histamine or inhibit its production in the body. — *n.* An antihistaminic drug.

an·ti·hu·man globulin (ăn′tē-hyoo′mən, ăn′tī-) *n.* See **Coombs′ serum.**

an·ti·hy·per·ten·sive (ăn′tē-hī′pər-tĕn′sĭv, ăn′tī-) *adj.* Reducing high blood pressure. — *n.* A drug or treatment that reduces high blood pressure.

an·ti-in·fec·tive (ăn′tē-ĭn-fĕk′tĭv, ăn′tī-) *adj.* Capable of preventing or counteracting infection.

an·ti-in·flam·ma·to·ry or **an·ti-in·flam·ma·to·ry** (ăn′tē-ĭn-flăm′ə-tôr′ē, ăn′tī-) *adj.* Reducing inflammation by acting on body mechanisms. — **an′ti-in·flam′ma·to·ry** *n.*

an·ti·lym·pho·cyte serum (ăn′tē-lĭm′fə-sīt′, ăn′-tī-) *n.* The globulin fraction of serum from a horse or another animal, usually used in conjunction with other immunosuppressive agents to suppress rejection of grafts or organ transplants.

an·ti·ly·sin (ăn′tē-lī′sĭn, ăn′tī-) *n.* An antibody that inhibits or prevents the effects of lysin.

an·ti·ma·lar·i·al (ăn′tē-mə-lâr′ē-əl, ăn′tī-) *adj.* Preventing or relieving the symptoms of malaria.

an·ti·mere (ăn′tī-mēr′) *n.* **1.** One of the corresponding parts of a bilaterally symmetrical organism. **2.** The right or left half of the body. — **an′ti·mer′ic** (-mēr′ĭk) *adj.*

an·ti·me·tab·o·lite (ăn′tē-mĭ-tăb′ə-līt′, ăn′tī-) *n.* A substance that closely resembles an essential metabolite and competes with, interferes with, or replaces it in physiological reactions.

an·ti·mi·cro·bi·al (ăn′tē-mī-krō′bē-əl, ăn′tī-) or **an·ti·mi·cro·bic** (-bĭk) *adj.* Tending to destroy microbes, prevent their development, or inhibit their pathogenic action.

an·ti·mo·ny (ăn′tə-mō′nē) *n.* An element with atomic number 51 and having several allotropes, the most common of which is a brittle, silver-white crystalline metal.

an·ti·mu·ta·gen (ăn′tē-myoo′tə-jən, -jĕn′, ăn′tī-) *n.* A substance that reduces or interferes with the mutagenic effects of a mutagen. — **an′·ti·mu′ta·gen′ic** *adj.*

an·ti·ne·o·plas·tic (ăn′tē-nē′ə-plăs′tĭk, ăn′tī-) *adj.* Preventing the development, spread, or maturation of neoplastic cells. — **an′ti·ne′o·plas′tic** *n.*

an·ti·nu·cle·ar antibody (ăn′tē-noo′klē-ər, -nyoo′-, ăn′tī-) *n.* An antibody that attacks cell nuclei.

an·ti·on·co·gene (ăn′tē-ŏng′kə-jēn, ăn′tī-) *n.* A tumor-suppressing gene that is involved in controlling cellular growth.

an·ti·par·a·sit·ic (ăn′tē-păr′ə-sĭt′ĭk, ăn′tī-) *adj.* Destroying or inhibiting the growth and reproduction of parasites. — **an′ti·par′a·sit′ic** *n.*

an·ti·per·ni·cious anemia factor (ăn′tē-pər-nĭsh′əs, ăn′tī-) *n.* See **vitamin B₁₂.**

an·ti·per·spi·rant (ăn′tē-pûr′spər-ənt, ăn′tī-) *n.* An astringent preparation applied to the skin to decrease perspiration.

an·ti·plas·min (ăn′tē-plăz′mĭn, ăn′tī-) *n.* A substance that inhibits or prevents the effects of plasmin.

an·ti·pro·throm·bin (ăn′tē-prō-thrŏm′bĭn, ăn′tī-) *n.* An anticoagulant that inhibits or prevents the conversion of prothrombin into thrombin.

an·ti·pru·rit·ic (ăn′tē-proo-rĭt′ĭk, ăn′tī-) *adj.* Preventing or relieving itching. — **an′ti·pru·rit′ic** *n.*

an·ti·psy·chot·ic (ăn′tē-sī-kŏt′ĭk, ăn′tī-) *adj.* Counteracting or diminishing the symptoms of a psychotic disorder such as schizophrenia, paranoia, or manic-depressive psychosis. — **an′ti·psy·chot′ic** *n.*

an·ti·py·ret·ic (ăn′tē-pī-rĕt′ĭk, ăn′tī-) *n.* An agent that reduces or prevents fever. — **an′ti·py·re′sis** (-rē′sĭs) *n.* Reducing or preventing fever. — **an′ti·py·re′sis** (-rē′sĭs) *n.*

an·ti·sep·sis (ăn′tī-sĕp′sĭs) *n.* Destruction of pathogenic organisms to prevent infection.

an·ti·sep·tic (ăn′tī-sĕp′tĭk) *adj.* **1.** Of, relating to, or producing antisepsis. **2.** Capable of preventing infection by inhibiting the growth of infectious agents. — *n.* A substance that inhibits the proliferation of infectious agents.

antiseptic dressing *n.* A sterile dressing of gauze impregnated with an antiseptic.

an·ti·se·rum (ăn′tī-sēr′əm) *n.* A serum having antibodies that are specific for one or more antigens.

antiserum anaphylaxis *n.* See **passive anaphylaxis.**

an·ti·si·al·a·gogue (ăn′tē-sī-ăl′ə-gôg′, a-′tī-) *n.*

An agent that slows or halts the flow of saliva.

an·ti·so·cial (ăn′tē-sō′shəl, ăn′tī-) *adj.* Behaving in violation of the social or legal norms of society. — **an′ti·so′cial·ly** *adv.*

antisocial personality disorder *n.* A personality disorder characterized by a history of continuous and chronic antisocial behavior that is not attributable to severe mental retardation, schizophrenia, or manic episodes.

an·ti·spas·mod·ic (ăn′tē-spăz-mŏd′ĭk, ăn′tī-) *adj.* Preventing or relieving convulsions or spasms. — *n.* An antispasmotic agent.

an·ti·su·dor·if·ic (ăn′tē-sōō′də-rĭf′ĭk, ăn′tī-) *adj.* Anhidrotic.

an·ti·tox·ic (ăn′tē-tŏk′sĭk) *adj.* **1.** Neutralizing the action of a toxin or poison. **2.** Of, relating to, or containing an antitoxin.

an·ti·tox·in (ăn′tē-tŏk′sĭn) *n.* **1.** An antibody formed in response to and capable of neutralizing a specific biological toxin. **2.** A serum containing antitoxins, used to prevent or treat diseases caused by biological toxins, such as tetanus, botulism, and diptheria.

an·ti·tryp·sin (ăn′tē-trĭp′sĭn, ăn′tī-) *n.* A serum protein that inhibits the activity of trypsin and other proteolytic enzymes.

antitrypsin deficiency *n.* An inherited deficiency of a trypsin-inhibiting serum protein, believed to increase the body's susceptibility to emphysema and cirrhosis.

an·ti·tus·sive (ăn′tē-tŭs′ĭv, ăn′tī-) *adj.* Capable of relieving or suppressing coughing. — **an′ti·tus′sive** *n.*

an·ti·ven·in (ăn′tē-věn′ĭn, ăn′tī-) *n.* An antitoxin active against the venom of a snake, spider, or other venomous organism.

an·ti·vi·ral (ăn′tē-vī′rəl, ăn′tī-) *adj.* Destroying or inhibiting the growth and reproduction of viruses. — **an′ti·vi′ral** *n.*

antiviral protein *n.* A human or animal factor that is induced by interferon in virus-infected cells and mediates interferon inhibition of virus replication.

an·ti·vi·ta·min (ăn′tē-vī′tə-mĭn, ăn′tī-) *n.* A substance that prevents a vitamin from exerting its typical metabolic effects.

an·trec·to·my (ăn-trĕk′tə-mē) *n.* Surgical excision of an antrum, such as removal of the pyloric antrum of the stomach.

an·tro·du·o·de·nec·to·my (ăn′trō-dōō′ō-də-nĕk′tə-mē, -dyōō′-, -dōō-ŏd′n-ĕk′tə-mē, -dyōō-) *n.* Surgical removal of the antrum of the stomach and the ulcer-bearing part of the duodenum.

an·tro·scope (ăn′trə-skōp′) *n.* An instrument for examining a cavity or antrum, especially the maxillary sinus.

an·tros·co·py (ăn-trŏs′kə-pē) *n.* Examination by means of an antroscope.

an·tros·to·my (ăn-trŏs′tə-mē) *n.* The surgical formation of an opening into an antrum.

an·trot·o·my (ăn-trŏt′ə-mē) *n.* Incision through the wall of an antrum.

an·trum (ăn′trəm) *n., pl.* **-tra** (-trə). **1.** A nearly closed cavity or chamber, especially in a bone. **2.** The pyloric end of the stomach, partially shut off during digestion from the cardiac end by the prepyloric sphincter. — **an′tral** (-trəl) *adj.*

an·u·re·sis (ăn′yə-rē′sĭs) *n.* The inability to pass urine. — **an′u·ret′ic** (-rĕt′ĭk) *adj.*

a·nu·ri·a (ə-nŏŏr′ē-ə, ə-nyŏŏr′-) *n.* The absence of urine formation. — **a·nu′ric** (ə-nŏŏr′ĭk, ə-nyŏŏr′-) *adj.*

a·nus (ā′nəs) *n., pl.* **a·nus·es.** The opening at the lower end of the alimentary canal through which solid waste is eliminated from the body.

an·vil (ăn′vĭl) *n.* See incus.

anx·i·e·ty (ăng-zī′ĭ-tē) *n.* **1.** A state of uneasiness and apprehension, as about future uncertainties. **2.** A cause of anxiety. **3.** A state of intense apprehension, uncertainty, and fear resulting from the anticipation of a threatening event or situation, often to a degree that the normal physical and psychological functioning of the affected individual is disrupted. **4.** Eager, often agitated desire.

anxiety disorder *n.* Any of various disorders in which anxiety is either the primary disturbance or is the result of confronting a feared situation or object.

anxiety hysteria *n.* Hysteria characterized by manifest anxiety.

anxiety neurosis *n.* A disorder characterized by feelings of persistent apprehension, fear, or impending doom, which, when acute, manifest themselves in attacks that are unpredictable, usually of short duration, and occur in situations that are not life threatening.

anxiety reaction *n.* A psychological state or experience involving the apprehension of danger, accompanied by a feeling of dread and such physical symptoms as restlessness and rapid heartbeat, occurring in the absence of any clearly identifiable fear stimulus.

anxiety state *n.* See anxiety neurosis.

anx·i·o·lyt·ic (ăng′zē-ō-lĭt′ĭk, -sē-, ăngk′sē-) *n.* A drug that relieves anxiety. — **anx′i·o·lyt′ic** *adj.*

a·or·ta (ā-ôr′tə) *n., pl.* **-tas** or **-tae** (-tē). The large artery that is the main trunk of the systemic arterial system and whose parts are the ascending aorta, the aortic arch, and the descending aorta. — **a·or′tal, a·or′tic** *adj.*

a·or·tal·gi·a (ā′ôr-tăl′jē-ə) *n.* Pain thought to be due to aneurysm or another pathologic condition of the aorta.

aortic arch *n.* **1.** The curved portion between the ascending and descending portions of the aorta, giving rise to the brachiocephalic trunk, the left common carotid, and the left subclavian arteries. **2.** Any of several pairs of arterial channels encircling the embryonic pharynx in the mesenchyme of the branchial arches.

aortic arch syndrome *n.* Obstruction of the branches of the aortic arch caused by thrombosis.

aortic atresia *n.* The congenital absence of the normal valvular orifice into the aorta.

aortic bulb *n.* The dilated first part of the aorta

containing the aortic semilunar valves and the aortic sinuses.

aortic insufficiency *n.* Valvular insufficiency involving the aortic valve.

aortic murmur *n.* An obstructive or regurgitant murmur produced at the aortic orifice.

aortic notch *n.* A slight notch in a sphygmographic tracing caused by rebound from the closure of the aortic valves.

aortic septal defect *n.* A small congenital opening between the aorta and pulmonary artery just above the semilunar valves.

aortic sinus *n.* The space between each semilunar valve and the wall of the aorta.

aortic stenosis *n.* Pathological narrowing of the orifice of the aortic valve.

aortic valve *n.* The valve between the left ventricle of the heart and the ascending aorta, consisting of three semilunar cusps.

a·or·ti·tis (ā′ôr-tī′tĭs) *n.* The inflammation of the aorta.

a·or·to·gram (ā-ôr′tə-grăm′) *n.* An x-ray image of the aorta made after the injection of a radiopaque substance.

a·or·tog·ra·phy (ā′ôr-tŏg′rə-fē) *n.* The radiographic visualization of the aorta and its branches by injection of a radiopaque substance.

a·or·to·il·i·ac bypass (ā-ôr′tō-ĭl′ē-ăk′) *n.* A shunt uniting the aorta and iliac artery to relieve obstruction of the lower abdominal aorta.

a·or·top·a·thy (ā′ôr-tŏp′ə-thē) *n.* Disease of the aorta.

a·or·to·plas·ty (ā-ôr′tə-plăs′tē) *n.* Surgical repair of the aorta.

a·or·to·re·nal bypass (ā-ôr′tō-rē′nəl) *n.* A shunt between the aorta and the distal renal artery to circumvent an obstruction of the renal artery.

a·or·tor·rha·phy (ā′ôr-tôr′ə-fē) *n.* Suture of the aorta.

a·or·to·scle·ro·sis (ā-ôr′tō-sklə-rō′sĭs) *n.* Arteriosclerosis of the aorta.

a·or·tot·o·my (ā′ôr-tŏt′ə-mē) *n.* Surgical incision into the aorta.

APA *abbr.* antipernicious anemia factor

ap·a·thet·ic (ăp′ə-thĕt′ĭk) *adj.* Lacking interest or concern; indifferent. — **ap′a·thet′i·cal·ly** *adv.*

ap·a·thism (ăp′ə-thĭz′əm) *n.* Sluggishness in reacting to stimuli.

ap·a·thy (ăp′ə-thē) *n.* Lack of interest, concern, or emotion; indifference.

APC *abbr.* acetylsalicylic acid, phenacetin, and caffeine (combined as an antipyretic and analgesic); antigen-presenting cell

a·pe·ri·od·ic (ā′pēr-ē-ŏd′ĭk) *adj.* Not occurring periodically. — **a′pe·ri·od′i·cal·ly** *adv.* — **a·pe′·ri·o·dic′i·ty** (-ə-dĭs′ĭ-tē) *n.*

a·per·i·stal·sis (ā-pĕr′ĭ-stôl′sĭs, -stăl′-) *n.* The absence of peristalsis.

ap·er·ture (ăp′ər-chər) *n.* **1.** An opening, such as a hole, gap, or slit. **2.** The diameter of the objective of a telescope or microscope. — **ap′er·tur′al** *adj.*

a·pex (ā′pĕks) *n.*, *pl.* **a·pex·es** or **a·pi·ces** (ā′pĭ-

sēz′, ăp′ĭ-). The pointed end of a conical or pyramidal structure.

apex beat *n.* A pulsation, either visible or palpable or both, made by the apex of the left ventricle of the heart as it strikes the chest wall in systole.

Ap·gar score (ăp′gär) *n.* A system of evaluating a newborn infant's general physical condition by assigning a numerical value (0, 1, or 2) to each of five criteria: heart rate, respiratory effort, muscle tone, response to stimuli, and skin color.

a·pha·gi·a (ə-fā′jē-ə, -jə) *n.* See **dysphagia.**

a·pha·ki·a (ə-fā′kē-ə) *n.* The absence of the crystalline lens of the eye. — **a·pha′ki·al, a·pha′kic** (ə-fā′kĭk) *adj.*

aphakic eye *n.* An eye having no lens.

aph·a·lan·gi·a (ăf′ə-lăn′jē-ə, ā′fə-) *n.* Absence of a digit or of one or more of the phalanges of a finger or toe.

a·pha·sia (ə-fā′zhə) *n.* Partial or total loss of the ability to articulate ideas or comprehend spoken or written language, resulting from brain damage due to injury or disease. — **a·pha′si·ac′** (-zē-ăk′) *n.* — **a·pha′sic** (-zĭk, -sĭk) *adj. & n.*

a·phe·mi·a (ə-fē′mē-ə) *n.* A form of motor aphasia in which the ability to express ideas in spoken words is lost.

aph·e·re·sis (ăf′ə-rē′sĭs) *n.* A procedure in which blood is drawn from a donor and separated into its components, some of which are retained, such as plasma or platelets, and the remainder returned by transfusion to the donor.

a·pho·ni·a (ā-fō′nē-ə) *n.* Loss of the voice resulting from disease, injury to the vocal cords, or psychological causes, such as hysteria. — **a·phon′ic** (ā-fŏn′ĭk, ā-fō′nĭk) *adj.*

a·phra·si·a (ə-frā′zē-ə, -zhə) *n.* The inability to speak.

aph·ro·dis·i·ac (ăf′rə-dĭz′ē-ăk′, -dē′zē-) *adj.* Arousing or intensifying sexual desire. — *n.* An aphrodisiac drug or food. — **aph′ro·di·si′a·cal** (-dī-zī′ĭ-kəl) *adj.*

aph·tha (ăf′thə) *n., pl.* **-thae** (-thē′). A minute painful ulcer on a mucous membrane of the mouth, often covered by a gray or white exudate.

aph·thae (ăf′thē′) *pl.n.* Canker sores.

a·phy·lax·is (ā′fə-lăk′sĭs, ăf′ə-) *n.* Lack of protection against disease. — **a′phy·lac′tic** (-lăk′tĭk) *adj.*

a·pi·cal (ā′pĭ-kəl, ăp′ĭ-) *adj.* Of, relating to, or situated nearer to the apex of a structure in relation to a specific reference point. — **a′pi·cal·ly** *adv.*

a·pi·cec·to·my (ā′pĭ-sĕk′tə-mē, ăp′ĭ-) *n.* Surgical removal of the apex of the petrous part of the temporal bone.

ap·i·ci·tis (ăp′ĭ-sī′tĭs, ā′pĭ-) *n.* Inflammation of the apex of a structure or organ.

ap·i·co·ec·to·my (ăp′ĭ-kō-ĕk′tə-mē, ā′pĭ-) *n.* Surgical removal of a dental root apex.

ap·i·col·y·sis (ăp′ĭ-kŏl′ĭ-sĭs) *n.* Surgical collapse of the apex of the lung.

ap·i·cot·o·my (ăp′ĭ-kŏt′ə-mē, ā′pĭ-) *n.* Surgical incision into an apical structure.

a·pla·si·a (ə-plā′zē-ə, -zhə) *n.* **1.** Congenital absence of an organ or tissue. **2.** Incomplete, retarded, or defective development of an organ or tissue. **3.** Cessation of the usual regenerative process in an organ or tissue.

aplasia cu·tis con·gen·i·ta (kyōō′tĭs kən-jĕn′ĭ-tə) *n.* The congenital absence or deficiency of a localized area of skin, usually on the scalp, with the base of the defect covered by a thin translucent membrane.

a·plas·tic (ā-plăs′tĭk, ə-plăs′-) *adj.* **1.** Unable to form or regenerate tissue. **2.** Of, relating to, or characterized by aplasia.

aplastic anemia *n.* A form of anemia in which the capacity of the bone marrow to generate red blood cells is defective, caused by bone marrow disease or exposure to toxic agents, such as radiation, chemicals, or drugs.

aplastic lymph *n.* Lymph containing a relatively large number of white blood cells but comparatively little fibrinogen and manifesting only a slight tendency to become organized.

ap·ne·a (ăp′nē-ə, ăp-nē′ə) *n.* Temporary absence or cessation of breathing. ⸺ **ap·ne′ic** *adj. & n.*

apneic pause *n.* Cessation of air flow in respiration for more than ten seconds.

ap·neu·mi·a (ăp-nōō′mē-ə, -nyōō′-) *n.* Congenital absence of the lungs.

ap·o·crine (ăp′ə-krĭn, -krīn′, -krēn′) *adj.* Of or relating to an apocrine gland or its secretions. ⸺ *n.* The apocrine gland.

apocrine carcinoma *n.* **1.** A carcinoma composed predominantly of anaplastic cells resembling those of apocrine epithelium, often found in the breast. **2.** A carcinoma of the apocrine glands.

apocrine chromesthesia *n.* The excretion of colored sweat, usually black, from apocrine glands of the face.

apocrine gland *n.* **1.** A coiled, tubular gland whose secretory cells accumulate their products on their apical surfaces that are then pinched off to become the secretion, as in the mammary glands. **2.** Apocrine sweat gland.

apocrine sweat gland *n.* Any of numerous sweat glands found primarily in the skin of the armpit, pubic region, and areolae of the breasts that produce a secretion that is more viscous than that formed by the eccrine glands; secretions from these glands occur most frequently during periods of emotional stress or sexual excitement.

ap·o·dal (ăp′ə-dl) or **ap·o·dous** (-dəs) *adj.* Having no feet or footlike appendages.

a·po·di·a (ā-pō′dē-ə, ə-pō′-) or **ap·o·dy** (ăp′ə-dē) *n.* Congenital absence of feet.

ap·o·en·zyme (ăp′ō-ĕn′zīm) *n.* The protein component of an enzyme that combines with the coenzyme to form the active enzyme and determine the specificity of the enzyme substrate.

ap·o·fer·ri·tin (ăp′ə-fĕr′ĭ-tĭn) *n.* A protein present in the intestinal mucosa that binds and stores iron by combining with a ferric hydroxide-phosphate compound to form ferritin.

ap·o·lip·o·pro·tein (ăp′ə-lĭp′ō-prō′tēn′, -tē-ĭn, -lī′pō-) *n.* The protein component that combines with a lipid to form a lipoprotein.

ap·o·mor·phine (ăp′ə-môr′fēn′) *n.* A poisonous white crystalline alkaloid derived from morphine and used medicinally to induce vomiting.

ap·o·neu·rec·to·my (ăp′ə-nōō-rĕk′tə-mē, -nyōō-) *n.* Excision of an aponeurosis.

ap·o·neu·ror·rha·phy (ăp′ə-nōō-rôr′ə-fē, -nyōō-) *n.* See **fasciorrhaphy.**

ap·o·neu·ro·sis (ăp′ə-nōō-rō′sĭs, -nyōō-) *n.* A sheetlike fibrous membrane resembling a flattened tendon that serves as a fascia to bind muscles together or to connect muscle to bone. ⸺ **ap′o·neu·rot′ic** (-rŏt′ĭk) *adj.*

ap·o·neu·ro·si·tis (ăp′ə-nōōr′ə-sī′tĭs, -nyōōr′-) *n.* Inflammation of an aponeurosis.

ap·o·neu·rot·o·my (ăp′ə-nōō-rŏt′ə-mē, -nyōō-) *n.* Surgical incision into an aponeurosis.

a·poph·y·sis (ə-pŏf′ĭ-sĭs) *n., pl.* **-ses** (-sēz′). An outgrowth or projection of an organ or part, especially from a bone that lacks an independent center of ossification. ⸺ **ap′o·phys′i·al** (ăp′ə-fĭz′ē-əl), **a·poph′y·se′al** (-sē′əl) *adj.*

ap·o·plec·tic (ăp′ə-plĕk′tĭk) *adj.* Relating to, suffering from, or predisposed to apoplexy. ⸺ **ap′o·plec′ti·cal·ly** *adv.*

ap·o·plex·y (ăp′ə-plĕk′sē) *n.* **1.** Sudden impairment of neurological function, especially from a cerebral hemorrhage; a stroke. **2.** An effusion of blood into a tissue or organ.

ap·o·pro·tein (ăp′ə-prō′tēn′, -tē-ĭn) *n.* A polypeptide that combines with a prosthetic group to form a conjugated protein.

ap·o·re·pres·sor (ăp′ə-rĭ-prĕs′ər) *n.* A repressor that combines with a specific corepressor to inhibit transcription of certain genes; it acts to regulate repressible enzyme systems.

ap·o·stax·is (ăp′ə-stăk′sĭs) *n.* Slight bleeding; bleeding by drops.

a·pos·thi·a (ə-pŏs′thē-ə) *n.* Congenital absence of the prepuce.

a·poth·e·car·ies′ measure (ə-pŏth′ĭ-kĕr′ēz) *n.* A system of liquid volume measure used in pharmaceutics.

apothecaries′ weight *n.* A system of weights used in pharmaceutics and based on an ounce equal to 480 grains and a pound equal to 12 ounces.

ap·pa·ra·tus (ăp′ə-rā′təs, -răt′əs) *n., pl.* **apparatus** or **-tus·es. 1.** An integrated group of materials or devices used for a particular purpose. **2.** A group or system of organs that collectively performs a specific function or process.

ap·pend·age (ə-pĕn′dĭj) *n.* A part or organ attached to a main structure and subordinate in function or size.

ap·pen·dec·to·my (ăp′ən-dĕk′tə-mē) *n.* Surgical removal of the vermiform appendix.

ap·pen·di·cec·to·my (ə-pĕn′dĭ-sĕk′tə-mē) *n.* See **appendectomy.**

ap·pen·di·ci·tis (ə-pĕn′dĭ-sī′tĭs) *n.* Inflammation of the vermiform appendix.

ap·pen·di·col·y·sis (ə-pĕn′dĭ-kŏl′ĭ-sĭs) *n.* Surgical freeing of the appendix from adhesions.

ap·pen·di·cos·to·my (ə-pĕn′dĭ-kŏs′tə-mē) *n*. Surgical opening of the tip of the veriform appendix to irrigate the bowel.

ap·pen·dic·u·lar (ăp′ən-dĭk′yə-lər) *adj*. **1.** Relating to an appendix. **2.** Relating to the limbs.

appendicular skeleton *n*. The bones of the limbs including those of the pectoral and pelvic girdles.

ap·pen·dix (ə-pĕn′dĭks) *n., pl*. **-dix·es** or **-di·ces** (-dĭ-sēz′). **1.** A supplementary or accessory part of a bodily organ or structure. **2.** The vermiform appendix.

ap·per·cep·tion (ăp′ər-sĕp′shən) *n*. **1.** Conscious perception with full awareness. **2.** The process of understanding by which newly observed qualities of an object are related to past experience. — **ap′per·cep′tive** (-sĕp′tĭv) *adj*.

ap·pe·stat (ăp′ĭ-stăt′) *n*. The area in the brain that is believed to regulate appetite and food intake.

ap·pe·tite (ăp′ĭ-tīt′) *n*. An instinctive physical desire, as for food or sex.

ap·pla·na·tion (ăp′lə-nā′shən) *n*. **1.** The flattening of the cornea by pressure, as with a tonometer. **2.** Undue flatness, as of the cornea.

ap·pla·nom·e·try (ăp′lə-nŏm′ĭ-trē) *n*. The use of a tonometer to measure pressure within the eye.

ap·pli·ance (ə-plī′əns) *n*. A dental or surgical device designed to perform a therapeutic or corrective function.

ap·pli·ca·tor (ăp′lĭ-kā′tər) *n*. An instrument for applying something, such as a medication.

ap·po·si·tion (ăp′ə-zĭsh′ən) *n*. **1.** The putting in contact of two parts or substances. **2.** The condition of being placed or fitted together. **3.** The growth of successive layers of a cell wall. — **ap′po·si′tion·al** *adj*. — **ap′po·si′tion·al·ly** *adv*.

appositional growth *n*. Growth by the addition of new layers on those previously formed, characteristic of tissues formed of rigid materials.

apposition suture *n*. A superficial suture of the skin only.

ap·prox·i·mate (ə-prŏk′sə-māt′) *v*. **-mat·ed, -mat·ing, -mates**. To bring together, as cut edges of tissue.

ap·prox·i·ma·tion (ə-prŏk′sə-mā′shən) *n*. Bringing tissue edges into desired apposition for suturing.

approximation suture *n*. A suture that pulls together the deep tissues in a wound.

a·prax·i·a (ā-prăk′sē-ə) *n*. **1.** A disorder of voluntary movement consisting of the partial or complete inability to execute purposeful movements without the impairment of muscular power and coordination. **2.** A psychomotor defect characterized by the inability to make proper use of a known object.

a·proc·ti·a (ā-prŏk′shē-ə, ə-prŏk′-) *n*. The congenital absence or imperforation of the anus.

a·pro·so·pi·a (ā′prə-sō′pē-ə, ăp′rə-) *n*. The congenital absence of part or all of the face, usually associated with other malformations.

ap·ti·tude test (ăp′tĭ-tōōd′, -tyōōd′) *n*. An occupation-oriented test for evaluating intelligence, achievement, and interest.

APUD cell (ā′pəd) *n*. A cell capable of amine precursor uptake and decarboxylation and of synthesizing and secreting polypeptide hormones.

a·py·ret·ic (ā′pī-rĕt′ĭk, ăp′ə-) *adj*. Having no fever; afebrile.

a·py·rex·i·a (ā′pī-rĕk′sē-ə, ăp′ə-) *n*. The absence of fever.

aq·ua·pho·bi·a (ăk′wə-fō′bē-ə) *n*. An abnormal fear of water.

aq·ue·duct (ăk′wĭ-dŭkt′) *n*. A channel or passage in a body part or an organ.

a·que·ous (ā′kwē-əs, ăk′wē-) *adj*. Relating to, similar to, containing, or dissolved in water.

aqueous chamber *n*. Either of the anterior or posterior chambers of the eye, containing the aqueous humor.

aqueous humor *n*. The clear, watery fluid circulating in the chamber of the eye between the cornea and the lens.

a·rach·nid·ism (ə-răk′nĭ-dĭz′əm) *n*. Systemic poisoning following the bite of a spider.

a·rach·no·dac·ty·ly (ə-răk′nō-dăk′tə-lē) *n*. A condition in which the hands and fingers, and often the feet and toes, are abnormally long and slender, characteristic of Marfan's syndrome.

arachnoid membrane *n*. A delicate fibrous membrane forming the middle of the three coverings of the brain and spinal cord, closely attached to the dura mater.

a·rach·no·pho·bi·a (ə-răk′nə-fō′bē-ə, -nō-) or **a·rach·ne·pho·bi·a** (ə-răk′nə-) *n*. An abnormal fear of spiders.

ar·bor (är′bər) *n., pl*. **ar·bo·res** (är′bə-rēz′). A treelike anatomical structure.

ar·bo·res·cent (är′bə-rĕs′ənt) *n*. See **dendriform**.

ar·bo·ri·za·tion (är′bər-ĭ-zā′shən) *n*. **1.** The treelike terminal branching of nerve fibers or blood vessels. **2.** The leaflike pattern formed under certain conditions by a dried smear of cervical mucus.

ar·bo·rize (är′bə-rīz′) *v*. **-rized, -riz·ing, -riz·es**. See **ramify**.

ar·bo·vi·rus (är′bə-vī′rəs) or **ar·bor·vi·rus** (är′bər-) *n*. Any of a large group of viruses transmitted by arthropods, such as mosquitoes and ticks, that include the causative agents of encephalitis, yellow fever, and dengue.

arc (ärk) *n*. A curved line or segment of a circle.

ARC *abbr*. AIDS-related complex

arch (ärch) *n*. An organ or structure having a curved or bowlike appearance, especially either of two arched sections of the bony structure of the foot.

ar·chen·ter·on (är-kĕn′tə-rŏn′, -tər-ən) *n*. See **gastrocele** (sense 1).

ar·che·type (är′kĭ-tīp′) *n*. **1.** An original model or type after which other similar things are patterned. **2.** In Jungian psychology, an inherited pattern of thought or symbolic image that is derived from the past collective experience of humanity and is present in the unconscious of the individual. — **ar′che·typ′al** (-tī′pəl), **ar′che·typ′-**

ic (-tĭp′ĭk), ar′che·typ′i·cal *adj.* — ar′che·typ′i·cal·ly *adv.*

arch of aorta *n.* See aortic arch (sense 1).

arc·ta·tion (ärk-tā′shən) *n.* A narrowing, contraction, or stricture of a canal or opening.

ar·cu·ate (är′kyōō-ĭt, -āt′) *adj.* Formed in the shape of an arc. — ar′cu·ate·ly *adv.*

ar·cu·a·tion (är′kyōō-ā′shən) *n.* A bending or curvature.

ar·cus (är′kəs) *n., pl.* **arcus.** A structure resembling a bent bow or an arch.

ar·e·a (âr′ē-ə) *n., pl.* **-as** or **-ae** (-ē-ē′). **1.** A circumscribed surface or space. **2.** All of the part supplied by a given artery or nerve. **3.** A part of an organ having a special function.

area of cardiac dullness *n.* A triangular area determined by percussion of the front of the chest that corresponds to the part of the heart not covered by lung tissue.

a·re·flex·i·a (ā′rī-flĕk′sē-ə) *n.* The absence of reflexes.

Ar·e·na·vi·rus (ăr′ə-nə-vī′rəs, ə-rē′nə-) *n.* The single genus of viruses in the family Arenaviridae that includes the viruses that cause lymphocytic choriomeningitis and Lassa fever.

a·re·o·la (ə-rē′ə-lə) *n., pl.* **-las** or **-lae** (-lē′). **1.** A small area. **2.** Any of numerous spaces or interstices in areolar tissue. **3.** Areola mammae. **4.** A pigmented, depigmented, or erythematous zone surrounding a papule, pustule, wheal, or cutaneous neoplasm. — a·re′o·lar, a·re′o·late (-lĭt) *adj.*

areola mam·mae (măm′ē) *n.* The circular pigmented area surrounding the nipple of the breast, having small projections from the glands beneath.

areolar gland *n.* Any of several cutaneous glands forming small, rounded projections from the surface of the areola of the breast.

areolar tissue *n.* Loose, irregularly arranged connective tissue that consists of collagenous and elastic fibers, a protein polysaccharide ground substance, and connective tissue cells.

ar·gi·nase (är′jə-nās′, -nāz) *n.* An enzyme found primarily in the liver that catalyzes the hydrolysis of arginine to urea and ornithine.

ar·gi·nine (är′jə-nēn′) *n.* An amino acid obtained from the hydrolysis or digestion of plant and animal protein.

ar·gi·ni·no·suc·cin·ic acid (är′jə-nĭ-nō-sək-sĭn′ĭk, är′jə-nē′-) *n.* An acid formed as an intermediate during the urea cycle.

ar·gi·ni·no·suc·cin·ic·ac·i·du·ri·a (är′jə-nĭ-nō-sək-sĭn′ĭk-ăs′ĭ-dŏŏr′ē-ə, -dyŏŏr′-, är′jə-nē′-) *n.* A disorder characterized by excessive excretion of argininosuccinic acid in the urine, epilepsy, ataxia, mental retardation, liver disease, and friable, tufted hair.

ar·gon (är′gŏn′) *n.* A colorless, inert gaseous element with atomic number 18 and constituting approximately one percent of Earth's atmosphere.

Ar·gy·rol (är′jə-rôl′, -rōl′) A trademark used for a silver-protein compound used as a local antiseptic.

a·rhin·i·a (ə-rĭn′ē-ə, ə-rī′nē-ə) *n.* See arrhinia.

a·ri·bo·fla·vin·o·sis (ā-rī′bō-flā′və-nō′sĭs) *n.* A condition caused by a riboflavin deficiency, characterized by cheilosis or angular stomatitis and magenta-colored tongue.

arm (ärm) *n.* An upper limb of the human body, connecting the hand and wrist to the shoulder.

ar·ma·men·tar·i·um (är′mə-měn-târ′ē-əm) *n., pl.* **-i·ums** or **-i·a** (-ē-ə). The complete equipment of a physician or medical institution.

arm·pit (ärm′pĭt′) *n.* The hollow under the upper part of the arm below the shoulder joint.

Arndt's law (ärnts) *n.* The principle stating that weak stimuli excite physiological activity, moderately strong stimuli favor it, strong stimuli retard it, and very strong stimuli arrest it.

Ar·nold-Chiari deformity (är′nəld-, -nōlt′-) *n.* A congenital deformity at the base of the brain, often associated with spina bifida, in which the cerebellar tissue is elongated and extends into the fourth ventricle.

a·ro·ma·ther·a·py (ə-rō′mə-thěr′ə-pē) *n.* The use of selected fragrant substances in lotions and inhalants in an effort to affect mood and promote health.

ar·o·mat·ic (är′ə-măt′ĭk) *adj.* **1.** Having an agreeable, somewhat pungent, spicy odor. **2.** Of, relating to, or containing one or more six-carbon rings. — *n.* Any of a group of vegetable drugs having a fragrant odor and slightly stimulant properties. — ar′o·mat′i·cal·ly *adv.*

ar·rec·tor (ə-rĕk′tər, ă-rĕk′-) *n., pl.* **ar·rec·to·res** (är′ĕk-tôr′ēz). See **erector.**

ar·rest (ə-rĕst′) *v.* **-rest·ed, -rest·ing, -rests. 1.** To stop; check. **2.** To undergo cardiac arrest. — *n.* **1.** A stoppage; an interference with or a checking of the regular course of a disease or symptom. **2.** Interference with the performance of a function. **3.** The inhibition of a developmental process, usually the ultimate stage of development.

ar·rhin·i·a (ə-rĭn′ē-ə, ə-rī′nē-ə) *n.* The congenital absence of the nose.

ar·rhyth·mi·a (ə-rĭth′mē-ə) *n.* An irregularity in the force or rhythm of the heartbeat.

ar·rhyth·mic (ə-rĭth′mĭk) *adj.* Lacking rhythm or regularity of rhythm.

ar·se·ni·a·sis (är′sə-nī′ə-sĭs) *n.* Chronic arsenic poisoning.

ar·se·nic (är′sə-nĭk) *n.* A poisonous metallic element with atomic number 33. Compounds containing arsenic are used in insecticides and solid-state doping agents.

ar·te·ri·al (är-tîr′ē-əl) *adj.* **1.** Of or relating to one or more arteries or to the entire system of arteries. **2.** Of, relating to, or being the bright red blood in the arteries that has absorbed oxygen in the lungs. — ar·te′ri·al·ly *adv.*

arterial blood *n.* Blood that is oxygenated in the lungs, is found in the left chambers of the heart and in the arteries, and is relatively bright red.

arterial forceps *n.* Locking forceps with sloping

blades for grasping the end of a blood vessel until a ligature is applied.

arterial line *n*. An intra-arterial catheter.

arterial spider *n*. A telangiectatic arteriole in the skin having capillary branches that radiate from a central area in a manner similar to legs from the body of a spider.

arterial tension *n*. The blood pressure within an artery.

ar·te·ri·arc·ti·a (är-tēr′ē-ärk′shē-ə, -tē-ə) *n*. Vasoconstriction of the arteries.

ar·te·ri·ec·ta·sis (är-tēr′ē-ĕk′tə-sĭs) or **ar·te·ri·ec·ta·si·a** (-ĕk-tā′zē-ə, -zhə) *n*. Vasodilation of the arteries.

ar·te·ri·ec·to·my (är-tēr′ē-ĕk′tə-mē) *n*. Surgical excision of part of an artery.

ar·te·ri·og·ra·phy (är-tēr′ē-ŏg′rə-fē) *n*. Examination of the arteries using x-rays following injection of a radiopaque substance. — **ar·te′ri·o·gram′** (-ə-grăm′) *n*. — **ar·te′ri·o·graph′ic** (-ə-grăf′ĭk) *adj*.

ar·te·ri·ole (är-tîr′ē-ōl′) *n*. A minute artery, especially a terminal artery continuous with the capillary network. — **ar·te′ri·o′lar** (-ō′lər, -ə-lər) *adj*.

ar·te·ri·o·lith (är-tēr′ē-ō-lĭth′) *n*. A calcareous deposit in an arterial wall or thrombus.

ar·te·ri·o·li·tis (är-tēr′ē-ō-lī′tĭs) *n*. Inflammation of the arterioles.

ar·te·ri·o·lo·scle·ro·sis (är-tēr′ē-ō′lō-sklə-rō′sĭs) *n*. Arteriosclerosis mainly affecting the arterioles.

ar·te·ri·op·a·thy (är-tēr′ē-ŏp′ə-thē) *n*. A disease of the arteries.

ar·te·ri·o·plas·ty (är-tēr′ē-ə-plăs′tē) *n*. Surgical reconstruction of the wall of an artery.

ar·te·ri·or·rha·phy (är-tēr′ē-ôr′ə-fē) *n*. Suture of an artery.

ar·te·ri·or·rhex·is (är-tēr′ē-ō-rĕk′sĭs) *n*. Rupture of an artery.

ar·te·ri·o·scle·ro·sis (är-tēr′ē-ō-sklə-rō′sĭs) *n*. Any of a group of chronic diseases in which thickening, hardening, and loss of elasticity of the arterial walls result in impaired blood circulation. — **ar·te′ri·o·scle·rot′ic** (-rŏt′ĭk) *n*.

ar·te·ri·o·spasm (är-tēr′ē-ō-spăz′əm) *n*. Spasm of one or more arteries.

ar·te·ri·o·ste·no·sis (är-tēr′ē-ō-stə-nō′sĭs) *n*. A temporary or permanent narrowing of an artery, as by vasoconstriction or arteriosclerosis.

ar·te·ri·ot·o·my (är-tēr′ē-ŏt′ə-mē) *n*. Surgical incision into the lumen of an artery.

ar·te·ri·ot·o·ny (är-tēr′ē-ŏt′ə-nē) *n*. See **blood pressure**.

ar·te·ri·o·ve·nous (är-tēr′ē-ō-vē′nəs) *adj*. Of, relating to, or connecting both arteries and veins.

arteriovenous carbon dioxide difference *n*. The difference in carbon dioxide content, in milliliters per 100 milliliters blood, between the arterial and venous bloods.

arteriovenous nicking *n*. A constriction of a vein in the retina of the eye at an artery-vein crossing.

arteriovenous oxygen difference *n*. The difference in the oxygen content, in milliliters per 100 milliliters blood, between arterial and venous blood.

arteriovenous shunt *n*. The passage of blood directly from arteries to veins, without going through the capillary network.

ar·te·ri·tis (är′tə-rī′tĭs) *n*. Inflammation of an artery or arteries.

ar·ter·y (är′tə-rē) *n*. Any of a branching system of muscular, elastic blood vessels that, except for the pulmonary and umbilical arteries, carry red or aerated blood away from the heart to the cells, tissues, and organs of the body.

ar·thral·gia (är-thrăl′jə, -jē-ə) *n*. Severe pain in a joint. — **ar·thral′gic** (-jĭk) *adj*.

ar·threc·to·my (är-thrĕk′tə-mē) *n*. The surgical excision of a joint.

ar·thri·tis (är-thrī′tĭs) *n*., *pl*. **-thrit·i·des** (-thrĭt′ĭ-dēz′). Inflammation of a joint or joints resulting in pain and swelling. — **ar·thrit′ic** (-thrĭt′ĭk) *adj*. *& n*. — **ar·thrit′i·cal·ly** *adv*.

ar·thro·cele (är′thrə-sēl′) *n*. **1**. Hernia of the synovial membrane through the capsule of a joint. **2**. Swelling of a joint.

ar·thro·cen·te·sis (är′thrō-sĕn-tē′sĭs) *n*. The surgical puncture and aspiration of a joint.

ar·thro·chon·dri·tis (är′thrō-kŏn-drī′tĭs) *n*. Inflammation of an articular cartilage.

ar·thro·cla·si·a (är′thrō-klā′zē-ə, -zhə) *n*. A forcible breaking up of the adhesions in an ankylosis to allow more mobility in the joint.

ar·throd·e·sis (är-thrŏd′ĭ-sĭs, är′thrə-dē′sĭs) *n*. The surgical fixation of a joint to promote bone fusion.

ar·thro·di·a (är-thrō′dē-ə) *n*. See **plane joint**. — **ar·thro′di·al** *adj*.

arthrodial joint *n*. See **plane joint**.

ar·thro·dyn·i·a (är′thrō-dĭn′ē-ə) *n*. See **arthralgia**. — **ar′thro·dyn′ic** (-dĭn′ĭk) *adj*.

ar·thro·dys·pla·sia (är′thrō-dĭs-plā′zhə, -zē-ə) *n*. Abnormal joint development.

ar·thro·en·dos·co·py (är′thrō-ĕn-dŏs′kə-pē) *n*. See **arthroscopy**.

ar·throg·ra·phy (är-thrŏg′rə-fē) *n*. Examination of the interior of a joint using x-rays following the injection of a radiopaque substance. — **ar′·thro·gram′** (är′thrə-grăm′) *n*.

ar·thro·gry·po·sis (är′thrə-grə-pō′sĭs) *n*. **1**. The permanent fixation of a joint in a contracted position. **2**. A congenital disorder marked by generalized stiffness of the joints, often accompanied by muscle and nerve degeneration, which results in severely impaired mobility of the limbs.

ar·thro·lith (är′thrə-lĭth′) *n*. A concretion within a joint.

ar·throl·y·sis (är-thrŏl′ĭ-sĭs) *n*. The surgical restoration of mobility in ankylosed joints.

ar·throm·e·ter (är-thrŏm′ĭ-tər) *n*. A calibrated device for measuring the arc or range of mobility of a joint.

ar·throm·e·try (är-thrŏm′ĭ-trē) *n*. The measurement of the range of movement in a joint.

ar·throp·a·thy (är-thrŏp′ə-thē) *n*. A disease or an abnormality of a joint.

ar·thro·plas·ty (är′thrə-plăs′tē) *n.* **1.** The creation of an artificial joint. **2.** The surgical restoration of the integrity and functional power of a joint.

ar·thro·pod (är′thrə-pŏd′) *n.* Any of numerous invertebrate animals of the phylum Arthropoda, including the insects, crustaceans, and arachnids.

Ar·throp·o·da (är-thrŏp′ə-də) *n.* A phylum of the Metazoa that includes crustaceans, insects, arachnids, centipedes, and horseshoe crabs.

ar·thro·py·o·sis (är′thrō-pī-ō′sĭs) *n.* The formation of pus in a joint.

ar·thro·scle·ro·sis (är′thrō-sklə-rō′sĭs) *n.* Stiffness or hardening of the joints.

ar·thros·co·py (är-thrŏs′kə-pē) *n.* Examination of the interior of a joint, such as the knee, using an endoscope that is inserted into the joint through a small incision. — **ar′thro·scope′** (är′thrə-skōp′) *n.* — **ar′thro·scop′ic** (-skŏp′ĭk) *adj.*

ar·thro·sis (är-thrō′sĭs) *n., pl.* **-ses** (-sēz). **1.** An articulation between bones. **2.** A degenerative disease of a joint.

ar·thros·to·my (är-thrŏs′tə-mē) *n.* Surgical construction of a temporary opening into a joint cavity.

ar·thro·sy·no·vi·tis (är′thrō-sī′nə-vī′tĭs) *n.* Inflammation of the synovial membrane of a joint.

ar·throt·o·my (är-thrŏt′ə-mē) *n.* Surgical incision into a joint.

ar·throx·e·sis (är-thrŏk′sĭ-sĭs) *n.* The surgical removal of diseased tissue from a joint by scraping.

ar·tic·u·lar (är-tĭk′yə-lər) *adj.* Of or relating to a joint or joints.

articular corpuscle *n.* Any of the encapsulated nerve endings in a joint capsule.

ar·tic·u·late (är-tĭk′yə-lĭt) *adj.* **1.** Capable of speaking distinctly and connectedly. **2.** Consisting of sections united by joints; jointed. — *v.* **-lat·ed, -lat·ing, -lates.** (ä-tĭk′yə-lāt′). **1.** To speak distinctly and connectedly. **2.** To join or connect together loosely to allow motion between the parts. **3.** To unite by forming a joint or joints. **4.** To form a joint; be jointed.

articulated *adj.* Characterized by or having articulations; jointed.

ar·tic·u·la·tion (är-tĭk′yə-lā′shən) *n.* **1.** The place of anatomical union, usually movable, between two or more bones. **2.** Distinct connected speech or enunciation. **3.** The contact relationship of the occlusal surfaces of the teeth during jaw movement.

ar·ti·fact or **ar·te·fact** (är′tə-făkt′) *n.* **1.** A structure or substance not normally present but produced by an external agent or action, such as a structure seen in a microscopic specimen after fixation that is not present in the living tissue. **2.** A skin lesion produced or perpetuated by self-inflicted action. — **ar′ti·fac·ti′tious** (-făk-tĭsh′-əs), **ar′ti·fac′tu·al** (-făk′chŏŏ-əl) *adj.*

artificial heart *n.* A mechanical pump used to replace the function of a damaged heart, either temporarily or as a permanent internal prosthesis.

artificial insemination *n.* Introduction of semen into the vagina or uterus without sexual contact.

artificial kidney *n.* See **hemodialyzer.**

artificial pacemaker *n.* An electronic device that substitutes for the natural pacemaker of the heart. It may be surgically implanted or placed externally on the chest.

artificial radioactivity *n.* The radioactivity of isotopes that exist only because they have been artificially produced through the bombardment of naturally occurring isotopes by subatomic particles or by high levels of x-rays or gamma rays.

artificial respiration *n.* A procedure to mechanically or manually force air into and out of the lungs in a rhythmic manner to restore or maintain respiration in a person who has stopped breathing.

artificial selection *n.* Human intervention in animal or plant reproduction to ensure that certain desirable traits are represented in successive generations.

artificial ventilation *n.* See **artificial respiration.**

ARV *abbr.* AIDS-related virus

ar·y·te·noid (är′ĭ-tē′noid′, ə-rĭt′n-oid′) *n.* **1.** Either of two small pitcher-shaped cartilages at the back of the larynx to which the vocal cords are attached. **2.** A muscle connected to either of these cartilages. **3.** Any of several small mucous glands located in front of these cartilages. — *adj.* Of or relating to these cartilages or an associated muscle or gland. — **ar′y·te·noid′al** *adj.*

ar·y·te·noi·dec·to·my (är′ĭ-tē′noi-děk′tə-mē, ə-rĭt′n-oi-) *n.* The surgical excision of an arytenoid cartilage.

ar·y·te·noi·do·pexy (är′ĭ-tə-noi′də-pěk′sē, ə-rĭt′-n-oi′-) *n.* Surgical fixation of the arytenoid cartilages or muscles.

AS *abbr. Latin.* auris sinistra (left ear)

as·bes·tos or **as·bes·tus** (ăs-běs′təs, ăz-) *n.* Either of two incombustible, chemical-resistant, fibrous mineral forms of impure magnesium silicate, used for fireproofing, electrical insulation, building materials, brake linings, and chemical filters. — *adj.* Of, made of, or containing one or the other of these two mineral forms.

as·bes·to·sis (ăs′běs-tō′sĭs, ăz′-) *n.* Pneumoconiosis due to prolonged inhalation of asbestos particles.

as·ca·ri·a·sis (ăs′kə-rī′ə-sĭs) *n.* A disease caused by infestation with worms of the genus *Ascaris.*

as·ca·rid (ăs′kə-rĭd) *n.* A worm of the family Ascarididae. — **as′ca·rid** *adj.*

ascending colon *n.* The part of the colon between the ileocecal orifice and the right colic flexure.

as·ci·tes (ə-sī′tēz) *n., pl.* **ascites.** The accumulation of serous fluid in the peritoneal cavity. — **as·cit′ic** (-sĭt′ĭk) *adj.*

as·co·my·cete (ăs′kō-mī′sēt′, -mī-sēt′) *n.* Any of a class (Ascomycetes) of fungi.

a·scor·bic acid (ə-skôr′bĭk) *n.* A white, crystalline vitamin found in citrus fruits, tomatoes, potatoes, and leafy green vegetables and used to prevent scurvy.

as·e·ma·si·a (ăs′ə-mā′zē-ə, -zhə) or **a·se·mi·a** (ə-sē′mē-ə) *n.* See **asymbolia** (sense 2).

a·sep·sis (ə-sĕp′sĭs, ā-) *n.* **1.** The state of being free of living pathogenic microorganisms. **2.** The process of removing pathogenic microorganisms or protecting against infection by such organisms.

a·sep·tic (ə-sĕp′tĭk, ā-) *adj.* Of, relating to, or characterized by asepsis.

aseptic necrosis *n.* Necrosis occurring in the absence of infection.

aseptic surgery *n.* Surgery performed under sterilized conditions.

a·sex·u·al (ā-sĕk′shoo-əl) *adj.* **1.** Having no evident sex or sex organs; sexless. **2.** Relating to, produced by, or involving reproduction that occurs without the union of male and female gametes, as in binary fission or budding. **3.** Lacking interest in or desire for sex. — **a·sex′u·al′i·ty** (-ăl′ĭ-tē) *n.* — **a·sex′u·al·ly** *adv.*

asexual dwarf *n.* A dwarf who is not developed sexually yet is beyond the age of puberty.

asexual generation *n.* Reproduction without the union of individuals or of the male and female germ cells.

a·si·a·lism (ə-sī′ə-lĭz′əm) or **a·si·a·li·a** (ā′sī-ā′lē-ə, -ăl′ē-ə) *n.* Diminished or arrested secretion of saliva.

A·sian influenza (ā′zhən, ā′shən) *n.* Influenza caused by a strain of influenza virus type A that was first isolated in China during the 1957 epidemic.

a·sleep (ə-slēp′) *adj.* **1.** In a state of sleep; sleeping. **2.** Numb, as of a limb. — *adv.* **1.** In or into a state of sleep. **2.** In or into a state of apathy or indifference.

Asn *abbr.* asparagine

a·so·cial (ā-sō′shəl) *adj.* **1.** Avoiding or averse to the society of others. **2.** Unable or unwilling to conform to normal standards of social behavior.

Asp *abbr.* aspartic acid

as·par·a·gin·ase (ə-spăr′ə-jə-nās′, -nāz′) *n.* An enzyme isolated from bacteria that catalyzes the hydrolysis of asparagine and is used in the chemotherapeutic treatment of leukemia.

as·par·a·gine (ə-spăr′ə-jēn′) *n.* An amino acid found in proteins.

as·par·tame (ăs′pər-tām′, ə-spär′-) *n.* A low-calorie, artificial sweetening agent derived from aspartic acid.

as·par·tic ac·id (ə-spär′tĭk) *n.* One of the nonessential amino acids that occur in proteins.

as·pect (ăs′pĕkt) *n.* The side of an object, such as an organ, that is facing in a particular direction.

as·per·gil·lo·ma (ăs′pər-jə-lō′mə) *n.* **1.** An infectious granuloma caused by fungi of the genus *Aspergillus.* **2.** A variety of bronchopulmonary aspergillosis characterized by a ball-like mass of the fungus *Aspergillus fumigatus* in a lung cavity.

as·per·gil·lo·sis (ăs′pər-jə-lō′sĭs) *n.* An infection or a disease caused by fungi of the genus *Aspergillus.*

As·per·gil·lus (ăs′pər-jĭl′əs) *n.* A genus of fungi that includes many common molds.

a·sper·ma·tism (ā-spûr′mə-tĭz′əm, ə-spûr′-) or

a·sper·mi·a (ā-spûr′mē-ə, ă-spûr′-) *n.* The inability to secrete or ejaculate semen.

as·phyx·i·a (ăs-fĭk′sē-ə) *n.* A condition in which an extreme decrease in the amount of oxygen in the body accompanied by an increase of carbon dioxide leads to loss of consciousness or death. — **as·phyx′i·al** *adj.*

as·phyx·i·ant (ăs-fĭk′sē-ənt) *adj.* Inducing or tending to induce asphyxia. — *n.* A substance, such as a toxic gas, or an event, such as drowning, that induces asphyxia.

as·phyx·i·ate (ăs-fĭk′sē-āt′) *v.* **-at·ed, -at·ing, -ates.** To induce or undergo asphyxia. — **as·phyx′i·a′tion** *n.*

as·pi·rate (ăs′pə-rāt′) *v.* **-rat·ed, -rat·ing, -rates.** To take in or remove by aspiration. — *n.* (-pər-ĭt). A substance removed by aspiration.

as·pi·ra·tion (ăs′pə-rā′shən) *n.* **1.** The removal of a gas or fluid by suction. **2.** The sucking of fluid or a foreign body into the airway when drawing breath. **3.** A surgical technique for treating cataracts of the eye, in which the lens is fragmented and aspirated by a needle.

aspiration biopsy *n.* See **needle biopsy.**

aspiration pneumonia *n.* Bronchopneumonia resulting from the entrance of foreign material, usually food particles or vomit, into the bronchi.

as·pi·ra·tor (ăs′pə-rā′tər) *n.* An apparatus for removing a substance from a body cavity, consisting usually of a hollow needle and a cannula, connected by tubing to a container in which a vacuum is created by a syringe or a suction pump.

as·pi·rin (ăs′pər-ĭn, -prĭn) *n.* A white, crystalline compound derived from salicylic acid and commonly used in tablet form to relieve pain and reduce fever and inflammation.

a·sple·ni·a (ə-splē′nē-ə) *n.* Congenital absence of the spleen. — **a·sple′nic** (ə-splē′nĭk, -splĕn′ĭk) *adj.*

as·say (ăs′ā′, ă-sā′) *n.* **1.** Qualitative or quantitative analysis of a substance, especially of a drug, to determine its components. **2.** A substance to be so analyzed. **3.** The result of such an analysis. **4.** An analysis or examination. — *v.* (ă-sā′, ăs′ā′). **1.** To subject a substance to chemical analysis. **2.** To examine a person's capability by trial or experiment; put to a test. **3.** To be shown by analysis to contain a certain proportion of atoms, molecules, compounds, or precious metal.

as·sim·i·late (ə-sĭm′ə-lāt′) *v.* **-lat·ed, -lat·ing, -lates.** **1.** To consume and incorporate nutrients into the body after digestion. **2.** To transform food into living tissue by the process of anabolism; metabolize constructively.

as·sim·i·la·tion (ə-sĭm′ə-lā′shən) *n.* **1.** The incorporation of digested substances from food into the tissues of an organism. **2.** The merging and change of newly perceived information and experiences into the existing cognitive structure.

as·sist-con·trol ventilation (ə-sĭst′kən-trōl′) *n.* A method of artificial respiration in which inspiration is produced automatically after a set interval if the person has not begun to inspire earlier.

as·sist·ed respiration (ə-sĭs'tĭd) *n.* A procedure for applying mechanically or manually generated positive pressure to gases in or surrounding the airway during inhalation to augment movement of gases into the lungs.

assisted ventilation *n.* See **assisted respiration**.

as·so·ci·a·tion (ə-sō'sē-ā'shən, -shē-) *n.* **1.** A connection of persons, things, or ideas by some common factor; union. **2.** A functional connection of two ideas, events, or psychological phenomena established through learning or experience.

association area *n.* See **association cortex**.

association constant *n.* A mathematical constant describing the bonding affinity of two molecules at equilibrium, especially of an antibody and an antigen.

association cortex *n.* Any of the expanses of the cerebral cortex that are not sensory or motor in the customary sense, but instead are thought to be involved in advanced stages of sensory information processing, multisensory integration, or sensorimotor integration.

association test *n.* A word association test used diagnostically in psychiatry and psychology in which a word is spoken to an individual who, in turn, is to immediately respond with whatever word comes to mind.

as·so·ci·a·tive aphasia (ə-sō'shē-ā'tĭv, -sē-, -shə-tĭv) *n.* See **conduction aphasia**.

associative learning *n.* A learning principle based on the belief that ideas and experiences reinforce one another and can be mentally linked to enhance the learning process.

associative neuron *n.* A nerve cell found within the central nervous system that links sensory and motor neurons.

as·sort·ment (ə-sôrt'mənt) *n.* The relationship between non-allelic genetic traits that are transmitted from parent to child randomly according to the linkage between the respective loci.

AST (ā'ĕs-tē') *n.* Aspartate aminotransferase; an enzyme that catalyzes the transfer of the amino group from glutamic acid to oxaloacetic acid forming alpha-ketoglutaric acid and aspartic acid.

a·sta·sia (ə-stā'zhə) *n.* The inability to stand due to muscular incoordination.

astasia-abasia *n.* Inability to stand or walk normally as a symptom of conversion hysteria.

as·ta·tine (ăs'tə-tēn', -tĭn) *n.* A radioactive halogen element with atomic number 85.

a·ste·a·to·sis (ə-stē'ə-tō'sĭs, ăs'tē-) *n.* Diminished or arrested action of the sebaceous glands.

as·ter (ăs'tər) *n.* See **astrosphere**.

a·ster·e·og·no·sis (ə-stĕr'ē-ŏg-nō'sĭs, -stĕr'-) *n.* The inability to determine the form of an object by touch.

a·ster·ni·a (ā-stûr'nē-ə, ə-stûr'-) *n.* The congenital absence of the sternum.

as·the·no·sper·mi·a (ăs'thə-nō-spûr'mē-ə) *n.* The loss or reduction of spermatozoan motility.

asth·ma (ăz'mə, ăs'-) *n.* Bronchial asthma. — **asth·mat'ic** (-măt'ĭk) *adj. & n.*

astigmatic lens *n.* See **cylindrical lens**.

a·stig·ma·tism (ə-stĭg'mə-tĭz'əm) *n.* A condition in which unequal curvatures in one or more of the refractive surfaces of the eye cause rays from a point to fail to focus at a single point on the retina. — **as'tig·mat'ic** (ăs'tĭg-măt'ĭk) *adj. & n.*

a·stig·ma·tom·e·ter (ə-stĭg'mə-tŏm'ĭ-tər) or **as·tig·mom·e·ter** (ăs'tĭg-mŏm'ĭ-tər) *n.* An instrument for measuring the degree of and determining the variety of astigmatism. — **a·stig'ma·tom'e·try** (-trē), **as'tig·mom'e·try** *n.*

as·tig·mat·o·scope (ăs'tĭg-măt'ə-skōp') or **a·stig·mo·scope** (ə-stĭg'mə-skōp') *n.* An instrument for detecting and measuring the degree of astigmatism. — **a·stig'ma·tos'co·py** (-tŏs'kə-pē), **as'tig·mos'co·py** (-mŏs'kə-pē)

a·stig·mi·a (ə-stĭg'mē-ə) *n.* See **astigmatism**.

a·sto·mi·a (ə-stō'mē-ə) *n.* Congenital absence of a mouth.

as·trag·a·lec·to·my (ə-străg'ə-lĕk'tə-mē) *n.* Surgical removal of the ankle bone.

as·trag·a·lus (ə-străg'ə-ləs) *n.* See **talus** (sense 1).

as·tra·pho·bi·a (ăs'trə-fō'bē-ə) *n.* An abnormal fear of lightning and thunder.

as·tric·tion (ə-strĭk'shən) *n.* **1.** Astringent action. **2.** Compression to arrest hemorrhage.

as·trin·gent (ə-strĭn'jənt) *adj.* Causing contraction of tissues, arrest of secretion, or control of bleeding. — *n.* A substance or preparation, such as alum, that draws together or constricts body tissues and is effective in stopping the flow of blood or other secretions. — **as·trin'gen·cy** *n.*

as·tro·blas·to·ma (ăs'trō-blă-stō'mə) *n.* A poorly differentiated tumor composed of astrocytes and arranged radially with short fibrils terminating on small blood vessels.

as·tro·cyte (ăs'trə-sīt') *n.* One of the large neuroglia cells of nervous tissue.

as·tro·cy·to·ma (ăs'trō-sī-tō'mə) *n., pl.* **-mas** or **-ma·ta** (-mə-tə). A malignant tumor of nervous tissue composed of well differentiated astrocytes.

as·trog·li·a (ăs-trŏg'lē-ə,) *n.* See **astrocyte**.

as·tro·sphere (ăs'trō-sfîr') *n.* A set of radiating fibrils extending outward from the centrosome and centrosphere of a dividing cell.

a·sy·lum (ə-sī'ləm) *n.* An institution for the care of people, especially those with physical or mental impairments, who require organized supervision or assistance.

a·sym·bo·li·a (ā'sĭm-bō'lē-ə) *n.* **1.** A loss of the ability to comprehend by touch the form and nature of an object. **2.** A phasia in which the significance of signs cannot be comprehended.

a·sym·met·ri·cal (ā'sĭ-mĕt'rĭkəl) or **a·sym·met·ric** (-rĭk) *adj.* Lacking symmetry between two or more like parts; not symmetrical.

a·sym·me·try (ā-sĭm'ĭ-trē) *n.* Disproportion between two or more like parts; lack of symmetry.

a·symp·to·mat·ic (ā'sĭmp-tə-măt'ĭk) *adj.* Exhibiting or producing no symptoms.

a·syn·cli·tism (ā-sĭn'klĭ-tĭz'əm, ə-sĭn'-) *n.* Absence of synclitism or parallelism between the axis of the presenting part of the fetus and the pelvic planes during childbirth.

a·syn·de·sis (ə-sǐn′dǐ-sǐs) *n.* A disorder in which separate ideas or thoughts cannot be joined into a coherent concept.

a·sy·ner·gi·a (ā′sə-nûr′jē-ə, -jə) or **a·syn·er·gy** (ā-sǐn′ər-jē) *n.* The lack of cooperation or working together of parts that normally act in unison. — **a′sy·ner′gic** *adj.*

a·sys·to·le (ā-sǐs′tə-lē, ə-sǐs′-) *n.* The absence of contractions of the heart; cardiac standstill. — **a′sys·tol′ic** (ā′sǐ-stŏl′ǐk) *adj.*

At·a·brine (ăt′ə-brǐn, -brēn′) A trademark used for an antimalarial preparation of quinacrine hydrochloride.

a·tac·tic abasia (ə-tăk′tǐk) or **a·tax·ic abasia** (ə-tăk′sǐk) *n.* Abasia due to ataxia of the legs.

at·a·vism (ăt′ə-vǐz′əm) *n.* The appearance of characteristics presumed to have been present in some remote ancestor; reversion to an earlier biological type. — **at′a·vist** *n.* — **at′a·vis′tic** *adj.* — **at′·a·vis′ti·cal·ly** *adv.*

a·tax·i·a (ə-tăk′sē-ə) or **a·tax·y** (ə-tăk′sē) *n.* Loss of the ability to coordinate muscular movement.

a·tax·i·a·pha·sia (ə-tăk′sē-ə-fā′zhə) *n.* Inability to form connected sentences.

ataxia telangiectasia *n.* A disease characterized by progressive ataxia due to disease in the cerebellum, oculocutaneous telangiectases, proneness to pulmonary infections, and immunodeficiency.

ataxic gait *n.* An unsteady or irregular gait.

a·tax·i·o·phe·mi·a (ə-tăk′sē-ō-fē′mē-ə) *n.* Incoordination of the speech muscles.

at·e·lec·ta·sis (ăt′l-ěk′tə-sǐs) *n.* **1.** The absence of gas from all or a part of the lungs, due to failure of expansion or resorption of gas from the alveoli. **2.** A congenital condition characterized by the incomplete expansion of the lungs at birth. — **at′e·lec·tat′ic** (-ěk-tăt′ǐk)

a·te·li·ot·ic dwarf (ə-tē′lē-ŏt′ǐk) *n.* A normally proportioned individual of unusually short stature.

a·ten·o·lol (ə-těn′ə-lôl′, -nŏl′) *n.* A beta-blocking agent used primarily in the treatment of angina pectoris and hypertension.

a·the·li·a (ə-thē′lē-ə) *n.* Congenital absence of the nipples.

ath·er·o·gen·e·sis (ăth′ər-ō-jěn′ǐ-sǐs) *n.* Formation of atheromatous deposits, especially on the innermost layer of arterial walls.

ath·er·o·ma (ăth′ə-rō′mə) *n., pl.* **-mas** or **-ma·ta** (-mə-tə). A deposit or degenerative accumulation of lipid-containing plaques on the innermost layer of the wall of an artery. — **ath′er·o·ma·to′sis** (-tō′sǐs) *n.* — **ath′er·om′a·tous** (-rŏm′ə-təs, -rō′-mə-) *adj.*

atheromatous degeneration *n.* The accumulation of lipid deposits on the inner surface of the arteries, eventually leading to thickening or calcification.

ath·er·o·scle·ro·sis (ăth′ə-rō-sklə-rō′sǐs) *n.* A form of arteriosclerosis characterized by the deposition of atheromatous plaques containing cho-

lesterol and lipids on the innermost layer of the walls of large and medium-sized arteries. — **ath′·er·o·scle·rot′ic** (-rŏt′ǐk) *adj.*

ath·lete's foot (ăth′lēts) *n.* A contagious fungal infection of the skin caused by a species of *Trichophyton* or *Epidermophyton* that usually affects the feet, especially the skin between the toes, and is characterized by itching, cracking, and scaling.

ath·let·ic heart (ăth-lět′ǐk) *n.* Enlargement of the heart observed in some athletes.

a·threp·si·a (ə-thrěp′sē-ə) or **ath·rep·sy** (ăth′rəp-sē) *n.* See **marasmus.** — **a·threp′tic** (-tǐk) *adj.*

a·thy·mi·a (ə-thī′mē-ə) *n.* **1.** The absence of emotion; morbid impassivity. **2.** The absence of the thymus gland or the suppression of its secretion.

a·thy·mism (ə-thī′mǐz′əm) *n.* Athymia (sense 2).

a·thy·roid·ism (ā-thī′roi-dǐz′əm, ə-thī′-) or **a·thy·re·a** (ā-thī′rē-ə, ə-thī′-) or **a·thy·ro·sis** (ā′thī-rō′sǐs, ăth′ī-) *n.* The absence of the thyroid gland or the suppression of its secretion. — **a′thy·rot′ic** (ā′thī-rŏt′ǐk, ăth′ī-) *adj.*

ATL *abbr.* adult T-cell lymphoma

at·las (ăt′ləs) *n.* The top or first cervical vertebra of the neck, supporting the skull and articulating with the occipital bone.

at·om (ăt′əm) *n.* A unit of matter, the smallest unit of an element, having all the characteristics of that element and consisting of a dense, central, positively charged nucleus surrounded by a system of electrons. — **a·tom′ic** (ə-tŏm′ǐk) *adj.*

atomic mass *n.* The mass of an atom, usually expressed in atomic mass units.

atomic number *n.* The number of protons in an atomic nucleus; it indicates the position of an element in the periodic table.

a·ton·ic (ā-tŏn′ǐk) *adj.* Relating to, caused by, or exhibiting lack of muscle tone. — **at′o·nic′i·ty** (ăt′ə-nǐs′ǐ-tē, ăt′n-ǐs-) *n.*

at·o·ny (ăt′ə-nē, ăt′n-ē) or **a·to·ni·a** (ā-tō′nē-ə) *n.* Lack of normal tone or tension; flaccidity.

at·o·pen (ăt′ə-pən, -pěn′) *n.* An agent that causes an atopic reaction.

atopic dermatitis *n.* Dermatitis characterized by intense itching, occurring in persons who are predisposed to certain hypersensitivity reactions.

a·top·og·no·si·a (ā-tŏp′ŏg-nō′zē-ə, -zhə, ə-tŏp′-) or **a·top·og·no·sis** (-nō′sǐs) *n.* The inability to discern the origin of a sensation.

at·o·py (ăt′ə-pē) *n.* A hereditary disorder marked by the tendency to develop an immediate allergic reaction to a substance and manifested by hay fever or similar allergic conditions. — **a·top′ic** (ā-tŏp′ǐk) *adj.*

ATP (ā′tē′pē′) *n.* Adenosine triphosphate; an adenosine-derived nucleotide that hydrolyzes to supply large amounts of energy to cells for various biochemical processes.

a·trau·mat·ic suture (ā′trô-măt′ǐk, -trou-, -trə-) *n.* A suture affixed to the end of a small eyeless needle.

a·tre·sia (ə-trē′zhə, -zhē-ə) *n.* **1.** The congenital absence or closure of a normal body orifice or tubular passage such as the anus or external ear canal.

2. The degeneration and resorption of one or more ovarian follicles before maturation.

a·tri·al (ā′trē-əl) *adj.* Of or relating to an atrium.

atrial complex *n.* The P wave in an electrocardiogram.

atrial extrasystole *n.* A premature contraction of the heart arising from an ectopic atrial focus.

atrial fibrillation *n.* Fibrillation in which the normal rhythmical contractions of the cardiac atria are replaced by rapid irregular twitchings of the muscular wall that cause the ventricles to respond irregularly.

atrial fusion beat *n.* A pulsation occurring when the atria of the heart are activated partly by a sinus impulse and partly by a retrograde impulse from the atrioventricular node or ventricle.

atrial natriuretic factor *n.* A peptide hormone released from cardiac atrial tissue that causes increased elimination of sodium by the kidney.

atrial septal defect *n.* A defect in the septum between the right and left atria of the heart, resulting from the failure of a foramen to close normally.

a·trich·i·a (ā-trĭk′ē-ə, ə-trĭk′-) *n.* The congenital or acquired absence of hair.

a·tri·o·meg·a·ly (ā′trē-ō-mĕg′ə-lē) *n.* Enlargement of the atrium of the heart.

a·tri·o·sep·to·pex·y (ā′trē-ō-sĕp′tə-pĕk′sē) *n.* Surgical repair of an atrial septal defect.

a·tri·o·sep·to·plas·ty (ā′trē-ō-sĕp′tə-plăs′tē) *n.* Repair of an atrial septal defect by plastic surgery.

a·tri·o·sep·tos·to·my (ā′trē-ō-sĕp-tŏs′tə-mē) *n.* The surgical establishment of a communication between the atria of the heart.

a·tri·o·ven·tri·cu·lar block (ā′trē-ō-vĕn-trĭk′yə-lər) *n.* Impairment of the normal conduction of impulses between atria and ventricles.

atrioventricular conduction *n.* Forward conduction of the cardiac impulse from the atria to ventricles via the atrioventricular node, represented in an electrocardiogram by the P-R interval.

atrioventricular extrasystole *n.* A premature contraction of the heart in which the stimulus arises from either the AV node or muscle-fiber bundle.

atrioventricular nodal extrasystole *n.* A premature beat arising from the AV node and leading to a simultaneous or almost simultaneous contraction of atria and ventricles.

atrioventricular nodal rhythm *n.* The cardiac rhythm that results when the heart is controlled by the atrioventricular node.

atrioventricular node *n.* A small mass of specialized cardiac muscle fibers, located near the ostium of the coronary sinus and giving rise to the bundle of muscle fibers integral to the conduction system of the heart.

atrioventricular septum *n.* The small part of the membranous septum of the heart separating the right atrium from the left ventricle.

a·tri·um (ā′trē-əm) *n., pl.* **-ums** or **a·tri·a** (ā′trē-ə). **1.** A chamber or cavity to which are connected several chambers or passageways. **2.** Either the right or the left upper chamber of the heart that receives blood from the veins and forces it into a ventricle. **3.** That part of the tympanic cavity that lies immediately deep to the eardrum. **4.** A subdivision of the alveolar duct in the lung from which the alveolar sacs open.

a·troph·e·de·ma (ə-trŏf′ĭ-dē′mə) *n.* See **angioneurotic edema**.

atrophic excavation *n.* An exaggeration of the normal or physiological cupping of the optic disk caused by atrophy of the optic nerve.

atrophic gastritis *n.* Chronic gastritis with atrophy of the mucous membrane and destruction of the peptic glands.

atrophic rhinitis *n.* Chronic rhinitis with thinning of the mucous membrane.

atrophic vaginitis *n.* Thinning and atrophy of the vaginal epithelium usually resulting from diminished endocrine stimulation and seen most commonly in postmenopausal women.

at·ro·phied (ăt′rə-fēd) *adj.* Characterized by atrophy.

at·ro·phy (ăt′rə-fē) *n.* A wasting or decrease in the size of an organ or tissue, as from death and reabsorption of cells, malnutrition, decreased function, or hormonal changes. — *v.* **-phied, -phy·ing, -phies.** To undergo atrophy. — **a·troph′ic** (ā-trŏf′ĭk) *adj.*

at·ro·pine (ăt′rə-pēn′, -pĭn) or **at·ro·pin** (-pĭn) *n.* An alkaloid obtained from belladonna and related plants, used to dilate the pupils of the eyes and as an antispasmodic, antisudorific, and an anticholinergic.

at·tached gingiva (ə-tăcht′) *n.* The portion of the oral mucous membrane bound to the tooth and to the alveolar arches of the jaw.

at·tack (ə-tăk′) *n.* An episode or onset of a disease, often sudden in nature. — **at·tack′** *v.*

at·tend·ing staff (ə-tĕn′dĭng) *n.* The physicians and surgeons who are members of a hospital staff and regularly attend their patients at the hospital.

at·ten·tion deficit disorder (ə-tĕn′shən) *n.* **1.** A childhood syndrome characterized by impulsiveness, hyperactivity, and short attention span, which often leads to learning disabilities and various behavioral problems. **2.** See **minimal brain dysfunction**.

at·ten·u·ate (ə-tĕn′yōō-āt′) *v.* **-at·ed, -at·ing, -ates.** **1.** To reduce in force, value, amount, or degree; weaken. **2.** To make bacteria or viruses less virulent.

at·ten·u·at·ed virus (ə-tĕn′yōō-ā′tĭd) *n.* A strain of a virus whose pathogenicity has been reduced so that it will initiate the immune response without producing the specific disease.

at·ten·u·a·tion (ə-tĕn′yōō-ā′shən) *n.* **1.** A dilution, thinning, or weakening of a substance, especially a reduction in the virulence of a virus or pathogenic organism through repeated inoculation, growth in a different culture medium, or exposure to heat, light, air or other weakening agents. **2.** The loss of energy of an ultrasonic beam as it passes through a material.

at·ti·cot·o·my (ăt'ĭ-kŏt'ə-mē) *n.* Surgical incision into the upper portion of the tympanic cavity.

at·ti·tude (ăt'ĭ-tood', -tyood') *n.* **1.** The position of the body and limbs; posture. **2.** A manner of acting. **3.** A relatively stable and enduring predisposition to behave or react in a characteristic way.

at·trac·tion (ə-trăk'shən) *n.* A force acting mutually between particles of matter to draw them together and to resist their separation.

attraction sphere *n.* See **astrosphere.**

at·tri·tion (ə-trĭsh'ən) *n.* A wearing away by friction or rubbing, such as the loss of tooth structure caused by abrasion or grinding.

a·typ·i·cal (ā-tĭp'ĭ-kəl) *adj.* Not corresponding to the normal form or type. — **a·typ'i·cal·ly** *adv.*

atypical lipoma *n.* A benign lipoma occurring primarily in older men on the posterior neck, shoulders, and back.

AU *abbr. Latin.* auris utraque (each ear)

au·di·o·an·al·ge·si·a (ô'dē-ō-ăn'əl-jē'zē-ə, -zhə) *n.* A deadening of pain produced by listening to a sound or sounds.

au·di·o·gen·ic epilepsy (ô'dē-ō-jĕn'ĭk) *n.* A form of reflex epilepsy induced by sound, usually a loud sudden noise.

au·di·o·gram (ô'dē-ə-grăm') *n.* A graphic record of hearing ability for various sound frequencies.

au·di·ol·o·gy (ô'dē-ŏl'ə-jē) *n.* The study of hearing disorders and the rehabilitation of people with hearing impairments. — **au'di·ol'o·gist** *n.*

au·di·om·e·ter (ô'dē-ŏm'ĭ-tər) *n.* An electrical instrument for measuring the threshold of hearing for pure tones of normally audible frequencies generally varying from 200 to 8000 Hz and recorded in decibels. — **au'di·o·met'ric** (-ō-mĕt'-rĭk) *adj.* — **au'di·o·me·tri'cian** (-ō-mə-trĭsh'ən) *n.* — **au'di·om'e·try** *n.*

au·di·tion (ô-dĭsh'ən) *n.* The sense or power of hearing.

au·di·to·ry (ô'dĭ-tôr'ē) *adj.* Of or relating to hearing, the organs of hearing, or the sense of hearing.

auditory aphasia *n.* Impairment of the ability to comprehend spoken language even though hearing is normal.

auditory brainstem response audiometry *n.* An electronic measure of auditory function using responses produced by the auditory nerve and the brainstem.

auditory canal *n.* Either of two passages of the ear, the internal or the external acoustic meatus.

auditory field *n.* The space or range within which a specified sound can be heard.

auditory hair *n.* Any of the cilia on the free surface of the auditory cells.

auditory nerve *n.* See **cochlear nerve.**

auditory receptor cell *n.* A columnar cell in the epithelium of the spiral organ having hairs.

auditory reflex *n.* A reflex occurring in response to a sound.

auditory tube *n.* See **eustachian tube.**

auditory vertigo *n.* See **Ménière's disease.**

auditory vesicle *n.* Either of the paired sacs of invaginated ectoderm in the embryo that develop into the labyrinth of the internal ear.

aug·men·ta·tion mammaplasty (ôg'mĕn-tā'-shən) *n.* Plastic surgery to enlarge the breast, often by insertion of an implant.

au·ra (ôr'ə) *n., pl.* **-ras** or **au·rae** (ôr'ē). A sensation, as of a cold breeze or a bright light, that precedes the onset of certain disorders, such as an epileptic seizure or an attack of migraine.

au·ral¹ (ôr'əl) *adj.* Of, relating to, or perceived by the ear.

au·ral² (ôr'əl) *adj.* Characterized by or relating to an aura.

au·ran·o·fin (ô-răn'ə-fĭn) *n.* A compound used to treat rheumatoid arthritis.

au·ran·ti·a·sis cu·tis (ôr'ăn-tī'ə-sĭs kyoo'tĭs) *n.* See **carotenosis cutis.**

Au·re·o·my·cin (ôr'ē-ō-mī'sĭn) A trademark used for chlortetracycline.

au·ri·cle (ôr'ĭ-kəl) *n.* **1.** Atrial auricle. **2.** The projecting shell-like structure on the side of the head constituting, with the external acoustic meatus, the external ear.

au·ric·u·lar (ô-rĭk'yə-lər) *adj.* **1.** Of or relating to the sense of hearing or the organs of hearing. **2.** Perceived by or spoken into the ear, as when testing hearing. **3.** Shaped like an ear or an earlobe; having earlike parts or extensions. **4.** Of or relating to an auricle of the heart.

auricular fibrillation *n.* See **atrial fibrillation.**

au·ris (ôr'ĭs) *n.* Ear.

au·ri·scope (ôr'ĭ-skōp') *n.* See **otoscope.**

aus·cul·tate (ô'skəl-tāt') or **aus·cult** (ô'skəlt) *v.* **-tat·ed, -tat·ing, -tates.** To examine by auscultation. — **aus'cul·ta'tive** *adj.* — **aus·cul'ta·to'ry** (ô-skŭl'tə-tôr'ē) *adj.*

aus·cul·ta·tion (ô'skəl-tā'shən) *n.* The act of listening for sounds made by internal organs, such as the heart and lungs, to aid in the diagnosis of certain disorders.

auscultatory alternans *n.* Alternation in the intensity of heart sounds or murmurs in the presence of regular cardiac rhythm.

auscultatory gap *n.* In measuring blood pressure by the auscultatory method, the period during which sounds indicating true systolic pressure fade away and reappear at a lower pressure point.

auscultatory percussion *n.* Auscultation performed at the same time that percussion is made.

Aus·tin Flint murmur (ô'stən flĭnt') *n.* See **Flint's murmur.**

Aus·tra·lia antigen (ô-strāl'yə) *n.* An antigen associated with the hepatitis B virus.

au·thor·i·tar·i·an personality (ə-thôr'ĭ-târ'ē-ən, ô-thôr'-) *n.* A personality pattern reflecting a desire for security, order, power, and status, with a desire for structured lines of authority, a conventional set of values or outlook, a demand for unquestioning obedience, and a tendency to be hostile toward or use as scapegoats individuals of minority or nontraditional groups.

au·thor·i·ty figure (ə-thôr′ĭ-tē, ô-thôr′-) *n.* A real or projected person in a position of power.

au·tism (ô′tĭz′əm) *n.* **1.** Abnormal introversion and egocentricity; acceptance of fantasy rather than reality. **2.** Infantile autism. — **au·tis′tic** (ô-tĭs′tĭk) *adj.*

au·to·ag·glu·ti·na·tion (ô′tō-ə-gloōt′n-ā′shən) *n.* **1.** Nonspecific agglutination or clumping together of cells due to physical-chemical factors. **2.** The agglutination of a person's red blood cells in his or her own serum as a consequence of specific autoantibody.

au·to·ag·glu·ti·nin (ô′tō-ə-gloōt′n-ĭn) *n.* An agglutinating autoantibody.

au·to·al·ler·gy (ô′tō-ăl′ər-jē) *n.* An altered reactivity in which antibodies (autoantibodies), produced against one's own tissues, exhibit a destructive effect. — **au′to·al·ler′gic** *adj.*

au·to·an·ti·bod·y (ô′tō-ăn′tĭ-bŏd′ē) *n.* An antibody that attacks the cells and tissues of the organism in which it was formed.

au·to·an·ti·gen (ô′tō-ăn′tĭ-jən) *n.* A tissue constituent that evokes an immune response to the host's tissues.

au·toc·la·sis (ô-tŏk′lə-sĭs) or **au·to·cla·si·a** (ô′tō-klā′zē-ə) *n.* **1.** A breaking up or rupturing from intrinsic or internal causes. **2.** Progressive, immunologically induced tissue destruction.

au·to·clave (ô′tō-klāv′) *n.* A pressurized, steam-heated vessel used for sterilization. — *v.* **-claved, -clav·ing, -claves.** To treat in an autoclave.

autocrine hypothesis *n.* The hypothesis that tumor cells containing viral oncogenes may have encoded a growth factor normally produced by other cell types, allowing them uncontrolled proliferation.

au·to·cy·tol·y·sin (ô′tō-sī-tŏl′ĭ-sĭn) *n.* See **autolysin.**

au·to·cy·tol·y·sis (ô′tō-sī-tŏl′ĭ-sĭs) *n.* See **autolysis** (sense 3).

au·to·cy·to·tox·in (ô′tō-sī′tə-tŏk′sĭn) *n.* A cytotoxic autoantibody.

au·to·der·mic graft (ô′tō-dûr′mĭk) *n.* A skin graft taken from the body receiving it.

au·to·di·ges·tion (ô′tō-dī-jĕs′chən, -dī′-) *n.* See **autolysis** (sense 2).

au·to·ech·o·la·li·a (ô′tō-ĕk′ō-lā′lē-ə) *n.* The repetition of some or all the words in one's own statements.

au·to·er·o·tism (ô′tō-ĕr′ə-tĭz′əm) or **au·to·e·rot·i·cism** (-ĭ-rŏt′ĭ-sĭz′əm) *n.* **1.** Self-satisfaction of sexual desire, as by masturbation. **2.** The arousal of sexual feeling without an external stimulus. — **au′to·e·rot′ic** (-ĭ-rŏt′ĭk) *adj.*

au·tog·a·my (ô-tŏg′ə-mē) *n.* Self-fertilization in which fission of the cell nucleus occurs without complete division of the cell itself. — **au·tog′a·mous** *adj.*

au·to·ge·ne·ic graft (ô′tō-jə-nē′ĭk) *n.* See **autograft.**

au·to·gen·e·sis (ô′tō-jĕn′ĭ-sĭs) *n.* **1.** The supposed development of living organisms from nonliving matter. **2.** The process by which a vaccine is made

from bacteria obtained from the patient's own body. — **au′to·ge·ne′tic** (-jə-nĕt′ĭk). — **au′to·ge·net′i·cal·ly** *adv.*

au·tog·e·nous (ô-tŏj′ə-nəs) or **au·to·gen·ic** (ô′tə-jĕn′ĭk) *adj.* **1.** Of or relating to autogenesis; self-generating. **2.** Of or relating to vaccines prepared from bacteria obtained from the infected person. — **au·tog′e·nous·ly** *adv.*

autogenous vaccine *n.* A vaccine made from a culture of bacteria taken from the person to be vaccinated.

au·to·graft (ô′tō-grăft′) *n.* A tissue or an organ grafted into a new position in or on the body of the same individual.

au·to·hem·ag·glu·ti·na·tion (ô′tō-hĕm′ə-gloōt′-n-ā′shən) *n.* Clumping of an individual's red blood cells by his or her own plasma.

au·to·he·mol·y·sin (ô′tō-hĭ-mŏl′ĭ-sĭn, -hē′mə-lī′-) *n.* An autoantibody that acts on the red blood cells in the same person or animal on whose body it is formed.

au·to·he·mol·y·sis (ô′tō-hĭ-mŏl′ĭ-sĭs, -hē′mə-lī′-sĭs) *n.* Hemolysis occurring in certain diseases through the action of an autohemolysin.

au·to·he·mo·ther·a·py (ô′tō-hē′mō-thĕr′ə-pē) *n.* Treatment of disease by the withdrawal and reinjection of the patient's own blood.

au·to·im·mune (ô′tō-ĭ-myoōn′) *adj.* Of or relating to an immune response against one of the body's own tissues or cells. — **au′to·im·mu′ni·ty** *n.* — **au′to·im′mu·ni·za′tion** (-ĭm′yə-nə-zā′shən) *n.*

autoimmune disease *n.* A disease resulting from an immune reaction produced by an individual's white blood cells or antibodies acting on the body's own tissues or extracellular proteins.

autoimmune hemolytic anemia *n.* Either of two forms of hemolytic anemia involving autoantibodies against red blood cell antigens; a cold-antibody type, and a warm-antibody type, caused by serum autoantibodies that react with a person's red blood cells, the antigenic specificity primarily in the Rh complex.

au·to·im·mu·no·cy·to·pe·ni·a (ô′tō-ĭm′yə-nō-sī′tō-pē′nē-ə) *n.* Anemia, thrombocytopenia, and leukopenia resulting from cytotoxic autoimmune reactions.

au·to·in·fec·tion (ô′tō-ĭn-fĕk′shən) *n.* **1.** Reinfection by microbes or parasitic organisms that are present on or within the body. **2.** Self-infection by direct contact with a contagious agent, as with parasite eggs transmitted by fingernails.

au·to·in·fu·sion (ô′tō-ĭn-fyoō′zhən) *n.* Forcing the blood from the extremities, as by the application of a bandage or pressure device, in order to raise the blood pressure and fill the vessels in the vital organs.

au·to·in·oc·u·la·tion (ô′tō-ĭ-nŏk′yə-lā′shən) *n.* A secondary infection originating from the site of an infection already present in the body.

au·to·in·tox·i·ca·tion (ô′tō-ĭn-tŏk′sĭ-kā′shən) *n.* Self-poisoning resulting from the absorption of waste products of metabolism, decomposed intestinal matter, or other toxins produced within the body.

au·to·i·sol·y·sin (ô′tō-ī-sŏl′ĭ-sĭn, -ī′sō-lī′-) *n.* An antibody that with complement causes lysis of cells in the organism in which the lysin is formed, as well as in others of the same species.

au·to·ker·a·to·plas·ty (ô′tō-kĕr′ə-tō-plăs′tē) *n.* The grafting of corneal tissue from one eye to the other eye.

au·to·ki·ne·sia (ô′tō-kĭ-nē′zhə, -kī-) or **au·to·ki·ne·sis** (-nē′sĭs) *n.* Voluntary movement. — **au′to·ki·net′ic** (-nĕt′ĭk) *adj.*

au·tol·o·gous (ô-tŏl′ə-gəs) *adj.* **1.** Of or relating to a natural, normal occurrence in a certain type of tissue or in a specific structure of the body. **2.** Of or relating to a graft in which the donor and recipient areas are in the same individual.

autologous graft *n.* See **autograft.**

au·tol·y·sate (ô-tŏl′ĭ-sāt′, -zāt′) *n.* An end product of autolysis.

au·tol·y·sin (ô-tŏl′ĭ-sĭn, ô′tə-lī′sĭn) *n.* A substance, such as an enzyme, that is capable of destroying the cells or tissues of an organism within which it is produced.

au·tol·y·sis (ô-tŏl′ĭ-sĭs) *n.* **1.** The destruction of tissues or cells of an organism by the action of substances that are produced within the organism. **2.** The hemolytic action of blood serum or plasma upon its own cells. — **au′to·lyt′ic** (ô′tə-lĭt′ĭk) *adj.*

autolytic enzyme *n.* An enzyme that digests the cell in which it is produced.

au·to·mat·ic beat (ô′tə-măt′ĭk) *n.* An ectopic beat that arises anew and is not precipitated by the preceding beat.

au·tom·a·tism (ô-tŏm′ə-tĭz′əm) *n.* **1.** The involuntary functioning of an organ or other body structure that is not under conscious control, such as the beating of the heart or the dilation of the pupil of the eye. **2.** The reflexive action of a body part. **3.** A condition in which one is consciously or unconsciously, but involuntarily, compelled to the performance of certain acts.

au·to·nom·ic (ô′tə-nŏm′ĭk) *adj.* **1.** Functionally independent; not under voluntary control. **2.** Relating to the autonomic nervous system. — **au′to·nom′i·cal·ly** *adv.*

autonomic ganglion *n.* Any of the various ganglia of the autonomic nervous system.

autonomic nervous system *n.* The part of the nervous system that regulates involuntary action, as of the intestines, smooth muscle, heart, and glands, and that is divided into two physiologically and anatomically distinct, mutually antagonistic systems, the sympathetic nervous system and the parasympathetic nervous system.

autonomic plexus *n.* Any of the plexuses of nerves in relation to blood vessels and viscera, whose component fibers are sympathetic, parasympathetic, and sensory.

au·to·pha·gia (ô′tə-fā′jə, -jē-ə) *n.* **1.** The biting of one's own flesh. **2.** or **autophagy** (-tŏf′ə-jē). The segregation and disposal of damaged organelles within a cell. **3.** or **autophagy.** The maintenance

of the nutrition of the whole body by metabolic consumption of some of the body tissues. — **au′to·phag′ic** (-făj′ĭk) *adj.*

autoplastic graft *n.* See **autograft.**

au·to·plas·ty (ô′tō-plăs′tē) *n.* Surgical repair or reconstruction of a body part using tissue taken from another part of the body. — **au′to·plas′tic** *adj.* — **au′to·plas′ti·cal·ly** *adv.*

au·top·sy (ô′tŏp′sē, ô′təp-) *n.* An examination of a cadaver in order to determine the cause of death or to study pathologic changes.

au·to·ra·di·o·graph (ô′tō-rā′dē-ō-grăf′) *n.* An image recorded on a photographic film or plate produced by the radiation emitted from a specimen that has been treated or injected with a radioactively labeled isotope or that has absorbed or ingested such an isotope. — **au′to·ra′di·o·graph′ic** *adj.* — **au′to·ra′di·og′ra·phy** (-ŏg′rə-fē) *n.*

au·to·reg·u·la·tion (ô′tō-rĕg′yə-lā′shən) *n.* **1.** The tendency of the blood flow toward an organ or part to remain at or return to the same level despite changes in arterial pressure. **2.** A biological system equipped with inhibitory feedback systems such that a given change tends to be largely or completely counteracted.

au·to·re·in·fec·tion (ô′tō-rē′ĭn-fĕk′shən) *n.* See **autoinfection** (sense 2).

au·to·re·pro·duc·tion (ô′tō-rē′prə-dŭk′shən) *n.* The capability of a gene, virus, or nucleoprotein molecule to bring about the synthesis of another molecule like itself from smaller molecules within the cell; replication.

au·to·sep·ti·ce·mi·a (ô′tō-sĕp′tĭ-sē′mē-ə) *n.* Septicemia thought to originate from microorganisms existing within the individual and not introduced from outside the organism.

au·to·se·rum (ô′tō-sēr′əm) *n.* Serum derived from an individual's own blood.

au·to·site (ô′tō-sīt′) *n.* The usually larger component of abnormal, unequally conjoined twins that is able to live independently and nourish the other parasitic component.

autosomal gene *n.* A gene on an autosome.

au·to·some (ô′tə-sōm′) *n.* A chromosome other than a sex chromosome, normally occurring in pairs in somatic cells and singly in gametes. — **au′to·so′mal** (-sō′məl) *adj.* — **au′to·so′mal·ly** *adv.*

au·to·sug·ges·tion (ô′tō-səg-jĕs′chən) *n.* **1.** The dwelling upon an idea or concept, thereby inducing some change in the mental or bodily functions. **2.** The process by which a person induces self-acceptance of an opinion, belief, or plan of action. — **au′to·sug·gest′** *v.* — **au′to·sug·gest′i·bil′i·ty** (-ə-bĭl′ĭ-tē) *n.* — **au′to·sug·gest′i·ble,** **au′to·sug·ges′tive** (-tĭv) *adj.*

au·to·tox·in (ô′tō-tŏk′sĭn) *n.* A poison that acts on the organism in which it is generated. — **au′to·tox′ic** *adj.*

au·to·trans·fu·sion (ô′tō-trăns-fyoō′zhən) *n.* Infusion of blood or blood products into the body of the person from whom they were withdrawn.

au·to·trans·plant (ô′tō-trăns′plănt′) *n.* See **autograft.**

au·to·trans·plan·ta·tion (ô′tō-trăns′plăn-tā′-shən) *n.* The transplantation of a tissue or an organ from one site to another on or in the body of the same person.

au·to·vac·ci·na·tion (ô′tō-văk′sə-nā′shən) *n.* Revaccination of a person using vaccine obtained from that person.

aux·e·sis (ôg-zē′sĭs, ôk-sē′-) *n.* Growth resulting from increase in cell size without cell division. — **aux·et′ic** (ôg-zĕt′ĭk) *adj.*

a·vas·cu·lar (ā-văs′kyə-lər) *adj.* Not associated with or supplied by blood vessels. — **a·vas′cu·lar′i·ty** (-lăr′ĭ-tē) *n.*

avascular graft *n.* A skin allograft that does not become vascularized.

a·vas·cu·lar·i·za·tion (ā-văs′kyə-lər-ĭ-zā′shən) *n.* **1.** The exclusion of blood from a part or a tissue. **2.** A loss of blood vessels, as in the tissue that forms in scarring.

a·ver·sion (ə-vûr′zhən, -shən) *n.* **1.** A fixed, intense dislike. **2.** A feeling of extreme repugnance accompanied by avoidance or rejection.

aversion therapy *n.* A type of behavior therapy designed to modify antisocial habits or addictions by creating a strong association with a disagreeable or painful stimulus.

a·vi·an leukosis-sarcoma complex (ā′vē-ən) *n.* **1.** A division of the RNA tumor viruses that causes a group of transmissable diseases of poultry. **2.** The group of diseases caused by this division of viruses.

avian leukosis-sarcoma virus *n.* See **avian leukosis-sarcoma complex** (sense 1).

av·i·din (ăv′ĭ-dĭn) *n.* A protein, found in uncooked egg white, that binds to and inactivates biotin.

a·vi·ta·min·o·sis (ā-vī′tə-mĭ-nō′sĭs) *n.* A disease, such as scurvy, beriberi, or pellagra, caused by deficiency of one or more essential vitamins.

AV nodal rhythm (ā′vē′) *n.* See **atrioventricular nodal rhythm.**

AV node *n.* See **atrioventricular node.**

av·oir·du·pois (ăv′ər-də-poiz′) *n.* A system of weights and measures based on a pound containing 16 ounces or 7,000 grains and equal to 453.59 grams.

avulsed wound *n.* A wound caused by avulsion.

a·vul·sion (ə-vŭl′shən) *n.* The forcible tearing away of a body part by trauma or surgery.

avulsion fracture *n.* A fracture occurring when a joint capsule, ligament, tendon, or muscle is pulled from a bone, taking with it a fragment of the bone to which it was attached.

ax·i·al (ăk′sē-əl) *adj.* **1.** Relating to or characterized by an axis; axile. **2.** Relating to or situated in the head and trunk region of the body.

axial muscle *n.* Any of the the skeletal muscles of the trunk or head.

axial plate *n.* The primitive streak of an embryo.

axial skeleton *n.* The bones of the head and trunk, excluding the pectoral and pelvic girdles.

ax·il·la (ăk-sĭl′ə) *n., pl.* **-il·lae** (-sĭl′ē). See **armpit.**

ax·il·lar·y (ăk′sə-lĕr′ē) *adj.* Relating to the axilla.

ax·is (ăk′sĭs) *n., pl.* **ax·es** (ăk′sēz′). **1.** A real or imaginary straight line about which a body or geometric object rotates or may be conceived to rotate. **2.** A center line to which parts of a structure or body may be referred. **3.** The second cervical vertebra. **4.** An artery that divides into many branches at its origin.

axis deviation *n.* The deflection of the electrical axis of the heart to the right or left of its normal position.

axis shift *n.* See **axis deviation.**

axis traction *n.* Traction upon the fetal head in the line of the birth canal by means of forceps.

axis-traction forceps *n.* Obstetrical forceps constructed to allow traction in the line in which the head must move along the pelvic axis.

ax·o·lem·ma (ăk′sō-lĕm′ə) *n.* The plasma membrane of an axon.

ax·ol·y·sis (ăk-sŏl′ĭ-sĭs) *n.* Degeneration and destruction of the axon of a nerve cell.

ax·om·e·ter (ăk-sŏm′ĭ-tər) *n.* An instrument for determining the position of the optical axes, used for adjusting eyeglasses.

ax·on (ăk′sŏn′) *n.* or **ax·one** (-sŏn′) *n.* The usually long process of a nerve fiber that generally conducts impulses away from the body of the nerve cell. — **ax′on·al** (ăk′sə-nəl, ăk-sŏn′əl) *adj.*

ax·o·nog·ra·phy (ăk′sə-nŏg′rə-fē) *n.* A procedure for recording electrical changes in axons.

ax·o·nom·e·ter (ăk′sə-nŏm′ĭ-tər) *n.* See **axometer.**

ax·on·ot·me·sis (ăk′sə-nŏt-mē′sĭs) *n.* Damage to nerve cells that destroys the axons but that does not destroy the supporting structures of the cells, making regeneration possible.

axon terminals *pl.n.* The somewhat enlarged, often club-shaped endings by which axons make synaptic contacts with other cells.

ax·o·plasm (ăk′sə-plăz′əm) *or* **ax·i·o·plasm** (ăk′-sē-ə-) *n.* The cytoplasm of an axon.

az·a·thi·o·prine (ăz′ə-thī′ə-prēn′) *n.* An immunosuppressive agent used especially to prevent organ rejection in kidney transplant recipients.

az·i·do·thy·mi·dine (ăz′ĭ-dō-thī′mĭ-dēn′) *n.* AZT.

az·lo·cil·lin sodium (ăz′lō-sĭl′ĭn) *n.* A derivative of penicillin used in treating infections caused by *Pseudomonas aeruginosa; Escherichia coli,* and *Haemophilus influenzae.*

az·ole (ăz′ōl′, ā′zōl′) *n.* A class of organic compounds having a five-membered heterocyclic ring with two double bonds; pyrrole.

a·zo·o·sper·mi·a (ā-zō′ə-spûr′mē-ə, ə-zō′-) *n.* **1.** Absence of live spermatozoa in the semen. **2.** Failure to form live spermatozoa.

az·o·pro·tein (ăz′ō-prō′tēn′, -tē-ĭn, ā′zō-) *n.* Any of various compounds formed by coupling proteins with diazonium compounds, often used as synthetic antigens.

az·o·te·mi·a (ăz′ə-tē′mē-ə, ā′zə-) *n.* See **uremia** (sense 1). — **az′o·te′mic** (-mĭk) *adj.*

az·o·tu·ri·a (ăz′ə-tŏŏr′ē-ə, -tyŏŏr′-) *n.* Increase of

nitrogenous substances, especially urea, in the urine.

AZT (ā′zē-tē′) *n.* Azidothymidine; an antiviral drug that inhibits replication of the retrovirus that causes AIDS.

az·tre·o·nam (ăz-trē′ə-năm′) *n.* A synthetic bacte-

ricidal antibiotic that acts against gram-negative aerobic pathogens.

az·y·gos vein (ăz′ĭ-gŏs′, ā-zī′gŏs′) *n.* An unpaired vein of the thorax that arises in the right lumbar region and terminates in the superior vena cava.

B

Ba·be·si·a (bə-bē′zē-ə, -zhə) *n.* A genus of parasitic protozoa of the family Babesiidae that infect the red blood cells of humans and other animals.

ba·be·si·o·sis (bə-bē′zē-ō′sĭs) or **bab·e·si·a·sis** (băb′ĭ-zī′ə-sĭs) *n.* A protozoan disease of the red blood cells caused by a species of *Babesia* that is transmitted by ticks and characterized by fever, malaise, and hemolytic anemia.

Ba·bin·ski's reflex (bə-bĭn′skēz) *n.* An extension of the great toe, sometimes with fanning of the other toes, in response to stroking of the sole of the foot; a normal reflex in only infants.

ba·by (bā′bē) *n.* A very young child; an infant.

baby tooth *n.* See **deciduous tooth.**

bac·am·pi·cil·lin hydrochloride (băk′ăm-pĭ-sĭl′-ĭn, bă-kăm′-) *n.* A semisynthetic penicillin that is effective against gram-negative and gram-positive bacteria and is used to treat infections of the intestinal, urinary, and respiratory tracts.

bac·il·lar·y (băs′ə-lĕr′ē, bə-sĭl′ə-rē) or **ba·cil·lar** (bə-sĭl′ər, băs′ə-lər) *adj.* **1.** Shaped like a rod. **2.** Consisting of small rods or rodlike structures. **3.** Caused by, relating to, or resembling bacilli.

bacillary dysentery *n.* Any of various severe infections of the colon caused by microorganisms, especially of the genus *Shigella*, that result in abdominal cramping, fever, and frequent passage of blood-stained stools or of material consisting of blood and mucus.

bac·il·le·mi·a (băs′ə-lē′mē-ə) *n.* The presence of bacilli in the blood.

ba·cil·lin (bə-sĭl′ĭn) *n.* An antibiotic substance produced by a species of *Bacillus*.

bac·il·lo·sis (băs′ə-lō′sĭs) *n.* An infection caused by bacilli.

bac·il·lu·ri·a (băs′ə-lŏŏr′ē-ə) *n.* The presence of bacilli in the urine.

ba·cil·lus (bə-sĭl′əs) *n., pl.* **-cil·li** (-sĭl′ī′). **1.** Any of various rod-shaped, usually gram-positive aerobic bacteria of the genus *Bacillus* that often occur in chains. **2.** Any of various bacteria, especially a rod-shaped bacterium.

Ba·cil·lus (bə-sĭl′əs) *n.* A genus of rod-shaped, usually gram-positive bacteria capable of producing endospores.

Bacillus Calmette–Guerin vaccine *n.* A vaccine containing attenuated human tubercle bacilli that is used for immunization against tuberculosis.

bac·i·tra·cin (băs′ĭ-trā′sĭn) *n.* A polypeptide anti-

biotic obtained from a strain of *Bacillus subtilis* and used as a topical ointment in the treatment of certain bacterial infections.

back (băk) *n.* **1.** The posterior portion of the trunk of the human body between the neck and the pelvis. **2.** The backbone or spine.

back·ache (băk′āk′) *n.* Discomfort or a pain in the region of the back or spine.

back·board (băk′bôrd′) *n.* **1.** A board placed under or behind something to provide firmness or support. **2.** A board placed beneath the body of a person with an injury to the neck or back, used especially in transporting the person in such a way as to avoid further injury.

backboard splint *n.* A board-rigid splint with slots for fixation by straps; shorter ones are used for neck injuries, longer ones for back injuries.

back·bone (băk′bōn′) *n.* See **spinal column.**

back·cross (băk′krôs′) *v.* **-crossed, -cross·ing, -cross·es.** To cross with a parent or with an individual genetically identical to one of its parents. — *n.* **1.** The act of making such a cross. **2.** An individual resulting from such a cross.

bac·te·re·mi·a (băk′tə-rē′mē-ə) or **bac·te·ri·e·mi·a** (băk-tēr′ē-ē′mē-ə) *n.* The presence of bacteria in the blood.

bac·te·ri·al food poisoning (băk-tîr′ē-əl) *n.* Enteritis or gastroenteritis caused by bacterial multiplication or by a soluble bacterial exotoxin in ingested foods.

bac·ter·id (băk′tər-ĭd) *n.* A recurrent or persistent eruption of pustules on the palms and soles, believed to be associated with a bacterial infection.

bac·ter·in (băk′tər-ĭn) *n.* A suspension of killed or weakened bacteria used as a vaccine.

bac·te·ri·o·gen·ic (băk-tēr′ē-ə-jĕn′ĭk) or **bac·te·ri·og·e·nous** (-ŏj′ə-nəs) *adj.* Caused by bacteria.

bac·te·ri·ol·o·gy (băk-tîr′ē-ŏl′ə-jē) *n.* The study of bacteria, especially in relation to medicine and agriculture. — **bac·te′ri·o·log′ic** (-ə-lŏj′ĭk) *adj.* — **bac·te′ri·ol′o·gist** *n.*

bac·te·ri·ol·y·sin (băk-tēr′ē-ŏl′ĭ-sĭn, -ə-lī′sĭn) *n.* A specific antibody that, together with other substances, destroys a bacterium.

bac·te·ri·ol·y·sis (băk-tēr′ē-ŏl′ĭ-sĭs) *n., pl.* **-ses** (-sēz′). Dissolution or destruction of bacteria. — **bac·te′ri·o·lyt′ic** (-ə-lĭt′ĭk) *adj.*

bac·te·ri·o·phage (băk-tēr′ē-ə-fāj′) *n.* A virus that has the ability to infect and lyse bacterial cells.

bac·te·ri·o·sis (băk-tēr′ē-ō′sĭs) *n*. An infection caused by bacteria.

bac·te·ri·o·stat (băk-tēr′ē-ə-stăt′) *n*. An agent that inhibits bacterial growth. — **bac·te′ri·o·stat′ic** *adj*.

bac·te·ri·um (băk-tēr′ē-əm) *n*., *pl*. **-te·ri·a** (-tēr′ē-ə). Any of the unicellular, prokaryotic microorganisms of the class Schizomycetes, which vary in terms of morphology, oxygen and nutritional requirements, and motility and may be free-living, saprophytic, or pathogenic, the latter causing disease in plants or animals.

bac·te·ri·u·ri·a (băk-tēr′ē-yŏŏr′ē-ə) *n*. The presence of bacteria in urine.

bag·as·so·sis (băg′ə-sō′sĭs) *n*. A respiratory disorder caused by breathing dust from waste sugar cane fiber.

bag of waters (băg) *n*. See **water bag**.

bak·ing soda (bā′kĭng) *n*. A white crystalline compound with a slightly alkaline taste, used as a gastric and systemic antacid, to alkalize urine, and for washes of body cavities.

bal·ance (băl′əns) *n*. **1**. A weighing device, especially one consisting of a rigid beam horizontally suspended by a low-friction support at its center, with identical weighing pans hung at either end, one of which holds an unknown weight while the effective weight in the other is increased by known amounts until the beam is level and motionless. **2**. A state of bodily equilibrium. **3**. The difference in magnitude between opposing forces or influences, such as for bodily parts or organs.

bal·anced anesthesia (băl′ənst) *n*. A technique of general anesthesia based on the concept that administration of a mixture of small amounts of several neuronal depressants provides the advantages but not the disadvantages of the individual components of the mixture.

balanced diet *n*. A diet that furnishes in proper proportions all of the nutrients necessary for adequate nutrition.

balanced polymorphism *n*. A system of genes in which two alleles are maintained in stable equilibrium because the heterozygote is more fit than either of the homozygotes.

balanced translocation *n*. Translocation of the long arm of an acrocentric chromosome to another chromosome, accompanied by loss of the small fragment containing the centromere.

bal·a·ni·tis (băl′ə-nī′tĭs) *n*. Inflammation of the penile or clitoral glans.

bal·a·no·plas·ty (băl′ə-nō-plăs′tē) *n*. Surgical repair of the penile glans.

bal·a·no·pos·thi·tis (băl′ə-nō-pŏs-thī′tĭs) *n*. Inflammation of the penile glans and the prepuce.

bal·a·nor·rha·gi·a (băl′ə-nō-rā′jē-ə, -jə) *n*. A continual discharge from the penile glans.

bald (bôld) *adj*. **bald·er**, **bald·est**. Lacking hair on the head.

bald·ness (bôld′nĭs) *n*. The lack of all or a significant part of the hair on the head and sometimes on other parts of the body.

Bal·kan frame (bôl′kən) *n*. An over-the-bed or free-standing horizontal pole, supported by uprights, from which a splinted limb can be suspended.

Balkan splint *n*. See **Balkan frame**.

ball (bôl) *n*. **1**. A spherical object or mass. **2**. A bezoar. **3**. A large pill or bolus.

ball-and-socket joint *n*. A joint in which a sphere on the head of one bone fits into a rounded cavity in the other bone, as in the hip joint.

bal·lis·mus (bə-lĭz′məs) *n*. Jerky or shaking movements of the arms or legs, especially such movements occurring in chorea.

bal·lis·to·car·di·o·graph (bə-lĭs′tō-kär′dē-ə-grăf′) *n*. A device used to determine the volume of blood passing through the heart in a specific period of time and the force of cardiac contraction by measuring the body's recoil as blood is ejected from the ventricles with each heartbeat. — **bal·lis′to·car′di·o·gram′** (-ə-grăm′) *n*, **bal·lis′to·car′di·og′ra·phy** (-ŏg′rə-fē) *n*.

ball of foot *n*. The padded portion of the sole of the human foot between the toes and the arch on which the weight of the body rests when the heel is raised.

bal·loon (bə-lōōn′) *n*. An inflatable spherical device that is inserted into a body cavity or structure and distended with air or gas.

balloon angioplasty *n*. A procedure in which a catheter equipped with a tiny balloon at the tip is inserted into an artery that has been narrowed by the accumulation of fatty deposits. The balloon is then inflated to clear the blockage and widen the artery.

bal·loon·sep·tos·to·my (bə-lōōn′sĕp-tŏs′tə-mē) *n*. The surgical creation of an artificial interatrial septal defect by cardiac catheterization during which an inflated balloon is pulled across the interatrial septum through the oval foramen.

balloon-tip catheter *n*. A tube with an inflatable balloon at its tip that, when inflated, can facilitate passage of the tube through a blood vessel.

bal·lotte·ment (bə-lŏt′mənt) *n*. **1**. A palpatory technique for detecting or examining an organ not near the surface of the body. **2**. The use of a finger to push sharply against the uterus and detect the presence or position of a fetus by its return impact.

ball valve *n*. A valve regulated by the position of a free-floating ball that moves in response to fluid or mechanical pressure.

balm (bäm) *n*. **1**. An aromatic salve or oil. **2**. A soothing, healing, or comforting agent.

Bam·ber·ger's sign (băm′bər-gərz, bäm′-) *n*. **1**. The jugular pulse occurring in tricuspid insufficiency of the heart. **2**. An indication of pericarditis with effusion in which the dullness of sound generated upon percussion at the angle of the scapula disappears as the patient leans forward.

ban·crof·ti·a·sis (băn′krôf-tī′ə-sĭs, băng′-) or **ban·crof·to·sis** (-tō′sĭs) *n*. A disease caused by infestation with *Wuchereria bancrofti*.

band·age (băn′dĭj) *n*. A strip of material such as gauze used to protect, immobilize, compress, or support a wound or injured body part. —*v.* -aged, -ag·ing, -ag·es. To apply a bandage to.

Band-Aid (bănd′ād′) A trademark used for an adhesive bandage with a gauze pad in the center, employed to protect minor wounds.

band cell *n.* Any of the blood granulocytic cells having a densely staining unsegmented nucleus.

band·ing (băn′dĭng) *n.* The staining of metaphase chromosomes in cultured cells to reveal their patterns in order to identify individual pairs.

Bandl's ring (băn′dlz) *n.* See **pathologic retraction ring.**

Banti's syndrome *n.* Chronic congestive enlargement of the spleen following venous hypertension, characterized by anemia, splenomegaly, ascites, jaundice, leukopenia, thrombocytopenia, and episodes of gastrointestinal bleeding.

bar·ag·no·sis (băr′ăg-nō′sĭs) *n.* Loss or impairment of the ability to differentiate varying weights or pressures.

Bá·rá·ny's caloric test (bä′răn′yəz) *n.* A test for assessing vestibular function in the ear.

bar·ber's itch (bär′bərz) *n.* Any of various skin eruptions on the face and neck, especially ringworm of the beard.

bar·bi·tal (bär′bĭ-tôl′, -tăl′) *n.* A white crystalline barbiturate that is used as a sedative and hypnotic, especially in the form of sodium barbital.

bar·bi·tu·rate (bär-bĭch′ər-ĭt, -ə-rāt′, bär′bĭ-tŏŏr′ĭt, -āt′, -tyŏŏr′-) *n.* Any of a group of barbituric acid derivatives that depress the central nervous system and are used as sedatives or hypnotics.

bar·bi·tu·rism (bär-bĭch′ə-rĭz′əm, bär′bĭ-tŏŏr′ĭz′-əm, -tyŏŏr′-) *n.* Chronic poisoning caused by any of the derivatives of barbituric acid.

bar·bo·tage (bär′-bə-täzh′) *n.* The production of spinal anesthesia in which a portion of the anesthetic solution is injected into the cerebral spinal fluid, which is then aspirated into the syringe and the process repeated until the contents of the syringe are injected.

Bar·det-Biedl syndrome (bär-dā′-bēd′l) *n.* An inherited disorder characterized by mental retardation, pigmentary retinopathy, polydactyly, obesity, and hypogenitalism.

bare·foot doctor (bâr′fŏŏt) *n.* A lay health care worker, especially in rural China, trained in such activities as first aid, childbirth assistance, the dispensing of drugs, and preventive medicine.

bar·es·the·sia (băr′ĕs-thē′zhə) *n.* See **pressure sense.**

bar·es·the·si·om·e·ter (băr′ĕs-thē′zē-ŏm′ĭ-tər) *n.* An instrument for measuring a person's sense of pressure.

bar·i·at·rics (băr′ē-ăt′rĭks) *n.* The branch of medicine that deals with the causes, prevention, and treatment of obesity. — **bar′i·at′ric** *adj.*

bar·i·um (bâr′ē-əm, băr′-) *n.* A soft alkaline-earth metal with atomic number 56.

barium enema The administration of barium in enema form for radiographic study of the lower intestinal tract.

barium sulfate *n.* A fine white powder used as a pigment and as a contrast medium in x-ray photography of the digestive tract.

Barnes curve (bärnz) *n.* The segment of a circle whose center is the promontory of the sacrum.

bar·o·re·cep·tor (băr′ō-rĭ-sĕp′tər) or **bar·o·cep·tor** (băr′ō-sĕp′tər) *n.* A sensory nerve ending in the walls of the auricles of the heart, vena cava, carotid sinus, and aortic arch, sensitive to stretching of the wall due to increased pressure from within, and functioning as the receptor of reflex mechanisms that tend to reduce that pressure.

bar·o·re·flex (băr′ō-rē′flĕks′) *n.* A reflex triggered by stimulation of a baroreceptor.

bar·o·si·nus·i·tis (băr′ō-sī′nə-sī′tĭs) *n.* See **aerosinusitis.**

bar·o·tax·is (băr′ō-tăk′sĭs) *n.* The response of living tissue to changes in pressure.

bar·o·ti·tis me·di·a (băr′ō-tī′tĭs mē′dē-ə) *n.* See **aerotitis media.**

bar·o·trau·ma (băr′ō-trou′mə, -trô′-) *n.* Injury caused by pressure, especially injury to the middle ear or paranasal sinuses because of an imbalance between the ambient pressure and pressure within the affected cavity.

Barr body (bär) *n.* The condensed, inactive, single X-chromosome found in the nuclei of somatic cells of most female mammals and whose presence is the basis of sex determination tests.

bar·rel chest (băr′əl) *n.* A large chest with increased anteroposterior diameter and usually some degree of kyphosis, sometimes seen in cases of emphysema.

bar·ren (băr′ən) *adj.* **1.** Not producing offspring. **2.** Incapable of producing offspring.

Barrett's syndrome *n.* Chronic peptic ulcer of the lower esophagus.

bar·ri·er (băr′ē-ər) *n.* **1.** A structure built to bar passage. **2.** A boundary or limit. **3.** An obstacle or impediment. **4.** Something that separates or holds apart. **5.** Something immaterial that obstructs or impedes behavior.

bar·tho·lin·i·tis (bär′tə-lə-nī′tĭs) *n.* Inflammation of the greater vestibular gland.

Bar·tho·lin's gland (bär′tl-ĭnz, -thə-lĭnz) *n.* See **greater vestibular gland.**

Bar·ton·el·la (bär′tn-ĕl′ə) *n.* A genus of bacteria found in humans and arthropods that multiply in red blood cells and reproduce by binary fission.

bar·ton·el·lo·sis (bär′tn-ĕl-ō′sĭs) *n.* A disease caused by *Bartonella bacilliformis* and transmitted by the bite of the sandfly.

Bar·ton's bandage (bär′tnz) *n.* A figure-of-8 bandage supporting a fractured mandible.

Bart's hemoglobin (bärts) *n.* An abnormal hemoglobin that is made up of gamma chains only and is not effective in oxygen transport.

ba·sal (bā′səl, -zəl) *adj.* **1.** Of, relating to, located at, or forming a base, usually of an organ or a tooth. **2.** Of, relating to, of situated at the lowest level, as of an organ.

basal anesthesia *n.* Parenteral administration of

one or more sedatives to depress consciousness but not produce general anesthesia.

basal body n. A cellular organelle associated with the formation of cilia and flagella and resembling the centriole in structure.

basal cell n. A type of cell found in the deepest layer of the epithelium.

basal cell carcinoma n. A slow-growing, locally invasive neoplasm of the skin derived from basal cells of the epidermis or hair follicles.

basal cell epithelioma n. See **basal cell carcinoma**.

basal cell nevus n. A hereditary disease characterized by lesions of the eyelids, nose, cheeks, neck, and armpits that are usually benign and that appear as uneroded papules histologically indistinguishable from basal cell carcinoma.

basal ganglia pl.n. The caudate and lentiform nuclei of the brain and the cell groups associated with them, considered as a group.

basal granule n. See **basal body**.

basal joint reflex n. A reflex of the thumb in which the metacarpophalangeal joint flexes and the interphalangeal joint extends in response to firm passive flexion of the third, fourth, or fifth finger.

basal layer n. **1.** The outermost layer of the endometrium, which undergoes only minimal changes during the menstrual cycle. **2.** The deepest layer of the epidermis.

basal metabolic rate n. The rate at which energy is used by an organism at complete rest, measured in humans by the heat given off per unit time, and expressed as the calories released per kilogram of body weight or per square meter of body surface per hour.

basal metabolism n. The minimum amount of energy required to maintain vital functions in an organism at complete rest, measured by the basal metabolic rate in an alert fasting individual.

base (bās) n. **1.** The part of an organ nearest its point of attachment. **2.** A fundamental ingredient; a chief constituent of a mixture.

base·ball finger (bās′bôl′) n. Permanent flexion of the terminal phalanx of a finger due to a break in the extensor tendon resulting from a blow from a ball or other object.

base deficit n. A decrease in the total concentration of bicarbonate indicative of metabolic acidosis or of compensated respiratory alkalosis.

base line n. **1.** A line corresponding to the base of the skull, passing through the external auditory meatus. **2.** A line serving as a basis, as for measurement, calculation, or location.

base·ment membrane (bās′mənt) n. A thin, delicate layer of connective tissue underlying the epithelium of many organs.

base of heart n. The part of the heart formed mainly by the left atrium and somewhat by the posterior part of the right atrium, separated from the vertebral column by the esophagus and aorta.

base of lung n. The lower concave part of the lung that rests upon the convexity of the diaphragm.

base of skull n. **1.** The interior aspect of the skull,

on which the brain rests. **2.** The inferior or external aspect of the skull.

base·plate (bās′plāt′) n. **1.** The portion of an artificial denture in contact with the jaw. **2.** A temporary form representing the base of a denture and used to help establish jaw relationships and the arrangement of teeth.

ba·sic (bā′sĭk) adj. **1.** Of, being, or serving as a starting point or basis. **2.** Producing, resulting from, or relating to a base. **3.** Containing a base, especially in excess of acid.

ba·sic·i·ty (bā-sĭs′ĭ-tē) n. **1.** The ability of an acid to react based on the number of replaceable hydrogen atoms it contains. **2.** The quality of being basic.

basic life support n. Emergency procedures performed to sustain life that include cardiopulmonary resuscitation, control of bleeding, treatment of shock and poisoning, stabilization of injuries and wounds, and first aid.

basic personality type n. **1.** An individual's unique, covert, or underlying personality characteristics. **2.** The shared behavioral traits of individuals raised in the same culture and experiencing similar child-rearing practices.

bas·i·lar (băs′ə-lər) adj. Of, relating to, or located at or near the base, especially the base of the skull.

ba·si·lem·ma (bā′sə-lĕm′ə) n. See **basement membrane**.

ba·sis (bā′sĭs) n., pl. **-ses** (-sēz′). The foundation upon which something, such as an anatomical part, rests.

bas·ket cell (băs′kĭt) n. **1.** Any of the neurons in the molecular layer of the cerebellum whose axons form a basketlike network around a Purkinje cell. **2.** A myoepithelial cell with branching processes that occurs basal to the secretory cells of certain salivary gland and lacrimal gland alveoli.

ba·so·e·ryth·ro·cyte (bā′sō-ĭ-rĭth′rə-sīt′, -zō-) n. A red blood cell that shows stippling associated with basic staining granules, representing a condition such as severe anemia, leukemia, lead poisoning, or malaria.

ba·so·phil (bā′sə-fĭl, -zə-) or **ba·so·phile** (-fīl′) n. A cell, especially a white blood cell, having granules that stain readily with basic dyes. — **ba′so·phil′ic** (-fĭl′ĭk) adj.

ba·so·phil·i·a (bā′sə-fĭl′ē-ə, -zə-) n. **1.** An increase in the number of basophils in the blood. **2.** An abnormal stippling of red blood cells with basic-staining granules.

basophilic leukopenia n. A condition characterized by a decrease in the number of basophilic granulocytes normally present in the blood.

Bas·sen–Korn·zweig syndrome (băs′ən-kôrn′-zwīg) n. See **abetalipoproteinemia**.

Bas·si·ni's operation (bə-sē′nēz, bä-) n. An operation for the radical correction of inguinal hernia.

bath (băth) n., pl. **baths** (băthz, băths). **1.** The act of soaking or cleansing the body or any of its parts, as in water or steam. **2.** The apparatus used in giving a bath.

bath·o·pho·bi·a (băth'ə-fō'bē-ə) *n.* An abnormal fear of depths.

bath pruritus *n.* Itching caused by inadequate rinsing off of soap or by overdrying of skin as a result of excessive bathing.

bath·y·an·es·the·sia (băth'ē-ăn'ĭs-thē'zhə) *n.* Loss of sensation in those parts of the body derived from the mesoderm.

bath·y·es·the·sia (băth'ē-ĭs-thē'zhə) *n.* The sensibility of the parts of the body located beneath the surface, such as muscle and joint sensibility.

bath·y·hy·per·es·the·sia (băth'ē-hī'pər-ĭs-thē'-zhə) *n.* The increased sensitivity of muscular tissues and other deep structures.

bath·y·hyp·es·the·sia (băth'ē-hĭp'ĭs-thē'zhə) *n.* The impaired sensitivity of muscular tissues and other deep structures.

bat·o·pho·bi·a (băt'ə-fō'bē-ə) *n.* An abnormal fear of being near an object of great height such as a skyscraper or mountain.

bat·tered child (băt'ərd) *n.* A child upon whom multiple, continuing, often serious nonaccidental injuries have been inflicted usually by parents, guardians, or other individuals.

bat·tered child syndrome (băt'ərd) *n.* A combination of continuing, often serious physical injuries, such as bruises, hematomas, or malnutrition, inflicted on a child through gross abuse usually by parents, guardians, or other caregivers.

battered woman syndrome *n.* A pattern of signs and symptoms, such as helplessness, constant fear, and a perceived inability to escape, commonly appearing in women who are physically and mentally abused over an extended period by a husband or other dominant individual.

bat·ter·ing parent syndrome (băt'ər-ĭng) *n.* A group of signs and symptoms characterizing a psychological disorder in a child's parent or other custodian, resulting in a tendency or disposition to abuse the child.

bat·ter·y (băt'ə-rē) *n.* An array of similar things intended for use together, such as achievement tests.

bat·tle·dore placenta (băt'l-dôr') *n.* A placenta in which the umbilical cord is attached at the border.

bat·tle fatigue or **bat·tle neurosis** (băt'l) *n.* See **war neurosis.**

Baude·locque's operation (bōd-lôks') *n.* In extra-uterine pregnancy, an incision through the posterior cul-de-sac of the vagina for the removal of the embryo.

Bau·er's syndrome (bou'ərz) *n.* Aortitis and aortic endocarditis as a manifestation of rheumatoid arthritis.

Bay·ley Scales of Infant Development (bā'lē) *pl.n.* Standardized tests used to assess the mental, motor, and behavioral progress of children over the first two and one-half years of life.

B cell *n.* **1.** See **beta cell. 2.** A type of lymphocyte that, when stimulated by a particular antigen, differentiates into plasma cells that synthesize the antibodies that circulate in the blood and react with the specific antigens.

BCG vaccine *n.* See **Bacillus Calmette–Guérin vaccine.**

B chain *n.* A polypeptide component of insulin containing 30 amino acids, the composition of which is species-specific.

BCL2 (bē'sē-ĕl-tōō') *n.* A gene associated with non-Hodgkin's lymphoma that normally helps regulate the life span of a white blood cell but which when mutated prevents such cells from dying, thus allowing possible further mutations and the development of cancer.

B complex *n.* See **vitamin B complex.**

beak·er cell (bē'kər) *n.* See **goblet cell.**

bear·ing down (bâr'ĭng) *n.* Forceful contraction of the abdominal muscles and diaphragm during the second stage of labor, either as a reflex or as a conscious effort.

bearing-down pain *n.* A uterine contraction accompanied by straining and tenesmus, usually appearing in the second stage of labor.

beat (bēt) *v.* **beat, beat·en** (bēt'n), **beat·ing, beats. 1.** To strike repeatedly. **2.** To pulsate; throb. —*n.* A stroke or blow, especially one that produces a sound as of the heart or pulse.

Bech·te·rew-Mendel reflex (běk'tə-rěf-, -rěv-) *n.* Flexion of the toes caused by percussion of the upper surface of the foot.

Beck·er's test (běk'ərz) *n.* A test for astigmatism that uses diagrams of sets of three lines radiating in different meridians.

bed (běd) *n.* **1.** A piece of furniture for reclining and sleeping, typically consisting of a flat, rectangular frame and a mattress resting on springs. **2.** Such a piece of furniture used for rest, recuperation, or treatment. **3.** A supporting, underlying, or securing base or structure, especially an anatomical one.

B.E.D. *abbr.* binge eating disorder

bed·bug (běd'bŭg') *n.* A wingless, odorous insect (*Cimex lectularius*) with a flat, reddish body that infests dwellings and bedding and feeds on human blood.

bed·pan (běd'păn') *n.* A metal, glass, or plastic receptacle for the urinary and fecal discharges of persons confined to bed.

bed·rid·den (běd'rĭd'n) or **bed·rid** (-rĭd') *adj.* Confined to bed because of illness or infirmity.

bed·side manner (běd'sīd') *n.* The attitude and conduct of a physician in the presence of a patient.

bed·sore (běd'sôr') *n.* A pressure-induced ulceration of the skin occurring in persons confined to bed for long periods of time.

bed·wet·ting (běd'wět'ĭng) *n.* Involuntary discharge of urine, especially when occurring nocturnally.

Beer's operation (bārz) *n.* A flap operation for cataract.

Bee·vor's sign (bē'vərz) *n.* An indication of paralysis of the lower portions of the abdominal straight muscles in which the navel moves upward.

be·hav·ior (bĭ-hāv′yər) *n.* **1.** The actions or reactions of persons or things in response to external or internal stimuli. **2.** The manner in which one behaves. — **be·hav′ior·al** *adj.*

behavior disorder *n.* **1.** Any of various forms of behavior that are considered inappropriate by members of the social group to which an individual belongs. **2.** A functional disorder or abnormality.

be·hav·ior·ism (bĭ-hāv′yə-rĭz′əm) *n.* A school of psychology that studies the observable and quantifiable aspects of behavior and excludes subjective phenomena, such as emotions or motives.

behavior modification *n.* **1.** The use of basic learning techniques, such as conditioning, biofeedback, reinforcement, or aversion therapy, to teach simple skills or alter undesirable behavior. **2.** See **behavior therapy.**

behavior therapy *n.* A form of psychotherapy that uses basic learning techniques to modify maladaptive behavior patterns by substituting new responses to given stimuli for undesirable ones. — **behavior therapist** *n.*

Beh·çet's syndrome (bĕch′ĕts′, bĕ-chĕts′) *n.* Recurrent attacks of genital and oral ulcerations and uveitis or iridocyclitis, often accompanied by arthritis.

bel (bĕl) *n.* A unit expressing the relative intensity of a sound, equal to ten decibels.

belch (bĕlch) *v.* **belched, belch·ing, belch·es.** To expel gas noisily from the stomach through the mouth; burp.

bel·la·don·na (bĕl′ə-dŏn′ə) *n.* **1.** A poisonous Eurasian perennial herb having usually solitary, purplish-brown, bell-shaped flowers and glossy black berries. **2.** An alkaloidal extract or tincture derived from this plant.

belladonna alkaloids *pl.n.* A group of alkaloids, including atropine and scopolamine, found in plants such as belladonna. They are used in medicine to dilate the pupils of the eyes, dry respiratory passages, prevent motion sickness, and relieve cramping of the intestines and bladder.

Bell's palsy (bĕlz) *n.* See **facial palsy.**

bel·ly (bĕl′ē) *n.* **1.** See **abdomen. 2.** *Informal.* The stomach. **3.** The womb; the uterus. **4.** The bulging, central part of a muscle.

bel·ly·ache (bĕl′ē-āk′) *n.* Pain in the stomach or abdomen; colic.

bel·ly·but·ton (bĕl′ē-bŭt′n) *n.* See **navel.**

bel·o·ne·pho·bi·a (bĕl′ə-nə-fō′bē-ə) *n.* An abnormal fear of sharply pointed objects, especially needles.

Bel·sey operation (bĕl′sē) *n.* A transthoracic procedure for the treatment of sliding hiatal hernia.

bend (bĕnd) *v.* **bent** (bĕnt), **bend·ing, bends.** To incline the body; stoop.

Ben·der gestalt test (bĕn′dər) *n.* A test of visuospatial and visuomotor coordination used to detect brain damage.

bend·ing fracture (bĕn′dĭng) *n.* A curving of a long bone due to multiple minute fractures.

bends (bĕndz) *n.* See **decompression sickness.**

Ben·e·dict's test (bĕn′ĭ-dĭkts′) *n.* A test for detecting glucose in urine.

be·nign (bĭ-nīn′) *adj.* Of no danger to health, especially relating to a tumorous growth.

benign dyskeratosis *n.* Dyskeratosis that often occurs in congenital or bullous skin diseases.

benign hypertension *n.* Essential hypertension that runs a relatively long and symptomless course.

benign inoculation reticulosis *n.* See **cat scratch disease.**

benign myalgic encephalomyelitis *n.* See **epidemic neuromyasthenia.**

benign tumor *n.* A tumor that does not metastasize or invade and destroy adjacent normal tissue.

ben·ox·a·pro·fen (bĕ-nŏk′sə-prō′fən) *n.* A nonsteroidal, anti-inflammatory, analgesic agent.

ben·tir·o·mide (bĕn-tēr′ə-mīd′) *n.* A peptide used as a screening test for exocrine pancreatic insufficiency and to monitor the adequacy of supplemental pancreatic therapy.

ben·ton·ite flocculation test (bĕn′tə-nīt′) *n.* A flocculation test for rheumatoid arthritis.

ben·zal·ko·ni·um chloride (bĕn′zăl-kō′nē-əm) *n.* A yellow-white powder prepared in an aqueous solution and used as a detergent, fungicide, bactericide, and spermicide.

benz·an·thra·cene (bĕn-zăn′thrə-sēn′) or **benz·an·threne** (-thrēn′) *n.* A crystalline, weakly carcinogenic cyclic hydrocarbon.

Ben·ze·drine (bĕn′zĭ-drēn′) A trademark used for a brand of amphetamine.

ben·zene (bĕn′zēn′, bĕn-zēn′) *n.* A clear, colorless, highly refractive flammable liquid derived from petroleum and used in or to manufacture a wide variety of chemical products.

benzene ring *n.* The hexagonal ring structure in the benzene molecule and its substitutional derivatives, each vertex of which is occupied and distinguished by a carbon atom.

ben·zo·caine (bĕn′zə-kān′) *n.* A white, odorless, tasteless crystalline substance used as a local anesthetic.

ben·zo·di·az·e·pine (bĕn′zō-dī-ăz′ə-pēn′, -pĭn) *n.* Any of a group of psychotropic agents used as antianxiety agents, muscle relaxants, sedatives, and hypnotics.

ben·zo·na·tate (bĕn-zō′nə-tāt′) *n.* A colorless to faintly yellow oil that is soluble in most organic solvents and is used as an antitussive drug.

ben·zo·thi·a·di·a·zide (bĕn′zō-thī′ə-dī′ə-zīd′) *n.* Any of a group of diuretics that increase excretion of sodium, chloride, and water.

benzoyl peroxide *n.* A flammable white granular solid used as a bleaching agent, a polymerization catalyst, and in pharmaceuticals.

ber·i·ber·i (bĕr′ē-bĕr′ē) *n.* A disease caused by a deficiency of thiamine, endemic in eastern and southern Asia and characterized by neurological symptoms, cardiovascular abnormalities, and edema.

ber·ke·li·um (bər-kē'lē-əm, bûrk'lē-əm) *n.* A synthetic radioactive element with atomic number 97.

Ber·nard–Cannon homeostasis (bĕr-när'-) *n.* The set of mechanisms by which cybernetic adjustment of physiological and biochemical states is made in postnatal life.

Bern·stein test (bûrn'stīn, -stēn) *n.* A test to establish that substernal pain is due to reflux esophagitis.

ber·ry aneurysm (bĕr'ē) *n.* A small saccular aneurysm of a cerebral artery that resembles a berry.

be·ryl·li·o·sis (bə-rĭl'ē-ō'sĭs) *n.* Beryllium poisoning characterized by the occurrence of granulomatous fibrosis, especially of the lungs, due to inhalation of beryllium salts.

be·ryl·li·um (bə-rĭl'ē-əm) *n.* A lightweight, corrosion-resistant metallic element with atomic number 4 and used as an aerospace structural material and in nuclear reactors.

Bes·nier–Boeck–Schaumann disease or **Bes·nier–Boeck–Schaumann syndrome** (bĕ-nyä'-) *n.* See **sarcoidosis**.

bes·ti·al·i·ty (bĕs'chē-ăl'ĭ-tē, bēs'-) *n.* **1.** The quality or condition of being an animal or like an animal. **2.** Conduct or an action marked by depravity or brutality. **3.** Sexual relations between a human and an animal.

be·ta (bā'tə, bē'-) *n.* The second item in a series or system of classification. — *adj.* Of or relating to the second position from a designated carbon atom in an organic molecule at which an atom or a radical may be substituted.

beta-adrenergic *adj.* Of, relating to, or being a beta-receptor.

be·ta·ad·re·ner·gic blocking agent (bā'tə-ăd'rə-nûr'jĭk, bē'-) *n.* See **beta-blocker**.

beta-adrenergic receptor *n.* Any of various cell membrane receptors that can bind with epinephrine and related substances that activate or block the actions of cells containing such receptors; these cells initiate physiological responses such as increasing the rate and force of contraction of the heart as well as relaxing bronchial and vascular smooth muscle.

beta-blocker *n.* A drug that opposes the excitatory effects of norepinephrine released from sympathetic nerve endings at beta-receptors and is used for the treatment of angina, hypertension, arrhythmia, and migraine.

beta carotene *n.* An isomer of carotene.

beta cell *n.* **1.** Any of the basophilic chromophil cells located in the anterior lobe of the pituitary gland. **2.** Any of the insulin-producing cells of the islets of Langerhans in the pancreas.

beta-endorphin *n.* An endorphin produced by the pituitary gland that is a potent pain suppressant.

beta globulin *n.* A type of globulin found in blood plasma.

beta-hemolytic streptococci *pl.n.* Streptococci that completely lyse red blood cells cultured on blood agar medium, producing a clear area around the cell colonies.

be·ta·ine (bē'tə-ēn', -ĭn) *n.* A sweet crystalline alkaloid found in sugar beets and other plants, used in the treatment of muscular degeneration.

beta-lipoprotein *n.* See **low-density lipoprotein**.

be·ta·meth·a·sone (bā'tə-mĕth'ə-sōn', bē'-) *n.* A synthetic glucocorticoid used as a topical anti-inflammatory agent for the treatment of dermatological conditions.

beta-receptor *n.* See **beta-adrenergic receptor**.

be·than·e·chol (bĕ-thăn'ĭ-kôl') *n.* A cholinergic drug that acts principally by stimulating the parasympathetic nervous system and is used in the form of its chloride to treat abdominal distention and urinary retention.

Betz cell (bĕts) *n.* Any of the large pyramidal cells in the motor area of the cerebral cortex.

Beuren syndrome (byŏor'ən) *n.* Supravalvular aortic stenosis with peripheral pulmonary arterial stenosis marked by mental retardation.

be·zoar (bē'zôr') *n.* A hard indigestible mass of material, such as hair, vegetable fibers, or the seeds and skins of fruits, formed in the alimentary canal of animals and humans.

BHA (bē'āch-ā') *n.* A white, waxy phenolic antioxidant used to preserve fats and oils.

BHT (bē'āch-tē') *n.* A crystalline phenolic antioxidant used to preserve fats and oils.

bi·ax·i·al joint (bī-ăk'sē-əl) *n.* A joint in which there are two principal axes of movement situated at right angles to each other.

bib. *abbr. Latin.* bibe (drink)

bib·li·o·ther·a·py (bĭb'lē-ō-thĕr'ə-pē) *n.* A form of supportive psychotherapy in which carefully selected reading materials are used to assist a subject in solving personal problems or for other therapeutic purposes.

bi·car·di·o·gram (bī-kär'dē-ə-grăm') *n.* The composite curve of an electrocardiogram showing the combined effects of the right and left ventricles.

bi·ceps (bī'sĕps') *n., pl.* **biceps** or **-ceps·es** (-sĕp'-sĭz). **1.** A muscle with two heads or points of origin. **2.** The large muscle at the front of the upper arm that flexes the forearm. **3.** The large muscle at the back of the thigh that flexes the knee joint and rotates the leg laterally. — **bi·cip'i·tal** (-sĭp'ĭ-tl) *adj.*

biceps reflex *n.* Contraction of the biceps muscle when its tendon is struck.

bi·clo·nal·i·ty (bī'klō-năl'ĭ-tē) *n.* A condition in which some cells have markers of one cell line and other cells have markers of another cell line, as in some leukemias. — **bi·clon'al** (-klō'nəl) *adj.*

bi·con·cave lens (bī'kŏn-kāv', bī-kŏn'kāv) *n.* A lens that is concave on two opposing surfaces.

bi·con·vex lens (bī'kŏn-vĕks', bī-kŏn'vĕks') *n.* A lens with both surfaces convex.

bi·cor·nate uterus (bī-kôr'nāt', -nĭt) *n.* A uterus that is divided into two lateral horns; the cervix may be single or double.

bi·cor·nu·ate (bī-kôr'nyŏo-ĭt, -āt') *adj.* **1.** Having two horns or horn-shaped parts. **2.** Shaped like a crescent. — **bi·cor′nu·ous** (-əs) *adj.*

bi·cus·pid valve (bī-kŭs′pĭd) *n.* See **mitral valve.**

bi·dac·ty·ly (bī-dăk′tə-lē) *n.* Congenital absence of all fingers or toes except the first and fifth digits.

bi·di·rec·tion·al ventricular tachycardia (bī′dĭ-rĕk′shə-nəl, dī-) *n.* Ventricular tachycardia in which the QRS complexes in the electrocardiogram are alternately positive and negative.

BIDS (bĭdz) *n.* A congenital condition resulting from a deficiency of high-sulfur protein and characterized by brittle hair, impaired intelligence, decreased fertility, and short stature.

Bier·nac·ki's sign (byĕr-nät′skēz) *n.* Analgesia of the ulnar nerve occurring in cases of tabes dorsalis and general paresis.

Bier's method (bērz) *n.* A method for administering anesthesia to a part, especially a limb, through intravenous injections of anesthesia after the part has been constricted and elevated.

bi·fid cranium (bī′fĭd) *n.* See **encephalocele.**

bifid tongue *n.* A tongue whose tip is divided longitudinally for a certain distance.

bi·fo·cal (bī-fō′kəl, bī′fō′-) *adj.* **1.** Having two focal lengths. **2.** Having one section that corrects for distant vision and another that corrects for near vision.

bifocal lens *n.* A lens having one section that corrects for distant vision and another section that corrects for near vision.

bi·fur·ca·tion (bī′fər-kā′shən) *n.* A division into two branches; a forking.

bi·gem·i·ny (bī-jĕm′ə-nē) *n.* **1.** An association in pairs. **2.** An abnormal pulse characterized by two beats in rapid succession followed by a pause. — **bi·gem·i·nal** (nəl) *adj.*

big toe *n.* The largest and innermost toe of the human foot.

bi·lat·er·al (bī-lăt′ər-əl) *adj.* **1.** Having or formed of two sides; two-sided. **2.** Having or marked by bilateral symmetry.

bilateral hermaphroditism *n.* Hermaphroditism with testicular and ovarian tissue occurring on both sides of the body.

bilateral symmetry *n.* Symmetrical arrangement, as of an organism or a part, along a central axis, so that it is divided into equivalent right and left halves by only one plane.

bi·lay·er (bī′lā′ər) *n.* A structure, such as a film or membrane, consisting of two molecular layers.

bile (bīl) *n.* A bitter, alkaline, brownish-yellow or greenish-yellow fluid that is secreted by the liver, stored in the gallbladder, and discharged into the duodenum and aids in the emulsification, digestion, and absorption of fats.

bile acid *n.* Any of several acids formed in the liver that commonly occur in the bile as sodium salts combined with an amino acid such as glycine.

bile duct or **biliary duct** *n.* Any of the excretory ducts in the liver that convey bile between the liver and the intestine.

bile pigment *n.* Any of the coloring materials in the bile derived from porphyrins, such as bilirubin and biliverdin.

bile salt *n.* **1.** Any of the sodium salts of the bile acids occurring in bile. **2.** A mixture, such as a commercial preparation derived from the bile of the ox, that is used medicinally as a hepatic stimulant or laxative.

bil·har·zi·al dysentery (bĭl-här′zē-əl) *n.* Intestinal damage or hemorrhage caused by passage of the spined eggs of certain trematode worms of the genus *Schistosoma.*

bil·i·ar·y (bĭl′ē-ĕr′ē) *adj.* **1.** Of or relating to bile, the bile ducts, or the gallbladder. **2.** Transporting bile.

biliary calculus *n.* See **gallstone.**

biliary cirrhosis *n.* Cirrhosis due to obstruction or infection of a hepatic bile duct.

biliary dyskinesia *n.* Spasms of the gallbladder or its ducts that impair filling or emptying and are caused by intrinsic or extrinsic disease.

bil·i·gen·e·sis (bĭl′ĭ-jĕn′ĭ-sĭs) *n.* The production of bile.

bil·ious (bĭl′yəs) *adj.* **1.** Of, relating to, or containing bile; biliary. **2.** Characterized by an excess secretion of bile. **3.** Relating to, characterized by, or experiencing gastric distress caused by a disorder of the liver or gallbladder. — **bil′ious·ness** *n.*

bil·i·ru·bin (bĭl′ĭ-rōō′bĭn, bĭl′ĭ-rōō′-) *n.* A reddish-yellow bile pigment derived from the degradation of heme during the normal or abnormal destruction of red blood cells.

bil·i·ru·bi·ne·mi·a (bĭl′ĭ-rōō′bə-nē′mē-ə) *n.* The presence of excess bilirubin in the blood.

bil·i·ru·bin·oid (bĭl′ĭ-rōō′bə-noid′) *n.* Any of various intermediate chemical substances, usually found in urine and feces, formed during the enzymatic conversion of bilirubin to stercobilin.

bil·i·ru·bi·nu·ri·a (bĭl′ĭ-rōō′bə-nŏŏr′ē-ə, -nyŏŏr′-) *n.* The presence of bilirubin in the urine.

bil·i·u·ri·a (bĭl′ĭ-yŏŏr′ē-ə) *n.* The presence of various bile salts or bile in the urine.

bil·i·ver·din (bĭl′ĭ-vûr′dĭn, bĭl′ĭ-vûr′-) *n.* A green pigment occurring in bile and sometimes formed by oxidation of bilirubin.

bill of health *n.* **1.** A certificate stating whether there is infectious disease aboard a ship or in a port of departure, given to the ship's master to present at the next port of arrival. **2.** An attestation as to condition, especially a favorable one.

Bill·roth's operation I (bĭl′rōts) *n.* Surgical excision of the pylorus with end-to-end anastomosis of the stomach and the duodenum.

Billroth's operation II *n.* The surgical resection of the pylorus to the stomach, followed by closure of the cut ends of the duodenum and gastrojejunostomy.

bi·man·u·al version (bī-măn′yōō-əl) *n.* A turning of the fetus in utero, performed by both internal and external manipulation with the hands.

bin·au·ral alternate loudness balance test or **alternate binaural loudness balance test** (bī-nôr′əl, bĭn-ôr′) *n.* A test for recruitment in one ear that compares the relative loudness of a series of intensities presented alternately to each ear.

binaural diplacusis *n.* A form of diplacusis in which the same sound is heard differently by the two ears.

bind·er (bīn′dər) *n.* A broad bandage, especially one encircling the abdomen.

Bi·net scale (bĭ-nā′) *n.* See **Binet–Simon scale.**

Binet–Simon scale *n.* An evaluation of the relative mental development of children by a series of psychological tests of intellectual ability.

Binet–Simon test *n.* See **Binet–Simon scale.**

binge eating disorder (bĭnj) *n.* A recurrent eating disorder characterized by the uncontrolled, excessive intake of any available food and often occurring following stressful events.

binge-eating syndrome *n.* See **bulimia.**

binge-purge syndrome *n.* See **bulimarexia.**

binge-vomit syndrome *n.* See **bulimarexia.**

bin·oc·u·lar microscope (bə-nŏk′yə-lər, bī) *n.* A microscope having two eyepieces, one for each eye, so that the object can be viewed with both eyes.

binocular vision *n.* Vision in which both eyes are used synchronously to produce a single image.

bi·no·mi·al nomenclature (bī-nō′mē-əl) *n.* The scientific naming of species whereby each species receives a Latin or Latinized name of two parts, the first indicating genus and the second species.

Bins·wang·er's disease (bĭn′swăng′ərz, bĭns′-väng′ərz) *n.* Organically caused dementia associated with chronic high blood pressure, characterized by recurrent edema of cerebral white matter with secondary demyelination.

bi·o·ac·tiv·i·ty (bī′ō-ăk-tĭv′ĭ-tē) *n.* The effect of a given agent, such as a vaccine, upon a living organism or on living tissue.

bi·o·a·vail·a·bil·i·ty (bī′ō-ə-vā′lə-bĭl′ĭ-tē) *n.* The physiological availability of a given amount of a drug, as distinct from its chemical potency.

biochemical profile *n.* An array of biochemical tests performed on persons admitted to a hospital or clinic.

bi·o·chem·is·try (bī′ō-kĕm′ĭ-strē) *n.* 1. The study of the chemical substances and vital processes occurring in living organisms. 2. The chemical composition of a particular living system or biological substance. — **bi′o·chem′i·cal** (-ĭ-kəl) *adj.*

bi·o·e·quiv·a·lent (bī′ō-ĭ-kwĭv′ə-lənt) *n.* A value indicating the rate at which a substance, such as a drug, enters the bloodstream and becomes available to the body.

bi·o·eth·ics (bī′ō-ĕth′ĭks) *n.* The study of the ethical and moral implications of new biological discoveries and biomedical advances, as in the fields of genetic engineering and drug research.

bi·o·feed·back (bī′ō-fēd′băk′) *n.* A training technique that enables a person to gain some voluntary control over autonomic body functions.

bi·o·gen·e·sis (bī′ō-jĕn′ĭ-sĭs) *n.* 1. The principle that life originates only from preexisting life and not from nonliving material. 2. See **biosynthesis.**

— **bi′o·ge·net′ic** (-jə-nĕt′ĭk), **bi′o·ge·net′i·cal** (-ĭ-kəl) *adj.*

bi·o·haz·ard (bī′ō-hăz′ərd) *n.* 1. A biological agent, such as an infectious microorganism, or a condition that constitutes a threat to humans, especially in biological research. 2. The potential danger, risk, or harm from exposure to such an agent or condition.

bi·o·in·stru·ment (bī′ō-ĭn′strə-mənt) *n.* A sensor or device attached to or embedded in body tissue to record and transmit physiological data to a receiving and monitoring station.

bi·o·log·ic (bī′ə-lŏj′ĭk) or **bi·o·log·i·cal** (-ĭ-kəl) *n.* A preparation, such as a drug, a vaccine, or an antitoxin, that is synthesized from living organisms or their products and used as a diagnostic, preventive, or therapeutic agent.

bi·o·log·i·cal (bī′ə-lŏj′ĭ-kəl) *adj.* 1. Of, relating to, caused by, or affecting life or living organisms. 2. Having to do with biology. 3. Related by blood, as in a child's biological parents.

biological clock *n.* An innate mechanism in living organisms that controls the periodicity or rhythm of various physiological functions or activities.

biological half-life *n.* See **half-life** (sense 2).

biological vector *n.* A vector that is essential in the life cycle of a pathogenic organism.

biological warfare *n.* The use of toxic biological products, disease-producing microorganisms, or organic biocides to cause death or injury to living organisms.

bi·ol·o·gy (bī-ŏl′ə-jē) *n.* 1. The science of life and of living organisms, including their structure, function, growth, origin, evolution, and distribution. 2. The life processes or characteristic phenomena of a group or category of living organisms. — **bi·ol′o·gist** *n.*

bi·ol·y·sis (bī-ŏl′ĭ-sĭs) *n.* 1. Death of a living organism or tissue caused or accompanied by lysis. 2. The decomposition of organic material by living organisms, such as microorganisms.

bi·o·mark·er (bī′ō-mär′kər) *n.* 1. See **marker.** 2. A specific physical trait that is used to measure or indicate the effects or progress of a disease or condition.

bi·o·mass (bī′ō-măs′) *n.* The total weight of all living things within a given area, biotic community, species population, or habitat.

bi·o·ma·te·ri·al (bī′ō-mə-tîr′ē-əl) *n.* A biocompatible material that is used to construct artificial organs, rehabilitation devices, or prostheses and replace natural body tissues.

bi·ome (bī′ōm′) *n.* The total complex of biotic communities occupying and characterizing a particular area or zone, such as a desert.

bi·o·me·chan·ics (bī′ō-mĭ-kăn′ĭks) *n.* 1. The study of the mechanics of a living body, especially of the forces exerted by muscles and gravity on the skeletal structure. 2. The mechanics of a part or function of a living body, such as of the heart.

bi·o·med·i·cal (bī′ō-mĕd′ĭ-kəl) *adj.* 1. Of or relating to biomedicine. 2. Of, relating to, or involving biological, medical, and physical sciences.

bi·o·med·i·cine (bī'ō-měd'ĭ-sĭn) *n.* **1.** The branch of medical science that deals with the ability of humans to tolerate environmental stresses and variations, as in space travel. **2.** The application of the principles of the natural sciences, especially biology and physiology, to clinical medicine.

bi·om·e·try (bī-ŏm'ĭ-trē) or **bi·o·met·rics** (bī'ō-mět'rĭks) *n.* The statistical analysis of biological data. — **bi·o·me·tri·cian** (bī'ō-mĭ-trĭsh'ən) *n.*

bi·o·mi·cro·scope (bī'ō-mī'krə-skōp') *n.* An instrument consisting of a microscope combined with a rectangular light source, used for examination of the cornea, aqueous humor, and retina of the eye.

bi·o·mi·cros·co·py (bī'ō-mī-krŏs'kə-pē) *n.* **1.** The microscopic examination of living tissue in the body. **2.** The examination of structures of the eye with a biomicroscope.

bi·o·ne·cro·sis (bī'ō-nə-krō'sĭs, nĕ-) *n.* See **necrobiosis** (sense 2).

bi·on·ic (bī-ŏn'ĭk) *adj.* **1.** Relating to or developed from bionics. **2.** Having anatomical structures or physiological processes that are replaced or enhanced by electronic or mechanical components.

bi·on·ics (bī-ŏn'ĭks) *n.* The science of biological functions and mechanisms as analogous to electronics, using knowledge of human and other animal systems to devise improvements in various machines, especially computers.

bi·o·pol·y·mer (bī'ō-pŏl'ə-mər) *n.* A macromolecule, such as a protein or nucleic acid, that is formed in a living organism.

bi·op·sy (bī'ŏp'sē) *n.* **1.** The removal and examination of a sample of tissue from a living body for diagnostic purposes. **2.** A specimen so obtained.

bi·o·rhythm (bī'ō-rĭth'əm) *n.* A biologically inherent cyclic variation or recurrence of an event or state, such as sleep cycles and circadian rhythms. — **bi·o·rhyth'mic** (-rĭphonth'mĭk) *adj.*

bi·o·sci·ence (bī'ō-sī'əns) *n.* See **life science.** — **bi·o·sci'en·tif'ic** (-sī'ən-tĭf'ĭk) *adj.* — **bi·o·sci'en·tist** *n.*

bi·o·sen·sor (bī'ō-sĕn'sər, -sôr) *n.* **1.** A device that detects, records, and transmits information regarding a physiological change or process. **2.** A device that uses biological materials to monitor the presence of various chemicals in a substance.

bi·o·so·cial (bī'ō-sō'shəl) *adj.* Of or relating to the interaction of biological and social influences.

bi·o·spec·trom·e·try (bī'ō-spĕk-trŏm'ĭ-trē) *n.* The spectroscopic determination of the types and amounts of various substances in living tissue or body fluids.

bi·o·spec·tros·co·py (bī'ō-spĕk-trŏs'kə-pē) *n.* The spectroscopic examination of specimens of living tissue or body fluids.

bi·o·sphere (bī'ə-sfēr') *n.* **1.** All the regions of the earth and its atmosphere in which living organisms are found or can live. **2.** The living organisms and their environment composing the biosphere. — **bi·o·spher'ic** (-sfēr'ĭk, -sfēr'-) *adj.*

bi·o·sta·tis·tics (bī'ō-stə-tĭs'tĭks) *n.* The science of

statistics applied to the analysis of biological or medical data.

bi·o·syn·the·sis (bī'ō-sĭn'thĭ-sĭs) *n.* Formation of a chemical compound by a living organism. — **bi·o·syn·thet'ic** (-thĕt'ĭk) *adj.*

bi·o·sys·tem (bī'ō-sĭs'təm) *n.* A living organism or a system of living organisms that can directly or indirectly interact with others.

bi·o·tech·nol·o·gy (bī'ō-tĕk-nŏl'ə-jē) *n.* **1.** The use of microorganisms, such as bacteria or yeasts, or biological substances, such as enzymes, to perform specific industrial or manufacturing processes. Applications include the production of certain drugs and the bioconversion of organic waste. **2.** The application of the principles of engineering and technology to the life sciences.

bi·o·te·lem·e·try (bī'ō-tə-lĕm'ĭ-trē) *n.* The monitoring, recording, and measuring of a living organism's basic physiological functions, such as heart rate, by the use of telemetry techniques.

bi·o·ther·a·py (bī'ō-thĕr'ə-pē) *n.* Treatment of disease with biologicals, such as certain drugs, vaccines, or antitoxins.

bi·o·tin (bī'ə-tĭn) *n.* A colorless crystalline vitamin of the vitamin B complex, essential for the activity of many enzyme systems and found in large quantities in liver, egg yolk, milk, and yeast.

bi·o·tox·in (bī'ō-tŏk'sĭn) *n.* A toxic substance produced by a living organism.

Bi·ot's respiration (bē-ōz', byōz) *n.* Abrupt and irregularly alternating periods of apnea with periods of breathing that are consistent in rate and depth, often occurring as a result of increased intracranial pressure.

bi·o·type (bī'ə-tīp') *n.* A population or group of individuals having the same genotype. — **bi'o·typ'ic** (-tĭp'ĭk) *adj.*

bi·phen·yl (bī-fĕn'əl, -fē'nəl) *n.* A colorless crystalline aromatic hydrocarbon used as a fungicides and in organic synthesis.

bi·po·lar (bī-pō'lər) *adj.* **1.** Having two poles; used especially of nerve cells in which the branches project from two usually opposite points. **2.** Of or relating to a major affective disorder that is characterized by episodes of mania and depression. — **bi'po·lar'i·ty** (-lăr'ĭ-tē) *n.*

bipolar II *n.* See **dysphoric hypomania.**

bipolar cautery *n.* Cauterization using high frequency electrical current passed through tissue from an active to a passive electrode.

bipolar cell *n.* A neuron having two processes.

bipolar disorder *n.* An affective disorder marked by alternating episodes of mania and depression.

bipolar lead (lēd) *n.* The electrical connection of two electrodes to a recording instrument and to two different places on the body, such as the chest and a limb.

bipolar version *n.* See **bimanual version.**

bi·po·ten·ti·al·i·ty (bī'pə-tĕn'shē-ăl'ĭ-tē) *n.* **1.** The capability of differentiating along two developmental pathways. **2.** The capacity to function either as a male or a female. **3.** The condition of having both male and female reproductive organs; hermaphroditism.

bird-breeder's lung *n.* Extrinsic allergic alveolitis caused by an acquired sensitivity to inhaled particles from bird excreta.

birth (bûrth) *n.* **1.** The emergence and separation of offspring from the body of the mother. **2.** The act or process of bearing young; parturition. **3.** The circumstances or conditions relating to this event, as its time or location.

birth amputation *n.* See **congenital amputation**.

birth canal *n.* The passage through which the fetus is expelled during parturition, leading from the uterus through the cervix, vagina, and vulva.

birth control *n.* Voluntary limitation or control of the number of children conceived, especially by planned use of contraceptive techniques.

birth control pill *n.* See **oral contraceptive**.

birth defect *n.* A physiological or structural abnormality that develops at or before birth and is present at the time of birth, especially as a result of faulty development, infection, heredity, or injury.

birth family *n.* A family consisting of one's biological as opposed to adoptive parents and their offspring.

birth father or **birthfather** *n.* A biological father.

birth·ing (bûr′thĭng) *adj.* Having to do with or used during birth. — *n.* The act of giving birth.

birthing center *n.* A medical facility, often associated with a hospital, that is designed to provide a comfortable, homelike setting during childbirth.

birthing room *n.* An area of a hospital or outpatient medical facility equipped for labor, delivery, and recovery and designed as a natural, homelike environment.

birth·mark (bûrth′märk′) *n.* A mole or blemish present on the skin from birth; a nevus.

birth mother or **birthmother** *n.* A biological mother.

birth palsy *n.* Paralysis due to cerebral hemorrhage occurring at birth or to anoxic injury of the fetal brain in utero.

birth pang *n.* One of the repetitive pains occurring in childbirth.

birth parent or **birthparent** *n.* A biological parent.

birthrate or **birth rate** *n.* The ratio of total live births to total population in a specified community or area over a specified period of time, often expressed as the number of live births per 1,000 of the population per year.

birth trauma *n.* **1.** A physical injury sustained by an infant during birth. **2.** The psychological shock an infant is said to experience during birth.

birth weight *n.* In humans, the first weight of an infant, obtained within the first hour after birth. An infant of birth weight 5½ lbs or more is considered full-sized.

bi·sex·u·al (bī-sĕk′shōō-əl) *adj.* **1.** Of or relating to both sexes. **2.** Having both male and female reproductive organs; hermaphroditic. **3.** Of, relating to, or having a sexual orientation to persons of either sex. — *n.* **1.** A bisexual organism; a

hermaphrodite. **2.** A bisexual person or organism. — **bi′sex·u·al′i·ty** (-ăl′ĭ-tē) *n.*

bis·muth (bĭz′məth) *n.* A highly diamagnetic metallic element with atomic number 83 and used in various low-melting alloys.

bis·tou·ry (bĭs′tə-rē) *n.* A long, narrow-bladed knife used for opening abscesses or for slitting sinuses and fistulas.

bite (bīt) *v.* **bit** (bĭt), **bit·ten** (bĭt′n) or **bit, bit·ing, bites.** **1.** To cut, grip, or tear with the teeth. **2.** To pierce the skin of with the teeth, fangs, or mouthparts. — *n.* **1.** The act of biting. **2.** A puncture or laceration of the skin by the teeth of an animal or the mouthparts of an insect or similar organism.

bite plane *n.* See **biteplate**.

biteplate or **bite plate** *n.* A removable dental appliance, made of wire and plastic, that is worn in the palate and used as a diagnostic or therapeutic aid in orthodontics or prosthodontics.

bite·wing (bīt′wĭng′) *n.* A dental x-ray film having a central projection on which the teeth can close, positioning it for the radiographic examination of several upper and lower teeth simultaneously.

bi·tol·ter·ol mes·y·late (bī-tōl′tə-rôl mĕs′ə-lāt′, -rōl′) *n.* A sympathomimetic bronchodilator used in the prophylaxis and treatment of bronchial asthma and reversible bronchospasm.

Bi·tot's spots (bē-tōz′) *pl.n.* Small grayish foamy triangular deposits on the conjunctiva, associated with vitamin A deficiency.

Black Death (blăk) *n.* A form of bubonic plague, caused by the bacillus *Yersinia* (or *Pasturella*) *pestis*, that was pandemic throughout Europe and much of Asia in the 14th century.

black eye *n.* A bruised discoloration of the flesh surrounding the eye.

black fly *n.* Any of various small dark humpbacked flies of the family Simuliidae, the females of which are aggressive biters and serve as vectors in the transmission of onchocerciasis.

black·head (blăk′hĕd′) *n.* A plug of keratin and sebum within a hair follicle that is blackened at the surface; a comedo.

black lung *n.* A form of pneumoconiosis common in coal miners, characterized by the deposit of carbon particles in the lungs.

black measles *n.* A severe form of measles characterized by dark, hemorrhagic skin eruptions.

black·out (blăk′out′) *n.* **1.** Temporary loss of consciousness due to decreased blood flow to the brain. **2.** Temporary loss of memory.

black tongue *n.* The presence of a blackish- to yellowish-brown patch or patches on the tongue, accompanied by elongation of the papillae.

black vomit *n.* **1.** Dark vomit consisting of digested blood and gastric contents. **2.** Severe yellow fever marked by dark vomit.

black·wa·ter fever (blăk′wô′tər) *n.* A serious, often fatal complication of falciparum malaria, characterized by the passage of bloody, dark red or black urine.

blad·der (blăd′ər) n. **1.** Any of various distensible membranous sacs, such as the urinary bladder, that serve as receptacles for fluid or gas. **2.** A blister, pustule, or cyst filled with fluid or air.

blain (blān) n. A skin swelling or sore; a blister; a blotch.

Blair–Brown graft (blâr′-broun′) n. A split-skin graft of intermediate thickness.

Bla·lock–Taussig operation (blā′lŏk-) n. Surgical anastomosis of a subclavian artery to a pulmonary artery in order to direct blood from the systemic circulation to the lungs in cases of congenital malformations of the heart.

bland diet n. A regular diet omitting foods that may irritate the gastrointestinal tract.

blan·ket suture (blăng′kĭt) n. A continuous lockstitch suture used to pull together the skin of a wound.

blast cell n. An immature precursor of a blood cell.

blas·te·ma (blă-stē′mə) n. **1.** The formative, undifferentiated material from which cells are formed. **2.** A mass of embryonic cells from which an organ or a body part develops or regenerates. — **blas·te′mal, blas·te·mat′ic** (blăs′tə-măt′ĭk), **blas·te′mic** (blă-stē′mĭk) adj.

blast injury n. The tearing of lung tissue or rupture of abdominal viscera without external injury, as by the force of an explosion.

blas·to·coel or **blas·to·cele** or **blas·to·coele** (blăs′-tə-sēl′) n. The fluid-filled cavity in the blastula. — **blas·to·coe′lic** adj.

blas·to·cyst (blăs′tə-sĭst′) n. The modified blastula stage of mammalian embryos, consisting of the inner cell mass and a thin trophoblast layer enclosing the blastocoel. — **blas′to·cys′tic** adj.

blas·to·cyte (blăs′tə-sīt′) n. An undifferentiated blastomere of the morula or blastula stage of an embryo.

blas·to·cy·to·ma (blăs′tō-sī-tō′mə) n. See **blastoma.**

blas·to·derm (blăs′tə-dûrm′) or **blas·to·der·ma** (blăs′tə-dûr′mə) n. The layer of cells formed by the cleavage of a fertilized mammalian egg, which divides into the three germ layers from which the embryo develops. — **blas′to·der′mal, blas′to·der′mic, blas′to·der·mat′ic** (-dər-măt′ĭk) adj.

blastodermic vesicle n. See **blastocyst.**

blas·to·disk or **blas·to·disc** (blăs′tə-dĭsk′) n. **1.** The disk of active cytoplasm at the animal pole of an egg. **2.** The blastoderm, especially in very early stages when its extent is small.

blas·to·gen·e·sis (blăs′tə-jĕn′ĭ-sĭs) n. **1.** Development of an embryo during cleavage and germ layer formation. **2.** Transformation of small lymphocytes of human peripheral blood into large, undifferentiated cells capable of undergoing mitosis. — **blas′to·ge·net′ic** (-jə-nĕt′ĭk), **blas′to·gen′ic** (-jĕn′ĭk) adj.

blas·to·ma (blă-stō′mə) n., pl. **-mas** or **-ma·ta** (-mə-tə). A neoplasm composed of immature, undifferentiated cells.

blas·to·mere (blăs′tə-mēr′) n. Any of the cells resulting from the cleavage of a fertilized ovum

during early embryonic development. — **blas′to·mer′ic** (-měr′ĭk, -měr′-) adj.

blas·to·my·co·sis (blăs′tō-mī-kō′sĭs) n. A chronic granulomatous and suppurative disease caused by Blastomyces dermatitidis, originating as a respiratory infection, and usually spreading to the lungs, bones, and skin.

blas·to·pore (blăs′tə-pôr′) n. The opening into the archenteron formed by the invagination of the blastula to form a gastrula. — **blas′to·por′ic, blas′to·por′al** (-pôr′əl) adj.

blas·tu·la (blăs′chə-lə) n., pl. **-las** or **-lae** (-lē′). An early embryonic form produced by cleavage of a fertilized ovum and consisting of a spherical layer of cells surrounding a fluid-filled cavity. — **blas′-tu·lar** adj. — **blas′tu·la′tion** (-lā′shən) n.

bleb (blĕb) n. A large flaccid vesicle.

bleed (blēd) v. **bled** (blĕd), **bleed·ing, bleeds. 1.** To lose blood as a result of rupture or severance of blood vessels. **2.** To take or remove blood from.

bleed·er (blē′dər) n. **1.** A person, such as a hemophiliac, who bleeds freely or is subject to frequent hemorrhages. **2.** A blood vessel from which there is uncontrolled bleeding. **3.** A blood vessel severed by trauma or surgery that requires cautery or ligature to arrest the flow of blood. **4.** A person who draws blood from another; a phlebotomist.

blem·ish (blĕm′ĭsh) n. A small circumscribed alteration of the skin considered to be unesthetic but insignificant.

blen·nad·e·ni·tis (blĕ-năd′n-ī′tĭs) n. Inflammation of the mucous glands.

blen·nor·rhe·a (blĕn′ə-rē′ə) n. A mucous discharge, especially from the urethra or vagina. — **blen′nor·rhe′al** adj.

blen·nos·ta·sis (blĕ-nŏs′tə-sĭs) n. The reduction or suppression of secretion from the mucous membranes. — **blen′no·stat′ic** (blĕn′ə-stăt′ĭk) adj.

blen·nu·ri·a (blĕ-nŏŏr′ē-ə, -nyŏŏr′-) n. The presence of mucus in the urine.

ble·o·my·cin sulfate (blē′ə-mī′sĭn) n. An antineoplastic antibiotic obtained from the bacterium Streptomyces verticillus.

bleph·a·rec·to·my (blĕf′ə-rĕk′tə-mē) n. Excision of all or part of an eyelid.

bleph·ar·e·de·ma (blĕf′ər-ĭ-dē′mə) n. Edema of the eyelids, causing swelling and often a baggy appearance.

bleph·a·ri·tis (blĕf′ə-rī′tĭs) n. Inflammation of the eyelids.

bleph·a·ro·con·junc·ti·vi·tis (blĕf′ə-rō-kən-jŭngk′tə-vī′tĭs) n. Inflammation of the eyelids and conjunctiva.

bleph·a·ro·ple·gi·a (blĕf′ə-rō-plē′jē-ə, -jə) n. Paralysis of an eyelid.

bleph·a·rop·to·sis (blĕf′ə-rŏp-tō′-sĭs, -rō-tō′-) n. Drooping of the upper eyelid.

bleph·a·ro·stat (blĕf′ə-rō-stăt′) n. An instrument used to hold the eyelids apart.

bleph·a·rot·o·my (blĕf′ə-rŏt′ə-mē) n. Surgical incision of an eyelid.

blind (blīnd) adj. **1.** Unable to see; without useful sight. **2.** Having a maximal visual acuity of the better eye, after correction by refractive lenses, of one-tenth normal vision or less (20/200 or less on the Snellen test). **3.** Of, relating to, or for sightless persons. **4.** Closed at one end, as a tube or sac. — **blind′ness** *n.*

blind fistula *n.* A fistula that is open at one end only.

blind gut *n.* See **cecum** (sense 1).

blind spot *n.* **1.** See **optic disk. 2.** The area of blindness in the visual field corresponding to the optic disk.

blis·ter (blĭs′tər) *n.* A local swelling of the skin that contains watery fluid and is caused by burning, infection, or irritation.

bloat (blōt) *n.* Abdominal distention due to swallowed air or intestinal gas production. — **bloat′ed** (blō′tĭd) *adj.*

block (blŏk) *n.* **1.** Interruption, especially obstruction, of a normal physiological function. **2.** Interruption, complete or partial, permanent or temporary, of the passage of a nervous impulse. **3.** Atrioventricular block. **4.** Sudden cessation of speech or a thought process without an immediate observable cause, sometimes considered a consequence of repression. — *v.* **blocked, blocking, blocks.** To arrest passage through; obstruct. — **block′age** (blŏk′ĭj) *n.*

block·ade (blŏ-kād′) *n.* **1.** Intravenous injection of large amounts of colloidal dyes in which the reaction of the reticuloendothelial cells to other influences is temporarily prevented. **2.** Arrest of nerve impulse transmission at autonomic synaptic junctions, autonomic receptor sites, or myoneural junctions through the action of a drug.

block anesthesia *n.* See **conduction anesthesia.**

block·ing activity (blŏk′ĭng) *n.* The repression or elimination of electrical activity in the brain because of the arrival of a sensory stimulus.

blocking agent *n.* A drug that blocks transmission of nerve impulses at an autonomic receptor site, autonomic synapse, or neuromuscular junction.

blocking antibody *n.* **1.** An antibody that combines with an antigen without a reaction but that blocks another antibody from later combining with that antigen. **2.** An immunoglobulin that combines specifically with an atopic allergen but does not elicit an allergic reaction.

Blocq's disease (blŏks) *n.* See **astasia-abasia.**

blood (blŭd) *n.* **1.** The fluid consisting of plasma, red blood cells, white blood cells, and platelets that is circulated by the heart through the arteries and veins, carrying oxygen and nutrients to and waste materials away from all body tissues. **2.** Descent from a common ancestor; parental lineage.

blood-air barrier *n.* The material intervening between alveolar air and the blood that consists of a nonstructural film or surfactant, alveolar epithelium, basement membrane, and endothelium.

blood albumin *n.* See **seralbumin.**

blood alcohol concentration *n.* The concentration of alcohol in the blood, expressed as the weight of alcohol in a fixed volume of blood and used as a measure of the degree of intoxication in an individual.

blood-aqueous barrier *n.* A membrane of the capillary bed of the ciliary body of the eye that permits two-way transfer of fluids between the aqueous chamber of the eye and the blood.

blood bank *n.* **1.** A place, usually a separate division of a hospital laboratory, in which blood is collected from donors, typed, and often separated into several components for future transfusion to recipients. **2.** Blood or plasma stored in such a place.

blood blister *n.* A blister containing blood, resulting from a pinch or a crushing injury.

blood-brain barrier *n.* A physiological mechanism that alters the permeability of brain capillaries so that some substances, such as certain drugs, are prevented from entering brain tissue, while other substances are allowed to enter freely.

blood capillary *n.* One of the minute blood vessels that connect arterioles and venules and are a part of an intricate network throughout the body for the interchange of oxygen, carbon dioxide, and other substances between blood and tissue cells.

blood cell *n.* Any of the cells contained in blood.

blood-cerebrospinal fluid barrier *n.* A barrier located at the tight cellular junctions of the cuboidal epithelium of the choroid plexus.

blood clot *n.* A semi-solid, gelatinous mass of blood that consists of red blood cells, white blood cells, and platelets in a fibrin network.

blood count *n.* **1.** Calculation of the number of red blood cells, white blood cells, and platelets in a cubic millimeter of blood by counting the cells in an accurate volume of diluted blood. **2.** The determination of the percentages of various types of white blood cells observed in a stained film of blood. **3.** Complete blood count.

blood count *n.* **1.** The number of red blood cells, white blood cells, and platelets in a definite volume of blood. **2.** Complete blood count.

blood crystal *n.* A crystal of hematoidin in the blood.

blood disk *n.* A platelet.

blood dyscrasia *n.* A diseased state of the blood, usually involving permanent abnormal cellular elements.

blood gas *n.* Any of the gases dissolved in blood plasma, including oxygen, nitrogen, and carbon dioxide.

blood gas analysis *n.* The measurement of the partial pressure of oxygen and carbon dioxide concentrations in blood.

blood group *n.* **1.** Any of several immunologically distinct, genetically determined classes of human blood (A, B, AB, and O) that are based on the presence or absence of certain antigens, are clinically identified by characteristic agglutination reactions, and are important with respect to blood transfusions and organ transplantation. **2.** Blood type.

blood group antigen *n.* Any of various inherited

antigens found on the surface of red blood cells that determine a blood grouping reaction with a specific antiserum.

blood grouping *n.* The process of identifying a person's blood group by serologic testing of a sample of blood.

blood group-specific substances A and B *n.* A solution of complexes of polysaccharides and amino acids that is used to render group O blood reasonably safe for transfusion into persons of group A, B, or AB.

blood heat *n.* The normal temperature (about 37.0°C or 98.6°F) of human blood.

blood·less operation (blŭd′lĭs) *n.* An operation performed with negligible loss of blood.

blood·let·ting (blŭd′lĕt′ĭng) *n.* The removal of blood, usually from a vein, for therapeutic purposes. — **blood′let′ter** *n.*

blood·line (blŭd′līn′) *n.* Direct line of descent; pedigree.

blood·mo·bile (blŭd′mə-bēl′) *n.* A motor vehicle equipped for collecting blood from donors.

blood plasma *n.* The pale yellow or gray-yellow, protein-containing fluid portion of the blood in which the blood cells and platelets are normally suspended.

blood plasma fraction *n.* The components of blood plasma separated by a technique such as electrophoresis.

blood platelet *n.* See **platelet**.

blood poisoning *n.* **1.** See **septicemia**. **2.** See **toxemia**.

blood pressure *n.* The pressure exerted by the blood against the walls of the blood vessels, especially the arteries.

blood profile *n.* See **complete blood count**.

blood relation *n.* A person who is related to another by birth rather than by marriage.

blood·shot (blŭd′shŏt′) *adj.* Red and inflamed as a result of locally congested blood vessels, as of he eyes.

blood·stream (blŭd′strēm′) *n.* The flow of blood through the circulatory system of an organism.

blood sugar *n.* **1.** See **glucose**. **2.** The concentration of glucose in the blood, measured in milligrams of glucose per 100 milliliters of blood.

blood test *n.* **1.** An examination of a sample of blood to determine its chemical, physical, or serologic characteristics. **2.** A serologic test for certain diseases, such as syphilis or AIDS.

blood type *n.* **1.** The specific reaction pattern of one's red blood cells to antisera of a blood group. **2.** Blood group.

blood typing *n.* See **blood grouping**.

blood urea nitrogen *n.* Nitrogen in the form of urea in the blood or serum, used as a indicator of kidney function.

blood vessel *n.* An elastic tubular channel, such as an artery, a vein, a sinus, or a capillary, through which the blood circulates.

blood·y (blŭd′ē) *adj.* **1.** -i·er, -i·est. Stained with blood. **2.** Of, characteristic of, or containing blood. **3.** Suggesting the color of blood; blood-red. — *v.* -ied, -y·ing, -ies. **1.** To stain, spot, or color with or as if with blood. **2.** To make bleed, as by injuring or wounding.

blot (blŏt) *n.* The Northern, Southern, or Western blot analysis.

blow·ing wound (blō′ĭng) *n.* See **open pneumothorax**.

blow-out fracture *n.* A fracture of the bone at the floor of the eye socket caused by the force produced by a blow to the globe of the eye.

blue baby *n.* An infant born with cyanosis as a result of a congenital cardiac or pulmonary defect that causes incomplete oxygenation of the blood.

blue·ber·ry muf·fin baby (blōō′bĕr′ē mŭf′ĭn) *n.* An infant that has jaundice and purpura, especially of the face, which may result from intrauterine viral infection.

blue line *n.* A bluish line along a border of the gums caused by chronic heavy metal poisoning.

blue nevus *n.* A dark-blue or blue-black smooth nevus formed by melanin-pigmented spindle cells in the lower dermis.

Blum·berg's sign (blŭm′bərgz, blōōm′-) *n.* An indication of peritonitis in which pain is felt upon sudden release of steadily applied pressure on a suspected area of the abdomen.

blush (blŭsh) *n.* A sudden and brief redness of the face and neck due to emotion; flush. — **blush** *v.*

B lymphocyte or **B-lymphocyte** *n.* See **B cell**.

board certification *n.* The process by which a person is tested and approved to practice in a specialty field, especially medicine, after successfully completing the requirements of a board of specialists in that field.

board·er baby (bôr′dər) *n.* An infant, often the offspring of a drug addict or an AIDS victim, who remains for months at the hospital where he or she was born, waiting for placement in a home.

bod·y (bŏd′ē) *n.* **1.** The entire material or physical structure of an organism, especially of a human. **2.** The physical part of a person. **3.** A corpse. **4.** The trunk or torso of a human, as distinguished from the head, neck, and extremities. **5.** The largest or principal part, as of an organ; corpus.

body clock *n.* An internal mechanism of the body that is thought to regulate physical and mental functions in rhythm with normal daily activities.

body fluid *n.* **1.** A natural bodily fluid or secretion of fluid such as blood, semen, or saliva. **2.** Total body water, contained principally in blood plasma and in intracellular and interstitial fluids.

body image *n.* **1.** The cerebral representation of all body sensation organized in the parietal cortex. **2.** The subjective concept of one's physical appearance based on self-observation and the reactions of others.

body louse *n.* A parasitic louse *(Pediculus humanus corporis)* that infests the body and clothes of humans.

body mass index *n.* A measurement of the relative percentages of fat and muscle mass in the human body, in which weight in kilograms is divided by height in meters squared and the result used as an index of obesity.

Boer·haa·ve's syndrome (boor'hä'vəz) *n.* Complete and spontaneous rupture of the lower esophagus.

Bohr effect (bôr) *n.* The influence of carbon dioxide on the oxygen dissociation curve of blood.

bohr·i·um (bôr'ē-əm) *n.* An artificially produced radioactive element with atomic number 107.

boil (boil) *n.* A painful, circumscribed pus-filled inflammation of the skin and subcutaneous tissue usually caused by a staphylococcal infection.

bo·lus (bō'ləs) *n.*, *pl.* **-lus·es. 1.** A round mass. **2.** A round medicinal preparation, such as a large pill or tablet, that is usually of a soft consistency and not prepackaged. **3.** A soft mass of chewed food within the mouth or alimentary canal.

bond (bŏnd) *n.* The linkage or force holding two neighboring atoms of a molecule in place and resisting their separation, usually accomplished by the transfer or sharing of one or more electrons or pairs of electrons between the atoms.

bone (bōn) *n.* **1.** The dense, semirigid, porous, calcified connective tissue forming the major portion of the skeleton of most vertebrates, consisting of a dense organic matrix and an inorganic, mineral component. **2.** Any of the more than 200 anatomically distinct structures making up the human skeleton. **3.** A piece of bone.

bone block *n.* A surgical procedure in which the bone next to the joint is modified to limit the motion of the joint.

bone canaliculus *n.* Any of various channels interconnecting bone lacunae or connecting them with a haversian canal.

bone conduction *n.* The process by which sound waves are transmitted to the inner ear by the cranial bones without traveling through the air in the ear canal.

bone forceps *n.* Strong forceps used for seizing or removing fragments of bone.

bone grafting *n.* See **osteoplasty** (sense 1).

bone marrow *n.* The soft fatty vascular tissue filling the cavities of bones, having a stroma of reticular fibers and cells.

bone marrow transplantation *n.* A technique in which bone marrow is removed from one person and transplanted in another so as to enhance or restore that person's immune response or supply of blood cells or to replace diseased or destroyed bone marrow.

bone matrix *n.* The intercellular substance of bone tissue consisting of collagen fibers, ground substance, and inorganic bone salts.

bon·y or **bon·ey** (bō'nē) *adj.* **-i·er** or **-ey·er, -i·est** or **-ey·est. 1.** Resembling or consisting of bone. **2.** Having an internal skeleton of bones. **3.** Having prominent or protruding bones. **4.** Lean.

bony labyrinth *n.* See **osseous labyrinth**.

bony palate *n.* A concave elliptical bony plate, constituting the roof of the oral cavity.

boost·er *n.* An additional dose of an immunizing agent, such as a vaccine or toxoid, given at a time after an initial dose to sustain the immune response elicited by the initial dose.

booster shot *n.* See **booster**.

bo·rax (bôr'ăks', -əks) *n.* Sodium borate.

bor·bo·ryg·mus (bôr'bə-rĭg'məs) *n.*, *pl.* **-mi** (-mī'). A rumbling noise produced by the movement of gas through the intestines.

bor·der (bôr'dər) *n.* The part of a surface that forms its outer boundary or edge.

bor·der·line personality disorder (bôr'dər-līn') *n.* A personality disorder characterized by a long-standing pattern of instability in interpersonal relationships, behavior, mood, and self-image that can interfere with social or occupational functioning or cause extreme emotional distress.

Bor·det–Gen·gou bacillus (bôr-dā'-zhän-goo') *n.* A gram-negative bacterium, *Bordetella pertussis,* that causes whooping cough in humans.

bo·ric acid (bôr'ĭk) *n.* A water-soluble white or colorless crystalline compound used as an antiseptic and preservative.

bo·ron (bôr'ŏn') *n.* A soft, amorphous or crystalline nonmetallic element with atomic number 5, used in flares and nuclear reactor control rods.

boron neutron capture therapy *n.* A treatment for cancers, especially virulent ones of the brain, in which a person who has been injected with a boron compound that concentrates in cancerous cells is exposed to neutron irradiation causing the boron compound to emit particles that destroy the cancer cells.

Bor·re·li·a (bə-rē'lē-ə, -rĕl'ē-ə) *n.* A genus of parasitic irregularly coiled helical spirochetes, some species of which cause relapsing fever in humans.

bor·re·li·o·sis (bə-rē'lē-ō'sĭs, -rĕl'ē-) *n.* Disease caused by bacteria of the genus *Borrelia.*

bos·om (booz'əm, boo'zəm) *n.* **1.** The chest of a human. **2.** A woman's breast or breasts.

Bos·ton's sign (bô'stənz) *n.* An indication of Graves' disease in which the lowering of the upper eyelid is jerky during the downward rotation of the eye.

bot·fly (bŏt'flī') *n.* A robust hairy fly of the order Diptera whose larvae produce a variety of myiasis conditions in humans.

bot·u·lin (bŏch'ə-lĭn) *n.* See **botulinus toxin**.

bot·u·li·num (bŏch'ə-lī'nəm) or **bot·u·li·nus** (-nəs) *n.* An anaerobic, rod-shaped bacterium (*Clostridium botulinum*) that secretes botulinus toxin and inhabits soils.

bot·u·li·nus toxin (bŏch'ə-lī'nəs) *n.* Any of several potent neurotoxins produced by the bacterium *Clostridium botulinum* and resistant to proteolytic digestion.

bot·u·lism (bŏch'ə-lĭz'əm) *n.* A severe, sometimes fatal food poisoning caused by ingestion of a toxin produced by the bacterium *Clostridium botulinum* in improperly canned or preserved food and characterized by nausea, vomiting, disturbed vision, and paralysis.

bou·bas (boo'bəz) *n.* See **yaws**.

bou·gie (boo'zhē, -jē) *n.* A cylindrical instrument, usually somewhat flexible and yielding, used for calibrating or dilating constricted areas in tubular organs, such as the urethra or rectum.

bou·gie·nage (bŏō'zhē-näzh') *n.* The examination or treatment of the interior of a canal by the passage of a bougie or cannula.

bou·ton (bŏō-tôn') *n.* A button, pustule, or knoblike swelling.

bou·ton·neuse fever (bŏō'tə-nœz') *n.* A tickborne typhus in tropical and South Africa, and Asia, caused by *Rickettsia conori.*

bovine growth hormone *n.* A naturally occurring or genetically engineered hormone of cattle that regulates growth and milk production.

Bow·ditch's law (bou'dĭch'ĭz) *n.* The principle that heart muscle, regardless of the strength of the stimulus it receives, will contract to its fullest extent or will not contract at all.

bow·el (bou'əl, boul) *n.* The intestine.

bowel bypass *n.* See jejunoileal bypass.

bowel bypass syndrome *n.* A syndrome following and resulting from bowel bypass surgery whose symptoms include fever, chills, malaise, and inflammatory cutaneous papules and pustules on the extremities and upper trunk.

bowel movement *n.* **1.** The discharge of waste matter from the large intestine; defecation. **2.** The waste matter discharged from the large intestine; feces.

Bow·en's disease (bō'ənz) *n.* A precancerous dermatosis or form of intraepidermal carcinoma characterized by the development of pinkish or brownish papules on the skin covered with a thickened horny layer.

bow·leg (bō'lĕg') *n.* A leg having an outward curvature in the region of the knee.

Bow·man's capsule (bō'mənz) *n.* A doublewalled, cup-shaped structure around the glomerulus of each nephron of the vertebrate kidney. It serves as a filter to remove organic wastes, excess inorganic salts, and water.

Boy·den meal (boid'n) *n.* A meal of egg yolks beaten into sweetened milk, used to test the evacuation time of the gallbladder.

Boze·man–Fritsch catheter (bōz'mən-frĭch') *n.* A slightly curved double-channel uterine catheter with several openings at the tip.

BP or **B.P.** *abbr.* blood pressure; boiling point.

brace (brās) *n.* **1.** An orthopedic appliance that supports or holds a movable part of the body in correct position while allowing motion of the part. **2.** *Often* **braces.** A dental appliance, constructed of bands and wires that is fixed to the teeth to correct irregular alignment.

bra·chi·al (brā'kē-əl) *adj.* Of or relating to the arm.

brachial artery *n.* **1.** An artery that is a continuation of the axillary artery, bifurcating at the elbow into the radial and the ulnar arteries. **2.** An artery that lies superficial to the median nerve in the arm; superficial brachial artery. **3.** An artery with its origin in the brachial artery, with distribution to the shoulder and the muscles and integument of the arm; deep brachial artery.

bra·chi·al·gia (brā'kē-ăl'jē-ə, -jə) *n.* Pain in the arm.

brachial plexus *n.* A network of nerves located in the neck and axilla, supplying the chest, shoulder, and arm.

brachial plexus neuropathy *n.* An acute syndrome of unknown cause marked by pain in the shoulder girdle, weakness of the muscles innervated by the brachial plexus, and mild sensory loss in the affected dermatomes, usually of limited duration with spontaneous recovery.

brachial vein *n.* Either of two veins in either arm accompanying the brachial artery and emptying into the axillary vein.

brachiocephalic trunk *n.* See innominate artery.

brachiocephalic vein *n.* Either of two veins formed by the union of the internal jugular and subclavian veins.

bra·chi·um (brā'kē-əm, brăk'ē-) *n., pl.* **bra·chi·a** (brā'kē-ə, brăk'ē-ə). **1.** The arm, especially between the shoulder and the elbow. **2.** An armlike structure.

Bracht maneuver (bräkt, bräkнt) *n.* Delivery of a fetus in breech position by extending the legs and trunk of the fetus over the pubic symphysis and abdomen of the mother, which leads to spontaneous delivery of the fetal head.

brach·y·car·di·a (brăk'ē-kär'dē-ə) *n.* See bradycardia.

brach·y·chei·li·a or **brach·y·chi·li·a** (brăk'ē-kī'lē-ə) *n.* Abnormally short lips.

brach·y·dac·ty·ly (brăk'ē-dăk'tə-lē) *n.* Abnormal shortness of the fingers.

brach·yg·na·thi·a (brăk'ĭg-nā'thē-ə) *n.* Abnormal shortness or recession of the mandible.

brach·y·mel·i·a (brăk'ē-mĕl'ē-ə, -mē'lē-ə) *n.* Disproportionate shortness of the limbs.

brach·y·mes·o·pha·lan·gi·a (brăk'ē-mĕz'ō-fə-lăn'jē-ə, -mĕs'-) *n.* Abnormal shortness of the middle phalanges.

brach·y·pha·lan·gi·a (brăk'ē-fə-lăn'jē-ə) *n.* Abnormal shortness of the phalanges.

brach·y·syn·dac·ty·ly (brăk'ē-sĭn-dăk'tə-lē) *n.* Abnormal shortness of fingers or toes combined with a webbing between the adjacent digits.

brach·y·tel·e·pha·lan·gi·a (brăk'ē-tĕl'ə-fə-lăn'jē-ə) *n.* Abnormal shortness of the distal phalanges.

brach·y·ther·a·py (brăk'ē-thĕr'ə-pē) *n.* Radiotherapy in which the source of irradiation is placed close to the surface of the body or within a body cavity.

Brad·ford frame (brăd'fərd) *n.* A rectangular metal frame having canvas or webbing straps and used to support individuals with diseases or fractures of the spine, hip, or pelvis.

brad·y·ar·rhyth·mi·a (brăd'ē-ə-rĭth'mē-ə) *n.* A disturbance of the heart's rhythm resulting in a rate under 60 beats per minute.

brad·y·ar·thri·a (brăd'ē-är'thrē-ə) *n.* A form of

dysarthria characterized by an abnormal slowness or deliberation in speech.

brad·y·car·di·a (brăd´ĭ-kär´dē-ə) *n.* A slowness of the heartbeat, usually defined as a rate under 60 beats per minute in adults. — **brad´y·car´dic** (-dĭk), **brad´y·car´di·ac´** (-dē-ăk´) *adj.*

bra·dy·di·as·to·le (brăd´ē-dī-ăs´tə-lē) *n.* The prolongation of the diastole of the heart.

brad·y·es·the·sia (brăd´ē-ĕs-thē´zhə) *n.* Retardation in the rate of transmission of sensory impressions.

brad·y·ki·ne·sia (brăd´ē-kĭ-nē´zhə, -kī-) *n.* Extreme slowness in movement. — **brad´y·ki·net´ic** (-nĕt´ĭk) *adj.*

brad·yp·ne·a (brăd´ĭp-nē´ə, brăd´ē-nē´ə) *n.* Abnormal slowness of respiration.

brad·y·to·ci·a (brăd´ē-tō´sē-ə) *n.* Long, slow childbirth.

brain (brān) *n.* The portion of the central nervous system that is enclosed within the cranium, continuous with the spinal cord, and composed of gray matter and white matter. It is the primary center for the regulation and control of bodily activities, receiving and interpreting sensory impulses, and transmitting information to the muscles and body organs. It is also the seat of consciousness, thought, memory, and emotion.

brain·case (brān´kās´) *n.* The part of the skull that encloses the brain; the cranium.

brain concussion *n.* A clinical syndrome occurring as the result of trauma to the head and characterized by immediate and transient impairment of neural function, such as loss of consciousness and disturbance of vision and equilibrium.

brain damage *n.* Injury to the brain that is caused by various conditions, such as head trauma or infection, and that may be associated with a behavioral or functional abnormality.

brain death *n.* Irreversible brain damage and loss of brain function, as evidenced by cessation of breathing and other vital reflexes, unresponsiveness to stimuli, absence of muscle activity, and a flat electroencephalogram for a specific length of time. — **brain´-dead´** *adj.*

brain fever *n.* Inflammation of the brain or meninges, as in encephalitis or meningitis.

brain hormone *n.* Any of various hormones produced in the hypothalamic region of the brain, especially those acting on the pituitary gland to release other hormones.

brain sand *n.* A gritty substance present in central nervous tissue or in the pineal gland.

brain stem or **brainstem** *n.* The portion of the brain, consisting of the medulla oblongata, pons Varolii, and mesencephalon, that connects the spinal cord to the forebrain and cerebrum.

brain sugar *n.* See **galactose**.

brain swelling *n.* A localized or generalized increase in the bulk of brain tissue due to congestion or edema.

brain·wash·ing (brān´wŏsh´ĭng) *n.* Inducing a person to modify his or her beliefs, attitudes, or behavior by conditioning through various forms of pressure or torture.

brain wave *n.* A rhythmic fluctuation of electric potential between parts of the brain, as seen on an electroencephalogram.

bran (brăn) *n.* The outer layers of a cereal grain such as wheat, used as a source of dietary fiber in cereals and bran products.

branch (brănch) *n.* An offshoot or a division of the main portion of a structure, especially that of a nerve, blood vessel, or lymphatic vessel.

Brandt–An·drews maneuver (brănt´ăn´drooz) *n.* A method of expressing the placenta by grasping the umbilical cord with one hand and placing the other hand on the abdomen.

Brax·ton–Hicks contraction or **Brax·ton Hicks contraction** (brăk´stən hĭks´) *n.* One of a series of usually painless uterine contractions that occur with increasing frequency during the course of a pregnancy.

Braxton Hicks sign *n.* Irregular uterine contractions after the third month of pregnancy.

BRCA1 (bē´är-sē´ā-wŭn´) *n.* A defective gene found to be associated with the development of familial breast cancer.

break·bone fever (brāk´bōn´) *n.* See **dengue**.

break·down (brāk´doun´) *n.* **1.** The act or process of failing to continue or continue. **2.** A typically sudden collapse in physical or mental health. **3.** Disintegration or decomposition into parts or elements.

break·ing point (brā´kĭng) *n.* **1.** The point at which physical, mental, or emotional strength gives way under stress. **2.** The point at which a condition or situation becomes critical.

breast (brĕst) *n.* **1.** Either of two milk-secreting, glandular organs on the chest of a woman. **2.** A corresponding rudimentary gland in the male. **3.** The superior ventral surface of the human body, extending from the neck to the abdomen.

breast·bone (brĕst´bōn´) *n.* See **sternum**.

breast-feed *v.* **-fed** (-fĕd´), **-feed·ing, -feeds.** To feed (a baby) mother's milk from the breast.

breast pump *n.* A suction device for withdrawing milk from the breast.

breath (brĕth) *n.* **1.** The air inhaled and exhaled in respiration. **2.** A single respiration.

breath-holding test *n.* A test used as a rough index of cardiopulmonary reserve, which is measured by the length of time that a person can hold his or her breath.

breath·ing (brē´thĭng) *n.* The alternate inhalation and exhalation of air in respiration.

breath·ing bag (brē´thĭng) *n.* A collapsible reservoir from which gases are inhaled and into which gases may be exhaled during general anesthesia or artificial ventilation.

breathing reserve *n.* The difference between the volume of air breathed under ordinary resting conditions and the maximum breathing capacity.

breech (brēch) *n.* The lower rear portion of the human trunk; the buttocks.

breech birth *n.* See **breech delivery**.

breech delivery *n.* Delivery of a fetus with the buttocks or feet appearing first.

breech presentation *n.* Presentation of the fetus during birth with the buttocks or less commonly the knees or feet first.

Bren·ner tumor (brĕn′ər) *n.* An infrequent benign neoplasm of the ovary consisting primarily of fibrous tissue with nests of cells resembling transitional type epithelium and glandlike structures containing mucin.

brew·er's yeast (broō′ərz) *n.* A yeast (genus *Saccharomyces*) used as a ferment in brewing and also as a source of B-complex vitamins.

Brick·er operation (brĭk′ər) *n.* An operation in which an isolated segment of ileum is used to collect urine and to conduct it to the skin surface.

bridge (brĭj) *n.* **1.** An anatomical structure resembling a bridge or span. **2.** The upper part of the ridge of the nose formed by the nasal bones. **3.** A fixed or removable replacement for one or several but not all of the natural teeth.

bridge·work (brĭj′wûrk′) *n.* See **partial denture.**

bri·dle suture (brīd′l) *n.* A suture passed through the superior rectus muscle to rotate the globe downward in eye surgery.

Brill–Zins·ser disease (brĭlz-zĭn′sər) *n.* A relatively mild recurrence of epidemic typhus in persons previously infected with the *Rickettsia prowazekii* bacterium.

brise·ment for·cé (brēz-mäN′ fôr-sā′) *n.* The forcible breaking or manipulation of a joint or joints.

brit·tle bones (brĭt′l) *n.* See **osteogenesis imperfecta.**

brittle diabetes *n.* Insulin-dependent diabetes in which there are wide unpredictable fluctuations in blood glucose concentrations.

Broad·bent's sign (brôd′bĕnts′) *n.* An indication of adherent pericardium in which the retraction of the thoracic wall is synchronous with cardiac systole and is visible in the left posterior axillary line.

broad spectrum antibiotic *n.* An antibiotic having a wide range of activity against both gram-positive and gram-negative organisms.

bro·me·lain (brō′mə-lān′) or **bro·me·lin** (-lĭn) *n.* A peptide hydrolase obtained from pineapple used in treating inflammation and edema of soft tissues associated with traumatic injury.

bro·mine (brō′mēn) *n.* A volatile nonmetallic liquid element with atomic number 35 and having a highly irritating vapor.

bro·mo·crip·tine (brō′mō-krĭp′tēn′) *n.* An ergot alkaloid that slows dopamine turnover and inhibits prolactin secretion, used in the treatment of Parkinson's disease.

bro·mo·der·ma (brō′mə-dûr′mə) *n.* An acneform or granulomatous eruption due to hypersensitivity to bromide.

brom·phen·ir·a·mine ma·le·ate (brŏm′fĕn-ĭr′ə-mēn) *n.* A white crystalline compound used as an antihistamine.

brom·phe·nol test (brŏm-fē′nôl′, -nōl′) *n.* A colorimetric test that measures amounts of protein, albumin, and globulin in urine by the use of reagent-saturated strips of paper.

Bromp·ton cocktail (brŏmp′tən, brŏm′-) *n.* A mixture of morphine and cocaine usually used for analgesia in terminal cancer patients.

bron·chi·al (brŏng′kē-əl) *adj.* Relating to the bronchi, the bronchial tubes, or the bronchioles.

bronchial asthma *n.* A condition of the lungs characterized by a widespread narrowing of the airways due to spasm of the smooth muscle, edema of the mucosa, and the presence of mucus in the lumen of the bronchi and bronchioles. It is caused by the local release of vasoactive substances during the course of an allergic reaction.

bronchial pneumonia *n.* See **bronchopneumonia.**

bronchial tube *n.* Any of the smaller divisions of the bronchi of the lung.

bron·chi·ec·ta·sis (brŏng′kē-ĕk′tə-sĭs) *n.* Chronic dilation of bronchi or bronchioles, often as a result of inflammatory disease or obstruction. — **bron′chi·ec·tat′ic** (-ĕk-tăt′ĭk), **bron′chi·ec·ta′sic** (-tā′sĭk, -zĭk) *adj.*

bron·chil·o·quy (brŏng-kĭl′ə-kwē) *n.* See **bronchophony.**

bron·chi·ole (brŏng′kē-ōl′) *n.* Any of the fine, thin-walled, tubular extensions of a bronchus.

bron·chi·o·lec·ta·sis (brŏng′kē-ō-lĕk′tə-sĭs) *n.* Chronic dilation of the bronchioles.

bron·chi·o·li·tis (brŏng′kē-ō-lī′tĭs) *n.* Inflammation of the bronchioles, often associated with bronchopneumonia.

bron·chi·o·lus (brŏng-kī′ə-ləs) *n., pl.* **-li** (-lī′). A bronchiole.

bron·chi·tis (brŏn-kī′tĭs, brŏng-) *n.* Inflammation of the mucous membrane of the bronchial tubes. — **bron·chit′ic** (-kĭt′ĭk) *adj.*

bron·cho·con·stric·tor (brŏng′kō-kən-strĭk′tər) *n.* An agent that causes a reduction in the caliber of a bronchus or bronchial tube.

bron·cho·di·la·tor (brŏng′kō-dī-lā′tər, -dī′lā′-, -dĭ-lā′-) *n.* An agent that causes an increase in the caliber of a bronchus or bronchial tube.

bron·cho·e·soph·a·gol·o·gy (brŏng′kō-ĭ-sŏf′ə-gŏl′ə-jē) *n.* The medical specialty concerned with peroral endoscopic examination of the esophagus, trachea, and bronchi.

bron·cho·e·soph·a·gos·co·py (brŏng′kō-ĭ-sŏf′ə-gŏs′kə-pē) *n.* Examination of the trachea, bronchi, or esophagus using an endoscope.

bron·cho·fi·ber·scope (brŏng′kō-fī′bər-skōp′) *n.* A fiberoptic endoscope specialized for viewing the trachea and bronchi.

bron·cho·gen·ic carcinoma (brŏng′kə-jĕn′ĭk) *n.* Squamous cell or oat cell carcinoma that develops in the mucosa of the large bronchi and produces a persistent productive cough or hemoptysis.

bron·chog·ra·phy (brŏng-kŏg′rə-fē) *n.* The radiographic examination of the trachea and bronchi following the injection of a radiopaque material.

bron·cho·li·thi·a·sis (brŏng′kō-lĭ-thī′ə-sĭs) *n.*

Bronchial inflammation or obstruction caused by broncholiths.

bron·cho·my·co·sis (brŏng'kō-mī-kō'sĭs) *n.* A fungus disease of the bronchial tubes or bronchi.

bron·choph·o·ny (brŏng-kŏf'ə-nē) *n.* Exaggerated vocal resonance heard over a bronchus surrounded by consolidated lung tissue.

bron·cho·plas·ty (brŏng'kə-plăs'tē) *n.* Surgical repair of a defect in the bronchus.

bron·cho·pneu·mon·ia (brŏng'kō-nŏŏ-mōn'yə, -nyŏŏ-) *n.* Acute inflammation of the walls of the smaller bronchial tubes, involving the peribronchiolar alveoli and the alveolar ducts of the lungs.

bron·chor·rha·phy (brŏng-kôr'ə-fē) *n.* The suture of a wound of a bronchus.

bron·chor·rhe·a (brŏng'kə-rē'ə) *n.* Excessive secretion of mucus from the bronchial mucous membranes.

bron·cho·scope (brŏng'kə-skōp') *n.* An endoscope for inspecting the interior of the trachea and bronchi, either for diagnostic purposes or for the removal of foreign bodies. — **bron'cho·scop'ic** (-skŏp'ĭk) *adj.* — **bron·chos'co·py** (-kŏs'kə-pē) *n.*

bron·cho·spasm (brŏng'kə-spăz'əm) *n.* A contraction of smooth muscle in the walls of the bronchi and bronchioles that narrows the lumen.

bron·cho·spi·rog·ra·phy (brŏng'kō-spī-rŏg'-rə-fē) *n.* The use of a single-lumen endobronchial tube for measuring the ventilatory function of one lung.

bron·cho·spi·rom·e·ter (brŏng'kō-spī-rŏm'ĭ-tər) *n.* A device for measuring rates and volumes of air flow into each lung separately using a double-lumen endobronchial tube. — **bron'cho·spi·rom'e·try** (-ĭ-trē) *n.*

bron·cho·stax·is (brŏng'kō-stăk'sĭs) *n.* Hemorrhage from the bronchi.

bron·cho·ste·no·sis (brŏng'kō-stə-nō'sĭs) or **bron·chi·o·ste·no·sis** (brŏng'kē-ō-) *n.* Chronic narrowing of a bronchus.

bron·chos·to·my (brŏng-kŏs'tə-mē) *n.* The surgical formation of a new opening into a bronchus.

bron·chot·o·my (brŏng-kŏt'ə-mē) *n.* Incision into a bronchus.

bron·chus (brŏng'kəs) *n., pl.* **-chi** (-kī', -kē'). Either of two main branches of the trachea, leading directly to the lungs.

bronzed disease (brŏnzd) *n.* **1.** See **Addison's disease. 2.** See **hemochromatosis.**

bronze diabetes *n.* A type of diabetes associated with hemochromatosis.

brow (brou) *n.* **1.** The eyebrow. **2.** See **forehead.**

brow·lift (brou'lĭft') *n.* Plastic surgery to elevate the eyebrows and thereby remove excess skin folds or fullness in the upper eyelids.

brown lung disease (broun) *n.* See **byssinosis.**

Brown–Séquard's syndrome *n.* A syndrome caused by damage to one side of the spinal cord, marked by on one side hemiparaplegia and hemianesthesia on the side opposite the damage.

brow presentation *n.* Head presentation of the fetus during birth in which the brow leads.

Bru·cel·la (brōō-sĕl'ə) *n.* A genus of encapsulated, nonmotile bacteria containing short, rod-shaped to coccoid gram-negative cells that are parasites in and pathogens for humans.

bru·cel·lo·sis (brōō'sə-lō'sĭs) *n.* An infectious disease caused by a species of *Brucella,* characterized by fever, sweating, weakness, and headache, and transmitted by direct contact with diseased animals or through ingestion of infested foods.

Bru·dzin·ski's sign (brōō-jĭn'skēz) *n.* **1.** An indication of meningitis in which passive flexion of the leg on one side causes a similar movement in the opposite leg. **2.** Such an indication in which passive flexion of the neck causes flexion of the legs.

bruise (brōōz) *n.* An injury to underlying tissues or bone in which the skin is not broken, often characterized by ruptured blood vessels and discolorations; a contusion.

bru·it (brōō'ē) *n.* A sound, especially an abnormal one, heard in auscultation.

Brunn's membrane (brōōnz) *n.* The epithelium of the olfactory region of the nose.

brush biopsy *n.* A biopsy obtained by passing a bristled catheter into suspected areas of disease and removing cells caught in the bristles.

brush border *n.* An epithelial cell surface consisting of microvilli, as on the cells of the proximal tubule of the kidney.

brush catheter *n.* A catheter with a finely bristled brush tip that is endoscopically passed into the ureter or renal pelvis in order to brush cells from the surface of suspected tumors.

brux·ism (brŭk'sĭz'əm) *n.* The habitual involuntary grinding or clenching of the teeth, usually during sleep, as from anger, or frustration.

Btu *abbr.* British thermal unit

bu·bas (bōō'bəz, byōō'-) *n.* See **yaws.**

bu·bo (bōō'bō, byōō'-) *n., pl.* **-boes.** Inflammatory swelling of one or more lymph nodes, especially in the groin.

bu·bon·ic plague (bōō-bŏn'ĭk, byōō-) *n.* A contagious, often fatal epidemic disease caused by the bacterium *Yersinia pestis,* transmitted from person to person or by the bite of fleas from an infected host, especially a rat, and characterized by chills, fever, vomiting, diarrhea, and the formation of buboes.

bu·bon·o·cele (bōō-bŏn'ə-sēl', byōō-) *n.* An inguinal hernia, especially one in which the knuckle of intestine has not yet emerged from the external abdominal ring.

buc·ca (bŭk'ə) *n.* The cheek.

buc·cal (bŭk'əl) *adj.* **1.** Of, relating to, adjacent to, or in the direction of the cheek. **2.** Of or relating to the mouth cavity.

buccal cavity *n.* The portion of the oral cavity bounded by the lips, cheeks, and gums.

buccal gland *n.* Any of the mixed glands situated in the mucous membrane of the cheeks.

buc·co·lin·gual (bŭk'ō-lĭng'gwəl) *adj.* Relating to the cheek and the tongue.

buc·co·pha·ryn·ge·al (bŭk'ō-fə-rĭn'jē-əl, -jəl,

-făr'ĭn-jē'əl) *adj.* Relating to the cheek or mouth and the pharynx.

Buck's extension (bŭks) *n.* An apparatus for applying skin traction on the leg through contact between the skin and adhesive tape connected to a suspended weight.

buff·er (bŭf'ər) *n.* A substance that minimizes change in the acidity of a solution when an acid or base is added to the solution. — *v.* **-ered, -ering, -ers.** To treat a solution with a buffer.

buf·fy coat (bŭf'ē) *n.* The upper, lighter portion of the blood clot occurring when coagulation is delayed or when blood has been centrifuged.

bug (bŭg) *n.* **1.** A disease-producing microorganism, such as a flu bug. **2.** The illness or disease so produced.

bulb (bŭlb) *n.* A globular or fusiform anatomical structure.

bul·bar myelitis (bŭl'bər, -bär) *n.* Inflammation of the medulla oblongata.

bul·bi·tis (bŭl-bī'tĭs) *n.* Inflammation of the bulbous portion of the urethra.

bulb of eye *n.* See **eyeball** (sense 1).

bulb of penis *n.* The expanded posterior part of the corpus spongiosum of the penis lying in the interval between the crura of the penis.

bul·bo·u·re·thral gland (bŭl'bō-yōō-rē'thrəl) *n.* Either of two small racemose glands in the male that are located below the prostate and discharge a component of the seminal fluid into the urethra.

bul·bous bougie (bŭl'bəs) *n.* A bougie with a bulb-shaped tip, sometimes shaped like an acorn or an olive.

bu·lim·a·rex·i·a (byōō-lĭm'ə-rĕk'sē-ə, -lē'mə-, bōō-) *n.* An eating disorder characterized by an alternation between episodes of excessive food intake and periods of fasting and self-induced vomiting or diarrhea.

bu·lim·i·a (byōō-lĭm'ē-ə, -lē'mē-ə, bōō-) *n.* A chronic eating disorder involving repeated and secretive episodes of eating, characterized by uncontrolled rapid ingestion of large quantities of food over a short period of time, followed by self-induced vomiting, purging, and anorexia and accompanied by feelings of guilt, depression, and self-disgust. — **bu·lim'ic** *adj. & n.*

bulimia ner·vo·sa (nûr-vō'sə) *n.* See **bulimia.**

bul·la (bŏŏl'ə) *n., pl.* **bul·lae** (bŏŏl'ē). **1.** A large blister or vesicle of pathological origin. **2.** A bublike structure.

bull·dog forceps (bŏŏl'dôg') *n.* A short spring forceps for grasping and occluding a blood vessel.

bul·let forceps (bŏŏl'ĭt) *n.* A forceps having thin curved blades with serrated grasping surfaces for extracting a bullet from tissues.

bul·lous (bŭl'əs) *adj.* Relating to or characterized by bullae.

bullous pemphigoid *n.* A chronic generally benign skin disease, most commonly of old age, characterized by subepidermal blisters that cause detachment of the entire epidermis but that tend to heal without scarring.

bu·met·a·nide (byōō-mĕt'ə-nīd') *n.* A diuretic used in the treatment of edema associated with congestive heart failure and liver and renal disease.

BUN *abbr.* blood urea nitrogen

bun·dle (bŭn'dl) *n.* A structure composed of a group of fibers, such as a fasciculus.

bun·ion (bŭn'yən) *n.* A localized swelling at either the medial or dorsal aspect of the first joint of the big toe, caused by an inflamed bursa.

bun·ion·ec·to·my (bŭn'yə-nĕk'tə-mē) *n.* Excision of a bunion.

Bun·ya·vi·rus (bŭn'yə-vī'rəs) *n.* A large genus of arboviruses.

bunyavirus encephalitis *n.* A form of encephalitis having an abrupt onset, with severe frontal headache and low-grade to moderate fever, caused by a virus of the genus *Bunyavirus.*

buph·thal·mi·a (bŏŏf-thăl'mē-ə, byŏŏf-) or **buph·thal·mos** (-məs, -mōs') or **buph·thal·mus** (-məs) *n.* A disease of infancy marked by an increase of intraocular fluid and consequent enlargement of the eyeball.

bu·piv·a·caine (byŏŏ-pĭv'ə-kān') *n.* A potent, long-acting local anesthetic used in regional anesthesia.

bu·pro·pi·on (byŏŏ-prō'pē-ŏn') *n.* A pale yellow oil whose crystalline hydrochloride form is used therapeutically as an antidepressant.

bur or **burr** (bûr) *n.* A drilling tool for enlarging a trephine hole in the cranium.

bur·ied flap (bĕr'ēd) *n.* A surgical flap denuded of both surface epithelium and superficial dermis and transferred into the subcutaneous tissues.

buried suture *n.* A suture placed entirely below the surface of the skin.

Bur·kitt's lymphoma (bûr'kĭts) *n.* An undifferentiated malignant lymphoma usually occurring among children in central Africa, characterized by a large osteolytic lesion in the mandible or by a mass in the retroperitoneal area and associated with the Epstein — Barr virus.

burn (bûrn) *v.* **burned** or **burnt** (bûrnt), **burn·ing, burns.** **1.** To undergo or cause to undergo combustion. **2.** To consume or use as fuel or energy. **3.** To damage or injure by fire, heat, radiation, electricity, or a caustic agent. **4.** To irritate or inflame, as by chafing or sunburn. **5.** To become sunburned or windburned. **6.** To metabolize (glucose, for example) in the body. — *n.* **1.** An injury produced by fire, heat, radiation, electricity, or a caustic agent. **2.** A burned place or area. **3.** The process or result of burning. **4.** A stinging sensation. **5.** A sunburn or windburn.

burn center *n.* A multidisciplinary health care facility in which victims of burns are treated.

burp (bûrp) *n.* The noisy expulsion of gas from the stomach through the mouth. — *v.* **burped, burp·ing, burps.** **1.** To expel gas noisily from the stomach through the mouth. **2.** To cause (a baby) to expel gas from the stomach, as by patting the back after feeding.

bur·sa (bûr'sə) *n., pl.* **-sas** or **-sae** (-sē). A sac or saclike bodily cavity, especially one containing a viscous lubricating fluid and located between a tendon and a bone or at points of friction between moving structures. — **bur′sal** *adj.*

bur·sec·to·my (bər-sĕk′tə-mē) *n.* Surgical removal of a bursa.

bur·si·tis (bər-sī′tĭs) *n.* Inflammation of a bursa, especially in the shoulder, elbow, or knee joint.

bur·so·lith (bûr′sə-lĭth′) *n.* A calculus formed in a bursa.

bur·sop·a·thy (bər-sŏp′ə-thē) *n.* A disease of a bursa.

bur·sot·o·my (bər-sŏt′ə-mē) *n.* Incision through the wall of a bursa.

bu·spi·rone hydrochloride (byoo-spī′rōn′) *n.* An agent used in the management of anxiety disorders or for short-term relief of the symptoms of anxiety.

Bus·se–Buschke disease (boos′ə-) *n.* See crypto-coccosis.

bu·sul·fan (byoo-sŭl′fən) *n.* An alkylating agent that is used as an antineoplastic drug in the treatment of chronic myelocytic leukemia.

bu·ta·caine sulfate (byoo′tə-kān′) *n.* A local topical anesthetic.

bu·to·con·a·zole nitrate (byoo′tə-kŏn′ə-zōl′) *n.* An antifungal agent used primarily in the treatment of vulvovaginal candidiasis.

but·ter·fly rash (bŭt′ər-flī′) *n.* A scaling lesion on each cheek joined by a narrow band across the nose, seen in lupus erythematosus and seborrheic dermatitis.

but·tock (bŭt′ək) *n.* **1.** Either of the two rounded prominences on the human torso that are posterior to the hips and formed by the gluteal muscles and underlying structures. **2. buttocks.** The rear pelvic area of the human body.

but·ton (bŭt′n) *n.* A knob-like structure, device, or lesion.

but·ton·hole (bŭt′n-hōl′) *n.* **1.** A short straight surgical cut made through the wall of a cavity or canal. **2.** The contraction of an orifice down to a narrow slit, as in mitral stenosis.

button suture *n.* A suture that is passed through a button to prevent the threads from cutting through the flesh, then tied.

but·tress plate (bŭt′rĭs) *n.* A metal plate used to support the internal fixation of a fracture.

butyl a·mi·no·ben·zo·ate (ə-mē′nō-bĕn′zō-āt′, ăm′ə-nō-) *n.* A local anesthetic, very insoluble and only slightly absorbed.

bu·tyr·ic acid (byoo-tĕr′ĭk) *n.* Either of two colorless isomeric acids occurring in animal milk fats and used in disinfectants, emulsifying agents, and pharmaceuticals.

bu·ty·ro·phe·none (byoo-tĭr′ō-fə-nōn′, byoo′tə-rō-) *n.* Any of a group of neuroleptic drugs, such as haloperidol, administered in the treatment of acute psychotic episodes, schizophrenia, and other psychiatric disorders.

by·pass (bī′păs′) *n.* **1.** An alternative passage created surgically to divert the flow of blood or other bodily fluid to or circumvent an obstructed or diseased organ. **2.** A surgical procedure to create such a channel.

bys·si·no·sis (bĭs′ĭ-nō′sĭs) *n.* A form of pneumoconiosis that affects cotton, flax, and hemp workers and is characterized by wheezing.

~ ~ ~ ~ ~ ~ C ~ ~ ~ ~ ~ ~

c *abbr.* blood capillary; small calorie

C *abbr.* Celsius; centigrade; cytosine

CA *abbr.* cancer; carcinoma.

ca·ble graft (kā′bəl) *n.* A multiple-strand nerve graft arranged as a pathway for the regeneration of axons.

Cab·ot's ring body (kăb′əts) *n.* A ring-shaped or figure-8 structure, staining red with Wright's stain, found in red blood cells in severe anemias.

ca·chec·tin (kə-kĕk′tĭn) *n.* A polypeptide hormone that releases fat and reduces the concentration of enzymes needed to produce and store fat.

ca·chet (kă-shā′) *n.* An edible wafer capsule used for enclosing an unpleasant-tasting drug.

ca·chex·i·a (kə-kĕk′sē-ə) *n.* Weight loss, wasting of muscle, loss of appetite, and general debility that can occur during a chronic disease.

cach·in·na·tion (kăk′ə-nā′shən) *n.* Loud, hard, or compulsive laughter without apparent cause, often found in schizophrenia.

cac·o·geu·si·a (kăk′ə-gyoo′zē-ə, -zhə, -joo′-) *n.* A bad taste not due to food, drugs, or other ingested matter.

cac·o·mel·i·a (kăk′ə-mĕl′ē-ə, -mē′lē-ə) *n.* Congenital deformity of one or more limbs.

ca·cos·mi·a (kă-kŏs′mē-ə, -kŏz′-) *n.* The imagining of unpleasant odors, particularly putrefactive odors.

ca·cu·men (kə-kyoo′mən) *n., pl.* **-mi·na** (-mə-nə). The top or apex, as of an anatomical structure. — **ca·cu′mi·nal** (-mə-nəl) *adj.*

ca·dav·er (kə-dăv′ər) *n.* A dead body, especially one intended for dissection. — **ca·dav′er·ic** (-ər-ĭk) *adj.*

ca·dav·er·ine (kə-dăv′ə-rēn′) *n.* A syrupy, colorless, fuming ptomaine formed by the carboxylation of lysine by bacteria in decaying flesh.

cad·mi·um (kăd′mē-əm) *n.* A soft metallic element with atomic number 48 occurring primarily in zinc, copper, and lead ores, used in solders, batteries, and electroplating.

ca·du·ce·us (kə-doo′sē-əs, -shəs, -dyoo′-) *n., pl.*

-ce·i (-sē-ī′). **1.** A winged staff with two serpents twined around it, carried by Hermes. **2.** A medical insignia modeled on Hermes' staff.

ca·fé au lait spots (kă-fā′ ō lā′) *pl.n.* Uniformly light brown, sharply defined, and usually oval-shaped patches of the skin characteristic of neurofibromatosis, though also found in healthy individuals.

caf·feine or **caf·fein** (kă-fēn′, kăf′ēn′, kăf′ē-ĭn) *n.* A bitter white alkaloid often derived from tea or coffee and used chiefly as a mild stimulant and in the treatment of certain kinds of headache.

Cain complex (kān) *n.* In psychoanalytic theory, extreme envy or jealousy of a brother, leading to hatred.

cai·no·to·pho·bi·a (kā-nō′tə-fō′bē-ə) *n.* An abnormal fear of newness.

cais·son disease (kā′sŏn′, -sən) *n.* See **decompression sickness**.

Cal·a·bar bean (kăl′ə-bär) *n.* The poisonous seed of a tropical western African woody vine in the pea family and source of the drug physostigmine.

cal·a·mine (kăl′ə-mīn′, -mĭn) *n.* A pink, odorless, tasteless powder of zinc oxide with a small amount of ferric oxide, dissolved in mineral oils and used in skin lotions.

cal·ca·ne·o·a·poph·y·si·tis (kăl-kā′nē-ō-ə-pŏf′-ĭ-sī′tĭs) *n.* Inflammation at the posterior part of the calcaneus, at the Achilles' tendon insertion.

cal·ca·ne·us (kăl-kā′nē-əs) or **cal·ca·ne·um** (-nē-əm) *n., pl.* **-ne·i** (-nē-ī′) or **-ne·a** (-nē-ə). The quadrangular bone at the back of the tarsus, the largest of the tarsal bones. — **cal·ca′ne·al** *adj.*

cal·car (kăl′kär′) *n., pl.* **cal·car·i·a** (kăl-kâr′ē-ə). **1.** A small spurlike projection from a structure. **2.** An internal septum at the level of division of arteries and confluence of veins when branches or roots form an acute angle. **3.** A dull spine or projection from a bone. **4.** A horny outgrowth from the skin.

cal·car·e·ous degeneration (kăl-kâr′ē-əs) *n.* The deposition of insoluble calcium salts in necrotized degenerated tissue.

cal·car·i·u·ri·a (kăl-kâr′ē-yŏŏr′ē-ə) *n.* Excretion of calcium salts in the urine.

cal·ci·co·sis (kăl′sĭ-kō′sĭs) *n.* Pneumoconiosis resulting from the inhalation of limestone dust.

cal·cif·er·ol (kăl-sĭf′ə-rôl′, -rōl′) *n.* See **vitamin D₂**.

cal·ci·fi·ca·tion (kăl′sə-fĭ-kā′shən) *n.* **1.** Impregnation with calcium or calcium salts, as with calcium carbonate. **2.** Hardening, as of tissue, by such impregnation. **3.** A calcified substance or part.

cal·ci·fy (kăl′sə-fī′) *v.* **-fied, -fy·ing, -fies.** To make or become stony or chalky by deposition of calcium salts.

cal·ci·no·sis (kăl′sə-nō′sĭs) *n.* The abnormal deposition of calcium salts in a part or tissue of the body.

cal·ci·to·nin (kăl′sĭ-tō′nĭn) *n.* A peptide hormone, produced by the thyroid gland in humans, that lowers plasma calcium and phosphate levels without augmenting calcium accretion.

cal·ci·um (kăl′sē-əm) *n.* A soft metallic element with atomic number 20 that is a basic component of animals and plants and constitutes approximately 3 percent of Earth's crust. It occurs naturally in limestone, gypsum, and fluorite.

calcium channel-blocking agent *n.* Any of a class of drugs that inhibit movement of calcium ions across a cell membrane, used in the treatment of cardiovascular disorders.

calcium cyclamate *n.* An artificially prepared salt of cyclamic acid formerly used as a nonnutritive low-calorie sweetener, now banned because of possible carcinogenic effects of its metabolites.

cal·ci·u·ri·a (kăl′sē-yŏŏr′ē-ə) *n.* The presence of calcium in the urine.

cal·co·dyn·i·a (kăl′kō-dĭn′ē-ə) or **cal·ca·ne·o·dyn·i·a** (kăl-kā′nē-ō-) *n.* A condition in which bearing weight on the heel causes pain of varying severity.

cal·co·sphe·rite (kăl′kō-sfēr′īt′, -sfēr′-) *n.* A tiny round laminated body containing calcium salts.

cal·cu·lus (kăl′kyə-ləs) *n., pl.* **-lus·es** or **-li** (-lī′). **1.** An abnormal concretion in the body, usually formed of mineral salts and most commonly found in the gallbladder, kidney, or urinary bladder. **2.** Dental tartar.

Cald·well–Luc operation (kôld′wĕl′-lük′, kŏld′-) *n.* An intraoral surgical opening into the maxillary antrum through the fossa above the maxillary premolar teeth.

calf (kăf) *n., pl.* **calves** (kăvz). The fleshy, muscular back part of the human leg between the knee and ankle, formed chiefly by the bellies of the gastrocnemius and soleus muscles.

calf bone *n.* See **fibula**.

cal·i·ber (kăl′ə-bər) *n.* The diameter of the inside of a round cylinder, such as a tube.

cal·i·brate (kăl′ə-brāt′) *v.* **-brat·ed, -brat·ing, -brates. 1.** To check, adjust, or determine the graduations of a quantitative measuring instrument by comparison with a standard. **2.** To determine the caliber of a tube. **3.** To make corrections in or adjust a procedure or process. — **cal′i·bra′tor** *n.*

cal·i·cec·ta·sis (kăl′ĭ-sĕk′tə-sĭs, kā′lĭ-) or **cal·i·ec·ta·sis** (kăl′ē-ĕk′tə-sĭs, kā′lē-) *n.* Dilation of the calices, usually due to obstruction or infection.

cal·i·cec·to·my (kăl′ĭ-sĕk′tə-mē, kā′lĭ-) or **cal·i·ec·to·my** (kăl′ē-ĕk′tə-mē, kā′lē-) *n.* Excision of a calix.

ca·li·co·plas·ty (kā′lĭ-kō-plăs′tē) *n.* Plastic surgery of a calix, usually designed to increase its lumen at the infundibulum.

ca·li·cot·o·my (kā′lĭ-kŏt′ə-mē) *n.* Incision into a calix, usually to remove a calculus.

ca·lic·u·lus (kə-lĭk′yə-ləs) *n., pl.* **-li** (-lī′). A budshaped or cup-shaped structure.

Cal·i·for·nia virus (kăl′ĭ-fôr′nyə, -fôr′nē-ə) *n.* A strain of *Bunyavirus* that causes encephalitis.

cal·i·for·ni·um (kăl′ə-fôr′nē-əm) *n.* A synthetic radioactive element with atomic number 98 produced by neutron bombardment of curium.

ca·li·or·rha·phy (kā′lē-ôr′ə-fē) *n.* **1.** The suturing of a calix. **2.** Reconstructive surgery on a dilated or obstructed calix to improve urinary drainage.

cal·i·per or **cal·li·per** (kăl′ə-pər) *n.* An instrument consisting essentially of two curved hinged legs, used to measure thickness and distances.

cal·is·then·ics (kăl′ĭs-thĕn′ĭks) *pl.n.* Gymnastic exercises, such as sit-ups, designed to develop muscular tone and promote physical fitness.

ca·lix or **ca·lyx** (kā′lĭks, kăl′ĭks) *n., pl.* **ca·li·ces** or **ca·ly·ces** (kā′lĭ-sēz′, kăl′ĭ-). **1.** A flower-shaped or funnel-shaped structure. **2.** Any of the branches or recesses of the pelvis of the kidney into which the orifices of the malpighian renal pyramids project.

cal·los·i·ty (kə-lŏs′ĭ-tē) *n.* A localized thickening and enlargement of the horny layer of the skin.

cal·lus (kăl′əs) *n., pl.* **-lus·es. 1.** See **callosity. 2.** The hard bony tissue that develops around the ends of a fractured bone during healing.

calm·a·tive (kä′mə-tĭv, kăl′mə-) *adj.* Having relaxing or pacifying properties. — *n.* A sedative.

Cal·mette-Gué·rin bacillus (kăl-mĕt′gā-răn′, kăl-mĕt′gā-răn′) *n.* An attenuated strain of tubercle bacillus grown in repeated cultures on medium containing bile and used in the preparation of tuberculosis vaccines.

cal·mod·u·lin (kăl-mŏj′ə-lĭn) *n.* A calcium-binding protein that regulates cellular processes by modifying the activity of specific calcium-sensitive enzymes.

cal·o·mel (kăl′ə-mĕl′, -məl) *n.* A colorless, white or brown tasteless compound used as a purgative and an insecticide.

cal·or (kăl′ôr, -ər, kā′lôr) *n.* The bodily heat indicating an inflammation.

ca·lor·ic (kə-lôr′ĭk) *adj.* **1.** Of or relating to calories. **2.** Of or relating to heat.

caloric test *n.* Bárány's caloric test.

cal·o·rie (kăl′ə-rē) *n.* **1.** A unit of energy-producing potential supplied by food and released upon oxidation by the body, equal to the amount of energy required to raise the temperature of 1 kilogram of water by 1°C at one atmosphere pressure. **2.** The unit of heat equal to the amount of heat required to raise the temperature of 1 kilogram of water by 1°C at 1 atmosphere pressure; large calorie. **3.** Any of several approximately equal units of heat, each measured as the quantity of heat required to raise the temperature of 1 gram of water by 1°C from a standard initial temperature at 1 atmosphere pressure; small calorie.

cal·var·i·a (kăl-vâr′ē-ə) *n., pl.* **-i·ae** (-ē-ē′). Roof of the skull; the upper domelike portion of the skull without the lower jaw and facial parts.

calx (kălks) *n., pl.* **calx·es** or **cal·ces** (kăl′sēz′). The posterior rounded extremity of the foot; the heel.

cam·er·a (kăm′ər-ə, kăm′rə) *n., pl.* **-er·ae** (-ə-rē). A chamber or cavity, such as one of the chambers of the heart or eye.

cam·phor (kăm′fər) *n.* An aromatic crystalline compound obtained from the wood or leaves of the camphor tree or synthesized and used as an insect repellent and in external preparations to relieve mild pain and itching.

cam·pim·e·ter (kăm-pĭm′ĭ-tər) *n.* A portable, hand-held device used to measure the visual field.

camp·to·cor·mi·a (kămp′tə-kôr′mē-ə) *n.* A hysterical condition in which the body is bent completely forward at the trunk and is unable to be straightened.

camp·to·dac·ty·ly (kămp′tə-dăk′tə-lē) *n.* See **campylodactyly.**

camp·to·mel·i·a (kămp′tō-mĕl′ē-ə, -mĕl′ē-ə) *n.* A bending of the limbs that produces a permanent curving or bowing. — **camp′to·mel′ic** *adj.*

camptomelic dwarfism *n.* Dwarfism caused by the shortening of the lower limbs as a result of the femur and tibia bending anteriorly.

camp·to·spasm (kămp′tə-spăz′əm) *n.* See **camptocormia.**

cam·py·lo·bac·ter·o·sis (kăm′pə-lō-băk′tə-rō′-sĭs) *n.* A gastrointestinal condition characterized by diarrhea, abdominal cramps, and fever, caused by eating raw meat or unpasteurized milk contaminated with *Campylobacter jejuni,* a bacterium that infects poultry, cattle, and sheep.

cam·py·lo·dac·ty·ly (kăm′pə-lō-dăk′tə-lē) *n.* Permanent flexion of one or more of the finger joints.

ca·nal (kə-năl′) *n.* A duct, channel, or tubular structure.

can·a·lic·u·li·za·tion (kăn′ə-lĭk′yə-lĭ-zā′shən) *n.* Formation of small canals or channels in tissue.

can·a·lic·u·lus (kăn′ə-lĭk′yə-ləs) *n., pl.* **-li** (-lī′). A small canal or duct in the body, as one of the minute channels in compact bone.

ca·na·lis (kə-nā′lĭs) *n., pl.* **-les** (-lēz′). A canal or channel.

can·a·li·za·tion (kăn′ə-lĭ-zā′shən) *n.* The formation of canals or channels in tissue.

can·cel·lous bone (kăn-sĕl′əs, kăn′sə-ləs) *n.* See **spongy bone** (sense 1).

cancellous tissue *n.* Lattice-like or spongy bone tissue.

can·cel·lus (kăn-sĕl′əs) *n., pl.* **-li** (-lī′). A latticelike structure, such as spongy bone.

can·cer (kăn′sər) *n.* **1.** Any of various malignant neoplasms characterized by the proliferation of anaplastic cells that tend to invade surrounding tissue and metastasize to new body sites. **2.** The pathological condition characterized by such growths. — **can′cer·ous** (kăn′sər-əs) *adj.*

cancer á deux (ä′ dœ′) *n.* Carcinomas occurring at approximately the same time, or in fairly close succession, in two persons who live together.

can·cer·o·pho·bi·a (kăn′sə-rō-fō′bē-ə) or **car·ci·no·pho·bi·a** (kär′sə-nō-) *n.* An abnormal fear of developing a malignant growth.

can·croid (kăng′kroid′) *adj.* **1.** Of or relating to squamous cell carcinoma. **2.** Of or resembling a cancer. — *n.* See **squamous cell carcinoma.**

can·crum (kăng′krəm) *n., pl.* **-cra** (-krə). A gangrenous, ulcerative, inflammatory lesion; canker.

can·di·ci·din (kăn′dĭ-sīd′n) *n.* An antibiotic agent derived from a soil actinomycete and active against some molds of the genus *Candida*.

Can·di·da (kăn′dĭ-də) *n.* A genus of pathogenic yeastlike fungi.

can·di·de·mi·a (kăn′dĭ-dē′mē-ə) *n.* The presence in the blood of any fungus of the genus *Candida*.

can·di·di·a·sis (kăn′dĭ-dī′ə-sĭs) or **can·di·do·sis** (-dō′sĭs) *n.* A fungal infection caused by a member of the genus *Candida*, especially *Candida albicans*, that can involve various parts of the body, such as the skin and mucous membranes.

can·dy striper (kăn′dē strī′pər) *n.* A volunteer worker in a hospital.

ca·nine spasm (kā′nīn) *n.* See risus caninus.

canine tooth *n.* Any of four teeth having a thick conical crown and a long conical root, adjacent to the distal surface of the lateral incisors, in both deciduous and permanent dentition.

ca·ni·ti·es (kə-nĭsh′ē-ēz′) *n.* The diminishing of pigment in hair producing a range of colors from normal to white that is perceived as gray.

can·ker (kăng′kər) *n.* **1.** Ulceration of the mouth and lips. **2.** Cancrum.

canker sore *n.* A small painful ulcer of the mucous membrane of the mouth; an aphtha.

can·nab·i·noid (kə-năb′ə-noid′) *n.* Any of various organic substances, such as THC, found in cannabis.

can·na·bis (kăn′ə-bĭs) *n.* Any of several mildly euphoriant, intoxicating hallucinogenic drugs, such as marijuana, prepared from various parts of the hemp plant (*Cannabis sativa*).

can·non·ball pulse (kăn′ən-bôl′) *n.* See waterhammer pulse.

can·nu·la or **can·u·la** (kăn′yə-lə) *n., pl.* **-las** or **-lae** (-lē′). A flexible tube, usually containing a trocar at one end, that is inserted into a bodily cavity, duct, or vessel to drain fluid or administer a substance such as a medication.

can·nu·la·tion (kăn′yə-lā′shən) or **can·nu·li·za·tion** (-yə-lĭ-zā′shən) *n.* Insertion of a cannula.

can·ter·ing rhythm (kăn′tə-rĭng) *n.* See gallop.

can·thec·to·my (kăn-thěk′tə-mē) *n.* Excision of a canthus.

can·thi·tis (kăn-thī′tĭs) *n.* Inflammation of a canthus.

can·thol·y·sis (kăn-thŏl′ĭ-sĭs) *n.* See canthoplasty (sense 1).

can·tho·plas·ty (kăn′thə-plăs′tē) *n.* **1.** The lengthening of the palpebral fissure of the eyelids by cutting through the external canthus. **2.** Surgical restoration of the canthus.

can·thor·rha·phy (kăn-thôr′ə-fē) *n.* The surgical shortening of the palpebral fissure of the eyelids by suturing the canthus.

can·thot·o·my (kăn-thŏt′ə-mē) *n.* Surgical incision of the canthus.

can·thus (kăn′thəs) *n., pl.* **-thi** (-thī′). Angle formed by the meeting of the upper and lower eyelids at either side of the eye. — **can′thal** (-thəl) *adj.*

cap (kăp) *n.* A protective cover or seal, especially one that closes off an end or a tip and that resembles a close-fitting head covering.

ca·pac·i·ta·tion (kə-păs′ĭ-tā′shən) *n.* The change undergone by spermatozoa in the female genital tract that enables them to penetrate and fertilize an egg.

ca·pac·i·ty (kə-păs′ĭ-tē) *n.* **1.** The measure of potential cubic contents of a cavity or receptacle; volume. **2.** Ability to perform or produce.

cap·ac·tin (kă-păk′tĭn) *n.* Any of a class of proteins capping the ends of actin filaments.

cap·e·line bandage (kăp′ə-lēn′, -lĭn) *n.* A caplike bandage covering the head or the stump from an amputation.

cap·il·lar·ec·ta·si·a (kăp′ə-lĕr′ĭk-tā′zē-ə, -zhə) *n.* Dilation of the capillary blood vessels.

cap·il·la·ri·tis (kăp′ə-lə-rī′tĭs) *n.* Inflammation of a capillary or capillaries.

cap·il·lar·i·ty (kăp′ə-lăr′ĭ-tē) *n.* The interaction between contacting surfaces of a liquid and a solid that distorts the liquid surface from a planar shape.

cap·il·la·rop·a·thy (kăp′ə-lə-rŏp′ə-thē) *n.* A disease of the capillaries.

cap·il·lary (kăp′ə-lĕr′ē) *adj.* **1.** Of or relating to the capillaries. **2.** Relating to or resembling a hair; fine and slender. — *n.* Blood capillary.

capillary attraction *n.* A surface force of adhesion that causes fluids to rise along or into solid materials.

capillary bed *n.* The capillaries of the blood system considered collectively with their capacity.

capillary drainage *n.* The use of a wick of gauze or other material to drain a cavity or wound.

capillary fracture *n.* See hairline fracture.

capillary vein *n.* See venule.

cap·i·stra·tion (kăp′ĭ-strā′shən) *n.* See paraphimosis (sense 1).

cap·i·tel·lum (kăp′ĭ-tĕl′əm) *n., pl.* **-tel·la** (-tĕl′ə). **1.** Capitulum. **2.** The rounded protuberance at the lower end of the humerus that articulates with the radius.

ca·pit·i·um (kă-pĭt′ē-əm) *n.* A bandage for the head.

cap·i·ton·nage (kăp′ĭ-tə-näzh′) *n.* Surgical closure of a cyst cavity.

ca·pit·u·lum (kə-pĭch′ə-ləm) *n., pl.* **-la** (-lə). A small head or rounded articular extremity of a bone. — **ca·pit′u·lar** *adj.*

cap·let (kăp′lĭt) *n.* A smooth, coated, oval-shaped medicine tablet intended to be tamper-resistant.

cap·re·o·my·cin (kăp′rē-ō-mī′sĭn) *n.* An antibiotic derived from a bacterium (*Streptomyces capreolus*) that is effective against the microorganism responsible for tuberculosis in humans.

cap·sa·i·cin (kăp-sā′ĭ-sĭn) *n.* A colorless, pungent, crystalline compound that is a strong irritant to skin and mucous membranes.

cap·sid (kăp′sĭd) *n.* The protein shell that surrounds a virus particle.

capsular antigen *n.* An antigen found only in the capsules of certain microorganisms.

cap·sule (kăp′səl, -sool) *n.* **1.** A fibrous, membranous, or fatty sheath that encloses an organ or part, such as the fibrous tissues surrounding a joint. **2.** A small soluble container, usually made of gelatin, that encloses a dose of an oral medicine or a vitamin. — **cap′su·lar** (kăp′sə-lər, -syōō-) *adj.*

capsule forceps *n.* A fine strong forceps for removing the capsule of the lens in extracapsular extraction of cataract.

cap·su·li·tis (kăp′sə-lī′tĭs, -syōō-) *n.* Inflammation of the capsule of an organ or part.

cap·su·lo·plas·ty (kăp′sə-lə-plăs′tē) *n.* The surgical repair of a capsule, especially a joint capsule.

cap·su·lor·rha·phy (kăp′sə-lôr′ə-fē) *n.* Suture of a tear in a capsule, especially of a joint capsule.

cap·su·lot·o·my (kăp′sə-lŏt′ə-mē) *n.* Incision into a capsule, especially that of the crystalline lens of the eye, as to remove cataracts.

cap·to·pril (kăp′tə-prĭl′) *n.* A drug used in the treatment of hypertension that functions by inhibiting the enzymes that activate angiotensin.

cap·ture beat (kăp′chər) *n.* The cardiac cycle resulting when, after atrioventricular dissociation, the atria regain control of the ventricles.

cap·ut (kăp′ŏot, -ət) *n., pl.* **cap·i·ta** (kăp′ĭ-tə). The head.

car·ba·maz·e·pine (kär′bə-măz′ə-pēn′) *n.* An anticonvulsant and analgesic drug used in the treatment of certain forms of epilepsy.

car·ba·mide (kär′bə-mīd′, kär-băm′īd) *n.* See **urea.**

carb·a·mi·no·he·mo·glo·bin (kärb′ə-mē′nō-hē′-mə-glō′bĭn, kär-băm′ə-nō-) *n.* A compound of carbon dioxide and hemoglobin; one of the forms in which carbon dioxide exists in the blood.

car·ben·i·cil·lin di·so·di·um (kär-běn′ĭ-sĭl′ĭn dī-sō′dē-əm) *n.* The disodium salt of a semisynthetic derivative of penicillin effective in the treatment of severe systemic infections and genitourinary, respiratory, and soft-tissue infections.

car·bo·hy·drase (kär′bō-hī′drās, -drāz′) *n.* Any of various enzymes, such as amylase, that catalyze the hydrolysis of a carbohydrate.

car·bo·hy·drate (kär′bō-hī′drāt′) *n.* Any of a group of organic compounds that includes sugars, starches, celluloses, and gums and serves as a major energy source in the diet of animals; they are produced by photosynthetic plants and contain only carbon, hydrogen, and oxygen.

carbohydrate loading *n.* A dietary practice that increases carbohydrate reserves in muscle tissue through the consumption of extra quantities of high-starch foods and is often followed by endurance athletes prior to competition.

car·bo·hy·dra·tu·ri·a (kär′bō-hī′drä-tŏor′ē-ə, -tyŏor′-) *n.* The presence of an abnormally large amount of carbohydrates in the urine.

car·bol·ic acid (kär-bŏl′ĭk) *n.* See **phenol** (sense 1).

car·bon (kär′bən) *n.* A nonmetallic element with atomic number 6 that occurs in many inorganic and in all organic compounds and exists freely as graphite and diamond and as a constituent of coal, limestone, and petroleum.

carbon dioxide *n.* A colorless, odorless, incombustible gas formed during respiration, combustion, and organic decomposition and used in inert atmospheres, fire extinguishers, and aerosols.

carbon monoxide *n.* A colorless, odorless, highly poisonous gas formed by the incomplete combustion of carbon or a carbonaceous material, such as gasoline.

carbon monoxide hemoglobin *n.* See **carboxyhemoglobin.**

carbon monoxide poisoning *n.* A potentially fatal condition caused by inhalation of carbon monoxide gas which competes favorably with oxygen for binding with hemoglobin and thus interferes with the transportation of oxygen and carbon dioxide by the blood.

carbon tetrachloride *n.* A poisonous, nonflammable, colorless liquid used in fire extinguishers and as a dry-cleaning fluid.

car·bo·prost tromethamine (kär′bō-prŏst′) *n.* A prostaglandin used as an abortifacient and in the treatment of refractory postpartum bleeding.

car·box·y·he·mo·glo·bin (kär-bŏk′sē-hē′mə-glō′bĭn) *n.* The compound that is formed when inhaled carbon monoxide combines with hemoglobin in the blood.

car·box·y·he·mo·glo·bi·ne·mi·a (kär-bŏk′sē-hē′mə-glō′bə-nē′mē-ə) *n.* See **carbon monoxide poisoning.**

car·box·yl·a·tion (kär-bŏk′sə-lā′shən) *n.* The introduction of a carboxyl group (COOH) into a compound or molecule.

car·bun·cle (kär′bŭng′kəl) *n.* **1.** A deep-seated pyogenic infection of several contiguous hair follicles, with formation of connecting sinuses, often preceded or accompanied by fever, malaise, and prostration. **2.** See **anthrax** (sense 1). — **car·bun′cu·lar** (-kyə-lar) *adj.*

car·bun·cu·lo·sis (kär-bŭng′kyə-lō′sĭs) *n.* The occurrence of several carbuncles simultaneously or within a short period of time.

car·ci·no·em·bry·on·ic antigen (kär′sə-nō-ěm′-brē-ŏn′ĭk) *n.* A glycoprotein present in fetal gastrointestinal tissue, generally absent from adult cells with the exception of some carcinomas.

car·cin·o·gen (kär-sĭn′ə-jən, kär′sə-nə-jěn′) *n.* A cancer-causing substance or agent. — **car′cin·o·gen′ic** (kär′sə-nə-jěn′ĭk) *adj.*

car·ci·no·gen·e·sis (kär′sə-nə-jěn′ĭ-sĭs) *n.* The production of cancer.

car·ci·noid (kär′sə-noid′) *n.* A small tumor, usually found in the gastrointestinal tract, that secretes serotonin.

carcinoid tumor *n.* A small slow-growing neoplasm composed of islands of rounded cells of medium size; it can occur in the gastrointestinal tract, lungs, and other sites.

car·ci·no·ma (kär′sə-nō′mə) *n., pl.* **-mas** or **-ma·ta** (-mə-tə). An invasive malignant tumor derived from epithelial tissue that tends to metastasize to other areas of the body.

carcinoma in situ *n.* A neoplasm whose cells are localized in the epithelium and show no tendency to invade or metastasize to other tissues.

car·ci·no·ma·to·sis (kär′sə-nō′mə-tō′sĭs) *n.* A pathological condition characterized by the presence of carcinomas that have metastasized to many parts of the body; carcinosis.

car·ci·no·sar·co·ma (kär′sə-nō-sär-kō′mə) *n.* A malignant neoplasm that contains elements of carcinoma and sarcoma.

car·di·a (kär′dē-ə) *n., pl.* **-di·as** or **-di·ae** (-dē-ē′). **1.** The opening of the esophagus into the stomach. **2.** The upper portion of the stomach that adjoins this opening.

car·di·ac (kär′dē-ăk′) *adj.* **1.** Of, near, or relating to the heart. **2.** Of, near, or relating to the cardia. — *n.* A person with a heart disorder.

cardiac arrest *n.* A sudden cessation of cardiac function, resulting in loss of effective circulation.

cardiac arrhythmia *n.* See **cardiac dysrhythmia**.

cardiac asthma *n.* An asthmatic attack due to bronchoconstriction caused by pulmonary congestion and failure of the left ventricle.

cardiac catheter *n.* A long, fine catheter that can be passed into the chambers of the heart via a vein or artery to withdraw samples of blood, measure pressures within the heart's chambers or great vessels, or inject contrast media.

cardiac cirrhosis *n.* An extensive fibrotic reaction within the liver as a result of prolonged congestive heart failure.

cardiac cycle *n.* A complete beat of the heart, including systole and diastole and the intervals between, beginning with any event in the heart's action to the moment when that same event is repeated.

cardiac decompression *n.* The relief of pressure on the heart caused by blood or fluid in the pericardial sac by means of an incision in the pericardium.

cardiac dysrhythmia *n.* Any abnormality in the rate, regularity, or sequence of cardiac activation.

cardiac edema *n.* Edema resulting from congestive heart failure.

cardiac gland *n.* A coiled tubular gland situated in the cardiac region of the stomach.

cardiac infarction *n.* See **myocardial infarction**.

cardiac insufficiency *n.* See **heart failure** (sense 1).

cardiac jelly *n.* The gelatinous noncellular material between the endothelial lining and the myocardial layer of the heart in very young embryos, later serving as a substratum for cardiac mesenchyme.

cardiac massage *n.* A resuscitative procedure that employs the rhythmic compression of the chest and heart in an effort to restore and maintain the circulation after cardiac arrest or ventricular fibrillation.

cardiac murmur *n.* A murmur produced within the heart.

cardiac muscle *n.* The muscle of the heart, consisting of anastomosing transversely striated muscle fibers formed of cells united at intercalated disks; the myocardium.

cardiac neurosis *n.* Anxiety concerning the state of the heart, as a result of palpitation, chest pain, or other symptoms not due to heart disease.

cardiac opening *n.* The opening of the esophagus into the stomach.

cardiac plexus *n.* A wide-meshed network of anastomosing cords from the sympathetic and vagus nerves that surrounds the arch of the aorta and the pulmonary artery and continues to the atria, ventricles, and coronary vessels.

cardiac reserve *n.* The work that the heart is able to perform beyond that required under ordinary circumstances.

cardiac souffle *n.* A soft puffing heart murmur.

cardiac sound *n.* See **heart sound**.

cardiac sphincter *n.* A physiological sphincter at the esophagogastric junction.

cardiac tamponade *n.* Compression of venous return to the heart because of increased volume of fluid in the pericardium.

cardiac valve *n.* Any of the valves regulating the flow of blood through and from the heart, consisting of the aortic valve, the left and right atrioventricular valves, and the pulmonary valve.

car·di·al·gia (kär′dē-ăl′jə, -jē-ə) *n.* **1.** See **heartburn**. **2.** Cardiodynia.

car·di·nal symptom (kär′dn-əl, kärd′nəl) *n.* The primary or major symptom by which a diagnosis is made.

car·di·o·ac·tive (kär′dē-ō-ăk′tĭv) *adj.* Affecting the heart.

car·di·o·cele (kär′dē-ə-sēl′) *n.* Herniation or protrusion of the heart through an opening in the diaphragm or through a wound.

car·di·o·cen·te·sis (kär′dē-ō-sĕn-tē′sĭs) *n.* Puncture of a chamber of the heart for diagnosis or therapy.

car·di·o·di·o·sis (kär′dē-ō-dē-ō′sĭs, -dī-ō′sĭs) *n.* Dilation of the cardiac end of the stomach by passing an instrument through the esophagus.

car·di·o·dy·nam·ics (kär′dē-ō-dī-năm′ĭks) *n.* The mechanics of the heart's action in pumping blood.

car·di·o·dyn·i·a (kär′dē-ō-dĭn′ē-ə) *n.* Localized pain in the region of the heart.

car·di·o·gen·ic shock (kär′dē-ō-jĕn′ĭk) *n.* Shock resulting from a decline in cardiac output that occurs as a result of serious heart disease, especially myocardial infarction.

car·di·o·gram (kär′dē-ə-grăm′) *n.* **1.** The curve traced by a cardiograph, used in the diagnosis of heart disorders. **2.** See **electrocardiogram**.

car·di·o·graph (kär′dē-ə-grăf′) *n.* **1.** An instrument used to record the mechanical movements of the heart. **2.** See **electrocardiograph**. — **car′di·og′ra·phy** (-ŏg′rə-fē) *n.*

car·di·o·ky·mo·gram (kär′dē-ō-kī′mə-grăm′) *n.* A tracing of the changes in the size of the heart.

car·di·o·ky·mo·graph (kär′dē-ō-kī′mə-grăf′) *n.* A noninvasive device, placed on the chest, capable of recording motion made by the anterior left ventricle segmental wall of the heart. — **car′di·o·ky·mog′ra·phy** (-mŏg′rə-fē) *n.*

car·di·o·lith (kär′dē-ə-lĭth′) *n.* A concretion in the heart, or an area of calcareous degeneration in its walls or valves.

car·di·ol·o·gy (kär′dē-ŏl′ə-jē) *n.* The medical study of the structure, function, and disorders of the heart. — **car′di·ol′o·gist** *n.*

car·di·ol·y·sis (kär′dē-ŏl′ĭ-sĭs) *n.* Surgery to break up cardiac adhesions.

car·di·o·ma·la·ci·a (kär′dē-ō-mə-lā′shē-ə, -shə) *n.* Pathological softening of the walls of the heart.

car·di·o·meg·a·ly (kär′dē-ō-mĕg′ə-lē) *n.* Enlargement of the heart.

car·di·o·mo·til·i·ty (kär′dē-ō-mō-tĭl′ĭ-tē) *n.* The movements of the heart.

car·di·o·my·op·a·thy (kär′dē-ō-mī-ŏp′ə-thē) *n.* A disease or disorder of the heart muscle, especially of unknown or obscure cause.

car·di·o·neu·ro·sis (kär′dē-ō-nŏŏ-rō′sĭs, -nyŏŏ-) *n.* See **cardiac neurosis.**

car·di·o·o·men·to·pexy (kär′dē-ō-ō-mĕn′tə-pĕk′sē) *n.* Surgical attachment of the omentum to the heart to improve its blood supply.

car·di·op·a·thy (kär′dē-ŏp′ə-thē) *n.* A disease or disorder of the heart.

car·di·o·per·i·car·di·o·pex·y (kär′dē-ō-pĕr′ĭ-kär′dē-ō-pĕk′sē) *n.* Surgery to increase the blood supply to the myocardium.

car·di·o·pho·bi·a (kär′dē-ə-fō′bē-ə) *n.* An abnormal fear of heart disease.

car·di·o·plas·ty (kär′dē-ə-plăs′tē) *n.* See **esophagogastroplasty.**

car·di·o·ple·gi·a (kär′dē-ō-plē′jē-ə, -jə) *n.* **1.** Paralysis of the heart, or cardiac arrest, as from direct blow or trauma. **2.** Elective, temporary stopping of cardiac activity, usually by using drugs.

car·di·op·to·si·a (kär′dē-ŏp-tō′sē-ə, -shə) *n.* Downward displacement of the heart; prolapse of the heart.

car·di·o·pul·mo·nar·y (kär′dē-ō-pŏŏl′mə-nĕr′ē, -pŭl′-) *adj.* Of, relating to, or involving both the heart and the lungs.

cardiopulmonary bypass *n.* A procedure to circulate and oxygenate the blood during heart surgery involving the diversion of blood from the heart and lungs through a heart-lung machine and the return of oxygenated blood to the aorta.

cardiopulmonary murmur *n.* A murmur, synchronous with the heart's beat but disappearing when the breath is held, due to air movement in a part of lung compressed by the contracting heart.

cardiopulmonary resuscitation *n.* Restoration of cardiac output and pulmonary ventilation by artificial respiration and closed-chest massage after cardiac arrest and apnea.

car·di·or·rha·phy (kär′dē-ôr′ə-fē) *n.* The suturing of the heart wall.

car·di·or·rhex·is (kär′dē-ə-rĕk′sĭs) *n.* A rupture of the heart wall.

car·di·os·chi·sis (kär′dē-ŏs′kĭ-sĭs) *n.* The surgical division of adhesions between the heart and the pericardium or the chest wall in adhesive pericarditis.

car·di·o·sphyg·mo·graph (kär′dē-ō-sfĭg′mə-grăf′) *n.* An instrument for recording graphically the movements of the heart and the radial pulse.

car·di·o·ta·chom·e·ter (kär′dē-ō-tă-kŏm′ĭ-tər, -tə-) *n.* An instrument for measuring the rapidity of the heartbeat.

car·di·ot·o·my (kär′dē-ŏt′ə-mē) *n.* **1.** Surgical incision of the heart wall. **2.** Surgical incision of the cardiac end of the stomach.

car·di·o·ton·ic (kär′dē-ō-tŏn′ĭk) *adj.* Relating to or having a favorable effect upon the action of the heart. — **car′di·o·ton′ic** *n.*

car·di·o·val·vot·o·my (kär′dē-ō-văl-vŏt′ə-mē) *n.* See **cardiovalvulotomy.**

car·di·o·val·vu·li·tis (kär′dē-ō-văl′vyə-lī′tĭs) *n.* Inflammation of the heart valves.

car·di·o·val·vu·lot·o·my (kär′dē-ō-văl′vyə-lŏt′-ə-mē) *n.* Surgical correction of valvular stenosis by cutting or excising a part of a heart valve.

car·di·o·vas·cu·lar (kär′dē-ō-văs′kyə-lər) *adj.* Relating to or involving the heart and blood vessels.

cardiovascular system *n.* The heart and blood vessels considered as a whole.

car·di·o·ver·sion (kär′dē-ō-vûr′zhən, -shən) *n.* Restoration of the heartbeat to normal by electrical countershock.

car·di·o·ver·ter (kär′dē-ō-vûr′tər) *n.* A device for administering an electric shock in cardioversion.

car·di·tis (kär-dī′tĭs) *n.* Inflammation of the muscle tissue of the heart.

care·giv·er (kâr′gĭv′ər) *n.* **1.** A person, such as a physician, nurse, or social worker, who assists in the identification, prevention, or treatment of an illness or disability. **2.** A person, such as a parent or head of a household, who attends to the needs of a child or dependent adult.

Car·ey Coombs murmur (kâr′ē kōōmz′) *n.* An apical mid-diastolic murmur occurring in the acute stage of rheumatic mitral valvulitis and disappearing as the valvulitis subsides.

car·ies (kâr′ēz) *n., pl.* **caries.** Decay of a bone or tooth, especially dental caries.

car·i·o·gen·e·sis (kâr′ē-ō-jĕn′ĭ-sĭs) *n.* The production of dental caries. — **car′i·o·gen′ic** (-jĕn′ĭk) *adj.*

car·i·o·ge·nic·i·ty (kâr′ē-ō-jə-nĭs′ĭ-tē) *n.* The quality of being conducive to the production of dental caries.

Car·len's tube (kär′lənz) *n.* A double-lumen flexible endobronchial tube used for bronchospirometry, for isolation of one lung to prevent contamination or secretions from the other lung, or for ventilation of one lung.

car·min·a·tive (kär-mĭn′ə-tĭv, kär′mə-nā′-) *adj.* Inducing the expulsion of gas from the stomach and intestines. — *n.* A drug or agent that induces the expulsion of gastric or intestinal gas.

car·o·tene (kăr′ə-tēn′) or **car·o·tin** (-tĭn) *n.* An orange-yellow to red crystalline pigment that exists in three isomeric forms designated alpha, beta, and gamma; it is converted to vitamin A in the liver and is found in animal tissue and certain plants, such as carrots and squash.

car·o·te·ne·mi·a (kăr′ə-tə-nē′mē-ə) *n.* The presence of excess carotene in the blood, often resulting in yellowing of the skin.

car·o·te·no·sis cu·tis (kăr′ə-tə-nō′sĭs kyōō′tĭs) *n.*
A yellow or golden coloration of the skin caused
by an excessive intake of carotene.

ca·rot·id (kə-rŏt′ĭd) *n.* Either of the two major arteries, one on each side of the neck, that carry
blood to the head.

carotid artery *n.* **1.** An artery that originates on
the right from the brachiocephalic artery and on
the left from the aortic arch, runs upward into the
neck and divides opposite the upper border of the
thyroid cartilage; common carotid artery. **2.** An
artery with its origin in the common carotid artery and terminations in the maxillary and superficial temporal arteries as its terminal branches;
external carotid artery. **3.** An artery that arises
from the common carotid artery opposite the upper border of the thyroid cartilage and terminates
in the middle cranial fossa; internal carotid artery.

carotid bruit *n.* A bruit produced by blood flow in
a carotid artery.

ca·rot·o·dyn·i·a (kə-rŏt′ə-dĭn′ē-ə) *n.* Pain caused
by pressure on the carotid artery.

car·pal joint (kär′pəl) *n.* Any of the joints between
the carpal bones.

carpal tunnel *n.* A passageway in the wrist through
which the median nerve and the flexor muscles of
the hands and fingers pass.

carpal tunnel syndrome *n.* Chronic pain and paresthesia in the hand in the area of distribution of
the median nerve, caused by compression of the
median nerve within the carpal tunnel. Carpal
tunnel syndrome is often associated with repetitive motion, as in typing.

car·pec·to·my (kär-pĕk′tə-mē) *n.* Surgical removal of all or part of the carpus.

car·phen·a·zine ma·le·ate (kär-fĕn′ə-zēn′ mā′lē-
āt′, mə-lē′ət) *n.* A yellow, powdered, phenothiazine antipsychotic agent often used to treat acute
or chronic schizophrenia.

car·po·met·a·car·pal joint (kär′pō-mĕt′ə-kär′-
pəl) *n.* Any of the joints between the carpal and
the metacarpal bones.

car·pus (kär′pəs) *n., pl.* **-pi** (-pī′). **1.** The group of
eight carpal bones and associated soft parts form-
ing the joint between the forearm and the hand.
2. The carpal bones considered as a group.

car·ra·geen·an or **car·ra·geen·in** (kär′ə-gē′nən)
n. Any of a group of closely related colloids derived from Irish moss and several other red algae,
widely used in industrial, pharmaceutical, and
food products.

car·ri·er (kär′ē-ər) *n.* **1.** A person or an animal that
shows no symptoms of a disease but harbors the
infectious agent of that disease and is capable of
transmitting it to others. **2.** A quantity of naturally occurring element added to a minute amount
of pure isotope, especially a radioactive one, to
facilitate the chemical handling of the isotope. **3.**
An individual that carries, but does not express, a
gene for a particular recessive trait, yet when
mated with another carrier, can produce offspring that do.

carrier screening *n.* Indiscriminate examination of
members of a population to detect heterozygotes
for serious disorders and to discourage sexual union and marriage with other carriers. Prenatal diagnosis is used for a married couple who are both
carriers.

car·sick·ness (kär′sĭk′nĭs) *n.* A form of motion
sickness caused by travel in a motor vehicle.

car·ti·lage (kär′tl-ĭj) *n.* A tough, elastic, fibrous
connective tissue that is a major constituent of
embryonic and young vertebrate skeletons, is
converted largely to bone with maturation, and is
found in various parts of the adult body, such as
the joints, outer ear, and larynx.

cartilage bone *n.* A bone that develops in the region of a cartilage after the cartilage is partially
or completely destroyed.

cartilage capsule *n.* The basophilic matrix in hyaline cartilage surrounding a lacunae and its enclosed cartilage cell.

car·ti·lag·i·nous joint (kär′tl-ăj′ə-nəs) *n.* See
movable joint (sense 2).

ca·run·cle (kə-rŭng′kəl, kăr′ŭng′-) *n.* A fleshy, naked outgrowth.

cas·cade (kă-skād′) *n.* A succession of actions, processes, or operations, as of a physiological process.

cascade stomach *n.* A stomach in which the upper
posterior wall is pushed forward, creating an upper portion that fills until sufficient volume is
present to spill into the antrum.

case (kās) *n.* An occurrence of a disease or disorder.

ca·se·a·tion (kā′sē-ā′shən) *n.* Necrotic degeneration of bodily tissue into a soft, cheeselike substance.

case fatality rate *n.* The proportion of individuals
contracting a disease who die of that disease.

case history *n.* A detailed account of the facts affecting the development or condition of a person
or group under treatment or study.

ca·sein (kā′sēn′, -sē-ĭn) *n.* A white, tasteless, odorless protein precipitated from cow's milk by rennin that is the basis of cheese and is used in foods.

case study *n.* A detailed analysis of a person or
group, especially as a model of medical, psychiatric, psychological, or social phenomena.

cast (kăst) *n.* **1.** A rigid dressing, usually made of
gauze and plaster of Paris, used to immobilize an
injured body part, as in a fracture or dislocation.
2. A mass of fibrous material, coagulated protein,
or exudate that has taken the form of the cavity
in which it has been molded, such as the bronchial, renal, or vaginal cavity, and that is found histologically and in urine or sputum samples.

cast brace *n.* A specially designed plaster cast incorporating hinges and other brace components
and used in the treatment of fractures to promote
activity and joint motion.

Cas·tle's intrinsic factor (kăs′əlz) *n.* See **intrinsic
factor.**

cas·tor oil (kăs′tər) *n.* A colorless or pale yellowish
oil extracted from the seeds of the castor-oil
plant, used pharmaceutically as a laxative.

cas·trate (kăs′trāt′) *v.* **-trat·ed, -trat·ing, -trates. 1.** To remove the testicles of a male; emasculate. **2.** To remove the ovaries of a female.

cas·tra·tion (kă-strā′shən) *n.* **1.** Removal of the testicles or ovaries; sterilization. **2.** A psychological disorder that is manifested in the female as the fantasized loss of the penis or in the male as fear of its actual loss.

castration complex *n.* **1.** In psychoanalytic theory, a child's fear of injury to the genitals by the parent of the same sex as punishment for unconscious guilt over oedipal feelings. **2.** An unconscious fear of injury from those in authority.

CAT *abbr.* computerized axial tomography

ca·tab·o·lism (kə-tăb′ə-lĭz′əm) *n.* The metabolic breakdown of complex molecules into simpler ones, often resulting in a release of energy. — **cat′a·bol′ic** (kăt′ə-bŏl′ĭk) *adj.*

ca·tab·o·lite (kə-tăb′ə-līt′) *n.* A substance produced by the process of catabolism.

catabolite gene activator *n.* See **catabolite gene activator protein.**

catabolite gene activator protein *n.* A protein that can be activated by cyclic AMP and, in turn affects the action of RNA polymerase.

ca·tac·ro·tism (kə-tăk′rə-tĭz′əm) *n.* A condition of the pulse in which there are one or more secondary expansions of the artery following the main beat, producing upward notches or waves on the downstroke of the pulse tracing. — **cat′a·crot′ic** (kăt′ə-krŏt′ĭk) *adj.*

cat·a·di·cro·tism (kăt′ə-dī′krə-tĭz′əm) *n.* A condition of the pulse marked by two expansions of the artery following the main beat. — **cat′a·di·crot′ic** (-krŏt′ĭk) *adj.*

cat·a·gen (kăt′ə-jən, -jĕn′) *n.* A transitional phase of the hair cycle between growth and resting of the hair follicle.

cat·a·gen·e·sis (kăt′ə-jĕn′ĭ-sĭs) *n.* See **involution** (sense 3).

cat·a·lase (kăt′l-ās′, -āz′) *n.* An enzyme found in most living cells that catalyzes the decomposition of hydrogen peroxide to water and oxygen.

cat·a·lep·sy (kăt′l-ĕp′sē) *n.* A condition that occurs in a variety of physical and psychological disorders and is characterized by lack of response to external stimuli and by muscular rigidity, so that the limbs remain in whatever position they are placed. — **cat′a·lep′tic** (kăt′l-ĕp′tĭk) *adj.* — **cat′a·lep′toid′** *adj.*

ca·tal·y·sis (kə-tăl′ĭ-sĭs) *n., pl.* **-ses** (-sēz′). The action of a catalyst, especially an increase in the rate of a chemical reaction.

cat·a·lyst (kăt′l-ĭst) *n.* A substance that modifies and increases the rate of a reaction without being consumed in the process. — **cat′a·lyt′ic** (kăt′l-ĭt′-ĭk) *adj.*

cat·a·lyze (kăt′l-īz′) *v.* **-lyzed, -lyz·ing, -lyz·es.** To modify, especially to increase, the rate of a chemical reaction by catalysis.

cat·am·ne·sis (kăt′ăm-nē′sĭs) *n.* The medical history of a patient following an illness; the follow-up history. — **cat′am·nes′tic** (-nĕs′tĭk) *adj.*

cat·a·pha·si·a (kăt′ə-fā′zē-ə, -zhə) *n.* A speech disorder in which the same word or series of words is repeated involuntarily.

ca·taph·o·ra (kə-tăf′ə-rə) *n.* **1.** Semicoma. **2.** Somnolence interrupted by periods of partial consciousness.

cat·a·pla·sia (kăt′ə-plā′zhə, -zhē-ə) or **cat·a·pla·sis** (-plā′sĭs) *n.* Degenerative reversion of cells or tissue to a less differentiated form.

cat·a·plex·y (kăt′ə-plĕk′sē) *n.* A sudden loss of muscle tone and strength, usually caused by an intense emotional stimulus. — **cat′a·plec′tic** (-plĕk′tĭk) *adj.*

cat·a·ract (kăt′ə-răkt′) *n.* Opacity of the lens or capsule of the eye, causing impairment of vision or blindness. — **cat′a·rac′tous** (-răk′təs) *adj.*

ca·tarrh (kə-tär′) *n.* Inflammation of mucous membranes, especially of the nose and throat. — **ca·tarrh′al** *adj.*

catarrhal gastritis *n.* Gastritis with excessive secretion of mucus.

catarrhal inflammation *n.* An inflammatory process that occurs in mucous membranes and is characterized by increased blood flow to the mucosal vessels, edema of the interstitial tissue, and profuse discharge of mucus and epithelial debris.

cat·a·stal·sis (kăt′ə-stŏl′sĭs, -stăl′-) *n.* A downward wave of contraction occurring in the gastrointestinal tract during digestion.

cat·a·stal·tic (kăt′ə-stŏl′tĭk, -stăl′-) *adj.* Restricting or inhibitory; restraining.

cat·a·stroph·ic reaction (kăt′ə-strŏf′ĭk) *n.* Disorganized behavior in response to a severe shock or threatening situation with which the person cannot cope.

cat·a·to·ni·a (kăt′ə-tō′nē-ə) *n.* An abnormal condition often associated with schizophrenia and variously characterized by stupor, stereotypy, mania, and either rigidity or extreme flexibility of the limbs. — **cat′a·ton′ic** (-tŏn′ĭk) *adj.*

catatonic schizophrenia *n.* A type of schizophrenia characterized by marked disturbances in activity resulting in either generalized inhibition or excessive activity.

cat·a·tri·cro·tism (kăt′ə-trī′krə-tĭz′əm) *n.* An abnormality of the pulse marked by three minor expansions of the artery following the main beat. — **cat′a·tri·crot′ic** (-krŏt′ĭk) *adj.*

cat-cry syndrome *n.* See **cri-du-chat syndrome.**

cat·e·cho·la·mine (kăt′ĭ-kō′lə-mēn′, -kô′-) *n.* Any of a group of amines composed of a pyrocatechol molecule and a portion of an amine that have important physiological effects as neurotransmitters and hormones.

cat·er·pil·lar flap (kăt′ər-pĭl′ər, kăt′ə-) *n.* A tubed flap transferred end-over-end in stages from the donor area to a distant recipient area.

cat·gut (kăt′gŭt′) *n.* A tough, thin cord made from the treated and stretched intestines of certain animals and used for surgical ligatures.

ca·thar·sis (kə-thär′sĭs) *n., pl.* **-ses** (-sēz). **1.** Purgation. **2.** A psychological technique used to relieve tension and anxiety by bringing repressed feelings and fears to consciousness. **3.** The therapeutic result of this process; abreaction.

ca·thar·tic (kə-thär′tĭk) *adj.* Inducing catharsis; purgative. — *n.* An agent for purging the bowels, especially a laxative.

cath·e·ter (kăth′ĭ-tər) *n.* A hollow, flexible tube inserted into a body cavity, duct, or vessel to allow the passage of fluids or distend a passageway; its many uses include the drainage of urine from the bladder through the urethra and the diagnosis of heart disorders when inserted through a blood vessel into the heart.

cath·e·ter·ize (kăth′ĭ-tə-rīz′) *v.* -ized, -iz·ing, -iz·es. To introduce a catheter into. — **cath′e·ter·i·za′tion** (-rĭ-zā′shən).

ca·thex·is (kə-thĕk′sĭs) *n., pl.* -thex·es (-thĕk′sēz). Concentration of emotional energy on an object or idea.

cat·i·on (kăt′ī′ən) *n.* An ion or group of ions having a positive charge and characteristically moving toward the negative electrode in electrolysis.

CAT scanner (kăt) *n.* A device that produces cross-sectional views of an internal body structure using computerized axial tomography.

cat scratch disease *n.* An infectious disease that may follow the scratch or bite of a cat, producing inflammation of the regional lymph nodes and a low-grade fever.

cau·da (kô′də) *n., pl.* -dae (-dē′). A tail or taillike structure, or a tapering or elongated extremity of an organ or other part.

cau·dal (kôd′l) *adj.* **1.** Of, at, or near the tail or hind parts; posterior. **2.** Situated beneath or on the underside; inferior. **3.** Taillike.

caudal anesthesia *n.* Regional anesthesia by injection of a local anesthetic into the epidural space via the sacral hiatus.

caul (kôl) *n.* **1.** A portion of the amnion, especially when it covers the head of a fetus at birth. **2.** See **greater omentum**.

cau·li·flow·er ear (kô′lĭ-flou′ər) *n.* An ear that is swollen, hardened, and deformed from extravasation of blood following repeated blows.

cau·mes·the·sia (kô′mĭs-thē′zhə, -zē-ə) *n.* A sensation of burning heat irrespective of the temperature of the air.

cau·sal·gi·a (kô-săl′jē-ə, -jə, -zăl′-) *n.* A persistent, severe burning sensation of the skin, usually following injury to a peripheral nerve.

cau·ter·ize (kô′tə-rīz′) *v.* -ized, -iz·ing, -iz·es. To burn or sear with a cautery. — **cau′ter·i·za′tion** (-tər-ĭ-zā′shən) *n.*

cau·ter·y (kô′tə-rē) *n.* **1.** An agent or instrument used to destroy tissue by burning, searing, cutting, or scarring, including caustic substances, electric currents, lasers, and very hot or very cold instruments. **2.** The act or process of cauterizing.

ca·ve·o·la (kā-vē′ə-lə) *n., pl.* -lae (-lē′). A small pocket, vesicle, or recess, especially one communicating with the outside of a cell and indenting both cytoplasm and membrane.

cav·er·nil·o·quy (kăv′ər-nĭl′ə-kwē) *n.* The low-pitched, resonant sound of the voice detected over a lung cavity.

cav·er·nos·to·my (kăv′ər-nŏs′tə-mē) *n.* Surgical opening and drainage of a cavity.

cavernous sinus syndrome *n.* A syndrome caused by thrombosis of the cavernous intracranial sinus and marked by edema of the eyelids and conjunctivae and by paralysis of the third, fourth, and sixth cranial nerves.

cav·i·ta·tion (kăv′ĭ-tā′shən) *n.* The formation of cavities in a body tissue or an organ, especially those formed in the lung in tuberculosis.

ca·vi·tis (kā-vī′tĭs) *n.* Inflammation of a vena cava.

cav·i·ty (kăv′ĭ-tē) *n.* **1.** A hollow area within the body, such as a sinus cavity. **2.** A pitted area in a tooth caused by caries.

ca·vo·gram or **ca·va·gram** (kā′və-grăm′) *n.* A radiographic depiction of a vena cava.

ca·vog·ra·phy (kā-vŏg′rə-fē) *n.* Angiography of a vena cava.

ca·vum (kā′vəm) *n., pl.* -va (-və). A hollow space, hole, or cavity.

CBC *abbr.* complete blood count

cc or **c.c.** *abbr.* cubic centimeter

CCU *abbr.* coronary care unit; critical care unit

CDC *abbr.* Centers for Disease Control and Prevention

cDNA (sē′dē′ĕn-ā′) *n.* Complementary DNA; single-stranded DNA that is complementary to mRNA in the presence of reverse transcriptase.

CEA *abbr.* carcinoembryonic antigen

ce·cec·to·my (sē-sĕk′tə-mē) *n.* Surgical excision of all or part of the cecum.

ce·ci·tis (sē-sī′tĭs) *n.* Inflammation of the cecum.

ce·co·cen·tral scotoma (sē′kō-sĕn′trəl) *n.* Any of three forms of scotoma involving the optic disk area and the papillomacular fibers.

ce·co·co·los·to·my (sē′kō-kə-lŏs′tə-mē) *n.* Surgical formation of an anastomosis between the cecum and the colon.

ce·co·il·e·os·to·my (sē′kō-ĭl′ē-ŏs′tə-mē) *n.* See **il·eocecostomy**.

ce·co·pex·y (sē′kə-pĕk′sē) *n.* Surgical operation for anchoring the cecum to the abdominal wall.

ce·co·pli·ca·tion (sē′kə-plĭ-kā′shən) *n.* Surgical reduction in size of a dilated cecum by making folds or tucks in its wall.

ce·cor·rha·phy (sē-kôr′ə-fē) *n.* Suture of the cecum.

ce·co·sig·moid·os·to·my (sē′kō-sĭg′moi-dŏs′tə-mē) *n.* Surgical formation of an anastomosis between the cecum and the sigmoid colon.

ce·cos·to·my (sē-kŏs′tə-mē) *n.* Surgical formation of a permanent artificial opening into the cecum.

ce·cot·o·my (sē-kŏt′ə-mē) *n.* Incision into the cecum.

ce·cum or **cae·cum** (sē′kəm) *n., pl.* -ca (-kə). **1.** The large blind pouch forming the beginning of the large intestine. **2.** A saclike cavity with only one opening.

cef·a·drox·il (sĕf′ə-drŏk′səl) *n.* A semisynthetic, broad-spectrum antibiotic derived from cephalosporin with action similar to the penicillins.

cef·o·per·a·zone sodium (sĕf′ō-pĕr′ə-zōn′) *n.* A semisynthetic, parenteral cephalosporin antibiotic effective against a wide range of aerobic and anaerobic, gram-positive and gram-negative pathogens.

cef·o·tax·ime sodium (sĕf′ō-tăk′sēm′) *n.* A semisynthetic, parenteral cephalosporin antibiotic that inhibits cell-wall synthesis and is effective against a wide range of infections.

ce·fox·i·tin (sə-fŏk′sĭ-tĭn) *n.* A broadspectrum, semisynthetic antibiotic used for lower respiratory and other infections and septicemia.

cef·taz·i·dime (sĕf-tăz′ĭ-dēm′) *n.* A cephalosporin antibiotic especially effective against enterobacteria and species of *Pseudomonas*.

cef·ti·zox·ime sodium (sĕf′tĭ-zŏk′sēm′) *n.* A broad-spectrum, semisynthetic cephalosporin antibiotic effective against a range of infections including gonorrhea and septicemia.

celiac disease *n.* A malabsorption disease characterized by sensitivity to gluten and atrophy of the mucosa of the upper small intestine, manifested by diarrhea, steatorrhea, and nutritional deficiencies.

celiac ganglion *n.* Any of the largest and highest group of sympathetic prevertebral ganglia, on the upper part of the abdominal aorta and innervating the stomach, liver, gallbladder, spleen, kidney, small intestine, and the ascending and transverse colon.

celiac gland *n.* Any of the various nodes situated along the celiac trunk that receive lymphatic drainage from the stomach, duodenum, pancreas, spleen, and biliary tract.

celiac plexus *n.* **1.** The largest of the autonomic plexuses, lying in front of the aorta and behind the stomach, and sending branches to all the abdominal viscera. **2.** A lymphatic plexus formed of the superior mesenteric lymph nodes and of the nodes behind the stomach, duodenum, and pancreas, with the connecting vessels.

celiac plexus reflex *n.* A fall in arterial blood pressure coincident with surgical manipulations in the upper abdomen during general anesthesia.

ce·li·o·en·ter·ot·o·my (sē′lē-ō-ĕn′tə-rŏt′ə-mē) *n.* An incision into the intestine through the abdominal wall.

ce·li·o·gas·trot·o·my (sē′lē-ō-gă-strŏt′ə-mē) *n.* An incision into the stomach through the abdomen.

ce·li·op·a·thy (sē′lē-ŏp′ə-thē) *n.* An abdominal disease.

ce·li·or·rha·phy (sē′lē-ôr′ə-fē) *n.* Suture of the abdominal wall.

ce·li·os·co·py (sē′lē-ŏs′kə-pē) *n.* See **peritoneoscopy**.

ce·li·ot·o·my (sē′lē-ŏt′ə-mē) *n.* Surgical incision of the abdomen.

ce·li·tis (sē-lī′tĭs) *n.* Inflammation of the abdomen.

cell (sĕl) *n.* **1.** The smallest structural unit of an organism that is capable of independent functioning, consisting of one or more nuclei, cytoplasm, and various organelles, all surrounded by a sem-

ipermeable cell membrane. **2.** A small enclosed cavity or space.

cell body *n.* The part of a neuron containing the nucleus; does not include the axon and dendrites.

cell culture *n.* **1.** The maintenance or growth of dispersed cells in a medium after removal from the body. **2.** A culture of such cells.

cell cycle *n.* The series of events involving the growth, replication, and division of a eukaryotic cell.

cell division *n.* The process by which a cell divides to form two daughter cells. Upon completion of the process, each daughter cell contains the same genetic material as the original cell and roughly half its cytoplasm.

cell-mediated immune response *n.* The immune response produced when sensitized T cells directly attack foreign antigens and secrete lymphokines that initiate an immune response.

cell-mediated immunity *n.* Immunity resulting from a cell-mediated immune response.

cell membrane *n.* The semipermeable membrane that encloses the cytoplasm of a cell.

cell-transfer therapy *n.* A therapeutic technique in which cells from a person with a disease, usually cancer, are removed and genetically modified to make them cytotoxic or to improve their cytotoxic abilities before they are returned to the donor.

cel·lu·lar (sĕl′yə-lər) *adj.* **1.** Of, relating to, or resembling a cell. **2.** Consisting of, composed of, or containing a cell or cells.

cellular immune response *n.* See **cell-mediated immune response**.

cellular immunity *n.* See **cell-mediated immunity**.

cellular immunodeficiency *n.* Any of a group of disorders associated with recurrent bacterial, fungal, protozoal, and viral infections and characterized by atrophy of the thymus gland, depressed cell-mediated immunity, and defective humoral immunity.

cellular infiltration *n.* The migration of cells from their sources of origin, or the direct extension of cells as a result of unusual growth and multiplication, into organs or tissues.

cel·lu·lar·i·ty (sĕl′yə-lăr′ĭ-tē) *n.* The state of a tissue or other mass with regard to the degree, quality, or condition of cells present in it.

cellular pathology *n.* The interpretation of disease origins in terms of cellular alterations or the failure of cells to maintain homeostasis.

cellular respiration *n.* The series of metabolic processes by which living cells produce energy through the oxidation of organic substances.

cel·lu·lite (sĕl′yə-līt′) *n.* A fatty deposit causing a dimpled or uneven appearance, as around the thighs and buttocks.

cel·lu·li·tis (sĕl′yə-lī′tĭs) *n.* A spreading inflammation of subcutaneous or connective tissue.

cel·lu·lose (sĕl′yə-lōs′, -lōz′) *n.* A complex carbohydrate that is composed of glucose units, forms the main constituent of the cell wall in most plants, and is important in the manufacture of pharmaceuticals.

cell wall *n.* The rigid outermost cell layer found in plants and certain algae, bacteria, and fungi but characteristically absent from animal cells.

ce·lo·phle·bi·tis (sē′lō-flĭ-bī′tĭs) *n.* See **cavitis**.

ce·lo·scope (sē′lə-skōp′) *n.* An optical device for examining the interior of a body cavity.

ce·los·co·py (sē-lŏs′kə-pē) *n.* The examination of a body cavity with a celoscope.

ce·lo·so·mi·a (sē′lō-sō′mē-ə) *n.* A congenital protrusion of the abdomen or thorax, usually accompanied by defects of the sternum and ribs as well as of the abdominal walls.

ce·lot·o·my (sē-lŏt′ə-mē) *n.* See **herniotomy**.

Cel·si·us (sĕl′sē-əs, -shəs) *adj.* Of or relating to a temperature scale that registers the freezing point of water as 0° and the boiling point as 100° under normal atmospheric pressure.

ce·ment·i·cle (sĭ-mĕn′tĭ-kəl) *n.* A spherical calcified body lying free within the periodontal membrane or fused with the cementum of the tooth.

ce·men·ti·fy·ing fibroma (sĭ-mĕn′tə-fī′ĭng) *n.* A form of cementoma occurring in the mandible of the elderly and consisting of cellular fibrous tissue containing round or lobulated calcified masses of cementum.

cement line *n.* The refractile boundary of an osteon in compact bone.

ce·men·to·blast (sĭ-mĕn′tə-blăst′) *n.* One of the cells that takes part in the formation of the cementum.

ce·men·to·blas·to·ma (sĭ-mĕn′tō-blă-stō′mə) *n.* A benign odontogenic tumor in which the cells are developing into cementoblasts and there is a small amount of cementum or cementumlike material at the tooth root.

ce·men·to·cla·si·a (sĭ-mĕn′tō-klā′zē-ə, -zhə) *n.* The destruction of cementum by cementoclasts.

ce·men·to·clast (sĭ-mĕn′tə-klăst′) *n.* One of the multinucleated giant cells, similar to osteoclasts, that destroy cementum.

ce·men·to·ma (sē′mĕn-tō′mə, sĭ-mĕn′-) *n.* A tumor composed of tissue resembling cementum.

ce·men·tum (sĭ-mĕn′təm) *n.* A bonelike substance covering the root of a tooth.

ce·nes·the·si·a (sē′nĭs-thē′zhə) *n.* The sensation caused by the normal functioning of the internal organs; a sense of conscious existence. — **ce′nes·the′sic** (-zĭk) *adj.*

cen·ter (sĕn′tər) *n.* **1.** A point or place in the body that is equally distant from its sides or outer boundaries; the middle. **2.** A group of neurons in the central nervous system that control a particular function.

cen·te·sis (sĕn-tē′sĭs) *n., pl.* **-ses** (-sēz′). See **puncture**.

cen·ti·grade (sĕn′tĭ-grād′) *adj.* See **Celsius**.

cen·ti·me·ter (sĕn′tə-mē′tər) *n.* A unit of length equal to one hundredth (10^{-2}) of a meter (0.3937 inch).

cen·tral cord syndrome (sĕn′trəl) *n.* A syndrome characterized by paraplegia most severely involving the upper extremities caused by injury to the central part of the cervical spinal cord.

central fovea *n.* See **fovea centralis**.

central ganglioneuroma *n.* A rare form of glioma composed of nearly mature, slowly growing, neuronlike cells, found in the optic chiasm or cerebral white matter.

central necrosis *n.* Necrosis involving the inner portions of a tissue or organ.

central nervous system *n.* The portion of the vertebrate nervous system consisting of the brain and spinal cord.

central paralysis *n.* Paralysis due to a lesion in the brain or spinal cord.

central scotoma *n.* A scotoma involving the fixation point.

central venous catheter *n.* A catheter passed through a peripheral vein and ending in the thoracic vena cava; it is used to measure venous pressure or to infuse concentrated solutions.

central vision *n.* Vision produced by light rays falling directly on the fovea centralis.

cen·trif·u·gal nerve (sĕn-trĭf′yə-gəl, -trĭf′ə-) *n.* See **efferent nerve**.

cen·tri·fuge (sĕn′trə-fyōōj′) *n.* An apparatus consisting essentially of a compartment spun about a central axis to separate contained materials of different specific gravities, or to separate colloidal particles suspended in a liquid. — *v.* **-fuged, -fug·ing, -fug·es.** To rotate (something) in a centrifuge or to separate, dehydrate, or test by means of this apparatus.

cen·tri·ole (sĕn′trē-ōl′) *n.* One of two cylindrical cellular structures that form the astrospheres during mitosis.

centripetal nerve *n.* See **afferent nerve**.

cen·tro·ki·ne·sia (sĕn′trō-kĭ-nē′zhə, -kĭ-) *n.* A movement occurring as a result of a stimulus of central origin. — **cen′tro·ki·net′ic** (-nĕt′ĭk) *adj.*

cen·tro·mere (sĕn′trə-mēr′) *n.* The most condensed and constricted region of a chromosome to which the spindle fiber is attached during mitosis.

cen·tro·some (sĕn′trə-sōm′) *n.* A cytoplasmic region adjacent to the nucleus that contains the centrioles and serves to organize microtubules.

cen·trum (sĕn′trəm) *n., pl.* **-trums** or **-tra** (-trə). **1.** A center of any kind, especially an anatomical center. **2.** The major part of a vertebra, exclusive of the bases of the neural arch.

ceph·al·al·gia (sĕf′ə-lăl′jə, -jē-ə) *n.* Pain in the head.

ceph·al·e·de·ma (sĕf′ə-lĭ-dē′mə) *n.* Edema of the head.

ceph·a·lex·in (sĕf′ə-lĕk′sĭn) *n.* A semisynthetic analogue of cephalosporin used in the treatment of respiratory and urinary tract infections.

ceph·al·he·ma·to·cele (sĕf′əl-hē′mə-tə-sēl′, -hĭ-măt′ə-) or **ceph·a·lo·he·ma·to·cele** (sĕf′ə-lō-) *n.* A cephalhematoma in contact with the cerebral sinuses.

ceph·al·he·ma·to·ma (sĕf′əl-hē′mə-tō′mə) or **ceph·a·lo·he·ma·to·ma** (sĕf′ə-lō-) *n.* A blood cyst, tumor, or swelling of the scalp in a newborn infant due to an effusion of blood beneath the pericranium usually as a result of injury.

ceph·al·hy·dro·cele (sĕf'əl-hī'drə-sēl') n. Effusion of cerebrospinal fluid beneath the scalp in fractures of the skull.

ce·phal·ic (sə-făl'ĭk) adj. **1.** Of or relating to the head. **2.** Located on, in, or near the head.

cephalic index n. The ratio of the maximum width of the head to its maximum length, multiplied by 100.

cephalic pole n. The head end of the fetus.

cephalic presentation n. Presentation of the fetus headfirst during birth.

cephalic vein n. A vein that arises in the dorsal venous rete of the hand and passes upward in front of the elbow and along the lateral side of the arm.

cephalic version n. Version in which the fetus is turned so that the head presents.

ceph·a·lin (sĕf'ə-lĭn) or **keph·a·lin** (kĕf'-) n. Any of a group of phospholipids having hemostatic properties and found especially in the nervous tissue of the brain and spinal cord.

ceph·a·li·tis (sĕf'ə-lī'tĭs) n. See **encephalitis**.

ceph·a·lo·cele (sĕf'ə-lō-sēl') n. See **encephalocele**.

ceph·a·lo·cen·te·sis (sĕf'ə-lō-sĕn-tē'sĭs) n. The passage of a hollow needle or a trocar and cannula into the brain to drain an abscess or the fluid of a hydrocephalus.

ceph·a·lo·dyn·i·a (sĕf'ə-lō-dĭn'ē-ə) n. Pain in the head; headache.

ceph·a·lo·meg·a·ly (sĕf'ə-lō-mĕg'ə-lē) n. Enlargement of the head.

ceph·a·lo·men·in·gi·tis (sĕf'ə-lō-mĕn'ĭn-jī'tĭs) n. Inflammation of the membranes of the brain.

ceph·a·lom·e·ter (sĕf'ə-lŏm'ĭ-tər) n. An instrument used to position the head for measurement and radiographic examination.

ceph·a·lom·e·try (sĕf'ə-lŏm'ĭ-trē) n. **1.** The scientific measurement of the bones of the cranium and the face. **2.** A scientific study of the measurement of the head with relation to specific reference points to assess facial growth and development for orthodontic applications. — **ceph'a·lo·met'ric** (-lō-mĕt'rĭk) adj. — **ceph'a·lo·met'rics** (-rĭks) n.

ceph·a·lop·a·thy (sĕf'ə-lŏp'ə-thē) n. See **encephalopathy**.

ceph·a·lo·spo·rin (sĕf-ə-lə-spôr'ĭn) n. Any of various broad-spectrum antibiotics, closely related to the penicillins, that were originally derived from the fungus *Cephalosporium acremonium*.

ceph·a·lo·stat (sĕf'ə-lō-stăt') n. See **cephalometer**.

cer·clage (sār-kläzh', sər-) n. **1.** The use of an encircling wire loop or ring to bring together the ends of an obliquely fractured bone or the fragments of a broken patella. **2.** The use of an encircling silicone band around the sclera of the eye to bring together the choroid and retinal pigment epithelium to correct retinal detachment. **3.** The placement of a nonabsorbable suture around a functionally incompetent uterine cervix.

ce·re·a flex·i·bil·i·tas (sĕr'ē-ə flĕk'sə-bĭl'ĭ-təs) n. The capacity to maintain the limbs or other bodily parts in whatever position they are placed, as in catalepsy.

cerebellar cortex n. The thin gray surface layer of the cerebellum, consisting of an outer molecular layer and an inner granular layer.

cerebellar gait n. A staggering gait, often with a tendency to fall.

cerebellar hemisphere n. Either of the two lobes of the cerebellum lateral to the vermis.

cer·e·bel·li·tis (sĕr'ə-bĕ-lī'tĭs) n. Inflammation of the cerebellum.

cer·e·bel·lum (sĕr'ə-bĕl'əm) n., pl. **-bel·lums** or **-bel·la** (-bĕl'ə). The trilobed structure of the brain, lying posterior to the pons and medulla oblongata and inferior to the occipital lobes of the cerebral hemispheres, responsible for the regulation and coordination of complex voluntary muscular movement and the maintenance of posture and balance. — **cer'e·bel'lar** (-bĕl'ər) adj.

cer·e·bral (sĕr'ə-brəl, sə-rē'-) adj. Of or relating to the brain or cerebrum.

cerebral accident n. See **stroke** (sense 2).

cerebral anesthesia n. Loss of sensation due to a lesion of the cerebral cortex or other part of the cerebrum.

cerebral death n. See **brain death**.

cerebral decompression n. The relief of intracranial pressure by surgical removal of a piece of the cranium, usually in the subtemporal region, and incision of the dura mater.

cerebral edema n. Brain swelling due to increased volume of the extravascular compartment from the uptake of water in the cerebellar nerve network and the white matter.

cerebral gigantism n. A syndrome of unknown cause characterized by large size at birth and an accelerated growth rate in infancy and early childhood without a similar increase in serum growth hormone levels; it is marked by acromegalic features and moderate mental retardation.

cerebral hemisphere n. Either of the two symmetrical halves of the cerebrum, as divided by the longitudinal cerebral fissure.

cerebral hemorrhage n. Bleeding into the substance of the cerebrum, usually in the region of the internal capsule.

cerebral hernia n. Protrusion of brain substance through a defect in the skull.

cerebral palsy n. A disorder usually caused by brain damage occurring at or before birth and marked by muscular impairment. Often accompanied by poor coordination, it sometimes involves speech and learning difficulties. — **cer'e·bral-pal'sied** (sĕr'ə-brəl-pôl'zēd, sə-rē'-) adj.

cerebral sphingolipidosis n. Any of a group of inherited diseases characterized by progressive spastic paralysis, blindness, convulsions, mental retardation, and, ultimately, death, and caused by abnormal phospholipid metabolism. The disease occurs almost exclusively in individuals of eastern European Jewish descent in four enzymatically distinct forms: infantile (Tay-Sachs disease); early juvenile (Jansky-Bielschowsky disease); late juvenile (Spielmeyer-Vogt disease); and adult (Kufs disease).

cer·e·bra·tion (sĕr'ə-brā'shən) *n.* Activity of the mental processes; thinking.

cer·e·bri·tis (sĕr'ə-brī'tĭs) *n.* Nonlocalized inflammation of the cerebrum.

cer·e·bro·ma·la·ci·a (sĕr'ə-brō-mə-lā'shē-ə, -shə) *n.* See encephalomalacia.

cer·e·bro·men·in·gi·tis (sĕr'ə-brō-mĕn'ĭn-jī'tĭs) *n.* See meningoencephalitis.

cer·e·brop·a·thy (sĕr'ə-brŏp'ə-thē) *n.* See encephalopathy.

cer·e·bro·scle·ro·sis (sĕr'ə-brō-sklə-rō'sĭs) *n.* Hardening of the substance of the cerebral hemispheres.

cer·e·bro·side (sĕr'ə-brə-sīd', sə-rē'-) *n.* Any of various lipid compounds containing glucose or galactose and glucose, and found in the brain and other nerve tissue, especially the myelin sheath.

cerebroside lipidosis *n.* See Gaucher's disease.

cer·e·bro·si·do·sis (sĕr'ə-brō-sĭ-dō'sĭs) *n.* See Gaucher's disease.

cer·e·bro·sis (sĕr'ə-brō'sĭs) *n.* See encephalosis.

cer·e·bro·spi·nal (sĕr'ə-brō-spī'nəl, sə-rē'brō-) *adj.* Relating to the brain and the spinal cord.

cerebrospinal fluid *n.* The serumlike fluid that circulates through the ventricles of the brain, the cavity of the spinal cord, and the subarachnoid space, functioning as a shock absorber.

cerebrospinal meningitis *n.* See meningococcal meningitis.

cerebrospinal pressure *n.* Tension of the cerebrospinal fluid when measured by an instrument such as a manometer.

cer·e·brot·o·my (sĕr'ə-brŏt'ə-mē) *n.* Incision of the brain substance.

cer·e·bro·vas·cu·lar (sĕr'ə-brō-văs'kyə-lər, sə-rē'brō-) *adj.* Relating to the blood supply to the brain.

cerebrovascular accident *n.* See stroke (sense 2).

cer·e·brum (sĕr'ə-brəm, sə-rē'-) *n., pl.* **-brums** or **-bra** (-brə). The largest portion of the brain, including mainly the cerebral hemispheres that are joined at the bottom by the corpus callosum. It controls and integrates motor, sensory, and higher mental functions, such as thought, reason, emotion, and memory.

ce·ri·um (sĕr'ē-əm) *n.* A lustrous, malleable metallic rare-earth element with atomic number 58 that is used in lighter flint alloys.

cer·ti·fi·ca·tion (sûr'tə-fĭ-kā'shən) *n.* **1.** The reporting to health authorities of those diseases legally required to be reported. **2.** The attainment of board certification in a specialty. **3.** The court procedure by which a patient is committed to a mental institution. **4.** Involuntary mental hospitalization. — **cer·ti·fi·a·ble** (-fī'ə-bəl) *adj.*

ce·ru·le·in (sə-rōō'lē-ən) *n.* A decapeptide that stimulates smooth muscle, especially gallbladder contraction, and increases digestive secretions.

ce·ru·lo·plas·min (sə-rōō'lō-plăz'mĭn) *n.* A blue, copper-containing globulin of blood plasma, be-

lieved to play a part in erythropoiesis and oxygen reduction.

ce·ru·men (sə-rōō'mən) *n.* The brownish yellow, waxy secretion of the ceruminous glands of the external auditory meatus; earwax. — **ce·ru'mi·nal** (-mə-nəl), **ce·ru'mi·nous** (-mə-nəs) *adj.*

ce·ru·mi·no·lyt·ic (sə-rōō'mə-nō-lĭt'ĭk) *n.* A substance instilled into the external auditory canal to soften earwax.

ce·ru·mi·no·sis (sə-rōō'mə-nō'sĭs) *n.* Excessive formation of cerumen.

ce·ru·mi·nous gland (sə-rōō'mə-nəs) *n.* Any of the modified sudoriferous glands in the external auditory canal that secrete a waxy substance.

cer·vi·cal (sûr'vĭ-kəl) *adj.* Of or relating to a neck or a cervix.

cervical canal *n.* A spindle-shaped canal extending from the isthmus of the uterus to the opening of the uterus into the vagina.

cervical cap *n.* A small, rubber, cup-shaped contraceptive device that fits over the uterine cervix to prevent the entry of sperm.

cervical in·tra·ep·i·the·li·al neoplasia (ĭn'trə-ĕp'ə-thē'lē-əl) *n.* Dysplastic changes in the uterine cervix that may be precursors of squamous cell carcinoma.

cervical nerve *n.* Any of the nerves whose nuclei of origin are in the cervical spinal cord.

cervical pregnancy *n.* An ectopic pregnancy developing in the cervical canal.

cervical rib *n.* A supernumerary rib articulating with a cervical vertebra, usually the seventh, but not reaching the sternum in front.

cervical rib syndrome *n.* A syndrome caused by pressure on the nerves of the brachial plexus by a cervical rib and manifested by pain and tingling along the forearm and hand.

cer·vi·cec·to·my (sûr'vĭ-sĕk'tə-mē) *n.* Excision of the cervix of the uterus.

cer·vi·ci·tis (sûr'vĭ-sī'tĭs) *n.* Inflammation of the mucous membrane of the uterine cervix, frequently affecting the deeper structures.

cer·vi·co·dyn·ia (sûr'vĭ-kō-dĭn'ē-ə) *n.* Neck pain.

cer·vi·cog·ra·phy (sûr'vĭ-kŏg'rə-fē) *n.* A technique, equivalent to colposcopy, for photographing part or all of the uterine cervix.

cer·vi·co·plas·ty (sûr'vĭ-kə-plăs'tē) *n.* Plastic surgery on the neck or on the cervix of the uterus.

cer·vi·co·thor·ac·ic ganglion (sûr'vĭ-kō-thə-răs'-ĭk) *n.* A sympathetic trunk ganglion behind the subclavian artery at the level of the seventh cervical vertebra.

cer·vi·cot·o·my (sûr'vĭ-kŏt'ə-mē) *n.* Incision into the cervix of the uterus.

cer·vix (sûr'vĭks) *n., pl.* **cer·vix·es** or **cer·vi·ces** (sûr'vĭ-sēz', sər-vī'sēz). **1.** The neck. **2.** A neck-shaped anatomical structure, such as the narrow outer end of the uterus.

cervix u·ter·i (yōō'tə-rī') *n.* The lower part of the uterus extending from the isthmus of the uterus into the vagina; neck of uterus; neck of womb.

ce·sar·e·an or **cae·sar·e·an** or **cae·sar·i·an** or **ce·sar·i·an** (sĭ-zâr'ē-ən) *n.* A cesarean section.

cesarean hysterectomy or **caesarean hysterectomy** *n.* A cesarean section followed by removal of the uterus.

cesarean operation *n.* See **cesarean section.**

cesarean section or **caesarean section** *n.* Surgical incision through the wall of the abdomen and uterus for the delivery of a fetus.

cesarean section or **caesarean section** *n.* A surgical incision through the abdominal wall and uterus, performed to deliver a fetus.

ce·si·um or **cae·si·um** (sē′zē-əm) *n.* A soft ductile metal with atomic number 55 that is liquid at room temperature and used in photoelectric cells.

Ces·tan–Che·nais syndrome (sĕ-stän′shə-nā′, sĕ-stän′-) *n.* A syndrome caused by lesions of the brain stem and resulting in hemianesthesia, paralysis of the larynx and soft palate, and ptosis.

ces·tode (sĕs′tōd′) or **ces·toid** (-toid′) *n.* Any of various parasitic flatworms of the class Cestoidea, including the tapeworms, having a long, flat body equipped with a specialized organ of attachment at one end. — **ces′tode, ces′toid′** *adj.*

CF *abbr.* cystic fibrosis

CFS *abbr.* chronic fatigue syndrome

CG *abbr.* chorionic gonadotropin

Chad·dock reflex (chăd′ək) *n.* See **Chaddock sign.**

Chaddock sign *n.* Extension of the big toe in response to irritation of the skin covering the malleolus of the ankle joint, observed in organic disease of the corticospinal reflex paths.

chafe (chāf) *v.* **chafed, chaf·ing, chafes.** To cause irritation of the skin by friction.

Cha·gas disease or **Cha·gas–Cruz disease** (shä′gəs-) *n.* See **South American trypanosomiasis.**

cha·go·ma (shə-gō′mə) *n.* The skin lesion in acute Chagas disease.

chain (chān) *n.* **1.** A group of atoms bonded in a spatial configuration like links in a chain. **2.** A linear arrangement of living things such as cells or bacteria.

chain reaction *n.* A series of events in which each induces or influences the next.

chain reflex *n.* A series of reflexes, each serving as a stimulus for the next.

cha·la·sia (kə-lā′zē-ə, -zhə) or **cha·la·sis** (-lā′sĭs) *n.* The inhibition and relaxation of a previously sustained contraction of a muscle or synergistic group of muscles, such as the cardiac sphincter of the esophagus.

cha·la·zi·on (ka- lā′zē-on) *n., pl.* **-zi·a** (-zē-ä). A chronic inflammatory granuloma in the tarsus of the eyelid, due to inflammation of a Meibomian gland.

chal·co·sis (kăl-kō′sĭs) *n.* **1.** Chronic copper poisoning. **2.** A deposit of fine particles of copper in the lungs or other tissues.

chal·i·co·sis (kăl′ĭ-kō′sĭs) *n.* Pneumoconiosis caused by the inhalation of dust, occuring especially in stone cutters.

chal·lenge diet (chăl′ənj) *n.* A diet in which one or more specific substances are included for the purpose of determining whether an abnormal reaction occurs.

cha·lone (kā′lōn′, kăl′ōn′) *n.* **1.** A hormone that inhibits rather than stimulates. **2.** Any of several polypeptides that are produced by a body tissue and that cause the reversible inhibition of mitosis in the cells of that tissue.

cham·ber (chām′bər) *n.* A compartment or enclosed space.

chan·cre (shăng′kər) *n.* The primary lesion of syphilis; a hard, nonsensitive, dull red papule or area of infiltration that begins at the site of infection after an interval of 10 to 30 days. — **chan′crous** (-krəs) *adj.*

chan·croid (shăng′kroid′) *n.* An infectious venereal ulcer at the site of infection by *Haemophilus ducreyi* beginning after an incubation period of 3 to 5 days. — **chan′croi′dal** (-kroid′l) *adj.*

change of life *n.* Menopause.

chapped (chăpt) *adj.* Having or relating to skin that is dry, scaly, and fissured, owing to excessive evaporation of moisture from the skin surface.

char·ac·ter (kăr′ək-tər) *n.* An attribute, trait, or distinct structural or functional feature.

character disorder *n.* Any of a group of personality disorders characterized by a persistent pattern of maladaptive behavior, emotional instability, immaturity, or addiction.

char·ac·ter·is·tic (kăr′ək-tə-rĭs′tĭk) *n.* See **character.** — **char′ac·ter·is′tic** *adj.*

character neurosis *n.* Any of various disorders in which a disturbed behavior pattern, such as compulsiveness, is part of a person's personality and not the result of intrapsychic conflicts.

Charcot-Ley·den crystals (-līd′n) *pl.n.* Crystals in the shape of elongated double pyramids, formed from eosinophils, found in the sputum in bronchial asthma and in the feces in some intestinal infections.

Char·cot's disease (shär-kōz′) *n.* See **amyotrophic lateral sclerosis.**

char·la·tan (shär′lə-tən) *n.* A person fraudulently claiming knowledge and skills not possessed; a quack.

char·ley horse (chär′lē hôrs′) *n.* Localized pain or stiffness in a muscle following excessive muscular exertion or the contusion of a muscle.

chart (chärt) *n.* **1.** A recording, in tabular form, of clinical data relating to a case. **2.** A group of symbols of graduated size used for measuring visual acuity.

check·up (chĕk′ŭp′) *n.* **1.** An examination or inspection. **2.** A general physical examination.

Ché·diak–Hi·ga·shi disease (shăd′yäk-hĭ-gä′shē) *n.* See **Chédiak–Steinbrinck–Higashi syndrome.**

Chédiak–Stein·brinck–Higashi anomaly (-stīn′brĭngk-, -shtīn′-) *n.* See **Chédiak–Steinbrinck–Higashi syndrome.**

Chédiak–Steinbrinck–Higashi syndrome *n.* An inherited syndrome marked by abnormalities of granulation and nuclear structure of all types of white blood cells, often accompanied by hepatosplenomegaly, lymphadenopathy, anemia, and susceptibility to infection.

cheek (chĕk) *n.* **1.** The fleshy part of either side of the face below the eye and between the nose and ear. **2.** Either of the buttocks.

cheek·bone (chēk′bōn′) *n.* See **zygomatic bone.**

cheese worker's lung *n.* Extrinsic allergic alveolitis caused by the inhalation of spores of *Penicillium casei* from moldy cheese.

chei·lal·gi·a or **chi·lal·gi·a** (kī-lăl′jē-ə, -jə) *n.* Pain in the lip.

chei·lec·to·my or **chi·lec·to·my** (kī-lĕk′tə-mē) *n.* **1.** Excision of a portion of the lip. **2.** The chiseling away of bony irregularities on the lips of a joint cavity that interfere with movements of the joint.

chei·li·tis or **chi·li·tis** (kī-lī′tĭs) *n.* Inflammation of the lips or of a lip, with redness and the production of fissures radiating from the angles of the mouth.

chei·lo·plas·ty or **chi·lo·plas·ty** (kī′lə-plăs′tē) *n.* Plastic surgery of the lips.

chei·lor·rha·phy or **chi·lor·rha·phy** (kī-lôr′ə-fē) *n.* Suturing of the lip.

chei·los·chi·sis or **chi·los·chi·sis** (kī-lŏs′kĭ-sĭs) *n.* See **cleft lip.**

chei·lo·sis or **chi·lo·sis** (kī-lō′sĭs) *n.* A disorder of the lips often due to riboflavin deficiency and other B-complex vitamin deficiencies and characterized by fissures, especially in the corners of the mouth.

chei·lo·sto·ma·to·plas·ty or **chi·lo·sto·ma·to·plas·ty** (kī′lō-stō′mə-tə-plăs′tē) *n.* Plastic surgery of the lips and mouth.

chei·lot·o·my or **chi·lot·o·my** (kī-lŏt′ə-mē) *n.* Incision into the lip.

chei·rog·nos·tic or **chi·rog·nos·tic** (kī′rəg-nŏs′-tĭk) *n.* Able to recognize the hand, or to distinguish between right and left.

chei·ro·kin·es·the·sia or **chi·ro·kin·es·the·sia** (kī′rō-kĭn′ĭs-thē′zhə, -kī′nĭs-) *n.* Subjective sensation of movement of the hands. — **chei′ro·kin′es·thet′ic** (-thĕt′ĭk) *adj.*

chei·ro·plas·ty or **chi·ro·plas·ty** (kī′rə-plăs′tē) *n.* Plastic surgery on the hand.

chei·ro·po·dal·gi·a or **chi·ro·po·dal·gi·a** (kī′rō-pō-dăl′jē-ə, -jə) *n.* Pain in the hands and the feet.

chei·ro·spasm or **chi·ro·spasm** (kī′rə-spăz′əm) *n.* Spasm of the muscles of the hand, as in writers' cramp.

che·late (kē′lāt′) *n.* A chemical compound in the form of a heterocyclic ring, containing a metal ion. — *v.* **-lat·ed, -lat·ing, -lates.** To remove a heavy metal, such as lead or mercury, from the bloodstream by means of a chelate, such as EDTA. — **che′late′** *adj.* — **che·la′tion** *n.*

chem·ex·fo·li·a·tion (kĕm′ĕks-fō′lē-ā′shən) *n.* A chemosurgical technique designed to remove acne scars or treat chronic skin defects caused by exposure to sunlight.

chem·i·cal (kĕm′ĭ-kəl) *adj.* **1.** Of or relating to chemistry. **2.** Of or relating to the properties or actions of chemicals. — *n.* **1.** A substance with a distinct molecular composition produced by or used in a chemical process. **2.** A drug, especially

an illicit or addictive one. — **chem′i·cal·ly** *adv.*

chemical abuse *n.* See **substance abuse.**

chemical antidote *n.* A substance that unites with a poison to form an innocuous chemical compound.

chemical attraction *n.* The force of attraction between atoms that causes them to form and maintain certain combinations.

chemical dependency *n.* A physical and psychological habituation to a mood- or mind-altering drug, such as alcohol or cocaine.

chemical energy *n.* Energy liberated by a chemical reaction or absorbed in the formation of a chemical compound.

Chemical Mace A trademark used for a temporarily disabling liquid packed in aerosol form and sprayed in self-defense into the face of an attacker, thereby causing dizziness, irritation of the eyes, and immobilization.

chemical repair *n.* Conversion of a free radical to a stable molecule.

chem·ist (kĕm′ĭst) *n.* A scientist specializing in chemistry.

chem·is·try (kĕm′ĭ-strē) *n.* **1.** The science of the composition, structure, properties, and reactions of matter, especially of atomic and molecular systems. **2.** The composition, structure, properties, and reactions of a substance.

che·mo (kē′mō, kĕm′ō) *n.* Chemotherapy or a chemotherapeutic treatment.

che·mo·bi·ot·ic (kē′mō-bī-ŏt′ĭk, kĕm′ō-) *n.* A combination of an antibiotic with a chemotherapeutic agent.

che·mo·cau·ter·y (kē′mō-kô′tə-rē, kĕm′ō-) *n.* A chemical substance that destroys tissue upon application.

che·mo·lu·mi·nes·cence (kē′mō-lōo′mə-nĕs′əns, kĕm′ō-) *n.* Emission of light as a result of a chemical reaction.

che·mo·pre·ven·tion (kē′mō-prī-vĕn′shən, kĕm′-ō-) *n.* The use of chemical agents, drugs, or food supplements to prevent disease.

che·mo·pro·tec·tion (kē′mō-prə-tĕk′shən, kĕm′-ō-) *n.* A therapeutic technique in which bone marrow cells are removed from a person with cancer and are genetically modified to withstand higher doses of chemotherapy before being returned to the donor.

che·mo·re·cep·tion (kē′mō-rĭ-sĕp′shən, kĕm′ō-) *n.* The physiological response of a sense organ to a chemical stimulus. — **che′mo·re·cep′tive** *adj.*

che·mo·re·cep·tor (kē′mō-rĭ-sĕp′tər, kĕm′ō-) *n.* A sensory nerve cell or sense organ, as of smell or taste, that responds to chemical stimuli.

che·mo·sen·si·tiz·er (kē′mō-sĕn′sĭ-tī′zər, kĕm′-ō-) *n.* Any of several compounds that inhibit the functioning of a particular cellular glycoprotein and make cells, especially tumor cells, sensitive to chemotherapeutic agents.

che·mo·sis (kē-mō′sĭs) *n.* Edema of the bulbar conjunctiva, forming a swelling around the cornea. — **che·mot′ic** (-mŏt′ĭk) *adj.*

che·mo·sur·ger·y (kē′mō-sûr′jə-rē, kĕm′ō-) *n.* Selective destruction of tissue by use of chemicals.

che·mo·tax·is (kē′mō-tăk′sĭs, kĕm′ō-) *n.* The characteristic movement or orientation of an organism or cell along a chemical concentration gradient, toward or away from the stimulus.

che·mo·ther·a·py (kē′mō-thĕr′ə-pē, kĕm′ō-) *n.* **1.** The treatment of cancer using specific chemical agents or drugs that are selectively destructive to malignant cells and tissues. **2.** The treatment of disease using chemical agents or drugs that are selectively toxic to the causative agent of the disease, such as a microorganism. — **che′mo·ther′-a·peu′tic** (-pyōō′tĭk) *adj.* — **che′mo·ther′a·peu′ti·cal·ly** *adv.* — **che′mo·ther′a·pist** *n.*

che·mot·ro·pism (kĭ-mŏt′rə-pĭz′əm) *n.* See **chemotaxis.**

cher·ub·ism (chĕr′ə-bĭz′əm) *n.* A hereditary disease characterized by an enlargement of the jawbones in young children, producing a cherublike facial appearance.

chest (chĕst) *n.* The part of the body between the neck and the abdomen, enclosed by the ribs and the breastbone; thorax.

chest lead (lēd) *n.* See **precordial lead.**

chest wall *n.* The system of structures outside the lungs that move as a part of breathing, including the rib cage, diaphragm, and abdomen.

Cheyne-Stokes respiration (chān′-, chā′nē-) *n.* An abnormal pattern of breathing characterized by a gradual increase in depth and sometimes in rate to a maximum depth, followed by a decrease resulting in apnea, usually seen in comatose persons having a disease affecting the nervous centers of respiration.

Chiari's syndrome *n.* Thrombosis of the hepatic vein with enlargement of the liver and extensive development of collateral vessels.

chi·as·ma (kī-ăz′mə) or **chi·asm** (kī′ăz′əm) *n., pl.* **-ma·ta** (-mə-tə). **1.** A crossing or intersection of two tracts, as of nerves or ligaments. **2.** The point of contact between paired chromatids during meiosis, representing the cytological manifestation of crossing over. — **chi·as′mal, chi·as′mic, chi′as·mat′ic** (-măt′ĭk) *adj.*

chick·en breast (chĭk′ən) *n.* See **pigeon breast.** — **chick′en-breast′ed** (-brĕs′tĭd) *adj.*

chicken fat clot *n.* A clot formed in vitro or postmortem from white blood cells and plasma of sedimented blood.

chick·en·pox or **chicken pox** *n.* An acute contagious disease, primarily of children, that is caused by the varicella-zoster virus and characterized by skin eruptions, slight fever, and malaise.

chickenpox immune globulin (human) *n.* Globulin fraction of serum from persons recently recovered from herpes zoster infection, used to inoculate high-risk children to prevent infection.

chickenpox virus *n.* See **varicella-zoster virus.**

chief cell *n.* **1.** The principle cell of the parathyroid gland, often divided into dark chief cells and light chief cells. **2.** See **zymogenic cell.**

chig·ger (chĭg′ər) *n.* **1.** The six-legged larva of mites of the family Trombiculidae, parasitic on humans, inflicting a bite that produces a wheal accompanied by intense itchiness. **2.** Chigoe.

chig·oe (chĭg′ō) *n.* A small tropical flea *(Tunga penetrans)* the fertilized female of which burrows under the skin, frequently under the toenails, causing intense irritation and sores that may become severely infected.

chil·blain (chĭl′blān′) *n.* Erythema, itching, and burning, especially of the dorsa of the fingers and toes, and of the heels, nose, and ears, resulting from exposure to moist cold.

child (chīld) *n.* **1.** A person between birth and puberty. **2.** An unborn infant; a fetus. **3.** An infant; a baby. **4.** One who is childish or immature. **5.** A son or daughter; an offspring.

child·bear·ing (chīld′bâr′ĭng) *n.* Pregnancy and parturition. — **child′bear′ing** *adj.*

child·bed fever (chīld′bĕd′) *n.* See **puerperal fever.**

child·birth (chīld′bûrth′) *n.* Parturition.

child·hood (chīld′hōōd′) *n.* The period of life between infancy and puberty.

chill (chĭl) *n.* A feeling of cold, with shivering and pallor, sometimes accompanied by an elevation of temperature in the interior of the body.

chi·me·ra (kī-mēr′ə, kĭ-) *n.* **1.** One who has received a transplant of genetically and immunologically different tissue, such as bone marrow. **2.** Twins with two immunologically different types of red blood cells.

chi·mer·ic (kī-mēr′ĭk, -mēr′-) *adj.* **1.** Relating to a chimera. **2.** Composed of parts of different origin.

chin (chĭn) *n.* The prominence formed by the anterior projection of the lower jaw.

Chi·nese restaurant syndrome (chī-nēz′, -nēs′) *n.* A group of symptoms, including dizziness and headache, that may occur after ingesting of food containing large amounts of monosodium glutamate.

chin muscle *n.* A muscle with origin from the incisor fossa of the mandible, with insertion into the skin of the chin, and whose action raises and wrinkles the skin of the chin and the pushes up the lower lip.

chip graft *n.* A graft in which small pieces of cartilage or bone are packed into a bone defect.

chi·rop·o·dy (kĭ-rŏp′ə-dē, shĭ-) *n.* See **podiatry.** — **chi·rop′o·dist** *n.*

chi·ro·prac·tic (kī′rə-prăk′tĭk) *n.* A system of therapy that uses the recuperative powers of the body and the relationship between the musculoskeletal structures and the functions of the body, particularly of the spinal column and the nervous system, in the restoration and maintenance of health. — **chi′ro·prac′tor** *n.*

chi·tin (kīt′n) *n.* A tough, protective, semitransparent substance, primarily a nitrogen-containing polysaccharide, forming the cell walls of certain fungi. — **chi′tin·ous** *adj.*

chla·myd·i·a (klə-mĭd′ē-ə) *n., pl.* **-i·ae** (-ē-ē′). Any of several common, often asymptomatic, sexually transmitted diseases caused by the microorganism *Chlamydia trachomatis,* including nonspecific urethritis in men. **— chla·myd′i·al** *adj.*

Chla·myd·i·a (klə-mĭd′ē-ə) *n.* A genus of gram-negative, coccoid microorganisms that are pathogenic to humans, causing diseases such as trachoma, nonspecific urethritis, and proctitis.

chla·myd·i·o·sis (klə-mĭd′ē-ō′sĭs) *n.* Any of the diseases caused by *Chlamydia psittaci* and *C. trachomatis.*

chlo·as·ma (klō-ăz′mə) *n., pl.* **-ma·ta** (-mə-tə). A patchy brown discoloration of the face often associated with hormonal changes, as in pregnancy.

chlor·ac·ne (klôr-ăk′nē) *n.* An acnelike skin disorder caused by prolonged exposure to chlorinated hydrocarbons.

chlor·am·bu·cil (klôr-ăm′byə-sĭl) *n.* An anticancer drug that is a derivitive of nitrogen mustard and is used to depress the proliferation and maturation of lymphocytes in diseases such as leukemia.

chlor·am·phen·i·col (klôr′ăm-fĕn′ĭ-kôl′, -kōl′) *n.* A broad-spectrum oral antibiotic derived from the soil bacterium *Streptomyces venezuelae* or produced synthetically.

chlor·dane (klôr′dān′) *n.* A chlorinated hydrocarbon used as an insecticide that may be absorbed through the skin, causing severe toxic effects.

chlor·di·az·e·pox·ide (klôr′dī-ăz′ə-pŏk′sīd, -klôr′) *n.* A benzodiazepine drug whose hydrochloride is used as an antianxiety agent.

chlo·re·mi·a (klôr-ē′mē-ə) *n.* **1.** See **chlorosis. 2.** See **hyperchloremia.**

chlor·hy·dri·a (klôr-hī′drē-ə) *n.* See **hyperchlorhydria.**

chlo·ri·du·ri·a (klôr′ĭ-dŏŏr′ē-ə, -dyŏŏr′-) *n.* See **chloruresis.**

chlo·ri·nate (klôr′ə-nāt′) *v.* **-nat·ed, -nat·ing, -nates.** To treat or combine with chlorine or a chlorine compound. **— chlo′ri·na′tion** *n.*

chlo·rine (klôr′ēn′, -ĭn) *n.* A highly irritating poisonous halogen with atomic number 17 used widely to purify water and as a disinfectant and bleaching agent.

chlorine acne *n.* See **chloracne.**

chlo·ro·form (klôr′ə-fôrm′) *n.* A clear, colorless, heavy, sweet-smelling liquid used sometimes as a general anesthetic; it has generally been replaced by less toxic, more easily controlled agents.

chlo·ro·phe·nol (klôr′ō-fē′nôl′, -nōl′) *n.* One of several products obtained by the action of chlorine on phenol and used as an antiseptic.

chlo·ro·phyll or **chlo·ro·phyl** (klôr′ə-fĭl) *n.* Any of a group of green pigments in the photosynthetic cells of green plants, algae, and certain bacteria that convert light energy into ATP and other forms of energy needed for biochemical processes.

chlo·rop·si·a (klə-rŏp′sē-ə) *n.* A condition in which all objects appear to be colored green, as may occur in digitalis intoxication.

chlo·ro·quine (klôr′ə-kwīn′, -kwĕn′) *n.* An antimalarial also used in the treatment of hepatic amebiasis and certain skin diseases.

chlo·ro·sis (klə-rō′sĭs) *n.* A form of chronic iron-deficiency anemia, primarily of young women,

characterized by a greenish-yellow discoloration of the skin and usually associated with deficiency in iron and protein. **— chlo·rot′ic** (-rŏt′ĭk) *adj.*

chlor·phen·ox·a·mine (klôr′fĕn-ŏk′sə-mēn′) *n.* A hydrochloride used to treat idiopathic, arteriosclerotic, and postencephalitic parkinsonism, usually with concomitant administration of other anti-parkinsonian agents.

chlor·prom·a·zine (klôr-prŏm′ə-zēn′, -prō′mə-) *n.* A phenothiazine antipsychotic agent with antiadrenergic and anticholinergic actions.

chlor·pro·pa·mide (klôr-prō′pə-mīd′) *n.* An orally effective hypoglycemic agent used in controlling hyperglycemia in certain cases of diabetes mellitus.

chlor·pro·thix·ene (klôr′prō-thĭk′sēn′) *n.* An antipsychotic having antiemetic, adrenolytic, spasmolytic, and antihistaminic actions.

chlor·tet·ra·cy·cline (klôr′tĕt-rə-si′klēn′, -klĭn) *n.* A broad-spectrum antibiotic obtained from *Streptomyces aureofaciens.*

chlor·u·re·sis (klôr′yə-rē′sĭs) *n.* Excretion of chloride in the urine.

chlor·u·ri·a (klôr-yŏŏr′ē-ə) *n.* See **chloruresis.**

choke (chōk) *v.* **choked, chok·ing, chokes. 1.** To interfere with the respiration by compression or obstruction of the larynx or trachea. **2.** To have difficulty in breathing, swallowing, or speaking.

chokes (chōks) *n.* A manifestation of caisson disease or altitude sickness characterized by dyspnea, coughing, and choking.

cho·lan·gi·ec·ta·sis (kō-lăn′jē-ĕk′tə-sĭs) *n.* Dilation of a bile duct.

cho·lan·gi·o·car·ci·no·ma (kō-lăn′jē-ō-kär′-sə-nō′mə) *n.* An adenocarcinoma of the intrahepatic bile ducts.

cho·lan·gi·o·en·ter·os·to·my (kō-lăn′jē-ō-ĕn′tə-rŏs′tə-mē) *n.* The surgical connection of a bile duct to the intestine.

cho·lan·gi·o·fi·bro·sis (kō-lăn′jē-ō-fī-brō′sĭs) *n.* Fibrosis of the bile ducts.

cho·lan·gi·o·gas·tros·to·my (kō-lăn′jē-ō-gă-strŏs′tə-mē) *n.* The surgical formation of a communication between a bile duct and the stomach.

cho·lan·gi·og·ra·phy (kō-lăn′jē-ŏg′rə-fē) *n.* A radiographic examination of the bile ducts following administration of a radiopaque contrast medium. **— cho·lan′gi·o·gram′** (-ə-grăm′) *n.*

cho·lan·gi·ole (kō-lăn′jē-ōl′) *n.* A ductule occurring between a bile canaliculus and an interlobular bile duct.

cho·lan·gi·o·li·tis (kō-lăn′jē-ə-lī′tĭs) *n.* Inflammation of the small bile radicles or cholangioles.

cho·lan·gi·o·ma (kō-lăn′jē-ō′mə) *n.* A neoplasm of bile duct origin, especially within the liver.

cho·lan·gi·o·pan·cre·a·tog·ra·phy (kō-lăn′jē-ō-păng′krē-ə-tŏg′rə-fē, -păn′-) *n.* Radiographic examination of the bile ducts and pancreas following administration of a radiopaque contrast medium.

cho·lan·gi·os·co·py (kō-lăn′jē-ŏs′kə-pē) *n.* The examination of bile ducts using a cystoscope or fiberoptic endoscope.

cho·lan·gi·os·to·my (kō-lăn′jē-ŏs′tə-mē) *n.* The surgical formation of a fistula into a bile duct.

cho·lan·gi·ot·o·my (kō-lăn′jē-ŏt′ə-mē) *n.* Incision into a bile duct.

cho·lan·gi·tis or **cho·lan·gei·tis** (kō′lăn-jī′tĭs) *n.* Inflammation of a bile duct.

cho·lan·o·poi·e·sis (kō-lăn′ō-poi-ē′sĭs) *n.* Synthesis of cholic acid or its conjugates and bile salts by the liver. — **cho·lan′o·poi·et′ic** (-ĕt′ĭk) *adj.*

cho·le·cal·cif·er·ol (kō′lĭ-kăl-sĭf′ə-rôl′, -rōl′) *n.* See **vitamin D₃**.

cho·le·cys·tec·ta·si·a (kō′lĭ-sĭs′tĭk-tā′zē-ə, -zhə) *n.* Dilation of the gallbladder.

cho·le·cys·tec·to·my (kō′lĭ-sĭs-stĕk′tə-mē) *n.* Surgical removal of the gallbladder.

cho·le·cyst·en·ter·os·to·my (kō′lĭ-sĭ-stĕn′tə-rŏs′tə-mē) *n.* The surgical formation of a direct communication between the gallbladder and the intestine.

cho·le·cys·ti·tis (kō′lĭ-sĭ-stī′tĭs) *n.* Inflammation of the gallbladder.

cho·le·cys·to·co·los·to·my (kō′lĭ-sĭs′tō-kə-lŏs′tə-mē) or **co·lo·cho·le·cys·tos·to·my** (kō′lō-kō′lĭ-sĭ-stŏs′tə-mē) *n.* The surgical formation of a communication between the gallbladder and the colon.

cho·le·cys·to·du·o·de·nos·to·my (kō′lĭ-sĭs′tō-dōō′ə-də-nŏs′tə-mē, -dyōō′-, -dōō-ŏd′n-ŏs′-, -dyōō-) *n.* The surgical formation of a communication between the gallbladder and the duodenum.

cho·le·cys·to·gas·tros·to·my (kō′lĭ-sĭs′tō-gă-strŏs′tə-mē) *n.* The surgical formation of a communication between the gallbladder and the stomach.

cho·le·cys·tog·ra·phy (kō′lĭ-sĭs-stŏg′rə-fē) *n.* Visualization of the gallbladder by x-rays after the administration of a radiopaque substance. — **cho·le·cys′to·gram′** (-sĭs′tə-grăm′) *n.*

cho·le·cys·to·il·e·os·to·my (kō′lĭ-sĭs′tō-ĭl′ē-ŏs′tə-mē) *n.* The surgical formation of a communication between the gallbladder and the ileum.

cho·le·cys·to·je·ju·nos·to·my (kō′lĭ-sĭs′tō-jə-jōō′nŏs′tə-mē, -jē′jōō-, -jĕj′ōō-) *n.* The surgical formation of a communication between the gallbladder and the jejunum.

cho·le·cys·to·li·thi·a·sis (kō′lĭ-sĭs′tō-lĭ-thī′ə-sĭs) *n.* The presence of one or more gallstones in the gallbladder.

cho·le·cys·top·a·thy (kō′lĭ-sĭ-stŏp′ə-thē) *n.* Disease of the gallbladder.

cho·le·cys·to·pex·y (kō′lĭ-sĭs′tə-pĕk′sē) *n.* Suture of the gallbladder to the abdominal wall.

cho·le·cys·tor·rha·phy (kō′lĭ-sĭ-stôr′ə-fē) *n.* Suture of an incised or ruptured gallbladder.

cho·le·cys·to·so·nog·ra·phy (kō′lĭ-sĭs′tō-sə-nŏg′rə-fē) *n.* Ultrasonic examination of the gallbladder.

cho·le·cys·tos·to·my (kō′lĭ-sĭ-stŏs′tə-mē) *n.* The establishment of a fistula into the gallbladder.

cho·le·cys·tot·o·my (kō′lĭ-sĭ-stŏt′ə-mē) *n.* Surgical incision into the gallbladder.

cho·led·o·chec·to·my (kə-lĕd′ə-kĕk′tə-mē, kō′lĭ-dō-) *n.* Surgical removal of a portion of the common bile duct.

cho·led·o·chi·tis (kə-lĕd′ə-kī′tĭs, kō′lĭ-dō-) *n.* Inflammation of the common bile duct.

cho·led·o·cho·du·o·de·nos·to·my (kə-lĕd′ə-kō-dōō′ō-də-nŏs′tə-mē, dyōō′-, dōō-ŏd′n-ŏs′-, dyōō-) *n.* The surgical formation of a communication between the common bile duct and the duodenum.

cho·led·o·cho·en·ter·os·tomy (kə-lĕd′ə-kō-ĕn′tə-rŏs′tə-mē) *n.* The surgical formation of a communication between the common bile duct and any part of the intestine.

cho·led·o·cho·je·ju·nos·to·my (kə-lĕd′ə-kō-jə-jōō′nŏs′tə-mē, -jē′jōō-) *n.* The surgical formation of a communication between the common bile duct and the jejunum.

cho·led·o·cho·li·thi·a·sis (kə-lĕd′ə-kō-lĭ-thī′ə-sĭs) *n.* The presence of a gallstone in the common bile duct.

cho·led·o·cho·li·thot·o·my (kə-lĕd′ə-kō-lĭ-thŏt′ə-mē) *n.* Incision of the common bile duct for the extraction of an impacted gallstone.

cho·led·o·cho·plas·ty (kə-lĕd′ə-kō-plăs′tē) *n.* Plastic surgery on the common bile duct.

cho·led·o·chor·rha·phy (kə-lĕd′ə-kôr′ə-fē) *n.* The suturing together of the divided ends of the common bile duct.

cho·led·o·chos·to·my (kə-lĕd′ə-kŏs′tə-mē) *n.* The establishment of a fistula into the common bile duct.

cho·led·o·chot·o·my (kə-lĕd′ə-kŏt′ə-mē) *n.* Incision into the common bile duct.

cho·le·ic acid (kō-lē′ĭk) *n.* Any of several compounds formed of bile acids and sterols.

cho·le·li·thi·a·sis (kō′lə-lĭ-thī′ə-sĭs) *n.* The presence or formation of gallstones in the gallbladder or bile ducts.

cho·le·li·thot·o·my (kō′lə-lĭ-thŏt′ə-mē) *n.* Surgical removal of a gallstone.

cho·le·lith·o·trip·sy (kō′lə-lĭth′ə-trĭp′sē) *n.* The crushing of a gallstone.

cho·lem·e·sis (kō-lĕm′ĭ-sĭs) *n.* The vomiting of bile.

cho·le·mi·a (kō-lē′mē-ə) *n.* The presence of bile salts in the blood. — **cho·le′mic** (-mĭk)

cho·le·per·i·to·ne·um (kō′lə-pĕr′ĭ-tn-ē′əm) *n.* The presence of bile in the peritoneum.

cho·le·poi·e·sis (kō′lə-poi-ē′sĭs) *n.* Formation of bile. — **cho′le·poi·et′ic** (-ĕt′ĭk) *adj.*

chol·er (kŏl′ər) *n.* Anger; irritability.

chol·er·a (kŏl′ər-ə) *n.* An acute epidemic infectious disease caused by *Vibrio cholerae,* characterized by profuse watery diarrhea, extreme loss of fluid and electrolytes, and prostration. — **chol′e·ra′ic** (-ə-rā′ĭk) *adj.*

cho·le·re·sis (kō′lə-rē′sĭs) *n.* The secretion of bile by the liver into the gallbladder.

cho·ler·rha·gi·a (kō′lə-rā′jē-ə, -jə) *n.* Excessive flow of bile.

cho·le·sta·si·a (kō′lĭ-stā′zē-ə, -zhə) or **cho·le·sta·sis** (-stā′sĭs) *n.* An arrest in the flow of bile. — **cho′le·stat′ic** (-stăt′ĭk) *adj.*

cho·les·ter·in (kə-lĕs′tər-ĭn) *n.* Cholesterol.

cho·les·ter·ol (kə-lĕs′tə-rôl′, -rōl′) *n.* A white crystalline substance found in animal tissues and various foods, normally synthesized by the liver and important as a constituent of cell membranes and a precursor to steroid hormones.

cho·les·ter·ol·e·mi·a (kə-lĕs′tər-ə-lē′mē-ə) or **cho·les·ter·e·mi·a** (kə-lĕs′tə-rē′mē-ə) *n.* The presence of elevated levels of cholesterol in the blood.

cho·les·ter·ol·o·sis (kə-lĕs′tər-ə-lō′sĭs) or **cho·les·ter·o·sis** (kə-lĕs′tə-rō′sĭs) *n.* A condition marked by abnormal deposition of cholesterol, as in tissues or blood vessels.

cho·les·ter·ol·u·ri·a (kə-lĕs′tər-ə-lŏŏr′ē-ə, -lyŏŏr′-) *n.* Excretion of cholesterol in the urine.

cho·le·styr·a·mine (kō′lĭ-stĕr′ə-mēn′, kō-lĕs′tə-răm′ēn) *n.* A drug that binds to bile acids and promotes their excretion, used to lower serum cholesterol levels and treat itching associated with jaundice.

cho·lic acid (kō′lĭk) *n.* An abundant crystalline bile acid derived from cholesterol.

cho·line (kō′lēn′) *n.* A natural amine often classed in the vitamin B complex and a constituent of many other biologically important molecules, such as acetylcholine and lecithin.

cho·lin·er·gic (kō′lə-nûr′jĭk) *adj.* **1.** Relating to nerve cells or fibers that employ acetylcholine as their neurotransmitter. **2.** Relating to an agent that mimics the action of acetylcholine.

cholinergic receptor *n.* Any of the chemical sites in effector cells or at synapses through which acetylcholine exerts its action.

cho·lin·es·ter·ase (kō′lə-nĕs′tə-rās′, -rāz′) *n.* An enzyme that catalyzes the hydrolysis of choline esters chiefly at nerve terminals, where it inactivates acetylcholine.

cholinesterase inhibitor *n.* A drug, such as neostigmine, that restores myoneural function by inhibiting the biodegradation of acetylcholine in cases of myasthenia gravis.

chon·dral·gi·a (kŏn-drăl′jē-ə, -jə) *n.* See **chondrodynia**.

chon·drec·to·my (kŏn-drĕk′tə-mē) *n.* Excision of cartilage.

chon·dri·fi·ca·tion center (kŏn′drə-fĭ-kā′shən) *n.* Any of the various aggregations of embryonic mesenchymal cells at sites of future cartilage formation.

chon·dri·fy (kŏn′drə-fī′) *v.* **-fied, -fy·ing, -fies.** To change into or become cartilage.

chon·dri·tis (kŏn-drī′tĭs) *n.* Inflammation of cartilage.

chon·dro·blast (kŏn′drə-blăst′) *n.* A cell of growing cartilage tissue.

chon·dro·blas·to·ma (kŏn′drō-blă-stō′mə) *n.* A tumor arising in the epiphyses of long bones in young males, consisting of highly cellular tissue resembling fetal cartilage.

chon·dro·cal·ci·no·sis (kŏn′drō-kăl′sə-nō′sĭs) *n.* The calcification of cartilage.

chon·dro·clast (kŏn′drə-klăst′) *n.* A multinucleated cell involved in the reabsorption of cartilage.

chon·dro·cra·ni·um (kŏn′drō-krā′nē-əm) *n.* The cartilaginous parts of the developing skull.

chon·dro·cyte (kŏn′drə-sīt′) *n.* A connective tissue cell that occupies a lacuna within the cartilage matrix.

chon·dro·dyn·i·a (kŏn′drō-dĭn′ē-ə) *n.* Pain in cartilage.

chon·dro·dys·pla·sia (kŏn′drō-dĭs-plā′zhə, -zhē-ə) *n.* See **chondrodystrophy**.

chon·dro·dys·tro·phi·a (kŏn′drō-dĭ-strō′fē-ə) *n.* See **chondrodystrophy**.

chon·dro·dys·tro·phy (kŏn′drə-dĭs′trə-fē) *n.* A disturbance in the development of the cartilage of the long bones, involving especially the region of the epiphysial plates, and resulting in arrested growth of the long bones.

chon·dro·gen·e·sis (kŏn′drō-jĕn′ĭ-sĭs) *n.* The formation of cartilage.

chon·droid tissue (kŏn′droid′) *n.* **1.** Tissue resembling cartilage and occurring in adults. **2.** An early form of cartilage occurring in an embryo.

chon·drol·y·sis (kŏn-drŏl′ĭ-sĭs) *n.* The disappearance of articular cartilage as the result of lysis or dissolution of the cartilage matrix and cells.

chon·dro·ma (kŏn-drō′mə) *n., pl.* **-mas** or **-ma·ta** (-mə-tə). A benign neoplasm derived from mesodermal cells that form cartilage.

chon·dro·ma·la·cia (kŏn′drō-mə-lā′shə) *n.* Abnormal softening or degeneration of cartilage of the joints, especially of the knee.

chon·dro·ma·to·sis (kŏn′drō-mə-tō′sĭs) *n.* The presence of multiple chondromas.

chon·dro·mere (kŏn′drə-mēr′) *n.* A cartilage unit of the embryonic vertebral column.

chon·drop·a·thy (kŏn-drŏp′ə-thē) *n.* Disease of a cartilage.

chon·dro·phyte (kŏn′drə-fīt′) *n.* An abnormal cartilaginous mass that develops at the articular surface of a bone.

chon·dro·plast (kŏn′drə-plăst′) *n.* See **chondroblast**.

chon·dro·plas·ty (kŏn′drə-plăs′tē) *n.* Reparative or plastic surgery of cartilage.

chon·dro·po·ro·sis (kŏn′drō-pə-rō′sĭs) *n.* A state of cartilage in which spaces appear, occurring in the normal process of ossification or in pathological conditions.

chon·dro·sar·co·ma (kŏn′drō-sär-kō′mə) *n.* A malignant neoplasm derived from cartilage cells and occurring most frequently in pelvic bones or near the ends of long bones.

chon·dro·sis (kŏn-drō′sĭs) *n.* See **chondrogenesis**.

chon·dro·ster·no·plas·ty (kŏn′drō-stûr′nə-plăs′-tē) *n.* The surgical correction of malformations of the sternum.

chon·drot·o·my (kŏn-drŏt′ə-mē) *n.* The surgical division of a cartilage.

chor·dee (kôr′dē′, -dā′, kôr-dā′) *n.* **1.** Painful erection and curvature of the penis in gonorrhea. **2.** Ventral curvature of the penis, most apparent on erection, as seen in hypospadias.

chor·di·tis (kôr-dī′tĭs) *n.* Inflammation of a cord, usually a vocal cord.

chor·do·skel·e·ton (kôr′dō-skĕl′ĭ-tn) *n.* The part of the skeleton in the embryo that develops in relation with the notochord.

cho·re·a (kô-rē′ə, kə-) *n.* Irregular, spasmodic, involuntary movements of the limbs or facial muscles. — **cho·re′ic, cho·re′al** *adj.*

choreic abasia *n.* Abasia due to abnormal movements of the legs.

cho·re·o·phra·si·a (kôr′ē-ō-frā′zē-ə, -zhə) *n.* The continual repetition of meaningless phrases.

cho·ri·o·am·ni·o·ni·tis (kôr′ē-ō-ăm′nē-ə-nī′tĭs) *n.* Inflammation of the amniotic membranes caused by infection.

cho·ri·o·an·gi·o·ma (kôr′ē-ō-ăn′jē-ō′mə) *n.* A benign tumor of placental blood vessels.

cho·ri·o·an·gi·o·sis (kôr′ē-ō-ăn′jē-ō′sĭs) *n.* An abnormal increase in the number of vascular channels in placental villi; associated with a high incidence of neonatal death and fetal malformations.

cho·ri·o·car·ci·no·ma (kôr′ē-ō-kär′sə-nō′mə) *n.* A malignant tumor of syncytial trophoblasts and cytotrophoblasts, almost always occurring in the uterus.

cho·ri·o·cele (kôr′ē-ə-sēl′) *n.* A hernia of the choroid coat of the eye through a defect in the sclera.

cho·ri·o·ma (kôr′ē-ō′mə) *n.* A benign or malignant tumor of chorionic tissue.

cho·ri·o·men·in·gi·tis (kôr′ē-ō-mĕn′ĭn-jī′tĭs) *n.* Cerebral meningitis in which there is marked cellular infiltration of the meninges, often with a lymphocytic infiltration of the choroid plexuses.

cho·ri·on (kôr′ē-ŏn′) *n.* The outer membrane enclosing the embryo; in placental mammals it contributes to the development of the placenta. — **cho′ri·on′ic** (-ŏn′ĭk) *adj.*

chorionic gonadotropin *n.* A glycoprotein produced by the placenta and excreted in the urine of pregnant women, which stimulates ovarian secretion of the estrogen and progesterone required to maintain the conceptus and is used as an aid for conception.

chorionic growth hormone-prolactin *n.* See **human placental lactogen.**

chorionic villus *n.* Any of the various fingerlike projections of the chorion of the embryo that contain fetal blood vessels and grow into the intervillous lacuna of the placenta.

chorionic villus sampling *n.* A prenatal test to detect birth defects that is performed at an early stage of pregnancy and involves retrieval and examination of tissue from the chorionic villi.

cho·ri·o·ret·i·ni·tis (kôr′ē-ō-rĕt′n-ī′tĭs) *n.* Inflammation of the choroid and retina.

cho·roid (kôr′oid′) or **cho·ri·oid** (kôr′ē-oid′) *n.* The dark-brown vascular coat of the eye between the sclera and the retina.

cho·roid·e·re·mi·a (kôr′oi-də-rē′mē-ə, kô-) *n.* **1.** Congenital absence of the choroid of the eye. **2.** The progressive degeneration of the choroid in

males leading to progressive constriction of visual fields and complete blindness.

cho·roid·i·tis (kôr′oi-dī′tĭs) *n.* Inflammation of the choroid.

cho·roi·do·cy·cli·tis (kə-roi′dō-sĭ-klī′tĭs, -sī-, kô-) *n.* Inflammation of the choroid and the ciliary body.

cho·roi·dop·a·thy (kôr′oi-dŏp′ə-thē) *n.* Noninflammatory degeneration of the choroid.

cho·roi·do·ret·i·ni·tis (kə-roi′dō-rĕt′n-ī′tĭs, kô-) *n.* See **chorioretinitis.**

Christ·church chromosome (krīst′chûrch′) *n.* An abnormal small acrocentric chromosome with complete or almost complete deletion of the short arm; it is found in the leukocytes in some cases of chronic lymphocytic leukemia.

Christ·mas disease (krĭs′məs) *n.* See **hemophilia B.**

Christmas factor *n.* See **factor IX.**

chro·maf·fin body (krō′mə-fĭn) *n.* See **paraganglion.**

chromaffin cell *n.* A cell that stains readily with chromium salts, especially a cell of the adrenal medulla.

chro·maf·fin·o·ma (krō′mə-fə-nō′mə, krō-măf′-ə-) *n.* A tumor composed of chromaffin cells.

chro·maf·fi·nop·a·thy (krō-măf′ə-nŏp′ə-thē) *n.* A pathological condition of chromaffin tissue.

chromaffin tissue *n.* A cellular tissue, vascular and well supplied with nerves, made up chiefly of chromaffin cells and found in the medulla of the adrenal glands and in the paraganglia.

chromaffin tumor *n.* See **chromaffinoma.**

chro·mat·ic aberration (krō-măt′ĭk) *n.* Color distortion in an image produced by a lens, caused by the inability of the lens to bring the various colors of light to focus at a single point.

chromatic vision *n.* See **chromatopsia.**

chro·ma·tid (krō′mə-tĭd) *n.* Either of the two daughter strands of a duplicated chromosome that are joined by a single centromere and separate during cell division to become individual chromosomes.

chro·ma·tin (krō′mə-tĭn) *n.* A complex of nucleic acids and proteins in the cell nucleus that stains readily with basic dyes and condenses to form chromosomes during cell division.

chro·ma·tism (krō′mə-tĭz′əm) *n.* **1.** Abnormal pigmentation. **2.** See **chromatic aberration.**

chro·ma·tog·e·nous (krō′mə-tŏj′ə-nəs) *adj.* Producing color; causing pigmentation.

chro·mat·o·gram (krō-măt′ə-grăm′) *n.* The pattern of separated substances obtained by chromatography.

chro·ma·tog·ra·phy (krō′mə-tŏg′rə-fē) *n.* Any of various techniques for the separation of complex mixtures that rely on the differential affinities of substances for a gas or liquid mobile medium and for a stationary adsorbing medium through which they pass, such as paper, gelatin, or magnesia. — **chro′ma·tog′ra·pher** *n.*

chro·ma·tol·y·sis (krō′mə-tŏl′ĭ-sĭs) *n.* The disintegration of chromophil substance in a nerve cell body; it may occur after damage to its peripheral process. — **chro·mat′o·lyt′ic** (-măt′l-ĭt′ĭk) adj.

chro·mat·o·phore (krō-măt′ə-fôr′) n. A pigment-bearing phagocyte found chiefly in the skin, mucous membrane, and choroid coat of the eye, as well as in melanomas. — **chro·mat′o·phor′ic** (-fôr′ĭk) adj.

chro·ma·top·si·a (krō′mə-tŏp′sē-ə) n. A condition in which objects appear to be abnormally colored or tinged with color.

chro·ma·tu·ri·a (krō′mə-tŏŏr′ē-ə, -tyŏŏr′-) n. Abnormal coloration of the urine.

chro·mes·the·sia (krō′mĕs-thē′zhə) n. A condition in which another sensation, such as taste or smell, is stimulated by the perception of color.

chro·mi·dro·sis (krō′mĭ-drō′sĭs) or **chrom·hi·dro·sis** (krŏm′hĭ-drō′sĭs, -hī-) n. The excretion of sweat containing pigment.

chro·mi·um (krō′mē-əm) n. A lustrous hard metallic element with atomic number 24 that is resistant to tarnish and is used to harden steel alloys, in decorative platings, and as a pigment in glass.

chro·mo·blast (krō′mə-blăst′) n. An embryonic cell having the potential to develop into a pigment cell.

chro·mo·cys·tos·co·py (krō′mō-sĭ-stŏs′kə-pē) n. See **cystochromoscopy.**

chro·mo·cyte (krō′mə-sīt′) n. A pigmented cell, such as a red blood corpuscle.

chro·mo·gen·ic (krō′mə-jĕn′ĭk) adj. Of or relating to a chromogen or to chromogenesis.

chro·mol·y·sis (krō-mŏl′ĭ-sĭs) n. See **chromatolysis.**

chro·mo·mere (krō′mə-mēr′) n. **1.** A condensed segment of a chromonema. **2.** See **granulomere.**

chro·mo·my·co·sis (krō′mō-mī-kō′sĭs) n. A localized chronic mycosis of skin, characterized by lesions so rough and irregular as to present a cauliflower-like appearance.

chro·mo·ne·ma (krō′mə-nē′mə) n., pl. **-ma·ta** (-mə-tə). The coiled filament that extends the entire length of a chromosome and on which the genes are located.

chro·mo·phil (krō′mə-fĭl′) or **chro·mo·phile** (-fīl′) or **chro·mat·o·phil** (krō-măt′ə-fĭl′, krō′mə-tō-) n. A cell or other histologic element that stains readily. — adj. or **chro·mo·phil·ic** (krō′mə-fĭl′-ĭk). Staining readily. Used of a cell or cell structure.

chro·mo·phil·i·a (krō′mə-fĭl′ē-ə, -fēl′yə) or **chro·mat·o·phil·i·a** (krō-măt′ə-, krō′mə-tō-) n. The property possessed by most cells of staining readily with appropriate dyes.

chro·mo·pho·bi·a (krō′mə-fō′bē-ə) or **chro·mat·o·pho·bi·a** (krō-măt′ə-, krō′mə-tō-) n. **1.** Resistance to stains. Used of certain cells and histologic structures. **2.** An abnormal fear of colors or a color.

chro·mo·phor·ic (krō′mə-fôr′ĭk) adj. Of or relating to certain microorganisms that produce or carry color.

chromosomal map n. A representation of the karyotype and of the positioning and ordering on it of those loci that have been localized by any of several mapping methods.

chromosomal region n. The part of a chromosome defined either by anatomical details, especially by banding, or by its linkage groups.

chromosomal syndrome n. Any of a number of syndromes attributable to a chromosomal aberration and typically associated with mental retardation and multiple congenital anomalies.

chromosomal trait n. A trait dependent on a chromosomal aberration.

chro·mo·some (krō′mə-sōm′) n. **1.** A threadlike linear strand of DNA and associated proteins in the nucleus of animal and plant cells that carries the genes and functions in the transmission of hereditary information. **2.** A circular strand of DNA in bacteria that contains the hereditary information necessary for life. — **chro′mo·so′mal** (-sō′məl), **chro′mo·so′mic** (-sō′mĭk) adj.

chromosome aberration n. A deviation in the normal number of chromosomes or in their morphology.

chromosome mapping n. The process of determining the position of specific genes on specific chromosomes and constructing a diagram of each chromosome showing the relative positions of genes.

chron·ic (krŏn′ĭk) adj. Of long duration. Used of a disease of slow progress and long continuance.

chronic adrenocortical insufficiency n. See **Addison's disease.**

chronic alcoholism n. See **alcoholism** (sense 2).

chronic bronchitis n. Inflammation of the bronchial mucous membrane characterized by cough, hypersecretion of mucus, and expectoration of sputum over a long period of time, associated with increased vulnerability to bronchial infection.

chronic fatigue syndrome n. A syndrome characterized by sleep disorders and disruption of the immune system.

chronic inflammation n. Inflammation that may have a rapid or slow onset but is characterized primarily by its persistence; it occurs when tissues cannot overcome the effects of the injuring agent.

chronic malaria n. Malaria that develops after repeated attacks of one of the acute forms, usually falciparum malaria, and is characterized by profound anemia, enlargement of the spleen, emaciation, and muscular weakness.

chronic obstructive pulmonary disease n. A chronic lung disease, such as asthma or emphysema, in which breathing becomes slowed or forced.

chronic shock n. The state of subnormal blood volume that develops in a person with a debilitating disease, especially in the elderly, and that makes the person susceptible to hemorrhagic shock if moderate blood loss occurs.

chronic ulcer n. A longstanding ulcer with fibrous scar tissue at its base.

chron·o·bi·ol·o·gy (krŏn′ō-bī-ŏl′ə-jē) n. The study of the effect of time on biological events, especially repetitive or cyclic phenomena in individual organisms.

chron·o·log·i·cal age (krŏn′ə-lŏj′ĭ-kəl) *n.* The number of years a person has lived, used especially in psychometrics as a standard against which certain variables, such as behavior and intelligence, are measured.

chron·o·on·col·o·gy (krŏn′ō-ŏn-kŏl′ə-jē, -ŏng-) *n.* **1.** The study of the influence of biological rhythms on neoplastic growth. **2.** Anti-cancer treatment based on the timing of drug administration.

chro·not·ro·pism (krə-nŏt′rə-pĭz′əm) *n.* The modification of the rate of a periodic movement, such as heartbeat, by some external influence.

chry·si·a·sis (krĭ-sī′ə-sĭs) *n.* A permanent slate-gray discoloration of the skin and sclera resulting from deposition of gold in the connective tissue of the skin and eye after chrysotherapy.

chrys·o·der·ma (krĭs′ō-dûr′mə) *n.* See **chrysiasis.**

chrys·o·ther·a·py (krĭs′ə-thĕr′ə-pē) *n.* The treatment of disease by the administration of gold salts.

Chvos·tek's sign (vô′stĕks, кнə-vô′-) *n.* An indication of tetany in which a unilateral spasm of the oris muscle is initiated by a slight tap over the facial nerve anterior to the external auditory canal.

chyl·an·gi·o·ma (kī-lăn′jē-ō′mə) *n.* A tumor composed of prominent, dilated lacteals and larger intestinal lymphatic vessels.

chyle (kīl) *n.* A turbid, white or pale yellow fluid taken up by the lacteals from the intestine during digestion and carried by the lymphatic system via the thoracic duct into the circulation. — **chy·la′ceous** (kī-lā′shəs), **chy′lous** (kī′ləs) *adj.*

chy·le·mi·a (kī-lē′mē-ə) *n.* The presence of chyle in the circulating blood.

chy·li·fac·tion (kī′lə-făk′shən) *n.* See **chylopoiesis.** — **chy′li·fac′tive** (-făk′tĭv) *adj.*

chy·li·fi·ca·tion (kī′lə-fĭ-kā′shən) *n.* See **chylopoiesis.**

chy·lo·me·di·as·ti·num (kī′lō-mē′dē-ə-stī′nəm) *n.* An abnormal presence of chyle in the mediastinum.

chy·lo·mi·cron (kī′lō-mī′krŏn) *n.* One of the microscopic particles of fat occurring in chyle and in the blood, especially in great numbers after a meal high in fat.

chy·lo·mi·cro·ne·mi·a (kī′lō-mī′krə-nē′mē-ə) *n.* The presence of chylomicrons, especially an increased number, in the circulating blood.

chy·lo·phor·ic (kī′lə-fôr′ĭk) *adj.* Conveying chyle.

chy·lo·poi·e·sis (kī′lō-poi-ē′sĭs) *n.* The formation of chyle in the intestine and its absorption by the lacteals. — **chi′lo·poi·et′ic** (-poi-ĕt′ĭk) *adj.*

chy·lo·sis (kī-lō′sĭs) *n.* The formation of chyle from the food in the intestine, its absorption by the lacteals, and its mixture with the blood and conveyance to the tissues.

chy·lo·tho·rax (kī′lō-thôr′ăks′) *n.* An accumulation of chyle in the thoracic cavity.

chy·lu·ri·a (kī-lŏŏr′ē-ə, -lyŏŏr′-) *n.* The presence of chyle in the urine.

chyme (kīm) *n.* The thick semifluid mass of partly digested food that is passed from the stomach to the duodenum. — **chy′mous** (kī′məs) *adj.*

chy·mi·fi·ca·tion (kī′mə-fĭ-kā′shən) *n.* See **chymopoiesis.**

chy·mo·poi·e·sis (kī′mō-poi-ē′sĭs) *n.* The conversion of food to chyme, brought about by digestion in the stomach.

chy·mo·sin (kī′mə-sĭn) *n.* See **rennin.**

CIB *abbr. Latin.* cibus (food)

cic·a·trec·to·my (sĭk′ə-trĕk′tə-mē) *n.* The excision of a scar.

cic·a·trix (sĭk′ə-trĭks′, sĭ-kā′trĭks) *n., pl.* **cic·a·tri·ces** (sĭk′ə-trī′sēz, sĭ-kā′trĭ-sēz′). A scar left by the formation of new connective tissue over a healing sore or wound. — **cic′a·tri′cial** (sĭk′ə-trĭsh′əl), **ci·cat′ri·cose′** (sĭ-kăt′rĭ-kōs′) *adj.*

cic·a·tri·za·tion (sĭk′ə-trĭ-zā′shən) *n.* The process of scar formation.

cic·a·trize (sĭk′ə-trīz′) *v.* **-trized, -triz·ing, -triz·es.** To heal or become healed by the formation of scar tissue.

cic·lo·pir·ox ol·a·mine (sĭk′lō-pēr′ŏks′ ō′lə-mēn′, sī′klō-) *n.* A broad-spectrum antifungal agent used to treat a variety of fungus and yeast infections of the skin.

cig·a·rette drain (sĭg′ə-rĕt′, sĭg′ə-rĕt′) *n.* A drain made of gauze surrounded by a rubber tissue, rubber dam, or rubber tubing.

cil·i·a·rot·o·my (sĭl′ē-ə-rŏt′ə-mē) *n.* Surgical division of the ciliary zone of the iris.

cil·i·ar·y (sĭl′ē-ĕr′ē) *adj.* **1.** Of, relating to, or resembling cilia. **2.** Of or relating to the ciliary body and associated structures of the eye.

ciliary body *n.* A thickened portion of the vascular tunic of the eye located between the choroid and the iris.

ciliary gland *n.* Any of several modified sudoriferous glands in the margins of the eyelids producing secretions that lubricate the eyeball and having ducts that open into the follicles of the eyelashes.

ciliary muscle *n.* A smooth muscle of the ciliary body of the eye whose action changes the shape of lens in the process of accommodation.

ciliary reflex *n.* Contraction of the pupil in the accommodation reflex.

cil·i·at·ed epithelium (sĭl′ē-ā′tĭd) *n.* Epithelium having cilia on the surface not attached to another cell or structure.

cil·i·ec·to·my (sĭl′ē-ĕk′tə-mē) *n.* See **cyclectomy.**

cil·i·um (sĭl′ē-əm) *n., pl.* **-i·a** (-ē-ə). **1.** See **eyelash** (sense 1). **2.** A microscopic hairlike process extending from the surface of a cell or unicellular organism that produces a rhythmical motion and locomotion.

ci·met·i·dine (sĭ-mĕt′ĭ-dēn′, -dĭn′) *n.* A histamine analogue and antagonist used to treat peptic ulcer by inhibiting gastric acid secretion.

cin·cho·na (sĭng-kō′nə, sĭn-chō′-) *n.* **1.** Any of several trees and shrubs of the genus *Cinchona,* native chiefly to the Andes and cultivated for bark that yields the medicinal alkaloids quinine and quinidine, which are used to treat malaria. **2.** The dried bark of any of these plants.

cin·cho·nine (sĭng′kə-nēn′, sĭn′chə-) *n.* An alkaloid derived from the bark of various cinchona trees and used as an antimalarial agent.

cin·e·an·gi·o·car·di·og·ra·phy (sĭn′ē-ăn′jē-ō-kär′dē-ŏg′rə-fē) *n.* The use of a movie camera to film the passage of a contrast medium through chambers of the heart and great vessels for diagnostic purposes.

cin·e·an·gi·og·ra·phy (sĭn′ē-ăn′jē-ŏg′rə-fē) *n.* The use of a movie camera to film the passage of a contrast medium through blood vessels for diagnostic purposes.

cin·e·fluo·rog·ra·phy (sĭn′ē-flŏŏ-rŏg′rə-fē, -flô-) *n.* The use of a movie camera to obtain fluoroscopic views of organs after the administration of a contrast medium.

cin·e·ra·di·og·ra·phy (sĭn′ə-rā′dē-ŏg′rə-fē) *n.* The use of a movie camera to film an organ in motion.

cin·gu·lec·to·my (sĭng′gyə-lĕk′tə-mē) *n.* Surgical removal of a portion of the cortical hemisphere.

cin·gu·lot·o·my (sĭng′gyə-lŏt′ə-mē) *n.* Electrolytic destruction of the cortex and white matter of the cortical hemisphere and its connections.

cin·ox·a·cin (sĭ-nŏk′sə-sĭn) *n.* A synthetic organic acid used as an antibacterial to treat urinary tract infections.

cip·ro·flox·a·cin hydrochloride (sĭp′rō-flŏk′sə-sĭn) *n.* A synthetic broad-spectrum antibiotic with activity against a wide range of gram-negative and gram-positive organisms.

cir·ca·di·an (sər-kā′dē-ən, -kăd′ē-, sûr′kə-dī′ən, -dē′-) *adj.* Relating to biological variations or rhythms with a cycle of about 24 hours.

circadian rhythm *n.* A daily rhythmic activity cycle, based on 24-hour intervals, that is exhibited by many organisms.

cir·cle absorption anesthesia (sûr′kəl) *n.* Inhalation anesthesia in which a circuit with carbon dioxide absorbent is used for the complete or partial rebreathing of exhaled gases.

cir·cu·lar fold (sûr′kyə-lər) *n.* Any of the numerous folds of the mucous membrane of the small intestine.

circular psychosis *n.* Manic-depressive illness.

cir·cu·la·tion (sûr′kyə-lā′shən) *n.* Movement in a circle or circuit, especially the movement of blood through bodily vessels as a result of the heart's pumping action.

cir·cu·la·to·ry (sûr′kyə-lə-tôr′ē) *adj.* **1.** Of or relating to circulation. **2.** Of or relating to the circulatory system.

circulatory system *n.* The system of structures, consisting of the heart, blood vessels, and lymphatics, by which blood and lymph are circulated throughout the body.

cir·cum·a·nal gland (sûr′kəm-ā′nəl) *n.* Any of several sebaceous and apocrine sweat glands situated in the skin surrounding the anus.

cir·cum·cise (sûr′kəm-sīz′) *v.* **-cised, -cis·ing, -cis·es.** To perform a circumcision.

cir·cum·ci·sion (sûr′kəm-sĭzh′ən) *n.* **1.** The surgical removal of part or all of the prepuce. **2.** The cutting around an anatomical part.

cir·cum·duc·tion (sûr′kəm-dŭk′shən) *n.* Movement of a part in a circular direction.

cir·cum·scribed myxedema (sûr′kəm-skrībd′) *n.* Nodules and plaques of mucoid edema of the skin occurring in some patients with hyperthyroidism.

cir·cum·stan·ti·al·i·ty (sûr′kəm-stăn′shē-ăl′ĭ-tē) *n.* A disturbance in the thought process characterized by an excessive amount of detail that is often tangential, elaborate, and irrelevant.

cir·rho·sis (sĭ-rō′sĭs) *n.* **1.** A chronic disease of the liver characterized by the replacement of normal tissue with fibrous tissue and the loss of functional liver cells. It can result from alcohol abuse or infection especially by the hepatitis virus. **2.** Chronic interstitial inflammation of any tissue or organ. **—cir·rhot′ic** (-rŏt′ĭk) *adj.*

cir·sec·to·my (sər-sĕk′tə-mē) *n.* Excision of a section of a varicose vein.

cis·ter·na (sĭ-stûr′nə) *n., pl.* **-nae** (-nē′). **1.** A cavity or enclosed space serving as a reservoir, especially for chyle, lymph, or cerebrospinal fluid. **2.** An ultramicroscopic space or channel occurring between the membranes of the flattened sacs of the endoplasmic reticulum, the Golgi complex, or the two membranes of the nuclear envelope. **— cis·ter′nal** *adj.*

cisternal puncture *n.* Passage of a hollow needle through the membrane of the first cervical vertebra into the cerebellomedullary cistern.

cis·ter·nog·ra·phy (sĭs′tər-nŏg′rə-fē) *n.* The radiographic study of the basal cisterns of the brain after the introduction of an opaque contrast medium.

cis·tron (sĭs′trŏn′) *n.* The smallest functional unit of heredity; a length of chromosomal DNA associated with a single biochemical function and essentially equivalent to a gene. **— cis·tron′ic** *adj.*

cit·ric acid (sĭt′rĭk) *n.* A colorless translucent crystalline acid derived by fermentation of carbohydrates or from lemon, lime, and pineapple juices, and a necessary intermediate in metabolism.

citric acid cycle *n.* See Krebs cycle.

cit·rul·line (sĭt′rə-lēn′) *n.* An amino acid produced as an intermediate in the conversion of ornithine to arginine during urea formation in the liver.

cit·rul·li·ne·mi·a (sĭt′rə-lə-nē′mē-ə, sĭ-trŭl′ə-) *n.* A disease of amino acid metabolism in which there are elevated levels of citrulline in the blood, urine, and cerebrospinal fluid; it is manifested by mental retardation beginning in infancy.

cit·rul·li·nu·ri·a (sĭt′rə-lə-nŏŏr′ē-ə, -nyŏŏr-, sĭ-trŭl′ə-) *n.* Enhanced urinary excretion of citrulline; a manifestation of citrullinemia.

clad·o·spo·ri·o·sis (klăd′ə-spôr′ē-ō′sĭs) *n.* Infection with a fungus of the genus *Cladosporium.*

clair·voy·ance (klâr-voi′əns) *n.* The perception of objects or events that cannot be perceived by the senses.

clamp (klămp) *n.* An instrument for the compression or grasping of a structure.

clang association *n.* Psychic associations resulting from sounds, often observed in the manic phase of manic-depressive psychosis.

clap (klăp) *n.* Gonorrhea. Often used with *the*.

Clap·ton's line (klăp′tənz) *n.* A greenish discoloration of the dental margin of the gums occurring in chronic copper poisoning.

Clark's level (klärks) *n.* Any of four levels that mark the invasion of malignant melanoma through the skin layers to the subcutaneous fat layer, each successive level indicating a worsening prognosis.

Clark's weight rule *n.* A rule for determining the approximate dose of medicine appropriate for a child two years of age or older by dividing the child's weight in pounds by 150 and multiplying the result by the adult dose.

clasp (klăsp) *n.* A part of a removable partial denture that acts as a direct retainer or stabilizer for the denture.

clasp-knife rigidity *n.* See **clasp-knife spasticity**.

clasp-knife spasticity *n.* Rigidity of the extensor muscles of a joint that gives way abruptly to allow easy flexion, resulting from an exaggeration of the stretch reflex.

clas·si·fi·ca·tion (klăs′ə-fĭ-kā′shən) *n.* **1.** A systematic arrangement into groups. **2.** The systematic grouping of organisms into categories on the basis of evolutionary or structural relationships between them; taxonomy.

clau·di·ca·tion (klô′dĭ-kā′shən) *n.* A halt or lameness in a person's walk; a limp.

claus·tro·pho·bi·a (klô′strə-fō′bē-ə) *n.* An abnormal fear of being in narrow or enclosed spaces. — **claus′tro·phobe′** *n.* — **claus′tro·pho′bic** *adj.*

clav·i·cle (klăv′ĭ-kəl) *n.* Either of two slender bones that extend from the manubrium of the sternum to the acromion of the scapula. — **cla·vic′u·lar** (klə-vĭk′yə-lər) *adj.* — **cla·vic′u·late′** (-lāt′) *adj.*

clav·i·cot·o·my (klăv′ĭ-kŏt′ə-mē) *n.* Surgical division of the clavicle.

cla·vus (klā′vəs, klā′-) *n., pl.* **-vi** (-vī′). **1.** See **corn**. **2.** A condition resulting from healing of a granuloma of the foot in yaws, in which a core falls out, leaving an erosion.

claw foot *n.* A deformity of the foot characterized by an exaggerated arch and downward flexion of the toes.

claw-hand or **claw hand** *n.* Atrophy of the interosseous muscles of the hand with hyperextension of the joints of the metacarpus and flexion of the fingers.

clear·ance (klēr′əns) *n.* The removal of a substance from the blood, expressed as the volume of blood or plasma that is cleared of the substance per unit time.

clear·ing factor (klēr′ĭng) *n.* Any of the lipoprotein lipases that appear in plasma during lipemia and catalyze the hydrolysis of triglycerides.

cleav·age (klē′vĭj) *n.* **1.** A series of cell divisions in an ovum immediately following fertilization. **2.** The linear clefts in the skin indicating the general direction of the fibers in the dermis.

cleft (klĕft) *n.* A split or fissure between two parts.

cleft hand *n.* A congenital deformity in which the division between the fingers, especially between the third and fourth fingers, extends into the metacarpal region.

cleft lip *n.* A congenital facial deformity of the lip (usually the upper) due to a mesodermal deficiency or to a failure of merging in one or more of the embryologic processes that form the lip.

cleft palate *n.* A congenital fissure in the roof of the mouth, resulting from incomplete fusion of the palate during embryonic development. It may involve only the uvula or extend through the entire palate.

cleft spine *n.* See **spondyloschisis**.

cleft tongue *n.* See **bifid tongue**.

clenched fist sign *n.* An indication of the pain of angina pectoris in which a person presses a clenched fist against the chest as a means of showing its constricting, pressing quality.

click (klĭk) *n.* A slight sharp sound, such as that heard from the heart during systole.

cli·ent-cen·tered therapy (klī′ənt-sĕn′tərd) *n.* A system of psychotherapy based on the assumption that the patient has the internal resources to improve and is in the best position to resolve his or her own personality dysfunction.

cli·mac·ter·ic (klī-măk′tər-ĭk, klī′măk-tĕr′ĭk) *n.* A period of life characterized by physiological and psychic change that marks the end of the reproductive capacity of women and terminates with the completion of menopause. **2.** A corresponding period sometimes occurring in men that may be marked by a reduction in sexual activity, although fertility is retained.

cli·max (klī′măks′) *n.* **1.** The height of a disease; the stage of greatest severity. **2.** See **orgasm**.

clin·ic (klĭn′ĭk) *n.* **1.** A facility, often associated with a hospital or medical school, that is devoted to the diagnosis and care of outpatients. **2.** A medical establishment run by several specialists working in cooperation and sharing the same facilities. **3.** A group session offering counsel or instruction in a particular field or activity. **4.** A seminar or meeting of physicians and medical students in which medical instruction is conducted in the presence of the patient, as at the bedside. **5.** A place where such instruction occurs. **6.** A class or lecture of medical instruction conducted in this manner.

clin·i·cal (klĭn′ĭ-kəl) *adj.* **1.** Relating to the bedside treatment of a patient or to the course of the disease. **2.** Relating to the observed symptoms and course of a disease.

clinical diagnosis *n.* Diagnosis based on a study of the signs and symptoms of a disease.

clinical fitness *n.* The absence of clinically evident disease or of subclinical precursors to disease.

clinical medicine *n.* The study and practice of medicine based on direct observation of patients.

clinical nurse specialist *n.* A nurse with advanced knowledge and competence in a particular area of nursing practice, as in cardiology, oncology, or psychiatry.

clinical pathology *n.* **1.** The practice of pathology as it pertains to the care of patients. **2.** The subspecialty in pathology concerned with the theoretical and technical aspects of laboratory technology that pertain to the diagnosis and prevention of disease.

clinical psychology *n.* The branch of psychology that studies and treats emotional or behavioral disorders.

clinical thermometer *n.* A thermometer having a graduated glass tube with a bulb containing a liquid that expands and rises in the tube as the temperature increases.

cli·ni·cian (klĭ-nĭsh′ən) *n.* A physician, psychologist, or psychiatrist specializing in clinical studies or practice.

cli·no·dac·ty·ly (klī′nō-dăk′tə-lē) *n.* Permanent deflection of one or more fingers.

cli·no·scope (klī′nə-skōp′) *n.* An instrument for measuring strabismus in the eyes.

clip (klĭp) *n.* A fastener used in surgery to hold skin or other tissue in position or to control hemorrhage.

clip forceps *n.* A small forceps with a spring catch to hold a bleeding vessel.

clith·ro·pho·bi·a (klĭth′rə-fō′bē-ə) *n.* An abnormal fear of being locked in.

clit·o·ri·dec·to·my (klĭt′ər-ĭ-děk′tə-mē, klī′tər-) *n.* Excision of the clitoris.

clit·o·ri·di·tis (klĭt′ər-ĭ-dī′tĭs, klī′tər-) or **clit·o·ri·tis** (klĭt′ə-rī′tĭs, klī′tə-) *n.* Inflammation of the clitoris.

clit·o·ris (klĭt′ər-ĭs, klī′tər-) *n., pl.* **cli·to·ri·des** (klĭ-tôr′ĭ-dēz′). A small erectile body situated at the anterior portion of the vulva and projecting between the branched extremities of the labia minora forming its prepuce and frenulum. — **clit′o·ral** (-ər-əl) *adj.*

clit·o·rism (klĭt′ə-rĭz′əm, klī′tə-) *n.* Prolonged and usually painful erection of the clitoris.

clit·o·ro·meg·a·ly (klĭt′ə-rō-měg′ə-lē) *n.* An enlarged clitoris.

clo·fi·brate (klō-fī′brāt, -fĭb′rāt) *n.* A synthetic drug used primarily to reduce abnormally elevated levels of plasma cholesterol and triglyceride.

clom·i·phene (klŏm′ə-fēn, klō′mə-) *n.* A synthetic drug that is used in its citrate form to stimulate ovulation.

clone (klōn) *n.* **1.** A group of genetically identical cells descended from a single common ancestor, such as a bacterial colony whose members arose from a single original cell as a result of binary fission. **2.** An organism descended asexually from a single ancestor. **3.** A replica of a DNA sequence, such as a gene, produced by genetic engineering. — *v.* **cloned, clon·ing, clones. 1.** To make multiple identical copies of a DNA sequence. **2.** To establish and maintain pure lineages of a cell under laboratory conditions. **3.** To reproduce or propagate asexually. — **clon′al** (klō′nəl) *adj.*

clo·nic·i·ty (klō-nĭs′ĭ-tē, klō-) *n.* The state of being clonic.

clon·i·dine (klŏn′ĭ-dēn′, klō′nĭ-) *n.* A synthetic drug used in the treatment of hypertension and for the prevention of migraine headaches.

clon·ing (klō′nĭng) *n.* The transplantation of a nucleus from a somatic cell into an ovum, which then develops into an embryo.

clo·nism (klō′nĭz′əm, klŏn′ĭz′-) *n.* A succession of clonic spasms.

clo·nor·chi·a·sis (klō′nôr-kī′ə-sĭs) *n.* A disease caused by infestation with the liver fluke, *Clonorchis sinensis,* and affecting the distal bile ducts.

clon·o·spasm (klŏn′ə-spăz′əm) *n.* See **clonus.**

clo·nus (klō′nəs) *n., pl.* **-nus·es.** A form of movement marked by contractions and relaxations of a muscle, occurring in rapid succession, after forcible extension or flexion of a part. — **clon′ic** (-ĭk, klō′nĭk) *adj.*

closed anesthesia (klōzd) *n.* Inhalation anesthesia in which there is complete rebreathing of all exhaled gases, except for carbon dioxide.

closed chest massage *n.* Cardiac massage in which pressure is applied over the sternum.

closed circuit method *n.* A method for measuring oxygen consumption in which an initial quantity of oxygen is rebreathed through a carbon dioxide absorber and any decrease in the volume of oxygen taken in is noted.

closed comedo *n.* See **whitehead** (sense 1).

closed drainage *n.* The use of a water- or air-tight system to drain a body cavity.

closed fracture *n.* A bone fracture that causes little or no damage to the surrounding soft tissues.

closed hospital *n.* A hospital in which only physicians who are members of the attending and consulting staff may admit and treat patients.

closed reduction *n.* Reduction of a fractured bone by manipulation without incision into the skin.

closed surgery *n.* Surgery that is performed without an incision into skin, as in closed reduction.

clos·ing snap (klō′zĭng) *n.* The accentuated first heart sound of mitral stenosis, related to closure of the abnormal valve.

closing volume *n.* The amount of air in the lungs at which the flow from the lower parts of the lungs becomes severely reduced or stops during expiration.

Clos·trid·i·um (klō-strĭd′ē-əm) *n.* A genus of rod-shaped, spore-forming, chiefly anaerobic bacteria including those causing botulism and tetanus.

clo·sure principle (klō′zhər) *n.* In psychology, the principle that, when one views fragmentary stimuli forming a nearly complete figure, one ignores the missing parts and perceives the figure as whole.

clot (klŏt) *n.* A soft, nonrigid, insoluble mass formed when blood or lymph gels. — *v.* **clot·ted, clot·ting, clots.** To coagulate.

clot·tage (klŏt′ĭj) *n.* The blocking of a canal or duct by a blood clot.

clotting factor *n.* Any of various plasma components involved in the clotting of blood, including fibrinogen, prothrombin, thromboplastin, and calcium ion.

cloud·y swelling (klou′dē) *n.* A degenerative change in cells, in which the cells swell due to injury to the membranes affecting ionic transfer, causing the cytoplasm to appear cloudy and water to accumulate between cells.

clove oil *n.* An aromatic oil obtained from the buds, stems, or leaves of the clove tree, used as a temporary anesthetic for toothaches.

clox·a·cil·lin (klŏk′sə-sĭl′ĭn) *n.* A semisynthetic antibiotic of the penicillin group that is used primarily to treat infections caused by staphylococci, streptococci, or pneumococci.

club·bing (klŭb′ĭng) *n.* A condition affecting the fingers and toes in which the extremities are broadened and the nails are shiny and abnormally curved.

club·foot (klŭb′fŏŏt′) *n.* A congenital deformity of the foot, usually marked by a curled shape or twisted position of the ankle, heel, and toes.

club hair *n.* A hair before normal shedding, in which the bulb has become a club-shaped mass.

clus·ter headache (klŭs′tər) *n.* A recurring headache characterized by severe pain in the eye or temple on one side of the head, and watering of the eye and runny nose on one side of the head.

cly·sis (klī′sĭs) *n., pl.* **-ses** (-sēz′). An infusion of fluid, usually subcutaneous, for therapeutic purposes.

clys·ter (klĭs′tər) *n.* An enema.

cm *abbr.* centimeter

CMA *abbr.* Certified Medical Assistant

CMV *abbr.* cytomegalovirus

CNM *abbr.* Certified Nurse Midwife

CNS *abbr.* central nervous system

Co·A (kō′ā′) *n.* See **coenzyme A.**

co·ad·ap·ta·tion (kō′ăd-ăp-tā′shən) *n.* The joint correlated changes in two or more interdependent organs.

co·ag·glu·ti·nin (kō′ə-glŏŏt′n-ĭn) *n.* A substance that does not agglutinate an antigen, but induces the agglutination of an antigen that is coated with univalent antibody.

co·ag·u·lant (kō-ăg′yə-lənt) *n.* An agent that causes a sol or liquid, especially blood, to coagulate. — **co·ag′u·lant** *adj.*

co·ag·u·late (kō-ăg′yə-lāt′) *v.* **-lat·ed, -lat·ing, -lates.** To change from the liquid state to a solid or gel; clot; curdle. — **co·ag′u·la·bil′i·ty** *n.* — **co·ag′u·la′tor** *n.*

co·ag·u·la·tion (kō-ăg′yə-lā′shən) *n.* **1.** The change, caused by clotting, of blood, from liquid to solid; clotting. **2.** A clot; coagulum.

coagulation factor *n.* See **clotting factor.**

coagulation necrosis *n.* Necrosis in which the affected cells or tissue are converted into a dry, dull, fairly homogeneous eosinophilic mass as a result of the coagulation of protein.

co·ag·u·la·tive (kō-ăg′yə-lā′tĭv, -lə-tĭv) *adj.* Coagulant.

co·ag·u·lum (kō-ăg′yə-ləm) *n., pl.* **-la** (-lə). **1. 2.** A soft insoluble mass formed when a sol or liquid is coagulated.

co·a·les·cence (kō′ə-lĕs′əns) *n.* See **concrescence.**

coal tar *n.* A viscous black liquid containing numerous organic compounds that is obtained by the destructive distillation of coal and used as a raw material for many dyes and drugs.

co·ap·ta·tion (kō′ăp-tā′shən) *n.* The joining together or fitting of two surfaces, such as the edges of a wound or the ends of a broken bone.

coaptation splint *n.* A short splint designed to prevent overriding of the ends of a fractured bone; it is usually supplemented by a longer splint to fix the entire limb.

co·arct (kō-ärkt′) *v.* To restrict or press together, as a blood vessel.

co·arc·ta·tion (kō′ärk-tā′shən) *n.* A constriction, stricture, or stenosis.

coat (kōt) *n.* The outer covering or enveloping layer or layers of an organ or part.

coat·ed tongue (kō′tĭd) *n.* The presence of a whitish layer on the upper surface of the tongue, composed of epithelial debris, food particles, and bacteria.

co·bal·a·min (kō-băl′ə-mĭn) or **co·bal·a·mine** (-mēn′) *n.* See **vitamin B₁₂.**

co·balt (kō′bôlt′) *n.* A metallic element with atomic number 27 used for magnetic and high-temperature alloys and in the form of its salts for blue glass and ceramic pigments.

cob·bler's suture (kŏb′lərz) *n.* See **doubly armed suture.**

Cobb syndrome (kŏb) *n.* A syndrome caused by vascular abnormality of the spinal cord and resulting in neurologic symptoms and cutaneous angiomas.

co·caine (kō-kān′, kō′kān′) *n.* A colorless or white crystalline alkaloid extracted from coca leaves, sometimes used as a local anesthetic especially for the eyes, nose, or throat and widely used as an illicit drug for its euphoric and stimulating effects.

co·cain·ism (kō-kā′nĭz′əm) *n.* The habitual or excessive use of cocaine.

co·car·cin·o·gen (kō′kär-sĭn′ə-jən, kō-kär′sĭn-ə-jĕn′) *n.* A substance that works in combination with a carcinogen in the production of cancer.

coc·cid·i·oi·do·ma (kŏk-sĭd′ē-oi-dō′mə) *n.* A benign localized residual granulomatous lesion or scar in a lung following coccidioidomycosis.

coc·cid·i·oi·do·my·co·sis (kŏk-sĭd′ē-oi′dō-mī-kō′sĭs) *n.* An infectious respiratory disease of humans and other animals caused by inhaling the fungus *Coccidioides immitis;* it is characterized by fever and various respiratory symptoms.

coc·cid·i·o·sis (kŏk-sĭd′ē-ō′sĭs) *n.* A disease caused by a coccidium.

coc·cid·i·um (kŏk-sĭd′ē-əm) *n., pl.* **-i·a** (-ē-ə). Any of various protozoan parasites belonging to the order Coccidia and responsible for a disease of the alimentary canal in livestock, fowl, and humans. — **coc·cid′i·al** *adj.*

coc·cus (kŏk′əs) *n., pl.* **coc·ci** (kŏk′sī, kŏk′ī). A bacterium of round, spheroidal, or ovoid form. — **coc′coid′** (kŏk′oid′), **coc′cal** (kŏk′əl) *adj.*

coc·cy·al·gi·a (kŏk′sē-ăl′jē-ə, -jə) *n.* See **coccygodynia.**

coc·cy·dyn·i·a (kŏk′sĭ-dĭn′ē-ə) *n.* See **coccygodynia.**

coccygeal nerve *n.* The lowest of the spinal nerves, entering the formation of the coccygeal plexus.

coc·cy·gec·to·my (kŏk′sə-jĕk′tə-mē) *n.* Surgical removal of the coccyx.

coc·cy·go·dyn·i·a (kŏk′sĭ-gō-dĭn′ē-ə) *n.* Pain in the region of the coccyx.

coc·cy·got·o·my (kŏk′sĭ-gŏt′ə-mē) *n.* An operation for freeing the coccyx from its attachments.

coc·cy·o·dyn·i·a (kŏk′sē-ō-dĭn′ē-ə) *n.* See **coccygodynia.**

coc·cyx (kŏk′sĭks) *n., pl.* **coc·cy·ges** (kŏk-sī′jēz, kŏk′sĭ-jēz′). The small triangular bone located at the base of the spinal column, formed by the fusion of four rudimentary vertebrae, and articulating above with the sacrum.

coch·i·neal (kŏch′ə-nēl′, kŏch′ə-nēl′, kō′chə-, kō′chə-) *n.* A red dye made of the dried and pulverized bodies of female cochineal insects and used as a biological stain and as an indicator in acid-base titrations.

coch·le·a (kŏk′lē-ə, kō′klē-ə) *n., pl.* **-le·as** or **-le·ae** (-lē-ē′). A spiral-shaped cavity in the petrous portion of the temporal bone of the inner ear, containing the nerve endings essential for hearing and forming one of the divisions of the labyrinth. — **coch′le·ar** (-ər)

cochlear hair cell *n.* A sensory cell in the spiral organ in synaptic contact with sensory as well as efferent fibers of the auditory nerve.

cochlear nerve *n.* The cochlear part of the vestibulocochlear nerve, composed of nerve processes with terminals on the hair cells and the bipolar neurons of the spiral ganglion.

coch·le·o·pal·pe·bral reflex (kŏk′lē-ō-păl′-pə-brə, -păl-pē′-) *n.* A form of the wink reflex in which there is a contraction of the palpebral part of the orbicular muscle of the eye when a sudden noise is made close to the ear.

coch·li·tis (kŏk-lī′tĭs) or **coch·le·i·tis** (kŏk′lē-ī′tĭs) *n.* Inflammation of the cochlea.

Cock·ayne′s syndrome (kŏ-kānz′) *n.* A hereditary syndrome characterized by dwarfism, precociously senile appearance, optic atrophy, deafness, and mental retardation.

co·deine (kō′dēn′, -dē-ĭn) *n.* An alkaloid narcotic derived from opium or morphine and used as a cough suppressant, analgesic, and hypnotic.

cod-liver oil *n.* An oil obtained from the liver of cod and related fishes and used as a dietary source of vitamins A and D.

co·don (kō′dŏn′) *n.* A sequence of three adjacent nucleotides in DNA or in RNA constituting the genetic code that specifies the insertion of an amino acid in a specific structural position in a polypeptide chain during protein synthesis.

coe– *n.* For words beginning with *coe–* that are not found here, see under *ce–*.

co·en·zyme (kō-ĕn′zīm′) *n.* A thermostable nonprotein organic substance that usually contains a vitamin or mineral and combines with the apoenzyme to form an active enzyme system.

coenzyme A *n.* A coenzyme present in all living cells that is necessary for fatty acid synthesis and oxidation, pyruvate oxidation, and other acetylation reactions.

coenzyme Q *n.* Ubiquinone.

coeur en sa·bot (kûr′ ŏn sə-bō′, kœr än sä-bō′) *n.* A heart having an elevated apex combined with a transverse rectangular enlargement, giving it the radiographic appearance of a wooden shoe.

co·fac·tor (kō′făk′tər) *n.* A substance, such as a metallic iron or coenzyme, that must be associated with an enzyme for the enzyme to function.

Cof·fin–Sir·is syndrome (kô′fĭn-sĭr′ĭs) *n.* An inherited syndrome that in males causes mental retardation with wide bulbous nose and low nasal bridge, moderate hirsutism, and digital anomalies with nail hypoplasia. In females the syndrome may cause digital abnormalities and mild mental retardation.

cog·ni·tion (kŏg-nĭsh′ən) *n.* The mental faculty of knowing, which includes perceiving, recognizing, conceiving, judging, sensing, reasoning, and imagining.

cog·ni·tive (kŏg′nĭ-tĭv) *adj.* **1.** Of, characterized by, involving, or relating to cognition. **2.** Having a basis in or reducible to empirical factual knowledge.

cognitive therapy *n.* Any of a variety of techniques in psychotherapy that utilize guided self-discovery, imaging, self-instruction, symbolic modeling, and related forms of elicited cognitions as the principal mode of treatment.

cog·wheel respiration (kŏg′wēl′) *n.* Respiration in which the inspiratory sound is punctuated by two or three silent intervals.

cogwheel rigidity *n.* Rigidity in which the muscles respond with cogwheel-like jerks to the use of force in bending the limb, as occurs in Parkinson's disease.

co·he·sion (kō-hē′zhən) *n.* The intermolecular attraction that holds molecules and masses together.

co·hort (kō′hôrt′) *n.* A defined population group followed prospectively in an epidemiological study.

coin lesion of lungs *n.* Any of various solitary, round, circumscribed shadows appearing in radiographic examinations of the lungs that are believed to be caused by tuberculosis, carcinoma, cysts, infarcts, or vascular anomalies.

co·i·tion (kō-ĭsh′ən) *n.* See **coitus.**

co·i·tus (kō′ĭ-təs, kō-ē′-) *n.* Sexual union between a male and a female involving insertion of the penis into the vagina. — **co′i·tal** *adj.*

coitus in·ter·rup·tus (ĭn′tə-rŭp′təs) *n.* Sexual intercourse deliberately interrupted by withdrawal of the penis from the vagina prior to ejaculation.

coitus res·er·va·tus (rĕz′ər-vā′təs) *n.* Coitus in which ejaculation is delayed or suppressed.

cold (kōld) *n.* A viral infection characterized by inflammation of the mucous membranes lining the upper respiratory passages and usually accompanied by malaise, fever, chills, coughing, and sneezing.

cold abscess *n.* An abscess not accompanied by heat or other usual signs of inflammation.

cold agglutination *n.* The clumping of red blood cells by their own serum or by any other serum when the blood is cooled below body temperature.

cold-blooded *adj.* Ectothermic.

cold pack *n.* A compress of gauze, cloth, or plastic filled or moistened with a cold fluid and applied externally to swollen or injured body parts to relieve pain and swelling.

cold sore *n.* A small blister occurring on the lips and face and caused by a herpes simplex virus; fever blister.

cold stage *n.* The stage of chill in a malarial paroxysm.

cold sweat *n.* A reaction to nervousness, fear, pain, or shock, characterized by simultaneous perspiration and chill and cold moist skin.

cold ulcer *n.* A small gangrenous ulcer on the extremities, due to defective circulation.

co·lec·to·my (kə-lĕk′tə-mē) *n.* Surgical removal of part or all of the colon.

col·ic (kŏl′ĭk) *n.* **1.** Spasmodic pains in the abdomen. **2.** Paroxysms of pain with crying and irritability in young infants, due to a variety of causes, such as swallowing air or overfeeding. — *adj.* (also kō′lĭk). Relating to the colon.

col·i·cin (kŏl′ĭ-sĭn, kō′lĭ-) *n.* Any of various antibacterial proteins produced by certain strains of the colon bacillus that are lethal to other closely related strains of bacteria.

col·ick·y (kŏl′ĭ-kē) *adj.* Relating to or affected by colic.

co·li·form (kō′lə-fôrm′, kŏl′ə-) *adj.* Of or relating to the bacilli that commonly inhabit the intestines of humans and other vertebrates, especially the colon bacillus. — **co′li·form′** *n.*

co·lis·tin (kə-lĭs′tĭn, kō-) *n.* An antibiotic produced by the bacterium *Bacillus polymyxa* or *B. colistinus* that is effective against a wide range of gram-negative bacteria, used especially in the treatment of infections of the gastrointestinal tract.

co·li·tis (kə-lī′tĭs) *n.* Inflammation of the colon.

co·li·tox·e·mi·a (kō′lĭ-tŏk-sē′mē-ə) *n.* A condition resulting from the toxic effects of *Escherichia coli* in the circulating blood.

col·la·gen (kŏl′ə-jən) *n.* The fibrous protein constituent of bone, cartilage, tendon, and other connective tissue that converts into gelatin by boiling.

col·lag·e·nase (kə-lăj′ə-nās′, -nāz′, kŏl′ə-jə-) *n.* Any of various enzymes that catalyze the hydrolysis of collagen and gelatin.

col·lag·e·na·tion (kə-lăj′ə-nā′shən, kŏl′ə-jə-) *n.* **1.**

The replacement of normal tissue by collagenous connective tissue. **2.** The production of collagen by fibroblasts.

collagen disease or **collagen-vascular disease** *n.* Any of a group of diseases affecting connective tissue and frequently characterized by fibrinoid necrosis or vasculitis and including such diseases as lupus erythematosus, rheumatoid arthritis, rheumatic fever, and dermatomyositis.

collagen fiber or **collagenous fiber** *n.* An individual scleroprotein fiber composed of fibrils and usually arranged in branching bundles of indefinite length.

col·la·gen·ic (kŏl′ə-jĕn′ĭk) *adj.* Collagenous.

col·lag·e·no·sis (kə-lăj′ə-nō′sĭs, kŏl′ə-jə-) *n.* See **collagen disease.**

col·lag·e·nous (kə-lăj′ə-nəs) *adj.* Producing or containing collagen.

collagenous colitis *n.* Colitis occurring mostly in middle-aged women and characterized by persistent watery diarrhea and a deposit of a band of collagen beneath the basement membrane of the colon surface epithelium.

col·lapse (kə-lăps′) *v.* **-lapsed, -laps·ing, -laps·es.** **1.** To break down suddenly in strength or health and thereby fall into a condition of extreme prostration. **2.** To fall together or inward suddenly. — *n.* **1.** A condition of extreme prostration. **2.** A falling together of the walls of a structure. **3.** The failure of a physical system.

collapse therapy *n.* Surgical treatment of pulmonary tuberculosis in which the diseased lung is caused to collapse and is then immobilized.

col·lar·bone (kŏl′ər-bōn′) *n.* See **clavicle.**

col·lat·er·al circulation (kə-lăt′ər-əl) *n.* Circulation maintained in small anastomosing vessels when the main artery is obstructed.

collateral vessel *n.* A branch of an artery running parallel with the parent trunk.

col·lect·ing tubule (kə-lĕk′tĭng) *n.* Any of the various straight tubules of the kidney, present in the medulla and the medullary ray of the cortex.

col·lec·tive unconscious (kə-lĕk′tĭv) *n.* In Jungian psychology, a part of the unconscious mind that is shared by a society, a people, or all humankind. The product of ancestral experience, it contains such concepts as science, religion, and morality.

Col·les′ fracture (kŏl′ēz, ĭs) *n.* A bone fracture of the radius of the wrist in which the lower fragment is displaced dorsally.

col·lic·u·lec·to·my (kə-lĭk′yə-lĕk′tə-mē) *n.* Excision of the seminal colliculus.

col·lic·u·li·tis (kə-lĭk′yə-lī′tĭs) *n.* Inflammation of the urethra in the region of the seminal colliculus.

col·lic·u·lus (kə-lĭk′yə-ləs) *n., pl.* **-li** (-lī′). A small elevation above the surrounding parts of a structure.

col·li·ma·tion (kŏl′ə-mā′shən) *n.* **1.** The process of restricting and confining an x-ray beam to a given area. **2.** In nuclear medicine, the process of restricting the detection of emitted radiations to a given area of interest.

col·li·qua·tion (kŏl′ĭ-kwā′shən) *n.* **1.** Excessive

discharge of fluid. **2.** Softening of tissue. **3.** Degeneration of tissue to a liquid state.

colliquative necrosis *n.* See **liquefactive necrosis.**

col·lo·di·on (kə-lō′dē-ən) *n.* A highly flammable, colorless or yellowish syrupy solution of pyroxylin, ether, and alcohol, used as an adhesive to close small wounds and hold surgical dressings and in topical medications.

collodion baby *n.* An infant born with skin that is bright red, shiny, translucent, and drawn tight, giving the appearance the face is immobilized.

col·loid (kŏl′oid′) *n.* **1.** A suspension of finely divided particles in a continuous medium in which the particles do not settle out of the substance rapidly and are not readily filtered. **2.** The particulate matter so suspended. **3.** The gelatinous stored secretion of the thyroid gland, consisting mainly of thyroglobulin. **4.** Gelatinous material resulting from colloid degeneration in diseased tissue. — *adj.* Of, relating to, containing, or having the nature of a colloid. — **col·loi′dal** (kə-loid′l, kŏ-) *adj.*

col·lyr·i·um (kə-lēr′ē-əm) *n., pl.* **-i·ums** or **-i·a** (-ē-ə). **1.** A medicinal lotion applied to the eye; eyewash. **2.** Any preparation for the eye.

co·lo·cen·te·sis (kō′lə-sĕn-tē′sĭs) *n.* Surgical puncture of the colon to relieve distention.

co·lo·co·los·to·my (kō′lə-kə-lŏs′tə-mē) *n.* The surgical formation of a communication between two noncontinuous segments of the colon.

co·lo·en·ter·i·tis (kō′lə-ĕn′tə-rī′tĭs) *n.* See **enterocolitis.**

co·lon (kō′lən) *n., pl.* **-lons** or **-la** (-lə). The division of the large intestine extending from the cecum to the rectum. — **co·lon′ic** (kə-lŏn′ĭk) *adj.*

co·lon·al·gi·a (kō′lə-năl′jē-ə, -jə) *n.* Pain in the colon.

colon bacillus *n.* A rod-shaped bacterium, especially *Escherichia coli,* a generally nonpathogenic commensal found in all vertebrate intestinal tracts, but which can be virulent, causing diarrhea and other dysenteric symptoms.

co·lon·op·a·thy (kō′lə-nŏp′ə-thē) or **co·lop·a·thy** (kə-lŏp′ə-thē) *n.* Disease of the colon.

co·lon·o·scope (kō-lŏn′ə-skōp′, kə-) *n.* A long flexible endoscope, often equipped with a device for obtaining tissue samples, that is used for visual examination of the colon.

co·lon·os·co·py (kō′lə-nŏs′kə-pē) *n.* Examination of the inner surface of the colon by means of a colonoscope.

col·o·ny (kŏl′ə-nē) *n.* A discrete group of organisms, such as a group of cells growing on a solid nutrient surface.

co·lo·pex·os·to·my (kō′lə-pĕk-sŏs′tə-mē) *n.* The surgical formation of an artificial anus by creation of an opening into the colon after its fixation to the abdominal wall.

co·lo·pex·ot·o·my (kō′lə-pĕk-sŏt′ə-mē) *n.* Incision into the colon after its fixation to the abdominal wall.

col·o·pex·y (kŏl′ə-pĕk′sē, kō′lə-) *n.* The attach-

ment of a portion of the colon to the abdominal wall.

co·lo·pli·ca·tion (kō′lə-plĭ-kā′shən) *n.* The surgical reduction of the lumen of a dilated colon by making folds or tucks in its walls.

co·lo·proc·ti·tis (kō′lə-prŏk-tī′tĭs) *n.* Inflammation of the colon and the rectum.

co·lo·proc·tos·to·my (kō′lə-prŏk-tŏs′tə-mē) *n.* The surgical formation of a communication between the rectum and a segment of the colon.

co·lop·to·sis (kō′lŏp-tō′sĭs) or **co·lop·to·si·a** (-tō′sē-ə, -zē-ə) *n.* Downward displacement or prolapse of the colon, especially of the transverse portion.

co·lo·punc·ture (kō′lə-pŭngk′chər) *n.* See **colocentesis.**

col·or (kŭl′ər) *n.* **1.** That aspect of the appearance of objects and light sources that may be specified in terms of hue, lightness, and saturation. **2.** That portion of the visible electromagnetic spectrum specified in terms of wavelength, luminosity, and purity. **3.** The general appearance of the skin; complexion.

Col·o·ra·do tick fever (kŏl′ə-răd′ō, -rä′dō) *n.* A viral infection transmitted to humans by the tick *Dermacentor andersoni* and characterized by mild symptoms and intermittent fever.

col·or·blind or **col·or-blind** (kŭl′ər-blīnd′) *adj.* Partially or totally unable to distinguish certain colors.

color blindness *n.* Deficiency of color perception, whether hereditary or acquired, partial or complete.

color chart *n.* An assembly of chromatic samples used in checking color vision.

co·lo·rec·tal (kō′lə-rĕk′təl) *adj.* Relating to the colon and the rectum, or to the entire large bowel.

co·lo·rec·ti·tis (kō′lə-rĕk-tī′tĭs) *n.* See **coloproctitis.**

co·lo·rec·tos·to·my (kō′lə-rĕk-tŏs′tə-mē) *n.* See **coloproctostomy.**

color hearing *n.* The imaginary perception of colors in response to the actual perception of sounds.

co·lor·rha·gi·a (kŭl′ə-rā′jē-ə, -jə) or **co·lon·or·rha·gi·a** (kō′lə-nō-rā′jē-ə, -jə) *n.* An abnormal discharge from the colon.

co·lor·rha·phy (kə-lôr′ə-fē) *n.* Suture of the colon.

co·lor·rhe·a (kō′lə-rē′ə) or **co·lon·or·rhe·a** (kō′lə-nō-rē′ə) *n.* Diarrhea thought to originate from a process confined to or affecting chiefly the colon.

color scotoma *n.* An area of depressed color vision in the visual field.

co·lo·scope (kō′lə-skōp′) *n.* See **colonoscope.**

co·los·co·py (kə-lŏs′kə-pē) *n.* See **colonoscopy.**

co·lo·sig·moid·os·to·my (kō′lə-sĭg′moi-dŏs′tə-mē) *n.* The surgical formation of an anastomosis between the sigmoid colon and another part of the colon.

co·los·to·my (kə-lŏs′tə-mē) *n.* **1.** Surgical construction of an artificial excretory opening from the colon. **2.** The opening created by such a surgical procedure.

colostomy bag *n.* A receptacle worn over the stoma to collect feces following a colostomy.

co·los·tror·rhea (kə-lŏs′trə-rē′ə) *n.* An abnormally profuse secretion of colostrum.

co·los·trum (kə-lŏs′trəm) *n.* The first milk secreted at the time of parturition, differing from the milk secreted later by containing more lactalbumin and lactoprotein, and also being rich in antibodies that confer passive immunity to the newborn. — **co·los′tral** (-trəl) *adj.*

co·lot·o·my (kə-lŏt′ə-mē) *n.* Incision into the colon.

col·pal·gi·a (kŏl-păl′jē-ə, -jə) *n.* See **vaginodynia**.

col·pa·tre·sia (kŏl′pə-trē′zhə, -zhē-ə) *n.* See **vaginal atresia**.

col·pec·ta·sis (kŏl-pĕk′tə-sĭs) or **col·pec·ta·sia** (kŏl′-pĕk-tā′zhə, -zē-ə) *n.* Distention of vagina.

col·pec·to·my (kŏl-pĕk′tə-mē) *n.* See **vaginectomy**.

col·pi·tis (kŏl-pī′tĭs) *n.* See **vaginitis**.

col·po·cele (kŏl′pə-sēl′) *n.* **1.** A hernia projecting into the vagina. **2.** See **colpoptosis**.

col·po·clei·sis (kŏl′pō-klī′sĭs) *n.* Surgical obliteration of the lumen of the vagina.

col·po·cys·ti·tis (kŏl′pō-sĭ-stī′tĭs) *n.* Inflammation of the vagina and the bladder.

col·po·cys·to·cele (kŏl′pō-sĭs′tə-sēl′) *n.* See **cystocele**.

col·po·cys·to·plas·ty (kŏl′pō-sĭs′tə-plăs′tē) *n.* Plastic surgery to repair the vesicovaginal wall.

col·po·dyn·i·a (kŏl′pō-dĭn′ē-ə) *n.* See **vaginodynia**.

col·po·hy·per·pla·sia (kŏl′pō-hī′pər-plā′zhə) *n.* A thickening of the vaginal mucous membrane.

col·po·mi·cros·co·py (kŏl′pō-mī-krŏs′kə-pē) *n.* Direct observation and study of cells in the vagina and cervix using a special microscope.

col·po·per·i·ne·o·plas·ty (kŏl′pō-pĕr′ə-nē′ə-plăs′tē) *n.* See **vaginoperineoplasty**.

col·po·per·i·ne·or·rha·phy (kŏl′pō-pĕr′ə-nē-ôr′ə-fē) *n.* See **vaginoperineorrhaphy**.

col·po·pex·y (kŏl′pə-pĕk′sē) *n.* See **vaginofixation**.

col·po·plas·ty (kŏl′pə-plăs′tē) *n.* See **vaginoplasty**.

col·po·poi·e·sis (kŏl′pə-poi-ē′sĭs) *n.* Surgical construction of an artificial vagina.

col·po·pto·sis (kŏl′pō-tō′sĭs, -pŏp-tō′-) or **col·po·pto·si·a** (-tō′sē-ə, -zē-ə) *n.* Prolapse of the vaginal walls.

col·por·rha·gi·a (kŏl′pō-rā′jē-ə, -jə) *n.* Vaginal hemorrhage.

col·por·rha·phy (kŏl-pôr′ə-fē) *n.* Repair of a rupture of the vagina by suturing the edges of the tear.

col·por·rhex·is (kŏl′pō-rĕk′sĭs) *n.* A tearing of the vaginal wall; vaginal laceration.

col·po·scope (kŏl′pə-skōp′) *n.* An endoscopic instrument that magnifies the epithelia of the vagina and cervix in vivo to allow direct observation. — **col′po·scop′ic** (-skŏp′ĭk) *adj.*

col·pos·co·py (kŏl-pŏs′kə-pē) *n.* Examination of the vaginal and cervical epithelia by means of a colposcope.

col·po·spasm (kŏl′pə-spăz′əm) *n.* A spasmodic contraction of the vagina.

col·po·ste·no·sis (kŏl′pō-stə-nō′sĭs) *n.* A narrowing of the lumen of the vagina.

col·po·ste·not·o·my (kŏl′pō-stə-nŏt′ə-mē) *n.* Surgical correction of colpostenosis.

col·pot·o·my (kŏl-pŏt′ə-mē) *n.* See **vaginotomy**.

col·po·xe·ro·sis (kŏl′pō-zĭ-rō′sĭs) *n.* Abnormal dryness of the vaginal mucous membrane.

Co·lum·bi·a Mental Maturity scale (kə-lŭm′-bē-ə) *n.* A test for assessing the intellectual ability of children ranging from 3 to 12 years old.

col·umn (kŏl′əm) *n.* Any of various tubular or pillarlike supporting structures in the body, such as the spinal column, each generally having a single tissue origin and function.

co·lum·nar cell (kə-lŭm′nər) *n.* A cell, usually epithelial, that is tall, narrow, and somewhat cylindrical.

columnar epithelium *n.* Epithelium made up of cells that are taller than they are wide and that form a single layer.

co·ma (kō′mə) *n.* A state of profound unconsciousness in which a person is incapable of sensing or responding to external stimuli.

coma aberration *n.* The distortion in the formation of an image created when a bundle of light rays enters an optical system that is not parallel to the optic axis.

coma scale *n.* A clinical test for assessing impaired consciousness in which motor responsiveness, verbal performance, eye opening, and sometimes the function of cranial nerves are assessed.

co·ma·tose (kō′mə-tōs′, kŏm′ə-) *adj.* **1.** Of, relating to, or affected with coma. **2.** Marked by lethargy; torpid.

com·bat fatigue (kŏm′băt′) *n.* See **war neurosis**.

com·bi·na·tion therapy (kŏm′bə-nā′shən) *n.* Method of treating disease through the simultaneous use of a variety of drugs to eliminate or control the biochemical cause of the disease.

com·bined version (kəm-bīnd′) *n.* See **bimanual version**.

com·e·do (kŏm′ĭ-dō′) *n.*, *pl.* **-dos** or **-do·nes** (-dō′-nēz). A dilated hair follicle filled with keratin and sebum and often blackened at the surface; a blackhead.

com·e·do·car·ci·no·ma (kŏm′ĭ-dō-kär′sə-nō′mə) *n.* A form of carcinoma of the breast in which plugs of necrotic malignant cells may be expressed from the ducts.

com·e·do·gen·ic (kŏm′ĭ-dō-jĕn′ĭk) *adj.* Tending to produce or aggravate acne.

com·fort zone (kŭm′fərt) *n.* The temperature range between 28° and 30° C or 82½° and 86° F at which the unclothed body is able to maintain heat balance without shivering or sweating.

com·ma bacillus (kŏm′ə) *n.* See **Koch's bacillus**.

com·man·do procedure (kə-măn′dō) *n.* A surgical operation for the removal of malignant tumors of the floor of the oral cavity.

com·men·sal·ism (kə-mĕn′sə-lĭz′əm) *n*. A symbiotic relationship in which one organism derives benefit and the other is unharmed.

com·mi·nute (kŏm′ə-noōt′, -nyoōt′) *v*. **-nut·ed, -nut·ing, -nutes.** To reduce to powder; pulverize. — **com′mi·nu′tion** *n*.

com·mi·nut·ed (kŏm′i-nū-tĕd) *adj*. Broken into fragments. Used of a fractured bone.

comminuted fracture *n*. A fracture in which the bone is splintered, crushed, or broken.

commissural cheilitis *n*. See **angular cheilitis**.

com·mis·sure (kŏm′ə-shoōr′) *n*. **1.** A line or place at which two things are joined. **2.** A tract of nerve fibers passing from one side to the other of the spinal cord or brain. **3.** The point, angle, or surface where two parts, such as the eyelids, lips, or cardiac valves, join or form a connection. — **com′mis·su′ral** *adj*.

com·mis·sur·ot·o·my (kŏm′ə-shoō-rŏt′ə-mē, -soō-) *n*. **1.** Surgical division of a commissure, fibrous band, or ring. **2.** See **midline myelotomy.**

com·mit (kə-mĭt′) *v*. **-mit·ted, -mit·ting, -mits.** To place officially in confinement or custody, as in a mental health facility.

com·mon bile duct (kŏm′ən) *n*. The duct that is formed by the union of the hepatic and cystic ducts and discharges into the duodenum.

common cold *n*. See **cold.**

common-cold virus *n*. Any of numerous strains of viruses associated with the common cold, especially the rhinoviruses, and also including strains of adenovirus, and parainfluenza virus.

common hepatic duct *n*. The part of the biliary duct system that is formed by the junction of the right and left hepatic ducts and is joined by the cystic duct to form the common bile duct.

common iliac vein *n*. A vein that is formed by union of the external and internal iliac veins at the brim of the pelvis.

com·mu·ni·ca·ble (kə-myoō′nĭ-kə-bəl) *adj*. Transmittable between persons or species; contagious.

communicable disease *n*. A disease that is transmitted through direct contact with an infected individual or indirectly through a vector.

communicating branch *n*. A bundle of nerve fibers passing from one nerve to join another.

com·mu·ni·ca·tion (kə-myoō′nĭ-kā′shən) *n*. **1.** The exchange of thoughts, messages, or information, as by speech, signals, writing, or behavior. **2.** An opening or a connecting passage between two structures. **3.** A joining or connecting of solid fibrous structures, such as tendons and nerves.

com·mu·ni·ty medicine (kə-myoō′nĭ-tē) *n*. Public health services emphasizing preventive medicine and epidemiology for members of a given community or region.

community psychiatry *n*. Psychiatry focusing on the detection, prevention, early treatment, and rehabilitation of emotional and behavioral disorders as they develop in the community.

Co·mol·li·'s sign (kə-mō′lēz, kô-mô′lēz) *n*. An indication of fracture of the scapula in which a tri-

angular cushionlike swelling appears that corresponds to the outline of that bone.

co·mor·bid·i·ty (kō′môr-bĭd′ĭ-tē) *n*. A concomitant but unrelated pathological or disease process.

com·pact bone (kəm-păkt′, kŏm-, kŏm′păkt′) *n*. The compact noncancellous portion of bone that consists largely of concentric lamellar osteons and interstitial lamellae.

com·pat·i·ble (kəm-păt′ə-bəl) *adj*. Capable of being grafted, transfused, or transplanted from one individual to another without rejection.

com·pen·sat·ed acidosis (kŏm′pən-sā′tĭd) *n*. Acidosis in which the pH of body fluids is normal due to compensation by respiratory or renal mechanisms.

compensated alkalosis *n*. A rise in alkalinity that is compensated for by physiological changes to the pH of body fluids.

com·pen·sa·tion (kŏm′pən-sā′shən) *n*. **1.** A process in which a tendency for a change in a given direction is counteracted by another change so that the original change is not evident. **2.** An unconscious psychological mechanism by which one tries to make up for imagined or real deficiencies in personality or physical ability.

compensation neurosis *n*. A neurosis whose symptoms are believed to be associated with a real or presumed disability that may bring financial compensation.

com·pen·sa·to·ry circulation (kəm-pĕn′sə-tôr′ē) *n*. Circulation established in dilated collateral vessels when the main artery of the part is obstructed.

compensatory polycythemia *n*. Polycythemia resulting from anoxia, as in congenital heart disease, pulmonary emphysema, or prolonged residence at a high altitude.

com·pe·tence (kŏm′pĭ-təns) *n*. **1.** The quality of being competent or capable of performing an allotted function. **2.** The quality or condition of being legally qualified to perform an act. **3.** The mental ability to distinguish right from wrong and to manage one's own affairs. **4.** The ability to respond immunologically to bacteria, viruses, or other antigenic agents. **5.** Integrity, especially the normal tight closure of a cardiac valve. — **com′pe·tent** (-tənt) *adj*.

com·pe·ti·tion (kŏm′pĭ-tĭsh′ən) *n*. The process by which the activity or presence of one substance interferes with or suppresses the activity of another substance with similar affinities, as of antigens.

com·pet·i·tive bind·ing assay (kəm-pĕt′ĭ-tĭv bīn′dĭng) *n*. An assay in which a biologically specific binding agent competes for radioactively labeled or radioactively unlabeled compounds, used especially in tests for measuring the concentration of hormone receptors in a sample by introducing a radioactively labeled hormone.

competitive inhibition *n*. Blockage of the action of an enzyme on its substrate by replacement of the substrate with a similar but inactive compound that can combine with the active site of the enzyme but is not acted upon or split by it.

com·plaint (kəm-plānt′) *n.* **1.** A bodily disorder or disease; a malady or an ailment. **2.** The symptom or distress about which a patient seeks medical assistance.

com·ple·ment (kŏm′plə-mənt) *n.* A group of proteins found in normal blood serum and plasma that are activated sequentially in a cascadelike mechanism that allows them to combine with antibodies and destroy pathogenic bacteria and other foreign cells.

com·ple·men·tar·i·ty (kŏm′plə-měn-tăr′ĭ-tē) *n.* **1.** The correspondence or similarity between nucleotides or strands of nucleotides of DNA and RNA molecules that allows precise pairing. **2.** The affinity that an antigen and an antibody have for each other as a result of the chemical arrangement of their combining sites.

com·ple·men·ta·ry air (kŏm′plə-měn′tə-rē, -trē) *n.* See **inspiratory capacity.**

complementary DNA *n.* cDNA.

com·ple·men·ta·tion (kŏm′plə-mən-tā′shən, -měn-) *n.* **1.** Functional interaction between two defective viruses permitting replication under conditions inhibitory to the single virus. **2.** Interaction between two genetic units, one or both of which are defective, permitting the organism containing these units to function normally, whereas it could not do so if one unit were absent.

complement binding assay *n.* An assay for detecting immune complexes.

complement fixation *n.* The binding of active serum complement to a specific antigen-antibody pair used in diagnostic tests, such as the Wasserman test, to detect the presence of a specific antigen or antibody.

complement-fixation test *n.* An immunological test for determining the presence of a particular antibody in which serum is treated in a manner that allows existing antibodies to accept and bind to a known amount of antigen, so that if binding occurs the presence of the antibody is verified and its concentration in the serum can be calculated.

complement-fixing antibody *n.* An antibody that combines with and sensitizes an antigen, leading to the activation of complement and sometimes resulting in lysis.

complement protein *n.* Substance that is produced by a predecessor protein or in response to the presence of foreign material in the body and that triggers or participates in a complement reaction.

complement reaction *n.* A physiological reaction to the presence of a foreign microorganism in which a cascade of enzymatic reactions, triggered by molecular features of the microorganism, result in its lysis or phagocytosis.

com·plete antibody (kəm-plēt′) *n.* See **saline agglutinin.**

complete antigen *n.* An antigen capable of stimulating the formation of an antibody with which it then reacts.

complete blood count *n.* A combination of the determinations of the red blood cell count and indices, white blood cell count, hematocrit, and differential blood count.

complete denture *n.* A dental prosthesis that replaces all the natural teeth and their associated maxillary and mandibular structures.

com·plex (kŏm′plĕks′) *n.* **1.** A group of related, often repressed memories, thoughts, and impulses that compel characteristic or habitual patterns of thought, feelings, and behavior. **2.** A composite of chemical or immunological structures. **3.** An entity made up of three or more interrelated components. **4.** A group of individual structures known or believed to be anatomically, embryologically, or physiologically related. **5.** The combination of factors, symptoms, or signs of a disease or disorder that forms a syndrome. — *adj.* (kəm-plĕks′, kŏm′plĕks′). **1.** Consisting of interconnected or interwoven parts; composite. **2.** Composed of two or more units. **3.** Of or relating to group of individual structures known or believed to be anatomically, embryologically, or physiologically related.

com·plex·ion (kəm-plĕk′shən) *n.* The natural color, texture, and appearance of the skin, especially of the face.

com·pli·ance (kəm-plī′əns) *n.* **1.** A measure of the ease with which a structure or substance may be deformed, especially a measure of the ease with which a hollow organ may be distended. **2.** The degree of constancy and accuracy with which a patient follows a prescribed regimen.

com·pli·ca·tion (kŏm′plĭ-kā′shən) *n.* A pathological process or event occurring during a disease that is not an essential part of the disease; it may result from the disease or from other causes.

com·po·nent of complement (kəm-pō′nənt) *n.* Any one of the nine distinct protein units that are responsible for the immunological activities associated with complement.

com·pos·ite flap (kəm-pŏz′ĭt) *n.* A skin flap incorporating underlying muscle, bone, or cartilage.

composite graft *n.* A graft composed of multiple structures, such as skin and cartilage.

com·pos men·tis (kŏm′pəs mĕn′tĭs) *adj.* Of sound mind; sane.

com·pound (kŏm′pound′) *n.* **1.** A combination of two or more elements or parts. **2.** A pure, macroscopically homogeneous substance consisting of atoms or ions of two or more different elements in definite proportions that cannot be separated by physical means, and having properties unlike those of its constituent elements. — *adj.* (kŏm′-pound′, kŏm-pound′, kəm-). Consisting of two or more substances, ingredients, elements, or parts. — *v.* -**pound·ed**, -**pound·ing**, -**pounds.** (kŏm-pound′, kəm-, kŏm′pound′). **1.** To combine so as to form a whole; mix. **2.** To produce or create by combining two or more ingredients or parts, as for a prescription.

compound flap *n.* See **composite flap.**

compound fracture *n.* See **open fracture.**

compound gland *n.* A gland composed of a branching system of ducts that combine, eventually opening into a secretory duct.

compound joint *n.* A joint composed of three or more skeletal elements.

com·pre·hen·sion (kŏm′prĭ-hĕn′shən) *n.* See **apperception** (sense 1).

com·press (kŏm′prĕs′) *n.* A soft pad of gauze or other material applied with pressure to a part of the body to control hemorrhage or to supply heat, cold, moisture, or medication to alleviate pain or reduce infection. — *v.* **-pressed, -press·ing, -press·es.** (kəm-prĕs′). To press or squeeze together.

com·pres·sion (kəm-prĕsh′ən) *n.* **1.** See **condensation. 2.** The state of being compressed.

compression paralysis *n.* Paralysis due to compression of a nerve, as by prolonged pressure.

compression syndrome *n.* See **crush syndrome.**

com·pres·sor (kəm-prĕs′ər) *n.* A muscle that causes compression of a structure upon contraction.

com·pul·sion (kəm-pŭl′shən) *n.* An uncontrollable impulse to perform an act, often repetitively, as an unconscious mechanism to avoid unacceptable ideas and desires which arouse anxiety.

com·pul·sive (kəm-pŭl′sĭv) *adj.* Caused or conditioned by compulsion or obsession. — *n.* A person with behavior patterns governed by a compulsion.

compulsive neurosis *n.* Obsessive-compulsive neurosis.

compulsive personality *n.* A personality pattern characterized by rigidity, perfectionistic standards, meticulous attention to order and detail, and excessive concern with conformity, duty, and adherence to standards of conscience.

com·put·ed tomography (kəm-pyōō′tĭd) *n.* See **computerized axial tomography.**

com·put·er·ized axial tomography (kəm-pyōō′tə-rīzd′) *n.* Tomography used in diagnostic studies of internal bodily structures in which computer analysis of a series of cross-sectional scans made along a single axis of a bodily structure or tissue is used to construct a three-dimensional image of that structure.

co·na·tion (kō-nā′shən) *n.* The aspect of mental processes or behavior directed toward action or change and including impulse and desire. — **co′na·tive** (kō′nə-tĭv, kŏn′ə-) *adj.*

con·ceive (kən-sēv′) *v.* **-ceived, -ceiv·ing, -ceives. 1.** To become pregnant. **2.** To apprehend mentally; understand.

con·cen·tra·tion (kŏn′sən-trā′shən) *n.* **1.** An increase of the strength of a pharmaceutical preparation by the extraction, precipitation, and drying of its crude active agent. **2.** The amount of a specified substance in a unit amount of another substance.

con·cept (kŏn′sĕpt′) *n.* **1.** An abstract idea or notion. **2.** An explanatory principle in a scientific system.

concept formation *n.* The development of ideas based on the common properties of objects, events, or qualities using the processes of abstraction and generalization.

con·cep·tion (kən-sĕp′shən) *n.* **1.** The act of forming a general idea or notion. **2.** The formation of a viable zygote by the union of a spermatozoon and an ovum; fertilization. **3.** See **concept** (sense 2).

con·cep·tus (kən-sĕp′təs) *n., pl.* **-tus·es.** The products of conception; that is, the embryo, chorionic sac, placenta, and fetal membranes.

con·cha (kŏng′kə) *n., pl.* **-chae** (-kē′). Any of various structures, such as the external ear, that resemble a shell in shape. — **con′chal** (-kəl) *adj.*

con·cor·dance (kən-kôr′dns) *n.* The presence of a given trait in both members of a pair of twins. — **con·cor′dant** *adj.*

concordant alternans *n.* See **concordant alternation.**

concordant alternation *n.* An alternation in the mechanical or electrical activity of the heart, occurring in both systemic and pulmonary circuits.

con·cres·cence (kən-krĕs′əns) *n.* The growing together of originally separate parts.

con·cre·ti·o cor·dis (kən-krē′shē-ō kôr′dĭs) *n.* Extensive adhesion between parietal and visceral layers of the pericardium with partial or complete obliteration of the pericardial cavity.

con·cre·tion (kən-krē′shən) *n.* A solid mass, usually composed of inorganic material, formed in a cavity or tissue of the body; a calculus.

con·cus·sion (kən-kŭsh′ən) *n.* **1.** A violent shaking or jarring. **2.** An injury to a soft structure, especially the brain, produced by a violent blow and followed by a temporary or prolonged loss of function.

con·den·sa·tion (kŏn′dĕn-sā′shən, -dən-) *n.* **1.** The act of making more solid or dense. **2.** The process by which a gas or vapor changes to a liquid. **3.** The liquid formed when a gas is condensed. **4.** The psychological process by which a single symbol or word is associated with the emotional content of a group of ideas, feelings, memories, or impulses, especially as expressed in dreams.

con·di·tion (kən-dĭsh′ən) *n.* **1.** A disease or physical ailment. **2.** A state of health or physical fitness. — *v.* **-tioned, -tion·ing, -tions.** To cause an organism to respond in a specific manner to a conditioned stimulus in the absence of an unconditioned stimulus.

con·di·tioned (kən-dĭsh′ənd) *adj.* **1.** Exhibiting or trained to exhibit a conditioned response. **2.** Physically fit.

conditioned reflex *n.* See **conditioned response.**

conditioned response *n.* A new or modified response elicited by a stimulus after conditioning.

conditioned stimulus *n.* A previously neutral stimulus that, after repeated association with an unconditioned stimulus, elicits the response produced by the unconditioned stimulus itself.

con·di·tion·ing (kən-dĭsh′ə-nĭng) *n.* A process of behavior modification by which a subject comes to associate a desired behavior with a previously unrelated stimulus.

con·dom (kŏn′dəm, kŭn′-) *n.* A flexible sheath, usually made of thin rubber or latex, designed to cover the penis during sexual intercourse for contraceptive purposes or as a means of preventing sexually transmitted diseases.

con·duct (kən-dŭkt′) *v.* **-duct·ed, -duct·ing, -ducts.** To act as a medium for conveying something such as heat or electricity. — *n.* (kŏn′dŭkt′). The way a person acts, especially from the standpoint of morality. — **con·duc′tive** *adj.*

con·duct disorder (kŏn′dŭkt′) *n.* A behavior disorder of childhood or adolescence characterized by a pattern of conduct in which either the basic rights of others or the societal norms or rules appropriate for a certain age are violated.

con·duc·tion (kən-dŭk′shən) *n.* The transmission or conveying of something through a medium or passage, especially the transmission of electric charge or heat through a conducting medium without perceptible motion of the medium itself.

conduction analgesia *n.* The pharmacological deactivation of sensory nerves in a portion of the body.

conduction anesthesia *n.* Regional anesthesia in which a local anesthetic solution is injected about the nerves to inhibit nerve transmission.

conduction aphasia *n.* A form of aphasia in which there is ability to speak and write but words are skipped, repeated, or substituted for one another.

conductive deafness *n.* Hearing loss or impairment caused by a defect in part of the ear that conducts sound, specifically the external canal or the middle ear.

conductive hearing impairment *n.* Hearing impairment caused by an interference with the apparatus conducting sound to the inner ear.

conductive heat *n.* Heat transmitted to the body by direct contact, as by an electric pad or hot water bottle.

con·duc·tiv·i·ty (kŏn′dŭk-tĭv′ĭ-tē) *n.* **1.** The ability or power to conduct or transmit heat, electricity, or sound. **2.** The ability of a body structure to transmit an electric impulse, especially the ability of a nerve to transmit a wave of excitation.

con·duc·tor (kən-dŭk′tər) *n.* **1.** A substance or medium that conducts heat, light, sound, or especially an electric charge. **2.** An instrument or probe having a groove along which a knife is passed in slitting open a sinus or fistula.

condylar joint *n.* See **ellipsoidal joint.**

con·dy·lar·thro·sis (kŏn′dl-är-thrō′sĭs) *n.* A joint formed by condylar surfaces, such as the knee.

con·dyle (kŏn′dīl′, -dl) *n.* A rounded prominence at the end of a bone, most often for articulation with another bone.

con·dy·lec·to·my (kŏn′dl-ĕk′tə-mē) *n.* Excision of a condyle.

con·dy·lo·ma (kŏn′dl-ō′mə) *n., pl.* **-mas** or **-ma·ta** (-mə-tə). A wartlike growth on the skin or mucous membrane, usually in the area of the anus or external genitalia. — **con′dy·lo′ma·tous** (-mə-təs) *adj.*

condyloma a·cu·mi·na·tum (ə-kyōō′mə-nā′təm) *n.* See **genital wart.**

con·dy·lot·o·my (kŏn′dl-ŏt′ə-mē) *n.* Surgical incision or division of a condyle.

cone (kōn) *n.* See **cone cell.**

cone cell *n.* One of the photoreceptors in the retina of the eye that is responsible for daylight and color vision; they are concentrated in the fovea centralis, creating the area of greatest visual acuity.

cone granule *n.* The nucleus of a retinal cell connecting with one of the cones.

cone of light *n.* The bright triangular area of reflected light on the tympanic membrane during examination.

con·fab·u·la·tion (kən-făb′yə-lā′shən) *n.* The unconscious filling of gaps in one's memory by fabrications that one accepts as facts. — **con·fab′u·late′** *v.*

con·fec·tion (kən-fĕk′shən) *n.* A sweetened medicinal compound; an electuary.

con·fi·den·ti·al·i·ty (kŏn′fĭ-dĕn′shē-ăl′ĭ-tē) *n.* The ethical principle or legal right that a physician or other health professional will hold secret all information relating to a patient unless the patient gives consent permitting disclosure.

con·fine·ment (kən-fīn′mənt) *n.* Lying-in.

con·flict (kŏn′flĭkt′) *n.* A psychic struggle between opposing or incompatible impulses, desires, or tendencies.

con·flu·ence (kŏn′flōō-əns) *n.* A flowing or meeting together; a joining.

con·flu·ent (kŏn′flōō-ənt) *adj.* **1.** Flowing together; blended into one. **2.** Merging or running together so as to form a mass, as sores in a rash.

confluent and re·tic·u·late papillomatosis (rĭ-tĭk′yə-lĭt, -lāt′) *n.* A genetically determined skin condition occurring predominantly in females with onset at puberty, characterized by discrete and confluent papules that spread along the anterior and posterior mid-chest.

con·fu·sion (kən-fyōō′zhən) *n.* Impaired orientation with respect to time, place, or person; a disturbed mental state.

con·ge·ner (kŏn′jə-nər) *n.* **1.** A member of the same kind, class, or group. **2.** One of two or more muscles having the same function.

con·gen·i·tal (kən-jĕn′ĭ-tl) *adj.* **1.** Existing at or before birth usually through heredity, as a disorder or deformity. **2.** Acquired at birth or during uterine development usually as a result of environmental influences.

congenital afibrinogenemia *n.* A hereditary disorder of blood coagulation in which little or no fibrinogen is present in the plasma.

congenital amputation *n.* Loss of a fetal limb, usually a result of an intrinsic deficiency of embryonic tissue.

congenital anemia *n.* See **erythroblastosis fetalis.**

congenital anomaly *n.* See **birth defect.**

congenital ectodermal defect *n.* The incomplete development of the epidermis and skin appendages, causing the skin to be hairless and sweating to be deficient.

congenital generalized fibromatosis *n.* A rare disorder often fatal in the first week of life, although sometimes undergoing spontaneous remission, characterized by multiple subcutaneous and visceral fibrous tumors that are present at birth.

congenital glaucoma *n.* See **buphthalmia**.

congenital nevus *n.* A melanocytic nevus that is visible at birth, is often larger than an acquired nevus, and usually involves deeper dermal structures than an acquired nevus.

congenital stridor *n.* Stridor occurring at birth or within the first few months of life. It may be due to abnormal flaccidity of the epiglottis or arytenoids.

congenital syphilis *n.* Syphilis acquired by the fetus in utero.

con·gest (kən-jĕst′) *v.* **-gest·ed, -gest·ing, -gests**. To cause the accumulation of excessive blood or tissue fluid in a vessel or an organ.

con·gest·ed (kən-jĕs′tĭd) *adj.* Affected with or characterized by congestion.

con·ges·tion (kən-jĕs′chən) *n.* The presence of an abnormal amount of fluid in a vessel or organ; especially excessive accumulation of blood due either to increased afflux or to obstruction of return flow.

con·ges·tive (kən-jĕs′tĭv) *adj.* Characterized by congestion.

congestive heart failure *n.* See **heart failure**.

congestive splenomegaly *n.* Enlargement of the spleen due to passive congestion.

con·glom·er·ate (kən-glŏm′ər-ĭt) *adj.* Gathered or aggregated into a mass. — **con·glom′er·a′tion** (-ə-rā′shən) *n.*

con·glu·ti·na·tion (kən-glŏot′n-ā′shən, kŏn-) *n.* **1.** Agglutination of the antigen-antibody-complement complex by normal bovine serum and other colloidal materials. **2.** See **adhesion** (sense 4).

conidium *n., pl.* **-i·a** (-ē-ə). An asexually produced fungal spore.

co·ni·o·fi·bro·sis (kō′nē-ō-fī-brō′sĭs) *n.* Fibrosis, especially of the lungs, caused by dust.

co·ni·o·sis (kō′nē-ō′sĭs) *n.* Any of various diseases or pathological conditions caused by dust.

con·i·za·tion (kŏn′ĭ-zā′shən, kō′nĭ-) *n.* The excision of a cone of tissue, such as the mucosa of the uterine cervix.

con·joined twins (kən-joind′) *pl.n.* Identical twins born with their bodies joined at some point and having varying degrees of residual duplication, a result of the incomplete division of the ovum from which the twins developed.

con·ju·gate (kŏn′jə-gāt) *v.* **-gat·ed, -gat·ing, -gates**. To undergo conjugation. — *adj.* (-gĭt, -gāt′). Joined together, especially in a pair or pairs; coupled.

conjugated protein *n.* A compound, such as hemoglobin, made up of a protein molecule and a nonprotein prosthetic group.

conjugate paralysis *n.* Paralysis of one or more of the external muscles of the eye, resulting in loss of conjugate movement of the eyes.

con·junc·ti·va (kŏn′jŭngk-tī′və) *n., pl.* **-vas** or **-vae** (-vē). The mucous membrane that lines the inner surface of the eyelid and the exposed surface of the eyeball.

con·junc·ti·val (kŏn′jŭngk-tī′vəl) *adj.* Relating to the conjunctiva.

conjunctival reflex *n.* Closing of the eyes in response to irritation of the conjunctiva.

conjunctival test *n.* A test in which an allergen is placed on the conjunctiva.

con·junc·ti·vi·tis (kən-jŭngk′tə-vī′tĭs) *n.* Inflammation of the conjunctiva, characterized by redness and often accompanied by a discharge.

con·junc·ti·vo·ma (kən-jŭnk′tə-vō′mə) *n.* A tumor of the conjunctiva made up of conjunctival tissue.

con·junc·ti·vo·plas·ty (kŏn′jŭngk-tī′və-plăs′tē) *n.* Plastic surgery of the conjunctiva.

con·nec·tion (kə-nĕk′shən) *n.* **1.** The act of connecting or the state of being connected. **2.** Something that connnects.

con·nec·tive tissue (kə-nĕk′tĭv) *n.* The supporting or framework tissue of the body, arising chiefly from the embryonic mesoderm and including collagenous, elastic and reticular fibers, adipose tissue, cartilage, and bone.

connective-tissue disease *n.* A group of diseases affecting connective tissue that are believed to be noninheritable, such as rheumatic fever and rheumatoid arthritis, and that are generally characterized by fever, pain, stiffness, and inflammation.

connective tumor *n.* A tumor formed from connective tissue, such as an osteoma, fibroma, or sarcoma.

con·san·guin·i·ty (kŏn′săn-gwĭn′ĭ-tē, -săng-) *n.* Relationship by blood or by a common ancestor.

con·science (kŏn′shəns) *n.* **1.** The awareness of a moral or ethical aspect to one's conduct together with the urge to prefer right over wrong. **2.** The part of the superego in psychoanalysis that judges the ethical nature of one's actions and thoughts and then transmits such determinations to the ego for consideration.

con·scious (kŏn′shəs) *adj.* **1.** Having an awareness of one's environment and one's own existence, sensations, and thoughts. **2.** Intentionally conceived or done; deliberate. — *n.* In psychoanalysis, the component of waking awareness perceptible by a person at any given instant. — **con′scious·ly** *adv.*

con·scious·ness (kŏn′shəs-nĭs) *n.* **1.** The state or condition of being conscious. **2.** A sense of one's personal or collective identity, especially the complex of attitudes, beliefs, and sensitivities held by or considered characteristic of an individual or a group. **3.** In psychoanalysis, the conscious.

consciousness-raising *n.* A process, as by group therapy, of achieving greater awareness of one's needs so as to fulfill one's potential as a person.

con·sec·u·tive anophthalmia (kən-sĕk′yə-tĭv) *n.*

Anopthalmia due to atrophy or degeneration of the optic vesicle.

con·sen·su·al (kən-sĕn'shōō-əl) *adj.* **1.** Of or relating to a reflexive response of one body structure following stimulation of another, such as the concurrent constriction of one pupil in response to light shined in the other. **2.** Of or relating to involuntary movement of a body part accompanying voluntary movement of another. — **con·sen'su·al·ly** *adv.*

con·ser·va·tive (kən-sûr'və-tĭv) *adj.* Of or relating to treatment by gradual, limited, or well-established procedures; not radical. — **con·ser'va·tive·ly** *adv.*

con·sis·ten·cy principle (kən-sĭs'tən-sē) *n.* In psychology, the desire to be consistent, especially in attitudes and beliefs.

con·sol·i·da·tion (kən-sŏl'ĭ-dā'shən) *n.* The process of becoming a firm solid mass, as in an infected lung when the alveoli are filled with exudate in pneumonia.

con·stant positive pressure breathing (kŏn'stənt) *n.* Inhalation and exhalation of respiratory gases that are under a small constant positive pressure relative to the ambient pressure.

con·sti·pate (kŏn'stə-pāt') *v.* **-pat·ed, -pat·ing, -pates.** To cause constipation in the bowels.

con·sti·pat·ed (kŏn'stə-pā'tĭd) *adj.* Suffering from constipation.

con·sti·pa·tion (kŏn'stə-pā'shən) *n.* Difficult, incomplete, or infrequent evacuation of dry, hardened feces from the bowels.

con·sti·tu·tion (kŏn'stĭ-tōō'shən, -tyōō'-) *n.* The physical makeup of the body, including its functions, metabolic processes, reactions to stimuli, and resistance to the attack of pathogenic organisms.

con·sti·tu·tion·al (kŏn'stĭ-tōō'shə-nəl, -tyōō'-) *adj.* **1.** Of or relating to one's physical makeup. **2.** Of or proceeding from the basic structure or nature of a person or thing; inherent.

constitutional disease *n.* A disease involving the entire body or having a widespread array of symptoms.

constitutional reaction *n.* **1.** A generalized or systemic reaction to a stimulus. **2.** An allergic or immune response occurring at sites remote from that of the introduction of an antigen.

constitutional symptom *n.* A symptom indicating that a disease or disorder is affecting the whole body.

con·strict (kən-strĭkt') *v.* **-strict·ed, -strict·ing, -stricts.** To make smaller or narrower by binding or squeezing.

con·stric·tion (kən-strĭk'shən) *n.* **1.** The act of constricting or the state of being constricted. **2.** A feeling of tightness or pressure, as in the chest. **3.** A constricted or narrow part.

constriction ring *n.* True spastic stricture of the uterine cavity caused by a zone of muscle undergoing tetanic contraction and forming a tight constriction about some part of the fetus.

con·stric·tive pericarditis (kən-strĭk'tĭv) *n.* Tu-

berculous or other infection of the pericardium, with thickening of the membrane and constriction of the cardiac chambers.

con·stric·tor (kən-strĭk'tər) *n.* One that constricts, especially a muscle that contracts or compresses a part or organ of the body.

con·sult·ant (kən-sŭl'tənt) *n.* **1.** A physician or surgeon who does not take actual charge of a patient, but acts in an advisory capacity to the patient's primary physician. **2.** A member of a hospital staff who has no patients, but stands ready to advise the physician or surgeon.

con·sul·ta·tion (kŏn'səl-tā'shən) *n.* A meeting of two or more health professionals to discuss the diagnosis, prognosis, and treatment of a particular case.

con·sult·ing staff (kən-sŭl'tĭng) *n.* The body of specialists affiliated with a hospital who serve in an advisory capacity to the attending staff.

con·sump·tion (kən-sŭmp'shən) *n.* **1.** The act or process of using up something. **2.** A progressive wasting of body tissue. **3.** Pulmonary tuberculosis. No longer in technical use.

con·tact (kŏn'tăkt') *n.* **1.** A coming together or touching, as of bodies or surfaces. **2.** A person recently exposed to a contagious disease, usually through close association with an infected individual. — *v.* (kŏn'tăkt', kən-tăkt'). To bring, be, or come in contact. — *adj.* **1.** Of, sustaining, or making contact. **2.** Caused or transmitted by touching, as a rash.

con·tac·tant (kən-tăk'tənt) *n.* Any of a group of allergens that elicit manifestations of induced sensitivity by direct contact with the skin or mucosa.

contact cheilitis *n.* Inflammation of the lips resulting from contact with a specific allergen.

contact dermatitis *n.* An acute or chronic skin inflammation resulting from contact with an irritating substance or allergen.

contact lens *n.* A thin plastic or glass lens that is fitted over the cornea of the eye to correct various vision defects.

contact splint *n.* A slotted plate, held by screws, used in the treatment of fracture of long bones.

contact with reality *n.* The ability to understand or interpret external phenomena in relation to the norms of one's societal or cultural milieu.

con·ta·gion (kən-tā'jən) *n.* **1.** Disease transmission by direct or indirect contact. **2.** A disease that is or may be transmitted by direct or indirect contact; a contagious disease. **3.** See **contagium**.

con·ta·gious (kən-tā'jəs) *adj.* **1.** Of or relating to contagion. **2.** Transmissible by direct or indirect contact, as a disease; communicable. **3.** Capable of transmitting disease, as an infected patient; carrying a disease. — **con·ta'gious·ness** *n.*

contagious disease *n.* See **communicable disease**.

con·ta·gium (kən-tā'jəm) *n., pl.* **-gia** (-jə). The direct cause, such as a bacterium or virus, of a communicable disease.

con·tam·i·nate (kən-tăm'ə-nāt') *v.* **-nated, -nating, -nates. 1.** To make impure or unclean by contact or mixture. **2.** To expose to or permeate with radioactivity.

con·tam·i·na·tion (kən-tăm′ə-nā′shən) *n.* **1.** The act or process of rendering something harmful or unsuitable, as by the presence of radioactive substances. **2.** The presence of extraneous material that renders a substance or preparation impure or harmful.

con·tent (kŏn′tĕnt′) *n.* **1.** *Often* **contents**. Something contained, as in a receptacle. **2.** The proportion of a specified substance present in something else, as of protein in a food. **3.** The subject matter or essential meaning of something, especially a dream.

content analysis *n.* Any of various techniques for classifying and studying the verbalizations of normal or psychologically impaired individuals.

con·ti·nence (kŏn′tə-nəns) *n.* **1.** Self-restraint; moderation. **2.** Voluntary control over urinary and fecal discharge. **3.** Partial or complete abstention from sexual activity. — **con′ti·nent** *adj.*

con·tin·ued fever (kən-tĭn′yōōd) *n.* A fever of some duration in which there are no intermissions or marked remissions in the temperature.

con·tin·u·ous bar retainer (kən-tĭn′yōō-əs) *n.* A metal bar, usually resting on lingual surfaces of teeth, to aid in their stabilization and to act as an indirect retainer after orthodontic treatment.

continuous murmur *n.* A murmur heard throughout systole and into diastole.

continuous positive airway pressure *n.* A technique of respiratory therapy for either spontaneously breathing or mechanically ventilated patients in which airway pressure is maintained above atmospheric pressure by pressurization of the ventilatory circuit.

continuous positive pressure breathing *n.* See **controlled mechanical ventilation.**

continuous positive pressure ventilation *n.* See **controlled mechanical ventilation.**

con·tra·ap·er·ture (kŏn′trə-ăp′ər-chər) *n.* See **counteropening.**

con·tra·cep·tion (kŏn′trə-sĕp′shən) *n.* Intentional prevention of conception or impregnation through the use of various devices, agents, drugs, sexual practices, or surgical procedures.

con·tra·cep·tive (kŏn′trə-sĕp′tĭv) *adj.* Capable of preventing conception. — *n.* A device, drug, or chemical agent that prevents conception.

contraceptive device *n.* Any of various devices used to prevent pregnancy, including the diaphragm, condom, and intrauterine device.

contraceptive sponge *n.* A small absorbent contraceptive pad that contains a spermicide and is placed against the cervix of the uterus before sexual intercourse.

con·tract (kən-trăkt′, kŏn′trăkt′) *v.* **-tract·ed, -tract·ing, -tracts. 1.** To reduce in size by drawing together; shrink. **2.** To become reduced in size by or as if by being drawn together, as the pupil of the eye. **3.** To acquire or incur by contagion or infection.

con·trac·tile (kən-trăk′təl, -tīl′) *adj.* Capable of

contracting or causing contraction, as a tissue. — **con′trac·til′i·ty** (kŏn′trăk-tĭl′ĭ-tē) *n.*

con·trac·tion (kən-trăk′shən) *n.* **1.** The act of contracting or the state of being contracted. **2.** The shortening and thickening of functioning muscle or muscle fiber.

con·trac·tu·al psychiatry (kən-trăk′chōō-əl) *n.* An arrangement in which a person undergoing psychiatric treatment retains control over his or her participation with the psychiatrist and decides when to seek help.

con·trac·ture (kən-trăk′chər) *n.* An abnormal, often permanent shortening, as of muscle or scar tissue, that results in distortion or deformity, especially of a joint of the body.

con·tra·in·di·cate (kŏn′trə-ĭn′dĭ-kāt′) *v.* **-cat·ed, -cat·ing, -cates.** To indicate the inadvisability of something, such as a medical treatment.

con·tra·in·di·ca·tion (kŏn′trə-ĭn′dĭ-kā′shən) *n.* A factor that renders the administration of a drug or the carrying out of a medical procedure inadvisable. — **con′tra·in′di·cate′** *v.*

con·trast bath (kŏn′trăst′) *n.* A bath in which a part of the body is immersed alternately in hot and cold water.

contrast enema *n.* See **barium enema.**

contrast medium *n.* A substance, such as barium or air, used in radiography to increase the contrast of an image. A positive contrast medium absorbs x-rays more strongly than the tissue or structure being examined; a negative contrast medium, less strongly.

contrast stain *n.* A dye used to color a portion of a tissue or cell that remained uncolored when the other part was stained by a dye of different color.

con·tre·coup (kŏn′trə-kōō′) *n.* Injury to a part opposite the site of the primary injury, as an injury to the skull opposite the site of a blow.

con·trol (kən-trōl′) *v.* **-trolled, -trol·ling, -trols. 1.** To verify or regulate a scientific experiment by conducting a parallel experiment or by comparing with another standard. **2.** To hold in restraint; check. — *n.* **1.** A standard of comparison for checking or verifying the results of an experiment. **2.** An individual or group used as a standard of comparison in a control experiment.

control experiment *n.* An experiment that isolates the effect of one variable on a system by holding constant all variables but the one under observation.

controlled hypotension *n.* See **induced hypotension.**

controlled mechanical ventilation *n.* A method of artificial ventilation in which all inspirations occur as a result of positive pressure applied to the airway.

controlled respiration *n.* See **controlled ventilation.**

controlled substance *n.* Any of various drugs or chemical substances, including stimulants, depressants, and hallucinogens, whose possession and use are regulated under the Controlled Substances Act.

controlled ventilation *n.* Intermittent application of positive pressure to a gas or gases in or about the airway in order to force gas into the lungs in the absence of spontaneous ventilatory efforts.

con·tuse (kən-tōōz′, -tyōōz′) *v.* **-tused, -tus·ing, -tus·es.** To injure without breaking the skin; bruise.

contused wound *n.* A bruise.

con·tu·sion (kən-tōō′zhən, -tyōō′-) *n.* An injury in which the skin is not broken, often characterized by ruptured blood vessels and discolorations; a bruise.

con·va·lesce (kŏn′və-lĕs′) *v.* **-lesced, -lesc·ing, -lesc·es.** To return to health and strength after illness; recuperate.

con·va·les·cence (kŏn′və-lĕs′əns) *n.* **1.** Gradual return to health and strength after an illness, an injury, or a surgical operation. **2.** The period needed for returning to health after an illness, an injury, or a surgical operation.

con·va·les·cent (kŏn′və-lĕs′ənt) *adj.* Relating to convalescence. — *n.* A person who is recovering from an illness, an injury, or a surgical operation.

con·vec·tive heat (kən-vĕk′tĭv) *n.* Heat conveyed to the body by a moving warm medium, such as air or water.

con·ven·tion·al thoracoplasty (kən-vĕn′shə-nəl) *n.* Surgical removal of part of the ribs to allow inward retraction of the chest wall and collapse of a diseased lung.

con·ver·gence (kən-vûr′jəns) *n.* **1.** The process of coming together or the state of having come together toward a common point. **2.** Such a gathering at a single preganglionic motor neuron of several postganglionic motor neurons. **3.** The coordinated turning of the eyes inward to focus on an object at close range. **4.** The movement of cells from the periphery of the embryo toward the midline during gastrulation. — **con·verge′** *v.* — **con·ver′gent** *adj.*

convergence excess *n.* That condition in which an esophoria or esotropia is greater for near vision than for far vision.

convergent strabismus *n.* See **esotropia.**

con·ver·sion (kən-vûr′zhən, -shən) *n.* A defense mechanism in which repressed ideas, conflicts, or impulses are manifested by various bodily symptoms, such as paralysis or breathing difficulties, that have no physical cause. — **con·ver′sive** *adj.*

conversion disorder *n.* A disorder involving the loss or alteration of physical functioning, such as paralysis, voice loss, tunnel vision, or seizures, that is the result of a psychological involvement or need rather than a physical illness or disease.

con·ver·sive heat (kən-vûr′sĭv) *n.* Heat produced in the body by the absorption of waves, such as the sun's rays or infrared radiation, which are not in themselves hot.

con·vo·lut·ed tubule (kŏn′və-lōō′tĭd) *n.* The highly convoluted segments of nephron in the renal labyrinth of the kidney made up of the proximal tubule leading from the Bowman's capsule to the descending limb of Henle's loop and the distal tubule leading from the ascending limb of Henle's loop to a collecting tubule.

con·vo·lu·tion (kŏn′və-lōō′shən) *n.* **1.** A form or part that is folded or coiled. **2.** One of the convex folds of the surface of the brain.

con·vulse (kən-vŭls′) *v.* **-vulsed, -vuls·ing, -vuls·es.** To affect with irregular and involuntary muscular contractions; throw into convulsions.

con·vul·sion (kən-vŭl′shən) *n.* An intense, paroxysmal, involuntary muscular contraction.

con·vul·sive (kən-vŭl′sĭv) *adj.* **1.** Characterized by or having the nature of convulsions. **2.** Having or producing convulsions.

Coo·ley's anemia (kōō′lēz) *n.* See **thalassemia major.**

Coombs' serum (kōōmz) *n.* Serum from a rabbit or other animal previously immunized with purified human globulin to prepare antibodies directed against IgG and complement, used in the direct and indirect Coombs' tests.

Coombs' test *n.* Either of two tests for detecting red blood cell antibodies: the direct test, for detecting sensitized red blood cells in erythroblastosis fetalis and in acquired hemolytic anemia; and the indirect test, for cross-matching blood or investigating transfusion reactions.

co·or·di·na·tion (kō-ôr′dn-ā′shən) *n.* **1.** The harmonious adjustment or interaction of parts. **2.** Harmonious functioning of muscles or groups of muscles in the execution of movements.

COPD *abbr.* chronic obstructive pulmonary disease

cope (kōp) *v.* **coped, cop·ing, copes.** To contend with difficulties with the intent to overcome them.

cop·per (kŏp′ər) *n.* A ductile malleable metallic element with atomic number 29 that is an excellent conductor of heat and electricity. It is essential to nutrition and a component of various enzymes; several of its salts are used in medicine.

cop·rem·e·sis (kŏ-prĕm′ĭ-sĭs) *n.* See **fecal vomiting.**

cop·ro·an·ti·bod·y (kŏp′rō-ăn′tĭ-bŏd′ē) *n.* Any of various antibodies occurring in the intestinal tract and found in feces that are formed by plasma cells in the intestinal mucosa and consist chiefly of the IgA class.

cop·ro·lag·ni·a (kŏp′rə-lăg′nē-ə) *n.* A form of sexual perversion in which pleasure is obtained from the thought, sight, or touching of excrement.

cop·ro·la·lia (kŏp′rə-lā′lē-ə) *n.* The uncontrolled or involuntary use of obscene or scatological language that may accompany certain mental disorders, such as schizophrenia or Tourette's syndrome.

cop·ro·lith (kŏp′rə-lĭth′) *n.* A hard mass of fecal matter in the intestine.

cop·ro·ma (kŏ-prō′mə) *n.* The accumulation of hardened feces in the colon or rectum giving the appearance of an abdominal tumor.

cop·roph·a·gy (kŏ-prŏf′ə-jē) *n.* See **scatophagy.** — **cop·roph′a·gous** (-gəs) *adj.*

cop·ro·phil·i·a (kŏp′rə-fĭl′ē-ə) *n.* An abnormal, often obsessive interest in excrement, especially the use of feces for sexual excitement. — **cop′ro·phil′i·ac′** (-ē-ăk′) n.

cop·ro·pho·bi·a (kŏp′rə-fō′bē-ə) n. An abnormal abhorrence of defecation and feces.

cop·ro·por·phy·rin (kŏp′rə-pôr′fə-rĭn) n. Either of two porphyrin compounds found normally in feces as a decomposition product of bilirubin.

cop·ros·ta·sis (kŏ-prŏs′tə-sĭs, kŏp′rə-stā′-) n. The impaction of feces in the intestine.

cop·u·la (kŏp′yə-lə) n. A narrow part connecting two structures.

cop·u·late (kŏp′yə-lāt′) v. **-lat·ed, -lat·ing, -lates.** To engage in coitus or sexual intercourse.

cop·u·la·tion (kŏp′yə-lā′shən) n. See **coitus.**

cor (kôr) n., pl. **cor·da** (kôr′də). Heart.

cor·al calculus (kôr′əl) n. See **stag-horn calculus.**

cord or **chord** (kôrd) n. A long ropelike bodily structure, such as a nerve or tendon.

cord blood n. Blood present in the umbilical vessels at the time of delivery.

cor·dec·to·my (kôr-dĕk′tə-mē) n. Excision of all or a part of a cord, as of a vocal cord.

cor·don sa·ni·taire (kôr-dôɴ′sä-nē-târ′) n. A barrier designed to prevent a disease or other undesirable condition from spreading.

cor·do·pex·y (kôr′də-pĕk′sē) n. The surgical fixation of a cord, as of one or both vocal cords for the relief of laryngeal stenosis.

cor·dot·o·my or **chor·dot·o·my** (kôr-dŏt′ə-mē) n. **1.** An operation on the spinal cord. **2.** Surgical division of tracts of the spinal cord, as for the relief of severe pain.

core (kôr) n. **1.** The hard or fibrous central part of certain fruits, such as the apple, containing the seeds. **2.** The central or innermost part. **3.** The part of a nuclear reactor where fission occurs.

cor·ec·to·me·di·al·y·sis (kôr-ĕk′tə-mē-dī-ăl′ĭ-sĭs) n. A peripheral iridectomy to form an artificial pupil.

co·rel·y·sis (kô-rĕl′ĭ-sĭs) n. Surgical detachment of the adhesions between the capsule of the lens and the iris.

cor·e·o·plas·ty (kôr′ē-ə-plăs′tē) n. Plastic surgery to correct a deformed or occluded pupil.

cor·e·pex·y (kôr′ə-pĕk′sē) n. See **corepraxy.**

cor·e·prax·y (kôr′ə-prăk′sē) n. An operation to centralize a pupil that is abnormally situated.

co·re·pres·sor (kō′rĭ-prĕs′ər) n. A substance that combines with and activates a genetic repressor, thus preventing gene transcription and inhibiting protein synthesis.

Co·ri cycle (kôr′ē) n. The phases in the metabolism of carbohydrates in which muscles convert glycogen to lactic acid, which is carried by the blood to the liver where it is converted to glycogen then broken down to glucose that, in turn, is carried by the blood to muscles, where it is converted to glycogen and used as an energy source for muscular activity.

co·ri·um (kôr′ē-əm) n., pl. **co·ri·a** (kôr′ē-ə). See **dermis.**

corn (kôrn) n. A small conical callosity caused by pressure over a bony prominence, as on a toe.

cor·ne·a (kôr′nē-ə) n. The transparent, convex, anterior portion of the outer fibrous coat of the eyeball that covers the iris and the pupil and is continuous with the sclera. — **cor′ne·al** (-əl) adj.

corneal astigmatism n. Astigmatism due to a defect in the curvature of the corneal surface.

corneal graft n. See **keratoplasty.**

corneal margin n. The margin of the cornea overlapped by the sclera.

corneal reflex n. Contraction of the eyelids when the cornea is lightly touched.

corneal staphyloma n. See **anterior staphyloma.**

cor·ne·o·scle·ra (kôr′nē-ō-sklîr′ə) n. The cornea and sclera considered as the external coat of the eyeball. — **cor′ne·o·scler′al** adj.

cor·nic·u·lum (kôr-nĭk′yə-ləm) n., pl. **-la** (-lə). A small cornu or hornlike process.

cor·ni·fi·ca·tion (kôr′nə-fĭ-kā′shən) n. See **keratinization.**

cor·ni·fy (kôr′nə-fī′) v. **-fied, -fy·ing, -fies.** To undergo cornification.

co·ro·na (kə-rō′nə) n., pl. **-nas** or **-nae** (-nē). The crownlike upper portion of a body part or structure, such as the top of the head.

cor·o·na·rism (kôr′ə-nə-rĭz′əm) n. **1.** Coronary insufficiency. **2.** Angina pectoris.

cor·o·na·ri·tis (kôr′ə-nə-rī′tĭs) n. Inflammation of the coronary arteries.

cor·o·nar·y (kôr′ə-nĕr′ē) adj. **1.** Of, relating to, or being the coronary arteries or coronary veins. **2.** Of or relating to the heart. —n. A coronary thrombosis.

coronary artery n. **1.** An artery with its origin in the right aortic sinus, passing around the right side of the heart, and branching to the right atrium and ventricle; right coronary artery. **2.** An artery with its origin in the left aortic sinus, and dividing into two major branches, the anterior interventricular and the circumflex branch; left coronary artery.

coronary bypass n. See **coronary bypass surgery.**

coronary bypass surgery n. A surgical procedure performed to improve blood supply to the heart by creating new routes for blood flow when one or more of the coronary arteries become obstructed. The surgery involves removing a healthy blood vessel from another part of the body, such as the leg, and grafting it onto the heart to circumvent the blocked artery.

coronary care unit n. A hospital unit that is specially equipped to treat and monitor patients with serious heart conditions, such as coronary thrombosis.

coronary failure n. Acute coronary insufficiency.

coronary heart disease n. A disease of the heart and the coronary arteries that is characterized by atherosclerotic arterial deposits that block blood flow to the heart, causing myocardial infarction.

coronary insufficiency n. Inadequate coronary circulation leading to anginal pain.

coronary occlusion n. Blockage of a coronary vessel, usually by thrombosis or atheroma and often leading to myocardial infarction.

coronary thrombosis *n.* Obstruction of a coronary artery by a thrombus, often leading to destruction of heart muscle.

coronary valve *n.* A fold of endocardium where the coronary sinus opens into the right atrium.

coronary vein *n.* Any of the veins that drain blood from the muscular tissue of the heart and empty into the coronary sinus.

co·ro·na·vi·rus (kə-rō′nə-vī′rəs) *n.* Any of various single-stranded, RNA-containing viruses that cause respiratory infection in humans and resemble a crown when viewed under an electron microscope.

cor·o·ner (kôr′ə-nər) *n.* A public officer whose primary function is to investigate by inquest any death thought to be of other than natural causes.

cor·o·noid·ec·to·my (kôr′ə-noi-děk′tə-mē) *n.* Surgical removal of the coronoid process of the mandible.

cor·o·plas·ty (kôr′ə-plăs′tē) *n.* See coreoplasty.

co·rot·o·my (kô-rŏt′ə-mē) *n.* See iridotomy.

cor·po·re·al (kôr-pôr′ē-əl) *adj.* Of, relating to, or characteristic of the body.

corpse (kôrps) *n.* **1.** A dead body, especially the dead body of a human. **2.** A cadaver.

cor pul·mo·na·le (pŏŏl′mə-nä′lē, pŭl′-) *n.* Acute strain or hypertrophy of the right ventricle caused by a disorder of the lungs or of the pulmonary blood vessels.

cor·pus (kôr′pəs) *n., pl.* **-po·ra** (-pər-ə). **1.** The human body, consisting of the head, neck, trunk, and limbs. **2.** The main part of a bodily structure or organ. **3.** A distinct bodily mass or organ having a specific function.

corpus al·bi·cans (ăl′bǐ-kănz′) *n.* See albicans.

corpus cal·lo·sum (kə-lō′səm) *n.* The commissural plate of nerve fibers connecting the two cerebral hemispheres.

cor·pus·cle (kôr′pə-səl, -pŭs′əl) *n.* **1.** An unattached body cell, such as a blood or lymph cell. **2.** A rounded, globular mass of cells, such as the pressure receptor on certain nerve endings. **— cor·pus′cu·lar** (kôr-pŭs′kyə-lər) *adj.*

corpuscular lymph *n.* See aplastic lymph.

corpuscular radiation *n.* Radiation consisting of streams of subatomic particles such as protons, electrons, and neutrons.

corpus lu·te·um (lōō′tē-əm) *n.* A yellow, progesterone-secreting mass of cells that forms from a Graafian follicle after the release of a mature egg.

corpus luteum hormone *n.* See progesterone (sense 1).

corpus spon·gi·o·sum (spən′jē-ō′səm, -spän′) The longitudinal column of erectile tissue of the penis, containing the urethra.

cor·rect (kə-rĕkt′) *v.* **-rect·ed, -rect·ing, -rects.** To remove, remedy, or counteract something, such as a malfunction or defect. *— adj.* Free from error or fault; true or accurate.

cor·re·spon·dence (kôr′ĭ-spŏn′dəns) *n.* A relationship between corresponding points on each retina such that sensory stimulation produces a single image.

cor·ro·sive (kə-rō′sĭv, -zĭv) *adj.* Causing or tending to cause the gradual destruction of a substance by chemical action. *— n.* A substance having the capability or tendency to cause slow destruction.

cor·tex (kôr′těks′) *n., pl.* **-tex·es** or **-ti·ces** (-tǐ-sēz′). **1.** The outer layer of an internal organ or body structure, as of the kidney or adrenal gland. **2.** The cerebral cortex.

cor·ti·cal (kôr′tǐ-kəl) *adj.* **1.** Of, relating to, derived from, or consisting of cortex. **2.** Of, relating to, associated with, or depending on the cerebral cortex.

cortical audiometry *n.* Measurement of the electric potentials that arise in the auditory system above the level of the brainstem.

cortical hormone *n.* See adrenocortical hormone.

cor·ti·cec·to·my (kôr′tǐ-sěk′tə- mē) *n.* See topectomy.

cor·ti·coid (kôr′tǐ-koid′) *n.* A corticosteroid.

cor·ti·co·spi·nal (kôr′tǐ-kō-spī′nəl) *adj.* Of or relating to the cerebral cortex and the spinal cord.

cor·ti·co·ste·roid (kôr′tǐ-kō-stěr′oid′, -stěr′-) *n.* Any of the steroid hormones produced by the adrenal cortex or their synthetic equivalents, such as cortisol and aldosterone.

cor·ti·cos·ter·one (kôr′tǐ-kǒs′tə-rōn′) *n.* A corticosteroid produced in the adrenal cortex that functions in the metabolism of carbohydrates and proteins.

cor·ti·co·troph (kôr′tǐ-kō-trŏf′) *n.* Any of the cells of the anterior lobe of the pituitary gland that produce adrenocorticotropic hormone.

cor·ti·co·tro·pin (kôr′tǐ-kō-trō′pən) or **cor·ti·co·tro·phin** (-trō′fǐn) *n.* See ACTH.

cor·ti·sol (kôr′tǐ-sôl′, -zôl′, -sôl′, -zôl′) *n.* See hydrocortisone (sense 1).

cor·ti·sone (kôr′tǐ-sōn′, -zōn′) *n.* A naturally occurring corticosteroid that functions primarily in carbohydrate metabolism and is used in the treatment of rheumatoid arthritis, adrenal insufficiency, certain allergies, and gout.

Cor·ti's tunnel (kôr′tēz) *n.* The spiral canal in the ear's spiral organ that is filled with fluid and occasionally crossed by nonmedullated nerve fibers.

cor·us·ca·tion (kôr′ə-skā′shən) *n.* A sensation of a flash of light before the eyes.

Cor·vi·sart's facies (kôr′vē-särz′) *n.* The characteristic appearance seen in cardiac insufficiency or aortic regurgitation, consisting of a swollen, cyanotic face with shiny eyes and puffy eyelids.

co·ry·ne·bac·te·ri·um (kôr′ə-nē-băk-tēr′ē-əm, kə-rǐn′ə-) *n.* Any of various gram-positive, rod-shaped bacteria of the genus *Corynebacterium*, which includes many animal and plant pathogens, such as the causative agent of diphtheria.

co·ry·za (kə-rī′zə) *n.* See cold.

co·ry·za·vi·rus (kə-rī′zə-vī′rəs) *n.* See rhinovirus.

cos·met·ic (kŏz-mět′ĭk) *n.* A preparation designed to beautify the body by direct application. *— adj.* **1.** Serving to beautify the body. **2.** Serving to modify or improve the appearance of a physical feature, defect, or irregularity.

cosmetic surgery *n.* Surgery that modifies or improves the appearance of a physical feature, defect, or irregularity.

cos·ta (kŏs′tə) *n.*, *pl.* **-tae** (-tē). Rib. — **cos′tal** *adj.*

costal arch *n.* The portion of the lower opening of the chest formed by the cartilages of the seventh to tenth ribs.

costal cartilage *n.* The cartilage forming the anterior continuation of a rib.

cos·tal·gi·a (kŏ-stăl′jē-ə, -jə) *n.* Pain in the ribs; pleurodynia.

cos·tec·to·my (kŏ-stĕk′tə-mē) *n.* Surgical excision of a rib.

Cos·ten's syndrome (kŏs′tənz) *n.* A complex of symptoms that includes loss of hearing, tinnitus, dizziness, headache, and a burning sensation of the throat, tongue, and side of the nose; its anatomical and physiological causes are uncertain.

cos·tive (kŏs′tĭv) *adj.* **1.** Suffering from constipation. **2.** Causing constipation.

cos·to·chon·dri·tis (kŏs′tō-kŏn-drī′tĭs) *n.* Inflammation of one or more of the costal cartilages, characterized by pain of the anterior chest wall that may radiate.

cos·to·ster·no·plas·ty (kŏs′tō-stûr′nə-plăs′tē) *n.* Surgical correction of a malformation of the anterior chest wall.

cos·tot·o·my (kŏ-stŏt′ə-mē) *n.* Surgical division of a rib.

cos·to·trans·ver·sec·to·my (kŏs′tō-trăns′vûr-sĕk′tə-mē, -trănz′-) *n.* Surgical excision of part of a rib and the articulating transverse process.

Cotte's operation (kŏts, kôts) *n.* See **presacral neurectomy.**

cot·y·le·don (kŏt′l-ēd′n) *n.* One of the lobules constituting the uterine side of the placenta, consisting mainly of a rounded mass of villi.

couch·ing (kou′chĭng) *n.* An operation formerly used in treating cataract, in which the lens is displaced out of the line of vision.

cough (kôf) *v.* **coughed, cough·ing, coughs.** To expel air from the lungs suddenly and noisily, often to keep the respiratory passages free of irritating material. — *n.* **1.** The act of coughing. **2.** An illness marked by frequent coughing.

cough drop *n.* A small, often medicated and sweetened lozenge taken orally to ease coughing or soothe a sore throat.

cough reflex *n.* The reflex which initiates coughing in response to irritation of the larynx or tracheobronchial tree.

cough syrup *n.* A sweetened medicated liquid taken orally to ease coughing.

count (kount) *v.* **count·ed, count·ing, counts.** To name or list the units of a group or collection one by one in order to determine a total. — *n.* **1.** The act of counting or calculating. **2.** The totality of specific items in a particular sample.

count·er (koun′tər) *n.* One that counts, especially an electronic or mechanical device that automatically counts occurrences or repetitions of phenomena or events.

coun·ter·con·di·tion·ing (koun′tər-kən-dĭsh′ə-nĭng) *n.* Conditioning used to replace a negative conditioned response to a stimulus with a positive response.

coun·ter·ex·ten·sion (koun′tər-ĭk-stĕn′shən) *n.* See **countertraction.**

coun·ter·im·mu·no·e·lec·tro·pho·re·sis (koun′-tər-ĭm′yə-nō-ĭ-lĕk′trə-fə-rē′sĭs, -ĭ-myoō′-) *n.* A modification of immunoelectrophoresis in which antigen and antibody move in opposite directions and form precipitates in the area between the cells where they meet in concentrations of optimal proportions.

coun·ter·in·ci·sion (koun′tər-ĭn-sĭzh′ən) *n.* A second incision made adjacent to a primary incision.

coun·ter·ir·ri·ta·tion (koun′tər-ĭr′ĭ-tā′shən) *n.* Irritation or mild inflammation produced to relieve inflammation of underlying or adjacent tissues.

coun·ter·o·pen·ing (koun′tər-ō′pə-nĭng) *n.* A second opening made at the lowest part of an abscess or other fluid-containing cavity to assist in drainage.

coun·ter·punc·ture (koun′tər-pŭngk′chər) *n.* See **counteropening.**

count·er·shock (koun′tər-shŏk′) *n.* An electric shock applied to the chest to restore normal rhythm of the heart.

coun·ter·trac·tion (koun′tər-trăk′shən) *n.* Traction used to offset or oppose another traction in the reduction of fractures.

coun·ter·trans·fer·ence (koun′tər-trăns-fûr′əns, -trăns′fər-) *n.* The surfacing of a psychotherapist's own repressed feelings through identification with the emotions, experiences, or problems of a person undergoing treatment.

cou·ple (kŭp′əl) *n.* **1.** Two items of the same kind; a pair. **2.** A pair of forces of equal magnitude acting in parallel but opposite directions. — *v.* **-pled, -pling, -ples.** To unite sexually; copulate.

cou·pling (kŭp′lĭng) *n.* **1.** The act of uniting sexually. **2.** The configuration of two different mutant genes on the same chromosome, leading to the likelihood that they will both either be inherited or omitted in the next generation.

cou·vade (koō-väd′) *n.* A practice in certain non-Western cultures in which the husband of a woman in labor takes to his bed as though he were bearing the child.

Cou·ve·laire uterus (koō-və-lĕr′) *n.* Extravasation of blood into the uterine musculature and beneath the uterine peritoneum in association with premature detachment of the placenta.

co·vert sensitization (kŭv′ərt, kō′vərt, kō-vûrt′) *n.* Aversive conditioning or training during which a person is taught to imagine unpleasant consequences while engaging in an unwanted habit.

cov·er-un·cov·er test (kŭv′ər-ŭn-kŭv′ər) *n.* A test to detect strabismus in which one eye focusing on a given point is covered.

Cow·den's disease (koud′nz) *n.* An inherited condition characterized by benign tissue masses that form on the skin, hair follicles, and gums during infancy, and in the breasts following puberty, and are associated with a higher risk for developing malignancies later in life.

cow·per·i·tis (kōō′pə-rī′tĭs, kou′-, kōōp′ə-) *n.* Inflammation of the bulbourethral glands.

Cow·per's gland (kou′pərz, kōō′-) *n.* See **bulbourethral gland.**

cow·pox (kou′pŏks′) *n.* A mild, contagious skin disease of cattle that is caused by a virus and characterized by the eruption of a pustular rash. When the virus is transmitted to humans, as by vaccination, it can confer immunity to smallpox.

cox·a (kŏk′sə) *n., pl.* **cox·ae** (kŏk′sē′). **1.** See **hipbone. 2.** See **hip joint.**

cox·al·gi·a (kŏk-săl′jē-ə, -jə) *n.* Pain in or disease of the hip or hip joint.

Cox·i·el·la (kŏk′sē-ĕl′ə) *n.* A genus of filterable parasitic bacteria containing small rod-shaped or coccoid, gram-negative cells; it includes the species that causes Q fever in humans.

cox·i·tis (kŏk-sī′tĭs) *n.* Inflammation of the hip joint.

cox·o·dyn·i·a (kŏk′sə-dĭn′ē-ə) *n.* Pain in the hip joint.

cox·sack·ie·vi·rus or **Cox·sack·ie virus** (kōōk-sä′- kē-vī′rəs, kŏk-săk′ē-) *n.* Any of a group of *Enteroviruses* associated with a variety of illnesses including a disease resembling poliomyelitis but without paralysis.

CPR *abbr.* cardiopulmonary resuscitation

crab louse *n.* A sucking louse *(Pthirus pubis)* that generally infests the pubic region and causes severe itching.

cra·dle (krād′l) *n.* **1.** A small low bed for an infant, often furnished with rockers. **2.** A frame used to keep the bedclothes from pressing on an injured part.

cradle cap *n.* A form of dermatitis that occurs in infants and is characterized by heavy, yellow, crusted lesions on the scalp.

cramp (krămp) *n.* **1.** A sudden, involuntary, spasmodic muscular contraction causing severe pain, often occurring in the leg or shoulder as the result of strain or chill. **2.** A temporary partial paralysis of habitually or excessively used muscles. **3.** **cramps.** Spasmodic contractions of the uterus, such as those occurring during menstruation or labor, usually causing pain in the abdomen that may radiate to the lower back and thighs. — *v.* **cramped, cramp·ing, cramps.** To affect with or experience a cramp or cramps.

Cramp·ton test (krămp′tən) *n.* A test for physical condition and resistance in which one's pulse and blood pressure are recorded both in the recumbent and in the standing position, and the difference is graded from theoretical perfection (100) downward.

cra·ni·al (krā′nē-əl) *adj.* Of or relating to the skull or cranium.

cranial bone *n.* Any of the bones surrounding the brain, comprising the paired parietal and tempo-

ral bones and the unpaired occipital, frontal sphenoid, and ethmoid bones.

cranial cavity *n.* The space or hollow within the skull.

cranial nerve *n.* Any of 12 pairs of nerves that emerge from or enter the brain, comprising the olfactory, optic, oculomotor, trochlear, trigeminal, abducent, facial, vestibulocochlear, glossopharyngeal, vagus, accessory, and hypoglossal nerves.

cranial root *n.* Any of the roots of the accessory nerve that arise from the medulla.

cranial suture *n.* Any of the sutures between the bones of the skull.

cra·ni·ec·to·my (krā′nē-ĕk′tə-mē) *n.* Surgical removal of a portion of the cranium.

cra·ni·o·cele (krā′nē-ə-sēl′) *n.* See **encephalocele.**

cra·ni·o·fa·cial dysostosis (krā′nē-ō-fā′shəl) *n.* An inherited cranial deformity characterized by widening of the skull and high forehead, abnormal width between and protrusion of the eyes, a beaked nose, and hypoplasia of the maxilla.

cra·ni·ol·o·gy (krā′nē-ŏl′ə-jē) *n.* The scientific study of the characteristics of the skull, such as size and shape, especially in humans.

cra·ni·o·ma·la·ci·a (krā′nē-ō-mə-lā′shē-ə, -shə) *n.* Softening of the bones of the skull.

cra·ni·o·plas·ty (krā′nē-ə-plăs′tē) *n.* Surgical repair of a defect or deformity of the skull.

cra·ni·o·punc·ture (krā′nē-ō-pŭngk′chər) *n.* Surgical puncture of the skull.

cra·ni·o·scle·ro·sis (krā′nē-ō-sklə-rō′sĭs) *n.* Thickening of the skull.

cra·ni·o·ste·no·sis (krā′nē-ō-stə-nō′sĭs) *n.* Premature closure of the cranial sutures, resulting in malformation of the skull.

cra·ni·ot·o·my (krā′nē-ŏt′ə-mē) *n.* Surgical incision into the skull.

cra·ni·um (krā′nē-əm) *n., pl.* **-ni·ums** or **-ni·a** (-nē-ə). **1.** The bones of the head considered as a group; skull. **2.** The bony case enclosing the brain, excluding the bones of the face; braincase.

crap·u·lence (krăp′yə-ləns) *n.* Sickness caused by excessive eating or drinking.

cra·vat bandage (krə-văt′) *n.* A bandage made by bringing the point of a triangular bandage to the middle of the base and then folding lengthwise to the desired width.

cream (krēm) *n.* A pharmaceutical preparation consisting of a semisolid emulsion of either the oil-in-water or the water-in-oil type, ordinarily intended for topical use.

cre·a·tine (krē′ə-tēn′, -tĭn) or **cre·a·tin** (-tĭn) *n.* A nitrogenous organic acid that is found in the muscle tissue of vertebrates mainly in the form of phosphocreatine and supplies energy for muscle contraction.

cre·a·ti·ne·mi·a (krē′ə-tə-nē′mē-ə) *n.* The presence of excessive creatine in the blood.

creatine phosphate *n.* See **phosphocreatine.**

cre·at·i·nine (krē-ăt′n-ēn′, -ĭn) *n.* A creatine anhydride formed by the metabolism of creatine and found in muscle tissue and blood and normally excreted in the urine as metabolic waste.

creatinine clearance *n.* The volume of serum or plasma that would be cleared of creatinine by one minute's excretion of urine.

cre·a·ti·nu·ri·a (krē′ə-tə-no͞or′ē-ə, -nyo͞or′-) *n.* An increase in the amount of creatine in the urine.

Cre·dé's method (krā-dāz′) *n.* **1.** A method for preventing ophthalmia neonatorum by administering one drop of a 2 percent solution of silver nitrate into each eye of a newborn infant. **2.** A method for expressing urine by pressing the hand on the bladder.

creep·ing eruption (krē′pĭng) *n.* A skin disorder characterized by itchiness and a progressive net-like tunneling in the skin caused by the burrowing larvae of various parasites, especially a type of hookworm.

cre·mas·ter·ic reflex (krē′mă-stĕr′ĭk) *n.* A drawing up of the scrotum and the testicle in response to scratching of the skin over Scarpa's triangle or on the inner side of the thigh on the same side of the body.

cre·mas·ter muscle (krə-măs′tər, krē) *n.* A muscle that arises from the internal oblique muscle and whose action raises the testicles.

cre·na·tion (krĭ-nā′shən) *n.* A process resulting from osmosis in which red blood cells, in a hypertonic solution, undergo shrinkage and acquire a notched or scalloped surface.

cre·no·cyte (krē′nə-sīt′, krĕn′ə-) *n.* A red blood cell with notched edges.

crep·i·tant rale (krĕp′ĭ-tənt) *n.* A fine bubbling or crackling sound heard on auscultation, produced by the presence of a very thin secretion in the smaller bronchial tubes.

crep·i·tate (krĕp′ĭ-tāt′) *v.* **-tat·ed, -tat·ing, -tates.** To make a crackling or popping sound; crackle.

crep·i·ta·tion (krĕp′ĭ-tā′shən) *n.* **1.** A rattling or crackling sound like that made by rubbing hair between the fingers close to the ear. **2.** The sensation felt on placing the hand over the seat of a fracture when the broken ends of the bone are moved, or over tissue in which gas gangrene is present. **3.** The noise produced by rubbing bone or irregular cartilage surfaces together, as by movement of the patella against the femoral condyles in arthritis.

crep·i·tus (krĕp′ĭ-təs) *n.* **1.** Crepitation. **2.** A noisy discharge of gas from the intestine.

cres·cen·do murmur (krə-shĕn′dō) *n.* A murmur that increases in intensity and suddenly ceases.

crest (krĕst) *n.* A projection or ridge, especially of bone; cresta.

CREST syndrome (krĕst) *n.* A form of scleroderma that is a combination of calcinosis, Raynaud's phenomenon, esophageal motility disorders, sclerodactyly, and telangiectasia.

cre·tin (krēt′n) *n.* A person afflicted with cretinism. — **cre′tin·oid′** (-oid′) *adj.* — **cre′tin·ous** (-əs) *adj.*

cre·tin·ism (krēt′n-ĭz′əm) *n.* A congenital condition caused by a deficiency of thyroid hormone during prenatal development and characterized

in childhood by dwarfed stature, mental retardation, dystrophy of the bones, and a low basal metabolism.

Creutz·feldt–Jakob disease (kroits′fĕlt-) *n.* A rare, usually fatal disease of the brain, characterized by progressive dementia and gradual loss of muscle control, that occurs most often in middle age and is caused by a slow virus.

CRH *abbr.* corticotropin-releasing hormone

crib death *n.* See **sudden infant death syndrome.**

cri·bra·tion (krə-brā′shən) *n.* The condition of being perforated like a sieve.

crick (krĭk) *n.* A painful cramp or muscle spasm, as in the back or neck. — *v.* **cricked, crick·ing, cricks.** To cause a painful cramp or muscle spasm in by turning or wrenching.

cri·coid cartilage (krī′koid′) *n.* The lowermost of the laryngeal cartilages, expanded into a nearly quadrilateral plate.

cri·coi·dec·to·my (krī′koi-dĕk′tə-mē) *n.* Surgical excision of the cricoid cartilage.

cri·co·thy·rot·o·my (krī′kō-thī-rŏt′ə-mē) *n.* Incision through the skin and the cricothyroid membrane for emergency relief of upper respiratory obstruction.

cri·cot·o·my (krī-kŏt′ə-mē) *n.* Incision of the cricoid cartilage.

cri-du-chat syndrome (crē-do͞o-shä′) *n.* A congenital chromosomal disorder marked by microcephaly, epicanthal folds, micrognathia, strabismus, mental and physical retardation, and a characteristic catlike whine.

Crig·ler-Naj·jar syndrome (krĭg′lər-nä′jär′) *n.* An inherited defect in the ability to form bilirubin glucuronide, characterized by familial nonhemolytic jaundice and, in its severe form, by irreversible brain damage that resembles kernicterus.

crim·i·nal abortion (krĭm′ə-nəl) *n.* Abortion performed illegally.

cri·noph·a·gy (krə-nŏf′ə-jē) *n.* The disposal of excess secretory granules by lysosomes.

crip·ple (krĭp′əl) *n.* One that is partially disabled or unable to use a limb or limbs. — *v.* **-pled, -pling, -ples.** To cause to lose the use of a limb or limbs.

cri·sis (krī′sĭs) *n., pl.* **-ses** (-sēz). **1.** A sudden change in the course of a disease or fever, toward either improvement or deterioration. **2.** An emotionally stressful event or change in a person's life.

crisis center *n.* A center staffed especially by volunteers who give support and advice to people experiencing personal crises.

cris·pa·tion (krĭs-pā′shən) *n.* A slight involuntary muscular contraction, often producing a crawling sensation of the skin.

cris·ta (krĭs′tə) *n., pl.* **-tae** (-tē). **1.** A ridge, crest, or elevated line projecting from a level or evenly rounded surface; crest. **2.** One of the inward projections or folds of the inner membrane of a mitochondrion.

crit·i·cal (krĭt′ĭ-kəl) *adj.* **1.** Of or relating to a medical crisis. **2.** Being or relating to a grave physical condition especially of a patient. **3.** Of or relating to the value of a measurement, such as temperature, at which an abrupt change in a chemical of physical quality, property, or state occurs.

critical care unit *n.* See **intensive care unit**.

critical organ *n.* The organ or physiological system that would first be subjected to radiation in excess of the maximum permissible amount as the dose of a radioactive material is increased.

CRNA *abbr.* Certified Registered Nurse Anesthetist

croc·o·dile tears syndrome (krŏk′ə-dīl′) *n.* A syndrome caused by a lesion of the seventh cranial nerve central to the geniculate ganglion and resulting in residual facial paralysis with profuse lacrimation during eating.

Crohn's disease (krōnz) *n.* See **regional enteritis**.

Crooke's granule (krōoks) *n.* One of the lumpy masses of basophilic material in the basophil cells of the anterior lobe of the pituitary gland, associated with Cushing's disease.

cross·bite (krôs′bīt′) *n.* An abnormal relation of one or more teeth of one arch to the opposing tooth or teeth of the other arch, caused by deviation of tooth position or abnormal jaw position.

crossed eyes *n.* See **esotropia**.

crossed reflex *n.* A reflex movement on one side of the body in response to a stimulus applied to the opposite side.

cross-eye (krôs′ī′) *n.* A form of strabismus in which one or both eyes deviate toward the nose. — **cross′-eyed′** *adj.*

cross flap *n.* A skin flap transferred between corresponding body parts, as from one arm, breast, or eyelid to the other.

cross infection *n.* An infection spread from one organism to another.

cross·ing over (krô′sĭng) or **crossing-over** *n.* The exchange of genetic material between homologous chromosomes that occurs during meiosis and contributes to genetic variability.

cross matching or **crossmatching** *n.* **1.** A test for determining the compatibility between the blood of a donor and that of a recipient before transfusion. **2.** A test for determining tissue compatibility between a transplant donor and the recipient before transplantation, in which the recipient's serum is tested for antibodies that may react with the lymphocytes or other cells of the donor. **3.** The process of performing one of these tests.

cross-reacting antibody *n.* An antibody that reacts with an antigen other than the one that induced its production.

cross re·ac·tion (krôs′rē-ăk′shən) *n.* The reaction between an antigen and an antibody that was generated against a different but similar antigen.

cross tolerance *n.* Resistance to an effect or effects of a compound as a result of tolerance previously developed to a pharmacologically similar compound.

crotch (krŏch) *n.* The angle or region of the angle formed by the junction of two parts or members, such as two branches, limbs, or legs.

croup (krōop) *n.* **1.** See **laryngotracheobronchitis**. **2.** A pathological condition of the larynx, espe-

cially in infants and children, that is characterized by respiratory difficulty and a hoarse, brassy cough. — **croup′ous** (krōo′pəs), **croup′y** *adj.*

croupous membrane *n.* See **false membrane**.

Crou·zon's disease (krōo-zŏnz′, -zôN′) *n.* See **craniofacial dysostosis**.

crown (kroun) *n.* **1.** The top or highest part of bodily structure, especially the head. **2.** The part of a tooth that is covered by enamel and projects beyond the gum line. **3.** An artificial substitute for the natural crown of a tooth. — *v.* **crowned, crown·ing, crowns. 1.** To put a crown on a tooth. **2.** To reach a stage in labor when a large segment of the fetal scalp is visible at the vaginal orifice. Used of a fetus or the head of a fetus.

CRST syndrome (sē′är-ĕs-tē′) *n.* A form of scleroderma that is a combination of calcinosis cutis, Raynaud's phenomenon, sclerodactyly, and telangiectasia.

cru·ci·ate ligament of the knee (krōo′shē-āt′) *n.* Either of two ligaments, anterior and posterior, that pass from the intercondylar area of the tibia to the intercondylar fossa of the femur.

cruciate muscle *n.* A muscle in which the bundles of muscle fibers cross in an x-shaped configuration.

crus (krōos, krŭs) *n., pl.* **cru·ra** (krōor′ə). **1.** The section of the leg between the knee and foot. **2.** A body part consisting of elongated masses or diverging bands that resemble legs or roots. **3.** **crura.** A pair of diverging bands or elongated masses.

crush syndrome *n.* A severe shocklike condition that follows release of a limb or other large body part after a prolonged period of compression, as by a heavy object, characterized by edema, hematuria, and renal failure.

crust (krŭst) *n.* An outer layer or coating formed by the drying of a bodily exudate such as pus or blood; a scab. — *v.* **crust·ed, crust·ing, crusts.** To cover with, become covered with, or harden into a crust.

crutch (krŭch) *n.* A staff or support used by the physically injured or disabled as an aid in walking, usually designed to fit under the armpit and often used in pairs.

Cru·veil·hier–Baum·gar·ten murmur (krōo-vāl-yā′boum′gär′tn, krü-vě-) *n.* A murmur heard over the collateral veins in the abdominal wall that connect the portal and caval venous systems.

Cruveilhier–Baumgarten sign *n.* An indication of hepatic cirrhosis with portal hypertension in which a murmur is heard over a Medusa head.

Cruveilhier–Baumgarten syndrome *n.* Cirrhosis of the liver associated with patent umbilical or paraumbilical veins and varicose periumbilical veins.

Cruveilhier's sign *n.* See **Medusa head**.

crux (krŭks, krōoks) *n., pl.* **crux·es** or **cru·ces** (krōo′sēz). A cross or a crosslike structure.

cry·al·ge·si·a (krī′əl-jē′zē-ə, -zhə) *n.* Pain caused by cold.

cry·an·es·the·sia (krī′ăn-ĭs-thē′zhə) *n.* The loss of sensation or perception of cold.

cry·es·the·sia (krī′ĭs-thē′zhə) *n.* **1.** The ability to sense cold. **2.** Extreme sensitivity to cold.

cry·mo·ther·a·py (krī′mō-thĕr′ə-pē) *n.* See **cryotherapy.**

cry·o·an·es·the·sia (krī′ō-ăn′ĭs-thē′zhə) *n.* Localized application of cold as means of producing regional anesthesia.

cry·o·bank (krī′ə-bangk′) *n.* A place of storage that uses very low temperatures to preserve semen or transplantable tissues.

cry·o·cau·ter·y (krī′ō-kô′tə-rē) *n.* A substance or an instrument that causes the destruction of tissue by freezing.

cry·o·ex·trac·tion (krī′ō-ĭk-străk′shən) *n.* The removal of a cataract by the adhesion of a freezing probe to the lens.

cry·o·fi·brin·o·gen (krī′ō-fī-brĭn′ə-jən) *n.* An abnormal type of fibrinogen rarely found in human plasma.

cry·o·gen (krī′ə-jən) *n.* A liquid, such as liquid nitrogen, that boils at a temperature below about 110 Kelvin (−160°C) and is used to obtain very low temperatures; a refrigerant.

cry·o·gen·ic (krī′ə-jĕn′ĭk) *adj.* **1.** Relating to or producing low temperatures. **2.** Requiring or suitable for storage at low temperatures. — **cry′·o·gen′i·cal·ly** *adv.*

cry·o·glob·u·lin (krī′ō-glŏb′yə-lĭn) *n.* Any of various abnormal globulins that precipitate from plasma when cooled.

cry·ol·y·sis (krī-ŏl′ĭ-sĭs) *n.* Destruction by cold.

cry·o·pex·y (krī′ə-pĕk′sē) *n.* Surgical attachment of the sensory retina to the pigment epithelium and choroid using a cryoprobe.

cry·o·pre·cip·i·tate (krī′ō-prĭ-sĭp′ĭ-tāt′, -tĭt) *n.* A precipitate that forms when soluble material is cooled, especially a precipitate rich in factor VIII that is formed when normal blood plasma is cooled.

cry·o·pres·er·va·tion (krī′ō-prĕz′ər-vā′shən) *n.* Maintenance of the viability of excised tissues or organs by freezing at extremely low temperatures. — **cry′o·pre·serve′** (krī′ō-prĭ-zûrv′) *v.*

cry·o·probe (krī′ə-prōb′) *n.* A surgical instrument used to apply extreme cold to tissues during cryosurgery.

cry·o·pro·tec·tant (krī′ō-prə-tĕk′tənt) *n.* A substance used to protect cells or tissues from damage during freezing. — **cry′o·pro·tec′tant** *adj.* — **cry′o·pro·tec′tive** *adj.*

cry·o·pro·tein (krī′ō-prō′tēn′, -tē-ĭn) *n.* A protein, such as cryoglobulin, that precipitates from solution when cooled and redissolves upon warming.

cry·o·scope (krī′ə-skōp′) *n.* An instrument used to measure the freezing point of a liquid.

cry·os·co·py (krī-ŏs′kə-pē) *n.* A technique for determining the molecular weight of a solute, such as blood or urine, by dissolving a known quantity of it in a solvent and recording the amount by which the freezing point of the solvent drops.

cry·o·sur·ger·y (krī′ō-sûr′jə-rē) *n.* The exposure of tissues to extreme cold to bring about the destruction or elimination of abnormal cells.

cry·o·ther·a·py (krī′ō-thĕr′ə-pē) *n.* The use of low temperatures in medical therapy.

crypt (krĭpt) *n.* A small pit, recess, or glandular cavity in the body.

cryp·tec·to·my (krĭp-tĕk′tə-mē) *n.* Surgical excision or obliteration of a crypt, especially a tonsillar crypt.

cryptesthesia or **crypt·aes·the·sia** (krĭp′təs-thē′zhə, -zhē-ə) *n.* A mode of paranormal perception, such as clairvoyance.

cryp·tic (krĭp′tĭk) *adj.* **1.** Hidden or concealed. **2.** Tending to conceal or camouflage, as the coloring of an animal.

cryp·ti·tis (krĭp-tī′tĭs) *n.* Inflammation of a crypt or crypts, particularly in the rectum.

cryp·to·coc·co·sis (krĭp′tə-kŏ-kō′sĭs) *n.* A systemic infection caused by the fungus *Cryptococcus neoformans* that can affect the lungs, skin, or other body organs but that occurs most often in the brain and meninges.

Cryp·to·coc·cus (krĭp′tə-kŏk′əs) *n.* Any of a genus of yeastlike fungi commonly occurring in the soil and including certain pathogenic species.

cryp·to·lith (krĭp′tə-lĭth′) *n.* A concretion in a crypt.

cryp·to·men·or·rhe·a (krĭp′tō-mĕn′ə-rē′ə) *n.* Occurrence of the menses without any external flow of blood, as in cases of imperforate hymen.

cryp·tor·chi·dec·to·my (krĭp-tôr′kĭ-dĕk′tə-mē) *n.* Surgical removal of an undescended testicle.

cryp·tor·chi·do·pexy (krĭp-tôr′kĭ-dō-pĕk′sē) *n.* See **orchiopexy.**

cryp·tor·chism (krĭp-tôr′kĭz′əm) or **crypt·or·chi·dism** (-kĭ-dĭz′əm) *n.* A developmental defect marked by failure of the testes to descend into the scrotum.

cryp·to·spo·rid·i·o·sis (krĭp′tō-spə-rĭd′ē-ō′sĭs) *n.* Infection caused by protozoa of the genus *Cryptosporidium,* characterized in humans by chronic diarrhea.

Cryp·to·spo·rid·i·um (krĭp′tō-spô-rĭd′ē-əm) *n.* A genus of parasitic coccidian protozoans that infect the epithelial cells of the gastrointestinal tract in vertebrates and flourish in humans under conditions of intense immunosuppression.

crys·tal·line (krĭs′tə-lĭn, -līn′, -lēn′) *adj.* **1.** Being, relating to, or composed of crystal or crystals. **2.** Resembling crystal, as in transparency or distinctness of structure or outline.

crys·tal·lu·ri·a (krĭs′tə-lŏŏr′ē-ə, -lyŏŏr′-) *n.* The excretion of crystals in the urine.

C-section *n.* A cesarean section.

CSF *abbr.* cerebrospinal fluid

cu·bic centimeter (kyōō′bĭk) *n.* A unit of volume equal to one thousandth (10^{-3}) of a liter or one milliliter.

cu·bi·tus (kyōō′bĭ-təs) *n., pl.* **cubitus. 1.** See **elbow** (sense 1). **2.** See **ulna.**

cu·boid (kyōō′boid′) *adj.* Having the approximate shape of a cube. — *n.* A tarsal bone on the outer side of the foot, articulating with the calcaneus and lateral cuneiform and the fourth and fifth metatarsal bones. — **cu·boi′dal** (kyōō-boid′l) *adj.*

cuboidal epithelium *n.* Epithelium made up of cells that look like cubes in a vertical section but appear to be polyhedral when viewed on their surface.

cuff (kŭf) *n.* **1.** A bandlike structure encircling a part. **2.** An inflatable band, usually wrapped around the upper arm, that is used along with a sphygmomanometer in measuring arterial blood pressure.

cul-de-sac (kŭl′dĭ-săk′, kōōl′-) *n., pl.* **culs-de-sac** (kŭlz′-, kōōlz′-) or **cul-de-sacs.** A saclike cavity or tube open only at one end.

cul·do·cen·te·sis (kŭl′dō-sĕn-tē′sĭs, kōōl′-) *n.* Aspiration of fluid from the rectouterine space by puncture of the vaginal vault near the midline between the uterosacral ligaments.

cul·do·plas·ty (kŭl′də-plăs′tē, kōōl′-) *n.* A surgical procedure to remedy relaxation of the posterior fornix of the vagina.

cul·dos·co·py (kŭl-dŏs′kə-pē, kōōl-) *n.* The visual examination of the rectovaginal pouch and pelvic viscera by the introduction of an endoscope through the posterior vaginal wall.

cu·li·cide (kyōō′lĭ-sīd′) *n.* An agent that destroys mosquitoes.

Cul·len's sign (kŭl′ənz) *n.* An indication of intraperitoneal hemorrhage, especially in ruptured ectopic pregnancy, in which blood causes periumbilical darkening of the skin.

cul·ture (kŭl′chər) *n.* **1.** The growing of microorganisms, tissue cells, or other living matter in a specially prepared nutrient medium. **2.** Such a growth or colony, as of bacteria. — *v.* **-tured, -tur·ing, -tures.** **1.** To grow microorganisms or other living matter in a specially prepared nutrient medium. **2.** To use a substance as a medium for culture.

culture medium *n.* A liquid or gelatinous substance containing nutrients in which microorganisms or tissues are grown for scientific purposes.

culture shock *n.* A condition of confusion and anxiety affecting a person suddenly exposed to an unfamiliar culture or milieu.

cu·mu·la·tive effect (kyōōm′yə-lā′tĭv, -yə-lə-tĭv) *n.* The state at which repeated administration of a drug may produce effects that are more pronounced than those produced by the first dose.

cu·ne·i·form bone (kyōō′nē-ə-fôrm′, kyōō-nē′-) *n.* **1.** A wedge-shaped bone, especially any of the three bones located in the tarsus of the foot. **2.** See **triquetrum.**

cu·nic·u·lus (kyōō-nĭk′yə-ləs) *n., pl.* **-li** (-lī′). The burrow of the itch mite in the skin.

cun·ni·lin·gus (kŭn′ə-lĭng′gəs) *n.* Oral stimulation of the clitoris or vulva.

cup (kŭp) *n.* **1.** A cup-shaped structure or organ. **2.** See **cupping glass. 3.** A unit of capacity or volume equal to 16 tablespoons or 8 fluid ounces (237 milliliters).

cup biopsy forceps *n.* A slender flexible forceps with movable cup-shaped jaws used to obtain biopsy specimens.

cup·ping (kŭp′ĭng) *n.* The formation of a hollow or cup-shaped excavation.

cu·pu·lo·gram (kyōō′pyə-lə-grăm′) *n.* A graphic representation of vestibular function relative to normal performance.

cur·a·ble (kyōōr′ə-bəl) *adj.* Capable of being cured or healed.

cu·ra·re or **cu·ra·ri** (kōō-rä′rē, kyōō-) *n.* A purified preparation or alkaloid obtained from a tropical American woody plant, *Chondrodendron tomentosum,* used to relax skeletal muscles.

cu·ra·tive (kyōōr′ə-tĭv) *adj.* **1.** Serving or tending to cure. **2.** Of or relating to the cure of disease. — *n.* Something that cures; a remedy.

curative dose *n.* The dose required to eliminate the symptoms of a disease or to correct the manifestations of a deficiency in the diet.

curb tenotomy *n.* Excision of the tendon of the shortened muscle in strabismus, and fixation of it farther back on the aponeurosis of the globe.

cure (kyōōr) *n.* **1.** Restoration of health; recovery from disease. **2.** A method or course of treatment used to restore health. **3.** An agent, such as a drug, that restores health; a remedy. — *v.* **cured, cur·ing, cures.** **1.** To restore a person to health. **2.** To effect a recovery from a disease or disorder.

cure-all (kyōōr′ôl′) *n.* A remedy that cures all diseases or evils; a panacea.

cu·ret·tage (kyōōr′ĭ-täzh′) *n.* The removal of tissue or growths from the interior of a body cavity, such as the uterus, by scraping with a curette.

cu·rette or **cu·ret** (kyōō-rĕt′) *n.* A surgical instrument shaped like a scoop or spoon, used to remove tissue or growths from a body cavity. — *v.* **-rett·ed, -rett·ing, -rettes** or **-rets.** To scrape tissue or a body part with a curette.

cu·rette·ment or **cu·ret·ment** (kyōō-rĕt′mənt) *n.* See **curettage.**

cu·ri·um (kyōōr′ē-əm) *n.* A metallic synthetic radioactive transuranic element with atomic number 96.

Cur·ling's ulcer (kûr′lĭngz) *n.* An ulcer of the duodenum in a patient with extensive superficial burns or severe bodily injury.

cur·rant jelly clot (kûr′ənt, kûr′-) *n.* A jellylike mass of red blood cells and fibrin formed by the in vitro or postmortem clotting of whole or sedimented blood.

cur·rent (kûr′ənt, kŭr′-) *n.* **1.** A stream or flow of a liquid or gas. **2.** The amount of electric charge flowing past a specified circuit point per unit time.

Cursch·mann's spirals (kûrsh′mənz, kōōrsh′-mänz) *n.* Spirally twisted masses of mucus occurring in the sputum in bronchial asthma.

cur·va·ture (kûr′və-chōōr′, -chər) *n.* A curving or bending, especially an abnormal one.

curvature aberration *n.* A lack of spatial correspondence that causes the visual image of a straight extended object to appear curved.

curve (kûrv) *n.* **1.** A line or surface that deviates from straightness in a smooth, continuous fashion. **2.** Something characterized by such a line or surface, especially a rounded line or contour of the human body. **3.** A curved line representing variations in data on a graph. —v. **curved, curving, curves.** To move in or take the shape of a curve.

Cush·ing's basophilism (kōōsh′ĭngz) n. See **Cushing's syndrome.**

Cushing's syndrome n. A syndrome caused by an increased production of ACTH from a tumor of the adrenal cortex or of the anterior lobe of the pituitary gland. It is characterized by obesity and weakening of the muscles.

cush·ion (kōōsh′ən) n. A padlike body part.

cusp (kŭsp) n. **1.** A pointed or rounded projection on the chewing surface of a tooth. **2.** A triangular fold or flap of a heart valve.

cut (kŭt) v. **cut, cut·ting, cuts. 1.** To penetrate with a sharp edge; strike a narrow opening in. **2.** To separate into parts with or as if with a sharp-edged instrument; sever. **3.** To make an incision or a separation. **4.** To have a new tooth grow through the gums. **5.** To form or shape by severing or incising. **6.** To separate from a body; detach. **7.** To lessen the strength of; dilute. —n. **1.** The act of cutting. **2.** The result of cutting, especially an opening or wound made by a sharp edge.

cu·ta·ne·ous (kyōō-tā′nē-əs) adj. Of, relating to, or affecting the skin.

cutaneous larva migrans n. See **creeping eruption.**

cutaneous leishmaniasis n. An endemic disease in northern Africa and western and central Asia, caused by infection with the protozoan *Leishmania tropica* and transmitted by the bite of a sandfly of the genus *Phlebotomus.* It begins as a papule that enlarges to a nodule and then breaks down into an ulcer that leaves an indented scar.

cutaneous reaction n. See **cutireaction.**

cutaneous tuberculosis n. Pathologic skin lesions caused by *Mycobacterium tuberculosis.*

cut·down (kŭt′doun′) n. The incision of a vein to facilitate the insertion of a cannula or needle, as for the administration of intravenous medication.

cu·ti·cle (kyōō′tĭ-kəl) n. **1.** The strip of hardened skin at the base and sides of a fingernail or toenail. **2.** The outermost layer of the skin; epidermis. **3.** Dead or cornified epidermis.

cu·ti·re·ac·tion (kyōō′ĭ-rē-ăk′shən) n. An inflammatory reaction to a skin test.

cu·tis (kyōō′tĭs) n., pl. **-tis·es** or **-tes** (-tēz). Dermis.

cutis an·se·ri·na (ăn′sə-rī′nə) n. See **goose bumps.**

cu·ti·sec·tor (kyōō′tĭ-sĕk′tər) n. **1.** An instrument for cutting small pieces of skin for grafting. **2.** An instrument used to remove a section of skin for microscopic examination.

cy·a·nide (sī′ə-nīd) or **cy·a·nid** (-nĭd) n. Any of various salts or esters of hydrogen cyanide containing a CN group, especially the extremely poisonous compounds potassium cyanide and sodium cyanide.

cy·a·no·co·bal·a·min (sī′ə-nō′kō-băl′ə-mĭn, sī-ăn′ō-) n. See **vitamin B₁₂.**

cy·an·o·phil (sī-ăn′ə-fĭl′, sī′ə-nō-fĭl′) n. A cell or tissue element that is capable of being colored by a blue stain.

cy·a·no·sis (sī′ə-nō′sĭs) n. A bluish discoloration of the skin and mucous membranes resulting from inadequate oxygenation of the blood.

cy·a·not·ic (sī′ə-nŏt′ĭk) adj. Relating to or characterized by cyanosis.

cy·ber·net·ics (sī′bər-nĕt′ĭks) n. The theoretical study of communication and control processes in biological, mechanical, and electronic systems, especially the comparison of these processes in biological and artificial systems.

cy·cla·mate (sī′klə-māt′, sĭk′lə-) n. A salt or ester of cyclamic acid formerly used as a sweetening agent, especially calcium cyclamate or sodium cyclamate.

cy·cle (sī′kəl) n. **1.** An interval of time during which a characteristic, often regularly repeated event or sequence of events occurs. **2.** A single complete execution of a periodically repeated phenomenon. **3.** A periodically repeated sequence of events.

cy·clec·to·my (sī-klĕk′tə-mē, sĭ-klĕk′-) n. Excision of a portion of the ciliary body.

cy·clic (sī′klĭk, sĭk′lĭk) or **cy·cli·cal** (sī′klĭ-kəl, sĭk′-lĭ-kəl) adj. **1.** Of, relating to, or characterized by cycles. **2.** Recurring or moving in cycles. **3.** Of or relating to chemical compounds having atoms arranged in a ring or closed-chain structure. —**cy′cli·cal′i·ty** (sĭk′lə-kăl′ĭ-tē, sī′klə-) n. —**cy′cli·cal·ly** adv.

cyclic AMP n. A cyclic nucleotide of adenosine that acts at the cellular level as a regulator of various metabolic processes.

cyclic GMP n. A cyclic nucleotide of guanosine thought to act at the cellular level as a regulator of various metabolic processes, possibly as an antagonist to cyclic AMP.

cy·clo·ben·za·prine hydrochloride (sī′klō-bĕn′-zə-prēn′, sĭk′lō-) n. A skeletal muscle relaxant used to relieve acute muscular spasms.

cy·clo·cry·o·ther·a·py (sī′klō-krī′ō-thĕr′ə-pē) n. Application of a freezing probe to the sclera in the region of the ciliary body in the treatment of glaucoma.

cy·clo·di·al·y·sis (sī′klō-dī-ăl′ĭ-sĭs) n. Surgical opening of a passage between the anterior chamber and the suprachoroidal space in order to reduce pressure within the eye in glaucoma.

cy·clo·di·a·ther·my (sī′klō-dī′ə-thûr′mē) n. The destruction of part of the ciliary body of the eye by diathermy, performed in the treatment of glaucoma.

cy·clo·pho·to·co·ag·u·la·tion (sī′klō-fō′tō-kō-ăg′yə-lā′shən) n. Photocoagulation by directing a laser through the pupil to destroy individual ciliary processes, used in treating glaucoma.

cy·clo·pi·a (sī-klō′pē-ə) n. A congenital defect in which the two orbits merge to form a single cavity containing one eye. —**cy·clo′pi·an** adj.

cy·clo·ple·gia (sī'klə-plē'jə) *n.* Paralysis of the ciliary muscles of the eye, resulting in the loss of visual accommodation.

cy·clo·spor·ine (sī'klə-spôr'ēn, -ĭn) or **cy·clo·spor·in A** (-ĭn) *n.* A cyclic oligopeptide immunosuppressant produced by the fungus *Tolypocladium inflatum Gams,* used to inhibit organ transplant rejection.

cy·clo·thyme (sī'klə-thīm') *n.* A person afflicted with cyclothymia.

cy·clo·thy·mi·a (sī'klə-thī'mē-ə) *n.* A mild affective disorder characterized by alternating periods of elation and depression.

cy·clo·thy·mic disorder (sī'klə-thī'mĭk) *n.* A chronic mood disturbance generally lasting at least two years and characterized by mood swings including periods of hypomania and depression.

cyclothymic personality *n.* A personality disorder characterized by frequently alternating periods of elation and depression, usually occurring spontaneously and not from external circumstances.

cy·clot·o·my (sī-klŏt'ə-mē) *n.* Surgical incision of the ciliary muscle.

cy·e·sis (sī-ē'sĭs) *n.* See **pregnancy** (sense 2).

cyl·in·der (sĭl'ən-dər) *n.* **1.** A rodlike renal cast. **2.** A cylindrical lens. **3.** A metal container for gases stored under high pressure.

cy·lin·dri·cal lens (sə-lĭn'drĭ-kəl) *n.* A lens in which one of the surfaces is curved in one meridian and less curved in the opposite meridian.

cyl·in·dro·ma (sĭl'ən-drō'mə) *n.* A type of epithelial tumor characterized by islands of neoplastic cells embedded in a hyalinized stroma formed from ducts of glands; it occurs especially in the salivary glands, skin, and bronchi and is frequently malignant.

cyl·in·dru·ri·a (sĭl'ən-drŏŏr'ē-ə) *n.* The presence of renal casts in the urine.

cy·no·pho·bi·a (sī'nə-fō'bē-ə) *n.* An abnormal fear of dogs.

cy·pro·hep·ta·dine (sī'prō-hĕp'tə-dēn') *n.* An antihistamine used to relieve the symptoms of various allergic reactions, such as itching and skin rash.

cy·prot·er·one (sī-prŏt'ə-rōn') *n.* A synthetic steroid that inhibits the secretion of androgens.

Cys *abbr.* cysteine

cyst (sĭst) *n.* **1.** An abnormal membranous sac containing a gaseous, liquid, or semisolid substance. **2.** A sac or vesicle in the body. **3.** A small capsulelike sac that encloses certain organisms in their dormant or larval stage.

cyst·ad·e·no·ma (sĭ-stăd'n-ō'mə) *n.* A benign tumor derived from glandular tissue, in which secretions are retained and accumulate in cysts.

cys·tal·gi·a (sĭs'tăl'jē-ə, -jə) *n.* Pain in the bladder.

cys·ta·thi·o·nine (sĭs'tə-thī'ə-nēn', -nĭn') *n.* An intermediate in the conversion of methionine to cysteine.

cys·tec·ta·si·a (sĭs'tĭk-tā'zē-ə, -zhə) or **cys·tec·ta·sy** (sī-stĕk'tə-sē) *n.* Dilation of the bladder.

cys·tec·to·my (sĭ-stĕk'tə-mē) *n.* **1.** Surgical removal of a cyst. **2.** Surgical removal of all or a part of the gallbladder. **3.** Surgical removal of all or part of the urinary bladder.

cys·te·ine (sĭs'tē-ēn', -ĭn, sĭ-stē'ĭn) *n.* An alpha-amino acid found in most proteins and especially abundant in keratin.

cys·tic (sĭs'tĭk) *adj.* **1.** Of, relating to, or having the characteristic of a cyst. **2.** Having or containing cysts or a cyst. **3.** Enclosed in a cyst. **4.** Of, relating to, or involving the gallbladder or urinary bladder.

cystic acne *n.* Acne in which the predominant lesions are cysts and deep-seated scars.

cystic disease of breast *n.* See **fibrocystic disease of breast.**

cystic duct *n.* The duct that leads from the gallbladder and joins the hepatic duct to form the common bile duct.

cys·ti·cer·co·sis (sĭs'tĭ-sər-kō'sĭs) *n.* Infection with cysticerci in subcutaneous, muscle, or central nervous system tissues.

cys·ti·cer·cus (sĭs'tĭ-sûr'kəs) *n., pl.* **-ci** (-sī'). The larval stage of many tapeworms.

cystic fibrosis *n.* A hereditary metabolic disorder of the exocrine glands, usually developing during early childhood and affecting mainly the pancreas, respiratory system, and sweat glands. It is characterized by the production of abnormally viscous mucus by the affected glands, usually resulting in chronic respiratory infections and impaired pancreatic function.

cys·tine (sĭs'tēn') *n.* A white crystalline amino acid that is found in many proteins, especially keratin.

cystine calculus *n.* A soft type of urinary calculus composed of cystine.

cys·ti·ne·mi·a (sĭs'tə-nē'mē-ə) *n.* The presence of cystine in blood.

cys·ti·no·sis (sĭs'tə-nō'sĭs) *n.* A hereditary dysfunction of the renal tubules characterized by the presence of carbohydrates and amino acids in the urine, excessive urination, and low blood levels of potassium ions and phosphates, and caused by the abnormal metabolism of cystine and the accumulation of cystine crystals in tissues; it occurs in young children.

cys·ti·nu·ri·a (sĭs'tə-nŏŏr'ē-ə, -nyŏŏr'-) *n.* A hereditary condition characterized by excessive urinary excretion of cystine, lysine, arginine, and ornithine, caused by a defect in the renal tubules that impairs reabsorption of these acids.

cys·ti·tis (sĭ-stī'tĭs) *n.* Inflammation of the urinary bladder.

cys·to·cele (sĭs'tə-sēl') *n.* Herniation of bladder.

cys·to·chro·mos·co·py (sĭs'tō-krə-mŏs'kə-pē) *n.* Examination of the interior of the bladder after administration of a colored dye to aid in the identification or study of the function of the ureteral orifices.

cys·to·fi·bro·ma (sĭs'tō-fī-brō'mə) *n.* A fibroma in which cysts have formed.

cys·to·gram (sĭs'tə-grăm') *n.* An x-ray image produced by cystography.

cys·tog·ra·phy (sĭ-stŏg'rə-fē) *n.* Radiographic visualization of the bladder following injection of a radiopaque substance.

cys·to·li·thec·to·my (sĭs′tō-lĭ-thĕk′tə-mē) *n.* See cystolithotomy.

cys·to·li·thi·a·sis (sĭs′tō-lĭ-thī′ə-sĭs) *n.* The presence of a urinary calculus in the bladder.

cys·to·li·thot·o·my (sĭs′tō-lĭ-thŏt′ə-mē) *n.* Surgical removal of a urinary calculus from the bladder through an incision in its wall.

cys·to·ma (sĭ-stō′mə) *n., pl.* -mas or -ma·ta (-mə-tə). A cystic tumor.

cys·tom·e·ter (sĭ-stŏm′ĭ-tər) *n.* A device for studying bladder function by measuring capacity, sensation, internal pressure, and residual urine.

cys·to·pan·en·dos·co·py (sĭs′tō-păn′ĕn-dŏs′kə-pē) *n.* Examination of the interior of the bladder and urethra by an endoscope introduced through the urethra.

cys·to·pex·y (sĭs′tə-pĕk′sē) *n.* Surgical attachment of the gallbladder or of the urinary bladder to the abdominal wall or to other supporting structures.

cys·to·plas·ty (sĭs′tə-plăs′tē) *n.* Surgical repair of a defect in the urinary bladder.

cys·to·ple·gi·a (sĭs′tə-plē′jē-ə, -jə) *n.* Paralysis of the bladder.

cys·to·proc·tos·to·my (sĭs′tō-prŏk-tŏs′tə-mē) *n.* See vesicorectostomy.

cys·to·pto·sis (sĭs′tō-tō′sĭs, sĭs′tŏp-tō′-) or **cys·to·pto·si·a** (-tō-tō′sē-ə, -zē-ə, -tŏp-tō′-) *n.* Prolapse of the mucous membrane of the bladder into the urethra.

cys·to·py·e·li·tis (sĭs′tō-pī′ə-lī′tĭs) *n.* Inflammation of the bladder and the pelvis of the kidney.

cys·to·py·e·lo·ne·phri·tis (sĭs′tō-pī′ə-lō-nĭ-frī′-tĭs) *n.* Inflammation of the bladder, the pelvis of the kidney, and the kidney itself.

cys·to·rec·tos·to·my (sĭs′tō-rĕk-tŏs′tə-mē) *n.* See vesicorectostomy.

cys·tor·rha·phy (sĭ-stôr′ə-fē) *n.* Suturing of a wound or defect in the urinary bladder.

cys·tor·rhe·a (sĭs′tə-rē′-ə) *n.* A mucous discharge from the bladder.

cys·to·sar·co·ma (sĭs′tō-sär-kō′mə) *n.* A sarcoma in which cysts have formed.

cys·to·scope (sĭs′tə-skōp′) *n.* A tubular instrument equipped with a light and used to examine the interior of the urinary bladder and ureter. — **cys′to·scop′ic** (-skŏp′ĭk) *adj.* — **cys·tos′co·py** (sĭ-stŏs′kə-pē) *n.*

cystoscopic urography *n.* See retrograde urography.

cys·tos·to·my (sĭ-stŏs′tə-mē) *n.* The surgical formation of an opening into the urinary bladder.

cys·to·tome (sĭs′tə-tōm′) *n.* **1.** An instrument for cutting into the urinary bladder. **2.** An instrument for cutting into the capsule of a lens.

cys·tot·o·my (sĭ-stŏt′ə-mē) *n.* Surgical incision into the urinary bladder.

cys·to·u·re·ter·o·gram (sĭs′tō-yŏŏ-rē′tə-rō-grăm′, -yŏŏr′ĭ-tə-rō-) *n.* A radiograph of the bladder and the ureter.

cys·to·u·re·ter·og·ra·phy (sĭs′tō-yŏŏ-rē′tə-rŏg′-rə-fē, -yŏŏr′ĭ-tə-) *n.* Radiography of the bladder and the ureter.

cys·to·u·re·thro·gram (sĭs′tō-yŏŏ-rē′thrə-grăm′) *n.* A radiograph of the urinary bladder and urethra made after a contrast medium has been introduced.

cys·to·u·re·throg·ra·phy (sĭs′tō-yŏŏr′ĭ-thrŏg′-rə-fē) *n.* Radiography of the bladder and the urethra after the introduction of a radiopaque substance.

cys·to·u·re·thro·scope (sĭs′tō-yŏŏ-rē′thrə-skōp′) *n.* An instrument for visually examining the bladder and urethra.

cy·ta·phe·re·sis (sī′tə-fə-rē′sĭs) *n.* A procedure in which various cells can be separated from withdrawn blood and retained, with the plasma and other elements retransfused into the donor.

cy·ti·dine (sī′tĭ-dēn′) *n.* A white crystalline nucleoside composed of one molecule each of cytosine and ribose.

cy·to·cen·trum (sī′tō-sĕn′trəm) *n.* See centrosome.

cy·to·chrome (sī′tə-krōm′) *n.* Any of a class of iron-containing proteins important in cell respiration as catalysts of oxidation-reduction reactions.

cy·to·cide (sī′tə-sīd′) *n.* An agent that is destructive to cells. — **cy·to·cid′al** (-sīd′l) *adj.*

cy·toc·la·sis (sī-tŏk′lə-sĭs) *n.* The destruction of cells by fragmentation.

cy·to·di·ag·no·sis (sī′tō-dī′əg-nō′sĭs) *n.* The diagnosis of a disease through the microscopic study of cells.

cy·to·gen·e·sis (sī′tō-jĕn′ĭ-sĭs) *n.* The formation, development, and variation of cells.

cy·tog·e·ny (sī-tŏj′ə-nē) *n.* See cytogenesis.

cy·to·glu·co·pe·ni·a (sī′tō-glŏŏ′kə-pē′nē-ə) *n.* Deficiency of glucose within cells.

cy·to·kine (sī′tə-kīn′) *n.* Any of several nonantibody proteins, such as lymphokines, that are released by a cell population on contact with a specific antigen and act as intercellular mediators, as in the generation of an immune response.

cy·to·ki·ne·sis (sī′tō-kə-nē′sĭs, -kī-) *n.* The division of the cytoplasm of a cell following the division of the nucleus. — **cy′to·ki·net′ic** (-nĕt′ĭk) *adj.*

cytologic smear *n.* A cytologic specimen made by smearing a sample, then fixing it and staining it, usually with 95% ethyl alcohol and Papanicolaou stain.

cy·tol·o·gist (sī-tŏl′ə-jĭst) *n.* One who specializes in cytology.

cy·tol·o·gy (sī-tŏl′ə-jē) *n.* The branch of biology that deals with the formation, structure, and function of cells. — **cy′to·log′ic** (-tə-lŏj′ĭk) *adj.*

cy·tol·y·sin (sī-tŏl′ĭ-sĭn) *n.* A substance, such as an antibody, capable of dissolving or destroying cells.

cy·tol·y·sis (sī-tŏl′ĭ-sĭs) *n.* The dissolution or destruction of a cell. — **cy′to·lyt′ic** (sī′tə-lĭt′ĭk) *adj.*

cy·to·me·gal·ic inclusion disease (sī′tō-mĭ-găl′-ĭk) *n.* A disease caused by infection with cytomegalovirus, characterized by the presence of inclusion bodies in infected cells, enlargement of the liver and spleen, jaundice, purpura, thrombocytopenia, and fever; it often occurs in newborn infants, acquired in the womb or when passing through the birth canal of an infected mother, and can also occur in individuals with impaired immune systems.

cy·to·meg·a·lo·vi·rus (sī′tə-měg′ə-lō-vī′rəs) *n.* Any of a group of herpes viruses that attack and enlarge epithelial cells.

cy·to·mem·brane (sī′tə-měm′brān) *n.* See **cell membrane.**

cy·to·met·a·pla·sia (sī′tō-mět′ə-plā′zhə, -zhē-ə) *n.* A change in the form or function of a cell other than that related to neoplasia.

cy·tom·e·ter (sī-tŏm′ĭ-tər) *n.* A standardized glass slide or small glass chamber of known volume, used in counting and measuring cells, especially blood cells.

cy·tom·e·try (sī-tŏm′ĭ-trē) *n.* The counting of cells, especially blood cells, using a cytometer or hemocytometer.

cy·to·mor·pho·sis (sī′tō-môr-fō′sĭs) *n.* The series of changes that a cell undergoes during the various stages of its existence.

cy·top·a·thy (sī-tŏp′ə-thē) *n.* A disorder of a cell.

cy·to·pe·ni·a (sī′tə-pē′nē-ə) *n.* A deficiency or lack of cellular elements in the circulating blood.

cy·toph·a·gy (sī-tŏf′ə-jē) *n.* The ingestion of cells by phagocytes.

cy·to·phil·ic antibody (sī′tə-fĭl′ĭk) *n.* See **cytotropic antibody.**

cy·to·pho·tom·e·ter (sī′tō-fō-tŏm′ĭ-tər) *n.* An instrument used to identify and locate the chemical compounds within a cell by measuring the intensity of light passing through stained sections of the cytoplasm.

cy·to·plasm (sī′tə-plăz′əm) *n.* The protoplasm outside the nucleus of a cell. — **cy′to·plas′mic** (-plăz′mĭk) *adj.*

cy·to·plast (sī′tə-plăst′) *n.* The living intact cytoplasm that remains after the cell nucleus has been removed. — **cy′to·plas′tic** (-plăs′tĭk) *adj.*

cy·to·re·duc·tive therapy (sī′tō-rĭ-dŭk′tĭv) *n.* Therapy to reduce the number of cells in a lesion, usually a malignancy.

cy·to·sine (sī′tə-sēn′) *n.* A pyrimidine base that is an essential constituent of RNA and DNA.

cy·to·sis (sī-tō′sĭs) *n.* A condition in which there is more than the usual number of cells.

cy·to·skel·e·ton (sī′tə-skěl′ĭ-tn) *n.* The internal framework of a cell, composed largely of actin filaments and microtubules.

cy·to·smear (sī′tō-smēr) *n.* See **cytologic smear.**

cy·to·sol (sī′tə-sôl′) *n.* The fluid component of cytoplasm, excluding organelles and the insoluble, usually suspended, cytoplasmic components. — **cy′to·sol′ic** *adj.*

cy·to·some (sī′tə-sōm′) *n.* **1.** The cell body exclusive of the nucleus. **2.** Any of the osmiophilic bodies that have concentric lamellae and occur in the great alveolar cells of the lung.

cy·to·sta·sis (sī′tə-stā′sĭs, -stăs′ĭs) *n.* **1.** The slowing of movement and accumulation of blood cells in the capillaries, as in a region of inflammation. **2.** Arrest of cellular growth and multiplication.

cy·to·tax·is (sī′tə-tăk′sĭs) *n.* The attraction or repulsion of cells for one another. — **cy′to·tac′tic** (-tăk′tĭk) *adj.*

cy·to·tax·on·o·my (sī′tō-tăk-sŏn′ə-mē) *n.* The classification of organisms based on cellular structure and function, especially on the structure and number of chromosomes. — **cy′to·tax′o·nom′ic** (-tăk′sə-nŏm′ĭk) *adj.* — **cy′to·tax·on′o·mist** *n.*

cy·to·tech·nol·o·gist (sī′tə-těk-nŏl′ə-jĭst) *n.* A technician trained in medical examination and identification of cellular abnormalities.

cy·toth·e·sis (sī-tŏth′ĭ-sĭs, sī′tə-thē′sĭs) *n.* The repair of injury in a cell.

cy·to·tox·ic reaction (sī′tə-tŏk′sĭk) *n.* An immunological reaction in which a noncytotropic antibody combines with a specific antigen on the surface of a cell and forms a complex that initiates the activation of complement, leading to cell lysis or other damage.

cytotoxic T cell *n.* See **killer cell.**

cy·to·tox·in (sī′tə-tŏk′sĭn) *n.* A substance having a specific toxic effect on certain cells.

cy·to·tro·pho·blast (sī′tə-trō′fə-blăst′) *n.* The inner layer of the trophoblast.

cy·to·trop·ic antibody (sī′tə-trŏp′ĭk, -trō′pĭk) *n.* An antibody that has an affinity for additional kinds of cells unrelated to its specific affinity for the antigen that induced it.

cy·tot·ro·pism (sī-tŏt′rə-pĭz′əm) *n.* Affinity for cells, especially the ability of viruses to localize in and damage specific cells.

cy·tu·ri·a (sī-tŏor′ē-ə, -tyŏor′-) *n.* The presence of cells in unusual numbers in the urine.

~ ~ ~ ~ ~ D ~ ~ ~ ~ ~

D. *abbr.* diopter; doctor (in academic degrees)

DA or **D.A.** *abbr.* developmental age

da·car·ba·zine (dă-kär′bə-zēn′, dā-) *n.* DTIC.

dac·ry·a·gogue (dăk′rē-ə-gôg′) *n.* An agent that stimulates a lacrimal gland to secrete, promoting the flow of tears.

dac·ry·o·ad·e·ni·tis (dăk′rē-ō-ăd′n-ī′tĭs) *n.* Inflammation of a lacrimal gland.

dac·ry·o·blen·nor·rhe·a (dăk′rē-ō-blĕn′ə-rē′ə) *n.* Chronic discharge of mucus from a lacrimal sac.

dac·ry·o·cele (dăk′rē-ə-sēl′) *n.* See **dacryocystocele**.

dac·ry·o·cyst (dăk′rē-ə-sĭst′) *n.* See **lacrimal sac**.

dac·ry·o·cys·tal·gi·a (dăk′rē-ō-sĭs′tăl′jē-ə, -jə) *n.* Pain in the lacrimal sac.

dac·ry·o·cys·tec·to·my (dăk′rē-ō-sĭ-stĕk′tə-mē) *n.* Surgical removal of the lacrimal sac.

dac·ry·o·cys·ti·tis (dăk′rē-ō-sĭ-stī′tĭs) *n.* Inflammation of the lacrimal sac.

dac·ry·o·cys·to·blen·nor·rhe·a (dăk′rē-ō-sĭs′tə-blĕn′ə-rē′ə) *n.* See **dacryoblennorrhea**.

dac·ry·o·cys·to·cele (dăk′rē-ō-sĭs′tə-sēl′) *n.* Protrusion of the lacrimal sac.

dac·ry·o·cys·to·rhi·nos·to·my (dăk′rē-ō-sĭs′tə-rī-nŏs′tə-mē) *n.* The surgical opening of a passage for drainage from the lacrimal sac into the nasal cavity.

dac·ry·o·cys·tot·o·my (dăk′rē-ō-sĭ-stŏt′ə-mē) *n.* Surgical incision of the lacrimal sac.

dac·ry·o·lith (dăk′rē-ə-lĭth′) *n.* A concretion in a lacrimal sac or duct.

dac·ry·o·ma (dăk′rē-ō′mə) *n.* **1.** A swelling caused by the accumulation of tears in an obstructed lacrimal duct. **2.** A tumor of the lacrimal apparatus.

dac·ry·ops (dăk′rē-ŏps′) *n.* **1.** Excess of tears in the eye. **2.** A swelling of a lacrimal duct caused by excess fluid.

dac·ry·o·py·or·rhea (dăk′rē-ō-pī′ə-rē′ə) *n.* The discharge of tears containing pus.

dac·ry·o·py·o·sis (dăk′rē-ō-pī-ō′sĭs) *n.* The formation of pus in a lacrimal sac or duct.

dac·ry·or·rhe·a (dăk′rē-ə-rē′ə) *n.* Excessive flow of tears.

dac·ry·o·scin·tig·ra·phy (dăk′rē-ō-sĭn-tĭg′rə-fē) *n.* Scintigraphy of the lacrimal ducts to determine whether or how much they are blocked.

dac·ry·o·ste·no·sis (dăk′rē-ō-stə-nō′sĭs) *n.* Stricture or narrowing of a lacrimal duct.

dac·ti·no·my·cin (dăk′tə-nō-mī′sĭn) *n.* An antibiotic of the actinomycin group isolated from bacteria and used as an antineoplastic agent in the treatment of certain cancers.

dac·tyl (dăk′təl) *n.* A finger or toe; digit.

dac·ty·li·tis (dăk′tə-lī′tĭs) *n.* Inflammation of a finger or toe.

dac·tyl·o·gram (dăk-tĭl′ə-grăm′) *n.* A fingerprint.

dac·ty·lol·o·gy (dăk′tə-lŏl′ə-jē) *n.* The use of the fingers and hands to communicate and convey ideas, as in the manual alphabet used by hearing-impaired and speech-impaired people.

dac·ty·lo·meg·a·ly (dăk′tə-lō-mĕg′ə-lē) *n.* Abnormally large fingers or toes.

Dal·rym·ple's sign (dăl-rĭm′pəlz, dăl′rĭm-) *n.* An indication of Graves disease in which there is abnormal wideness of the palpebral fissures with retraction of the upper lid of the eye.

dam (dăm) *n.* A barrier against the passage of liquid or loose material, especially a rubber sheet used in dentistry to isolate one or more teeth from the rest of the mouth.

D and C *n.* Dilation and curettage.

D & C *abbr.* dilation and curettage

D & E *abbr.* dilation and evacuation

dan·der (dăn′dər) *n.* Small scales from the skin, hair, or feathers of an animal, often causing an allergic reaction in sensitive individuals.

dan·druff (dăn′drəf) *n.* A scaly scurf formed on and shed from the scalp, sometimes caused by seborrhea.

Dan·dy operation (dăn′dē) *n.* **1.** A suboccipital trigeminal rhizotomy. **2.** See **third ventriculostomy** (sense 2).

Dane particle (dān) *n.* Any of the larger spherical forms of hepatitis-associated antigens comprising the virion of hepatitis B virus.

DANS (dē′ā-ĕn-ĕs′) *n.* 1-dimethylaminonaphthalene-5-sulfonic acid; a green fluorescing compound used in immunohistochemistry to detect antigens.

dap·sone (dăp′sōn′, -zōn′) *n.* An antibacterial drug used primarily to treat leprosy and some forms of dermatitis.

dark adaptation (därk) *n.* The adjustment of the eye under reduced illumination, in which the sensitivity to light is greatly increased.

dark-adapted eye *n.* An eye that has been in darkness or semidarkness for some time and has undergone changes that render it more sensitive to low illumination.

Dar·von (där′vŏn) A trademark used for a mild, nonnarcotic analgesic drug.

dar·win·i·an reflex (där-wĭn′ē-ən) *n.* The tendency of young infants to grasp a bar and hang suspended.

daugh·ter cell (dô′tər) *n.* Either of the two identical cells that form when a cell divides.

Da·viel's operation (dăv′ē-ĕlz′, dä-vyĕlz′) *n.* An extracapsular cataract extraction.

dawn phenomenon *n.* The occurrence of abrupt increases in fasting levels of plasma glucose concentrations between the hours of 5 and 9 a.m., without preceding hypoglycemia, especially in diabetic patients receiving insulin therapy.

dB *abbr.* decibel

D.C. *abbr.* Doctor of Chiropractic

DDC (dē′dē-sē′) *n.* Dideoxycytidine; a nucleoside analogue drug that is similar to AZT in action.

DDI (dē′dē-ī′) *n.* Dideoxyinosine; a nucleoside analogue drug that is similar to AZT in action.

D.D.S. *abbr.* Doctor of Dental Science; Doctor of Dental Surgery

DDT (dē′dē-tē′) *n.* Dichlorodiphenyltrichloroethane; a colorless contact insecticide, toxic to humans and animals when swallowed or absorbed through the skin, that has been banned in the United States for most uses since 1972.

dead (dĕd) *adj.* **1.** Having lost life; no longer alive. **2.** Lacking feeling or sensitivity; numb or unresponsive.

dead-end host *n.* A host from which infectious agents are not transmitted to other susceptible hosts.

dead·ly nightshade (dĕd′lē) *n.* See **belladonna** (sense 1).

deaf (dĕf) *adj.* **1.** Partially or completely lacking in the sense of hearing. **2. Deaf.** Of or relating to the Deaf or their culture. — *n.* **1.** Deaf people considered as a group. **2. Deaf.** The community of deaf people who use American Sign Language as a primary means of communication.

deaf·en (dĕf′ən) *v.* **-ened, -en·ing, -ens.** To make deaf, especially momentarily by a loud noise.

de·af·fer·en·ta·tion (dē-ăf′ər-ən-tā′shən) *n.* The elimination or interruption of sensory nerve impulses by destroying or injuring the sensory nerve fibers.

deaf-mute (dĕf′myo͞ot′) *adj.* Unable to speak or hear.

deaf·ness (dĕf′nĭs) *n.* The lack or loss of the ability to hear.

de·ar·te·ri·al·i·za·tion (dē′är-tēr′ē-ə-lĭ-zā′shən) *n.* The deoxygenation of arterial blood to blood resembling venous blood.

death (dĕth) *n.* The end of life; the permanent cessation of vital bodily functions, as manifested in humans by the loss of heartbeat, the absence of spontaneous breathing, and brain death.

death instinct *n.* A primitive impulse for destruction, decay, and death, manifested by a turning away from pleasure, postulated as coexisting with and opposing the life instinct.

death rate *n.* The ratio of total deaths to total population in a specified community or area over a specified period of time. The death rate is often expressed as the number of deaths per 1,000 of the population per year.

death rattle *n.* A gurgling or rattling sound sometimes made in the throat of a dying person, caused by loss of the cough reflex and passage of the breath through accumulating mucus.

death wish *n.* **1.** A desire for self-destruction, often accompanied by feelings of depression, hopelessness, and self-reproach. **2.** A suicidal urge thought to drive certain people to put themselves consistently into dangerous situations.

de·band·ing (dē-bănd′dĭng) *n.* The removal of fixed orthodontic appliances.

de·bil·i·tat·ing (dĭ-bĭl′ĭ-tā′tĭng) *adj.* Causing a loss of strength or energy.

de·bil·i·ty (dĭ-bĭl′ĭ-tē) *n.* The state of being weak or feeble; infirmity.

dé·bride·ment (dā′brēd-mäN′, dĭ-brēd′mənt) *n.* The removal of dead, devitalized, or contaminated tissue and foreign matter from a wound, especially by surgical excision.

debt (dĕt) *n.* Something that is deficient or required to restore a normal state.

de·bulk·ing operation (dē-bŭl′kĭng) *n.* Excision of a major part of a malignant tumor which cannot be completely removed, so as to enhance the effectiveness of subsequent radiation therapy or chemotherapy.

de·ca·pac·i·ta·tion (dē′kə-păs′ĭ-tā′shən) *n.* The prevention of capacitation by spermatozoa, and thus of their ability to fertilize egg cells.

de·cap·i·ta·tion (dĭ-kăp′ĭ-tā′shən) *n.* The removal of a head, as of an animal, a fetus, or a bone.

de·cap·su·la·tion (dē-kăp′sə-lā′shən, -syo͞o-) *n.* Surgical removal of a capsule or enveloping membrane, as of the kidney.

de·cay (dĭ-kā′) *n.* **1.** The destruction or decomposition of organic matter as a result of bacterial or fungal action; rot. **2.** Dental caries. **3.** The loss of information that was registered by the senses and processed into the short-term memory system. **4.** Radioactive decay. — *v.* **-cayed, -cay·ing, -cays. 1.** To break down into component parts; rot. **2.** To disintegrate or diminish by radioactive decay. **3.** To decline in health or vigor; waste away.

decay theory *n.* The theory of memory loss that holds that an engram deteriorates progressively during the time when it is not activated.

de·cer·e·bra·tion (dē-sĕr′ə-brā′shən) *n.* The elimination of cerebral function in an animal by removing the cerebrum, cutting across the brain stem, or severing certain arteries in the brain stem, as for experimentation.

de·cho·les·ter·ol·i·za·tion (dē′kə-lĕs′tə-rôl′ĭ-zā′shən) *n.* The therapeutic reduction of cholesterol in the blood.

de·cid·u·a (dĭ-sĭj′o͞o-ə) *n., pl.* **-u·as** or **-u·ae** (-o͞o-ē′). A mucous membrane lining the uterus, modified during pregnancy and shed at parturition or during menstruation. — **de·cid′u·al** *adj.*

decidua ba·sa·lis (bə-sā′lĭs) *n.* The area of endometrium between the implanted chorionic vesicle and the myometrium, which becomes the maternal part of the placenta.

decidual cell *n.* An enlarged, ovoid, connective tissue cell in the uterine mucous membrane that enlarges and specializes during pregnancy.

de·cid·u·a·tion (dĭ-sĭj′o͞o-ā′shən) *n.* The shedding of endometrial tissue during menstruation.

de·cid·u·o·ma (dĭ-sĭj′o͞o-ō′mə) *n.* An intrauterine mass of decidual tissue, probably the result of hyperplasia of decidual cells retained in the uterus after parturition.

de·cid·u·ous (dĭ-sĭj′o͞o-əs) *adj.* **1.** Falling off or shed at a specific stage of growth, as teeth of the first dentition. **2.** Of, relating to, or being the first or primary dentition.

deciduous dentition *n.* See **primary dentition.**

deciduous tooth *n.* Any of the teeth of the primary dentition.

de·clamp·ing phenomenon (dē-klăm′pĭng) *n.* The occurrence of shock or hypotension following the abrupt release of clamps from a large portion of the vascular bed, such as the aorta, that is believed to be caused by transient pooling of blood in a previously ischemic area.

declamping shock *n.* See **declamping phenomenon.**

dec·li·na·tion (dĕk′lə-nā′shən) *n.* **1.** A bending, sloping, or other deviation from a normal vertical position. **2.** A deviation of the vertical meridian of the eye to one or the other side due to rotation of the eyeball about its anteroposterior axis.

de·com·pen·sa·tion (dē′kŏm-pən-sā′shən) *n.* **1.** Failure of the heart to maintain adequate blood circulation, marked by labored breathing, engorged blood vessels, and edema. **2.** The appearance or exacerbation of a mental disorder due to failure of defense mechanisms.

de·com·po·si·tion (dē-kŏm′pə-zĭsh′ən) *n.* **1.** The act or result of decomposing; disintegration. **2.** Separation into constituents by chemical reaction. **3.** Breakdown or decay of organic materials; decay; lysis. — **de·com′po·si′tion·al** *adj.*

de·com·pres·sion (dē′kəm-prĕsh′ən) *n.* **1.** The relief of pressure on a body part by surgery. **2.** The restoration of deep sea divers and caisson workers to atmospheric pressure by means of a decompression chamber.

decompression chamber *n.* A compartment in which atmospheric pressure can be gradually raised or lowered, used in readjusting divers or underwater workers to normal atmospheric pressure or in treating decompression sickness.

decompression sickness *n.* A disorder, seen especially in deep-sea divers or in caisson and tunnel workers, caused by the formation of nitrogen bubbles in the blood following a rapid drop in pressure and characterized by severe pains in the joints and chest, skin irritation, cramps, and paralysis.

de·con·gest (dē′kən-jĕst′) *v.* -gest·ed, -gest·ing, -gests. To relieve congestion, as of the sinuses.

de·con·ges·tant (dē′kən-jĕs′tənt) *n.* A medication or treatment that breaks up congestion, as of the sinuses, by reducing swelling. — *adj.* Capable of relieving congestion.

de·cor·ti·ca·tion (dē-kôr′tĭ-kā′shən) *n.* The removal of the surface layer, membrane, or fibrous cover of an organ or a structure. — **de·cor′ti·cate′** *v.*

de·cru·des·cence (dē′krōō-dĕs′əns) *n.* Abatement of the symptoms of a disease.

de·cu·bi·tus (dĭ-kyōō′bĭ-təs) *n.* **1.** The position of a patient in bed. **2.** A bedsore.

decubitus calculus *n.* A calculus of the urinary tract formed as a result of long immobilization.

decubitus paralysis *n.* A form of compression paralysis due to pressure on a limb during sleep.

decubitus ulcer *n.* See **bedsore.**

de·cus·sate (dĭ-kŭs′āt′, dĕk′ə-sāt′) *v.* -sat·ed, -sat·ing, -sates. To cross or become crossed so as to form an X; intersect. — *adj.* Intersected or crossed in the form of an X.

dec·us·sa·tion (dĕk′ə-sā′shən, dē′kə-) *n.* An X-shaped crossing, especially of nerves or bands of nerve fibers connecting corresponding parts on opposite sides of the brain or spinal cord.

de·dif·fer·en·ti·a·tion (dē′dĭf-ə-rĕn′shē-ā′shən) *n.* Regression of a specialized cell or tissue to a simpler unspecialized form, often preliminary to a major change. — **de·dif·fer·en′ti·ate′** *v.*

de·ep·i·car·di·al·i·za·tion (dē-ĕp′ĭ-kär′dē-ə-lĭ-zā′shən) *n.* The surgical destruction of the epicardium designed to promote collateral circulation to the myocardium.

deep reflex *n.* An involuntary muscular contraction following percussion of a tendon or bone.

def·e·cate (dĕf′ĭ-kāt′) *v.* -cat·ed, -cat·ing, -cates. To void feces from the bowels.

def·e·ca·tion (def-ĕ-kā′shŭn) *n.* The discharge of feces from the rectum.

de·fect (dē′fĕkt′, dĭ-fĕkt′) *n.* A lack of or abnormality in something necessary for normal functioning; a deficiency or imperfection.

de·fec·tive (dĭ-fĕk′tĭv) *n.* **1.** Having an imperfection or malformation. **2.** Lacking or deficient in some physical or mental function.

de·fense (dĭ-fĕns′) *n.* A means or method that helps protect the body or mind, as against disease or anxiety. — **de·fen′sive** (-fĕn′sĭv) *adj.*

defense mechanism *n.* **1.** Any of a variety of usually unconscious mental processes used to protect oneself from shame, anxiety, conflict, loss of self-esteem, or other unacceptable feelings or thoughts, and including behaviors such as repression, projection, denial, and rationalization. **2.** See **immunological mechanism.**

de·fen·sive circle (dĭ-fĕn′sĭv) *n.* The addition of a secondary disease that limits or arrests the progress of the primary disease, the two diseases exerting a reciprocally antagonistic action.

defensive medicine *n.* Diagnostic or therapeutic measures conducted primarily as a safeguard against possible malpractice liability.

deferent duct *n.* See **vas deferens.**

def·er·en·tec·to·my (dĕf′ər-ən-tĕk′tə-mē) *n.* See **vasectomy.**

def·er·en·tial (dĕf′ə-rĕn′shəl) *adj.* Of or relating to the vas deferens.

def·er·en·ti·tis (dĕf′ər-ən-tī′tĭs) *n.* Inflammation of the vas deferens.

de·fer·ves·cence (dē′fər-vĕs′əns, dĕf′ər-) *n.* The abatement of a fever.

de·fib·ril·la·tion (dē-fĭb′rə-lā′shən, -fī′brə-) *n.* The stopping of the fibrillation of the heart muscle and the restoration of normal contractions through the use of drugs or an electric shock. — **de·fib′ril·late′** *v.*

de·fib·ril·la·tor (dē-fĭb′rə-lā′tər, -fī′brə-) *n.* An electrical device used to counteract fibrillation of the heart muscle and restore normal heartbeat by applying a brief electric shock.

de·fi·bri·na·tion (dē-fī′brə-nā′shən, -fĭb′rə-) *n.* The removal of fibrin from blood. — **de·fi′bri·nate′** *v.*

de·fi·cien·cy (dĭ-fĭsh′ən-sē) *n.* A lack or shortage of something essential to health; an insufficiency.

deficiency disease *n.* A disease, such as rickets or scurvy, that is caused by a dietary deficiency of specific nutrients, especially a vitamin or mineral, and may stem from insufficient intake, digestion, absorption, or utilization of a nutrient.

de·fi·cient (dĭ-fĭsh′ənt) *adj.* **1.** Lacking an essential quality or element. **2.** Inadequate in amount or degree; insufficient.

def·i·cit (dĕf′ĭ-sĭt) *n.* **1.** A lack or deficiency of a substance. **2.** A lack or impairment in mental or physical functioning.

de·flec·tion (dĭ-flĕk′shən) *n.* **1.** A turning aside or deviation. **2.** The deviation of an indicator in a measuring instrument.

de·flu·vi·um (dē-flōo'vē-əm) *n.* Defluxion.

de·flux·ion (dē-flŭk'shən) *n.* **1.** A falling down or out, as of the hair. **2.** A flowing down or discharge of fluid.

de·for·ma·tion (dē'fôr-mā'shən, dĕf'ər-) *n.* **1.** An alteration in shape or structure of a previously normally formed part. **2.** A deformity.

de·formed (dĭ-fôrmd') *adj.* Distorted in form; misshapen.

de·for·mi·ty (dĭ-fôr'mĭ-tē) *n.* **1.** The state of being deformed. **2.** A deviation from the normal shape or size of a body part, resulting in disfigurement.

deg or **deg.** *abbr.* degree

de·gen·er·ate (dĭ-jĕn'ər-ĭt) *adj.* Characterized by degeneration, as of tissue, a cell, or an organ. — *v.* **-at·ed, -at·ing, -ates.** (-ə-rāt'). To undergo degeneration.

de·gen·er·a·tion (dĭ-jĕn'ə-rā'shən) *n.* The gradual deterioration of specific tissues, cells, or organs with impairment or loss of function, caused by injury, disease, or aging.

de·gen·er·a·tive (dĭ-jĕn'ər-ə-tĭv) *adj.* Of, relating to, causing, or characterized by degeneration.

degenerative joint disease *n.* See **osteoarthritis.**

de·glov·ing (dē-glŭv'ĭng) *n.* The surgical exposure of the front part of the mandible while working from within the mouth, as used in plastic surgery.

deglut *abbr. Latin.* degluttiatur (let be swallowed; swallow)

de·glu·ti·tion (dē'glōo-tĭsh'ən) *n.* The act of swallowing.

deg·ra·da·tion (dĕg'rə-dā'shən) *n.* Progressive decomposition of a chemical compound into a less complex compound.

de·gree (dĭ-grē') *n.* **1.** A unit of measure on a temperature scale. **2.** A division of a circle, equal to ¹⁄₃₆₀ of its circumference. **3.** A position or rank within a graded series.

de·gus·ta·tion (dē'gŭ-stā'shən) *n.* **1.** The act or function of tasting. **2.** The sense of taste.

de·hisce (dĭ-hĭs') *v.* **-hisced, -hisc·ing, -hisc·es.** To rupture or break open, as a surgical wound.

de·his·cence (dē-hĭs'əns) *n.* A bursting open or splitting along natural or sutured lines.

dehydrate *v.* **-drat·ed, -drat·ing, -drates. 1.** To remove water from; make anhydrous. **2.** To preserve by removing water from something, such as vegetables. **3.** To deplete the body's fluids.

de·hy·dra·tion (dē'hī-drā'shən) *n.* **1.** Excessive loss of water from the body or from an organ or a body part, as from illness or fluid deprivation. **2.** The process of removing water from a substance or compound.

de·in·sti·tu·tion·al·i·za·tion (dē-ĭn'stī'tōo'shə-nə-lī-zā'shən, -tyōo'-) *n.* The release of institutionalized people, especially mental health patients, from an institution for placement and care in the community. — **de·in'sti·tu'tion·al·ize'** *v.*

dé·já vu (dā'zhä vü') *n.* See **déjà vu phenomenon.**

déjà vu phenomenon *n.* **1.** The illusion of having already experienced something actually being ex-

perienced for the first time. **2.** An impression of having seen or experienced something before.

de·jec·tion (dĭ-jĕk'shən) *n.* **1.** Lowness of spirits; depression; melancholy. **2.** The evacuation of the bowels; defecation. **3.** Feces; excrement.

de·lac·ri·ma·tion (dē-lăk'rə-mā'shən) *n.* The excessive secretion of tears.

de·lam·i·na·tion (dē-lăm'ə-nā'shən) *n.* **1.** A splitting or separation into separate layers. **2.** The splitting of the blastoderm into two layers of cells to form a gastrula.

de Lang·e's syndrome (də lăng'ēz, läng'əz) or **Cor·ne·lia de Lang·e's syndrome** (kôr-nēl'yə) *n.* A syndrome of unknown cause characterized by mental retardation, short stature, characteristic facies with thick eyebrows and low hairline, and flat, spadelike hands with short tapering fingers.

delayed flap *n.* A flap raised in its donor area in two or more stages to increase its chances of survival after transfer.

delayed graft *n.* The application of a skin graft after waiting several days for healthy granulations to form.

delayed reaction *n.* An allergic or immune response that begins 24 to 48 hours after exposure to an antigen to which the individual has been sensitized.

Del·bet's sign (dĕl-bāz') *n.* An indication of aneurysm of a main artery in which the pulse disappears although collateral circulation remains efficient and nutrition of the part below the main artery is well maintained.

del·e·te·ri·ous (dĕl'ĭ-tĕr'ē-əs) *adj.* Having a harmful effect; injurious.

de·le·tion (dĭ-lē'shən) *n.* The loss, as through mutation, of one or more nucleotides from a chromosome.

de·lim·it·ing keratotomy (dĭ-lĭm'ĭ-tĭng) *n.* Incision in the cornea along the margin of an advancing ulcer.

de·lir·i·ous (dĭ-lĕr'ē-əs) *adj.* Of, suffering from, or characteristic of delirium.

de·lir·i·um (dĭ-lĕr'ē-əm) *n.* **-i·ums** or **-i·a** (-ē-ə). A temporary state of mental confusion resulting from high fever, intoxication, shock, or other causes, and characterized by anxiety, disorientation, memory impairment, hallucinations, trembling, and incoherent speech.

delirium tre·mens (trē'mənz) *n.* An acute, sometimes fatal episode of delirium usually caused by withdrawal or abstinence from alcohol following habitual excessive drinking and characterized by sweating, trembling, anxiety, confusion, and hallucinations.

de·liv·er (dĭ-lĭv'ər) *v.* **-ered, -er·ing, -ers. 1.** To assist a woman in giving birth to a baby. **2.** To extract something from an enclosed place, as a foreign body or a tumor.

de·liv·er·y (dĭ-lĭv'ə-rē, -lĭv'rē) *n.* The expulsion or extraction of a child and the fetal membranes through the genital canal into the external world; parturition.

delivery room *n.* A room or an area in a hospital that is equipped for delivering babies.

del·le (dĕl′ə) *n.* The lighter-colored area in the center of a stained red blood cell.

del·ta (dĕl′tə) *n.* **1.** The fourth one in a series. **2.** A surface or part that resembles a triangle, such as the terminus of a pattern in a fingerprint or the shape of a muscle. — *adj.* **1.** Of or characterizing the atom or radical group that is fourth in position from the functional group of atoms in an organic molecule, such as any of the delta-hydroxy acids. **2.** Of or relating to one of four closely related chemical substances. **3.** Relating to or characterizing a polypeptide chain that is one of five types of such chains in immunoglobins.

delta rhythm *n.* A brain wave pattern originating from the forward portion of the brain; it is associated with deep sleep in normal adults.

delta wave *n.* **1.** A slurring of the initial upstroke of the R wave in an electrocardiogram. **2.** See **delta rhythm.**

deltoid muscle *n.* A muscle with its origin from the clavicle, the acromion process, and the spine of the scapula, with insertion to the humerus, and whose action causes the abduction, flexion, extension, and rotation of the arm.

de·lu·sion (dĭ-lōō′zhən) *n.* A false belief strongly held in spite of invalidating evidence, especially as a symptom of mental illness.

de·lu·sion·al (dĭ-lōō′zhə-nəl) *adj.* Of, relating to, or characterized by a delusion or delusions.

delusion of gran·deur (grăn′jər, -jŏōr′) *n.* A delusion in which one believes oneself possessed of great importance, power, intellect, or ability.

delusion of negation *n.* A depressive delusion in which one imagines that the world has ceased to exist.

delusion of persecution *n.* A delusion that one is being persecuted or conspired against, characteristic of paranoid schizophrenia.

de·mand pacemaker (dĭ-mănd′) *n.* An artificial pacemaker usually implanted into cardiac tissue because its output of electrical stimuli can be inhibited by endogenous cardiac electrical activity.

de·ment·ed (dĭ-mĕn′tĭd) *adj.* **1.** Mentally ill; insane. **2.** Suffering from dementia.

de·men·tia (dĭ-mĕn′shə) *n.* Deterioration of intellectual faculties, such as memory, concentration, and judgment, due to an organic disease or a disorder of the brain, and often accompanied by emotional disturbance and personality changes.

Dem·er·ol (dĕm′ə-rôl′, -rŏl′, -rōl′) A trademark used for a sedative and analgesic agent.

dem·i·gaunt·let bandage (dĕm′ē-gônt′lĭt, -gänt′-) *n.* A gauntlet bandage that covers the hand but leaves the fingers exposed.

Dem·o·dex (dĕm′ə-dĕks′, dē′mə-) *n.* A genus of parasitic, usually nonpathogenic mites of the family Demodicidae that invade the skin and are usually found in the sebaceous glands and hair follicles of humans and animals.

de·mu·co·sa·tion (dē-myōō′kə-sā′shən) *n.* Surgical removal of a mucous membrane from a part of the body.

de·mul·cent (dĭ-mŭl′sənt) *adj.* Relieving irritation; soothing. — *n.* A soothing, usually mucilaginous or oily substance, such as lanolin, used to relieve pain in inflamed or irritated mucous membranes.

de·my·e·lin·at·ing disease (dē-mī′ə-lə-nā′tĭng) *n.* Any of a group of diseases of unknown cause in which there is extensive loss of the myelin sheaths of nerve fibers, as in multiple sclerosis.

de·my·e·lin·a·tion (dē-mī′ə-lə-nā′shən) or **de·my·e·lin·i·za·tion** (-lə-nĭ-zā′shən, -lĭn′ĭ-) *n.* The destruction or removal of the myelin sheath of a nerve fiber, as through disease.

de·na·ture (dē-nā′chər) *v.* **-tured, -tur·ing, -tures.** **1.** To change the nature or natural qualities of. **2.** To render unfit to eat or drink without destroying usefulness in other applications, especially adding methyl alcohol to ethyl alcohol. **3.** To alter the chemical structure of a protein, as with heat, alkali, or acid, so that some of its original properties, especially its biological activity, are diminished or eliminated. — **de·na′tur·a′tion** *n.*

den·dri·form (dĕn′drə-fôrm′) *adj.* Tree-shaped, branching.

den·drite (dĕn′drīt′) *n.* Any of the various branched protoplasmic extensions of a nerve cell that conducts impulses from adjacent cells inward toward the cell body.

den·drit·ic (dĕn-drĭt′ĭk) *adj.* Relating to the dendrites of nerve cells.

dendritic calculus *n.* See **stag-horn calculus.**

dendritic cell *n.* **1.** A cell that has branching processes. **2.** Any of the cells in the neural crest of the embryonic ectoderm having extensive processes and developing early as producers of melanin.

dendritic corneal ulcer *n.* Keratitis caused by herpes simplex virus.

dendritic process *n.* See **dendrite.**

den·droid (dĕn′droid′) *n.* See **dendriform.**

den·dron (dĕn′drŏn′) *n.* See **dendrite.**

de·ner·vate (dē-nûr′vāt) *v.* **-va·ted, -va·ting, -vates.** To deprive an organ or body part of a nerve supply, as by surgically removing or cutting a nerve or by blocking a nerve connection with drugs. — **de′ner·va′tion** *n.*

den·gue (dĕng′gē, -gā) *n.* An acute, infectious tropical disease that is caused by an arbovirus transmitted by mosquitoes, and characterized by high fever, rash, headache, and severe muscle and joint pain.

dengue virus *n.* A virus of the genus *Flavivirus* that is transmitted by a mosquito and is the cause of dengue.

de·ni·al (dĭ-nī′əl) *n.* An unconscious defense mechanism characterized by refusal to acknowledge painful realities, thoughts, or feelings.

den·i·da·tion (dĕn′ĭ-dā′shən) *n.* The detachment and expulsion of the endometrium of the uterus during menstruation.

Den·is Browne splint (dĕn′ĭs broun′) *n.* A light

aluminum splint applied to the lateral aspect of the leg and foot, used for clubfoot.

Den·nie's fold (děn'ēz) *n*. See **Dennie's line**.

Dennie's line *n*. An accentuated line below the margin of the lower eyelid, characteristic of atopic dermatitis.

den·tal (děn'tl) *adj*. **1.** Of, relating to, or for the teeth. **2.** Of, relating to, or intended for dentistry.

dental abscess *n*. See **alveolar abscess**.

dental calculus *n*. See **tartar** (sense 2).

dental caries *n*. Deterioration of the teeth and formation of cavities by the enzymatic action of bacteria on carbohydrates; tooth decay.

dental floss *n*. A waxed or unwaxed thread used to remove food particles and plaque from the teeth.

dental hygiene *n*. The practice of keeping the mouth, teeth, and gums clean and healthy to prevent disease, as by regular brushing and flossing and visits to a dentist.

dental hygienist *n*. A person trained and licensed to provide preventive dental services, such as cleaning the teeth and taking x-rays, usually in conjunction with a dentist.

dental implant *n*. An artificial tooth that is anchored in the gums or jawbone to replace a missing tooth.

dental plaque *n*. A film of mucus and bacteria on a tooth surface.

dental pulp *n*. The soft tissue forming the inner structure of a tooth and containing nerves and blood vessels.

dental surgeon *n*. A general practitioner of dentistry having a DDS or DMD degree.

dental technician *n*. A person who makes dental appliances and restorative devices, such as bridges or dentures, to the specifications of a dentist.

den·tin (děn'tǐn) or **den·tine** (-tēn') *n*. The main, calcareous part of a tooth, beneath the enamel and surrounding the pulp chamber and root canals.

dentin dysplasia *n*. A hereditary disorder of both the primary and permanent teeth characterized by short roots, obliteration of the pulp chambers and canals, and mobility and premature loss.

den·ti·no·gen·e·sis (děn'tə-nō-jěn'ĭ-sĭs) *n*. The formation of dentin.

den·tist (děn'tĭst) *n*. A person who is trained and licensed to practice dentistry.

den·tist·ry (děn'tĭ-strē) *n*. The science concerned with the prevention, diagnosis, and treatment of diseases of the teeth, gums, and related structures of the mouth and including the repair or replacement of defective teeth.

den·ti·tion (děn-tĭsh'ən) *n*. **1.** The natural teeth, considered collectively, in the dental arch. **2.** The type, number, and arrangement of a set of teeth. **3.** The process of growing new teeth; teething.

den·ture (děn'chər) *n*. **1.** A partial or complete set of artificial teeth for either the upper or lower jaw. **2.** *Often* **dentures**. A complete set of removable artificial teeth for both jaws.

de·nu·da·tion (dē'noō-dā'shən, -nyoō-, děn'yoō-) *n*. The removal of a covering or surface layer.

de·nude (dĭ-noōd', -nyoōd') *v*. **-nud·ed, -nud·ing, -nudes**. To divest of a covering, as of tissue or myelin.

de·o·dor·ant (dē-ō'dər-ənt) *n*. A substance that masks, suppresses, or neutralizes odors, especially a preparation applied to the skin to mask body odors. — *adj*. Capable of masking, suppressing, or neutralizing odors.

de·o·dor·ize (dē-ō'də-rīz') *v*. **-ized, -iz·ing, -iz·es**. To mask or neutralize the odor of. — **de·o'dor·i·za'tion** (-dər-ĭ-zā'shən) *n*.

de·os·si·fi·ca·tion (dē-ŏs'ə-fĭ-kā'shən) *n*. The loss or removal of the mineral constituents of bone.

de·ox·y·gen·a·tion (dē-ŏk'sə-jə-nā'shən) *n*. The process of removing dissolved oxygen from a liquid, such as water.

de·ox·y·ri·bo·nu·cle·ase (dē-ŏk'sē-rī'bō-noō'klē-ās', -āz', -nyoō'-) *n*. DNase.

de·ox·y·ri·bo·nu·cle·ic acid (dē-ŏk'sē-rī'bō-noō-klē'ĭk, -klā'-, -nyoō-) *n*. DNA.

de·ox·y·ri·bo·nu·cle·o·side (dē-ŏk'sē-rī'bō-noō'klē-ə-sīd', -nyoō'-) *n*. A nucleoside containing deoxyribose that is a constituent of DNA.

de·ox·y·ri·bo·nu·cle·o·tide (dē-ŏk'sē-rī'bō-noō'klē-ə-tīd', -nyoō'-) *n*. A nucleotide containing deoxyribose that is a constituent of DNA.

de·ox·y·ri·bose (dē-ŏk'sē-rī'bōs') *n*. A sugar that is a constituent of DNA.

de·ox·y sugar (dē-ŏk'sē) *n*. A sugar containing fewer oxygen atoms than carbon atoms, resulting in one or more carbons in the molecule lacking an attached hydroxyl group.

de·pend·ence (dĭ-pěn'dəns) *n*. **1.** The state of being dependent. **2.** Subordination to someone or something needed or greatly desired. **3.** A compulsive or chronic need; an addiction. — **de·pend'en·cy** (-sē) *n*.

de·pend·ent (dĭ-pěn'dənt) *adj*. **1.** Contingent on or subordinate to another. **2.** Relying on or requiring the aid of another for support. **3.** Hanging down. — *n*. One who relies on another especially for financial support.

dependent drainage *n*. A procedure for draining a cavity or structure from its lowest part into a receptacle positioned at yet a level lower.

dependent edema *n*. A clinically detectable increase in extracellular fluid volume localized in a dependent area such as a limb, characterized by swelling or pitting.

dependent personality *n*. A personality disorder characterized by a long-term pattern of passively allowing others to take responsibility for major areas of life, by a lack of self-confidence and independence, and of subordinating personal needs to the needs of others.

de·per·son·al·i·za·tion (dē-pûr'sə-nə-lĭ-zā'shən) *n*. A state in which the normal sense of personal identity and reality is lost, characterized by feelings that one's actions and speech cannot be controlled. — **de·per'son·al·ize'** (-līz') *v*.

de·pig·men·ta·tion (dē-pĭg'mən-tā'shən, -měn-) *n*. The loss or removal of normal pigmentation.

dep·i·late (děp'ə-lāt') *v*. **-lat·ed, -lat·ing, -lates**. To remove hair from the body by mechanical or chemical means or by electrolysis.

dep·i·la·tion (dĕp′ə-lā′shən) *n.* See **epilation.**

de·pil·a·to·ry (dĭ-pĭl′ə-tôr′ē) *adj.* Having the capability to remove hair. — *n.* A preparation in the form of a liquid or cream that is used to remove unwanted hair from the body.

de·plete (dĭ-plēt′) *v.* **-plet·ed, -plet·ing, -pletes. 1.** To use up something, such as an essential nutrient. **2.** To empty something out, as the body of electrolytes.

de·ple·tion (dĭ-plē′shən) *n.* **1.** The act or process of depleting. **2.** The state of being depleted; exhaustion. **3.** Removal of or reduction in a body substance, such as blood, a fluid, or a nutrient.

de·plu·ma·tion (dē′plo͞o-mā′shən) *n.* The falling out or loss of the eyelashes.

de·po·lar·i·za·tion (dē-pō′lər-ĭ-zā′shən) *n.* The elimination or neutralization of polarity, as in nerve cells.

de·pos·it (dĭ-pŏz′ĭt) *v.* **-it·ed, -it·ing, -its. 1.** To lay down or leave behind by a natural process. **2.** To become deposited; settle. — *n.* **1.** An accumulation of organic or inorganic material, such as a lipid or mineral, in a body tissue, structure, or fluid. **2.** A sediment or precipitate that has settled out of a solution.

de·pot injection (dē′pō, dĕp′ō) *n.* An injection of a substance in a form that tends to keep it at the site of injection so that absorption occurs over a prolonged period.

de·press (dĭ-prĕs′) *v.* **1.** To lower in spirits; deject. **2.** To cause to drop or sink; lower. **3.** To press down. **4.** To lessen the activity or force of something; weaken.

de·pres·sant (dĭ-prĕs′ənt) *adj.* Tending to lower the rate of vital physiological activities. — *n.* An agent, especially a drug, that decreases the rate of vital physiological activities.

de·pressed (dĭ-prĕst′) *adj.* **1.** Lower in amount, degree, or position. **2.** Sunk below the surrounding area. **3.** Flattened along the dorsal and ventral surfaces. **4.** Low in spirits; dejected. **5.** Suffering from psychological depression.

depressed skull fracture *n.* A fracture in which bone from part of the skull is pushed inward.

de·pres·sion (dĭ-prĕsh′ən) *n.* **1.** The act of depressing or the state of being depressed. **2.** A reduction in physiological vigor or activity. **3.** A lowering in amount, degree, or position. **4.** An inward displacement of a body part. **5.** A hollow or sunken area. **6.** The condition of feeling sad or despondent. **7.** A psychotic or neurotic condition characterized by an inability to concentrate and feelings of extreme sadness and hopelessness.

de·pres·sive (dĭ-prĕs′ĭv) *adj.* **1.** Tending to depress or lower. **2.** Depressing; gloomy. **3.** Of or relating to psychological depression. — *n.* A person suffering from psychological depression.

de·pres·sor (dĭ-prĕs′ər) *n.* **1.** Any of various muscles that serve to draw down a part of the body. **2.** Something that depresses or retards functional activity. **3.** An instrument used to push certain

structures out of the way during an operation or examination. **4.** An agent that lowers blood pressure. **5.** A nerve that when stimulated acts to lower arterial blood pressure.

depressor nerve *n.* A nerve that when stimulated acts to lower arterial blood pressure.

dep·ri·va·tion (dĕp′rə-vā′shən) *n.* The absence, loss, or withholding of something needed.

de·prive (dĭ-prīv′) *v.* **-prived, -priv·ing, -prives. 1.** To take something away from someone or something. **2.** To keep from possessing or enjoying something; deny.

de·pro·gram (dē-prō′grăm′, -grəm) *v.* **-grammed** or **-gramed, -gram·ming** or **-gram·ing, -grams** or **-grams.** To counteract or try to counteract the effect of an indoctrination, especially a religious or cult indoctrination.

depth of focus (dĕpth) *n.* See **focal depth.**

depth perception *n.* The ability to perceive spatial relationships, especially distances between objects, in three dimensions.

de·range (dĭ-rānj′) *v.* **-ranged, -rang·ing, -rang·es. 1.** To upset the normal condition or functioning of. **2.** To disturb mentally; make insane.

de·range·ment (dĭ-rānj′mənt) *n.* **1.** The disturbance of the regular order or arrangement of parts in a system. **2.** Mental disorder; insanity. — **de·range**′ *v.*

de·re·al·i·za·tion (dē-rē′ə-lĭ-zā′shən) *n.* The feeling that things in one's surroundings are unreal or somehow altered, as in schizophrenia.

de·re·pres·sion (dē′rĭ-prĕsh′ən) *n.* The activation of an operator gene by the deactivation of a repressor gene. — **de′re·press**′ (-prĕs′) *v.*

de·riv·a·tive (dĭ-rĭv′ə-tĭv) *n.* **1.** Something obtained or produced by modification of something else. **2.** A chemical compound that may be produced from another compound of similar structure in one or more steps. — *adj.* Resulting from or employing derivation.

der·ma (dûr′mə) *n.* See **dermis.**

der·ma·brad·er (dûr′mə-brā′dər) *n.* A motor-driven device used in dermabrasion.

der·ma·bra·sion (dûr′mə-brā′zhən) *n.* A surgical procedure designed to remove skin imperfections, such as scars, by abrading the surface of the skin with fine sandpaper or wire brushes.

Der·ma·cen·tor (dûr′mə-sĕn′tər) *n.* A genus of hard ticks in the family Ixodidae, including certain species that transmit disease.

der·mal (dûr′məl) or **der·mic** (-mĭk) *adj.* Of or relating to the skin or dermis.

dermal graft *n.* A skin graft made with a thin split-thickness graft of dermis.

dermal papilla *n.* Any of the superficial projections of the corium or dermis that interlock with recesses in the overlying epidermis, contain vascular loops and specialized nerve endings, and are arranged in ridgelike lines most prominent in the hand and foot.

der·mat·ic (dər-măt′ĭk) *n.* Dermal.

der·ma·ti·tis (dûr′mə-tī′tĭs) *n., pl.* **-ti·tis·es** or **-tit·i·des** (-tĭt′ĭ-dēz′). Inflammation of the skin.

der·ma·to·au·to·plas·ty (dûr′mə-tō-ô′tō-plǎs′tē) *n.* The grafting of skin from one part of the body to another.

der·ma·to·bi·a·sis (dûr′mə-tō-bī′ə-sĭs) *n.* The infection of humans and animals with larvae of the botfly *Dermatobia hominis.*

der·ma·to·fi·bro·ma (dûr′mə-tō-fī-brō′mə) *n.* A slow-growing benign skin nodule consisting mostly of fibrous tissue.

der·ma·tog·ra·phism (dûr′mə-tŏg′rə-fĭz′əm) *n.* A form of urticaria in which welts develop in the skin along the lines where one has been stroked or stratched.

der·ma·to·het·er·o·plas·ty (dûr′mə-tō-hĕt′ər-ə-plǎs′tē) *n.* The grafting of skin obtained from a member of a different species.

der·ma·tol·o·gist (dûr′mə-tŏl′ə-jĭst) *n.* A physician who specializes in the diagnosis and treatment of skin disorders.

der·ma·tol·o·gy (dûr′mə-tŏl′ə-jē) *n.* The branch of medicine that deals with the diagnosis and treatment of skin diseases. — **der·ma·to·log′i·cal** (-tə-lŏj′ĭ-kəl), **der′ma·to·log′ic** *adj.*

der·ma·tol·y·sis (dûr′mə-tŏl′ĭ-sĭs) *n.* Any of various disorders characterized by loosening or hanging of the skin.

der·ma·tome (dûr′mə-tōm′) *n.* **1.** An area of skin innervated by sensory fibers from a single spinal nerve. **2.** An instrument used in cutting thin slices of the skin, as for grafts. **3.** The part of a mesodermal somite from which the dermis develops.

der·ma·to·meg·a·ly (dûr′mə-tō-mĕg′ə-lē) *n.* A congenital defect in which the skin hangs in folds.

der·ma·to·my·co·sis (dûr′mə-tō-mī-kō′sĭs) *n.* An infection of the skin caused by dermatophytes or other fungi.

der·ma·to·my·o·si·tis (dûr′mə-tō-mī′ə-sī′tĭs) *n.* A progressive inflammatory condition characterized by muscular weakness, a skin rash, and edema of the eyelids and periorbital tissue.

der·ma·to·neu·ro·sis (dûr′mə-tō-nŏŏ-rō′sĭs, -nyŏŏ-) *n.* A skin eruption caused by emotional distress.

der·ma·to·path·ic lymphadenitis (dûr′mə-tō-pǎth′ĭk) *n.* See **dermatopathic lymphadenopathy.**

dermatopathic lymphadenopathy *n.* Enlargement of lymph nodes with proliferation of histiocytes and macrophages containing fat and melanin, secondary to various forms of dermatitis.

der·ma·to·pa·thol·o·gy (dûr′mə-tō-pǎ-thŏl′ə-jē) *n.* The histopathology of skin lesions.

der·ma·top·a·thy (dûr′mə-tŏp′ə-thē) *n.* A disease of the skin.

der·mat·o·phyte (dûr-mǎt′ə-fīt′, dûr′mə-tə-) *n.* Any of various fungi that can cause parasitic infections of the skin, hair, or nails. — **der·mat′o·phyt′ic** (-fīt′ĭk) *adj.*

der·ma·to·plas·ty (dûr′mə-tō-plǎs′tē) *n.* The use of skin grafts in plastic surgery to correct defects or replace skin destroyed by injury or disease. — **der′ma·to·plas′tic** (-plǎs′tĭk) *adj.*

der·ma·to·pol·y·neu·ri·tis (dûr′mə-tō-pŏl′ē-nŏŏ-rī′tĭs, -nyŏŏ-) *n.* See **acrodynia** (sense 1).

der·ma·to·scle·ro·sis (dûr′mə-tō-sklə-rō′sĭs) *n.* See **scleroderma.**

der·ma·to·sis (dûr′mə-tō′sĭs) *n., pl.* **-ses** (-sēz). A skin disease, especially one that is not accompanied by inflammation.

der·ma·to·ther·a·py (dûr′mə-tō-thĕr′ə-pē) *n.* The treatment of skin diseases.

der·mis (dûr′mĭs) *n.* The sensitive connective tissue layer of the skin located below the epidermis, containing nerve endings, sweat and sebaceous glands, and blood and lymph vessels.

der·mo·blast (dûr′mə-blǎst′) *n.* The part of the mesoderm that develops into the dermis.

der·moid cyst (dûr′moid′) *n.* A benign tumor resulting from abnormal embryonic development, occurring in the skin or ovary, and consisting of displaced ectodermal structures along the lines of embryonic fusion.

der·moid·ec·to·my (dûr′moi-dĕk′tə-mē) *n.* Surgical removal of a dermoid cyst.

dermoid tumor *n.* See **dermoid cyst.**

der·mo·plas·ty (dûr′mə-plǎs′tē) *n.* See **dermatoplasty.**

der·mo·vas·cu·lar (dûr′mō-vǎs′kyə-lər) *adj.* Of or relating to the blood vessels of the skin.

DES (dē′ē-ĕs′) *n.* Diethylstilbestrol; a synthetic nonsteroidal substance having estrogenic properties and once used to treat menstrual disorders.

De·sault's bandage (də-sōz′) *n.* A bandage that binds the elbow to a person's side and is used for fractures of the clavicle.

de·scend·ing colon (dĭ-sĕn′dĭng) *n.* The part of the colon extending from the left colic flexure to the pelvic brim.

de·scent (dĭ-sĕnt′) *n.* **1.** The process of descending or falling down from a higher position. **2.** The passage of the presenting part of the fetus into and through the birth canal.

de·sen·si·ti·za·tion (dē-sĕn′sĭ-tĭ-zā′shən) *n.* **1.** The reduction or abolition of allergic sensitivity or reactions to a specific allergen. **2.** The mitigation of one's emotional response to a distressing stimulus, such as a thought, by repeated exposure to or imagination of that stimulus.

de·sen·si·tize (dē-sĕn′sĭ-tīz′) *v.* **-tized, -tiz·ing, -tiz·es. 1.** To render insensitive or less sensitive, as a nerve or tooth. **2.** To make an individual nonreactive or insensitive to an antigen. **3.** To make a person emotionally insensitive or unresponsive, as by long exposure or repeated shocks.

de·sex (dē-sĕks′) *v.* **-sexed, -sex·ing, -sex·es.** To remove part or all of the reproductive organs of; neuter.

des·ic·cant (dĕs′ĭ-kənt) *n.* A substance, such as calcium oxide or silica gel, that has a high affinity for water and is used as a drying agent. — *adj.* Causing or promoting dryness.

des·ic·cate (dĕs′ĭ-kāt′) *v.* **-cat·ed, -cat·ing, -cates.** To dry thoroughly; render free from moisture.

des·ic·ca·tion (dĕs′ĭ-kā′shən) *n.* The process of being desiccated. — **des′ic·ca′tive** (-tĭv) *adj.*

de·sign·er drug (dĭ-zī′nər) *n.* A drug with properties and effects similar to a known hallucinogen or narcotic but having a slightly altered chemical structure, especially such a drug created in order to evade restrictions against illegal substances.

de·sip·ra·mine (dĭ-zĭp'rə-mēn, dĕz'ə-prăm'ĭn) *n.* A tricyclic antidepressant used in the treatment of psychological depression.

des·mi·tis (dĕz-mī'tĭs, dĕs-) *n.* Inflammation of a ligament.

des·mo·cra·ni·um (dĕz'mō-krā'nē-əm, dĕs'-) *n.* The mass of embryonic mesenchymal cells that develop into the cranium.

des·mo·lase (dĕz'mə-lās', -lāz') *n.* Any of various enzymes that break or form carbon-to-carbon bonds in a molecule and play a role in respiration and fermentation.

des·mop·a·thy (dĕz-mŏp'ə-thē, dĕs-) *n.* A disease of the ligaments.

des·mo·pla·si·a (dĕz'mə-plā'zē-ə, -zhə, dĕs'-) *n.* The formation and proliferation of fibroblasts and fibrous connective tissue, especially in tumors.

des·mo·plas·tic (dĕz'mə-plăs'tĭk, dĕs'-) *adj.* **1.** Producing or forming adhesions. **2.** Causing fibrosis in the vascular stroma of a neoplasm.

desmoplastic fibroma *n.* A benign fibrous tumor of bone affecting children and young adults.

de·spe·ci·a·tion (dē-spē'shē-ā'shən, -sē-) *n.* The removal of species-specific antigenic properties from a foreign protein.

des·qua·mate (dĕs'kwə-māt') *v.* **-mat·ed, -mat·ing, -mates.** To shed, peel, or come off in scales. Used of skin.

des·qua·ma·tion (dĕs'kwə-mā'shən) *n.* **1.** The shedding or peeling of the epidermis in scales. **2.** The shedding of the outer layer of a surface. — **des'qua·mate'** (-māt') *v.*

des·quam·a·tive (dĕs-kwăm'ə-tĭv, dĕs'kwə-mā'-tĭ) *adj.* Relating to or marked by desquamation.

det. *abbr. Latin.* detur (let there be given; give)

de·tach (dĭ-tăch') *v.* **-tached, -tach·ing, -tach·es.** **1.** To separate or unfasten; disconnect. **2.** To remove from association or union with something.

detached retina *n.* The separation of the sensory layer of the retina from the pigment layer.

de·tach·ment (dĭ-tăch'mənt) *n.* **1.** The act or process of disconnecting or detaching; separation. **2.** The state of being separate or detached. **3.** Indifference to or remoteness from the concerns of others; aloofness. **4.** Absence of prejudice or bias; disinterest.

de·ter·gent (dĭ-tûr'jənt) *n.* A cleansing substance that acts similarly to soap but is made from chemical compounds rather than fats and lye. — *adj.* Having cleansing power.

de·te·ri·o·rate (dĭ-tēr'ē-ə-rāt') *v.* **-rat·ed, -rat·ing, -rates.** **1.** To grow worse; degenerate. **2.** To weaken or disintegrate; decay.

de·te·ri·o·ra·tion (dĭ-tēr'ē-ə-rā'shən) *n.* The process or condition of becoming worse.

de·ter·mi·na·tion (dĭ-tûr'mə-nā'shən) *n.* **1.** A change for the better or for the worse in the course of a disease. **2.** A fixed movement or ten-

dency toward an object or end. **3.** The ascertaining or fixing of the quantity, quality, position, or character of something.

de·tox (dē-tŏks') *v.* **-toxed, -tox·ing, -tox·es.** To subject to detoxification. — *n.* (dē'tŏks'). A section of a hospital or clinic in which patients are detoxified.

de·tox·i·fy (dē-tŏk'sə-fī') *v.* **-fied, -fy·ing, -fies. 1.** To counteract or destroy the toxic properties of a substance. **2.** To remove the effects of poison from something, such as the blood. **3.** To treat a person for alcohol or drug dependence, usually under a medically supervised program designed to rid the body of intoxicating or addictive substances.

de·tri·tion (dĭ-trĭsh'ən) *n.* The act of wearing away by friction.

de·tri·tus (dĭ-trī'təs) *n., pl.* **detritus.** Loose matter resulting from the wearing away or disintegration of a tissue or substance.

de·tru·sor (dĭ-troō'sər, -zər) *n.* A muscle that pushes down, such as the muscle that expels urine from the bladder.

de·tu·mes·cence (dē'toō-mĕs'əns, -tyoō-) *n.* Reduction or lessening of a swelling, especially the restoration of a swollen organ or part to normal size.

deu·ter·o·plasm (doō'tə-rō-plăz'əm, dyoō'-) *n.* See **deutoplasm.**

deu·to·plasm (doō'tə-plăz'əm, dyoō'-) *n.* The nutritive substances in the cytoplasm, especially the yolk of an ovum.

de·vas·cu·lar·i·za·tion (dē-văs'kyə-lər-ĭ-zā'shən) *n.* The interruption of the blood supply to a part of the body by the blockage or destruction of blood vessels.

de·vel·op (dĭ-vĕl'əp) *v.* **-oped, -op·ing, -ops. 1.** To progress from earlier to later stages of a life cycle. **2.** To aid in the growth of; strengthen. **3.** To grow by degrees into a more advanced or mature state. **4.** To become affected with a disease; contract.

de·vel·op·ment (dĭ-vĕl'əp-mənt) *n.* **1.** The act of developing. **2.** The state of being developed. **3.** A significant event, occurrence, or change. **4.** The natural progression from a previous, simpler, or embryonic stage to a later, more complex, or adult stage. — **de·vel'op·men'tal** (-mĕn'tl) *adj.*

developmental age *n.* **1.** The age of a fetus from conception to any point in time prior to birth. **2.** An index of development stated as the age in years of an individual and determined by specified standardized measurements such as motor and mental tests and body measurements.

developmental anomaly *n.* An anomaly established during intrauterine life.

developmental disability *n.* A cognitive, emotional, or physical impairment, especially one related to abnormal sensory or motor development, that appears in infancy or childhood and involves a failure or delay in progressing through the normal developmental stages of childhood.

de·vi·ant (dē'vē-ənt) *adj.* Differing from a norm or from the accepted standards of a society. — *n.*

One that differs from a norm, especially a person whose behavior and attitudes differ from accepted social standards. — de'vi•ance, de'vi•an•cy n.

de·vi·a·tion (dē'vē-ā'shən) n. **1.** A turning away or aside from a normal course. **2.** An abnormality. **3.** Deviant behavior or attitudes.

de·vice (dĭ-vīs') n. A contrivance or an invention serving a particular purpose, especially a machine used to perform one or more relatively simple tasks.

dex·a·meth·a·sone (děk'sə-měth'ə-sōn', -zōn') n. A synthetic glucocorticoid used primarily in the treatment of inflammatory disorders.

Dex·e·drine (děk'sĭ-drĭn, -drēn') A trademark used for dextroamphetamine.

dex·tral·i·ty (děk-străl'ĭ-tē) n. Preference for the right hand in performing manual tasks; right-handedness.

dex·tran (děk'străn', -strən) n. Any of a group of long-chain polymers of glucose with various molecular weights that are used in isotonic sodium chloride solution for the treatment of shock, in distilled water for the relief of the edema of nephrosis, and as plasma volume expanders.

dex·tri·nu·ri·a (děk'strə-nŏŏr'ē-ə) n. The presence of dextrin in the urine.

dex·tro·am·phet·a·mine (děk'strō-ăm-fět'əmēn', -mĭn) n. A white crystalline compound that is an isomer of amphetamine and is used in the form of its phosphate or sulfate salt as a central nervous system stimulant.

dex·tro·car·di·a (děk'strō-kär'dē-ə) n. The displacement of the heart to the right, either as dextroposition, in which the heart is structurally normal, or as cardiac heterotaxia, in which the left and right chambers are transposed.

dex·tro·gas·tri·a (děk'strō-găs'trē-ə) n. The displacement of the stomach to the right.

dex·trose (děk'strōs') n. A form of glucose found naturally in animal and plant tissue and derived synthetically from starch.

dex·tro·ver·sion (děk'strə-vûr'zhən) n. **1.** A turning to the right, as of the eyes. **2.** Rotation of both eyes to the right.

di·a·be·tes (dī'ə-bē'tĭs, -tēz) n. Any of several metabolic disorders marked by excessive discharge of urine and persistent thirst, especially one of the two types of diabetes mellitus.

diabetes in·sip·i·dus (ĭn-sĭp'ĭ-dəs) n. A chronic metabolic disorder characterized by intense thirst and excessive urination, caused by a deficiency of the pituitary hormone vasopressin.

diabetes in·ter·mit·tens (ĭn'tər-mĭt'ənz) n. Diabetes mellitus in which there are periods of relatively normal carbohydrate metabolism followed by relapses to a diabetic state.

diabetes mel·li·tus (mə-lī'təs, měl'ĭ-) n. **1.** A severe, chronic form of diabetes caused by insufficient production of insulin and resulting in abnormal metabolism of carbohydrates, fats, and proteins. The disease, which typically appears in childhood or adolescence, is characterized by increased sugar levels in the blood and urine, exces-

sive thirst, frequent urination, acidosis, and wasting. **2.** A mild form of diabetes that typically appears first in adulthood and is exacerbated by obesity and an inactive lifestyle. This disease often has no symptoms, is usually diagnosed by tests that indicate glucose intolerance, and is treated with changes in diet and exercise.

di·a·bet·ic (dī'ə-bět'ĭk) adj. **1.** Of, relating to, having, or resulting from diabetes. **2.** Intended for use by a person with diabetes. — n. A person who has diabetes.

diabetic acidosis n. Decreased pH and bicarbonate concentration in the body fluids caused by accumulation of ketone bodies in uncontrolled diabetes mellitus.

diabetic coma n. A coma that develops in severe and inadequately treated cases of diabetes mellitus.

diabetic dermopathy n. A skin disorder most commonly occurring on the shins of people with diabetes mellitus, characterized by discolored patches and small papules that often become pigmented and ulcerated and result in scars.

diabetic diet n. A diet suitable for a diabetic person, with the aim of maintaining normal blood sugar levels.

diabetic neuropathy n. A combined sensory and motor neuropathy, usual symmetric and segmental and involving autonomic neurons, seen frequently in older diabetic patients.

diabetic retinopathy n. Retinal changes occurring in long-term diabetes and characterized by punctate hemorrhages, microaneurysms, and sharply defined waxy exudates.

di·a·be·tog·en·ous (dī'ə-bĭ-tŏj'ə-nəs) adj. Caused by diabetes.

di·a·ce·tyl·mor·phine (dī'ə-sēt'l-môr'fēn', dī-ăs'-ĭ-tl-) n. See **heroin**.

di·ac·la·sis (dī-ăk'lə-sĭs, dī'ə-klā'sĭs) n. See **osteoclasis**.

di·ad·o·cho·ki·ne·sia (dī-ăd'ə-kō-kĭ-nē'zhə, -kī-) or **di·ad·o·cho·ki·ne·sis** (-sĭs) n. The normal power of alternately bringing a limb into opposite positions, as flexion and extension. — **di·ad·o·cho·ki·net·ic** (-nět'ĭk) adj.

di·ag·nose (dī'əg-nōs', -nōz') v. **-nosed, -nosing, -nos·es.** To make a diagnosis.

di·ag·no·sis (dī'əg-nō'sĭs) n., pl. **-ses** (-sēz). **1.** The act or process of identifying or determining the nature and cause of a disease or injury through evaluation of patient history, examination, and review of laboratory data. **2.** The opinion derived from such an evaluation.

diagnosis by exclusion n. Diagnosis made by excluding all other known diseases.

di·ag·nos·tic (dī'əg-nōs'tĭk) adj. **1.** Of, relating to, or used in a diagnosis; **2.** Serving to identify a particular disease; characteristic. — n. **1.** Often **diagnostics.** The art or practice of medical diagnosis. **2.** A symptom or a distinguishing feature serving as supporting evidence in a diagnosis. **3.** An instrument or a technique used in medical diagnosis.

diagnostic diphtheria toxin *n.* See **Schick test toxin.**

di·ag·nos·ti·cian (dī′əg-nŏ-stĭsh′ən) *n.* A person who diagnoses, especially a physician specializing in medical diagnostics.

diagnostic specificity *n.* The probability that, given the absence of disease, a normal test result will exclude the disease.

diagnostic ultrasound *n.* Use of ultrasound to obtain images for medical diagnostic purposes.

di·a·ki·ne·sis (dī′ə-kə-nē′sĭs, -kī-) *n.* The final stage of the prophase in meiosis, characterized by shortening and thickening of the paired chromosomes, formation of the spindle fibers, disappearance of the nucleolus, and degeneration of the nuclear membrane.

di·al·y·sis (dī-ăl′ĭ-sĭs) *n., pl.* **-ses** (-sēz′). **1.** The separation of smaller molecules from larger molecules or of dissolved substances from colloidal particles in a solution by selective diffusion through a semipermeable membrane. **2.** Hemodialysis. — **di′a·lyt′ic** (-ə-lĭt′ĭk) *adj.* — **di′a·lyt′i·cal·ly** *adv.*

dialysis encephalopathy syndrome *n.* A degenerative disease of the brain occurring in some individuals on chronic hemodialysis and marked by the loss of intellectual abilities, involuntary muscular jerks, and personality changes.

di·a·lyze (dī′ə-līz′) *v.* **-lyzed, -lyz·ing, -lyz·es.** To subject to or undergo dialysis or hemodialysis. — **di′a·lyz′a·bil′i·ty** *n.* — **di′a·lyz′a·ble** *adj.*

di·a·lyz·er (dī′ə-lī′zər) *n.* **1.** A machine equipped with a semipermeable membrane and used for performing dialysis. **2.** A hemodialyzer.

di·am·e·ter (dī-ăm′ĭ-tər) *n.* **1.** A straight line connecting two opposite points on the surface of a spherical or cylindrical body, or at the boundary of an opening or foramen, passing through the center of such body or opening. **2.** The distance measured along such a line.

Di·an·a complex (dī-ăn′ə) *n.* In psychoanalytic theory, the adoption of perceived masculine traits and behavior in a female.

di·a·pe·de·sis (dī′ə-pĭ-dē′sĭs) *n.* The movement or passage of blood cells, especially white blood cells, through intact capillary walls into surrounding body tissue.

di·a·per rash (dī′ə-pər, dī′pər) *n.* A form of dermatitis that occurs where a diaper is in contact with the skin and is caused by exposure to feces and urine and possibly by the ammonia produced by decomposing urine.

di·aph·a·no·scope (dī-ăf′ə-nə-skōp′) *n.* An instrument for illuminating the interior of a body cavity to determine the translucency of its walls.

di·aph·a·nos·co·py (dī-ăf′ə-nŏs′kə-pē) *n.* Examination of a body part with a diaphanoscope.

di·a·pho·re·sis (dī′ə-fə-rē′sĭs, dī-ăf′ə-) *n.* Perspiration, especially when copious and medically induced.

di·a·phragm (dī′ə-frăm′) *n.* **1.** A musculomembranous partition separating the abdominal and thoracic cavities and functioning in respiration. **2.** A

membranous part that divides or separates. **3.** A contraceptive device consisting of a thin flexible disk, usually made of rubber, that is designed to cover the uterine cervix to prevent the entry of sperm during sexual intercourse. **4.** A disk having a fixed or variable opening used to restrict the amount of light traversing a lens or optical system. — **di′a·phrag·mat′ic** (-frăg-măt′ĭk) *adj.*

diaphragmatic ligament of mesonephros *n.* The segment of the embryonic urogenital ridge extending from the mesonephros to the diaphragm.

diaphragm phenomenon *n.* A lowering of the line of retraction on the side of the chest that marks the insertion of the diaphragm during inspiration followed by an elevation during expiration.

di·aph·y·sec·to·my (dī-ăf′ĭ-sĕk′tə-mē, dī′ə-fĭ-) *n.* The partial or complete removal of the shaft of a long bone.

di·aph·y·sis (dī-ăf′ĭ-sĭs) *n., pl.* **-ses** (-sēz′). The shaft of a long bone. — **di′a·phys′i·al** (dī′ə-fĭz′-ē-əl), **di·aph′y·se′al** (dī-ăf′ĭ-sē′əl, dī′ə-fĭz′ē-əl) *adj.*

di·aph·y·si·tis (dī-ăf′ĭ-sī′tĭs) *n.* Inflammation of the shaft of a long bone.

di·ar·rhe·a or **di·ar·rhoe·a** (dī′ə-rē′ə) *n.* Excessive and frequent evacuation of watery feces, usually indicating gastrointestinal disease or disorder. — **di′ar·rhe′al**, **di′ar·rhe′ic** (-ĭk), **di′ar·rhet′ic** (-rĕt′ĭk) *adj.*

di·ar·thro·di·al joint (dī′är-thrō′dē-əl) *n.* See **movable joint** (sense 1).

di·ar·thro·sis (dī′är-thrō′sĭs) *n.* See **movable joint** (sense 1).

di·as·chi·sis (dī-ăs′kĭ-sĭs) *n.* A sudden loss of function in a portion of the brain that is at a distance from the site of injury, but is connected to it by neurons.

di·a·scope (dī′ə-skōp′) *n.* A flat glass plate through which one can examine superficial skin lesions by means of pressure.

di·as·co·py (dī-ăs′kə-pē) *n.* Examination of the skin with a diascope.

di·a·stal·sis (dī′ə-stôl′sĭs, -stăl′-) *n.* Peristalsis in which a region of inhibition precedes the wave of contraction, as in the intestinal tract. — **di′a·stal′tic** (-stôl′tĭk, -stăl′-) *adj.*

di·as·ta·sis (dī-ăs′tə-sĭs) *n.* **1.** Separation of normally joined parts, such as the separation of certain abdominal muscles during pregnancy. **2.** The last stage of diastole in the heart, occurring just before contraction and during which little additional blood enters the ventricle.

di·a·su·ri·a (dī′ə-stā-sōōr′ē-ə, -syōōr′-) *n.* See **amylasuria.**

di·as·ter (dī-ăs′tər) *n.* See **amphiaster.**

di·as·to·le (dī-ăs′tə-lē) *n.* The normal rhythmically occurring relaxation and dilatation of the heart chambers, especially the ventricles, during which they fill with blood. — **di′a·stol′ic** (dī′ə-stŏl′ĭk) *adj.*

diastolic murmur *n.* A murmur heard during diastole.

diastolic pressure *n.* The lowest arterial blood pressure reached during a ventricular cycle.

di·a·ther·my (dī′ə-thûr′mē) *n.* The therapeutic generation of local heat in body tissues by high-frequency electromagnetic radiation, electric currents, or ultrasonic waves.

di·ath·e·sis (dī-ăth′ĭ-sĭs) *n., pl.* **-ses** (-sēz′). A hereditary predisposition of the body to a disease, a group of diseases, an allergy, or another disorder. — **di′a·thet′ic** (dī′ə-thĕt′ĭk) *adj.*

di·az·e·pam (dī-ăz′ə-păm′) *n.* A tranquilizer used in the treatment of anxiety and tension and as a sedative and an anticonvulsant.

di·bu·caine (dī-byōō′kān′) *n.* A local anesthetic used topically on the skin and mucous membranes or administered by injection into the subarachnoid space to produce spinal anesthesia.

di·chro·ma·tism (dī-krō′mə-tĭz′əm) *n.* **1.** The state of being dichromatic. **2.** A form of color-blindness in which only two of the three fundamental colors can be distinguished due to a lack of one of the retinal cone pigments.

di·chro·ma·top·si·a (dī-krō′mə-tŏp′sē-ə) *n.* See **dichromatism** (sense 2).

Dick test (dĭk) *n.* A skin test used to determine immunity or susceptibility to scarlet fever.

Dick test toxin *n.* See **streptococcus erythrogenic toxin.**

dicrotic notch *n.* The notch in a pulse tracing that precedes the dicrotic wave.

dicrotic pulse *n.* A pulse marked by a double beat, with the second beat weaker than the first.

dicrotic wave *n.* The second rise in the tracing of a dicrotic pulse.

di·cro·tism (dī′krə-tĭz′əm) *n.* A condition in which the pulse is felt as two beats per single heartbeat. — **di·crot′ic** (-krŏt′ĭk) *adj.*

dic·ty·o·ma (dĭk′tē-ō′mə) *n.* An epitheliomatous tumor of the nonpigmented layer of the ciliary epithelium.

dic·ty·o·tene (dĭk′tē-ə-tēn′) *n.* The stage of meiosis at which the primary oocyte is arrested in the female fetus during the period from late fetal life through birth and childhood until ovulation.

di·dac·tyl·ism (dī-dăk′tə-lĭz′əm) *n.* A congenital defect in which there are only two digits on a hand or a foot.

did·y·mal·gi·a (dĭd′ə-măl′jē-ə, -jə) *n.* See **orchialgia.**

did·y·mi·tis (dĭd′ə-mī′tĭs) *n.* See **orchitis.**

die (dī) *v.* **died, dy·ing** (dī′ĭng), **dies. 1.** To cease living; become dead; expire. **2.** To cease existing, especially by degrees; fade.

dieb. alt. *abbr. Latin.* diebus alternis (every other day)

di·en·ceph·a·lon (dī′ĕn-sĕf′ə-lŏn′, -lən) *n.* The posterior part of the prosencephalon, composed of the epithalamus, the dorsal thalamus, the subthalamus, and the hypothalamus.

di·es·trus (dī-ĕs′trəs) or **di·es·trum** (-trəm) *n.* The period of sexual quiescence intervening between two periods of estrus. — **di·es′trous** (-trəs) *adj.*

di·et (dī′ĭt) *n.* **1.** Food and drink in general. **2.** A prescribed course of eating and drinking in which the amount and kind of food, as well as the times at which it is to be taken, are regulated for therapeutic purposes. **3.** Reduction of caloric intake so as to lose weight. — *v.* **-et·ed, -et·ing, -ets.** To eat and drink according to a regulated system, especially so as to lose weight or control a medical condition.

di·e·tar·y (dī′ĭ-tĕr′ē) *adj.* Of or relating to diet.

dietary fiber *n.* Coarse, indigestible plant matter, consisting primarily of polysaccharides such as cellulose, that when eaten stimulates intestinal peristalsis.

di·e·tet·ic (dī′ĭ-tĕt′ĭk) *adj.* **1.** Of or relating to diet. **2.** Of or being a food that, naturally or through processing, has a low caloric content.

di·e·tet·ics (dī′ĭ-tĕt′ĭks) *n.* The branch of therapeutics concerned with diet in relation to health and disease.

di·eth·yl ether (dī-ĕth′əl) *n.* A pungent, volatile, highly flammable liquid derived from the distillation of ethyl alcohol with sulfuric acid and widely used as an inhalation anesthetic.

di·eth·yl·stil·bes·trol (dī-ĕth′əl-stĭl-bĕs′trôl, -trōl′) *n.* DES.

di·e·ti·tian or **di·e·ti·cian** (dī′ĭ-tĭsh′ən) *n.* A person specializing in dietetics.

dif·fer·ence (dĭf′ər-əns, dĭf′rəns) *n.* The magnitude or degree by which one quantity differs from another of the same kind.

dif·fer·en·tial blood count (dĭf′ə-rĕn′shəl) *n.* An estimate, based on cell counts in a representative sample, of the percentage of white blood cell types that make up the total white blood cell count.

differential diagnosis *n.* Determination of which one of two or more diseases with similar symptoms is the one from which the patient is suffering.

differential u·re·ter·al cath·e·ter·i·za·tion test (yōō-rē′tər-əl-kăth′ĭ-tər-ĭ-zā′shən) *n.* A test to determine various functional parameters of one kindney compared with the other kidney.

dif·fer·en·ti·a·tion (dĭf′ə-rĕn′shē-ā′shən) *n.* **1.** The acquisition or possession of a character or function different from that of the original type. **2.** See **differential diagnosis.**

dif·frac·tion halo (dĭ-frăk′shən) *n.* The hazy colorless region that surrounds red blood cells viewed under a microscope.

dif·fuse (dĭ-fyōōs′) *adj.* Not limited to one tissue or location; widespread. — *v.* **-fused, -fus·ing, -fus·es.** (dĭ-fyōōz′). To spread or be spread widely, as through a tissue or system. — **dif·fus′i·ble** (-fyōō′zə-bəl) *adj.*

diffuse cutaneous leishmaniasis *n.* A chronic form of leishmaniasis caused by *Leishmania aethiopia* in Ethiopia and Kenya and by various subspecies of *L. mexicana* in Central and South America, and characterized by non-ulcerating, non-necrotizing skin lesions that spread widely over the body.

diffusible stimulant *n.* A stimulant that produces a rapid but temporary effect.

dif·fu·sion (dĭ-fyōō′zhən) *n.* **1.** The process of diffusing or the condition of being diffused. **2.** See **dialysis** (sense 1).

diffusion anoxia *n.* See **diffusion hypoxia**.

diffusion hypoxia *n.* An abrupt transient decrease in alveolar oxygen tension when ambient air is inhaled at the conclusion of a nitrous oxide anesthesia.

diffusion respiration *n.* A procedure for maintaining oxygenation of the blood during apnea through the intratracheal insufflation of oxygen at high flow rates.

di·flo·ra·sone di·ac·e·tate (dī-flôr′ə-sōn′ dī-ăs′ĭ-tāt′) *n.* An anti-inflammatory corticosteroid used in topical preparations.

di·gen·e·sis (dī-jĕn′ĭ-sĭs) *n.* Reproduction in distinctive patterns in alternate generations, typically involving alternating sexual and asexual cycles in succeeding host organisms, as seen in malarial parasites and certain trematode flatworms. — **di′ge·net′ic** (-jə-nĕt′ĭk) *adj.*

di·gest (dī-jĕst′, dĭ-) *v.* **-gest·ed, -gest·ing, -gests. 1.** To convert food into simpler chemical compounds that can be absorbed and assimilated by the body, as by chemical and muscular action in the alimentary canal. **2.** To soften or disintegrate by means of chemical action, heat, or moisture. — **di·gest′i·bil′i·ty** *n.* — **di·gest′i·ble** *adj.*

di·ges·tion (dī-jĕs′chən, dĭ-) *n.* The process by which food is converted into substances that can be absorbed and assimilated by the body, especially that accomplished in the alimentary canal by the mechanical and enzymatic breakdown of foods into simpler chemical compounds.

di·ges·tive (dī-jĕs′tĭv, dĭ-) *adj.* Of or relating to digestion. — *n.* A digestant.

digestive gland *n.* A gland, such as the liver or pancreas, that secretes into the alimentary canal substances necessary for digestion.

digestive system *n.* The alimentary canal and digestive glands regarded as an integrated system responsible for the ingestion, digestion, and absorption of foodstuffs and the elimination of associated wastes.

digestive tract *n.* See **alimentary canal**.

dig·it (dĭj′ĭt) *n.* A finger or toe; dactyl.

dig·i·tal (dĭj′ĭ-tl) *adj.* **1.** Of or resembling a finger or toe or an impression made by them. **2.** Done or performed with a finger. — **dig′i·tal·ly** *adv.*

dig·i·tal·in (dĭj′ĭ-tăl′ĭn, -tā′lĭn) *n.* A standardized mixture of glycosides obtained from the leaves and seeds of the common foxglove and used as a cardiotonic.

dig·i·tal·is (dĭj′ĭ-tăl′ĭs) *n.* **1.** A plant of the genus *Digitalis,* which includes the foxgloves, several species of which are a source of cardioactive steroid glycosides used in the treatment of certain heart diseases. **2.** A drug prepared from the seeds and dried leaves of the purple foxglove, *Digitalis purpurea,* prescribed as a cardiac stimulant in the treatment of congestive heart failure and other cardiac disorders.

dig·i·tal·i·za·tion (dĭj′ĭ-tl-ĭ-zā′shən) *n.* The administration of digitalis by a dosage schedule until sufficient amounts are present in the body to produce the desired therapeutic effects.

digital joint *n.* Any of the hinge joints between the phalanges of the fingers or toes.

digital reflex *n.* See **Hoffmann's sign**.

digital sub·trac·tion angiography (səb-trăk′shən) *n.* A computer-assisted x-ray technique that subtracts images of bone and soft tissue to permit viewing of the cardiovascular system.

dig·i·tox·in (dĭj′ĭ-tŏk′sĭn) *n.* A secondary cardioactive glycoside that is derived from and similar in effect to digitalis but that is more completely absorbed from the gastrointestinal tract.

dig·ox·in (dĭj-ŏk′sĭn) *n.* A cardioactive steroid glycoside obtained from the leaves of a foxglove, *Digitalis lanata,* with pharmacological effects similar to digitalis.

di·hy·dro·pte·ro·ic acid (dī-hī′drō-tə-rō′ĭk) *n.* An intermediate formed during the biosynthesis of folic acid.

di·hy·dro·tes·tos·ter·one (dī-hī′drō-tĕs-tŏs′tə-rōn′) *n.* A derivative of testosterone having androgenic activity and anabolic and tumor-suppressing capabilities useful in the treatment of certain breast cancers.

di·hy·drox·y·ac·e·tone (dī′hī-drŏk′sē-ăs′ĭ-tōn′) *n.* An isomer of glyceraldehyde important in the metabolism of carbohydrates and used to darken the skin to simulate a tan.

dil. *abbr. Latin.* dilue (dilute)

di·lac·er·a·tion (dī-lăs′ə-rā′shən) *n.* Discission of a cataractous lens.

dil·a·ta·tion (dĭl′ə-tā′shən, dī′lə-) *n.* Physiological, pathological, or artificial enlargement of a cavity, canal, blood vessel, or opening.

dilatation and curettage *n.* See **dilation and curettage**.

dil·a·ta·tor (dĭl′ə-tā′tər, dī′lə-) *n.* See **dilator** (sense 2).

di·late (dī-lāt′, dī′lāt′) *v.* **-lat·ed, -lat·ing, -lates. 1.** To make or become wider or larger. **2.** To perform or undergo dilation or dilatation.

di·la·tion (dī-lā′shən, dĭ-) *n.* **1.** The act of dilating or the condition of being dilated. **2.** Dilatation.

dilation and curettage *n.* A surgical procedure in which the cervix is expanded using a dilator and the uterine lining scraped with a curette, performed for the diagnosis and treatment of various uterine conditions.

dilation and evacuation *n.* A surgical procedure in which the cervix is dilated and the early products of conception are removed from the uterus.

di·la·tor (dī-lā′tər, dī′lā′-, -dī-lā′-) *n.* **1.** An instrument or a substance for enlarging a cavity, canal, blood vessel, or opening. **2.** A muscle that dilates an orifice or a body part, such as a blood vessel or the pupil of the eye.

dil·do or **dil·doe** (dĭl′dō) *n.* or **-dos** or **-does** An object shaped like and used as a substitute for an erect penis.

dil·ti·a·zem hydrochloride (dĭl-tī′ə-zĕm′) *n.* A calcium channel blocking agent used as a coronary vasodilator.

di·lute (dī-lo͞ot′, dĭ-) *v.* **-lut·ed, -lut·ing, -lutes.** To reduce a solution or mixture in concentration, strength, quality, or purity, as by adding water. — *adj.* Thinned or weakened by diluting. — **di·lu′tive** *adj.*

di·lu·tion (dī-lo͞o′shən, dĭ-) *n.* **1.** The act of reducing the concentration of a mixture or solution. **2.** A diluted solution.

dim. *abbr. Latin.* dimidius (half)

di·mel·i·a (dī-mĕl′ē-ə, -mē′lē-ə) *n.* Congenital duplication of all or part of a limb.

di·men·hy·dri·nate (dī′mĕn-hī′drə-nāt′) *n.* An antihistamine used to treat motion sickness and allergic disorders.

di·men·sion (dĭ-mĕn′shən, dī-) *n.* **1.** A measure of spatial extent, especially width, height, or length. **2.** Scope or magnitude.

di·mer·cap·rol (dī′mər-kăp′rôl, -rōl) *n.* A chelating agent developed as an antidote for lewisite and other arsenical poisons, also used as an antidote for antimony, bismuth, chromium, mercury, gold, and nickel poisoning.

di·meth·yl·sulf·ox·ide (dī-mĕth′əl-sŭl-fŏk′sīd′) *n.* DMSO.

di·meth·yl·tryp·ta·mine (dī-mĕth′əl-trĭp′tə-mēn′) *n.* DMT.

dim·ple (dĭm′pəl) *n.* **1.** A small natural indentation in the chin, cheek, or sacral region, probably due to some developmental fault in subcutaneous connective tissue or in underlying bone. **2.** A similar depression resulting from trauma or the contraction of scar tissue. — **dim′ple** *v.*

dim·pling (dĭm′plĭng) *n.* A condition marked by the formation of natural or artificial dimples.

din·ner pad (dĭn′ər) *n.* A pad placed over the pit of the stomach before the application of a plaster jacket, and removed after the plaster has hardened, in order to leave space for varying conditions of abdominal distention.

di·nu·cle·o·tide (dī-no͞o′klē-ə-tīd′, -nyo͞o′-) *n.* A nucleotide molecule that consists of a combination of two nucleotide units.

di·ox·in (dī-ŏk′sĭn) *n.* Any of several carcinogenic or teratogenic heterocyclic hydrocarbons that occur as impurities in petroleum-derived herbicides.

di·pep·tide (dī-pĕp′tīd′) *n.* A peptide that, on hydrolysis, yields two amino acid molecules.

di·pha·sic (dī-fā′zĭk) *adj.* **1.** Having two phases or stages. **2.** Of or being a disorder, such as manic-depressive psychosis, characterized by two distinct phases.

di·phen·yl (dī-fĕn′əl, -fē′nəl) *n.* See biphenyl.

diph·the·ri·a (dĭf-thěr′ē-ə, dĭp-) *n.* An acute infectious disease caused by the bacillus *Corynebacterium diphtheriae,* characterized by the production of a systemic toxin and the formation of a false membrane on the lining of the mucous membrane of the throat and other respiratory passages, causing difficulty in breathing, high fever, and weakness. The toxin is particularly harmful to the tissues of the heart and central nervous system. — **diph′the·rit′ic** (-thə-rĭt′ĭk), **diph·ther·′ic** (-thěr′ĭk), **diph·the′ri·al** *adj.*

diphtheria, tetanus toxoids, and pertussis vaccine *n.* A vaccine available in three forms: diphtheria and tetanus toxoids plus pertussis vaccine (DTP); tetanus-diphtheria toxoids, adult type (Td); and tetanus toxoids (T); used for active immunization against diphtheria, tetanus, and whooping cough.

diphtheritic membrane *n.* A false membrane formed on mucous surfaces in diphtheria.

diph·the·roid (dĭf′thə-roid′) *n.* A local infection that resembles diphtheria, especially in the formation of a false membrane, but that is caused by a microorganism other than *Corynebacterium diphtheriae.* — **diph′the·roid′** *adj.*

di·phyl·lo·both·ri·a·sis (dī-fĭl′ō-bŏth-rī′ə-sĭs) *n.* Infection with the cestode tapeworm *Diphyllobothrium latum* following ingestion of raw or inadequately cooked fish infected with the larva.

Di·phyl·lo·both·ri·um (dī-fĭl′ō-bŏth′rē-əm) *n.* A large genus of tapeworms of which one species causes diphyllobothriasis in humans.

di·piv·e·frin hydrochloride (dī-pĭv′ə-frĭn) *n.* An ophthalmic adrenergic used in drop form in the initial therapy for controlling intraocular pressure in chronic open-angle glaucoma.

dip·la·cu·sis (dĭp′lə-ko͞o′sĭs) *n.* A difference in the perception of sound by the ears, either in time or in pitch, so that one sound is heard as two.

di·ple·gia (dī-plē′jə, -jē-ə) *n.* Paralysis of corresponding parts on both sides of the body. — **di·ple′gic** *adj. & n.*

dip·lo·co·ri·a (dĭp′lō-kôr′ē-ə) *n.* Presence of a double pupil in the eye.

dip·loi·dy (dĭp′loi′dē) *n.* The state or condition of being diploid.

dip·lo·ne·ma (dĭp′lə-nē′mə) *n., pl.* **-mas** or **-ma·ta** (-mə-tə). The doubled form of the chromosome strand visible at the diplotene stage of meiosis.

di·plo·pi·a (dĭ-plō′pē-ə) *n.* See double vision. — **di·plo′pic** (-plō′pĭk, -plŏp′ĭk) *adj.*

dip·lo·sis (dĭ-plō′sĭs) *n.* The formation of the diploid number of chromosomes during fertilization by the fusion of the nuclei of two haploid gametes.

dip·lo·some (dĭp′lə-sōm′) *n.* The pair of centrioles of mammalian cells.

dip·lo·tene (dĭp′lə-tēn′) *n.* A stage of meiotic prophase in which the paired homologous chromosomes begin to separate and chiasmata become visible.

di·pro·pyl·tryp·ta·mine (dī-prō′pĭl-trĭp′tə-mēn′) *n.* A hallucinogenic drug similar to DMT; DPT.

dip·se·sis (dĭp-sē′sĭs) *n.* Abnormal or excessive thirst.

dip·so·gen (dĭp′sə-jən, -jĕn′) *n.* A thirst-provoking agent. — **dip′so·gen′ic** (-jĕn′ĭk) *adj.*

dip·so·ma·ni·a (dĭp′sə-mā′nē-ə, -mān′yə) *n.* An insatiable craving for alcoholic beverages.

— dip·so·ma·ni·ac (-ăk′) *adj. & n.* — dip′so·ma·ni′a·cal (-mə-nī′ə-kəl) *adj.*

dip·so·sis (dĭp-sō′sĭs) *n.* See dipsesis.

dip·so·ther·a·py (dĭp′sə-thĕr′ə-pē) *n.* The treatment of certain diseases by controlled abstention from liquids.

di·pyr·id·a·mole (dī-pĭr′ĭ-də-mōl′, -pə-rĭd′ə-) *n.* A drug that acts as a coronary vasodilator and is used in the treatment of angina pectoris.

di·rect flap (dĭ-rĕkt′, dī) *n.* A surgical flap that is raised completely and transferred to its recipient site during the same procedure.

direct fracture *n.* A bone fracture, especially of the skull, occurring at the point of injury.

direct ophthalmoscope *n.* An instrument designed to visualize the interior of the eye, with the instrument relatively close to the subject's eye and the observer viewing an upright magnified image.

di·rec·tor (dĭ-rĕk′tər, dī-) *n.* A smoothly grooved instrument used with a knife to limit the incision of tissues.

direct percussion *n.* See immediate percussion.

direct transfusion *n.* Transfusion of blood from the donor directly to the recipient.

direct vision *n.* See central vision.

dirt-eating *n.* See geophagy.

dis·a·bil·i·ty (dĭs′ə-bĭl′ĭ-tē) *n.* A disadvantage or deficiency, especially a physical or mental impairment that prevents or restricts normal achievement.

dis·a·bled (dĭs-ā′bəld) *adj.* Impaired, as in physical functioning. — *n.* Physically impaired people considered as a group. Often used with *the.*

di·sac·cha·ride (dī-săk′ə-rīd′) *n.* Any of a class of carbohydrates, including lactose and sucrose, that yield two monosaccharides upon hydrolysis.

dis·ag·gre·ga·tion (dĭs-ăg′rĭ-gā′shən) *n.* **1.** A breaking up into component parts. **2.** An inability to coordinate various sensations and a failure to observe their mutual relations. — dis·ag′gre·gate′ *v.*

dis·as·so·ci·a·tion (dĭs′ə-sō′shē-ā′shən, -sē-) *n.* Dissociation.

disc·ec·to·my (dĭs-kĕk′tə-mē) *n.* The partial or complete excision of an intervertebral disk.

dis·charge (dĭs-chärj′) *v.* -charged, -charg·ing, -charg·es. **1.** To emit a substance, as by excretion or secretion. **2.** To release a patient from custody or care. **3.** To generate an electrical impulse. Used of a neuron. — *n.* (dĭs′chärj′, dĭs-chärj′). **1.** The act of releasing, emitting, or secreting. **2.** A substance that is excreted or secreted. **3.** The generation of an electrical impulse in a neuron.

dis·chro·na·tion (dĭs′krə-nā′shən) *n.* A disturbance in the consciousness of time.

dis·cis·sion (dĭ-sĭzh′ən) *n.* **1.** The incision of or cutting through a part. **2.** An operation for soft cataracts in which the crystalline capsule is opened and the substance of the crystalline lens is broken up to allow it to be absorbed.

dis·cli·na·tion (dĭs′klə-nā′shən) *n.* See extorsion (sense 2).

dis·clos·ing solution (dĭ-sklō′zĭng) *n.* A solution that selectively stains all soft debris, pellicle, and bacterial plaque on teeth.

dis·co·gram or dis·ko·gram (dĭs′kə-grăm′) *n.* An x-ray image produced by discography.

dis·cog·ra·phy (dĭs-skŏg′rə-fē) *n.* Examination of the intervertebral disk space using x-rays after injection of contrast media into the disk.

dis·coid lupus er·y·the·ma·to·sus (dĭs′koid′ ĕr′-ə-thē′mə-tō′səs, -thĕm′ə-) *n.* Lupus erythematosus in which only cutaneous lesions are present, commonly on the face, occurring as atrophic plaques with erythema, hyperkeratosis, follicular plugging, and telangiectasia.

dis·con·tin·u·a·tion test (dĭs′kən-tĭn′yōō-ā′shən) *n.* A test to determine whether a certain drug is responsible for a reaction; a positive result is obtained if symptoms stop after use of the drug is discontinued.

dis·cop·a·thy (dĭ-skŏp′ə-thē) *n.* Disease of a disk, especially of an intervertebral disk.

dis·co·pla·cen·ta (dĭs′kō-plə-sĕn′tə) *n.* A placenta having discoid shape.

dis·cor·dance (dĭ-skôr′dns) *n.* The presence of a given genetic trait in only one member of a pair of identical twins. — dis·cor′dant *adj.*

discordant alternation *n.* An alternation in heart activities that involve either the systemic or pulmonary circuit, but not both.

dis·cot·o·my (dĭ-skŏt′ə-mē) *n.* See discectomy.

dis·ease (dĭ-zēz′) *n.* A pathological condition of a body part, an organ, or a system resulting from various causes, such as infection, genetic defect, or environmental stress, and characterized by an identifiable group of signs or symptoms.

dis·eased (dĭ-zēzd′) *adj.* **1.** Affected with disease. **2.** Unsound or disordered.

disease determinant *n.* Any of a group of variables, such as specific disease agents and environmental factors, that directly or indirectly influence the frequency or distribution of a disease.

dis·en·gage·ment (dĭs′ĕn-gāj′mənt) *n.* The emergence of the presenting part of the fetus from the vaginal canal during childbirth. — dis′en·gage′ *v.*

dis·e·qui·lib·ri·um (dĭs-ē′kwə-lĭb′rē-əm, -ĕk′wə-) *n.* Loss or lack of stability or equilibrium.

dish·pan hands (dĭsh′păn′) *pl.n.* A rough, dry, scaly condition of the hands typically caused by sensitivity to or excessive use of household detergents or cleaning agents.

dis·in·fect (dĭs′ĭn-fĕkt′) *v.* -fect·ed, -fect·ing, -fects. To cleanse something so as to destroy or prevent the growth of disease-carrying microorganisms. — dis′in·fec′tion *n.*

dis·in·fec·tant (dĭs′ĭn-fĕk′tənt) *n.* An agent, such as heat, radiation, or a chemical, that disinfects by destroying, neutralizing, or inhibiting the growth of disease-carrying microorganisms. — *adj.* Serving to disinfect.

dis·in·fes·tant (dĭs′ĭn-fĕs′tənt) *n.* An agent that eradicates an infestation, as of vermin.

dis·in·hi·bi·tion (dĭs′ĭn-hə-bĭsh′ən, -ĭn-ə-, dĭs-ĭn′-)

n. **1.** A loss of inhibition, as through the influence of drugs or alcohol. **2.** A temporary loss of an inhibition caused by an unrelated stimulus, such as a loud noise.

dis·in·te·gra·tion (dĭs-ĭn'tĭ-grā'shən) *n.* **1.** The breaking up of the component parts of a substance, as in decay. **2.** The disorganization or disruption of mental processes in mental illness. **3.** The natural or induced transformation of an atomic nucleus from a more massive to a less massive configuration by the emission of particles or radiation. — **dis·in'te·grate'** *v.*

dis·joint (dĭs-joint') *v.* **-joint·ed, -joint·ing, -joints.** To put out of joint; dislocate.

dis·junc·tion (dĭs-jŭngk'shən) *n.* The separation of homologous chromosomes during meiosis.

disk or **disc** (dĭsk) *n.* **1.** A thin, flat, circular object or plate. **2.** See **lamella** (sense 2).

dis·ki·tis or **dis·ci·tis** (dĭs-kī'tĭs) *n.* A nonbacterial inflammation of an intervertebral disk or disk space.

disk syndrome *n.* A syndrome that is caused by a compressive radiculopathy from intervertebral disk pressure and combines symptoms of lower back pain, pain in the thigh, and sciatica with wasting and loss of Achilles and patellar reflexes.

dis·lo·cate (dĭs'lō-kāt', dĭs-lō'kāt) *v.* **-cat·ed, -cat·ing, -cates.** To displace a body part, especially to displace a bone from its normal position.

dis·lo·ca·tion (dĭs'lō-kā'shən) *n.* Displacement of a body part, especially the temporary displacement of a bone from its normal position; luxation.

dislocation fracture *n.* A bone fracture occurring near a joint and causing the bone to dislocate from the joint.

dis·mem·ber (dĭs-mĕm'bər) *v.* **-bered, -ber·ing, -bers.** To amputate a limb or a part of a limb. — **dis·mem'ber·ment** *n.*

dis·or·der (dĭs-ôr'dər) *n.* A disturbance or derangement that affects the function of mind or body, such as an eating disorder or the abuse of a drug. — *v.* **-dered, -der·ing, -ders.** To disturb the normal physical or mental health of; derange.

dis·or·gan·i·za·tion (dĭs-ôr'gə-nĭ-zā'shən) *n.* The destruction of an organ or tissue causing loss of function.

dis·o·ri·en·ta·tion (dĭs-ôr'ē-ĕn-tā'shən) *n.* **1.** Loss of one's sense of direction, position, or relationship with one's surroundings. **2.** A temporary or permanent state of confusion regarding place, time, or personal identity.

dis·pen·sa·ry (dĭ-spĕn'sə-rē) *n.* **1.** An office in a hospital, school, or other institution from which medical supplies, preparations, and treatments are dispensed. **2.** A public institution that dispenses medicines or medical aid.

dis·pense (dĭ-spĕns') *v.* **-pensed, -pens·ing, -pens·es.** To prepare and give out medicines.

dis·place·ment (dĭs-plās'mənt) *n.* **1.** Removal from the normal location or position. **2.** A defense mechanism in which there is an unconscious shift of emotions, affect, or desires from the original object to a more acceptable or immediate substitute.

dis·sect (dĭ-sĕkt', dī-, dī'sĕkt') *v.* **-sect·ed, -sect·ing, -sects.** **1.** To cut apart or separate tissue, especially for anatomical study. **2.** In surgery, to separate different anatomical structures along natural lines by dividing the connective tissue framework.

dissecting aneurysm *n.* The splitting or dissection of an arterial wall by blood entering through a tear of the inner lining or by interstitial hemorrhage.

dis·sec·tion (dĭ-sĕk'shən, dī-) *n.* **1.** The act or an instance of dissecting. **2.** Something that has been dissected, such as a tissue specimen under study.

dis·sem·i·nat·ed (dĭ-sĕm'ə-nā'tĭd) *adj.* Spread over a large area of a body, a tissue, or an organ.

disseminated intravascular coagulation *n.* A hemorrhagic disorder that occurs following the uncontrolled activation of clotting factors and fibrinolytic enzymes throughout small blood vessels, resulting in tissue necrosis and bleeding.

dis·sim·u·la·tion (dĭ-sĭm'yə-lā'shən) *n.* Concealment of the truth about a situation, especially about a state of health. — **dis·sim'u·late'** *v.*

dis·so·ci·at·ed anesthesia (dĭ-sō'shē-ā'tĭd, -sē-) *n.* Loss of sensation for pain and temperature without the loss of tactile sense.

dis·so·ci·a·tion (dĭ-sō'sē-ā'shən, -shē-) *n.* Separation of a group of related psychological activities into autonomously functioning units, as in the generation of multiple personalities. — **dis·so'ci·ate'** *v.* — **dis·so'ci·a'tive** *adj.*

dissociation sensibility *n.* Loss of the sensibility to pain and temperature with the preservation of the sense of touch.

dissociative anesthesia *n.* A form of general anesthesia characterized by catalepsy, catatonia, and amnesia, but not necessarily involving complete unconsciousness.

dissociative reaction *n.* A psychological reaction characterized by such dissociative behavior as amnesia, fugues, sleepwalking, and dream states.

dis·solve (dĭ-zŏlv') *v.* **-solved, -solv·ing, -solves.** **1.** To pass or cause to pass into a solution, as salt in water. **2.** To become or cause to become liquid; melt. **3.** To cause to disintegrate or become disintegrated.

dis·tance (dĭs'təns) *n.* The extent of space between two objects or places; an intervening space.

dis·tant flap (dĭs'tənt) *n.* A surgical flap in which the recipient area is distant from, and must be brought close to, the donor site.

dis·tem·per (dĭs-tĕm'pər) *n.* **1.** An infectious viral disease occurring in dogs, characterized by loss of appetite, a catarrhal discharge from the eyes and nose, vomiting, fever, lethargy, partial paralysis, and sometimes death. **2.** A similar viral disease of cats characterized by fever, vomiting, diarrhea, and sometimes death. **3.** Any of various similar mammalian diseases.

distend *v.* **-tend·ed, -tend·ing, -tends.** To swell out or expand or cause to swell out or expand from or as if from internal pressure.

dis·ten·tion or **dis·ten·sion** (dĭ-stĕn′shən) *n*. The act of distending or the state of being distended.

dis·to·mi·a·sis (dĭs′tō-mī′ə-sĭs) or **dis·to·ma·to·sis** (-mə-tō′sĭs) *n*. Infection by a trematode or fluke.

dis·tor·tion (dĭ-stôr′shən) *n*. **1.** A twisting out of normal shape or form. **2.** A psychological defense mechanism that helps to repress or disguise unacceptable thoughts. **3.** Parataxic distortion. — **dis·tor′tion·al, dis·tor′tion·ar′y** *adj*.

distortion aberration *n*. The faulty formation of an image arising because the magnification of the peripheral part of an object is different from that of the central part when viewed through a lens.

dis·trac·tion (dĭ-străk′shən) *n*. **1.** A condition or state of mind in which the attention is diverted from an original focus or interest. **2.** Separation of bony fragments or joint surfaces of a limb by extension.

dis·tress (dĭ-strĕs′) *n*. **1.** Mental or physical suffering or anguish. **2.** Severe strain resulting from exhaustion or trauma. — **dis·tress′** *adj*.

dis·tri·bu·tion (dĭs′trə-byōō′shən) *n*. **1.** The extension of the branches of arteries or nerves to the tissues and organs. **2.** The area in which the branches of an artery or a nerve terminate, or the area supplied by such an artery or nerve. — **dis′-tri·bu′tion·al** *adj*.

di·sul·fi·ram (dī-sŭl′fə-răm′) *n*. An antioxidant used in the treatment of chronic alcoholism that interferes with the normal metabolic degradation of alcohol in the body, producing an unpleasant reaction when a small quantity of alcohol is consumed.

Ditt·rich's plug (dĭt′rĭks) *n*. Any of the minute, grayish, ill-smelling masses of bacteria and fatty acid crystals in the sputum in pulmonary gangrene and fetid bronchitis.

di·u·re·sis (dī′ə-rē′sĭs) *n*. Discharge of urine, especially in unusually large amounts.

di·u·ret·ic (dī′ə-rĕt′ĭk) *adj*. Tending to increase the discharge of urine. — *n*. A substance or drug that tends to increase the discharge of urine.

di·ur·nal (dī-ûr′nəl) *adj*. **1.** Having a 24-hour period or cycle. **2.** Occurring or active during the daytime rather than at night. — **di·ur′nal·ly** *adv*.

di·val·pro·ex sodium (dī-văl′prō-ĕks′) *n*. An anticonvulsant used in petit mal and related seizure disorders.

di·ver·gence (dĭ-vûr′jəns, dī-) *n*. **1.** A moving or spreading apart in different directions from a common point. **2.** The degree by which things deviate or spread apart. **3.** A turning of both eyes outward from a common point or of one eye when the other is fixed. **4.** The spreading of branches of the neuron to form synapses with several other neurons. — **di·ver′gent** *adj*.

divergent strabismus *n*. See exotropia.

di·ver·tic·u·lec·to·my (dī′vûr-tĭk′yə-lĕk′tə-mē) *n*. Surgical excision of a diverticulum.

di·ver·tic·u·li·tis (dī′vûr-tĭk′yə-lī′tĭs) *n*. Inflam-

mation of a diverticulum, especially of the small pockets in the wall of the colon that fill with stagnant fecal material and become inflamed.

di·ver·tic·u·lo·ma (dī′vûr-tĭk′yə-lō′mə) *n*. A granulomatous mass in the wall of the colon.

di·ver·tic·u·lo·sis (dī′vûr-tĭk′yə-lō′sĭs) *n*. A condition characterized by the presence of numerous diverticula in the colon.

di·ver·tic·u·lum (dī′vûr-tĭk′yə-ləm) *n., pl.* **-la** (-lə). A pouch or sac branching out from a hollow organ or structure, such as the intestine. — **di′ver·tic′u·lar** *adj*.

divide *v*. **-vid·ed, -vid·ing, -vides. 1.** To separate or become separated into parts, sections, groups, or branches. **2.** To sector into units of measurement; graduate. **3.** To separate and group according to kind; classify. **4.** To branch out, as a blood vessel. **5.** To undergo cell division.

div·ing reflex (dī′vĭng) *n*. A reflexive response to diving in many aquatic mammals and birds, characterized by physiological changes that decrease oxygen consumption, such as slowed heart rate, until breathing resumes. Though less pronounced, the reflex also occurs in humans upon submersion in water.

di·vi·nyl ether (dī-vī′nəl) *n*. A rapidly acting inhalation anesthetic.

di·vi·sion (dĭ-vĭzh′ən) *n*. **1.** The act or process of dividing. **2.** The highest taxonomic category in botanical classification, corresponding to a phylum. **3.** Cell division.

di·vul·sion (dī-vŭl′shən) *n*. **1.** The removal of a part by tearing. **2.** The forcible dilation of the walls of a cavity or canal.

di·vul·sor (dī-vŭl′sər, -sôr′) *n*. An instrument for forcible dilation of the urethra or other canal or cavity.

di·xyr·a·zine (dī-zīr′ə-zēn′) *n*. A phenothiazine compound used as an antipsychotic agent.

diz·zi·ness (dĭz′ē-nĭs) *n*. A disorienting sensation such as faintness, giddiness, light-headedness, or unsteadiness.

DMD *abbr.* Doctor of Dental Medicine

DMSO (dē′ĕm-ĕs-ō′) *n*. Dimethyl sulfoxide; a colorless hygroscopic liquid obtained from lignin, used as an industrial solvent and in medicine as a penetrant to convey medications into the tissues.

DMT (dē′ĕm-tē′) *n*. Dimethyltryptamine; a synthetic hallucinogenic drug.

DNA (dē′ĕn-ā′) *n*. Deoxyribonucleic acid; a nucleic acid that consists of two long chains of nucleotides twisted together into a double helix and joined by hydrogen bonds between complementary bases adenine and thymine or cytosine and guanine; it carries the cell's genetic information and hereditary characteristics via its nucleotides and their sequence and is capable of self-replication and RNA synthesis.

DNA fingerprinting *n*. A method used to identify multilocus DNA banding patterns that are specific to an individual by exposing a sample of the person's DNA to molecular probes and analytical techniques such as Southern blot analysis.

DNA helix *n.* See **double helix.**

DNA polymorphism *n.* A condition in which one of two different but normal nucleotide sequences can exist at a particular site in a DNA molecule.

DNase (dē-ĕn′ās) or **DNAase** (dē′ĕn-ā′ās) *n.* An enzyme that catalyzes the hydrolysis of DNA.

DNA virus *n.* A virus whose nucleic acid core is composed of DNA, such as any of the adenoviruses, herpesviruses, or poxviruses.

DNR *abbr.* do not resuscitate

D.N.S. *abbr.* Director of Nursing Services; Doctor of Nursing Services

D.O. *abbr.* Doctor of Osteopathy

DOA *abbr.* dead on admission; dead on arrival

doc (dŏk) *n.* A physician, dentist, or veterinarian.

DOC (dē′ō-sē′) *n.* **1.** Deoxycorticosterone; a steroid hormone secreted by the adrenal cortex or produced synthetically and used to treat adrenal insufficiency. **2.** Deoxycholic acid; a bile acid used as a choleretic and digestant and in the synthesis of adrenocortical hormones such as cortisone.

doc·tor (dŏk′tər) *n.* **1.** A person, especially a physician, dentist, or veterinarian, trained in the healing arts and licensed to practice. **2.** A person who has earned the highest academic degree awarded by a college or university in a specified discipline.

Doerf·ler–Stewart test (dûrf′lər-) *n.* A test that differentiates between functional and organic hearing loss by examining a person's ability to respond to spondee words in the presence of a masking noise.

dol (dōl) *n.* A unit for the measurement of pain intensity.

dol·i·chol (dŏl′ĭ-kôl) *n.* Any of various long-chain unsaturated isoprenoid alcohols found either free or phosphorylated in membranes of the endoplasmic reticulum and Golgi apparatus.

do·lor (dō′lər) *n.* **1.** Pain. **2.** Sorrow; grief. — **do′·lo·rif′ic** *adj.*

do·lo·rim·e·try (dō′lə-rĭm′ĭ-trē, dŏl′ə-) *n.* The measurement of pain sensitivity or pain intensity.

DOM (dē′ō-ĕm′) *n.* 2,5-Dimethoxy-4-methylamphetamine; an hallucinogenic agent chemically related to amphetamine and mescaline.

do·main (dō-mān′) *n.* One of the homologous regions that make up an immunoglobulin's heavy and light chains; they contain approximately 110 to 120 amino acids and serve specific immunological functions.

dom·i·nance (dŏm′ə-nəns) *n.* The condition or state of being dominant.

dominance of genes *n.* A full phenotypic expression of a gene in both heterozygotes and homozygotes.

dom·i·nant (dŏm′ə-nənt) *adj.* **1.** Exercising the most influence or control. **2.** Of, relating to, or being an allele that produces the same phenotypic effect whether inherited with a homozygous or heterozygous allele. — *n.* **1.** A dominant allele or trait. **2.** An organism having a dominant trait.

dominant character *n.* An inherited character determined by a dominant gene.

dominant eye *n.* The eye customarily used for monocular tasks.

dominant gene *n.* A gene that is expressed phenotypically in heterozygous or homozygous persons.

dominant hemisphere *n.* The cerebral hemisphere that is more involved than the other in governing certain body functions, such as controlling the arm and leg used preferentially in skilled movements.

dominant inheritance *n.* Inheritance in which an allele produces the same phenotypic effect whether it is inherited with a homozygous or heterozygous allele.

Do·nath–Land·stei·ner phenomenon (dō′năth-länd′stī′nər, -nät-) *n.* The hemolysis that occurs in a sample of blood from a person with paroxysmal hemoglobinuria when the sample is cooled to around 5°C and then warmed.

Don·ders' law (dŏn′dərz) *n.* The principle that the rotation of the eyeball is determined by the distance of the object from the median plane and the line of the horizon.

Don Juan (dŏn wŏn′) *n.* A man who is an obsessive seducer of women, especially one who does so out of feelings of impotence or inferiority.

do·nor (dō′nər) *n.* One from whom blood, tissue, or an organ is taken for use in a transfusion or transplant.

donor card *n.* A card, usually carried on one's person, authorizing the use of one's bodily organs for transplantation in the event of one's death.

don·o·va·no·sis (dŏn′ə-və-nō′sĭs) *n.* A chronic destructive ulceration of the external genitalia caused by bacterial infection, which is observed intracellularly as encapsulated forms in the infected tissue.

do·pa (dō′pə) *n.* Dihydroxyphenylalanine; an amino acid formed in the liver from tyrosine and converted to dopamine in the brain.

do·pa·mine (dō′pə-mēn′) *n.* A monoamine neurotransmitter formed in the brain by the decarboxylation of dopa and essential to the normal functioning of the central nervous system. A reduction in its concentration within the brain is associated with Parkinson's disease.

dope (dōp) *n.* **1.** A narcotic, especially an addictive narcotic. **2.** An illicit drug, especially marijuana.

Dop·pler echocardiography (dŏp′lər) *n.* The use of Doppler ultrasonography techniques to augment two-dimensional echocardiograms by allowing velocities to be registered within the echocardiographic image.

Doppler effect *n.* An apparent change in the frequency of waves, as of sound or light, occurring when the source and observer are in motion relative to each other, with the frequency increasing when the source and observer approach each other and decreasing when they move apart.

Doppler ultrasonography *n.* Ultrasonography applying the Doppler effect, in which frequency-shifted ultrasound reflections produced by moving targets in the bloodstream, usually red blood cells, are used to determine the direction and velocity of blood flow.

dor·sad (dôr′săd′) *adv.* In the direction of the back; dorsally.

dor·sal (dôr′səl) *adj.* **1.** Of, toward, on, in, or near the back or upper surface of an organ, a part, or an organism. **2.** Lying on the back; supine.

dorsal column of spinal cord *n.* See **posterior column of spinal cord.**

dor·sal·gi·a (dôr-săl′jē-ə, -jə) *n.* Pain in the upper back.

dorsal horn *n.* See **posterior horn** (senses 1, 2).

dorsal root *n.* The sensory root of a spinal nerve.

dorsal root ganglion *n.* See **spinal ganglion.**

dor·si·flex·ion (dôr′sə-flĕk′shən) *n.* The turning of the foot or the toes upward.

dor·sum (dôr′səm) *n., pl.* **-sa** (-sə). **1.** The back. **2.** The upper, outer surface of an organ, an appendage, or a part.

dos·age (dō′sĭj) *n.* **1.** Administration of a therapeutic agent in prescribed amounts. **2.** Determination of the amount to be so administered. **3.** The amount so administered.

dose (dōs) *n.* **1.** A specified quantity of a therapeutic agent, such as a drug or medicine, prescribed to be taken at one time or at stated intervals. **2.** The amount of radiation administered as therapy to a given site. — *v.* **dosed, dos·ing, dos·es. 1.** To give or prescribe something, such as medicine, in specified amounts. **2.** To give someone a dose.

dot (dŏt) *n.* A tiny round mark made by or as if by a pointed instrument; a spot.

dot·age (dō′tĭj) *n.* The loss of previously intact mental powers; senility.

dou·ble blind experiment (dŭb′əl blīnd′) *n.* A testing procedure, designed to eliminate biased results, in which the identity of those receiving a test treatment is concealed from both administrators and subjects until after the study is completed.

double-channel catheter *n.* A catheter with two lumens, allowing injection and removal of fluid.

double contrast enema *n.* A procedure consisting of a barium enema followed after evacuation by the injection of air into the rectum, for finer radiographic study of rectal and colonic mucosa.

double fracture *n.* A fracture occurring in two sections of the same bone.

double helix *n.* The coiled structure of a double-stranded DNA molecule in which strands linked by hydrogen bonds form a spiral configuration.

double-jointed *adj.* Having unusually flexible joints, especially of the limbs or fingers.

double pneumonia *n.* Pneumonia affecting both lungs.

dou·blet (dŭb′lĭt) *n.* A pairing of two lenses to optically correct a chromatic and spherical aberration.

double vision *n.* A disorder of vision in which a single object appears double.

dou·bly armed suture (dŭb′lē) *n.* A suture performed with a needle at each end.

douche (do͞osh) *n.* **1.** A stream of water, often containing medicinal or cleansing agents, that is ap-

plied to a body part or cavity for hygienic or therapeutic purposes. **2.** An instrument for applying a douche. — *v.* **douched, douch·ing, douch·es.** To cleanse or treat by means of a douche.

douche bath *n.* Local application of water to the body in the form of a jet or stream.

Doug·las bag (dŭg′ləs) *n.* A receptacle for collecting expired air to determine oxygen consumption in humans under various work conditions.

dow·a·ger's hump (dou′ə-jərz) *n.* An abnormal curvature of the spine that is primarily manifested as a rounded hump in the upper back and that typically affects older women, with the curvature being the result of collapse of the spinal column because of osteoporosis.

down·er (dou′nər) *n.* A depressant or sedative drug, such as a barbiturate or tranquilizer.

Dow·ney cell (dou′nē) *n.* A type of atypical lymphocyte usually occurring in infectious mononucleosis and other viral diseases.

Down syndrome (doun) or **Down's syndrome** (dounz) *n.* A congenital disorder, caused by the presence of an extra 21st chromosome, and marked by mild to moderate mental retardation, short stature, and a flattened facial profile.

dox·o·ru·bi·cin (dŏk′sə-ro͞o′bĭ-sĭn) *n.* An antibiotic obtained from the bacterium *Streptomyces peuceticus,* used as an anticancer drug.

DP *abbr.* Doctor of Podiatry

DPH *abbr.* Diploma in Public Health; Doctor of Public Health; Doctor of Public Hygiene

DPM *abbr.* Doctor of Physical Medicine; Doctor of Podiatric Medicine

DPT (dē′pē-tē′) *n.* Dipropyltryptamine; a hallucinogenic drug similar to DMT.

dr *abbr.* dram

drac·on·ti·a·sis (drăk′ŏn-tī′ə-sĭs) *n.* See **dracunculiasis.**

dra·cun·cu·li·a·sis (drə-kŭng′kyə-lī′ə-sĭs) or **dra·cun·cu·lo·sis** (-lō′sĭs) *n.* Infestation with *Dracunculus medinensis.*

Dra·cun·cu·lus (drə-kŭng′kyə-ləs) *n.* A genus of nematodes that includes parasitic species such as *D. medinensis,* which migrates within subcutaneous tissues and forms chronic ulcers in the skin.

draft (drăft) *n.* A measured portion of a liquid or aerosol medication; a dose.

dra·gée (drä-zhā′) *n.* A small, often medicated candy.

drain (drān) *n.* A device, such as a tube, inserted into the opening of a wound or into a body or dental cavity to facilitate discharge of fluid or purulent material. — *v.* **drained, drain·ing, drains.** To draw off a liquid gradually as it forms.

drain·age (drā′nĭj) *n.* The removal of fluid or purulent material from a wound or body cavity.

drainage tube *n.* A tube inserted into a wound or cavity to facilitate fluid removal.

dram (drăm) *n.* **1.** A unit of weight in the U.S. Customary System equal to ¹⁄₁₆ of an ounce or 27.34 grains (1.77 grams). **2.** A unit of apothecary weight equal to ⅛ of an ounce or 60 grains (3.89 grams).

Dram·a·mine (drăm′ə-mēn′) A trademark used for dimenhydrinate.

drape (drāp) v. **draped, drap·ing, drapes.** To cover, dress, or hang with or as if with cloth in loose folds. — n. A cloth arranged over a patient's body during a medical examination or treatment or during surgery.

drawer sign (drôr) n. An indication of laxity or a tear in the anterior or posterior cruciate ligments of the knee in which there is a forward or backward sliding of the tibia.

drawer test n. See **drawer sign.**

dream (drēm) n. A series of images, ideas, emotions, and sensations occurring involuntarily in the mind during certain stages of sleep.

dream analysis n. Diagnosis of a patient's mental state by a study of his or her dreams.

dream·y state (drē′mē) n. The semiconscious state associated with an epileptic attack.

drep·a·no·cyte (drĕp′ə-nə-sīt′, drə-păn′ə-) n. See **sickle cell.** — **drep′a·no·cyt′ic** adj.

dress (drĕs) v. **dressed, dress·ing, dress·es.** To apply medication, bandages, or other therapeutic materials to an area of the body such as a wound.

dress·ing (drĕs′ĭng) n. A therapeutic or protective material applied to a wound.

dressing forceps n. A slender forceps for grasping gauze or sutures and removing fragments of necrosed tissue and small foreign bodies when dressing wounds.

drift (drĭft) n. **1.** A gradual deviation from an original course, model, method, or intention. **2.** Variation or random oscillation about a fixed setting, position, or mode of behavior.

Drin·ker respirator (drĭng′kər) n. An airtight metal tank that encloses all of the body except the head and forces the lungs to inhale and exhale through regulated changes in air pressure.

drip (drĭp) n. **1.** The process of forming and falling in drops. **2.** Moisture or liquid such as medication that falls in drops.

drip feed n. **1.** Administration of blood, plasma, saline, or sugar solutions, usually intravenously, a drop at a time. **2.** The device or tubes by which such a substance is administered. **3.** The substance administered.

drive (drīv) n. A strong motivating tendency or instinct, especially of sexual or aggressive origin, that prompts activity toward a particular end.

drom·o·graph (drŏm′ə-grăf′, drō′mə-) n. An instrument for recording the rate at which blood flows or circulates within the body.

drom·o·ma·ni·a (drŏm′ə-mā′nē-ə, drō′mə-) n. An uncontrollable impulse or desire to wander or travel.

dro·nab·i·nol (drō-năb′ə-nôl) n. The principal psychoactive substance present in *Cannabis sativa* used therapeutically to control nausea and vomiting associated with cancer chemotherapy.

drop (drŏp) n. **1.** The smallest quantity of liquid heavy enough to fall in a spherical mass. **2.** A volume of liquid equal to 1/76 of a teaspoon and regarded as a unit of dosage for medication. **3.** A

small globular piece of candy, usually readily dissolved in the mouth. — v. **dropped, drop·ping, drops.** To fall, be dispensed, or poured in drops.

drop foot n. See **foot-drop.**

drop hand n. See **wrist-drop.**

drop·per (drŏp′ər) n. A device that produces drops, especially a small tube with a suction bulb at one end for drawing in a liquid and releasing it in drops.

drop·sy (drŏp′sē) n. Edema. No longer in technical use.

drows·i·ness (drou′zē-nĭs) n. A state of impaired awareness associated with a desire or inclination to sleep.

Dr.P.H. abbr. Doctor of Pubic Health; Doctor of Public Hygiene

drug (drŭg) n. **1.** A substance used in the diagnosis, treatment, or prevention of a disease or as a component of a medication. **2.** Such a substance as recognized or defined by the U.S. Food and Drug Administration. **3.** A chemical substance, such as a narcotic, that affects the central nervous system, causing changes in behavior and often addiction. — v. **drugged, drug·ging, drugs. 1.** To administer a drug, especially in large quantity, to a person. **2.** To stupefy or dull with or as if with a drug; to narcotize.

drug abuse n. Habitual use of drugs to alter one's mood, emotion, or state of consciousness.

drug eruption n. An eruption caused by the ingestion, injection, inhalation, or insertion of a drug, often as a result of allergic sensitization.

drug·gist (drŭg′ĭst) n. **1.** A pharmacist. **2.** One who sells drugs.

drug in·ter·ac·tion (ĭn′tər-ăk′shən) n. The pharmacological result, either desirable or undesirable, of drugs interacting with themselves or with other drugs, with endogenous chemical agents, with components of the diet, or with chemicals used in or resulting from diagnostic tests.

drug tetanus n. A condition characterized by tonic spasms, caused by a tetanic drug.

drum (drŭm) n. See **eardrum.**

drunk·en·ness (drŭng′kə-nĭs) n. The condition of being delirious with or as if with an alcoholic beverage; intoxicated.

druse (drōōz) n., pl. **dru·sen** (drōō′zən). One of the small hyaline or colloid bodies sometimes occurring behind the retina of the eye.

dry abscess (drī) n. The remains of an abscess after the pus is absorbed.

dry cough n. A cough not accompanied by expectoration; a nonproductive cough.

dry gangrene n. Gangrene that develops as a result of arterial obstruction and is characterized by mummification of the dead tissue and absence of bacterial decomposition.

dry joint n. A joint affected with atrophic desiccating changes.

dry labor n. Labor after spontaneous loss of practically all of the amniotic fluid.

dry nurse n. A nurse employed to care for but not breast-feed an infant.

dry pleurisy *n.* Pleurisy characterized by a fibrinous exudation, resulting in adhesion between the opposing surfaces of the pleura.

dry rale *n.* An auscultative sound produced by a bronchial constriction or narrowing.

dry socket *n.* A painful inflamed condition at the site of extraction of a tooth that occurs when a blood clot fails to form properly or is dislodged.

dry synovitis *n.* Synovitis with little serous or purulent effusion.

dry vomiting *n.* See **vomiturition.**

DT *abbr.* delirium tremens; duration tetany

DTaP *abbr.* acellular pertussis vaccine

DTIC (dē'tē-ī-sē') *n.* Dacarbazine; an antineoplastic agent used in the treatment of malignant melanoma and Hodgkin's disease.

DTP *abbr.* diphtheria, tetanus toxoids, and pertussis vaccine

du·al·ism (dōō'ə-lĭz'əm, dyōō'-) *n.* The view in psychology that the mind and body function separately, without interchange.

Du·bin John·son syndrome (dōō'bĭn-jŏn'sən, dyōō'-) *n.* An inherited defect in hepatic excretory function characterized by an increase of serum bilirubin concentration, high urinary excretion of a form of coproporphyrin, retention of dark pigment by hepatocytes, and nonvisualization of gall bladder using cholecystogram.

dub·ni·um (dōōb'nē-əm) *n.* An artificially produced radioactive element with atomic number 105.

Du·bo·witz score (dōō'bə-wĭts', dyōō'-) *n.* A method of clinical assessment of a newborn from birth until five days old that includes neurological criteria for its maturity and other physical criteria to determine its gestational age.

Du·crey's bacillus (dōō-krāz') *n.* A gram-negative, rod-shaped bacterium *Haemophilus ducreyi* that causes chancroids in humans.

duct (dŭkt) *n.* A tubular bodily canal or passage, especially one for carrying a glandular secretion such as bile.

duc·tion (dŭk'shən) *n.* **1.** The act of leading, bringing, or conducting. **2.** The rotation of an eye on the vertical and horizontal axis.

duct·less (dŭkt'lĭs) *adj.* Lacking a duct, as glands that only secrete internally.

ductless gland *n.* See **endocrine gland.**

duc·tule (dŭk'tōōl', -tyōōl') *n.* A small duct.

Du·gas' test (dōō-gäz', dyōō-) *n.* A test performed to determine whether an injured shoulder is due to a dislocation or a fracture.

Dukes classification (dōōks, dyōōks) *n.* A classification into three stages of the extent of spread of operable carcinoma of the large intestine.

dull (dŭl) *adj.* **dull·er, dull·est. 1.** Lacking responsiveness or alertness; insensitive. **2.** Not intensely or keenly felt, as in pain. — **dullness** *n.*

dump·ing syndrome (dŭm'pĭng) *n.* A condition occurring after eating in patients with shunts of the upper alimentary canal and including flushing, sweating, dizziness, weakness, and vasomotor collapse.

du·o·de·nec·to·my (dōō'ō-də-nĕk'tə-mē, dyōō'-,

du·o·de·ni·tis (dōō'ō-də-nī'tĭs, dyōō'-, dōō-ŏd'n-ī'-, dyōō'-) *n.* Inflammation of the duodenum.

du·o·de·no·en·ter·os·to·my (dōō'ə-dē'nō-ĕn'tə-rŏs'tə-mē, dyōō'-, dōō-ŏd'n-ō-, dyōō'-) *n.* The surgical formation of a passage between the duodenum and another part of the intestinal tract.

du·o·de·no·je·ju·nos·to·my (dōō'ə-dē'nō-jə-jōō'nŏs'tə-mē, dyōō'-, dōō-ŏd'n-ō-, dyōō'-) *n.* The surgical formation of a passage between the duodenum and the jejunum.

du·o·de·nol·y·sis (dōō'ō-də-nŏl'ĭ-sĭs, dyōō'-, dōō-ŏd'n-ŏl'-, dyōō'-) *n.* The freeing of the duodenum from adhesions by means of surgery.

du·o·de·nor·rha·phy (dōō'ə-də-nôr'ə-fē, dyōō'-, dōō-ŏd'n-ôr'-, dyōō'-) *n.* Suture of a tear or incision in the duodenum.

du·o·de·nos·co·py (dōō'ə-də-nŏs'kə-pē, dyōō'-, dōō-ŏd'n-ŏs'-, dyōō'-) *n.* The examination of the interior of the duodenum through an endoscope.

du·o·de·nos·to·my (dōō'ə-də-nŏs'tə-mē, dyōō'-, dōō-ŏd'n-ŏs'-, dyōō'-) *n.* The surgical establishment of an opening into the duodenum.

du·o·de·not·o·my (dōō'ə-də-nŏt'ə-mē, dyōō'-, dōō-ŏd'n-ŏt'-, dyōō'-) *n.* Surgical incision of the duodenum.

du·o·de·num (dōō'ə-dē'nəm, dyōō'-, dōō-ŏd'n-əm, dyōō-) *n., pl.* **du·o·de·nums** or **du·o·de·na** (dōō'ə-dē'nə, dyōō'-, dōō-ŏd'n-ə, dyōō-). The beginning portion of the small intestine, starting at the lower end of the stomach and extending to the jejunum. — **du'o·de'nal** (dōō'ə-dē'nəl, dyōō'-, dōō-ŏd'n-əl, dyōō-) *adj.*

du·plex uterus (dōō'plĕks', dyōō'-) *n.* A uterus with a double lumen.

du·pli·ca·tion (dōō'plĭ-kā'shən, dyōō'-) *n.* The existence or growth into two corresponding parts.

duplication of chromosomes *n.* The repetition of a section of genetic material in a chromosome.

Du·puy-Du·temps operation (dü-pwē'-dü-tän') *n.* An operation for correcting stenosis of the lacrimal duct.

du·ra (dōōr'ə, dyōōr'ə) *n.* See **dura mater.** — **du'ral** *adj.*

dura ma·ter (mā'tər, mä-) *n.* The tough fibrous membrane covering the brain and spinal cord and lining the inner surface of the skull.

dur. dol. *abbr. Latin.* durante dolore (while the pain lasts)

Du·ro·ziez murmur (dōō-rō'zē-ā', dü-rô-zyā') *n.* See **Duroziez symptom.**

Duroziez symptom *n.* A double murmur heard over the femoral artery in cases of aortic insufficiency.

dwarf (dwôrf) *n., pl.* **dwarfs** or **dwarves** (dwôrvz). An abnormally small person, often having limbs and features not properly proportioned or formed.

dwarf·ism (dwôr'fĭz'əm) *n.* A pathological condition of arrested growth having various causes.

dy·ad (dī'ăd', -əd) *n.* **1.** Two individuals or units regarded as a pair, such as a mother and a daughter. **2.** One pair of homologous chromosomes resulting from the meiotic division of a tetrad.

dye (dī) *n.* A substance that is used to color materials or substances, such as cells and microorganisms.

dy·nam·ic refraction (dī-nām′ĭk) *n.* Refraction of the eye during accommodation.

dy·nam·ics (dī-nām′ĭks) *n.* Psychodynamics.

dynamic splint *n.* A splint that aids in initiating and performing movements by controlling the plane and range of motion of the injured part.

dy·na·mo·gen·e·sis (dī′nə-mō-jĕn′ĭ-sĭs) *n.* The generation of power, force, or energy, especially muscular or nervous energy.

dy·nam·o·graph (dī-nām′ə-grăf′) *n.* An instrument for recording the degree of muscular force.

dy·na·mom·e·ter (dī′nə-mŏm′ĭ-tər) *n.* A device for measuring the degree of muscular force.

dy·nein (dī′nēn′, -nē-ĭn) *n.* An ATPase associated with motile structures, especially the microtubules in cilia and flagella.

dys·a·cou·si·a or **dys·a·cu·si·a** (dĭs′ə-kōō′zē-ə, -zhə) *n.* A condition in which ordinary sounds produce discomfort or pain in the ear.

dys·a·cu·sis (dĭs′ə-kōō′sĭs) *n.* **1.** An impairment of hearing that is not primarily a loss of the ability to perceive sound. **2.** Dysacousia.

dys·a·phi·a (dĭs-ā′fē-ə) *n.* An impairment in the sense of touch.

dys·ar·te·ri·ot·o·ny (dĭs′är-tĕr′ē-ŏt′ə-nē) *n.* Abnormal blood pressure.

dys·ar·thri·a (dĭs-är′thrē-ə) *n.* Difficulty in articulating words due to emotional stress or to paralysis, incoordination, or spasticity of the muscles used in speaking. — **dys·ar′thric** *adj.*

dys·ar·thro·sis (dĭs′är-thrō′sĭs) *n.* **1.** Deformity, dislocation, or disease of a joint. **2.** False joint. **3.** Dysarthria.

dys·au·to·no·mi·a (dĭs-ô′tə-nō′mē-ə) *n.* Abnormal functioning of the autonomic nervous system.

dys·bar·ism (dĭs′bə-rĭz′əm) *n.* A complex of symptoms resulting from exposure to excessively low or rapidly changing air pressure that includes decompression sickness.

dys·ba·si·a (dĭs-bā′zē-ə, -zhə) *n.* **1.** Difficulty in walking, especially as the result of a nervous system disorder. **2.** Difficulty in or distortion of walking in persons with mental disorders.

dys·bu·li·a (dĭs-bōō′lē-ə, -byōō′-) *n.* A weakness and uncertainty of willpower. — **dys·bu′lic** *adj.*

dys·cal·cu·li·a (dĭs′kăl-kyōō′lē-ə) *n.* Impairment of the ability to solve mathematical problems, usually resulting from brain dysfunction.

dys·ce·pha·li·a (dĭs′sə-fā′lē-ə, -fāl′yə) or **dys·ceph·a·ly** (dĭs-sĕf′ə-lē) *n.* A congenital malformation of the cranium and the bones of the face.

dys·chei·ri·a or **dys·chi·ri·a** (dĭs-kī′rē-ə) *n.* The inability to tell which side of the body has been touched even though there is no apparent loss of sensation. — **dys·chei′ral** *adj.*

dys·che·zi·a (dĭs-kē′zē-ə, -zhə) *n.* The inability to defecate without pain or difficulty.

dys·chon·dro·gen·e·sis (dĭs-kŏn′drō-jĕn′ĭ-sĭs) *n.* Abnormal development of cartilage.

dys·chon·dro·pla·sia (dĭs-kŏn′drō-plā′zhə, -zhē-ə) *n.* See **enchondromatosis.**

dys·chon·dros·te·o·sis (dĭs′kŏn-drŏs′tē-ō′sĭs) *n.* A familial bone dysplasia characterized by bowing of the radius, dorsal dislocation of the distal ulna and proximal carpal bones, and mesomelic dwarfism.

dys·chro·ma·top·si·a (dĭs-krō′mə-tŏp′sē-ə) *n.* See **dichromatism** (sense 2).

dys·chro·mi·a (dĭs-krō′mē-ə) *n.* A discoloration, especially of the skin.

dys·co·ri·a (dĭs-kôr′ē-ə) *n.* An abnormality in the shape of the pupil.

dys·cra·sia (dĭs-krā′zhə, -zhē-ə) *n.* An abnormal state or disorder of the body, especially of the blood.

dys·en·ter·y (dĭs′ən-tĕr′ē) *n.* An inflammatory disorder of the lower intestinal tract, usually caused by a bacterial, parasitic, or protozoan infection and resulting in pain, fever, and severe diarrhea, often accompanied by the passage of blood and mucus. — **dys′en·ter′ic** *adj.*

dys·er·e·thism (dĭs-ĕr′ə-thĭz′əm) *n.* A condition in which a person responds slowly to stimuli.

dys·es·the·sia (dĭs′ĕs-thē′zhə) *n.* **1.** Impairment of sensation, especially that of touch. **2.** A condition in which an unpleasant sensation is produced by ordinary stimuli.

dys·fi·brin·o·ge·ne·mi·a (dĭs′fī-brĭn′ə-jə-nē′mē-ə, -fī′brə-nō-) *n.* A familial disorder in which fibrinogens function inadequately resulting in symptoms ranging from bleeding to thrombosis.

dys·func·tion or **dis·func·tion** (dĭs-fŭngk′shən) *n.* Abnormal or impaired functioning, especially of a bodily system or organ. — **dys·func′tion·al** *adj.*

dys·gam·ma·glob·u·li·ne·mi·a (dĭs-găm′ə-glŏb′yə-lə-nē′mē-ə) *n.* A disorder involving an abnormality in the structure, distribution, or frequency of serum gamma-globulins.

dys·gen·e·sis (dĭs-jĕn′ĭ-sĭs) *n.* Defective or abnormal embryonic development of an organ.

dys·gna·thi·a (dĭs-nā′thē-ə) *n.* An abnormality of the mouth that extends beyond the teeth and includes the maxilla, mandible, or both. — **dys·gnath′ic** (-năth′ĭk, -nā′thĭk) *adj.*

dys·gno·si·a (dĭs-nō′zē-ə, -zhə) *n.* A cognitive disorder, especially one resulting from a mental disorder or disease.

dys·graph·i·a (dĭs-grăf′ē-ə) *n.* Impairment of the ability to write, usually caused by brain dysfunction or disease.

dys·har·mon·ic diplacusis (dĭs′här-mŏn′ĭk) *n.* A form of diplacusis in which the same sound is heard with a different pitch in each ear.

dys·he·ma·to·poi·e·sis (dĭs-hē′mə-tō-poi-ē′sĭs, dĭs′hĭ-măt′ə-) or **dys·he·mo·poi·e·sis** (dĭs-hē′mə-) *n.* Abnormal formation of blood cells. — **dys·he′ma·to·poi·et′ic** (-ĕt′ĭk, -hĭ-măt′ō-) *adj.*

dys·ker·a·to·sis (dĭs-kĕr′ə-tō′sĭs) *n.* **1.** Premature keratinization in cells not in the keratinizing surface layer of skin. **2.** Keratinization of the corneal epithelium. — **dys·ker′a·tot′ic** (-tŏt′ĭk) adj.

dys·ki·ne·sia (dĭs′kə-nē′zhə, -kī-) n. An impairment in the ability to control movements, marked by spasmodic or repetitive motions or lack of coordination. — **dys′ki·net′ic** (-nĕt′ĭk) adj.

dyskinesia al·ger·a (ăl′jər-ə) n. A hysterical condition in which active movement causes pain.

dys·la·li·a (dĭs-lā′lē-ə, -lăl′ē-ə) n. An articulation disorder resulting from impaired hearing or structural abnormalities of the articulatory organs, such as the tongue.

dys·lex·i·a (dĭs-lĕk′sē-ə) n. A learning disorder marked by impairment of the ability to recognize and comprehend written words. — **dys·lec′tic** (-lĕk′tĭk) n.

dys·lex·ic (dĭs-lĕk′sĭk) adj. Of or relating to dyslexia. — n. A person affected by dyslexia.

dys·lo·gi·a (dĭs-lō′jē-ə, -jə) n. **1.** Difficulty in the expression of ideas or of the ability to speak. **2.** Impairment of the ability to reason or to think logically.

dys·men·or·rhe·a or **dys·men·or·rhoe·a** (dĭs′mĕn′ə-rē′ə) n. Painful menstruation.

dys·mim·i·a (dĭs-mĭm′ē-ə) n. **1.** An impairment of the ability to use gestures to express oneself. **2.** An inability to imitate.

dys·mor·phism (dĭs-môr′fĭz′əm) n. An anatomical malformation.

dys·mor·pho·gen·e·sis (dĭs-môr′fō-jĕn′ĭ-sĭs) n. The process of abnormal tissue formation.

dys·my·o·to·ni·a (dĭs′mī-ə-tō′nē-ə) n. Abnormal muscular tonicity.

dys·o·rex·i·a (dĭs-ə-rĕk′sē-ə) n. A diminished, disordered, or unnatural appetite.

dys·os·mi·a (dĭs-ŏz′mē-ə) n. An impairment or dysfunction of the sense of smell.

dys·os·te·o·gen·e·sis (dĭs-ŏs′tē-ə-jĕn′ĭ-sĭs) n. See **dysostosis.**

dys·os·to·sis (dĭs′ŏs-tō′sĭs) n. The defective formation of bone.

dys·pa·reu·ni·a (dĭs′pə-rōō′nē-ə) n. Difficult or painful sexual intercourse.

dys·pep·sia (dĭs-pĕp′shə, -sē-ə) n. Disturbed digestion; indigestion.

dys·pha·gia (dĭs-fā′jə, -jē-ə) or **dys·pha·gy** (dĭs′fə-jē) n. Difficulty in swallowing or inability to swallow. — **dys·phag′ic** (-fāj′ĭk) adj.

dys·pha·sia (dĭs-fā′zhə, -zhē-ə) n. Impairment of speech and verbal comprehension, especially when associated with brain injury.

dys·phe·mi·a (dĭs-fē′mē-ə) n. A speech disorder marked by stammering or stuttering, usually having an emotional or psychological basis.

dys·pho·ni·a (dĭs-fō′nē-ə) n. Difficulty in speaking, usually evidenced by hoarseness.

dys·pho·ri·a (dĭs-fôr′ē-ə) n. An emotional state characterized by anxiety, depression, and restlessness.

dys·phor·ic hypomania (dĭs-fôr′ĭk) n. An affective disorder in which a person who has had a major depressive episode undergoes an episode of illness having some manic symptoms although not so severe or of such duration as to be categorized as manic.

dys·phra·sia (dĭs-frā′zhə, -zē-ə) n. See **dysphasia.**

dys·pig·men·ta·tion (dĭs′pĭg-mən-tā′shən) n. An abnormality in the formation or distribution of pigment, especially in the skin.

dys·pla·sia (dĭs-plā′zhə, -zhē-ə) n. Abnormal development or growth of tissues, organs, or cells.

dys·plas·tic (dĭs-plăs′tĭk) adj. Relating to or characterized by dysplasia.

dysp·ne·a (dĭsp-nē′ə) n. Difficulty in breathing, often associated with lung or heart disease and resulting in shortness of breath. — **dysp·ne′ic** (-nē′ĭk) adj.

dys·prax·i·a (dĭs-prăk′sē-ə) n. The impairment or painful functioning of an organ.

dys·pro·si·um (dĭs-prō′zē-əm, -zhē-əm) n. A soft, silvery rare-earth element with atomic number 66 used in nuclear research.

dys·som·ni·a (dĭs-sŏm′nē-ə) n. A disturbance in the normal rhythm or pattern of sleep.

dys·sta·si·a (dĭs-stā′sē-ə, -zē-ə, -zhə) n. Difficulty in standing. — **dys·stat·ic** (-stăt′ĭk) adj.

dys·syn·er·gi·a (dĭs′sə-nûr′jē-ə) n. See **ataxia.**

dys·tax·i·a (dĭs-tăk′sē-ə) n. A mild ataxia.

dys·thy·mi·a (dĭs-thī′mē-ə) n. A mood disorder characterized by despondency or mild depression. — **dys·thy′mic** adj.

dysthymic disorder n. A chronic mood disturbance lasting at least two years in adults or one year in children, characterized by mild depression and symptoms such as insomnia, tearfulness, and pessimism.

dys·to·ci·a (dĭs-tō′sē-ə, -shē-ə, -shə) n. A slow or difficult labor or delivery.

dys·to·ni·a (dĭs-tō′nē-ə) n. Abnormal tonicity of tissue. — **dys·ton′ic** (-tŏn′ĭk) adj.

dystonic reaction n. A state of abnormal tension or muscle tone, similar to dystonia, produced as a side effect of certain antipsychotic medications.

dys·to·pi·a (dĭs-tō′pē-ə) n. An abnormal position, as of an organ or a body part. — **dys·top′ic** (-tŏp′ĭk) adj.

dys·tro·phin (dĭs′trə-fĭn) n. A structural protein found in small amounts in normal muscle but absent or present in abnormal amounts in persons with muscular dystrophy.

dys·troph·o·neu·ro·sis (dĭ-strŏf′ō-nŏō-rō′sĭs, -nyŏō-) n. A nervous disorder attributed to poor or improper nutrition.

dys·tro·phy (dĭs′trə-fē) or **dys·tro·phi·a** (dĭ-strō′-fē-ə) n. **1.** A degenerative disorder caused by inadequate or defective nutrition. **2.** Any of several disorders in which the muscles weaken and atrophy. — **dys·troph′ic** (-strŏf′ĭk, -strō′fĭk) adj.

dys·u·ri·a (dĭs-yŏŏr′ē-ə) n. Difficult or painful urination. — **dys·u′ric** (-yŏŏr′ĭk) adj.

dys·ver·sion (dĭs-vûr′zhən) n. A turning in any direction, but not a complete turning over.

E

ear (ĕr) *n.* **1.** The organ of hearing, responsible for maintaining equilibrium as well as sensing sound and divided into the external ear, the middle ear, and the inner ear. **2.** The part of this organ that is externally visible. **3.** The sense of hearing.

ear·ache (ĕr'āk') *n.* Pain in the ear; otalgia.

ear canal *n.* The narrow, tubelike passage through which sound enters the ear.

ear·drop (ĕr'drŏp') *n.* **eardrops.** Liquid medicine administered into the ear.

ear·drum (ĕr'drŭm') *n.* The thin, semitransparent, oval-shaped membrane that separates the middle ear from the external ear.

earlobe or **ear lobe** *n.* The soft, fleshy, pendulous lower part of the external ear.

ear·wax (ĕr'wăks') *n.* The yellowish, waxlike secretion of certain glands lining the canal of the external ear, cerumen.

eat (ēt) *v.* **ate** (āt), **eat·en** (ēt'n), **eat·ing, eats. 1.** To take into the body by the mouth for digestion or absorption. **2.** To consume, ravage, or destroy by or as if by ingesting, such as by a disease.

eating disorder *n.* A potentially life-threatening neurotic condition, such as anorexia nervosa or bulimia, usually seen in young women.

Eb·o·la virus (ĕb'ə-lə) *n.* A virus that causes viral hemorrhagic fever.

Eb·stein's anomaly (ĕb'stīnz, ĕp'shtīnz) *n.* Congenital downward displacement of the tricuspid valve into the right ventricle.

Ebstein's sign *n.* An indication of pericardial effusion.

EBV *abbr.* Epstein–Barr virus

EB virus (ē'bē') *n.* See **Epstein–Barr virus.**

ec·cen·tric (ĭk-sĕn'trĭk, ĕk-) *adj.* **1.** Departing from a recognized, conventional, or established norm or pattern. **2.** Situated or proceeding away from the center. — **ec·cen'tri·cal·ly** *adv.* — **ec'cen·tric'i·ty** (ĕk'sĕn-trĭs'ĭ-tē) *n.*

ec·chon·dro·ma (ĕk'ən-drō'mə) *n., pl.* **-mas** or **-ma·ta** (-mə-tə). A cartilaginous tumor arising as an overgrowth from normally situated cartilage, such as a mass protruding from the articular surface of a bone.

ec·chon·dro·sis (ĕk'ən-drō'sĭs) *n., pl.* **-ses** (-sēz). See **ecchondroma.**

ec·chy·mo·ma (ĕk'ĭ-mō'mə) *n., pl.* **-mas** or **-ma·ta** (-mə-tə). A slight hematoma following a bruise.

ec·chy·mo·sis (ĕk'ĭ-mō'sĭs) *n., pl.* **-ses** (-sēz'). The passage of blood from ruptured blood vessels into subcutaneous tissue, marked by a purple skin discoloration. — **ec'chy·mot'ic** (-mŏt'ĭk) *adj.*

ec·crine (ĕk'rĭn, -rīn', -rēn') *adj.* **1.** Relating to an eccrine gland or its secretion, especially sweat. **2.** Exocrine.

eccrine gland or **eccrine sweat gland** *n.* Any of the numerous small sweat glands distributed over the body's surface that produce a clear aqueous secretion important in temperature regulation.

eccrine poroma *n.* A poroma of the eccrine sweat glands on the sole of the foot.

ec·cri·sis (ĕk'rĭ-sĭs) *n.* **1.** The excretion of waste products from the body. **2.** A waste product.

ECG *abbr.* electrocardiogram; electrocardiograph

e·chi·no·coc·co·sis (ĭ-kī'nə-kə-kō'sĭs) *n., pl.* **-ses** (-sēz). **1.** Infestation with organisms of the genus *Echinococcus.* **2.** Hydatid disease.

e·chi·no·coc·cus (ĭ-kī'nə-kŏk'əs) *n., pl.* **-coc·ci** (-kŏk'sī', -kŏk'ī'). A parasitic tapeworm of the genus *Echinococcus.*

ech·o·a·cou·si·a (ĕk'ō-ə-kōō'zē-ə, -zhə) *n.* A subjective disturbance of hearing in which a sound heard appears to be repeated.

ech·o·a·or·tog·ra·phy (ĕk'ō-ā'ôr-tŏg'rə-fē) *n.* The use of ultrasound to diagnose and study the aorta, usually the abdominal aorta.

ech·o·car·di·o·gram (ĕk'ō-kär'dē-ə-grăm') *n.* A visual record produced by echocardiography.

ech·o·car·di·og·ra·phy (ĕk'ō-kär'dē-ŏg'rə-fē) *n.* The use of ultrasound in the diagnosis of cardiovascular lesions and in recording the size, motion, and composition of various cardiac structures. — **ech'o·car'di·o·graph'** (-ə-grăf') *n.* — **ech'o·car'di·o·graph'ic** *adj.*

ech·o diplacusis (ĕk'ō) *n.* A form of diplacusis in which the sound heard in the affected ear is repeated.

ech·o·en·ceph·a·lo·gram (ĕk'ō-ĕn-sĕf'ə-lə-grăm', -ə-lō-) *n.* A visual record produced by echoencephalography.

ech·o·en·ceph·a·log·ra·phy (ĕk'ō-ĕn-sĕf'ə-lŏg'rə-fē) *n.* The use of reflected ultrasound to create a detailed image of the brain. — **ech'o·en·ceph'a·lo·graph'** (-lə-grăf', -lō-) *n.* — **ech'o·en·ceph'a·lo·graph'ic** *adj.*

ech·o·gram (ĕk'ō-grăm') *n.* See **sonogram.**

e·chog·ra·phy (ĕ-kŏg'rə-fē) *n.* See **ultrasonography.**

ech·o·la·li·a (ĕk'ō-lā'lē-ə) *n.* **1.** The immediate and involuntary repetition of words or phrases just spoken by others, often a symptom of some types of schizophrenia. **2.** An infant's repetition of sounds made by others, a normal developmental occurrence. — **ech'o·la'lic** (-lĭk) *adj.*

e·chop·a·thy (ĕ-kŏp'ə-thē) *n.* A mental disorder in which the words or actions of another are imitated and repeated.

ech·o·prax·i·a (ĕk'ō-prăk'sē-ə) *n.* The involuntary imitation of movements made by another.

ech·o·vi·rus (ĕk'ō-vī'rəs) or **ECHO virus** (ĕk'ō) *n.* Any of a number of retroviruses of the family Picornaviridae, inhabiting the gastrointestinal tract and associated with various diseases, such as viral meningitis, mild respiratory infections, and severe diarrhea in newborns.

Eck fistula (ĕk) *n*. An anastomosis created between the vena cava and the portal vein to divert blood from the liver and to the heart.

ec·lamp·si·a (ĭ-klămp′sē-ə) *n*. Coma and convulsions during or immediately after pregnancy or parturition, characterized by edema, hypertension, and proteinuria. — **e·clamp′tic** (-tĭk) *adj*.

e·clipse period (ĭ-klĭps′) *n*. The period of time between infection by a virus and the appearance of the mature virus within the cell.

ec·mne·sia (ĕk-nē′zhə, -zē∍) *n*. Loss of memory for recent events.

E. co·li (ē kō′lī) *n*. A bacillus *(Escherichia coli)* normally found in the gastrointestinal tract of humans and animals and existing as numerous strains, some of which are responsible for diarrheal diseases.

e·con·a·zole (ĭ-kŏn′ə-zōl′) *n*. A broad-spectrum antifungal agent used in the treatment of athlete's foot and related fungal infections.

ec·o·tax·is (ĕk′ō-tăk′sĭs) *n*. The migration of lymphocytes from the thymus and bone marrow into specific lymphoid tissues.

é·cra·seur (ā-krä-zœr′) *n*. A surgical snare, especially one of great strength for cutting through the base or pedicle of a tumor.

ECT *abbr*. electroconvulsive therapy

ec·ta·si·a (ĕk-tā′zē-ə, -zhə) or **ec·ta·sis** (ĕk′tə-sĭs) *n*. Dilation or distention of a tubular structure or organ.

ec·thy·ma (ĕk-thī′mə) *n*. A pyogenic infection of the skin due to staphylococci or streptococci and characterized by adherent crusts beneath which ulceration occurs.

ec·to·an·ti·gen (ĕk′tō-ăn′tĭ-jən) *n*. A toxin or other inducer of antibody formation, separate or separable from its source.

ec·to·blast (ĕk′tə-blăst′) *n*. See **ectoderm**.

ec·to·car·di·a (ĕk′tō-kär′dē-ə) *n*. Congenital displacement of the heart.

ec·to·derm (ĕk′tə-dûrm′) *n*. The outermost of the three primary germ layers, from which the epidermis, nervous tissue, and sense organs develop. — **ec′to·der′mal, ec′to·der′mic** *adj*.

ec·to·der·mo·sis (ĕk′tō-dər-mō′sĭs) *n*., *pl*. **-ses** (-sēz). A disorder of an organ or tissue developed from the ectoderm.

ec·to·en·zyme (ĕk′tō-ĕn′zīm) *n*. **1.** An enzyme situated on the outer surface of a cell's membrane so that its active site is available to the exterior environment of the cell. **2.** Extracellular enzyme.

ec·to·mere (ĕk′tə-mēr′) *n*. Any of the blastomeres from which the ectoderm develops. — **ec′to·mer′ic** (-mēr′ĭk, -mĕr′-) *adj*.

ec·to·morph (ĕk′tə-môrf′) *n*. A person having a lean, slightly muscular build in which tissues derived from the embryonic ectoderm predominate. — **ec′to·mor′phic** *adj*. — **ec′to·mor′phy** *n*.

ec·to·par·a·site (ĕk′tə-păr′ə-sīt′) *n*. A parasite

that lives on the surface or exterior of the host organism. — **ec′to·par′a·sit′ic** (-sĭt′ĭk) *adj*. — **ec′-to·par′a·sit·ism** (-sĭ-tĭz′əm, -sī-) *n*.

ec·to·pi·a (ĕk-tō′pē-ə) or **ec·to·py** (ĕk′tə-pē) *n*. An abnormal location or position of an organ or a body part, occurring congenitally or as the result of injury. — **ec·top′ic** (-tŏp′ĭk) *adj*.

ec·top·ic (ĕk-tŏp′ĭk) *adj*. **1.** Out of place, as of an organ not in its proper position, or of a pregnancy occurring elsewhere than in the cavity of the uterus. **2.** Of or relating to a heartbeat that has its origin elsewhere than in the sinoatrial node.

ectopic beat *n*. A beat of the heart originating somewhere other than the sinoatrial node.

ectopic pregnancy *n*. Implantation and development of a fertilized ovum outside the uterus, as in a fallopian tube or the cervical canal.

ectopic tachycardia *n*. Tachycardia originating in a focus other than the sinus node.

ec·to·therm (ĕk′tə-thûrm′) *n*. An organism that regulates its body temperature largely by exchanging heat with its surroundings.

ec·trog·e·ny (ĕk-trŏj′ə-nē) *n*. Congenital absence of a body part. — **ec′tro·gen′ic** (-trə-jĕn′ĭk) *adj*.

ec·tro·me·li·a (ĕk′trō-mē′lē-ə) *n*. Congenital absence of one or more limbs. — **ec′tro·mel′ic** (-mĕl′ĭk, -mē′lĭk) *adj*.

ec·ze·ma (ĕk′sə-mə, ĕg′zə-, ĭg-zē′-) *n*. An acute or chronic noncontagious inflammation of the skin, characterized chiefly by redness, itching, and the outbreak of lesions that may discharge serous matter and become encrusted and scaly.

ED *abbr*. effective dose

e·de·ma (ĭ-dē′mə) *n*., *pl*. **-mas** or **-ma·ta** (-mə-tə). An accumulation of an excessive amount of watery fluid in cells, tissues, or serous cavities.

edema ne·o·na·to·rum (nē′ō-nā-tôr′əm) *n*. A diffuse, firm edema occurring in the newborn, beginning usually in the legs and spreading upward.

ed·ro·pho·ni·um chloride (ĕd′rə-fō′nē-əm) *n*. A competitive antagonist of skeletal muscle relaxants, such as curare derivatives, used as an antidote for curariform drugs, as a diagnostic agent in myasthenia gravis, and in myasthenic crisis.

EDTA (ē′dē-tē-ā′) *n*. Ethylenediaminetetraacetic acid; a crystalline acid that forms a sodium salt used as an antidote for metal poisoning, an anticoagulant, and an ingredient in a variety of industrial reagents.

EEG *abbr*. electroencephalogram

EENT *abbr*. eye, ear, nose, and throat

ef·fect (ĭ-fĕkt′) *n*. **1.** Something brought about by a cause or an agent; a result. **2.** The power to produce an outcome or achieve a result; influence. **3.** The condition of being in full force or execution. **4.** Something that produces a specific impression or supports a general design or intention. — *v*. **-fect·ed, -fect·ing, -fects. 1.** To bring into existence. **2.** To produce as a result. **3.** To bring about. — **ef·fect′er** *n*. — **ef·fect′i·ble** *adj*.

ef·fec·tor (ĭ-fĕk′tər) *n*. **1.** A muscle, a gland, or an organ capable of responding to a stimulus, especially a nerve impulse. **2.** A nerve ending that carries impulses to a muscle, a gland, or an organ and activates contraction or secretion.

ef·fem·i·na·tion (ĭ-fĕm'ə-nā'shən) n. The acquisition of feminine characteristics, either physiologically by women, or pathologically by persons of either sex.

ef·fer·ent (ĕf'ər-ənt) adj. Directed away from a central organ or section. — n. An efferent organ or body part, such as a blood vessel.

efferent duct n. Any of the small seminal ducts leading from the testis to the epididymis.

efferent nerve n. A nerve conveying impulses from the central nervous system to the periphery.

ef·fi·cien·cy (ĭ-fĭsh'ən-sē) n. The production of the desired effects or results with minimum waste of time, effort, or skill.

ef·flu·vi·um (ĭ-flōō'vē-əm) n., pl. **-vi·ums** or **-vi·a** (-vē-ə). A shedding, especially of hair.

ef·fu·sion (ĭ-fyōō'zhən) n. **1.** The escape of fluid from the blood vessels or lymphatics into the tissues or a cavity. **2.** The fluid so escaped.

e·flor·ni·thine hydrochloride (ĭ-flôr'nə-thēn') n. An antineoplastic and antiprotozoal orphan drug used in the treatment of *Pneumocystis carinii* pneumonia in AIDS and of sleeping sickness caused by *Trypanosoma brucei gambiense*.

e·gest (ē-jĕst') v. **e·gest·ed, e·gest·ing, e·gests.** To discharge or excrete from the body.

e·ges·ta (ē-jĕs'tə) pl.n. Unabsorbed food residues that are discharged from the digestive tract.

egg (ĕg) n. The female sexual cell or gamete; an ovum.

e·go (ē'gō, ĕg'ō) n. In psychoanalytic theory, the division of the psyche that is conscious, most immediately controls thought and behavior, and mediates between the person and external reality.

ego·bron·choph·o·ny (ē'gō-brŏng-kŏf'ə-nē) n. Egophony accompanied by bronchophony.

e·go·cen·tric (ē'gō-sĕn'trĭk, ĕg'ō-) adj. Marked by extreme concentration of attention upon oneself; self-centered. — **e'go·cen'tric n.**

ego ideal n. In psychoanalytic theory, the part of one's ego that contains an idealized self based on those people, especially parents and peers, one admires and wishes to emulate.

ego identity n. The sense of oneself as a distinct continuous entity.

e·go·ma·ni·a (ē'gō-mā'nē-ə, -mān'yə, ĕg'ō-) n. Extreme self-appreciation or preoccupation with the self.

e·goph·o·ny (ē-gŏf'ə-nē) n. A peculiar broken quality of the voice sounds, like the bleating of a goat, heard over lung tissue in cases of pleurisy with effusion.

e·go·trop·ic (ē'gō-trŏp'ĭk, -trō'pĭk, ĕg'ō-) n. Egocentric.

Eh·lers-Dan·los syndrome (ā'lərs-dän'lŏs, -dän-lōs') n. A hereditary disorder of the connnective tissue characterized by overelasticity and friability of the skin, excessive joint extensibility, and fragility of the cutaneous blood vessels.

ehr·lich·i·o·sis (âr-lĭk'ē-ō'sĭs) n. Infection with parasitic leukocytic rickettsiae of the genus *Ehr-*

lichia, especially by *E. sennetsu,* which produces manifestations in humans similar to those of Rocky Mountain spotted fever.

eighth cranial nerve n. See **vestibulocochlear nerve.**

ei·ko·nom·e·ter or **ei·co·nom·e·ter** (ī'kə-nŏm'-ĭ-tər) n. An instrument for detecting aniseikonia.

ein·stein·i·um (īn-stī'nē-əm) n. A radioactive transuranic element with atomic number 99, synthesized by neutron irradiation of plutonium.

e·jac·u·late (ĭ-jăk'yə-lāt') v. **-lat·ed, -lat·ing, -lates.** To eject or discharge abruptly, especially to discharge semen in orgasm. — n. (ĭ-jăk'yə-lĭt). Semen ejaculated in orgasm.

e·jac·u·la·tion (ĭ-jăk'yə-lā'shən) n. The act of ejaculating.

e·jac·u·la·ti·o pre·cox (ĭ-jăk'yə-lā'shē-ō prē'-kŏks') n. Premature ejaculation.

e·jac·u·la·to·ry duct (ĭ-jăk'yə-lə-tôr'ē) n. The duct that is formed by the union of the deferent duct and the excretory duct of the seminal vesicle and opens into the prostatic urethra.

e·jec·ta (ĭ-jĕk'tə) n. Something that has been ejected from the body.

e·jec·tion (ĭ-jĕk'shən) n. **1.** The act of driving or casting out by physical force from within. **2.** See **ejecta.**

ejection fraction n. The blood present in the ventricle at the end of diastole and expelled during the contraction of the heart.

ejection murmur n. A systolic murmur ending before the second heart sound, produced by ejection of blood into the aorta or pulmonary artery.

ejection sound n. A sharp sound that is heard on auscultation in early systole over the aortic or pulmonic area when the aorta or pulmonary artery is dilated.

EKG abbr. electrocardiogram; electrocardiograph

e·lab·o·ra·tion (ĭ-lăb'ə-rā'shən) n. **1.** The process of secreting a complex substance that has been synthesized from simpler substances. — **e·lab'o·rate'** v.

e·las·tance (ĭ-lăs'təns) n. A measure of the tendency of a hollow organ to recoil toward its original dimensions upon removal of a distending or compressing force. It is the reciprocal of compliance.

e·las·tase (ĭ-lăs'tās', -tāz') n. An enzyme found especially in pancreatic juice that catalyzes the hydrolysis of elastin.

e·las·tic (ĭ-lăs'tĭk) adj. Returning to the original shape after being distorted.

elastic bandage n. A stretchable bandage used to create localized pressure.

elastic cartilage n. A yellowish flexible cartilage in which the matrix is infiltrated by a network of elastic fibers; it occurs primarily in the external ear, eustachian tube, and some cartilages of the larynx and epiglottis.

e·las·ti·cin (ĭ-lăs'tĭ-sĭn) n. See **elastin.**

e·las·tic·i·ty (ĭ-lă-stĭs'ĭ-tē, ē'lă-) n. **1.** The condition or property of being elastic; flexibility. **2.** The property of returning to an initial form or state following deformation.

elastic membrane *n.* A membrane formed of elastic connective tissue fibers, such as that surrounding arteries.

elastic tissue *n.* Connective tissue in which elastic fibers predominate.

e·las·tin (ĭ-lăs′tĭn) *n.* A yellow, elastic, fibrous mucoprotein, similar to collagen, and the major connective tissue protein of elastic fibers.

e·las·to·fi·bro·ma (ĭ-lăs′tō-fī-brō′mə) *n.* A nonencapsulated slow-growing mass of poorly cellular, collagenous, fibrous tissue and elastic tissue, occurring usually in subscapular adipose tissue of elderly persons.

e·las·to·ma (ĭ-lă-stō′mə, ē′lă-) *n.* An inherited disorder of connective tissue characterized by slightly elevated yellowish plaques on the neck, armpits, abdomen, and thighs, associated with angioid streaks of the retina and similar elastic tissue degeneration in other organs.

e·las·tor·rhex·is (ĭ-lăs′tə-rĕk′sĭs) *n.* Fragmentation of elastic tissue in which the normal wavy strands appear shredded and clumped.

e·las·to·sis (ĭ-lă-stō′sĭs, ē′lă-) *n.* **1.** A degenerative change in elastic tissue. **2.** The degeneration of connective tissue in the skin, such that many tissues resemble elastin when stained.

El·a·vil (ĕl′ə-vĭl) A trademark used for a preparation of amitriptyline, an antidepressant drug.

el·bow (ĕl′bō′) *n.* **1.** The joint or bend of the arm between the forearm and the upper arm. **2.** The bony outer projection of this joint. **3.** Something having a bend or an angle similar to an elbow.

elbow bone *n.* See **ulna**.

el·bowed bougie (ĕl′bōd′) *n.* A bougie with a sharply angulated bend near its tip.

elbow joint *n.* A compound hinge joint between the humerus and the bones of the forearm.

eld·er·care (ĕl′dər-kâr′) *n.* Social and medical programs and facilities intended for the care and maintenance of the aged.

e·lec·tive mutism (ĭ-lĕk′tĭv) *n.* A form of childhood mutism characterized by the refusal to speak in social situations, although the ability to speak is intact.

E·lec·tra complex (ĭ-lĕk′trə) *n.* In psychoanalytic theory, a daughter's unconscious libidinal desire for her father.

e·lec·tri·cal alternation (ĭ-lĕk′trĭ-kəl) *n.* A varied alternation in the activity of the heart indicative of myocardial disease as measured by an electrocardiograph.

electrical failure *n.* Failure in which the cardiac inadequacy is secondary to disturbance of the electrical impulse.

e·lec·tro·an·al·ge·si·a (ĭ-lĕk′trō-ăn′əl-jē′zē-ə, -zhə) *n.* Analgesia induced by electric current.

e·lec·tro·an·es·the·sia (ĭ-lĕk′trō-ăn′ĭs-thē′zhə) *n.* Anesthesia produced by an electric current.

e·lec·tro·car·di·o·gram (ĭ-lĕk′trō-kär′dē-ə-grăm′) *n.* The curve traced by an electrocardiograph.

e·lec·tro·car·di·o·graph (ĭ-lĕk′trō-kär′dē-ə-grăf′) *n.* An instrument used in the detection and diagnosis of heart abnormalities that measures electrical potentials on the body surface and generates a record of the electrical currents associated with heart muscle activity. — **e·lec′tro·car′di·og′ra·phy** (-kär′dē-ŏg′rə-fē) *n.*

e·lec·tro·cau·ter·i·za·tion (ĭ-lĕk′trō-kô′tər-ĭ-zā′-shən) *n.* The cauterization of tissue by an electrocautery.

e·lec·tro·cau·ter·y (ĭ-lĕk′trō-kô′tə-rē) *n.* **1.** An instrument for directing a high-frequency current through a local area of tissue. **2.** A metal cauterizing instrument heated by electricity. **3.** The cauterization of tissue using such an instrument.

e·lec·tro·cer·e·bral silence (ĭ-lĕk′trō-sĕr′ə-brəl, -sə-rē′-) *n.* The absence of electrical activity in the brain measured by an electroencephalogram, indicating cerebral death.

e·lec·tro·co·ag·u·la·tion (ĭ-lĕk′trō-kō-ăg′yə-lā′-shən) *n.* Therapeutic use of a high-frequency electric current to bring about the coagulation and destruction of tissue.

e·lec·tro·coch·le·o·gram (ĭ-lĕk′trō-kŏk′lē-ə-grăm′, -kō′klē-) *n.* The record obtained by electrocochleography.

e·lec·tro·coch·le·og·ra·phy (ĭ-lĕk′trō-kŏk′lē-ŏg′rə-fē) *n.* A measurement of the electrical potentials generated in the inner ear as a result of sound stimulation.

e·lec·tro·con·trac·til·i·ty (ĭ-lĕk′trō-kŏn′trăk-tĭl′ĭ-tē) *n.* The power of contraction of muscular tissue in response to an electrical stimulus.

e·lec·tro·con·vul·sive therapy (ĭ-lĕk′trō-kən-vŭl′sĭv) *n.* Administration of electric current to the brain in order to induce unconsciousness and brief convulsions. Used in the treatment of certain mental disorders, especially acute depression.

e·lec·tro·cor·ti·co·gram (ĭ-lĕk′trō-kôr′tĭ-kə-grăm′) *n.* The tracing recorded during electrocorticography.

e·lec·tro·cor·ti·cog·ra·phy (ĭ-lĕk′trō-kôr′tĭ-kŏg′rə-fē) *n.* The technique of measuring the electrical activity of the cerebral cortex.

e·lec·trode (ĭ-lĕk′trōd′) *n.* A solid electric conductor through which an electric current enters or leaves an electrolytic cell or other medium.

e·lec·tro·der·mal audiometry (ĭ-lĕk′trō-dûr′-məl) *n.* A form of electrophysiologic audiometry used to determine hearing thresholds by measuring changes in skin resistance as a conditioned response to noise stimuli.

e·lec·tro·des·ic·ca·tion (ĭ-lĕk′trō-dĕs′ĭ-kā′shən) *n.* Destruction of lesions or sealing off of blood vessels by monopolar high-frequency electric current.

e·lec·tro·di·ag·no·sis (ĭ-lĕk′trō-dī′əg-nō′sĭs) *n.* Determination of the nature of a disease through observation of changes in electrical irritability.

e·lec·tro·di·al·y·sis (ĭ-lĕk′trō-dī-ăl′ĭ-sĭs) *n.* Dialysis at a rate increased by the application of an electric potential across the dialysis membrane, used especially to remove electrolytes from a colloidal suspension.

e·lec·tro·en·ceph·a·lo·gram (ĭ-lĕk′trō-ĕn-sĕf′ə-lə-grăm′) *n.* A graphic record of the electrical activity of the brain as recorded by an electroencephalograph.

e·lec·tro·en·ceph·a·lo·graph (ĭ-lĕk′trō-ĕn-sĕf′ə-lə-grăf′) *n.* An instrument that generates a record of the electrical activity of the brain by measuring electric potentials using electrodes attached to the scalp. — **e·lec′tro·en·ceph′a·lo·graph′ic** *adj.* — **e·lec′tro·en·ceph′a·log′ra·phy** (-lŏg′rə-fē) *n.*

e·lec·tro·en·dos·mo·sis (ĭ-lĕk′trō-ĕn′dŏz-mō′sĭs, -dŏs-) *n.* Endosmosis produced by an electric field.

e·lec·tro·gas·tro·gram (ĭ-lĕk′trō-găs′trə-grăm′) *n.* The graphic record obtained with the electrogastrograph.

e·lec·tro·gas·tro·graph (ĭ-lĕk′trō-găs′trə-grăf′) *n.* An instrument that produces a record of the electrical phenomena associated with gastric secretion and movement.

e·lec·tro·gram (ĭ-lĕk′trə-grăm′) *n.* A graphic record made from the measurement of electrical events in living tissues.

e·lec·tro·he·mo·sta·sis (ĭ-lĕk′trō-hē′mə-stā′sĭs, -hē-mŏs′tə-) *n.* The arrest of hemorrhage by means of a high frequency current to coagulate the bleeding part.

e·lec·tro·im·mu·no·dif·fu·sion (ĭ-lĕk′trō-ĭm′yə-nō-dĭ-fyōō′zhən, -ĭ-myōō′-) *n.* An immunochemical method that combines electrophoretic separation with immunodiffusion by incorporating antibody into the support medium.

e·lec·tro·ky·mo·gram (ĭ-lĕk′trō-kī′mə-grăm′) *n.* The graphic record produced by the electrokymograph.

e·lec·tro·ky·mo·graph (ĭ-lĕk′trō-kī′mə-grăf′) *n.* An apparatus for recording the movements of the heart and great vessels by observing changes in the x-ray silouettes.

e·lec·trol·y·sis (ĭ-lĕk-trŏl′ĭ-sĭs, ē′lĕk-) *n.* **1.** Chemical change, especially decomposition, produced in an electrolyte by an electric current. **2.** Destruction of living tissue, especially of hair roots, by means of an electric current.

e·lec·tro·lyte (ĭ-lĕk′trə-līt′) *n.* Any of various ions, such as sodium, potassium, or chloride, required by cells to regulate the electric charge and flow of water molecules across the cell membrane.

electrolyte balance *n.* The relative concentrations of ions in the body's extracellular and intracellular fluids, especially those produced from ionized salts such as sodium, potassium, or calcium.

e·lec·tro·lyt·ic (ĭ-lĕk′trə-lĭt′ĭk) *adj.* **1.** Of or relating to electrolysis. **2.** Produced by electrolysis. **3.** Of or relating to electrolytes.

e·lec·tro·mag·net·ic radiation (ĭ-lĕk′trō-măg-nĕt′ĭk) *n.* Radiation originating in a varying electromagnetic field, such as visible light, radio waves, x-rays, and gamma rays.

e·lec·tro·my·o·gram (ĭ-lĕk′trō-mī′ō-grăm′) *n.* A graphic record of the electrical activity of a muscle as recorded by an electromyograph.

e·lec·tro·my·o·graph (ĭ-lĕk′trō-mī′ə-grăf′) *n.* An instrument used in the diagnosis of neuromuscular disorders that produces an audio or visual record of the electrical activity of a skeletal muscle by means of an electrode inserted into the muscle or placed on the skin. — **e·lec′tro·my·og′ra·phy** (-mī-ŏg′rə-fē) *n.*

e·lec·tro·nar·co·sis (ĭ-lĕk′trō-när-kō′sĭs) *n.* An insensitivity to pain induced by the application of electric current to the body.

e·lec·tro·neu·rog·ra·phy (ĭ-lĕk′trō-nŏŏ-rŏg′rə-fē, -nyŏŏ-) *n.* A method of measuring and recording the electric changes and conduction velocities associated with impulses passing along peripheral nerves.

e·lec·tro·neu·ro·my·og·ra·phy (ĭ-lĕk′trō-nŏŏr′ō-mī-ŏg′rə-fē, -nyŏŏr′-) *n.* Electromyography in which the peripheral nerves to the muscle under study are stimulated with electric current.

e·lec·tron·ic fetal monitor (ĭ-lĕk-trŏn′ĭk, ē-lĕk-) *n.* An electronic device used to monitor fetal heartbeat and maternal uterine contractions.

e·lec·tron radiography (ĭ-lĕk′trŏn′) *n.* A radiographic imaging process in which the incident x-rays are converted to a latent charge image and developed by a special printing process to eliminate background fog and image noise.

e·lec·tro·nys·tag·mog·ra·phy (ĭ-lĕk′trō-nĭs′tăg-mŏg′rə-fē) *n.* A study of the recorded changes in corneoretinal potential caused by movements of the eye, used to assess nystagmus.

e·lec·tro·pho·re·sis (ĭ-lĕk′trō-fə-rē′sĭs) *n.* A method of separating substances, especially proteins, and analyzing molecular structure based on the rate of movement of each component in a colloidal suspension while under the influence of an electric field. — **e·lec′tro·pho·ret′ic** (-rĕt′ĭk) *adj.*

e·lec·tro·phren·ic respiration (ĭ-lĕk′trō-frĕn′ĭk) *n.* Respiration induced by rhythmic electrical stimulation at the motor points of the phrenic nerve, usually used in acute bulbar poliomyelitis.

e·lec·tro·ret·i·no·gram (ĭ-lĕk′trō-rĕt′n-ə-grăm′) *n.* A graphic record of the electrical activity of the retina. — **e·lec′tro·ret′i·nog′ra·phy** (-rĕt′n-ŏg′rə-fē) *n.*

e·lec·tro·scis·sion (ĭ-lĕk′trō-sĭzh′ən, -sĭsh′-) *n.* The cutting of tissues by an electrocautery knife.

e·lec·tro·shock (ĭ-lĕk′trō-shŏk′) *n.* See **electroconvulsive therapy.** — *v.* **-shocked, -shock·ing, -shocks.** To administer electroconvulsive therapy to an individual.

electroshock therapy *n.* See **electroconvulsive therapy.**

e·lec·tro·sur·ger·y (ĭ-lĕk′trō-sûr′jə-rē) *n.* The surgical use of high-frequency electric current for cutting or destroying tissue.

e·lec·tro·tax·is (ĭ-lĕk′trō-tăk′sĭs) *n.* Movement of organisms or cells in response to an electric current.

e·lec·tro·ther·a·peu·tics (ĭ-lĕk′trō-thĕr′ə-pyōō′tĭks) *n.* See **electrotherapy.**

e·lec·tro·ther·a·py (ĭ-lĕk′trō-thĕr′ə-pē) *n.* Medical therapy using electric currents.

e·lec·trot·ro·pism (ĭ-lĕk′trŏt′rə-pĭz′əm, ē′lĕk-, ĭ-lĕk′trō-trō′-) *n.* See **electrotaxis.**

el·e·doi·sin (ĕl′ĭ-doi′sĭn) *n.* A protein formed in the venom gland of several species of octopuses and used as a vasodilator and a contraction agent of extravascular smooth muscle.

el·e·ment (ĕl′ə-mənt) *n.* **1.** A substance that cannot be reduced to simpler substances by normal chemical means and that is composed of atoms having an identical number of protons in each nucleus. **2.** A fundamental, essential, or irreducible constituent of a composite entity.

element 110 *n.* An artificially produced radioactive element with atomic number 110.

element 111 *n.* An artificially produced radioactive element with atomic number 111.

element 112 *n.* An artificially produced radioactive element with atomic number 112.

el·e·phan·ti·a·sis (ĕl′ə-fən-tī′ə-sĭs) *n.* Chronic, often extreme enlargement and hardening of cutaneous and subcutaneous tissue, especially of the legs and external genitals, resulting from lymphatic obstruction and usually caused by infestation of the lymph glands and vessels with a filarial worm. — **el′e·phan·ti′ac′** (-tī′ăk′) *adj.*

elephantiasis neu·ro·ma·to·sa (nŏo-rō′mə-tō′-sə, nyŏo-) *n.* Enlargement of a limb due to diffuse neurofibromatosis of the skin and subcutaneous tissue.

el·e·phan·toid fever (ĕl′ə-făn′toid′, ĕl′ə-fən-toid′) *n.* Lymphangitis and fever marking the beginning of endemic elephantiasis.

el·e·va·tor (ĕl′ə-vā′tər) *n.* A surgical instrument used to elevate tissues or to raise a sunken part, such as a depressed fragment of bone.

e·lev·enth cranial nerve (ĭ-lĕv′ənth) *n.* See **accessory nerve.**

e·lim·i·na·tion (ĭ-lĭm′ə-nā′shən) *n.* The process of expelling or removing, especially of waste products from the body.

elimination diet *n.* A diet designed to detect the foods causing allergic reactions by separate and successive withdrawal of foods from the diet.

ELISA (ĭ-lī′zə, -sə) *n.* Enzyme-linked immunosorbent assay; a sensitive immunoassay that uses an enzyme linked to an antibody or antigen as a marker for the detection of a specific protein, especially an antigen or antibody; often used to determine exposure to a particular infectious agent, such as HIV, by identifying antibodies present in a blood sample.

e·lix·ir (ĭ-lĭk′sər) *n.* A sweetened aromatic solution of alcohol and water, used as a vehicle for medicine.

El·li·ot's operation (ĕl′ē-əts) *n.* A surgical procedure in which the eyeball is trephined at the corneoscleral margin to relieve tension in glaucoma.

el·lip·soi·dal joint (i-lĭp-soid′l, ĕl′ĭp-, ē′lĭp-) *n.* A modified biaxial ball-and-socket joint in which the joint surfaces are elongated or ellipsoidal.

el·lip·to·cyte (ĭ-lĭp′tə-sīt′) *n.* An elliptical red blood cell.

e·ma·ci·a·tion (ĭ-mā′shē-ā′shən) *n.* The process of losing so much flesh as to become extremely thin.

em·a·na·tion (ĕm′ə-nā′shən) *n.* Something that issues from a source; an emission.

e·mas·cu·la·tion (ĭ-măs′kyə-lā′shən) *n.* The surgical removal of the testes and penis of a male; castration.

em·balm (ĕm-bäm′) *v.* **-balmed, -balm·ing, -balms.** To treat a corpse with preservatives in order to prevent decay.

Emb·den–Mey·er·hof pathway (ĕm′dən-mī′ər-hŏf′) *n.* The anaerobic metabolic pathway by which glucose, especially the glycogen in human muscle, is converted to lactic acid.

em·bo·le (ĕm′bə-lē) *n.* Emboly.

em·bo·lec·to·my (ĕm′bə-lĕk′tə-mē) *n.* Surgical removal of an embolus.

em·bo·lism (ĕm′bə-lĭz′əm) *n.* **1.** Obstruction or occlusion of a blood vessel by an embolus. **2.** An embolus.

em·bo·li·za·tion (ĕm′bə-lĭ-zā′shən) *n.* **1.** The process by which a blood vessel or organ is obstructed by an embolus or other mass. **2.** The surgical introduction of various substances into the circulatory system to obstruct specific blood vessels, used to control hemorrhage.

em·bo·lo·la·li·a (ĕm′bə-lō-lā′lē-ə) *n.* A speech disorder in which meaningless words or sounds are interjected into sentences.

em·bo·lus (ĕm′bə-ləs) *n., pl.* **-li** (-lī′). A mass, such as an air bubble, a detached blood clot, or a foreign body, that travels through the bloodstream and lodges so as to obstruct or occlude a blood vessel.

em·bo·ly (ĕm′bə-lē) *n.* The formation of a gastrula from a blastula by invagination.

em·bro·ca·tion (ĕm′brə-kā′shən) *n.* **1.** The act or process of moistening and rubbing a part of the body with a liniment or lotion. **2.** A liniment or lotion.

em·bry·ec·to·my (ĕm′brē-ĕk′tə-mē) *n.* Surgical removal of an embryo, especially one implanted outside of the uterus.

em·bry·o (ĕm′brē-ō′) *n., pl.* **-os. 1.** An organism in its early stages of development, especially before it has reached a distinctively recognizable form. **2.** An organism at any time before full development or birth. **3.** In humans, the prefetal product of conception from implantation through the eighth week of development.

em·bry·o·gen·e·sis (ĕm′brē-ō-jĕn′ĭ-sĭs) or **em·bry·og·e·ny** (-ŏj′ə-nē) *n.* The development and growth of an embryo, especially the period from the second week through the eighth week following conception. — **em′bry·o·gen′ic** (-jĕn′ĭk) *adj.*

em·bry·ol·o·gist (ĕm′brē-ŏl′ə-jĭst) *n.* A specialist in embryology.

em·bry·ol·o·gy (ĕm′brē-ŏl′ə-jē) *n.* **1.** The branch of biology that deals with the formation, early growth, and development of living organisms. **2.** The embryonic structure or development of a particular organism.

em·bry·o·ma (ĕm′brē-ō′mə) *n.* See **embryonal tumor.**

em·bry·on·al carcinoma (ĕm′brē-ə-nəl) *n.* A malignant neoplasm of the testis.

embryonal carcinosarcoma *n.* See **blastoma**.

embryonal rhabdomyosarcoma *n.* A form of rhabdomyosarcoma occurring in infants and children and characterized by malignant tumors of loose, spindle-celled tissue in many parts of the body in addition to skeletal muscles.

embryonal tumor or **embryonic tumor** *n.* A usually malignant tumor arising during intrauterine or early postnatal development from the rudiments of an organ or from immature tissue and forming immature structures characteristic of the part from which it arises.

em·bry·on·ic (ĕm′brē-ŏn′ĭk) or **em·bry·on·al** (ĕm′brē-ə-nəl) *adj.* Of, relating to, or being an embryo. — **em′bry·on′ic·al·ly** *adv.*

embryonic disk *n.* A flattened, disklike region of cells from which the embryo develops in the second week of pregnancy.

embryonic membrane *n.* See **fetal membrane**.

em·bry·op·a·thy (ĕm′brē-ŏp′ə-thē) *n.* A developmental disorder in an embryo, especially one caused by a disease such as rubella.

em·bry·ot·o·my (ĕm′brē-ŏt′ə-mē) *n.* The cutting of the fetus while in the uterus to aid its removal when delivery is impossible by natural means.

em·bry·o·tox·ic·i·ty (ĕm′brē-ō-tŏk-sĭs′ĭ-tē) *n.* The state of being toxic to an embryo, resulting in death or in abnormal development.

em·bry·o·tox·on (ĕm′brē-ō-tŏk′sŏn′, -ən) *n.* A congenital opacity of the cornea's marginal ring.

embryo transfer *n.* After artificial insemination, the process by which the fertilized ovum is transferred as a blastocyst to the recipient's uterus.

em·bry·o·troph (ĕm′brē-ə-trŏf′) *n.* The nutritive material supplied to the embryo of a placental mammal during development. — **em′bry·o·troph′ic** (-trŏf′ĭk) *adj.*

em·bry·ot·ro·phy (ĕm′brē-ŏt′rə-fē) *n.* The nutrition of the embryo.

e·med·ul·late (ĭ-mĕd′l-āt′, ĭ-mĕd′yə-lāt′) *v.* **-lat·ed, -lat·ing, -lates.** To extract marrow or pith.

e·mer·gen·cy medical technician (ĭ-mûr′jən-sē) *n.* A person trained and certified to appraise and initiate the administration of emergency care for victims of trauma or acute illness before or during transportation of the victims to a health care facility via ambulance or aircraft.

emergency medicine *n.* The branch of medicine that deals with evaluation and initial treatment of medical conditions caused by trauma or sudden illness.

emergency room *n.* The section of a health care facility intended to provide rapid treatment for victims of sudden illness or trauma.

emergency theory *n.* See **fight-or-flight reaction**.

em·e·sis (ĕm′ĭ-sĭs) *n., pl.* **-ses** (-sēz′). The act of vomiting.

e·met·ic (ĭ-mĕt′ĭk) *n.* An agent that causes vomiting. — *adj.* Causing vomiting.

EMG *abbr.* electromyogram

EMG syndrome *n.* A hereditary disorder characterized by exomphalos, macroglossia, and gigantism, often with neonatal hypoglycemia.

e·mic·tion (ĭ-mĭk′shən) *n.* See **urination**.

em·i·gra·tion (ĕm′ĭ-grā′shən) *n.* The passage of white blood cells through the walls of small blood vessels.

em·i·nence (ĕm′ə-nəns) *n.* The projecting prominent part of an organ, especially a bone.

e·mis·sion (ĭ-mĭsh′ən) *n.* A discharge of fluid from a living body, usually a seminal discharge.

em·men·a·gogue (ĭ-mĕn′ə-gôg′) *n.* A drug or an agent that induces or hastens menstrual flow. — **em·men′a·gog′ic** (-gŏj′ĭk) *adj.*

em·men·i·a (ĭ-mĕn′ē-ə, ĭ-mē′nē-ə) *n.* See **menses**. — **em·men′ic** (ĭ-mĕn′ĭk) *adj.*

em·me·tro·pi·a (ĕm′ĭ-trō′pē-ə) *n.* The condition of the normal eye when parallel rays are focused exactly on the retina and vision is perfect. — **em′·me·trop′ic** (-trŏp′ĭk, -trō′pĭk) *adj.*

em·o·din (ĕm′ə-dĭn′) *n.* An orange crystalline compound found in plants, and used as a laxative.

e·mol·lient (ĭ-mŏl′yənt) *adj.* Softening and soothing, especially to the skin. — *n.* An agent that softens or soothes the skin.

e·mo·tion (ĭ-mō′shən) *n.* An intense mental state that arises subjectively rather than through conscious effort, often accompanied by physiological changes. — **e·mo′tion·al** (ĭ-mō′shə-nəl) *adj.*

emotional deprivation *n.* The lack of adequate and appropriate interpersonal and environmental interaction, usually in the early developmental years.

emotional disorder *n.* An emotional illness.

emotional illness *n.* A psychological disorder characterized by irrational and uncontrollable fears, persistent anxiety, or extreme hostility.

e.m.p. *abbr. Latin.* ex modo praescripto (in the manner prescribed)

em·pa·thize (ĕm′pə-thīz′) *v.* **-thized, -thiz·ing, -thiz·es.** To feel empathy in relation to another.

em·pa·thy (ĕm′pə-thē) *n.* **1.** Direct identification with, understanding of, and vicarious experience of another person's situation, feelings, and motives. **2.** The projection of one's own feelings or emotional state onto an object or animal. — **em′pa·thet′ic** (-thĕt′ĭk), **em·path′ic** (-păth′ĭk) *adj.*

em·phy·se·ma (ĕm′fĭ-sē′mə, -zē′-) *n.* **1.** A pathological condition of the lungs marked by an abnormal increase in the size of the air spaces, resulting in labored breathing and an increased susceptibility to infection. It can be caused by irreversible alveolar expansion or by destruction of alveolar walls. **2.** An abnormal distention of body tissues caused by retention of air. — **em′phy·sem′a·tous** (-sĕm′ə-təs, -sē′mə-, -zĕm′ə-, -zē′mə-) *adj.* — **em′phy·se′mic** *adj. & n.*

em·pir·i·cism (ĕm-pĕr′ĭ-sĭz′əm) *n.* **1.** Employment of empirical methods, as in science. **2.** The practice of medicine that disregards scientific theory and relies solely on practical experience. — **em·pir′i·cist** *n.*

em·py·e·ma (ĕm′pī-ē′mə) *n., pl.* **-ma·ta** (-mə-tə).

The presence of pus in a body cavity, especially the pleural cavity. — **em′py·e′mic** *adj.*

em·py·e·sis (ĕm′pī-ē′sĭs) *n., pl.* **-ses** (-sēz). A pustular eruption.

EMS *abbr.* electrical muscle stimulation

EMT *abbr.* emergency medical technician

e·mul·sion (ĭ-mŭl′shən) *n.* A suspension of small globules of one liquid in a second liquid with which the first will not mix. — **e·mul′sive** *adj.*

e·nal·a·pril ma·le·ate (ĭ-năl′ə-prĭl mā′lē-āt′, mə-lē′ət) *n.* An angiotensin-converting enzyme inhibitor used as an antihypertensive agent.

e·nam·el (ĭ-năm′əl) *n.* The hard, calcareous substance covering the exposed portion of a tooth.

e·nam·e·lo·gen·e·sis (ĭ-năm′ə-lō-jĕn′ĭ-sĭs) *n.* See **amelogenesis**.

enarthrodial joint *n.* See **ball-and-socket joint**.

en·ar·thro·sis (ĕn′är-thrō′sĭs) *n.* See **ball-and-socket joint**.

en·cap·su·late (ĕn-kăp′sə-lāt′) *v.* **-lat·ed, -lat·ing, -lates. 1.** To form a capsule or sheath around. **2.** To become encapsulated. — **en·cap′su·la′tion** *n.*

en·ceph·a·lal·gi·a (ĕn-sĕf′ə-lăl′jē-ə, -jə) *n.* Pain in the head; headache.

en·ceph·a·lat·ro·phy (ĕn-sĕf′ə-lăt′rə-fē) *n.* Atrophy of the brain. — **en·ceph′a·la·troph′ic** (-lə-trŏf′ĭk) *adj.*

en·ceph·a·li·tis (ĕn-sĕf′ə-lī′tĭs) *n., pl.* **-lit·i·des** (-lĭt′ĭ-dēz). Inflammation of the brain. — **en·ceph′a·lit′ic** (-lĭt′ĭk) *adj.*

encephalitis le·thar·gi·ca (lə-thär′jĭ-kə) *n.* A viral epidemic encephalitis marked by apathy, paralysis of an eye muscle, and extreme weakness.

en·ceph·a·lo·cele (ĕn-sĕf′ə-lō-sēl′) *n.* A congenital gap in the skull, usually with protrusion of brain material.

en·ceph·a·lo·fa·cial angiomatosis (ĕn-sĕf′ə-lō-fā′shəl) *n.* See **Sturge-Weber syndrome**.

en·ceph·a·lo·gram (ĕn-sĕf′ə-lə-grăm′, -ə-lō-) *n.* **1.** An x-ray picture of the brain taken by encephalography. **2.** An electroencephalogram.

en·ceph·a·lo·graph (ĕn-sĕf′ə-lə-grăf′, -ə-lō-) *n.* **1.** An encephalogram. **2.** An electroencephalogram.

en·ceph·a·log·ra·phy (ĕn-sĕf′ə-lŏg′rə-fē) *n.* Radiographic examination of the brain in which some of the cerebrospinal fluid is replaced with air or another gas that acts as a contrasting medium. — **en·ceph′a·lo·graph′ic** (-ə-lə-grăf′ĭk, -ə-lō-) *adj.* — **en·ceph′a·lo·graph′i·cal·ly** *adv.*

en·ceph·a·lo·ma (ĕn-sĕf′ə-lō′mə) *n., pl.* **-mas** or **-ma·ta** (-mə-tə). A tumor or swelling of the brain.

en·ceph·a·lo·ma·la·ci·a (ĕn-sĕf′ə-lō-mə-lā′shē-ə, -shə) *n.* Softening of brain tissue, usually due to vascular insufficiency or degenerative changes.

en·ceph·a·lo·men·in·gi·tis (ĕn-sĕf′ə-lō-mĕn′ĭn-jī′tĭs) *n.* See **meningoencephalitis**.

en·ceph·a·lo·my·e·li·tis (ĕn-sĕf′ə-lō-mī′ə-lī′tĭs) *n.* An acute inflammation of the brain and spinal cord.

en·ceph·a·lo·my·e·lo·cele (ĕn-sĕf′ə-lō-mī′ə-lə-sēl′) *n.* A congenital defect in the occipital region with herniation of the meninges, medulla, and spinal cord.

en·ceph·a·lo·my·e·lo·neu·rop·a·thy (ĕn-sĕf′ə-lō-mī′ə-lō-nŏō-rŏp′ə-thē, -nyŏō-) *n.* Any of various diseases involving the brain, spinal cord, and peripheral nervous system.

en·ceph·a·lo·my·e·lop·a·thy (ĕn-sĕf′ə-lō-mī′ə-lŏp′ə-thē) *n.* Any of various diseases involving both the brain and spinal cord.

en·ceph·a·lo·my·e·lo·ra·dic·u·lop·a·thy (ĕn-sĕf′ə-lō-mī′ə-lō-rə-dĭk′yə-lŏp′ə-thē) *n.* Any of various diseases involving the brain, spinal cord, and spinal roots.

en·ceph·a·lo·my·o·car·di·tis (ĕn-sĕf′ə-lō-mī′ō-kär-dī′tĭs) *n.* An acute viral disease characterized by inflammation and degeneration of skeletal and cardiac muscle and lesions of the central nervous system.

en·ceph·a·lon (ĕn-sĕf′ə-lŏn′) *n., pl.* **-la** (-lə). See **brain**. — **en·ceph′a·lous** *adj.*

en·ceph·a·lop·a·thy (ĕn-sĕf′ə-lŏp′ə-thē) *n.* Any of various diseases of the brain. — **en·ceph′a·lo·path′ic** (-lə-păth′ĭk) *adj.*

en·ceph·a·lo·scle·ro·sis (ĕn-sĕf′ə-lō-sklə-rō′sĭs) *n.* A hardening of the brain.

en·ceph·a·lo·sis (ĕn-sĕf′ə-lō′sĭs) *n.* Any of various organic diseases of the brain.

en·ceph·a·lot·o·my (ĕn-sĕf′ə-lŏt′ə-mē) *n.* Dissection or incision of the brain.

en·ceph·a·lo·tri·gem·i·nal angiomatosis (ĕn-sĕf′ə-lō-trī-jĕm′ə-nəl) *n.* See **Sturge-Weber syndrome**.

en·chon·dro·ma (ĕn′kŏn-drō′mə) *n.* A benign cartilaginous growth starting within the medullary cavity of a bone originally formed from cartilage. — **en′chon·dro′ma·tous** (-drō′mə-təs, -drŏm′ə-) *adj.*

en·chon·dro·ma·to·sis (ĕn-kŏn′drō-mə-tō′sĭs, ĕn′kŏn-drō′-) *n.* A congenital but nonfamilial disorder involving tubular bones, especially of the hands and feet, and characterized by proliferation of cartilage in the metaphyses that cause distorted lengthening or fractures.

en·chon·dro·sar·co·ma (ĕn′kŏn′drō-sär-kō′mə) *n.* A malignant neoplasm of cartilage cells derived from an enchondroma or occurring in the same locations.

en·clave (ĕn′klāv′, ŏn′-) *n.* A detached mass of tissue enclosed in tissue of another kind.

en·cod·ing (ĕn-kō′dĭng) *n.* The first of three stages in the memory process, involving processes associated with receiving or briefly registering stimuli through one or more of the senses and modifying that information; loss of information from this stage occurs rapidly unless the next stages, storage and retrieval, are activated.

en·co·pre·sis (ĕn′kŏ-prē′sĭs) *n.* The uncontrolled or involuntary passage of feces for psychological reasons.

en·coun·ter group (ĕn-koun′tər) *n.* A psychotherapy group in which participants try to increase their sensitivity and gain insight into their emotions by expressing their own emotions and responding to emotions of others in the group.

en·cyst (ĕn-sĭst′) *v.* **-cyst·ed, -cyst·ing, -cysts.** To enclose or become enclosed in a cyst. — **en·cyst'-ment, en'cys·ta'tion** *n.*

encysted calculus *n.* A urinary calculus enclosed in a sac developed from the wall of the bladder.

end·ar·ter·ec·to·my (ĕn'där-tə-rĕk'tə-mē) *n.* Surgical excision of the inner lining of an artery that is clogged with atherosclerotic buildup.

end·ar·te·ri·tis (ĕn'där-tə-rī'tĭs) or **en·do·ar·te·ri·tis** (ĕn'dō-är'tə-) *n.* Inflammation of the intima of an artery.

end artery *n.* An artery with insufficient anastomoses to maintain viability of the tissue supplied if occlusion of the artery occurs.

end·brain (ĕnd'brān') *n.* See **telencephalon.**

end-diastolic volume *n.* The amount of blood in the ventricle immediately before a cardiac contraction begins; used as a measurement of diastolic function.

en·dem·ic (ĕn-dĕm'ĭk) *adj.* Prevalent in or restricted to a particular region, community, or group of people. Used of a disease. — **en·dem'i·cal·ly** *adv.* — **en·dem'ism** *n.*

endemic stability *n.* A situation in which all factors influencing disease occurrence are relatively stable, resulting in little fluctuation in disease incidence over time.

endocardial fibroelastosis *n.* A congenital condition characterized by thickening of the inner lining of the left ventricle, thickening and malformation of the cardiac valves, and hypertrophy of the heart.

en·do·car·di·tis (ĕn'dō-kär-dī'tĭs) *n.* Inflammation of the endocardium. — **en'do·car·dit'ic** (-dĭt'ĭk) *adj.*

en·do·car·di·um (ĕn'dō-kär'dē-əm) *n., pl.* **-di·a** (-dē-ə). The thin serous membrane, composed of endothelial and subendothelial tissue, that lines the interior of the heart. — **en'do·car'di·al** *adj.*

en·do·cer·vix (ĕn'dō-sûr'vĭks) *n.* The mucous membrane of the uterine cervical canal.

en·do·chon·dral bone (ĕn'dō-kŏn'drəl) *n.* See **cartilage bone.**

en·do·cra·ni·um (ĕn'dō-krā'nē-əm) *n., pl.* **-ni·a** (-nē-ə). **1.** The outermost layer of the dura mater. **2.** The inner surface of the skull.

en·do·crine (ĕn'də-krĭn, -krēn', -krīn') *adj.* **1.** Secreting internally, most commonly into the systemic circulation. **2.** Of or relating to endocrine glands or the hormones secreted by them. — *n.* **1.** The secretion of an endocrine gland; a hormone. **2.** An endocrine gland.

endocrine gland *n.* Any of various ductless glands, such as the thyroid, adrenal, or pituitary, producing hormonal secretions that pass directly into the bloodstream.

en·do·cri·nol·o·gy (ĕn'də-krə-nŏl'ə-jē) *n.* The study of the glands and hormones of the body and their related disorders. — **en'do·cri'no·log'ic** (-krĭn'ə-lŏj'ĭk), **en'do·crin'o·log'i·cal** *adj.* — **en'do·cri·nol'o·gist** *n.*

en·do·cri·no·ma (ĕn'də-krə-nō'mə) *n.* A tumor with endocrine tissue that retains the function of the parent organ, usually to an excessive degree.

en·do·cri·nop·a·thy (ĕn'də-krə-nŏp'ə-thē) *n.* A disorder in the function of an endocrine gland and the consequences thereof.

en·do·cy·to·sis (ĕn'dō-sī-tō'sĭs) *n.* A process of cellular ingestion by which the plasma membrane folds inward to bring substances into the cell. — **en'do·cyt'ic** (-sĭt'ĭk), **en'do·cy·tot'ic** (-sī-tŏt'-ĭk) *adj.* — **en'do·cy·tose'** (-tōs') *v.*

en·do·derm (ĕn'də-dûrm') or **en·to·derm** (ĕn'tə-) *n.* The innermost of the three primary germ layers, developing into the gastrointestinal tract, lungs, and associated structures. — **en'do·der'-mal** *adj.*

en·do·en·ter·i·tis (ĕn'dō-ĕn'tə-rī'tĭs) *n.* Inflammation of the intestinal mucous membrane.

en·do·en·zyme (ĕn'dō-ĕn'zīm') *n.* An enzyme that acts on or is retained within the cell producing it.

en·dog·e·nous (ĕn-dŏj'ə-nəs) *adj.* **1.** Originating or produced within an organism, a tissue, or a cell. **2.** Caused by factors within the body. Used of a disease. — **en·dog'e·nous·ly** *adv.* — **en·dog'e·ny** *n.*

endogenous depression *n.* A group of symptoms that resemble depression but are not precipitated by a stressful experience, especially psychomotor agitation or retardation, insomnia and early morning awakening, weight loss, excessive guilt, and a lack of reactivity to one's environment.

endogenous infection *n.* An infection caused by an infectious agent that was already present in the body but had previously been inapparent or dormant.

en·do·in·tox·i·ca·tion (ĕn'dō-ĭn-tŏk'sĭ-kā'shən) *n.* Poisoning by an endogenous toxin.

en·do·lymph (ĕn'də-lĭmf') *n.* The fluid contained in the membranous labyrinth of the inner ear. — **en'do·lym·phat'ic** (-lĭm-făt'ĭk) *adj.*

en·do·me·tri·oid tumor (ĕn'dō-mē'trē-oid') *n.* A tumor of the ovary containing epithelial or stromal elements resembling endometrial tissue.

en·do·me·tri·o·ma (ĕn'dō-mē'trē-ō'mə) *n.* A circumscribed mass of endometrial tissue occurring outside the uterus in endometriosis.

en·do·me·tri·o·sis (ĕn'dō-mē'trē-ō'sĭs) *n.* A condition, usually resulting in pain and dysmenorrhea, characterized by the abnormal occurrence of functional endometrial tissue outside the uterus, frequently in the form of cysts containing altered blood.

en·do·me·tri·tis (ĕn'dō-mĭ-trī'tĭs) *n.* Inflammation of the endometrium.

en·do·me·tri·um (ĕn'dō-mē'trē-əm) *n., pl.* **-tri·a** (-trē-ə). The glandular mucous membrane comprising the inner layer of the uterine wall. — **en'-do·me'tri·al** *adj.*

en·do·morph (ĕn'də-môrf') *n.* A person having a build characterized by relative prominence of the abdomen and other soft body parts developed from the embryonic endodermal layer. — **en'do·mor'phic** *adj.* — **en'do·mor'phy** *n.*

en·do·my·o·car·di·tis (ĕn'dō-mī'ō-kär-dī'tĭs) *n.*

Inflammation of the endocardium and the myocardium.

en·do·my·o·me·tri·tis (ĕn′dō-mī′ō-mĭ-trī′tĭs) n. Sepsis involving the tissues of the uterus occurring after a cesarean section.

en·do·mys·i·um (ĕn′dō-mĭs′ē-əm, -mĭz′-) n. The fine connective tissue sheathing a muscle fiber.

en·do·neu·ri·um (ĕn′dō-nŏōr′ē-əm, -nyŏōr′-) n., pl. **-neu·ri·a** (-nŏōr′ē-ə, -nyŏōr′-). The delicate connective tissue enveloping individual nerve fibers within a peripheral nerve.

en·do·par·a·site (ĕn′dō-păr′ə-sīt′) n. A parasite living within the body of its host. — **en′do·par·a·sit′ic** (-sĭt′ĭk) adj. — **en′do·par′a·sit·ism** (-sĭ-tĭz′-əm) n.

en·do·per·i·car·di·tis (ĕn′dō-pĕr′ĭ-kär-dī′tĭs) n. Simultaneous inflammation of the endocardium and the pericardium.

en·do·per·i·to·ni·tis (ĕn′dō-pĕr′ĭ-tn-ī′tĭs) n. Superficial inflammation of the peritoneum.

en·do·plas·mic reticulum (ĕn′də-plăz′mĭk) n. The cytoplasmic network composed of tubules or cisternae. Some membranes carry ribosomes on their surfaces while others are smooth.

en·do·rec·tal pull-through procedure (ĕn′dō-rĕk′təl) n. Removal of diseased rectal mucosa along with resection of the lower bowel, followed by anastomosis of the proximal stump to the anus, in order to spare rectal muscle function.

end organ n. The encapsulated termination of a sensory nerve.

en·dor·phin (ĕn-dôr′fĭn) n. Any of a group of peptide hormones that bind to opiate receptors and are found mainly in the brain. Endorphins reduce the sensation of pain and affect emotions.

en·do·scope (ĕn′də-skōp′) n. An instrument for examining visually the interior of a bodily canal or hollow organ such as the colon. — **en′do·scop′ic** (-skŏp′ĭk) adj. — **en′do·scop′ic·al·ly** adv.

endoscopic biopsy n. A biopsy obtained by instruments passed through an endoscope or by a needle introduced under endoscopic guidance.

endoscopic retrograde cholangiopancreatography n. The use of an endoscope to inspect the pancreatic duct and common bile duct. It may also involve biopsy or the introduction of contrast material for radiographic examination.

en·dos·co·pist (ĕn-dŏs′kə-pĭst) n. A specialist in the use of an endoscope.

en·dos·co·py (ĕn-dŏs′kə-pē) n. Examination of the interior of a canal or hollow organ by means of an endoscope.

en·do·skel·e·ton (ĕn′dō-skĕl′ĭ-tn) n. An internal supporting skeleton, derived from the mesoderm, that is characteristic of vertebrates and certain invertebrates. — **en′do·skel′e·tal** (-ĭ-tl) adj.

en·dos·mo·sis (ĕn′dŏz-mō′sĭs, -dŏs-) n. The passage of a fluid inward through a permeable membrane, as of a cell, toward a fluid of higher concentration. — **en′dos·mot′ic** (-mŏt′ĭk) adj. — **en′dos·mot′i·cal·ly** adv.

en·do·so·nos·co·py (ĕn′dō-sə-nŏs′kə-pē) n. A sonographic study carried out by transducers in-

serted into the body as miniature probes in the urethra, bladder, or rectum.

en·dos·te·o·ma (ĕn′dŏ-stē-ō′mə) or **en·dos·to·ma** (ĕn′dŏ-stō′mə) n. A benign tumor of bone tissue in the medullary cavity of a bone.

en·dos·te·um (ĕn-dŏs′tē-əm) n., pl. **-te·a** (-tē-ə). The thin layer of cells lining the medullary cavity of a bone. — **en·dos′te·al** adj.

en·do·the·li·o·ma (ĕn′dō-thē′lē-ō′mə) n., pl. **-mas** or **-ma·ta** (-mə-tə). Any of various benign or occasionally malignant neoplasms derived from the endothelial tissue of blood or lymph vessels.

en·do·the·li·o·sis (ĕn′dō-thē′lē-ō′sĭs) n. Proliferation of endothelium.

en·do·the·li·um (ĕn′dō-thē′lē-əm) n., pl. **-li·a** (-lē-ə). A thin layer of flat epithelial cells that lines serous cavities, lymph vessels, and blood vessels. — **en′do·the′li·al** adj.

en·do·therm (ĕn′də-thûrm) n. An organism that generates heat to maintain its body temperature.

en·do·ther·mic (ĕn′dō-thûr′mĭk) or **en·do·ther·mal** (-məl) adj. **1.** Of or relating to a chemical reaction during which there is absorption of heat. **2.** Of or relating to an endotherm; warm-blooded. — **en′do·ther′my** n.

en·do·tox·e·mi·a (ĕn′dō-tŏk-sē′mē-ə) n. The presence of endotoxins in the blood, which, if from gram-negative rod-shaped bacteria, may cause hemorrhages, renal necrosis, and shock.

en·do·tox·i·co·sis (ĕn′dō-tŏk′sĭ-kō′sĭs) n. Poisoning by an endotoxin.

en·do·tox·in (ĕn′dō-tŏk′sən) n. A toxin that forms an integral part of the cell wall of certain bacteria and is only released upon destruction of the bacterial cell. — **en′do·tox′ic** adj.

en·do·tra·che·al anesthesia (ĕn′də-trā′kē-əl) n. An inhalation anesthetic technique in which anesthetic and respiratory gases pass through a tube placed in the trachea via the mouth or nose.

endotracheal intubation n. The passage of a tube through the nose or mouth into the trachea for maintenance of the airway.

endotracheal tube n. A tube inserted into the trachea to provide a passageway for air.

end plate or **endplate** n. The area of synaptic contact between a motor nerve and a muscle fiber.

end stage n. The late, fully developed phase of a disease.

end-systolic volume n. The amount of blood in the ventricle at the end of the cardiac ejection period and immediately preceding ventricular relaxation; used as a measure of systolic function.

en·e·ma (ĕn′ə-mə) n., pl. **-mas.** Injection of liquid into the rectum through the anus for cleansing, for stimulating evacuation of the bowels, or for other therapeutic or diagnostic purposes.

en·er·gy (ĕn′ər-jē) n. The capacity for work or vigorous activity; vigor; power.

enervate v. **-vat·ed, -vat·ing, -vates.** To remove a nerve or part of a nerve. — **en′er·va′tion** n.

ENG abbr. electronystagmography

en·gage·ment (ĕn-gāj′mənt) n. The entrance of

the fetal head or presenting part into the upper opening of the maternal pelvis.

en·gorge (ĕn-gôrj′) v. **-gorged, -gorg·ing, -gorg·es.** To fill to excess, as with blood or other fluid. — **en·gorge′ment** n.

en·gram (ĕn′grăm′) n. A physical alteration thought to occur in neural tissue in response to stimuli, posited as an explanation for memory.

en·graph·i·a (ĕn-grăf′ē-ə) n. The formation of engrams.

en·keph·a·lin (ĕn-kĕf′ə-lĭn) n. Either of two closely related pentapeptides having opiate qualities and occurring in the brain, spinal cord, and other parts of the body.

en·oph·thal·mos (ĕn′ŏf-thăl′məs, -mŏs′, -ŏp-) n. Recession of the eyeball within the orbit.

ENT abbr. ear, nose, and throat

en·ta·me·ba or **en·ta·moe·ba** (ĕn′tə-mē′bə) or **en·da·me·ba** or **en·da·moe·ba** (ĕn′də-) n. A parasitic ameba of the genus Entamoeba.

en·tam·e·bi·a·sis or **en·tam·oe·bi·a·sis** (ĕn′tă-mə-bī′ə-sĭs) n. Infection with Entamoeba histolytica.

en·ter·al (ĕn′tər-əl) adj. **1.** Within or by way of the intestine, as distinguished from parenteral. **2.** Enteric. — **en′ter·al·ly** adv.

en·ter·al·gi·a (ĕn′tə-răl′jē-ə, -jə) n. Severe abdominal pain accompanying spasms of the intestine. — **en′ter·al′gic** (-jĭk) adj.

en·ter·ec·to·my (ĕn′tə-rĕk′tə-mē) n. Surgical removal of a segment of the intestine.

en·ter·el·co·sis (ĕn′tər-əl-kō′sĭs) n. Ulceration of the intestine.

en·ter·ic (ĕn-tĕr′ĭk) adj. **1.** Of, relating to, or within the intestine. **2.** By way of the intestine.

enteric coated tablet n. A tablet coated with a substance to delay release of the medication until the tablet has passed through the stomach and into the intestine.

enteric fever n. **1.** See typhoid fever. **2.** See paratyphoid fever.

enteric virus n. See enterovirus.

en·ter·i·tis (ĕn′tə-rī′tĭs) n. Inflammation of the intestinal tract, especially of the small intestine.

en·ter·o·a·nas·to·mo·sis (ĕn′tə-rō-ə-năs′tə-mō′-sĭs) n. See enteroenterostomy.

en·ter·o·bac·ter·i·um (ĕn′tə-rō-băk-tēr′ē-əm) n., pl. **-i·a** (-ē-ə). Any of various gram-negative rod-shaped bacteria of the family Enterobacteriaceae that includes some pathogens of animals, such as the colon bacillus and salmonella.

en·ter·o·bi·a·sis (ĕn′tə-rō-bī′ə-sĭs) n. Infestation of the intestine with the pinworm Enterobius vermicularis.

En·ter·o·bi·us (ĕn′tə-rō′bē-əs) n. A genus of nematode worms including the common pinworm E. vermicularis, an intestinal parasite.

en·ter·o·cele (ĕn′tə-rō-sēl′) n. **1.** A hernial protrusion through a defect in the rectovaginal or vesicovaginal pouch. **2.** An intestinal hernia.

en·ter·o·cen·te·sis (ĕn′tə-rō-sĕn-tē′sĭs) n. Surgical puncture of the intestine with a hollow needle to withdraw gas or fluid.

en·ter·oc·ly·sis (ĕn′tə-rŏk′lĭ-sĭs) n. See high enema.

en·ter·o·co·li·tis (ĕn′tə-rō-kō-lī′tĭs, -kə-) n. Inflammation of the mucous membrane of both the small and large intestine.

en·ter·o·co·los·to·my (ĕn′tə-rō-kə-lŏs′tə-mē) n. **1.** The surgical formation of a connection between the small intestine and colon. **2.** The connection itself.

en·ter·o·cyst (ĕn′tə-rō-sĭst′) n. A cyst of the wall of the intestine.

en·ter·o·cys·to·cele (ĕn′tə-rō-sĭs′tə-sēl′) n. A hernia of the intestine and the bladder wall.

en·ter·o·cys·to·ma (ĕn′tə-rō-sĭ-stō′mə) n. See enterocyst.

en·ter·o·en·ter·os·to·my (ĕ′tə-rō-ĕn′tə-rŏs′-tə-mē) n. A surgical connection between two segments of intestine.

en·ter·o·gas·tric reflex (ĕn′tə-rō-găs′trĭk) n. Peristaltic contraction of the small intestine induced by the entrance of food into the stomach.

en·ter·o·gas·tri·tis (ĕn′tə-rō-gă-strī′tĭs) n. See gastroenteritis.

en·ter·o·gas·trone (ĕn′tə-rō-găs′trōn′) n. A hormone released by the upper intestinal mucosa that inhibits gastric motility and secretion.

en·ter·o·he·pat·ic circulation (ĕn′tə-rō-hĭ-păt′-ĭk) n. Circulation of substances such as bile salts, which are absorbed from the intestine and carried to the liver, where they are secreted into the bile and again enter the intestine.

en·ter·o·hep·a·ti·tis (ĕn′tə-rō-hĕp′ə-tī′tĭs) n. Inflammation of the intestine and the liver.

en·ter·o·ki·ne·sis (ĕn′tə-rō-kə-nē′sĭs, -kī-) n. Muscular contraction of the alimentary canal, as in peristalsis. — **en′ter·o·ki·net′ic** (-nĕt′ĭk) adj.

en·ter·o·lith (ĕn′tə-rō-lĭth′) n. An intestinal calculus formed of layers surrounding a nucleus of a hard indigestible substance.

en·ter·o·li·thi·a·sis (ĕn′tə-rō-lĭ-thī′ə-sĭs) n. The presence of calculi in the intestine.

en·ter·ol·o·gy (ĕn′tə-rŏl′ə-jē) n. The branch of medical science concerned with disorders of the intestinal tract.

en·ter·o·my·co·sis (ĕn′tə-rō-mī-kō′sĭs) n. An intestinal disease of fungal origin.

en·ter·on (ĕn′tə-rŏn′) n. The alimentary canal.

en·ter·o·path·o·gen (ĕn′tə-rō-păth′ə-jən, -jĕn′) n. An organism capable of producing intestinal disease. — **en′ter·o·path′o·gen′ic** (-jĕn′ĭk) adj.

en·ter·op·a·thy (ĕn′tə-rŏp′ə-thē) n. A disease of the intestinal tract.

en·ter·o·pex·y (ĕn′tə-rō-pĕk′sē) n. The surgical fixation of a segment of the intestine to the abdominal wall.

en·ter·o·plas·ty (ĕn′tə-rō-plăs′tē) n. Reconstructive surgery of the intestine.

en·ter·op·to·sis (ĕn′tə-rŏp-tō′sĭs) or **en·ter·op·to·si·a** (-tō′sē-ə, -zē-ə) n. The abnormal descent of the intestines in the abdominal cavity, usually associated with downward displacement of the other viscera.

en·ter·or·rha·phy (ĕn'tə-rôr'ə-fē) *n.* Suture of the intestine.

en·ter·o·sep·sis (ĕn'tə-rō-sĕp'sĭs) *n.* Sepsis occurring or originating in the intestine.

en·ter·o·stat·in (ĕn'tə-rō-stăt'n) *n.* A substance produced in the pancreas that initiates a sensation of fullness, which may lead to decreased food consumption and weight loss.

en·ter·o·ste·no·sis (ĕn'tə-rō-stə-nō'sĭs) *n.* A narrowing or stricture of the lumen of the intestine.

en·ter·os·to·my (ĕn'tə-rŏs'tə-mē) *n.* **1.** Surgical construction of an opening into the intestine through an incision in the abdominal wall. **2.** The opening itself. — **en'ter·os'to·mal** *adj.*

en·ter·ot·o·my (ĕn'tə-rŏt'ə-mē) *n.* Surgical incision of the intestine.

en·ter·o·tox·in (ĕn'tə-rō-tŏk'sĭn) *n.* A cytotoxin produced by bacteria that is specific for the mucous membrane of the intestine and causes the vomiting and diarrhea of food poisoning.

en·ter·o·vi·rus (ĕn'tə-rō-vī'rəs) *n.* A virus of the genus *Enterovirus,* which includes polioviruses and coxsackieviruses and can infect the gastrointestinal tract and spread to other areas, especially the nervous system.

en·the·sis (ĕn'thĭ-sĭs) *n., pl.* **-ses** (-sēz). The surgical insertion of synthetic or other inorganic material to replace lost tissue.

en·the·sop·a·thy (ĕn'thĕ-sŏp'ə-thē) *n.* A disease occurring at the site of attachment of muscle tendons and ligaments to bones or joint capsules. — **en·the'so·path'ic** (ĕn-thē'sə-păth'ĭk) *adj.*

en·to·cele (ĕn'tə-sēl') *n.* An internal hernia.

en·trails (ĕn'trālz', -tralz) *pl.n.* The internal organs, especially the intestines; viscera.

en·tro·pi·on (ĕn-trō'pē-ŏn', -ən) *n.* **1.** The inversion or turning inward of a part. **2.** The infolding of the margin of an eyelid.

e·nu·cle·ate (ĭ-nōō'klē-āt', ĭ-nyōō'-) *v.* **-at·ed, -at·ing, -ates. 1.** To remove something, such as a tumor or an eye, whole and without rupture from an enveloping cover or sac. **2.** To remove the nucleus of a cell. — *adj.* (-ĭt, -āt'). Lacking a nucleus. — **e·nu'cle·a'tion** *n.*

en·u·re·sis (ĕn'yə-rē'sĭs) *n.* The uncontrolled or involuntary discharge of urine.

en·ve·lope (ĕn'və-lōp', ŏn'-) *n.* An enclosing structure or cover, such as a membrane or the outer coat of a virus.

en·ven·om·a·tion (ĕn-vĕn'ə-mā'shən) *n.* The injection of a poisonous material by sting, spine, bite, or other similar means.

en·vi·ron·ment (ĕn-vī'rən-mənt, -vī'ərn-) *n.* The totality of circumstances surrounding an organism or group of organisms, especially the combination of external physical conditions that affect and influence their growth, development, and survival. — **en·vi'ron·men'tal** (-mĕn'tl) *adj.*

en·zyme (ĕn'zīm) *n.* Any of numerous proteins or conjugated proteins produced by living organisms and functioning as specialized catalysts for biochemical reactions. — **en'zy·mat'ic** (-zə-măt'ĭk) *adj.*

enzyme-linked immunosorbent assay *n.* ELISA.

en·zy·mol·y·sis (ĕn'zə-mŏl'ĭ-sĭs) *n.* Chemical change or cleavage of a substance by enzymatic action.

en·zy·mop·a·thy (ĕn'zə-mŏp'ə-thē) *n.* Any of various disturbances of enzyme function, such as the genetic deficiency of a specific enzyme.

e·o·sin (ē'ə-sən) *n.* Any of a class of red acid dyes used as cytoplasmic stains and as counterstains in histology, especially the sodium and potassium salts of certain of these dyes.

e·o·sin·o·pe·ni·a (ē'ə-sĭn'ə-pē'nē-ə) *n.* A reduction in the normal number of eosinophils present in the blood.

e·o·sin·o·phil (ē'ə-sĭn'ə-fĭl') or **e·o·sin·o·phile** (-fīl') *n.* **1.** A type of white blood cell containing cytoplasmic granules that are easily stained by eosin or other acid dyes. **2.** A microorganism, cell, or histological element easily stained by eosin or other acid dyes. — **e'o·sin'o·phil'ic** *adj.*

eosinophil chemotactic factor of anaphylaxis *n.* A peptide that is chemotactic for eosinophilic white blood cells and is released from disrupted mast cells.

e·o·sin·o·phil·i·a (ē'ə-sĭn'ə-fĭl'ē-ə) *n.* An increase in the number of eosinophils in the blood.

eosinophilic granuloma *n.* A lesion characterized by numerous histiocytes that may contain Langerhans granules, eosinophils, and pockets of necrosis; it usually occurs as a solitary lesion in a bone, although it may develop in the lung.

eosinophilic leukocyte *n.* See **eosinophil** (sense 1).

eosinophilic leukopenia *n.* A condition characterized by a decrease in the number of eosinophilic granulocytes normally present in the blood.

e·o·sin·o·phil·u·ri·a (ē'ə-sĭn'ə-fĭl-yŏŏr'ē-ə) *n.* The presence of eosinophils in the urine.

ep·en·dy·mal cell (ĭ-pĕn'də-məl) *n.* **1.** A type of neuroglia cell lining the central canal of the spinal cord or the brain. **2.** A cell of the ependymal area of the developing neural tube.

ep·en·dy·mi·tis (ĭ-pĕn'də-mī'tĭs) *n.* Inflammation of the epithelial membrane of the spinal cord or neural ventricles.

ep·en·dy·mo·ma (ĭ-pĕn'də-mō'mə) *n., pl.* **-mas** or **-ma·ta** (-mə-tə). A central nervous system neoplasm made up of relatively undifferentiated ependymal cells.

e·phe·bi·at·rics (ĭ-fē'bē-ăt'rĭks) *n.* See **adolescent medicine.**

e·phed·rine (ĭ-fĕd'rĭn, ĕf'ĭ-drēn') *n.* A white, odorless, powdered or crystalline alkaloid used in the treatment of allergies and asthma.

ep·i·bleph·a·ron (ĕp'ə-blĕf'ə-rŏn') *n.* A congenital horizontal fold of skin near the margin of the upper or lower eyelid caused by the abnormal insertion of muscle fibers.

ep·i·can·thic fold (ĕp'ĭ-kăn'thĭk) *n.* A fold of skin of the upper eyelid that partially covers the inner corner of the eye.

ep·i·can·thus (ĕp'ĭ-kăn'thəs) *n., pl.* **-thi** (-thī). See **epicanthic fold.**

ep·i·car·di·a (ĕp'ĭ-kär'dē-ə) *n.* The lower portion

of the esophagus extending through the diaphragm to the stomach.

ep·i·car·di·um (ĕp'ĭ-kär'dē-əm) *n., pl.* **-di·a** (-dē-ə). The inner layer of the pericardium that is in contact with the surface of the heart. — **ep'i·car'di·al** *adj.*

ep·i·con·dyle (ĕp'ĭ-kŏn'dīl, -dĭl) *n.* A rounded projection at the end of a bone, located on or above a condyle and usually serving as a place of attachment for ligaments and tendons.

ep·i·con·dy·li·tis (ĕp'ĭ-kŏn'dl-ī'tĭs) *n.* Infection or inflammation of an epicondyle.

ep·i·cra·ni·um (ĕp'ĭ-krā'nē-əm) *n., pl.* **-ni·ums** or **-ni·a** (-nē-ə). The structures that cover the cranium. — **ep'i·cra'ni·al** *adj.*

ep·i·cri·sis (ĕp'ĭ-krī'sĭs, ĕp'ĭ-krī'sĭs) *n.* A secondary crisis in the course of a disease.

ep·i·cys·tot·o·my (ĕp'ĭ-sĭ-stŏt'ə-mē) *n.* See **suprapubic cystotomy.**

ep·i·dem·ic (ĕp'ĭ-dĕm'ĭk) or **ep·i·dem·i·cal** (-ĭ-kəl) *adj.* Spreading rapidly and extensively by infection and simultaneously affecting many people in an area or a population, as of a disease or illness. — *n.* An outbreak or unusually high occurrence of a disease or illness in a population or area.

epidemic hemorrhagic fever *n.* An acute viral hemorrhagic fever characterized by headache, high fever, sweating, thirst, photophobia, coryza, cough, myalgia, arthralgia, and abdominal pain with nausea and vomiting. This phase lasts from three to six days and is followed by capillary hemorrhages, edema, oliguria, and shock.

ep·i·de·mic·i·ty (ĕp'ĭ-də-mĭs'ĭ-tē) *n.* The ability to spread from one host to others.

epidemic keratoconjunctivitis *n.* A highly infectious follicular conjunctivitis of the eye caused by an adenovirus and characterized by inflammation but little exudate.

epidemic neuromyasthenia *n.* An epidemic disease characterized by stiffness of the neck and back, headache, diarrhea, fever, and localized muscular weakness.

epidemic nonbacterial gastroenteritis *n.* An epidemic, communicable, but mild disease of sudden onset caused by epidemic gastroenteritis virus and marked by fever, abdominal cramps, nausea, vomiting, diarrhea, and headache.

epidemic pleurodynia *n.* An epidemic disease caused by a coxsackievirus, characterized by paroxysmal pain in the lower chest and accompanied by fever, headache, and malaise.

epidemic typhus *n.* A form of typhus characterized by high fever, mental and physical depression, and macular and papular eruptions; it is caused by *Rickettsia prowazekii* and transmitted by body lice.

ep·i·de·mi·ol·o·gy (ĕp'ĭ-dē'mē-ŏl'ə-jē, -dĕm'ē-) *n.* The branch of medicine that deals with the study of the causes, distribution, and control of disease in populations. — **ep'i·de'mi·ol'o·gist** *n.*

epidermal cyst *n.* A cyst formed of a mass of epidermal cells that has been pushed beneath the epidermis as a result of trauma.

ep·i·der·mis (ĕp'ĭ-dûr'mĭs) *n.* The nonvascular outer protective layer of the skin, covering the dermis. — **ep'i·der'mal** (-məl), **ep'i·der'mic** *adj.*

ep·i·der·mi·tis (ĕp'ĭ-dər-mī'tĭs) *n.* Inflammation of the epidermis.

ep·i·der·mo·dys·pla·sia ver·ru·ci·for·mis (ĕp'ĭ-dûr'mō-dĭs-plā'zhə, zhē-ə və-rōō'sə-fôr'mĭs) *n.* The occurrence of numerous flat warts on the hands, face, neck, and feet.

ep·i·der·moid (ĕp'ĭ-dûr'moid') *adj.* Composed of or resembling epidermal tissue. — *n.* A cystic tumor made up of abnormal epidermal cells.

ep·i·der·mol·y·sis (ĕp'ĭ-dər-mŏl'ĭ-sĭs) *n.* A condition in which the epidermis is loosely attached to the dermis and readily detaches or forms blisters.

epidermolysis bul·lo·sa (bə-lō'sə) *n.* Any of a group of inherited chronic noninflammatory skin diseases in which large blisters and erosions develop after slight trauma.

ep·i·did·y·mec·to·my (ĕp'ĭ-dĭd'ə-mĕk'tə-mē) *n.* Surgical removal of the epididymis.

ep·i·did·y·mis (ĕp'ĭ-dĭd'ə-mĭs) *n., pl.* **ep·i·di·dym·i·des** (ĕp'ĭ-dĭ-dĭm'ĭ-dēz'). A long narrow convoluted tube that is part of the spermatic duct system and lies on the posterior aspect of each testicle, connecting it to the vas deferens.

ep·i·did·y·mi·tis (ĕp'ĭ-dĭd'ə-mī'tĭs) *n.* Inflammation of the epididymis.

ep·i·did·y·mo·or·chi·tis (ĕp'ĭ-dĭd'ə-mō-ôr-kī'tĭs) *n.* Inflammation of both the epididymis and the testis.

ep·i·did·y·mo·plas·ty (ĕp'ĭ-dĭd'ə-mō-plăs'tē) *n.* Surgical repair of the epididymis.

ep·i·did·y·mot·o·my (ĕp'ĭ-dĭd'ə-mŏt'ə-mē) *n.* Incision into the epididymis.

ep·i·did·y·mo·vas·ec·to·my (ĕp'ĭ-dĭd'ə-mō-və-sĕk'tə-mē, -vă-zĕk'-) *n.* Surgical removal of the epididymis and the vas deferens.

ep·i·did·y·mo·va·sos·to·my (ĕp'ĭ-dĭd'ə-mō-vă-sŏs'tə-mē) *n.* The surgical severing of the vas deferens with anastomosis to the epididymis, usually to avoid an obstruction causing sterility.

ep·i·du·ral (ĕp'ĭ-dŏŏr'əl, -dyŏŏr'-) *adj.* Located on or over the dura mater. — *n.* An injection into the epidural space of the spine.

epidural anesthesia *n.* Regional anesthesia produced by injection of a local anesthetic solution into the epidural space of the lumbar or sacral region of the spine.

epidural block *n.* Obstruction of the epidural space by compression, hematoma, or scar tissue.

epidural space *n.* The space between the walls of the vertebral canal and the dura mater of the spinal cord.

ep·i·du·rog·ra·phy (ĕp'ĭ-dŏŏ-rŏg'rə-fē, -dyŏŏ-) *n.* Radiographic visualization of the epidural space following the instillation of a radiopaque contrast medium.

ep·i·gas·tral·gia (ĕp'ĭ-gă-străl'jē-ə, -jə) *n.* Pain in the epigastric region.

ep·i·gas·tri·um (ĕp'ĭ-găs'trē-əm) *n., pl.* **-tri·a** (-trē-ə). The highest of the three median regions of the abdomen, lying above the umbilical region and between the hypochondriac regions. — **ep′i‧gas′tric** (-trĭk) *adj.*

ep·i·gas·tro·cele (ĕp′ĭ-găs′trə-sēl′) *n.* A hernia located in the epigastric region.

ep·i·gen·e·sis (ĕp′ə-jĕn′ĭ-sĭs) *n.* The theory that a person is developed by successive differentiation of an unstructured egg rather than by a simple enlarging of a preformed entity. — **ep′i‧ge‧net′ic** (-jə-nĕt′ĭk) *adj.*

ep·i·glot·ti·dec·to·my (ĕp′ĭ-glŏt′ĭ-dĕk′tə-mē) *n.* Excision of all or a part of the epiglottis.

ep·i·glot·tis (ĕp′ĭ-glŏt′ĭs) *n., pl.* **-glot·tis·es** or **-glot·ti·des** (-glŏt′ĭ-dēz′). The thin elastic cartilaginous structure located at the root of the tongue that folds over the glottis to prevent food and liquid from entering the trachea during the act of swallowing. — **ep′i‧glot′tic** *adj.*

ep·i·glot·ti·tis (ĕp′ĭ-glŏ-tī′tĭs) *n.* Inflammation of the epiglottis.

ep·i·ker·a·to·pha·ki·a (ĕp′ĭ-kĕr′ə-tō-fā′kē-ə) *n.* A surgical procedure that modifies optical refractive error through the addition of a donated cornea to the anterior surface of the faulty cornea.

ep·i·late (ĕp′ə-lāt′) *v.* **-lat·ed, -lat·ing, -lates.** To remove a hair from a part of the body by forcible extraction, electrolysis, or loosening at the root by chemical means.

ep·i·la·tion (ĕp′ə-lā′shən) *n.* The removal of hair, as by mechanical or chemical means.

ep·i·lep·sy (ĕp′ə-lĕp′sē) *n.* Any of various neurological disorders characterized by sudden, recurring attacks of motor, sensory, or psychic malfunction with or without loss of consciousness or convulsive seizures.

ep·i·lep·tic (ĕp′ə-lĕp′tĭk) *n.* One who has epilepsy. — *adj.* **1.** Affected with epilepsy. **2.** Of, relating to, or associated with epilepsy.

ep·i·lep·to·gen·ic zone (ĕp′ə-lĕp′tə-jĕn′ĭk) *n.* A cortical region of the brain that, when stimulated, produces spontaneous seizure or aura.

ep·i·mor·pho·sis (ĕp′ə-môr-fō′sĭs) *n.* Regeneration of a body part by extensive cell proliferation and differentiation at the cut surface.

ep·i·mys·i·ot·o·my (ĕp′ə-mĭz′ē-ŏt′ə-mē, -mĭzh′ē-) *n.* Surgical incision or sectioning of a muscle within its sheath.

ep·i·mys·i·um (ĕp′ə-mĭz′ē-əm, -mĭzh′ē-) *n., pl.* **-mys·i·a** (-mĭz′ē-ə, -mĭzh′-). The sheath of connective tissue surrounding a muscle.

ep·i·neph·rine or **ep·i·neph·rin** (ĕp′ə-nĕf′rĭn) *n.* **1.** A catecholamine hormone of the adrenal medulla that is the most potent stimulant of the sympathetic nervous system, resulting in increased heart rate and force of contraction, vasoconstriction or vasodilation, relaxation of bronchiolar and intestinal smooth muscle, and other metabolic effects. **2.** A white to brownish crystalline compound used in medicine as a heart stimulant, vasoconstrictor, and bronchial relaxant.

ep·i·phar·ynx (ĕp′ə-făr′ĭngks) *n.* See **nasopharynx.**

ep·i·phe·nom·e·non (ĕp′ə-fĭ-nŏm′ə-nŏn′) *n.* An additional condition or symptom during the course of a disease, not necessarily connected with it.

e·piph·o·ra (ĭ-pĭf′ər-ə) *n.* Watering of the eyes due to a blockage of the lacrimal ducts or the excessive secretion of tears.

ep·i·phys·i·ol·y·sis (ĕp′ə-fĭz′ē-ŏl′ĭ-sĭs) *n.* The loosening or separation, either partial or complete, of an epiphysis from the shaft of a bone.

e·piph·y·sis (ĭ-pĭf′ĭ-sĭs) *n., pl.* **-ses** (-sēz′). **1.** The end of a long bone that is originally separated from the main bone by a layer of cartilage but that later becomes united to the main bone through ossification. **2.** See **pineal body.** — **ep′i‧phys′i·al** (ĕp′ə-fĭz′ē-əl), **ep′i·physe·al** *adj.*

e·piph·y·si·tis (ĭ-pĭf′ĭ-sī′tĭs) *n.* Inflammation of an epiphysis.

e·pip·lo·on (ĭ-pĭp′lō-ŏn′) *n., pl.* **-lo·a** (-lō-ə). See **greater omentum.**

ep·i·scle·ra (ĕp′ĭ-sklĕr′ə) *n.* The layer of connective tissue between the sclera and the conjunctiva of the eye.

e·pis·i·o·per·i·ne·or·rha·phy (ĭ-pĭz′ē-ō-pĕr′ə-nē-ôr′ə-fē, ĭ-pē′zē-) *n.* Suture of the perineum and vulva.

e·pis·i·o·plas·ty (ĭ-pĭz′ē-ō-plăs′tē, ĭ-pē′zē-) *n.* Surgical repair of a defect of the vulva.

e·pis·i·or·rha·phy (ĭ-pĭz′ē-ôr′ə-fē, ĭ-pē′zē-) *n.* Suture of a lacerated vulva.

e·pis·i·o·ste·no·sis (ĭ-pĭz′ē-ō-stə-nō′sĭs, ĭ-pē′zē-) *n.* Contraction or narrowing of the vulvar orifice.

e·pis·i·ot·o·my (ĭ-pĭz′ē-ŏt′ə-mē, ĭ-pē′zē-) *n.* Surgical incision of the perineum during childbirth to facilitate delivery.

ep·i·spa·di·as (ĕp′ĭ-spā′dē-əs) or **ep·i·spa·di·a** (-dē-ə) *n.* A congenital defect in which the urethra opens on the upper surface of the penis. — **ep′i‧spa′di·al** *adj.*

e·pis·ta·sis (ĭ-pĭs′tə-sĭs) *n., pl.* **-ses** (-sēz′). **1.** A film that forms on the surface of a urine specimen. **2.** An interaction between nonallelic genes, especially in which one gene suppresses the expression of another. **3.** The suppression of a bodily discharge or secretion. — **ep′i·stat′ic** (ĕp′ĭ-stăt′ĭk) *adj.*

ep·i·stax·is (ĕp′ĭ-stăk′sĭs) *n., pl.* **-stax·es** (-stăk′sēz′). A nosebleed.

ep·i·ster·num (ĕp′ĭ-stûr′nəm) *n.* The broad upper segment of the sternum occasionally fused with the body of the sternum and forming the sternal angle.

ep·i·ten·din·e·um (ĕp′ĭ-tĕn-dĭn′ē-əm) *n.* The white fibrous sheath surrounding a tendon.

ep·i·the·li·al·i·za·tion (ĕp′ə-thē′lē-ə-lĭ-zā′shən) or **ep·i·the·li·za·tion** (-thē′lĭ-zā′shən) *n.* The process of covering a denuded surface with epithelium.

ep·i·the·li·al·ize (ĕp′ə-thē′lē-ə-līz′) or **ep·i·the·lize** (-thē′līz) *v.* **-ized** or **-lized, -iz·ing** or **-liz·ing, -iz·es** or **-liz·es.** To become covered with epithelial tissue, as of a wound.

epithelial pearl *n.* See **keratin pearl.**

epithelial plug *n.* A mass of epithelial cells temporarily occluding an embryonic opening, most commonly of the nostrils.

ep·i·the·li·oid cell (ĕp′ə-thē′lē-oid′) *n.* A nonepithelial cell, especially one derived from a macrophage, having certain characteristics that cause it to resemble an epithelial cell, often found in granulomas associated with tuberculosis.

ep·i·the·li·o·ma (ĕp′ə-thē′lē-ō′mə) *n., pl.* **-mas** or **-ma·ta** (-mə-tə). A benign or malignant tumor derived from epithelium.

ep·i·the·li·um (ĕp′ə-thē′lē-əm) *n., pl.* **-li·ums** or **-li·a** (-lē-ə). Membranous tissue composed of one or more layers of cells separated by very little intercellular substance and forming the covering of most internal and external surfaces of the body and its organs. — **ep′i·the′li·al** *adj.*

ep·i·tope (ĕp′ĭ-tōp′) *n.* The molecular grouping on the surface of an antigen capable of eliciting an immune response and of combining with the antibody produced to counter that response.

ep·o·nych·i·a (ĕp′ə-nĭk′ē-ə) *n.* An infection affecting the proximal nail fold.

Ep·som salts (ĕp′səm) *pl.n.* Hydrated magnesium sulfate, used as a cathartic and as an agent to reduce inflammation.

Ep·stein–Barr virus (ĕp′stīn-) *n.* A herpesvirus that is the causative agent of infectious mononucleosis. It is also associated with various types of human cancers.

e·qua·to·ri·al staphyloma (ē′kwə-tôr′ē-əl, ĕk′-wə-) *n.* A staphyloma occurring in the area of exit of the vortex veins of the eyeball.

e·quil·i·bra·tion (ĭ-kwĭl′ə-brā′shən) *n.* The development or maintenance of an equilibrium.

e·qui·lib·ri·um (ē′kwə-lĭb′rē-əm, ĕk′wə-) *n.* **1.** A condition in which all acting influences are canceled by others, resulting in a balanced or unchanging system. **2.** Mental or emotional balance.

er·bi·um (ûr′bē-əm) *n.* A soft rare-earth element with atomic number 68, used in nuclear research.

Erb's palsy *n.* Birth palsy in which there is paralysis of the muscles of the upper arm due to a lesion of the brachial plexus or the roots of the fifth and sixth cervical nerves.

Erb's sign *n.* An indication of tetany in which the electric excitability of the muscles increases.

ERCP *abbr.* endoscopic retrograde cholangiopancreatography

e·rect (ĭ-rĕkt′) *adj.* **1.** Vertical or upright. **2.** In a state of physiological erection.

e·rec·tile (ĭ-rĕk′təl, -tīl′) *adj.* **1.** Of or relating to tissue that is capable of filling with blood and becoming rigid. **2.** Capable of being raised to an upright position.

erectile tissue *n.* Tissue with numerous vascular spaces that may become engorged with blood.

e·rec·tion (ĭ-rĕk′shən) *n.* **1.** The firm and enlarged condition of a body organ or part when the erectile tissue surrounding it becomes filled with blood, especially such a condition of the penis or clitoris. **2.** The process of filling with blood.

e·rec·tor (ĭ-rĕk′tər) *n.* A muscle that makes a body part erect.

erector muscle of hair *n.* Any of the bundles of smooth muscle fibers, attached to the deep part of hair follicles, passing outward alongside the sebaceous glands to the papillary layer of the corium, whose action erects hairs.

erector muscle of spine *n.* A muscle with its origin from the sacrum, ilium, and spines of the lumbar vertebrae, dividing into three columns that insert into the ribs and vertebrae, and whose action extends the vertebral column.

e·rep·sin (ĭ-rĕp′sən) *n.* An enzyme complex in intestinal and pancreatic juices that catalyzes the breakdown of polypeptides into amino acids.

er·e·thism (ĕr′ə-thĭz′əm) *n.* Abnormal irritability or sensitivity of an organ or a body part to stimulation.

ERG *abbr.* electroretinogram

er·ga·si·a (ûr-gā′zē-ə, -zhə) *n.* The sum of the mental, behavioral, and physiological functions and reactions that make up a person.

er·gas·to·plasm (ûr-găs′tə-plăz′əm) *n.* See **granular endoplasmic reticulum.**

er·go·cal·cif·er·ol (ûr′gō-kăl-sĭf′ə-rôl′, -rōl′) *n.* See **vitamin D₂.**

er·go·graph (ûr′gə-grăf′) *n.* A device for measuring work capacity of a muscle or group of muscles during contraction. — **er′go·graph′ic** *adj.*

er·gom·e·ter (ûr-gŏm′ĭ-tər) *n.* See **dynamometer.**

er·go·nom·ics (ûr′gə-nŏm′ĭks) *n.* The applied science of equipment design, as for the workplace, intended to maximize productivity by reducing operator fatigue and discomfort.

er·gos·ter·ol (ûr-gŏs′tə-rôl′, -rōl′) *n.* A crystalline sterol synthesized by yeast from sugars or derived from ergot and converted to vitamin D₂ when exposed to ultraviolet radiation.

er·got (ûr′gət, -gŏt′) *n.* **1.** A fungus (*Claviceps purpurea*) that infects various cereal plants and forms compact black masses of branching filaments. **2.** The dried sclerotia of ergot, usually obtained from rye seed and used as a source of several medicinally important alkaloids and as the basic source of lysergic acid.

er·got·a·mine (ûr-gŏt′ə-mēn′, -mĭn) *n.* A crystalline alkaloid derived from ergot that induces vasoconstriction, used especially in treating migraine.

e·rode (ĭ-rōd′) *v.* **e·rod·ed, e·rod·ing, e·rodes. 1.** To wear away by or as if by abrasion. **2.** To eat into; ulcerate.

e·rog·e·nous zone (ĭ-rŏj′ə-nəs) *n.* A part of the body that excites sexual feelings when touched or stimulated.

Eros (ē′rŏs, âr′ŏs) or **eros** *n.* **1.** In psychoanalytic theory, the sum of all instincts for self-preservation. **2.** Sexual drive; libido.

E-rosette test *n.* A test to identify T lymphocytes by mixing purified human blood lymphocytes with serum and sheep red blood cells.

e·ro·sion (ĭ-rō′zhən) *n.* The superficial destruction of a surface by friction, pressure, ulceration, or trauma.

e·rot·i·cism (ĭ-rŏt′ĭ-sĭz′əm) *n.* Sexual excitement.

er·o·tism (ĕr′ə-tĭz′əm) *n.* Eroticism.

e·ro·to·gen·ic zone (ĭ-rō'tə-jĕn'ĭk, ĭ-rŏt'ə-) *n*. See **erogenous zone.**

e·ro·to·ma·ni·a (ĭ-rō'tə-mā'nē-ə, ĭ-rŏt'ə-) *n*. Excessive sexual desire.

er·o·top·a·thy (ĕr'ə-tŏp'ə-thē) *n*. An abnormality of sexual desire. — **e·ro'to·path'ic** (ĭ-rō'tə-păth'ĭk, ĭ-rŏt'ə-) *adj*.

e·ro·to·pho·bi·a (ĭ-rō'tə-fō'bē-ə, ĭ-rŏt'ə-) *n*. An abnormal fear of love, especially sexual feelings and their physical expression.

er·ror (ĕr'ər) *n*. A defect or insufficiency in structure or function.

e·ruc·ta·tion (ĭ-rŭk-tā'shən, ē'rŭk-) *n*. The act or an instance of belching.

e·rupt (ĭ-rŭpt') *v*. **e·rupt·ed, e·rupt·ing, e·rupts. 1.** To break through the gums. Used of teeth. **2.** To appear on the skin. Used of a rash or blemish.

e·rup·tion (ĭ-rŭp'shən) *n*. **1.** An appearance of a rash or blemish on the skin. **2.** The emergence of a tooth through the gums. — **e·rup'tive** (-tĭv) *adj*.

eruptive xanthoma *n*. A condition affecting individuals with severe hyperlipemia in which groups of waxy yellow or yellowish-brown lesions appear suddenly, especially over extensors of the elbows and knees and on the back and buttocks.

er·y·sip·e·las (ĕr'ĭ-sĭp'ə-ləs, ĕr'-) *n*. An acute disease of the skin and subcutaneous tissue caused by a species of hemolytic streptococcus and marked by localized inflammation and fever.

er·y·sip·e·loid (ĕr'ĭ-sĭp'ə-loid', ĭr'ə-) *n*. An infectious disease of the skin that is contracted by handling fish or meat infected with the bacterium *Erysipelothrix rhusiopathiae* and characterized by red lesions on the hands.

Er·y·sip·e·lo·thrix (ĕr'ĭ-sĭp'ə-lō-thrĭks', -sə-pĕl'ə-, ĕr'ĭ-) *n*. A genus of gram-positive rod-shaped bacteria that are parasitic on mammals, birds, and fish.

er·y·the·ma (ĕr'ə-thē'mə) *n*. Redness of the skin caused by dilatation and congestion of the capillaries, often a sign of inflammation or infection. — **er'y·them'a·tous** (-thĕm'ə-təs, -thē'mə-) *adj*.

erythema an·nu·lar·e (ăn'yə-lâr'ē) *n*. Erythema characterized by ringed or rounded lesions.

erythema chron·i·cum mi·grans (krŏn'ĭ-kəm mī'grănz') *n*. A raised erythematous ring on the skin having hard borders and a central clearing, and radiating from the site of an insect bite; it is the characteristic lesion of Lyme disease.

erythema dose *n*. The minimum amount of x-rays or other form of radiation sufficient to produce redness of the skin after application, regarded as the dose that is safe to give at one time.

erythema in·fec·ti·o·sum (ĭn-fĕk'shē-ō'səm) *n*. A mild infectious disease occurring mainly in early childhood, marked by a rosy-red rash on the cheeks, often spreading to the trunk and limbs. Fever and arthritis may also be present.

erythema mul·ti·for·me (mŭl'tə-fôr'mē) *n*. A skin disease believed to be caused by allergies, seasonal changes, or drug sensitivities, marked by the acute eruption of red macules, papules, or subdermal vesicles on the skin and mucous membranes; the characteristic lesion consists of a papule surrounded by a concentric ring.

erythema no·do·sum (nō-dō'səm) *n*. A skin disease associated with joint pain, fever, hypersensitivity, or infection, and characterized by small, painful, pink to blue nodules under the skin and on the shins that tend to recur.

er·y·thral·gi·a (ĕr'ə-thrăl'jē-ə, -jə) *n*. A mottled reddening of the skin, usually accompanied by throbbing pain.

er·y·thras·ma (ĕr'ə-thrăz'mə) *n*. A bacterial skin infection marked by reddish brown, slightly raised patches, especially in armpits and groin.

e·ryth·re·de·ma (ĭ-rĭth'rĭ-dē'mə) *n*. See **acrodynia** (sense 1).

er·y·thre·mi·a (ĕr'ə-thrē'mē-ə) *n*. A chronic form of polycythemia of unknown cause, characterized by an increase in blood volume and red blood cells, bone marrow hyperplasia, redness or cyanosis of the skin, and splenic enlargement.

er·y·threm·ic myelosis (ĕr'ə-thrĕm'ĭk, -thrē'mĭk) *n*. A neoplastic process involving the erythropoietic tissue, characterized by anemia, irregular fever, splenomegaly, hepatomegaly, hemorrhagic disorders, and the presence in the blood of numerous erythroblasts in all stages of maturation.

er·y·thrism (ĕr'ə-thrĭz'əm) *n*. Redness of the hair with a ruddy freckled complexion. — **er'y·thris'·tic** (-thrĭs'tĭk) *adj*.

e·ryth·ro·blast (ĭ-rĭth'rə-blăst') *n*. Any of the nucleated cells normally found only in bone marrow that develop into red blood cells. — **e·ryth'·ro·blast'ic** *adj*.

e·ryth·ro·blas·to·sis (ĭ-rĭth'rō-blă-stō'sĭs) *n*., *pl*. **-ses** (-sēz). The abnormal presence of erythroblasts in the blood.

erythroblastosis fe·ta·lis (fē-tā'lĭs) *n*. A severe hemolytic disease of a fetus or newborn caused by the production of maternal antibodies against the fetal red blood cells, usually involving Rh incompatibility between the mother and fetus.

er·y·throc·la·sis (ĕr'ə-thrŏk'lə-sĭs) *n*. The fragmentation or breaking down of red blood cells.

e·ryth·ro·cy·a·no·sis (ĭ-rĭth'rō-sī'ə-nō'sĭs) *n*. A condition caused by exposure to cold and characterized by swelling of the limbs and the appearance of irregular red-blue patches on the skin, occurring especially in girls and women.

e·ryth·ro·cyte (ĭ-rĭth'rə-sīt') *n*. See **red blood cell.** — **e·ryth'ro·cyt'ic** (-sĭt'ĭk) *adj*.

erythrocyte fragility test *n*. See **fragility test.**

erythrocyte indices *pl.n*. Calculations for determining the average size, hemoglobin content, and concentration of red blood cells, including mean cell volume, mean cell hemoglobin, and mean cell hemoglobin concentration.

erythrocyte sedimentation rate *n*. The rate at which red blood cells settle in anticoagulated blood.

erythrocytic series *n*. The cells in various stages of hematopoiesis in the red bone marrow.

e·ryth·ro·cy·tol·y·sin (ĭ-rĭth'rō-sī-tŏl'ĭ-sĭn) *n*. See **hemolysin.**

e·ryth·ro·cy·tol·y·sis (ĭ-rĭth'rō-sī-tŏl'ĭ-sĭs) *n.* See hemolysis.

e·ryth·ro·cy·tor·rhex·is (ĭ-rĭth'rō-sī'tə-rĕk'sĭs) *n.* The rupture of red blood cells causing the escape of particles of protoplasm.

e·ryth·ro·cy·tos·chi·sis (ĭ-rĭth'rō-sī-tŏs'kĭ-sĭs) *n.* The fragmentation or breaking up of red blood cells into small particles that contain hemoglobin but that morphologically resemble platelets.

e·ryth·ro·cy·to·sis (ĭ-rĭth'rō-sī-tō'sĭs) *n.* An abnormal increase in the number of circulating red blood cells.

e·ryth·ro·der·ma (ĭ-rĭth'rō-dûr'mə) *n.* A skin disease characterized by intense, widespread reddening of the skin, often preceding or associated with exfoliation.

e·ryth·ro·don·tia (ĭ-rĭth'rō-dŏn'shə, -shē-ə) *n.* A reddish or reddish-brown discoloration of the teeth.

erythrogenic toxin *n.* See streptococcus erythrogenic toxin.

e·ryth·ro·ker·a·to·der·ma (ĭ-rĭth'rō-kĕr'ə-tō-dûr'mə) *n.* A skin condition in which papules and scaly skin form as a result of injury.

er·y·throl·y·sin (ĕr'ə-thrōl'ĭ-sĭn) *n.* See hemolysin.

er·y·throl·y·sis (ĕr'ə-thrōl'ĭ-sĭs) *n.* See hemolysis.

e·ryth·ro·me·lal·gi·a (ĭ-rĭth'rō-mə-lăl'jē-ə, -jə) *n.* Paroxysmal throbbing and burning pain in the skin, affecting one or both legs and feet, sometimes one or both hands, accompanied by a dusky mottled redness of the parts and associated with polycythemia vera, thrombocytemia, gout, neurological disease, or heavy-metal poisoning.

e·ryth·ro·my·cin (ĭ-rĭth'rə-mī'sĭn) *n.* An antibiotic obtained from a strain of the actinomycete *Streptomyces erythreus,* effective against many gram-positive and some gram-negative bacteria.

e·ryth·ro·ne·o·cy·to·sis (ĭ-rĭth'rō-nē'ō-sī-tō'sĭs) *n.* The presence of regenerative forms of red blood cells in the blood.

e·ryth·ro·pe·ni·a (ĭ-rĭth'rō-pē'nē-ə) *n.* A deficiency in the number of red blood cells.

e·ryth·ro·pla·ki·a (ĭ-rĭth'rō-plā'kē-ə) *n.* A red, velvety, plaquelike lesion of the mucous membrane, often indicating a precancerous condition.

e·ryth·ro·pla·sia (ĭ-rĭth'rō-plā'zhə, -zhē-ə) *n.* Erythema and dysplasia of the epithelium.

e·ryth·ro·poi·e·sis (ĭ-rĭth'rō-poi-ē'sĭs) *n.* The formation or production of red blood cells. — e·ryth'ro·poi·et'ic (-ĕt'ĭk) *adj.*

erythropoietic protoporphyria *n.* A benign inherited disorder of porphyrin metabolism characterized by enhanced fecal excretion of protoporphyrin and elevated quantities of protoporphyrin in red blood cells, plasma, and feces, with acute solar urticaria or chronic solar eczema appearing quickly upon exposure to sunlight.

e·ryth·ro·poi·e·tin (ĭ-rĭth'rō-poi-ē'tĭn) *n.* A glycoprotein hormone that stimulates the production of red blood cells by bone marrow; it is produced mainly by the kidneys and released in response to decreased levels of oxygen in body tissue.

e·ryth·ro·pros·o·pal·gi·a (ĭ-rĭth'rō-prŏs'ə-păl'-jē-ə, -jə) *n.* See cluster headache.

e·ryth·ror·rhex·is (ĭ-rĭth'rə-rĕk'sĭs) *n.* See erythrocytorrhexis.

es·cape (ĭ-skāp') *n.* **1.** A gradual effusion from an enclosure; a leakage. **2.** A cardiological situation in which one pacemaker defaults, or an atrioventricular conduction fails, and another pacemaker sets the heart's pace for one or more beats.

escape beat *n.* An automatic beat, usually arising from the atrioventricular node or ventricle, but occurring after an expected normal beat has defaulted.

escape rhythm *n.* Three or more consecutive impulses occurring at a rate that does not exceed the upper limit of the inherent pacemaker of the heart.

es·cap·ism (ĭ-skā'pĭz'əm) *n.* The tendency to escape from daily reality or routine by indulging in daydreaming, fantasy, or entertainment.

es·char (ĕs'kär') *n.* A dry scab or slough formed on the skin as a result of a burn or by the action of a corrosive or caustic substance.

es·cha·rot·ic (ĕs'kə-rŏt'ĭk) *n.* A caustic or corrosive substance or drug. — *adj.* Producing an eschar.

es·cha·rot·o·my (ĕs'kə-rŏt'ə-mē) *n.* Surgical incision into a burn eschar to lessen its pull on the surrounding tissue.

Esch·e·rich·i·a (ĕsh'ə-rĭk'ē-ə) *n.* A genus of aerobic, gram-negative, rod-shaped bacteria widely found in nature; one species, *Escherichia coli,* which normally occurs in human and animal intestines, can cause urogenital tract infections and diarrhea in infants and adults.

es·mo·lol hydrochloride (ĕs'mə-lôl') *n.* A beta-blocker used to treat certain types of tachycardia.

es·o·eth·moi·di·tis (ĕs'ō-ĕth'moi-dī'tĭs) *n.* Inflammation of the lining membrane of the ethmoid sinuses.

es·o·gas·tri·tis (ĕs'ō-gă-strī'tĭs) *n.* Inflammation of the mucous membrane of the stomach.

e·soph·a·gal·gi·a (ĭ-sŏf'ə-găl'jē-ə, -jə) *n.* Pain in the esophagus.

esophageal reflux *n.* Reflux of stomach contents into the esophagus.

esophageal speech *n.* A technique for speaking after total laryngectomy involving the swallowing of air and its subsequent expulsion to produce a vibration in the hypopharynx.

e·soph·a·gec·ta·sis (ĭ-sŏf'ə-jĕk'tə-sĭs) or e·soph·a·gec·ta·si·a (-jĭk-tā'zē-ə, -zhə) *n.* Dilation of the esophagus.

e·soph·a·gec·to·my (ĭ-sŏf'ə-jĕk'tə-mē) *n.* Surgical excision of all or a part of the esophagus.

e·soph·a·gism (ĭ-sŏf'ə-jĭz'əm) *n.* Esophageal spasm causing dysphagia.

e·soph·a·gi·tis (ĭ-sŏf'ə-jī'tĭs) *n.* Inflammation of the esophagus.

e·soph·a·go·car·di·o·plas·ty (ĭ-sŏf'ə-gō-kär'dē-ō-plăs'tē) *n.* A reconstructive operation on the esophagus and cardiac end of the stomach.

e·soph·a·go·cele (ĭ-sŏf'ə-gō-sēl') *n.* Protrusion of

the mucous membrane of the esophagus through a rupture in the muscular coat.

e·soph·a·go·dyn·i·a (ĭ-sŏf′ə-gō-dĭn′ē-ə) *n.* See **esophagalgia.**

e·soph·a·go·en·ter·os·to·my (ĭ-sŏf′ə-gō-ĕn′tə-rŏs′tə-mē) *n.* The surgical formation of a communication between esophagus and intestine.

e·soph·a·go·gas·trec·to·my (ĭ-sŏf′ə-gō-gă-strĕk′tə-mē) *n.* The removal of a portion of the lower esophagus and proximal stomach for treatment of neoplasms or strictures, especially lesions near the cardioesophageal junction.

e·soph·a·go·gas·tro·a·nas·to·mo·sis (ĭ-sŏf′ə-gō-găs′trō-ə-năs′tə-mō′sĭs) *n.* See **esophagogastrostomy.**

e·soph·a·go·gas·tro·plas·ty (ĭ-sŏf′ə-gō-găs′trə-plăs′tē) *n.* Surgical repair of the cardiac sphincter of the stomach.

e·soph·a·go·gas·tros·to·my (ĭ-sŏf′ə-gō-gă-strŏs′tə-mē) *n.* Surgical anastomosis of the esophagus to the stomach, usually following esophagogastrectomy.

e·soph·a·go·gram (ĭ-sŏf′ə-gə-grăm′) *n.* A radiograph of the esophagus obtained during esophagography.

e·soph·a·gog·ra·phy (ĭ-sŏf′ə-gŏg′rə-fē) *n.* Radiographic visualization of the esophagus using a swallowed radiopaque contrast medium.

e·soph·a·go·ma·la·ci·a (ĭ-sŏf′ə-gō-mə-lā′shē-ə, -shə) *n.* Softening of the walls of the esophagus.

e·soph·a·go·my·ot·o·my (ĭ-sŏf′ə-gō-mī-ŏt′ə-mē) *n.* Treatment of esophageal achalasia by a longitudinal division of the lowest part of the esophageal muscle down to the submucosal layer; some muscle fibers of the cardia may also be divided.

e·soph·a·go·plas·ty (ĭ-sŏf′ə-gə-plăs′tē) *n.* Surgical repair of a defect in the wall of the esophagus.

e·soph·a·go·pli·ca·tion (ĭ-sŏf′ə-gō-plī-kā′shən) *n.* Surgery to narrow a dilated esophagus by making longitudinal folds or tucks in its walls.

e·soph·a·gop·to·sis (ĭ-sŏf′ə-gŏp-tō′sĭs, -gō-tō′sĭs) or **e·soph·a·gop·to·si·a** (-tō′sē-ə, -zē-ə) *n.* Relaxation and downward displacement of the walls of the esophagus.

e·soph·a·go·scope (ĭ-sŏf′ə-gə-skōp′) *n.* An endoscope for examining the interior of the esophagus.

e·soph·a·gos·co·py (ĭ-sŏf′ə-gŏs′kə-pē) *n.* Examination of the interior of the esophagus by means of an esophagoscope.

e·soph·a·go·spasm (ĭ-sŏf′ə-gə-spăz′əm) *n.* Spasm of the walls of the esophagus.

e·soph·a·go·ste·no·sis (ĭ-sŏf′ə-gō-stə-nō′sĭs) *n.* Stricture or narrowing of the esophagus.

e·soph·a·gos·to·my (ĭ-sŏf′ə-gŏs′tə-mē) *n.* The surgical formation of an opening directly into the esophagus.

e·soph·a·got·o·my (ĭ-sŏf′ə-gŏt′ə-mē) *n.* An incision through the wall of the esophagus.

e·soph·a·gus or **oe·soph·a·gus** (ĭ-sŏf′ə-gəs) *n., pl.* **-gi** (-jī′, -gī′). The portion of the digestive canal between the pharynx and stomach. — **e·soph′a·ge′al** (-jē′əl) *adj.*

es·o·pho·ri·a (ĕs′ə-fôr′ē-ə) *n.* A tendency of the eyes to deviate inward. — **es′o·phor′ic** (-fôr′ĭk, -fŏr′-) *adj.*

es·o·sphe·noid·i·tis (ĕs′ō-sfē′noi-dī′tĭs) *n.* Osteomyelitis of the sphenoid bone.

es·o·tro·pi·a (ĕs′ə-trō′pē-ə) *n.* Strabismus in which the visual axes converge. — **es′o·trop′ic** (-trŏp′ĭk, -trō′pĭk) *adj.*

ESP *abbr.* extrasensory perception

es·pun·di·a (ĭ-spŭn′dē-ə, ĕs-pōōn′dyä) *n.* A type of American leishmaniasis caused by *Leishmania braziliensis* that affects the mucous membranes, particularly of the nose and mouth, eventually resulting in grossly destructive changes.

ESR *abbr.* erythrocyte sedimentation rate; electron spin resonance

es·sen·tial (ĭ-sĕn′shəl) *adj.* **1.** Constituting or being part of the essence of something; inherent. **2.** Basic or indispensable; necessary. **3.** Of, relating to, or being a dysfunctional condition or a disease whose cause is unknown. **4.** Of, relating to, or being a substance that is required for normal functioning but cannot be synthesized by the body and therefore must be included in the diet. — *n.* **1.** Something fundamental. **2.** Something necessary or indispensable.

essential amino acid *n.* An alpha-amino acid that is required for protein synthesis but cannot be synthesized by humans and must be obtained in the diet.

essential hematuria *n.* Hematuria whose cause has not been determined.

essential hypertension *n.* Hypertension without known cause or preexisting renal disease.

essential tachycardia *n.* Persistent rapid action of the heart that cannot be attributed to any discernible organic lesion.

Es·ser graft (ĕs′ər) *n.* See **inlay graft.**

es·ter (ĕs′tər) *n.* Any of a class of organic compounds formed from an organic acid and an alcohol, usually with the elimination of water.

Est·lan·der operation (ĕst′lăn′dər, -län′-) *n.* Transfer of a full-thickness flap from one side of the lip to the same side of the opposite lip.

es·tra·di·ol (ĕs′trə-dī′ôl′, -ōl′) *n.* The most potent naturally occurring estrogen.

es·tra·mus·tine phosphate sodium (ĕs′trə-mŭs′tēn′) *n.* An antineoplastic agent that combines the actions of estrogen and nitrogen mustard in the treatment of carcinoma of the prostate.

es·tri·ol (ĕs′trī-ôl′, -ōl′, ĕ-strī′-) *n.* A metabolite of estradiol, usually the predominant estrogenic metabolite found in the urine of pregnant women.

es·tro·gen or **oes·tro·gen** (ĕs′trə-jən) *n.* Any of several natural or synthetic substances formed by the ovary, placenta, testis, and certain plants, that stimulate the female secondary sex characteristics, exert systemic effects such as the growth and maturation of long bones, and are used to treat disorders due to estrogen deficiency and to ameliorate cancers of the breast and prostate.

es·tro·gen·ic (ĕs′trə-jĕn′ĭk) *adj.* **1.** Causing estrus in animals. **2.** Having an action similar to that of an estrogen.

es·trone (ĕs′trōn′) *n.* A metabolite of estradiol having considerably less biological activity than estradiol but similar properties and uses.

es·trous cycle (ĕs′trəs) *n.* The recurrent set of physiological and behavioral changes that take place from one period of estrus to another.

es·trus or **oes·trus** (ĕs′trəs) *n.* The periodic state of sexual excitement in the female of most mammals, excluding humans, that immediately precedes ovulation and during which the female is most receptive to mating.

eth·am·bu·tol (ĕ-thăm′byə-tôl′, -tŏl′) *n.* An antibacterial drug used with other drugs in the treatment of pulmonary tuberculosis.

eth·a·nol (ĕth′ə-nôl′, -nŏl′) *n.* See **alcohol** (sense 2).

e·ther (ē′thər) *n.* An anesthetic ether, especially diethyl ether.

eth·i·cal (ĕth′ĭ-kəl) *adj.* **1.** Of, relating to, or dealing with ethics. **2.** Being in accordance with the accepted principles of right and wrong that govern the conduct of a profession.

eth·ics (ĕth′ĭks) *n.* The rules or standards governing the conduct of a person or the members of a profession.

eth·moi·dal crest (ĕth-moid′l) *n.* **1.** A ridge on the nasal surface of the upper jawbone that attaches to the middle nasal concha. **2.** A ridge on the palatine bone to which the middle nasal concha attaches.

ethmoidal sinus *n.* Any of the evaginations of the mucus membrane of the middle or superior canals of the nasal cavity.

eth·moid bone (ĕth′moid′) *n.* A light spongy bone located between the eye sockets, forming part of the walls and septum of the superior nasal cavity, and containing numerous perforations for the passage of the fibers of the olfactory nerves.

eth·moi·dec·to·my (ĕth′moi-dĕk′tə-mē) *n.* Removal of all or a part of the mucosal lining and bony partitions between the ethmoid sinuses.

eth·moid·i·tis (ĕth′moi-dī′tĭs) *n.* Inflammation of the ethmoid sinuses.

eth·no·cen·trism (ĕth′nō-sĕn′trĭz′əm) *n.* The tendency to evaluate other groups according to the values and standards of one's own ethnic group, especially with the conviction that one's own ethnic group is superior to the other groups. — **eth′-no·cen′tric** (-trĭk)

ethyl alcohol *n.* See **alcohol** (sense 2).

e·thy·no·di·ol (ĕ-thī′nə-dī′ôl′, -ŏl′) *n.* A semisynthetic steroid having similar effects as progesterone and administered with an estrogen as an oral contraceptive.

et·i·dro·nate di·so·di·um (ĕt′ĭ-drō′nāt′ dī-sō′-dē-əm) *n.* A drug that affects bone resorption and is used to treat of Paget's disease, heterotopic ossification, and hypercalcemia of malignancy.

e·ti·ol·o·gy or **ae·ti·ol·o·gy** (ē′tē-ŏl′ə-jē) *n.* **1.** The science and study of the causes or origins of dis-

ease. **2.** The cause or origin of a disease or disorder as determined by medical diagnosis.

e·to·po·side (ē′tə-pō′sīd′) *n.* A semisynthetic derivative of podophyllotoxin that is a mitotic inhibitor used in the treatment of refractory testicular tumors and small cell lung cancer.

e·tret·i·nate (ĭ-trĕt′n-āt′) *n.* A retinoid used in the treatment of severe recalcitrant psoriasis.

eu·chlor·hy·dri·a (yōō′klôr-hī′drē-ə) *n.* The presence of normal amounts of free hydrochloric acid in the gastric juice.

eu·cho·li·a (yōō-kō′lē-ə) *n.* A normal state of the bile in quantity and quality.

eu·chro·ma·tin (yōō-krō′mə-tĭn) *n.* Chromosomal material that consists of uncoiled dispersed threads during interphase, is genetically active, and stains lightly with basic dyes.

eu·cra·sia (yōō-krā′zhə, -zhē-ə) *n.* A condition of reduced susceptibility to certain drugs or nutritional elements.

eu·di·a·pho·re·sis (yōō-dī′ə-fə-rē′sĭs, dī-ăf′ə-) *n.* Normal, free sweating.

eu·gen·ic (yōō-jĕn′ĭk) *adj.* **1.** Of or relating to eugenics. **2.** Relating or adapted to the production of good or improved offspring.

eu·gen·ics (yōō-jĕn′ĭks) *n.* The study of hereditary improvement of the human race by controlled selective breeding.

eu·glob·u·lin (yōō-glŏb′yə-lĭn) *n.* A simple protein that is soluble in dilute salt solutions and insoluble in distilled water.

eu·gly·ce·mi·a (yōō′glī-sē′mē-ə) *n.* Normal concentration of glucose in the blood. — **eu′gly·ce′-mic** (-mĭk) *adj.*

eu·gna·thi·a (yōō-nā′thē-ə, -năth′ē-ə) *n.* Normal development and function of the system that includes the jaw and the teeth.

eu·kar·y·ote or **eu·car·y·ote** (yōō-kăr′ē-ōt, -ē-ət) *n.* A single-celled or multicellular organism whose cells contain a distinct membrane-bound nucleus. — **eu·kar′y·ot′ic** (-ŏt′ĭk) *adj.*

eu·me·tri·a (yōō-mē′trē-ə) *n.* A normal graduation of the strength of nerve impulses to match the intended voluntary movement.

eu·nuch (yōō′nək) *n.* A man or boy whose testes have been removed or have never developed.

eu·nuch·oid gigantism (yōō′nə-koid′) *n.* Gigantism in which testicular secretions are deficient or absent, causing deficient sexual development.

eu·nuch·oid·ism (yōō′nə-koi-dĭz′əm) *n.* A state in which testes are present but fail to function.

eu·pep·si·a (yōō-pĕp′sē-ə, -shə) *n.* Good digestion.

eu·pho·ri·a (yōō-fôr′ē-ə) *n.* A feeling of great happiness or well-being, commonly exaggerated and not necessarily well founded.

eu·plas·tic lymph (yōō-plăs′tĭk) *n.* Lymph containing relatively few white blood cells but a comparatively high concentration of fibrinogen, tending to organize with fibrous tissue.

eup·ne·a (yōōp-nē′ə) *n.* Easy, free respiration, as is observed normally under resting conditions. — **eup·ne′ic** *adj.*

eu·prax·i·a (yōō-prăk′sē-ə) *n*. Normal ability to perform coordinated movements.

eu·rhyth·mi·a (yōō-rĭ*th*′mē-ə) *n*. Harmonious relationships among the organs of the body.

eu·ro·pi·um (yōō-rō′pē-əm) *n*. A rare-earth element with atomic number 63, used as a neutron absorber in nuclear research.

eu·ry·o·pi·a (yōōr′ē-ō′pē-ə) *n*. Abnormally wide opening of the eyes.

eu·sta·chian tube (yōō-stā′shən, -shē-ən, -kē-ən) *n*. A slender tube that connects the tympanic cavity with the nasal part of the pharynx and equalizes air pressure on either side of the eardrum.

eu·tha·na·sia (yōō′thə-nā′zhə, -zhē-ə) *n*. **1.** The act or practice of ending the life of a person suffering from a terminal illness or an incurable condition, as by lethal injection or the suspension of extraordinary medical treatment. **2.** A quiet, painless death.

eu·then·ics (yōō-thĕn′ĭks) *n*. The science concerned with establishing optimum living conditions for plants, animals, or humans, especially through care for proper provisioning and environment.

eu·tro·phi·a (yōō-trō′fē-ə) *n*. A state of normal nourishment and growth.

e·vac·u·ate (ĭ-văk′yōō-āt′) *v*. **-at·ed, -at·ing, -ates. 1.** To empty or remove the contents of. **2.** To excrete or discharge waste matter, especially from the bowels.

e·vac·u·a·tion (ĭ-văk′yōō-ā′shən) *n*. Discharge of waste materials from the excretory passages of the body, especially from the bowels.

e·vac·u·a·tor (ĭ-văk′yōō-ā′tər) *n*. An instrument for removal of material from a body cavity.

e·vag·i·na·tion (ĭ-văj′ə-nā′shən) *n*. The protrusion of some part or organ from its normal position. — **e·vag′i·nate′** *v*.

e·vap·o·rate (ĭ-văp′ə-rāt′) *v*. **-rat·ed, -rat·ing, -rates. 1.** To convert or change into a vapor; volatilize. **2.** To produce vapor. **3.** To draw or pass off in the form of vapor. **4.** To draw moisture from, as by heating, leaving only the dry solid portion. — **e·vap′o·ra′tive** *adj*.

e·vap·o·ra·tion (ĭ-văp′ə-rā′shən) *n*. **1.** A change from liquid to vapor form. **2.** Loss of volume of a liquid by conversion into vapor.

e·ven·tra·tion (ē′vĕn-trā′shən) *n*. **1.** Protrusion of the omentum or intestine through an opening in the abdominal wall. **2.** Removal of the contents of the abdominal cavity.

eventration of the diaphragm *n*. Extreme elevation of part of the diaphragm, which is usually atrophic and abnormally thin.

e·ver·sion (ĭ-vûr′zhən, -shən) *n*. A turning outward, as of the eyelid.

e·vert (ĭ-vûrt′) *v*. **e·vert·ed, e·vert·ing, e·verts.** To turn inside out or outward.

e·vis·cer·a·tion (ĭ-vĭs′ə-rā′shən) *n*. **1.** Removal of the contents of the eyeball, leaving the sclera and sometimes the cornea. **2.** See **exenteration. 3.** Protrusion of the abdominal viscera, as through a defect created by dehiscence. — **e·vis′cer·ate′**

ev·o·ca·tion (ĕv′ə-kā′shən, ē′və-) *n*. The induction of a particular tissue produced by the action of an evocator during embryogenesis.

ev·o·ca·tor (ĕv′ə-kā′tər, ē′və-) *n*. The chemical factor discharged from an organizer, controlling morphogenesis in the early embryo.

e·voked response (ĭ-vōkt′) *n*. An alteration in the electrical activity of a part of the nervous system as a result of receiving a sensory stimulus.

ev·o·lu·tion (ĕv′ə-lōō′shən, ē′və-) *n*. **1.** A continuing process of change from one state, condition, or form to another. **2.** The theory that groups of organisms change with passage of time, mainly as a result of natural selection, so that descendants differ morphologically and physiologically from their ancestors.

e·vul·sion (ĭ-vŭl′shən) *n*. A forcible pulling out or extraction.

Ew·art's sign (yōō′ərts) *n*. An indication of a large pericardial effusion marked by an area of dullness below the left scapula, bronchial breathing, and bronchophony.

Ew·ing's tumor (yōō′ĭngz) *n*. A malignant tumor usually occurring before age 20 in males and involving the bones of the extremities; it usually affects the metaphysis of the bone.

ex·ac·er·ba·tion (ĭg-zăs′ər-bā′shən) *n*. An increase in the severity of a disease or in any of its signs or symptoms. — **ex·ac′er·bate′** *v*.

ex·am·i·na·tion (ĭg-zăm′ə-nā′shən) *n*. An investigation or inspection made for the purpose of diagnosis.

ex·am·ine (ĭg-zăm′ĭn) *v*. **1.** To study or analyze an organic material. **2.** To test or check the condition or health of. **3.** To determine the qualifications, aptitude, or skills of by means of questions or exercises.

ex·an·the·ma (ĕg′zăn-thē′mə) or **ex·an·them** (ĭg-zăn′thəm) *n*. **1.** A skin eruption occurring as a symptom of an acute viral or coccal disease. **2.** A disease, such as measles or scarlet fever, accompanied by a skin eruption. — **ex·an′the·mat′ic** (ĭg-zăn′-thə-măt′ĭk), **ex′an·them′a·tous** (ĕg′zăn-thĕm′ə-təs) *adj*.

exanthema su·bi·tum (sōō′bĭ-təm) *n*. A viral disease affecting infants and young children, characterized by fever lasting several days and a spotty rash that appears shortly after the fever subsides.

ex·ca·la·tion (ĕk′skə-lā′shən) *n*. The absence, suppression, or failure to develop one member of a series, such as a finger or vertebra.

ex·ca·va·tion (ĕk′skə-vā′shən) *n*. **1.** A natural cavity, pouch, or recess. **2.** A cavity formed artificially as the result of a pathological process.

ex·ca·va·tor (ĕk′skə-vā′tər) *n*. An instrument, such as a sharp spoon or curette, used in scraping out pathological tissue.

ex·ce·men·to·sis (ĕk′sĭ-mĕn-tō′sĭs) *n*. The outgrowth of cementum on the root surface of a tooth.

ex·cess (ĭk-sĕs′, ĕk′sĕs′) *n*. An amount or quantity beyond what is normal or sufficient; a surplus.

ex·change (ĭks-chānj′) v. To substitute one thing for another. — n. The act of substituting one thing for another.

exchange transfusion n. The removal of most of a patient's blood followed by introduction of an equal amount from donors.

ex·cise (ĭk-sīz′) v. **-cised, -cis·ing, -cis·es.** To remove by cutting.

ex·ci·sion (ĭk-sĭzh′ən) n. **1.** Surgical removal by cutting, as of a tumor or a portion of a structure or organ. **2.** A recombination event in which a genetic element is removed.

excision biopsy n. Excision of an entire lesion for gross and microscopic examination.

ex·cit·a·ble (ĭk-sī′tə-bəl) adj. **1.** Capable of reacting to a stimulus. Used of a tissue, cell, or cell membrane. **2.** Capable of emotional arousal. — **ex·cit′a·bil′i·ty, ex·cit′a·ble·ness** n.

excitable area n. See **motor cortex.**

ex·ci·ta·tion (ĕk′sī-tā′shən) n. **1.** The act of increasing the rapidity or intensity of the physical or mental processes; stimulation. **2.** The complete, all-or-none response of a nerve or muscle to an adequate stimulus, ordinarily including propagation of excitation along the membranes of the cell or cells involved.

ex·cite·ment (ĭk-sīt′mənt) n. An emotional state characterized by its potential for impulsive or poorly controlled activity.

ex·cit·ing eye (ĭk-sī′tĭng) n. The injured eye in sympathetic ophthalmia.

ex·ci·tor nerve (ĭk-sī′tər) n. A nerve conducting impulses that stimulate increased function.

ex·clave (ĕk′sklāv′) n. An outlying, detached portion of a gland or other part, as of the thyroid or pancreas; an accessory gland.

ex·clu·sion (ĭk-sklōō′zhən) n. Surgical isolation of a part or segment without removal from the body.

ex·co·ri·ate (ĭk-skôr′ē-āt′) v. **-at·ed, -at·ing, -ates.** To scratch or otherwise abrade the skin by physical means. — **ex·co′ri·a′tion** n.

ex·cre·ment (ĕk′skrə-mənt) n. Waste or excretions cast out of the body, especially feces.

ex·cres·cence (ĭk-skrĕs′əns) n. An outgrowth from a surface that may be normal, such as a fingernail, or abnormal, such as a wart.

ex·cre·ta (ĭk-skrē′tə) pl.n. See **excretion** (sense 2). — **ex·cre′tal** adj.

ex·crete (ĭk-skrēt′) v. **-cret·ed, -cret·ing, -cretes.** To eliminate waste material from the body.

ex·cre·tion (ĭk-skrē′shən) n. **1.** The act or process of discharging waste matter from the blood, tissues, or organs. **2.** The matter, such as urine or sweat, that is so excreted.

ex·cre·to·ry (ĕk′skrĭ-tôr′ē) adj. Of, relating to, or used in excretion.

excretory duct n. Any of various ducts carrying secretion from a gland or fluid from a reservoir.

excretory gland n. A gland separating waste material from the blood.

ex·cy·clo·duc·tion (ĭk-sī′klō-dŭk′shən) n. The outward rotation of the upper pole of a cornea.

ex·cy·clo·pho·ri·a (ĭk-sī′klō-fôr′ē-ə) n. The tendency of the eyes to rotate outward, prevented by the impulse of the eyes to act in coordination.

ex·cys·ta·tion (ĕk′sĭ-stā′shən) n. Escape from a cyst. Used of encysted parasites.

ex·e·mi·a (ĭk-sē′mē-ə) n. A condition in which a considerable portion of the blood is temporarily removed from circulation, as in shock when there is a great accumulation within the abdomen.

ex·en·ceph·a·ly (ĕk′sən-sĕf′ə-lē) n. A condition in which the skull is defective, causing exposure or extrusion of the brain. — **ex′en·ce·phal′ic** (-sə-făl′ĭk) adj.

ex·en·ter·a·tion (ĕk-sĕn′tə-rā′shən) n. The surgical removal of internal organs and tissues, usually the radical removal of the contents of a body cavity. — **ex·en′ter·ate′** v.

ex·en·ter·i·tis (ĕk-sĕn′tə-rī′tĭs) n. Inflammation of the peritoneal covering of the intestine.

ex·er·cise (ĕk′sər-sīz′) n. Active bodily exertion performed to develop or maintain fitness.

ex·er·e·sis (ĕk-sĕr′ĭ-sĭs) n. Surgical removal of any part or organ; excision.

ex·fo·li·a·tion (ĕks-fō′lē-ā′shən) n. **1.** Detachment and shedding of superficial cells of an epithelium or a tissue surface. **2.** Scaling or desquamation of the horny layer of epidermis. — **ex·fo′li·ate′** v.

ex·fo·li·a·tive (ĕks-fō′lē-ā′tĭv) adj. Marked by exfoliation, desquamation, or profuse scaling.

exfoliative dermatitis n. Widespread dermatitis characterized by scaling and shedding of the skin and usually accompanied by redness.

exfoliative gastritis n. Gastritis with excessive shedding of mucosal epithelial cells.

ex·ha·la·tion (ĕks′hə-lā′shən, ĕk′sə-) n. **1.** The act or an instance of breathing out. **2.** Something, such as air or vapor, that is exhaled.

ex·hale (ĕks-hāl′, ĕk-sāl′) v. **-haled, -hal·ing, -hales. 1.** To breathe out; expire. **2.** To emit a gas, vapor, or odor.

ex·haus·tion (ĭg-zôs′chən) n. **1.** The inability to respond to stimuli; extreme fatigue. **2.** The act or an instance of using up a supply of something. **3.** The extraction of the active constituents of a drug by treating with water or other solvent.

exhaustion psychosis n. A confused emotional state resulting from exhaustion.

ex·hi·bi·tion·ism (ĕk′sə-bĭsh′ə-nĭz′əm) n. An abnormal compulsion to expose the genitals with the intent of provoking sexual interest in the viewer. — **ex′hi·bi′tion·ist** n.

ex·o·an·ti·gen (ĕk′sō-ăn′tĭ-jən) n. See **ectoantigen.**

ex·o·car·di·a (ĕk′sō-kär′dē-ə) n. See **ectocardia.**

ex·o·crine (ĕk′sə-krĭn, -krēn, -krīn′) adj. **1.** Of or relating to a glandular secretion that is released externally through a duct to a surface. **2.** Relating to a gland that secretes through a duct or ducts.

exocrine gland n. A gland, such as a sebaceous gland or sweat gland, that releases its secretions to the body's cavities, organs, or surface through a duct.

ex·o·cy·to·sis (ĕk′sō-sī-tō′sĭs) n., pl. **-ses** (sēz′).

The appearance of migrating inflammatory cells in the epidermis.

ex·o·de·vi·a·tion (ĕk′sō-dē′vē-ā′shən) *n.* **1.** Exophoria. **2.** Exotropia.

ex·o·en·zyme (ĕk′sō-ĕn′zīm′) *n.* See **extracellular enzyme.**

ex·o·e·ryth·ro·cyt·ic stage (ĕk′sō-ĭ-rĭth′rə-sĭt′ĭk) *n.* The developmental stage of the malaria parasite in liver parenchyma cells of the vertebrate host before the red blood cells become infected.

ex·og·e·nous (ĕk-sŏj′ə-nəs) *adj.* **1.** Originating or produced outside of an organism, a tissue, or a cell. **2.** Having a cause external to the body. Used of diseases. — **ex·og′e·nous·ly** *adv.*

ex·om·pha·los (ĕk-sŏm′fə-lŏs′, -ləs) or **ex·um·bil·i·ca·tion** (ĕk′sŭm-bĭl′ĭ-kā′shən) *n.* **1.** Protrusion of the navel. **2.** See **umbilical hernia. 3.** See **omphalocele.**

ex·on (ĕk′sŏn) *n.* A nucleotide sequence in DNA that carries the code for the final mRNA molecule and thus defines the amino acid sequence during protein synthesis. — **ex·on′ic** *adj.*

ex·o·pho·ri·a (ĕk′sə-fôr′ē-ə) *n.* A tendency of the eyes to deviate outward. — **ex′o·phor′ic** (-fôr′ĭk, -fôr′ĭk) *adj.*

ex·oph·thal·mic (ĕk′səf-thăl′mĭk) *adj.* **1.** Relating to exophthalmos. **2.** Marked by prominence of the eyeball.

exophthalmic goiter *n.* Any of various forms of hyperthyroidism, such as Graves' disease, involving enlargement of the thyroid gland and protrusion of the eyeballs.

exophthalmic ophthalmoplegia *n.* Ophthalmoplegia with protrusion of the eyeballs due to orbital edema and contracture of the ocular muscles, incidental to thyroid disorders.

ex·oph·thal·mos (ĕk′səf-thăl′məs) *n.* Abnormal protrusion of the eyeball.

ex·o·se·ro·sis (ĕk′sō-sĭ-rō′sĭs) *n.* Serous oozing from the skin surface, as from eczema or abrasion.

ex·o·skel·e·ton (ĕk′sō-skĕl′ĭ-tn) *n.* All hard parts, such as hair, teeth, and nails that develop from the ectoderm or mesoderm in vertebrates.

ex·os·mo·sis (ĕk′sŏz-mō′sĭs, -sŏs-) *n.* The passage of a fluid through a semipermeable membrane toward a solution of lower concentration, especially the passage of water through a cell membrane into the surrounding medium. — **ex′os·mot′ic** (-mŏt′ĭk) *adj.*

ex·os·to·sis (ĕk′sŏ-stō′sĭs) *n.*, *pl.* **ex·os·to·ses** (-sēz). A cartilage-capped bony projection arising from a bone that develops from cartilage.

ex·o·tox·in (ĕk′sō-tŏk′sĭn) *n.* An toxin secreted by a microorganism and released into the environment in which it grows, where it is rapidly active in small amounts.

ex·o·tro·pi·a (ĕk′sə-trō′pē-ə) *n.* A form of strabismus in which the visual axis of one eye deviates from that of the other.

ex·pec·tant (ĭk-spĕk′tənt) *adj.* Pregnant.

ex·pec·to·rant (ĭk-spĕk′tər-ənt) *adj.* Promoting or facilitating the secretion or expulsion of phlegm, mucus, or other matter from the respiratory tract. — *n.* An expectorant medicine.

ex·pec·to·rate (ĭk-spĕk′tə-rāt′) *v.* **-rat·ed, -rat·ing, -rates. 1.** To eject saliva, mucus, or other body fluid from the mouth; spit. **2.** To clear out the chest and lungs by coughing up and spitting out matter. — **ex·pec′to·ra′tion** *n.*

ex·pe·ri·ence (ĭk-spēr′ē-əns) *n.* The feeling of emotions and sensations as opposed to thinking; involvement in what is happening rather than abstract reflection on an event or an encounter. — **ex·pe′ri·ence** *v.*

ex·per·i·ment (ĭk-spĕr′ə-mənt) *n.* **1.** A test under controlled conditions that demonstrates a known truth, examines the validity of a hypothesis, or determines the efficacy of something previously untried. **2.** The process of conducting such a test. **3.** An innovative act or procedure. **4.** The result of experimentation. — *v.* **-ment·ed, -ment·ing, -ments.** (-mĕnt′). **1.** To conduct an experiment. **2.** To try something new, especially in order to gain experience.

experimental medicine *n.* The scientific investigation of medical problems by experimentation upon animals or by clinical research.

ex·pi·ra·tion (ĕk′spə-rā′shən) *n.* See **exhalation** (sense 1).

ex·pi·ra·to·ry (ĭk-spī′rə-tôr′ē) *adj.* Of, relating to, or involving the expiration of air from the lungs.

expiratory stridor *n.* A singing sound during general anesthesia due to the semi-approximated vocal cords offering resistance to the escape of air.

ex·pire (ĭk-spīr′) *v.* **-pired, -pir·ing, -pires. 1.** To breathe one's last breath; die. **2.** To exhale.

expired gas *n.* A gas that has been expired from the lungs.

ex·plant (ĕk-splănt′) *v.* To transfer living tissue from an organism to an artificial medium for culture. — *n.* (ĕks′plănt′). Tissue so transferred.

ex·plo·ra·tion (ĕk′splə-rā′shən) *n.* An active examination, usually involving endoscopy or a surgical procedure, to determine conditions present as an aid in diagnosis. — **ex·plor′a·to′ry** (ĭk-splôr′ə-tôr′ē) *adj.*

explore *v.* **-plored, -plor·ing, -plores.** To examine for diagnostic purposes.

ex·plor·er (ĭk-splôr′ər) *n.* A sharp, pointed probe used to investigate tooth surfaces to detect caries or other defects.

ex·press (ĭk-sprĕs′) *v.* **-pressed, -press·ing, -press·es.** To press or squeeze out.

ex·pres·sion (ĭk-sprĕsh′ən) *n.* **1.** The act of pressing or squeezing out. **2.** The outward manifestation of a mood or disposition by mobility of the facial features; facies. **3.** The phenotype manifested by a genotype under a given set of environmental conditions.

ex·pul·sive pain (ĭk-spŭl′sĭv) *n.* A labor pain associated with contraction of the uterine muscle.

ex·qui·site (ĕk′skwĭ-zĭt, ĭk-skwĭz′ĭt) *adj.* Extremely intense, keen, or sharp. Used of pain or tenderness.

ex·sect (ĕk-sĕkt′) *v.* See **excise.**

ex·sec·tion (ĕk-sĕk′shən) *n.* See **excision.**

ex·sic·cate (ĕk′sĭ-kāt′) *v.* **-cat·ed, -cat·ing, -cates.** To dry up or cause to dry up; desiccate. — **ex′sic·ca′tor** *n.* — **ex′sic·ca′tive** *adj.*

ex·sic·ca·tion (ĕk′sĭ-kā′shən) *n.* **1.** The process of being dried up; desiccation. **2.** Removal of water of crystallization.

ex·sorp·tion (ĕk-sôrp′shən, -zôrp′-) *n.* The movement of substances from the blood into the lumen of the gut.

ex·stro·phy (ĕk′strə-fē) *n.* A congenital turning out or eversion of a hollow organ.

ex·tend (ĭk-stĕnd′) *v.* **-tend·ed, -tend·ing, -tends.** To straighten a limb; unbend.

extended family therapy *n.* Family therapy that involves family members who are outside the nuclear family but are closely associated with it.

extended radical mastectomy *n.* Surgical removal of the entire breast, the pectoral muscles, and the lymphatic-bearing tissues of the armpit and chest wall.

ex·ten·sion (ĭk-stĕn′shən) *n.* **1.** The act of straightening or extending a flexed limb. **2.** A pulling or dragging force exerted on a limb in a distal direction.

ex·ten·sor (ĭk-stĕn′sər) *n.* A muscle that extends or straightens a limb or body part.

ex·te·ri·or·ize (ĭk-stēr′ē-ə-rīz′) *v.* **-ized, -iz·ing, -iz·es. 1.** To turn outward; externalize. **2.** To direct a patient's interest, thoughts, or feelings into a channel leading outside himself or herself. **3.** To expose an internal organ temporarily for observation, or permanently for physiological experiment or surgery.

ex·tern (ĕk′stûrn′) *n.* An advanced student or recent graduate who assists in the medical or surgical care of hospital patients, but who lives outside the institution.

ex·ter·nal (ĭk-stûr′nəl) *adj.* Relating to, connected with, or existing on the outside; exterior.

external auditory canal *n.* See **ear canal.**

external ear *n.* The outer portion of the ear including the auricle and the passage leading to the eardrum.

external fistula *n.* A fistula between a body cavity and the skin.

external fixation *n.* The fixation of a fractured bone by a splint or plastic dressing.

external genitalia *n.* **1.** The vulva of the female. **2.** The penis and scrotum of the male.

external hemorrhoids *pl.n.* Hemorrhoids at the outer side of the external anal sphincter.

external iliac vein *n.* A continuation of the femoral vein uniting with the internal iliac vein to form the common iliac vein.

external respiration *n.* The exchange of respiratory gases in the lungs.

external traction *n.* A pulling force created by using fixed anchorage outside the oral cavity, as in the treatment of midfacial fractures.

external urethral opening *n.* **1.** The slitlike opening of the urethra in the glans penis. **2.** In the female, the external orifice of the urethra in the vestibule.

external urethrotomy *n.* A urethrotomy via an external opening in the perineum or penile skin.

external version *n.* Version of a fetus performed by external manipulation with both hands.

ex·ter·o·cep·tor (ĕk′stə-rō-sĕp′tər) *n.* One of the peripheral end organs of the afferent nerves in the skin or mucous membranes that respond to stimuli originating from outside the body. — **ex′ter·o·cep′tive** *adj.*

ex·ter·o·fec·tive (ĕk′stə-rō-fĕk′tĭv) *adj.* Relating to the response of the nervous system to external stimuli.

ex·ti·ma (ĕk′stə-mə) *n.* The outer coat of a blood vessel.

ex·tir·pa·tion (ĕk′stər-pā′shən) *n.* The surgical removal of an organ, a part of an organ, or a diseased tissue. — **ex′tir·pate′** *v.*

ex·tor·sion (ĭk-stôr′shən) *n.* **1.** The outward rotation of a limb or an organ. **2.** The outward divergent rotation of the upper poles of the vertical meridian of each eye.

ex·tra·cel·lu·lar (ĕk′strə-sĕl′yə-lər) *adj.* Located or occurring outside a cell or cells.

extracellular enzyme *n.* An enzyme, such as a digestive enzyme, that functions outside the cell from which it originates.

extracellular fluid *n.* **1.** The interstitial fluid and the plasma, constituting about 20 percent of the weight of the body. **2.** All fluid outside of cells, usually excluding transcellular fluid.

extracellular toxin *n.* See **exotoxin.**

ex·tra·cor·po·re·al (ĕk′strə-kôr-pôr′ē-əl) *adj.* Situated or occurring outside the body.

extracorporeal circulation *n.* Circulation of the blood outside the body, as through a heart-lung machine or artificial kidney.

ex·tract (ĭk-străkt′) *v.* **-tract·ed, -tract·ing, -tracts. 1.** To draw or pull out, using great force or effort. **2.** To obtain from a substance by chemical or mechanical action, as by pressure, distillation, or evaporation. — *n.* (ĕk′străkt′). **1.** A concentrated preparation of a drug obtained by removing the active constituents of the drug with suitable solvents, evaporating all or nearly all of the solvent, and adjusting the residual mass or powder to the prescribed standard. **2.** A concentrated preparation of the essential constituents of a food or a flavoring; a concentrate. — **ex·tract′a·ble, ex·tract′i·ble** *adj.* — **ex·trac′tor** *n.*

ex·trac·tion (ĭk-străk′shən) *n.* **1.** The act of extracting or the condition of being extracted. **2.** Something obtained by extracting; an extract. **3.** The removal by withdrawing or pulling out of a tooth from its socket. **4.** Removal of a baby from the genital canal in assisted delivery. **5.** The active portion of a drug.

extraction coefficient *n.* The percentage of a substance removed from the blood or plasma in a single passage through a tissue.

extraction ratio *n.* The fraction of a substance removed from blood flowing through the kidney, calculated using the ratio of the concentrations of the substance in arterial and renal venous plasma.

ex·trac·tor (ĭk-străk′tər) n. An instrument used for drawing or pulling out any natural part or a foreign body.

ex·tra·py·ram·i·dal (ĕk′strə-pĭ-răm′ĭ-dl) adj. Relating to or involving neural pathways situated outside or independent of the pyramidal tracts.

ex·tra·py·ram·i·dal disease (ĕk′strə-pĭ-răm′ĭ-dl) n. A degenerative disease, such as Parkinsonism or chorea, that affects the corpus striatum of the brain or other part of the extrapyramidal motor system and is manifested by tremor, muscular rigidity or weakness, and involuntary movements.

extrapyramidal motor system n. All of the brain structures affecting bodily movement but excluding the motor neurons, the motor cortex, and the pyramidal tract.

ex·tra·sen·so·ry (ĕk′strə-sĕn′sə-rē) adj. Being outside the normal range or bounds of the senses.

extrasensory perception n. Perception by means other than through the ordinary senses, as in telepathy, clairvoyance, or precognition.

ex·tra·sys·to·le (ĕk′strə-sĭs′tə-lē) n. An ectopic, usually premature contraction of the heart, resulting in momentary cardiac arrhythmia.

ex·trav·a·sate (ĭk-străv′ə-sāt′) v. -sat·ed, -sat·ing, -sates. To exude from or pass out of a vessel into the tissues. Used of blood, lymph, or urine. — **ex·trav′a·sate′, ex·trav′a·sa′tion** n.

ex·tra·vas·cu·lar fluid (ĕk′strə-văs′kyə-lər) n. All fluid outside the blood vessels, comprising both intracellular and transcellular fluids, constituting about 48 percent to 58 percent of body weight.

ex·trem·i·ty (ĭk-strĕm′ĭ-tē) n. **1.** An end of an elongated or pointed structure. **2.** A bodily limb or appendage.

ex·trin·sic (ĭk-strĭn′sĭk, -zĭk) adj. Of or relating to an organ or a structure, especially a muscle, originating outside of the part where it is found or upon which it acts. — **ex·trin′si·cal·ly** adv.

extrinsic factor n. See vitamin B₁₂.

ex·tro·ver·sion or **ex·tra·ver·sion** (ĕk′strə-vûr′zhən) n. **1.** A turning inside out, as of an organ or a part. **2.** Interest in one's environment or in others as opposed to or to the exclusion of oneself.

ex·tro·vert or **ex·tra·vert** (ĕk′strə-vûrt′) n. An individual interested in others or in the environment as opposed to or to the exclusion of self.

ex·trude (ĭk-strōōd′) v. -trud·ed, -trud·ing, -trudes. **1.** To thrust, force, or press out. **2.** To protrude or project.

ex·tru·sion (ĭk-strōō′zhən) n. **1.** A thrusting or forcing out of a normal position. **2.** The eruption or migration of a tooth beyond its normal occlusal position.

ex·tu·ba·tion (ĭn′tōō-bā′shən, -tyōō-) n. The removal of a tube from an organ, structure, or orifice; specifically, the removal of the tube after intubation of the larynx or trachea.

ex·u·date (ĕks′yōō-dāt′) n. A fluid that has exuded out of a tissue or its capillaries due to injury or inflammation.

ex·u·da·tion (ĕks′yōō-dā′shən) n. **1.** The act or process of exuding. **2.** An exudate.

ex·u·da·tive inflammation (ĕks′yōō-dā′tĭv) n. Inflammation in which the distinguishing feature is an exudate, which may be serous, serofibrinous, fibrinous, or mucous.

exudative retinitis n. A chronic inflammatory condition of the retina, characterized by the appearance of white or yellowish raised areas encircling the optic disk, due to the accumulation of edematous fluid beneath the retina.

ex·ude (ĭg-zōōd′, ĭk-sōōd′) v. -ud·ed, -ud·ing, -udes. To ooze or pass gradually out of a body structure or tissue.

eye (ī) n. **1.** An organ of vision or of light sensitivity. **2.** Either of a pair of hollow structures located in bony sockets of the skull, functioning together or independently, each having a lens capable of focusing incident light on an internal photosensitive retina from which nerve impulses are sent to the brain; the organ of vision. **3.** The external, visible portion of this organ together with its associated structures, especially the eyelids, eyelashes, and eyebrows. **4.** The pigmented iris of this organ.

eye·ball (ī′bôl′) n. **1.** The globe-shaped portion of the eye surrounded by the socket and covered externally by the eyelids. **2.** The eye itself.

eye bank n. A place where corneas of eyes removed immediately after death are preserved for subsequent keratoplasty.

eye bath n. See eyecup (sense 1).

eye·brow (ī′brou′) n. **1.** The bony ridge extending over the eye. **2.** The arch of short hairs covering this ridge.

eye chart n. A chart of letters and figures of various sizes, used to test visual acuity.

eye·cup (ī′kŭp′) n. A small cup with a rim contoured to fit the socket of the eye, used for applying a liquid medicine or wash to the eye.

eyed·ness (īd′nĭs) n. A preference for use of one eye rather than the other.

eye·drop·per (ī′drŏp′ər) n. A dropper for administering liquid medicines, especially one for dispensing medications into the eye.

eye·glass (ī′glăs′) n. **1.** eyeglasses. Glasses for the eyes. **2.** A single lens in a pair of glasses; a monocle. **3. 4.** See eyecup.

eye·ground (ī′ground′) n. The fundus of the eye as seen with the ophthalmoscope.

eye·lash (ī′lăsh′) n. **1.** Any of the short hairs fringing the edge of the eyelid. **2.** A row of the hairs fringing the eyelid.

eyelash sign n. An indication of unconsciousness due to functional disease rather than cranial trauma or a brain lesion, in which the stroking of the eyelashes will elicit movement of the eyelids.

eye·lid or **eye-lid** (ī′lĭd′) n. Either of two folds of skin and muscle that can be closed over the exposed portion of the eyeball.

eye·lift (ī′lĭft′) n. Cosmetic plastic surgery of the tissue surrounding the eye to reduce or eliminate folds, wrinkles, and sags.

eye·sight (ī'sīt') *n.* **1.** The faculty of sight; vision. **2.** Range of vision; view.

eye socket *n.* See orbital cavity.

eye·strain (ī'strān') *n.* Pain and fatigue of the eyes, often accompanied by headache, resulting from prolonged use of the eyes, uncorrected defects of vision, or an imbalance of the eye muscles.

eye·tooth (ī'tōōth') *n.* A canine tooth of the upper jaw.

eye·wash (ī'wŏsh') *n.* A soothing solution for bathing or medicating the eye.

~ ~ ~ ~ ~ ~ **F** ~ ~ ~ ~ ~ ~

F *abbr.* Fahrenheit

Fab fragment (ĕf'ā-bē') *n.* The portion of an immunoglobulin molecule that binds the antigen.

Fa·bry's disease (fä'brēz) *n.* A sex-linked disorder of glycolipid metabolism marked by progressive symptoms including fever, hypertension, and purple skin lesions, with death resulting from renal, cardiac, or cerebrovascular complications.

face (fās) *n.* **1.** The front portion of the head, from forehead to chin. **2.** Facies.

face-bow (fās'bō') *n.* A caliperlike device used in dentistry to record the relationship of the jaws to the temporomandibular joints.

face-lift (fās'lĭft') *n.* Plastic surgery to remove facial wrinkles, sagging skin, fat deposits, or other visible signs of aging for cosmetic purposes.

face presentation *n.* Head presentation of the fetus during birth in which the face is the presenting part.

fac·et (fās'ĭt) *n.* A small smooth area on a bone or other firm structure.

fac·e·tec·to·my (fās'ĭ-tĕk'tə-mē) *n.* Excision of a facet, as of a vertebra.

fa·cial (fā'shəl) *adj.* Relating to the face.

facial bone *n.* Any of the bones surrounding the mouth and nose and contributing to the eye sockets, including the upper jawbones, the zygomatic, nasal, lacrimal, and palatine bones, lower jawbone, and hyoid bone.

facial hemiplegia *n.* Paralysis of one side of the face.

facial muscle *n.* Any of the numerous muscles that are supplied by the facial nerve and are attached to and move the skin.

facial nerve *n.* Either of a pair of nerves that originate in the tegmentum of the lower portion of the pons, emerge from the brain at the posterior border of the pons, leave the cranial cavity through the internal acoustic meatus, reach the facial muscles through various branches, control facial muscles, and relay sensation from the taste buds of the front part of the tongue.

facial palsy *n.* Unilateral paralysis of the facial muscles supplied by the seventh cranial nerve.

facial spasm *n.* See facial tic.

facial tic *n.* Involuntary spasmodic movement of the facial muscles.

facial vein *n.* Any of four veins of the face: the anterior facial vein, common facial vein, deep facial vein, and retromandibular vein.

fa·ci·es (fā'shē-ēz', -shēz) *n., pl.* **facies. 1.** Face. **2.** The appearance or expression of the face, especially when typical of a certain disorder or disease.

fa·cil·i·ta·tion (fə-sĭl'ĭ-tā'shən) *n.* The enhancement or reinforcement of a reflex or other nerve activity by the arrival of other excitatory impulses at the reflex center.

fa·ci·o·plas·ty (fā'shē-ə-plăs'tē) *n.* Reparative or reconstructive surgery of the face.

fac·tor (fāk'tər) *n.* **1.** One that contributes in the cause of an action. **2.** A gene. **3.** A substance, such as a vitamin, that functions in a specific biochemical reaction or bodily process, such as blood coagulation.

factor VIII *n.* A factor in blood clotting, a deficiency of which is associated with hemophilia A.

factor IX *n.* A factor in blood clotting necessary for the formation of intrinsic blood thromboplastin; a deficiency of it causes hemophilia B or Christmas disease.

fac·ul·ta·tive (fāk'əl-tā'tĭv) *adj.* Capable of functioning under varying environmental conditions. Used of certain organisms, such as bacteria that can live with or without oxygen. — **fac'ul·ta'·tive·ly** *adv.*

fac·ul·ty (fāk'əl-tē) *n.* A natural or specialized power of a living organism.

Fahr·en·heit (fār'ən-hīt') *adj.* Of or relating to a temperature scale that registers the freezing point of water as 32°F and the boiling point as 212°F at one atmosphere of pressure.

fail·ure (fāl'yər) *n.* The inability to function or perform satisfactorily.

faint (fānt) *n.* An abrupt, usually brief loss of consciousness; a syncope attack. — *adj.* Extremely weak; threatened with syncope. — **faint** *v.*

faith healer *n.* One who treats disease with prayer.

fal·cip·a·rum malaria (fāl-sĭp'ər-əm, fôl-) *n.* Malaria caused by *Plasmodium falciparum* and characterized by severe paroxysms about every 48 hours and often by acute cerebral, renal, or gastrointestinal manifestations.

fall·en arch (fô'lən) *n.* A breaking down of the longitudinal or transverse arch of the foot, resulting in flat foot or spread foot.

fall·ing of the womb (fô′lĭng) *n.* See **prolapse of the uterus.**

fal·lo·pi·an tube or **Fallopian tube** (fə-lō′pē-ən) *n.* Either of a pair of slender tubes from each ovary to the side of the fundus of the uterus, through which the ova pass.

Fal·lot's tetralogy (fă-lōz′) *n.* A congenital malformation of the heart characterized by a defect in the ventricular septum, misplacement of the origin of the aorta, narrowing of the pulmonary artery, and enlargement of the right ventricle.

Fallot's triad *n.* Trilogy of Fallot.

false hermaphroditism *n.* See **pseudohermaphroditism.**

false image *n.* The image in the deviating eye in strabismus.

false joint *n.* A bony junction, usually the site of a poorly united fracture, that allows abnormal motion.

false knot *n.* A knotlike bulge in the umbilical vein causing apparent twisting of the cord.

false membrane *n.* A thick, tough, fibrinous exudate formed on the surface of a mucous membrane or the skin.

false-negative reaction *n.* An erroneous or mistakenly negative response.

false pain *n.* A uterine contraction, preceding and sometimes resembling a true labor pain, but distinguishable from it by the lack of progressive effacement and dilation of the cervix.

false-positive reaction *n.* An erroneous or mistakenly positive response.

false pregnancy *n.* See **pseudocyesis.**

false rib *n.* Any of the five pairs of lower ribs that do not articulate directly with the sternum.

false waters *pl.n.* A leakage of fluid before or at the beginning of labor, before the rupture of the amnion.

fal·si·fi·ca·tion (fôl′sə-fĭ-kā′shən) *n.* The deliberate act of misrepresentation so as to deceive.

falx (fălks, fôlks) *n., pl.* **fal·ces** (făl′sēz′, fôl′-). A sickle-shaped anatomical structure.

fa·mil·ial (fə-mĭl′yəl) *adj.* Occurring or tending to occur among members of a family, usually by heredity.

familial aggregation *n.* Occurrence of a trait in more members of a family than can be readily accounted for by chance.

familial hyperlipoproteinemia *n.* Any of several inherited disorders of lipoprotein metabolism characterized by changes in serum concentrations of low-density lipoproteins and the lipids associated with them. .

familial screening *n.* The screening of close relatives of individuals who have diseases that may be latent, as in age-dependent dominant traits, or that may involve risk to offspring, as X-linked traits.

fam·i·ly (făm′ə-lē, făm′lē) *n.* **1.** A group of blood relatives, especially parents and their children. **2.** A taxonomic category of related organisms ranking below an order and above a genus.

family doctor *n.* **1.** A physician who practices the specialty of family medicine. **2.** See **general practitioner.**

family medicine *n.* The branch of medicine that deals with provision of comprehensive health care to people regardless of age or sex while placing particular emphasis on the family unit.

family physician *n.* See **family doctor** (sense 1).

family planning *n.* A program to regulate the number and spacing of children in a family through the practice of contraception or other methods of birth control.

family practice *n.* See **family medicine.**

family practitioner *n.* See **family doctor** (sense 1).

family therapy *n.* A form of psychotherapy in which the interrelationships of family members are examined in group sessions in order to identify and alleviate the problems of one or more members of the family.

fa·mo·ti·dine (fə-mō′tĭ-dēn′) *n.* A drug that inhibits gastric secretion and is used in the treatment of duodenal ulcers.

FANA test *n.* See **fluorescent antinuclear antibody test.**

Fan·co·ni's anemia (făn-kō′nēz, făn-) *n.* A type of idiopathic refractory anemia characterized by pancytopenia, hypoplasia of the bone marrow, and congenital anomalies, occurring in members of the same family.

Fanconi's syndrome *n.* A group of renal tubular disorders that includes acquired or hereditary renal tubular disfunction and softening of bone.

fan·ta·sy (făn′tə-sē, -zē) *n.* Imagery that is more or less coherent, as in dreams and daydreams, yet unrestricted by reality.

far·del (fär-dĕl′) *n.* A measurement used in genetic counseling to determine the penalty incurred as a result of the occurrence of a genetic disease in an individual.

farm·er's lung (fär′mərz) *n.* An occupational disease characterized by fever and dyspnea, caused by inhalation of organic dust from moldy hay containing spores of actinomycetes and certain true fungi.

far point *n.* The farthest point of distinct vision.

far·sight·ed or **far-sight·ed** (fär′sī′tĭd) *adj.* **1.** Able to see distant objects better than objects at close range. **2.** Capable of seeing to a great distance.

far·sight·ed·ness (fär′sī′tĭd-nĭs) *n.* See **hyperopia.**

fas·ci·a (făsh′ē-ə) *n., pl.* **fas·ci·ae** (făsh′-ē-ē′, fă′-shē-ē). A sheet or band of fibrous connective tissue enveloping, separating, or binding together muscles, organs, and other soft structures of the body. — **fas′ci·al** *adj.*

fascia ad·her·ens (ăd-hēr′ənz, -hēr′-) *n.* A broad intercellular junction in the intercalated disk of cardiac muscle anchoring actin filaments.

fascia graft *n.* A graft of fibrous tissue, usually the broad fascia.

fas·ci·cle (făs′ĭ-kəl) *n.* See **fasciculus.**

fas·cic·u·lar graft (fə-sĭk′yə-lər) *n.* A nerve graft in which each bundle of fibers is approximated and sutured separately.

fas·cic·u·la·tion (fə-sĭk′yə-lā′shən) *n.* **1.** An arrangement of fasciculi. **2.** A coarser form of muscular contraction than fibrillation, consisting of involuntary contractions or twitchings of groups of muscle fibers. — **fas·cic′u·late′** v.

fas·cic·u·lus (fə-sĭk′yə-ləs) n., pl. **-li** (-lī′). A bundle of anatomical fibers, as of muscle or nerve.

fas·ci·ec·to·my (făsh′ē-ĕk′tə-mē, făs′-) n. Surgical excision of strips of fascia.

fas·ci·i·tis (făsh′ē-ī′tĭs, făs′-) n. **1.** Inflammation in a fascia. **2.** The proliferation of fibroblasts in a fascia.

fas·ci·od·e·sis (făsh′ē-ŏd′ĭ-sĭs, făs′-) n. Surgical attachment of a fascia to another fascia or to a tendon.

fas·ci·o·plas·ty (făsh′ē-ə-plăs′tē) n. Plastic surgery on a fascia.

fas·ci·or·rha·phy (făsh′ē-ôr′ə-fē) n. Suture of a fascia or of an aponeurosis.

fas·ci·ot·o·my (făsh′ē-ŏt′ə-mē) n. Surgical incision through a fascia.

fast v. **fast·ed, fast·ing, fasts. 1.** To abstain from food. **2.** To eat very little or abstain from certain foods, especially as a religious discipline. — n. **1.** The act or practice of abstaining from or eating very little food. **2.** A period of such abstention. **3.** A period of such abstention.

fas·tig·i·um (fă-stĭj′ē-əm) n. **1.** The summit of the roof of the fourth ventricle of the brain. **2.** The acme or period of full development of a disease.

fat (făt) n. **1.** Any of various soft, solid, or semisolid organic compounds constituting the esters of glycerol and fatty acids and their associated organic groups. **2.** A mixture of such compounds occurring widely in organic tissue, especially in the adipose tissue of animals. Fats and oils make up that class of foods known as simple lipids. **3.** Adipose tissue. **4.** Obesity; corpulence. — **fat** adj.

fa·tal (făt′l) adj. Causing or capable of causing death.

fa·tal·i·ty (fā-tăl′ĭ-tē, fə-) n. **1.** A death resulting from an accident or a disaster. **2.** One that is killed as a result of such an occurrence.

fa·tal·i·ty rate (fā-tăl′ĭ-tē, fə-) n. See **death rate.**

fat cell n. Any of various connective tissue cells found in adipose tissue, specialized for the storage of fat, and distended with one or more fat globules.

fat·i·ga·ble (făt′ĭ-gə-bəl) adj. Subject to fatigue. — **fat′i·ga·bil′i·ty** n.

fa·tigue (fə-tēg′) n. **1.** Physical or mental weariness resulting from exertion. **2.** A sensation of boredom and lassitude due to absence of stimulation, to monotony, or to lack of interest in one's surroundings. **3.** The decreased capacity or complete inability of an organism, an organ, or a part to function normally because of excessive stimulation or prolonged exertion.

fatigue fracture n. A fracture, usually transverse in orientation, that occurs as a result of repeated or unusual endogenous stress.

fat necrosis n. Necrosis of adipose tissue, characterized by the formation of small quantities of calcium soaps when fat is hydrolyzed into glycerol and fatty acids.

fat pad n. An accumulation of encapsulated adipose tissue.

fat-soluble adj. Soluble in fats or fat solvents.

fat-soluble vitamin n. Any of various vitamins soluble in fats or fat solvents.

fat·ty (făt′ē) adj. **1.** Containing or composed of fat. **2.** Characteristic of fat; greasy. **3.** Derived from or chemically related to fat.

fatty acid n. Any of a large group of long-chain monobasic organic acids hydrolytically derived from fats.

fatty acid oxidation cycle n. The series of reactions by which fatty acids are metabolized by the body to produce energy.

fatty degeneration n. The accumulation of fat globules within the cells of an organ, such as the liver or heart, resulting in deterioration of tissue and diminished functioning of the affected organ.

fatty heart n. **1.** Fatty degeneration of the myocardium. **2.** Accumulation of fatty tissue on the outer surface of the heart with occasional infiltration between muscle bundles of the heart wall.

fatty infiltration n. The abnormal accumulation of fat droplets in the cytoplasm of cells.

fau·ces (fô′sēz′) pl.n. The passage from the back of the mouth to the pharynx, bounded by the soft palate, the base of the tongue, and the palatine arches.

fau·ci·tis (fô-sī′tĭs) n. Inflammation of the fauces.

fault·y union (fôl′tē) n. Union of a fracture by fibrous tissue without bone formation.

fau·na (fô′nə) n., pl. **-nas** or **-nae** (-nē). Animals, especially the animals of a particular region or period, considered as a group.

fa·ve·o·lus (fə-vē′ə-ləs) n., pl. **fa·ve·o·li** (-lī′). A small pit or depression.

fa·vid (fā′vĭd) n. An allergic reaction in the skin observed in favus.

fa·vism (fā′vĭz′əm) n. An acute hereditary condition in which the ingestion of certain species of beans, or the inhalation of the pollen of their flowers, causes fever, headache, abdominal pain, severe anemia, prostration, and coma.

fa·vus (fā′vəs) n. A severe type of chronic ringworm of the scalp and nails caused by certain dermatophytes.

Fc fragment (ĕf-sē′) n. The portion of an immunoglobulin molecule that can be crystallized.

FDA abbr. Food and Drug Administration

fear (fēr) n. A feeling of agitation and dread caused by the presence or imminence of danger.

fe·bric·i·ty (fĭ-brĭs′ĭ-tē) n. The condition of having a fever.

feb·rile (fĕb′rəl, fē′brəl) adj. Of, relating to, or characterized by fever; feverish.

febrile convulsion n. A convulsion accompanying high fever in infants and young children.

fe·cal (fē′kəl) adj. Of, relating to, or composed of feces.

fecal abscess n. See **stercoral abscess.**

fecal fistula n. See **intestinal fistula.**

fecal impaction n. An immovable collection of

compressed or hardened feces in the colon or rectum.

fe·ca·lith (fē′kə-lĭth′) *n.* See **coprolith.**

fe·cal·u·ri·a (fē′kə-lōōr′ē-ə, -lyōōr′-) *n.* Commingling of feces with urine passed from the urethra in persons with a fistula connecting the intestinal tract and bladder.

fecal vomiting *n.* The vomiting of fecal matter that has been drawn into the stomach from the intestine by repeated spasmodic contractions of the gastric muscles.

fe·ces (fē′sēz) *pl.n.* The matter discharged from the bowel during defecation; excrement.

fe·cund (fē′kənd, fĕk′ənd) *adj.* Capable of producing offspring; fertile.

fe·cun·da·tion (fē′kən-dā′shən, fĕk′ən-) *n.* The act of fertilizing; fertilization. — **fe′cun·date′** *v.*

fe·cun·di·ty (fĭ-kŭn′dĭ-tē) *n.* The capacity for producing offspring, especially in abundance.

feed·back (fēd′băk′) *n.* **1.** The return of a portion of the output of a process or system to the input, especially when used to maintain performance or to control a system or process. **2.** The portion of the output so returned. **3.** The return of information about the result of a process or activity; an evaluative response.

feedback inhibition *n.* Inhibition of activity by an end product of the action.

feedback mechanism *n.* See **feedback inhibition.**

feed·ing (fē′dĭng) *n.* The taking or giving of food or nourishment.

feeding tube *n.* A flexible tube that is inserted through the pharynx and into the esophagus and stomach and through which liquid food is passed.

feel (fēl) *v.* **felt** (fĕlt), **feel·ing, feels. 1.** To perceive through the sense of touch. **2.** To perceive (pain or heat, for example) as a physical sensation. **3.** To be conscious of a particular physical, mental, or emotional state.

feel·ing (fē′lĭng) *n.* **1.** The sensation involving perception by touch. **2.** A physical sensation, as of pain. **3.** An affective state of consciousness, such as that resulting from emotions or desires.

fel·la·ti·o (fə-lā′shē-ō′, fĕ-) *n.* Oral stimulation of the penis.

fel·on (fĕl′ən) *n.* A purulent infection or abscess involving the bulbous distal end of a finger.

Fel·ty's syndrome (fĕl′tēz) *n.* A condition caused by hypersplenism and resulting in rheumatoid arthritis with splenomegaly and leukopenia.

fe·male (fē′māl′) *adj.* Of, relating to, or denoting the sex that produces ova or bears young. — *n.* **1.** A member of the sex that produces ova or bears young. **2.** A woman or girl.

female catheter *n.* A short, nearly straight catheter that can be passed into the bladder of the female.

fem·i·nin·i·ty complex (fĕm′ə-nĭn′ĭ-tē) *n.* In psychoanalytic theory, the unconscious fear, in boys and men, of castration at the hands of the mother, resulting in identification with the imagined aggressor and the desire for breasts and vagina.

fem·i·ni·za·tion (fĕm′ə-nĭ-zā′shən) *n.* The acquisition of female characteristics by the male. — **fem′i·nize′** (-nīz′) *v.*

fem·o·ral (fĕm′ər-əl) *adj.* Relating to the femur or thigh.

femoral artery *n.* An artery with its origin as the continuation of the external iliac artery and its termination in the popliteal artery at the upper part of the popliteal space.

femoral nerve *n.* A nerve that arises from the second, third, and fourth lumbar nerves in the substance of the internal loin muscle and supplies the muscles and skin of the anterior region of the thigh.

femoral vein *n.* A vein that accompanies the femoral artery in the same sheath and in the groin, becomes the external iliac vein.

fe·mur (fē′mər) *n., pl.* **fe·murs** or **fem·o·ra** (fĕm′-ər-ə). **1.** See **thigh. 2.** The long bone of the thigh, and the longest and strongest bone in the human body, situated between the pelvis and the knee and articulating with the hipbone and with the tibia and patella.

fe·nes·tra (fə-nĕs′trə) *n., pl.* **-trae** (-trē′). **1.** A small anatomical opening, often closed by a membrane. **2.** The opening in a bone made by surgical fenestration. **3.** A specialized opening, as in a surgical instrument. — **fe·nes′tral** *adj.*

fen·es·tra·tion (fĕn′ĭ-strā′shən) *n.* **1.** An opening in the surface of a structure, as in a membrane. **2.** The surgical creation of such an opening. **3.** The surgical creation of an artificial opening in the bony part of the inner ear to improve or restore hearing.

fen·flu·ra·mine (fĕn-flōōr′ə-mēn′) *n.* A fluorinated compound used in the treatment of refractory obesity.

fen·ta·nyl (fĕn′tə-nĭl) *n.* A narcotic analgesic used in combination with other drugs before, during, or following surgery.

fer·ment (fûr′mĕnt′) *n.* **1.** An agent, such as a yeast, a bacterium, a mold, or an enzyme, that causes fermentation. **2.** Fermentation. — *v.* **-ment·ed, -ment·ing, -ments.** (fər-mĕnt′). To cause or undergo fermentation.

fer·men·ta·tion (fûr′mən-tā′shən, -mĕn-) *n.* Any of a group of chemical reactions that split complex organic compounds into relatively simple substances, especially the anaerobic conversion of sugar to carbon dioxide and alcohol by yeast.

fer·mi·um (fûr′mē-əm, fĕr′-) *n.* A synthetic radioactive metallic element with atomic number 100.

fern·ing (fûr′nĭng) *n.* The formation of a fernlike pattern in a specimen of crystallized cervical mucus secreted at midcycle.

fern test *n.* A test for estrogenic activity in which cervical mucus smears form a fernlike pattern at times when estrogen secretion is elevated, as at the time of ovulation.

fer·ri·tin (fĕr′ĭ-tĭn) *n.* An iron-containing protein complex, found principally in the intestinal mucosa, spleen, and liver, that functions as the primary form of iron storage in the body.

fer·ro·cy·to·chrome (fĕr′ō-sī′tə-krōm′) n. A cytochrome containing ferrous iron.

fer·ro·pro·tein (fĕr′ō-prō′tēn′, -tē-ĭn) n. Any of the proteins, such as heme or cytochrome, that contain iron in a prosthetic group.

fer·ru·gi·na·tion (fə-rōō′jə-nā′shən, fĕ-) n. Deposition of ferric salts in the walls of small blood vessels, usually within the basal ganglia and cerebellum.

fer·tile (fûr′tl) adj. **1.** Capable of conceiving and bearing young. **2.** Fertilized. Used of an ovum.

fertile period n. The period in the menstrual cycle during which conception is most likely to occur, usually from days 10 to 18 after the onset of menstruation.

fer·til·i·ty (fər-tĭl′ĭ-tē) n. The state of being fertile, especially the ability to produce young.

fer·til·i·za·tion (fûr′tl-ĭ-zā′shən) n. The union of male and female gametes to form a zygote, a process that begins with the penetration of the secondary oocyte by the spermatozoon and is completed with the fusion of the male and female pronuclei.

fes·ter (fĕs′tər) v. -tered, -ter·ing, -ters. **1.** To ulcerate. **2.** To form pus; putrefy. — n. An ulcer.

fes·ti·na·tion (fĕs′tə-nā′shən) n. The acceleration of gait noted in Parkinsonism and other nervous disorders.

fe·tal (fēt′l) adj. Of, relating to, or being a fetus.

fetal age n. See **developmental age** (sense 1).

fetal alcohol syndrome n. A complex of birth defects including cardiac, cranial, facial, or neural abnormalities and physical and mental growth retardation, occurring in an infant as a result of excess alcohol consumption by the mother during pregnancy.

fetal aspiration syndrome n. A syndrome resulting from meconium aspiration by the fetus and often leading to aspiration pneumonia.

fetal distress syndrome n. An abnormal condition of a fetus during gestation or at the time of delivery, marked by altered heart rate or rhythm and leading to compromised blood flow or changes in blood chemistry.

fetal dystocia n. A difficult delivery due to an abnormality in fetal shape, size, or position.

fetal hemoglobin n. The predominant form of hemoglobin in a fetus and a newborn. Normally present in small amounts in an adult, it may be abnormally elevated in certain forms of anemia.

fetal medicine n. The branch of medicine that deals with the growth, development, care, and treatment of the fetus and with environmental factors that may harm the fetus.

fetal membrane n. A structure or tissue, such as the chorion, amnion, and allantois, developed from the fertilized ovum but not part of the embryo proper.

fetal placenta n. The chorionic portion of the placenta, containing the fetal blood vessels, from which the umbilical cord arises.

fetal souffle n. A blowing murmur, synchronous with the fetal heartbeat, sometimes only systolic and sometimes continuous, heard on auscultation over the pregnant uterus.

fe·ti·cide (fē′tĭ-sīd′) n. Destruction of the embryo or fetus in the uterus.

fet·ish (fĕt′ĭsh, fē′tĭsh) n. **1.** Something, such as an object or a nonsexual part of the body, that arouses sexual desire and may become necessary for sexual gratification. **2.** An abnormally obsessive preoccupation or attachment.

fet·ish·ism (fĕt′ĭ-shĭz′əm, fē′tĭ-) n. The act of using a fetish for sexual arousal and gratification.

fe·to·glob·u·lin (fē′tə-glŏb′yə-lĭn) n. Any of the plasma globulins of unknown function occurring in small amounts in normal adults and in larger amounts in the second-trimester fetus.

fe·tog·ra·phy (fē-tŏg′rə-fē) n. Radiography of the fetus within the uterus.

fe·tol·o·gy (fē-tŏl′ə-jē) n. The branch of medicine concerned with the study, diagnosis, and treatment of the fetus, especially within the uterus.

fe·tom·e·try (fē-tŏm′ĭ-trē) n. Estimation of fetal size, especially of the head, before delivery.

fe·to·pro·tein (fē′tə-prō′tēn, -tē-ĭn) n. Any of several antigens normally present in a fetus and occurring abnormally in adults as a result of certain neoplastic conditions or diseases of the liver.

fe·tor (fē′tər, -tôr′) n. A very offensive odor.

fetor ex o·re (ĕks ôr′ē) n. See **halitosis**.

fe·to·scope (fē′tə-skōp′) n. A flexible fiberoptic device used to view a fetus in utero. — **fe·tos′co·py** (fē-tŏs′kə-pē) n.

fe·to·tox·ic·i·ty (fē′tō-tŏk-sĭs′ĭ-tē) n. Injury to the fetus from a substance that enters the maternal and placental circulation and may cause death or retardation of growth and development.

fet·tle (fĕt′l) n. **1.** Proper or sound condition. **2.** Mental or emotional state; spirits.

fe·tus (fē′təs) n., pl. -tus·es. **1.** The unborn young of a viviparous vertebrate having a basic structural resemblance to the adult animal. **2.** In humans, the unborn young from the end of the eighth week after conception to the moment of birth.

fetus pap·y·ra·ce·us (păp′ə-rā′shē-əs, -shəs) n. One of twin fetuses that has died and been pressed flat against the uterine wall by the growth of the living fetus.

fe·ver (fē′vər) n. **1.** Body temperature above the normal of 98.6°F (37°C). **2.** Any of various diseases in which there is an elevation of the body temperature above normal.

fever blister n. A small blister occurring on the lips and face and caused by herpes simplex; cold sore.

fe·ver·ish (fē′vər-ĭsh) adj. **1.** Having a fever. **2.** Relating to or resembling a fever. **3.** Causing or tending to cause a fever.

FFP abbr. fresh frozen plasma

fi·ber (fī′bər) n. **1.** A slender thread or filament. **2.** Extracellular filamentous structures such as collagenic or elastic connective tissue fibers. **3.** The nerve cell axon with its glial envelope. **4.** An elongated threadlike cell, such as a muscle cell or lenticular epithelial cell. **5.** Coarse, indigestible plant matter, such as cellulose, that stimulates intestinal peristalsis when eaten.

fiber optics *n.* An optical system in which light or an image is conveyed by a compact, coherent bundle of fine flexible glass or plastic fibers. — **fi′ber·op′tic** *adj.*

fi·ber·scope (fī′bər-skōp′) *n.* A flexible fiber-optic instrument used to view an inaccessible object or area, such as a body cavity.

fi·bre·mi·a (fī-brē′mē-ə) *n.* The presence of formed fibrin in the blood, causing thrombosis or embolism.

fi·bril (fī′brəl, fīb′rəl) or **fi·bril·la** (fī-brĭl′ə) *n.* A minute fiber.

fi·bril·lar (fī′brə-lər, fīb′rə-) or **fi·bril·lar·y** (-lĕr′ē) *adj.* **1.** Relating to a fibril. **2.** Relating to the fine rapid contractions or twitchings of fibers or of groups of fibers in skeletal or cardiac muscle.

fibrillary tremor *n.* Isolated twitching of the fine strands or fasciculi of a muscle.

fib·ril·late (fĭb′rə-lāt′, fī′brə-) *v.* **-lat·ed, -lat·ing, -lates. 1.** To undergo or cause to undergo fibrillation. **2.** To make or to become fibrillar. — *adj.* Fibrillated.

fib·ril·la·tion (fĭb′rə-lā′shən, fī′brə-) *n.* **1.** Fine, rapid twitching of individual muscle fibers with little or no movement of the muscle as a whole. **2.** The formation of fibrils. **3.** Vermicular twitching, usually slow, of individual muscular fibers, usually in the atria or ventricles of the heart and in recently denervated skeletal muscle fibers.

fi·bril·lo·gen·e·sis (fī′brə-lō-jĕn′ĭ-sĭs, fīb′rə-, fī-brĭl′ō-) *n.* The development of fine fibrils normally present in collagen fibers of connective tissue.

fi·brin (fī′brĭn) *n.* An elastic, insoluble, whitish protein derived from fibrinogen and forming an interlacing fibrous network in the coagulation of blood. — **fi′brin·ous** *adj.*

fibrin calculus *n.* A urinary calculus formed primarily from blood fibrinogen.

fi·brin·o·gen (fī-brĭn′ə-jən) *n.* A protein in the blood plasma that is essential for the coagulation of blood and is converted to fibrin by thrombin and ionized calcium.

fi·brin·o·ge·ne·mi·a (fī-brĭn′ə-jə-nē′mē-ə) *n.* See **hyperfibrinogenemia.**

fi·bri·no·gen·e·sis (fī′brə-nō-jĕn′ĭ-sĭs) *n.* The formation or production of fibrin.

fi·brin·o·gen·ol·y·sis (fī-brĭn′ə-jə-nŏl′ĭ-sĭs, fī′-brə-nō-) *n.* The inactivation or dissolution of fibrinogen in the blood.

fi·brin·o·gen·o·pe·ni·a (fī-brĭn′ə-jĕn′ō-pē′nē-ə) *n.* A less than the normal concentration of fibrinogen in the blood.

fibrinoid degeneration or **fibrinous degeneration** *n.* A form of degeneration in which tissue, such as connective tissue or blood vessels, accumulates deposits of an acidophilic homogeneous material that resembles fibrin when stained.

fi·bri·nol·y·sis (fī′brə-nŏl′ĭ-sĭs) *n.*, *pl.* **-ses** (-sēz′). The breakdown of fibrin, usually by plasmin. — **fi′bri·no·lyt′ic** (-nə-lĭt′ĭk) *adj.*

fibrinolytic purpura *n.* Purpura in which the bleeding is associated with rapid fibrinolysis of the clot.

fibrinous bronchitis *n.* Inflammation of the bronchial mucous membrane, accompanied by a fibrinous exudation.

fibrinous cataract *n.* See **fibroid cataract.**

fibrinous inflammation *n.* Exudative inflammation in which there is a large amount of fibrin in the exudate.

fibrinous pericarditis *n.* Acute pericarditis with fibrinous exudate on the serous membrane.

fibrinous pleurisy *n.* See **dry pleurisy.**

fibrinous polyp *n.* A mass of fibrin retained within the uterine cavity after childbirth.

fibrinous rhinitis *n.* See **membranous rhinitis.**

fi·bri·nu·ri·a (fī′brə-nŏŏr′ē-ə, -nyŏŏr′-) *n.* The passage of urine that contains fibrin.

fi·bro·ad·e·no·ma (fī′brō-ăd′n-ō′mə) *n.* A benign tumor commonly occurring in breast tissue, derived from glandular epithelium and composed of dense epithelial and fibroblastic tissue.

fi·bro·blast (fī′brə-blăst′) *n.* A stellate or spindle-shaped cell with cytoplasmic processes present in connective tissue, capable of forming collagen fibers. — **fi′bro·blas′tic** *adj.*

fi·bro·car·ci·no·ma (fī′brō-kär′sə-nō′mə) *n.* A hard, slow-growing carcinoma composed primarily of fibrous tissue.

fi·bro·car·ti·lage (fī′brō-kär′tl-ĭj) *n.* Cartilage that contains thick bundles of collagen fibers.

fi·bro·chon·dri·tis (fī′brō-kŏn-drī′tĭs) *n.* Inflammation of a fibrocartilage.

fi·bro·chon·dro·ma (fī′brō-kŏn-drō′mə) *n.* A benign neoplasm of cartilaginous tissue, having an abnormally large amount of fibrous stroma.

fi·bro·cyst (fī′brə-sĭs′) *n.* A cystic lesion that is circumscribed by or situated within a conspicuous amount of fibrous connective tissue.

fibrocystic disease of breast *n.* A benign disease common in women aged 30–60, marked by formation of small fluid-containing cysts in one or both breasts, associated with stromal fibrosis and variable degrees of intraductal epithelial hyperplasia and sclerosing adenosis.

fibrocystic disease of the pancreas *n.* See **cystic fibrosis.**

fi·bro·cys·to·ma (fī′brō-sĭ-stō′mə) *n.* A benign neoplasm, usually derived from glandular epithelium, characterized by cysts within a conspicuous fibrous stroma.

fi·bro·dys·pla·sia (fī′brō-dĭs-plā′zhə, -zhē-ə) *n.* Abnormal development of fibrous connective tissue.

fi·bro·e·las·to·sis (fī′brō-ĭ-lăs′tō′sĭs) *n.* Excessive proliferation of collagenous and elastic fibrous tissue.

fi·bro·en·chon·dro·ma (fī′brō-ĕn′kŏn-drō′mə) *n.* An enchondroma having neoplastic cartilage cells within an abundant fibrous stroma.

fi·bro·ep·i·the·li·o·ma (fī′brō-ĕp′ə-thē′lē-ō′mə) *n.* A skin tumor composed of fibrous tissue intersected by thin anastomosing bands of basal cells of the epidermis.

fi·bro·fol·lic·u·lo·ma (fī'brō-fə-lĭk'yə-lō'mə) *n.* A neoplastic proliferation of the fibrous sheath of the hair follicle, with solid extensions of the epithelium of the follicular infundibulum.

fi·broid (fī'broid') *adj.* Composed of or resembling fibrous tissue. — *n.* **1.** A fibroma or myoma occurring especially in the uterine wall. **2.** See **fibroleiomyoma.**

fibroid adenoma *n.* See **fibroadenoma.**

fibroid cataract *n.* A sclerotic hardening of the lenticular capsule, following exudative iridocyclitis.

fi·broid·ec·to·my (fī'broi-děk'tə-mē) *n.* Surgical removal of a fibroid tumor.

fi·bro·lei·o·my·o·ma (fī'brō-lī'ō-mī-ō'mə) *n.* A leiomyoma containing nonneoplastic collagenous fibrous tissue.

fi·bro·li·po·ma (fī'brō-lĭ-pō'mə, -lī-) *n.* A lipoma having an abundant amount of fibrous tissue.

fi·bro·ma (fī-brō'mə) *n.*, *pl.* **-mas** or **-ma·ta** (-mə-tə). A benign neoplasm derived from fibrous connective tissue. — **fi·brom'a·tous** (-brŏm'ə-təs, -brō'mə-) *adj.*

fibroma mol·le grav·i·dar·um (mŏl'ē grăv'ĭ-dâr'əm) *n.* Skin tags or polyps that develop during pregnancy and often disappear at term.

fibroma myx·o·ma·to·des (mĭk-sō'mə-tō'dēz) *n.* See **myxofibroma.**

fi·bro·ma·to·sis (fī-brō'mə-tō'sĭs) *n.* **1.** The occurrence of multiple fibromas, with a relatively large distribution. **2.** Abnormal hyperplasia of a fibrous tissue.

fi·bro·my·ec·to·my (fī'brō-mī-ěk'tə-mē) *n.* Excision of a fibromyoma.

fi·bro·my·o·ma (fī'brō-mī-ō'mə) *n.* A benign tumor having a large amount of fibrous tissue.

fi·bro·my·o·si·tis (fī'brō-mī'ə-sī'tĭs) *n.* Chronic inflammation of a muscle with an overgrowth of the connective tissue.

fi·bro·nec·tin (fī'brə-něk'tĭn) *n.* A fibrous linking protein that functions as a reticuloendothelial mediated host defense mechanism and is impaired by surgery, burns, infection, neoplasia, and disorders of the immune system.

fi·bro·neu·ro·ma (fī'brō-nŏŏ-rō'mə, -nyŏŏ-) *n.* See **neurofibroma.**

fi·bro·pla·sia (fī'brə-plā'zhə, -zhē-ə) *n.* The formation of fibrous tissue, as in the healing of wounds. — **fi'bro·plas'tic** (-plăs'tĭk) *adj.*

fi·bro·sar·co·ma (fī'brō-sär-kō'mə) *n.* A malignant tumor derived from fibrous connective tissue, marked by immature proliferating fibroblasts or undifferentiated anaplastic spindle cells.

fi·bro·sis (fī-brō'sĭs) *n.* The formation of fibrous tissue as a reparative or reactive process. — **fi·brot'ic** (-brŏt'ĭk) *adj.*

fi·bro·si·tis (fī'brə-sī'tĭs) *n.* Inflammatory hyperplasia of white fibrous connective tissue, especially surrounding the muscles.

fi·brous (fī'brəs) *adj.* Composed of or containing fibers.

fibrous cortical defect *n.* A common small defect of a bone, in which the cortex is filled with fibrous tissue, occurring most frequently in the lower femoral shaft of a child.

fibrous joint *n.* See **immovable joint.**

fibrous tissue *n.* Tissue composed of bundles of collagenous white fibers between which are rows of connective tissue cells.

fibrous tubercle *n.* A tubercle in which fibroblasts proliferate about the periphery, eventually forming a rim or wall of cellular fibrous tissue or collagenous material.

fib·u·la (fĭb'yə-lə) *n.*, *pl.* **-las** or **-lae** (-lē'). The outer, narrower, and smaller of the two bones of the human lower leg, extending from the knee to the ankle, and articulating with the tibia above and the tibia and talus below. — **fib'u·lar** (-lər) *adj.*

fifth cranial nerve *n.* See **trigeminal nerve.**

fifth disease *n.* See **erythema infectiosum.**

fight-or-flight reaction *n.* A set of physiological changes, such as increases in heart rate, arterial blood pressure, and blood glucose, initiated by the sympathetic nervous system to mobilize body systems in response to stress.

figure eight suture *n.* A suture used to approximate fascial edges, made using crisscross stiches.

figure-of-8 bandage *n.* A bandage applied alternately to two parts, usually two segments of a limb above and below the joint.

fil·a·ment (fĭl'ə-mənt) *n.* A fibril, fine fiber, or threadlike structure. — **fil'a·men'tous** (-měn'təs), **fil'a·men'ta·ry** (-měn'tə-rē, -měn'trē) *adj.*

fi·lar·i·a (fə-lâr'ē-ə) *n.*, *pl.* **-i·ae** (-ē-ē'). Any of various threadlike nematode worms that are parasitic in vertebrates and are often transmitted as larvae by mosquitos and other biting insects. The adult form lives in the blood and lymphatic tissues, causing inflammation and obstruction. — **fi·lar'i·al** (-ē-əl), **fi·lar'i·an** (-ē-ən) *adj.*

fil·a·ri·a·sis (fĭl'ə-rī'ə-sĭs) *n.* Disease caused by the presence of filariae in the tissues of the body, often resulting in occlusion of the lymphatic channels that can lead to elephantiasis.

Fi·la·tov flap (fə-lä'təf) or **Filatov-Gil·lies flap** (-gĭl'ēz) *n.* See **tubed flap.**

fil·i·form bougie (fĭl'ə-fôrm', fī'lə-) *n.* A very slender bougie usually used for exploration of strictures or sinus tracts having small diameters.

fill·ing (fĭl'ĭng) *n.* Material, such as amalgam or gold, used to fill a cavity in a tooth.

filling defect *n.* A defect in the contour of part of the gastrointestinal tract, as seen by x-ray after contrast medium has been introduced, indicating the presence of a tumor or foreign body.

film (fĭlm) *n.* **1.** A light-sensitive or x-ray-sensitive substance used in taking photographs or radiographs. **2.** A thin layer or membranous coating.

fi·lo·pres·sure (fī'lō-prěsh'ər) *n.* Temporary pressure on a blood vessel by a ligature.

fil·ter (fĭl'tər) *n.* **1.** A porous material through which a liquid or gas is passed in order to separate the fluid from suspended particulate matter. **2.** A device containing such a substance. **3.** A translucent screen, used in both diagnostic and therapeutic radiology, that permits the passage of certain rays and inhibits the passage of others that have a lower and less desirable energy. — v. -tered, -ter·ing, -ters. 1. To pass a liquid or gas through a filter. 2. To remove by passing through a filter. 3. To pass through or as if through a filter. — fil′ter·er n. — fil′ter·less adj.

filtering operation n. In the treatment of glaucoma, the surgical creation of a fistula between the anterior chamber of the eye and the subconjunctival space.

fil·trate (fĭl′trāt′) v. -trat·ed, -trat·ing, -trates. To put or go through a filter. — n. Material, especially liquid, that has passed through a filter.

fil·tra·tion (fĭl-trā′shən) n. The process of passing a liquid through a filter.

fi·lum (fī′ləm) n., pl. -la (-lə). A threadlike anatomical structure; a filament.

fim·bri·a (fĭm′brē-ə) n., pl. -bri·ae (-brē-ē′). 1. A fringelike anatomical part or structure. 2. See pilus (sense 2). — fim′bri·al adj.

fim·bri·ate (fĭm′brē-ĭt, -āt) or **fim·bri·at·ed** (-ā′tĭd) adj. Having fimbriae. — fim′bri·a′tion n.

fin·ger (fĭng′gər) n. One of the five digits of the hand, especially one other than the thumb.

fin·ger·nail (fĭng′gər-nāl′) n. The nail on a finger.

finger-nose test n. A test of voluntary coordination of the arms and hands in which one is asked to touch the tip of his or her nose slowly with the index finger of an arm extended to the side.

fin·ger·print (fĭng′gər-prĭnt′) n. 1. An impression on a surface of the curves formed by the ridges on a fingertip, especially such an impression made in ink and used as a means of identification. 2. A distinctive or identifying mark or characteristic. 3. An analytical method capable of making fine distinctions between similar compounds. — v. -print·ed, -print·ing, -prints. 1. To take the fingerprints of. 2. To identify by means of a distinctive mark or characteristic.

finger-thumb reflex n. See basal joint reflex.

fin·ger·tip (fĭng′gər-tĭp′) n. The extreme end or tip of a finger.

finger-to-finger test n. A test for coordination of the arms and hands in which one is asked to bring the index fingers together.

fire (fīr) v. **fired, fir·ing, fires.** To generate an electrical impulse. Used of a neuron.

first aid n. Emergency treatment administered to an injured or sick person before professional medical care is available. — first′-aid′ adj.

first cranial nerve n. See olfactory nerve.

first-degree burn n. A mild burn that produces redness of the skin but no blistering.

first finger n. See index finger.

first heart sound n. The heart sound that occurs with ventricular systole and is produced mainly by closure of the atrioventricular valves.

Fish·berg concentration test (fĭsh′bərg) n. A test of renal water conservation in which urine samples are collected after a person has abstained from fluids overnight and the specific gravity of the urine is measured.

fishskin disease n. See ichthyosis.

fis·sion (fĭsh′ən) n. 1. The act or process of splitting into parts. 2. The amitotic division of a cell or its nucleus.

fis·sure (fĭsh′ər) n. 1. A deep furrow, cleft, or slit. 2. A developmental break or fault in the enamel of a tooth.

fissure of Syl·vi·us (sĭl′vē-əs) or **sylvian fissure** n. The deepest and most prominent of the cortical fissures of the brain, extending between the frontal and temporal lobes, then back and over the lateral aspect of the cerebral hemisphere.

fis·tu·la (fĭs′chə-lə) n., pl. -las or -lae (-lē′). An abnormal passage from a hollow organ to the body surface, or from one organ to another.

fis·tu·la·tion (fĭs′chə-lā′shən) or **fis·tu·li·za·tion** (-lĭ-zā′shən) n. Formation of a fistula in a part of the body.

fis·tu·lec·to·my (fĭs′chə-lĕk′tə-mē) n. Surgical removal of a fistula.

fis·tu·lot·o·my (fĭs′chə-lŏt′ə-mē) n. Incision or surgical enlargement of a fistula.

fit¹ (fĭt) v. **fit·ted** or **fit, fit·ted, fit·ting, fits.** To be the proper size and shape. — adj. **fit·ter, fit·test.** Physically sound; healthy. — n. The degree of precision with which surfaces are adjusted or adapted to each other in a machine, device, or collection of parts.

fit² (fĭt) n. 1. A seizure or a convulsion, especially one caused by epilepsy. 2. The sudden appearance of a symptom such as coughing or sneezing.

fit·ness (fĭt′nĭs) n. 1. The state of being physically sound and healthy, especially as the result of exercise and proper nutrition. 2. A state of general mental and physical well-being. 3. The state of being suitably adapted to an environment.

fitness walking n. The aerobic sport of brisk, rhythmic, vigorous walking.

fix·ate (fĭk′sāt′) -at·ed, -at·ing, -ates. v. 1. To make fixed or stable. 2. To focus one's eyes or attention on. 3. To form a fixation; become attached to in an immature or neurotic way.

fix·a·tion (fĭk-sā′shən) n. 1. The condition of being stabilized or firmly attached. 2. The act or process of stabilizing or attaching, especially a body part by surgery. 3. The rapid preservation of tissue elements to retain as nearly as possible the same characteristics they had in the living body. 4. The conversion of a gas into solid or liquid form by chemical reactions, either with or without the help of living tissue. 5. In psychoanalytic theory, a strong attachment to a person or thing, especially one formed in childhood or infancy and manifested in lifelong immature or neurotic behavior. 6. The coordinated focusing of both eyes on an object.

fixation point n. See point of fixation.

fix·a·tive (fĭk′sə-tĭv) adj. Serving to fix, bind, or make firm or stable. — n. A substance used for the preservation of tissue or cell specimens.

fix·a·tor (fĭk′sā′tər, fĭk-sā′tər) n. A device that provides rigid immobilization of a fractured bone by means of rods attached to pins that are placed in or through the bone.

fixator muscle *n.* A muscle that stabilizes one part of the body during movement of another part.

fixed macrophage *n.* See **histiocyte.**

fixed partial denture *n.* A denture that is permanently attached to natural teeth or tooth roots for support.

fixed-rate pacemaker *n.* An artificial pacemaker that emits electrical stimuli at a constant frequency regardless of the heart's rhythm.

fixed virus *n.* Rabies virus that has undergone serial passage through rabbits, thus stabilizing its virulence and incubation period.

flac·cid (flăk′sĭd, flăs′ĭd) *adj.* Lacking firmness, resilience, or muscle tone. — **flac·cid′i·ty** (-sĭd′ĭ-tē)

flag·el·late (flăj′ə-lĭt, -lāt′, flə-jĕl′ĭt) *adj.* **1.** Flagellated. **2.** Relating to or caused by a flagellate organism. — *n.* A member of the class Mastigophora, comprising organisms having a flagellum.

flag·el·la·tion (flăj′ə-lā′shən) *n.* **1.** Whipping oneself or another as a means of arousing or heightening sexual feeling. **2.** The flagellar arrangement on an organism.

flag·el·lo·sis (flăj′ə-lō′sĭs) *n.* Infection with flagellated protozoa in the intestinal or genital tract.

fla·gel·lum (flə-jĕl′əm) *n., pl.* **-gel·la** (-jĕl′ə). A long threadlike appendage, especially a whiplike extension of certain cells or unicellular organisms that functions as an organ of locomotion.

flail (flāl) *v.* **flailed, flail·ing, flails.** To move vigorously or erratically; thrash about.

flank (flăngk) *n.* **1.** The side of the body between the pelvis or hip and the last rib; the side. **2.** The section of flesh in that area.

flap (flăp) *n.* Tissue in a surgical graft that is only partially detached from its donor site so that it is nourished during transfer to the recipient site.

flap amputation *n.* Amputation in which flaps of muscular and cutaneous tissues are used to cover the end of the bone.

flap·less amputation (flăp′lĭs) *n.* An amputation that does not use tissue to cover the stump.

flash·back (flăsh′băk′) *n.* **1.** An unexpected recurrence of the effects of a hallucinogenic drug long after its original use. **2.** A recurring, intensely vivid mental image of a past traumatic experience.

flash blindness *n.* Temporary loss of vision produced when retinal light-sensitive pigments are bleached by light more intense than that to which the retina is adapted at that moment.

flat bone *n.* A bone having a thin, flattened shape, as the scapula.

flat chest *n.* A chest in which the anteroposterior diameter is less than the average.

flat condyloma *n.* A secondary syphilitic eruption of flat-topped papules, usually found wherever contiguous folds of skin produce heat and moisture and especially about the anus and genitals.

flat electroencephalogram *n.* An electroencephalogram characterized by the absence of electric potentials of cerebral origin, indicating a lack of brain-wave activity and under certain conditions cerebral death.

flat flap *n.* A surgical flap in which the pedicle is left flat or open during transfer rather than tubed.

flat·foot (flăt′fŏŏt′) *n., pl.* **-feet** (-fēt′). A condition in which the arch of the foot is abnormally flattened down so that the entire sole makes contact with the ground.

flat plate *n.* A survey radiograph, usually of the abdomen, without use of contrast media and obtained while the patient is recumbent.

flat·u·lence (flăch′ə-ləns) or **flat·u·len·cy** (flăch′ə-lən-sē) *n.* The presence of excessive gas in the digestive tract. — **flat′u·lent** *adj.*

fla·tus (flā′təs) *n.* Gas generated in or expelled from the digestive tract, especially from the stomach or intestines.

flat wart *n.* A small, flat, flesh-colored wart that occurs in groups, especially on the face of children.

flat·worm (flăt′wûrm′) *n.* Any of various worms of the phylum Platyhelminthes, including the parasitic tapeworms and flukes, characteristically having a soft, flat, bilaterally symmetrical body and no body cavity.

fla·vin (flā′vĭn) or **fla·vine** (-vēn′) *n.* Any of various water-soluble yellow pigments, including riboflavin, found in plant and animal tissue as coenzymes of flavoproteins.

flavin-adenine dinucleotide or **flavine-adenine dinucleotide** *n.* A derivative of riboflavin that functions in oxidation-reduction reactions as a coenzyme of various flavoproteins.

flavin mononucleotide or **flavine mononucleotide** *n.* A derivative of riboflavin that condenses with adenine nucleotide to form flavin adenine dinucleotide and that acts as a coenzyme of various flavoproteins.

Fla·vi·vi·rus (flā′və-vī′rəs) *n.* A genus of arboviruses, of which an important pathogen is the yellow fever virus.

fla·vo·en·zyme (flā′vō-ĕn′zīm′) *n.* An enzyme that possesses a flavin nucleotide as coenzyme.

fla·vo·pro·tein (flā′vō-prō′tēn′, -tē-ĭn) *n.* Any of a group of enzymes containing flavin bound to protein and acting as dehydrogenation catalysts in biological oxidations.

flea (flē) *n.* Any of various small, wingless, blood-sucking insects of the order Siphonaptera that have legs adapted for jumping and are parasitic in the hair and feathers of warm-blooded animals.

fle·cai·nide acetate (flĭ-kā′nīd′) *n.* A membrane-stabilizing drug with local anesthetic activity, used in the treatment of ventricular arrhythmias.

flesh (flĕsh) *n.* The soft tissue of the body of a vertebrate, covering the bones and consisting mainly of skeletal muscle and fat. — **flesh′y** *adj.*

flesh fly *n.* Any of various dipterous flies of the family Sarcophagidae whose larvae are parasitic in living animal tissue or feed on carrion.

flesh wound *n.* A wound that penetrates the flesh but does not damage underlying bones or vital organs.

flex (flĕks) *v.* **flexed, flex·ing, flex·es. 1.** To bend.

2. To contract a muscle. **3.** To move a joint so that the parts it connects approach each other.

flex·i·ble (flĕk'sə-bəl) *adj.* **1.** Capable of being bent or flexed; pliable. **2.** Capable of being bent repeatedly without injury or damage. — **flex'i·bil'i·ty, flex'i·ble·ness** *n.*

flex·ion (flĕk'shən) *n.* **1.** The act of bending a joint or limb in the body by the action of flexors. **2.** The condition of being flexed or bent.

flex·or (flĕk'sər) *n.* A muscle that when contracted acts to bend a joint or limb in the body.

flex·ure (flĕk'shər) *n.* **1.** A bend or curve, as in a tubular organ. **2.** The act or an instance of bending. — **flex'ur·al** *adj.*

Flint's murmur (flĭnts) *n.* A diastolic murmur, similar to that of mitral stenosis, heard at the cardiac apex in some cases of free aortic insufficiency.

float·ers (flō'tər) *pl.n.* Specks or small threads in the visual field, usually perceived to be moving, that are caused by minute aggregations of cells or proteins in the vitreous humor of the eye.

float·ing (flō'tĭng) *adj.* **1.** Completely or partially unattached. **2.** Out of the normal position; unduly movable. Used of certain organs such as the kidney.

floating cartilage *n.* A loose piece of cartilage within a joint cavity that is detached from the articular cartilage or from a meniscus.

floating kidney *n.* A kidney that is displaced and movable.

floating rib *n.* Any of the two lowest pairs of ribs with no anterior attachment to the sternum.

floating spleen *n.* A spleen that is palpable because of excessive mobility from a relaxed or lengthened pedicle.

floc·cil·la·tion (flŏk'sə-lā'shən) *n.* An aimless plucking at the bedclothes occurring especially in the delirium of a fever.

flocculation reaction *n.* A precipitation test characterized by a flocculent precipitate of antigen and antibody.

flocculation test *n.* See **flocculation reaction.**

floc·cu·lent (flŏk'yə-lənt) *adj.* **1.** Having a fluffy or wooly appearance. **2.** Containing numerous shreds or fluffy particles of grayish or white mucus or other material. Used of a fluid such as urine. **3.** Of or being a fluid bacterial culture in which there are numerous colonies either floating in the fluid medium or loosely deposited at the bottom. — **floc'cu·lence** *n.*

flood·ing (flŭd'ĭng) *n.* A form of desensitization used in behavior therapy in which the patient imagines or is exposed to anxiety-producing stimuli.

flo·ra (flôr'ə) *n., pl.* **flo·ras** or **flo·rae** (flôr'ē'). **1.** Plants considered as a group, especially those of a particular region or time. **2.** The microorganisms that normally inhabit a bodily organ or part.

flor·id (flôr'ĭd) *adj.* Of a bright red or ruddy color. Used of certain skin lesions. — **flo·rid'i·ty** (flə-rĭd'ĭ-tē, flô-), **flor'id·ness** *n.*

florid oral papillomatosis *n.* Diffuse involvement of the lips and oral mucosa with benign squamous papillomas.

flow (flō) *v.* **flowed, flow·ing, flows. 1.** To move or run smoothly with unbroken continuity. **2.** To circulate, as the blood in the body. **3.** To menstruate. — *n.* **1.** The smooth motion characteristic of fluids. **2.** Menstrual discharge.

fl oz or **fl. oz.** *abbr.* fluid ounce

flu (flōō) *n.* Influenza.

fluc·tu·ate (flŭk'chōō-āt') *v.* **-at·ed, -at·ing, -ates. 1.** To vary irregularly. **2.** To rise and fall in waves. — **fluc'tu·ant** (-ənt) *adj.* — **fluc'tu·a'tion** *n.*

flu·dro·cor·ti·sone acetate (flōō'drō-kôr'tĭ-sōn', -zōn') *n.* A synthetic mineralocorticoid used topically as an anti-inflammatory agent and systemically in the treatment of adrenocortical insufficiency.

flu·id (flōō'ĭd) *n.* An amorphous substance whose molecules move freely past one another; a liquid or gas. — *adj.* Of or characteristic of a fluid. — **flu·id'i·ty** (-ĭd'ĭ-tē), **flu'id·ness** *n.*

fluid balance *n.* The difference between the amount of water taken into the body and the amount excreted or lost.

flu·id·ex·tract (flōō'ĭd-ĕk'străkt') *n.* A concentrated alcohol solution of a vegetable drug of such strength that each milliliter contains the equivalent of one gram of the dry drug.

fluid ounce or **fluidounce** *n.* A unit of volume or capacity equal to 8 fluid drams or 29.57 milliliters.

fluke (flōōk) *n.* See **trematode.**

flu·nis·o·lide (flōō-nĭs'ə-līd') *n.* An anti-inflammatory corticosteroid administered by inhalation in the treatment of allergies and asthma.

flu·o·cin·o·nide (flōō'ə-sĭn'ə-nīd') *n.* A corticosteroid used topically as an anti-inflammatory agent.

fluo·res·ce·in (flōō-rĕs'ē-ĭn, flô-) *n.* An orange-red compound that exhibits intense fluorescence in alkaline solution and is used in ophthalmology to reveal corneal lesions.

fluo·res·cence (flōō-rĕs'əns, flô-) *n.* **1.** The emission of electromagnetic radiation, especially of visible light, stimulated in a substance by the absorption of incident radiation and persisting only as long as the stimulating radiation is continued. **2.** The property of emitting such radiation. — **fluo·res'cent** *adj.*

fluorescence microscopy *n.* Microscopy using naturally fluorescent or treated materials that emit visible light when they are irradiated with ultraviolet or violet-blue visible rays.

fluorescent antibody technique *n.* Either of two techniques used to test for antigen with a fluorescent antibody: direct, in which immunoglobulin conjugated with a fluorescent dye is added to tissue and combines with specific antigen; or indirect, in which unlabeled immunoglobulin is added to tissue and combines with specific antigen, after which the antigen-antibody complex may be labeled with a fluorescent antibody.

fluorescent antinuclear antibody test *n.* A test

for antinuclear antibody components, especially for diagnosis of collagen-vascular diseases.

fluor·i·da·tion (flo͞or′ĭ-dā′shən, flôr′-) *n.* The addition of a fluorine compound to a drinking water supply for the purpose of reducing tooth decay. — **fluor′i·date** *v.*

fluor·ide (flo͞or′īd′, flôr′-) *n.* A compound of fluorine with another element.

fluor·i·di·za·tion (flo͞or′ĭ-dī-zā′shən, flôr′-) *n.* The therapeutic use of fluorides to reduce the incidence of dental decay, as by topical application of fluoride agents to the teeth.

fluor·ine (flo͞or′ēn′, -ĭn, flôr′-) *n.* A highly corrosive poisonous gaseous halogen element with atomic number 9, the most reactive of the elements, used in a variety of industrial compounds.

fluor·ite (flo͞or′īt′, flôr′-) *n.* A mineral that is often fluorescent in ultraviolet light and occurs in light green, blue, yellow, brown, and colorless forms.

fluo·rog·ra·phy (flo͞o-rŏg′rə-fē, flô-) *n.* See **photofluorography**.

fluor·o·scope (flo͞or′ə-skōp′, flôr′-) *n.* A device equipped with a fluorescent screen on which the internal structures of an optically opaque object, such as the body, may be continuously viewed as shadowy images formed by the differential transmission of x-rays through the object. — *v.* **-scoped, -scop·ing, -scopes.** To examine the interior of a body with a fluoroscope. — **fluor′o·scop′ic** (-skŏp′ĭk) *adj.* — **fluor′o·scop′i·cal·ly** *adv.*

fluo·ros·co·py (flo͞o-rŏs′kə-pē, flô-) *n.* Examination by means of a fluoroscope. — **fluo·ros′co·pist** *n.*

fluo·ro·sis (flo͞o-rō′sĭs, flô-) *n.* An abnormal condition caused by excessive intake of fluorine, as from fluoridated drinking water, marked by mottling of the teeth. — **fluo·rot′ic** (-rŏt′ĭk) *adj.*

fluor·o·u·ra·cil (flo͞or′ō-yo͝or′ə-sĭl, flôr′-) *n.* An antineoplastic agent used especially in the treatment of cancers of the skin, breast, and digestive system.

flu·ox·e·tine hydrochloride (flo͞o-ŏk′sĭ-tēn′) *n.* An oral antidepressant that enhances serotonin activity by inhibiting its uptake by neurons of the central nervous system.

flu·raz·e·pam (flo͞o-răz′ə-păm′) *n.* A mild hypnotic drug used especially in the form of its hydrochloride in the treatment of insomnia.

flush (flŭsh) *v.* **flushed, flush·ing, flush·es.** 1. To turn red, as from fever, heat, or strong emotion; blush. 2. To clean, rinse, or empty with a rapid flow of a liquid, especially water. — *n.* 1. An act of cleansing or rinsing with a flow of water. 2. A reddening of the skin, as with fever, emotion, or exertion. 3. A brief sensation of heat over all or part of the body.

flut·ter (flŭt′ər) *n.* Abnormally rapid pulsation, especially of the atria or ventricles of the heart.

flux (flŭks) *n.* 1. The discharge of large quantities of fluid material from the body, especially the discharge of watery feces from the intestines. 2. Material thus discharged from the bowels.

flux density *n.* The rate of flow of fluid, particles, or energy per unit area.

fly (flī) *n.* Any of numerous two-winged insects of the order Diptera, especially any of the family Muscidae, which includes the housefly.

foam cell *n.* A cell containing lipids in small vacuoles, as seen in leprosy and xanthoma, often a histiocyte but may be some other cell such as a smooth muscle cell.

fo·cal (fō′kəl) *adj.* Of or relating to a focus. — **fo′cal·ly** *adv.*

focal distance *n.* See **focal length.**

focal epilepsy *n.* An epileptic attack in which an isolated disturbance of cerebral function causes the twitching of a limb, the occurrence of a somatosensory or special sense phenomenon, or a disturbance of complex mental functions.

focal infection *n.* A bacterial infection localized in a specific part of the body, such as the tonsils, that may spread to another part of the body.

focal length *n.* The distance from the surface of a lens or mirror to its focal point.

focal point *n.* See **focus** (sense 1).

focal reaction *n.* A limited reaction that occurs at the point of entrance of an infecting organism or an injection.

fo·cus (fō′kəs) *n., pl.* **-cus·es** or **-ci** (-sī′, -kī′). 1. A point at which rays of light or other radiation converge or from which they appear to diverge, as after refraction or reflection in an optical system. 2. See **focal length.** 3. The distinctness or clarity of an image rendered by an optical system. 4. The state of maximum distinctness or clarity of such an image. 5. The region of a localized bodily infection or disease. — *v.* **-cused** or **-cussed, -cus·ing** or **-cus·sing, -cus·es** or **-cus·ses.** 1. To cause light rays or other radiation to converge on or toward a central point; concentrate. 2. To render an object or image in clear outline or sharp detail by adjustment of one's vision or an optical device. 3. To adjust a lens or instrument to produce a clear image. 4. To converge on or toward a central point of focus; be focused.

Fo·gar·ty catheter (fō′gər-tē) *n.* A catheter with an inflatable balloon near its tip, used to remove emboli and thrombi from the cardiovascular system, and to remove stones from the biliary ducts.

fog·ging (fŏg′ĭng) *n.* A method of refracting the eye in which accommodation is relaxed by overcorrection with a convex spherical lens, used in testing vision.

fold (fōld) *n.* 1. A crease or ridge apparently formed by folding, as of a membrane; a plica. 2. In the embryo, a transient elevation or reduplication of tissue in the form of a lamina.

Fo·ley catheter (fō′lē) *n.* A catheter held in the bladder by an inflatable balloon.

fo·lic acid (fō′lĭk, fŏl′ĭk) *n.* A yellowish-orange compound of the vitamin B complex group, occurring in green plants, fresh fruit, liver, and yeast.

fo·lie á deux (fô-lē′ ä dœ′, fŏl′ē) *n.* A condition in which symptoms of a mental disorder, such as delusive beliefs or ideas, occur simultaneously in two persons who share a close relationship or association.

folie du doute (dü dōōt′, dōō) n. A mental disorder characterized by extreme indecision, especially concerning everyday matters, and a pathological preoccupation with minute details.

Fo·lin's test (fō′lĭnz) n. **1.** A test for determining the quantity of uric acid in urine. **2.** A test for determining the quantity of urea in urine.

folk medicine n. Traditional medicine as practiced by nonprofessional healers or embodied in local custom or lore, generally involving the use of natural and especially herbal remedies.

fol·li·cle (fŏl′ĭ-kəl) n. **1.** A small bodily cavity or sac. **2.** A crypt or minute cul-de-sac or lacuna, such as the depression in the skin from which the hair emerges. **3.** An ovarian follicle. **4.** A spherical mass of cells usually containing a cavity.

follicle mite n. Any of various tiny mites of the genus *Demodex* that infest the hair follicles of mammals.

follicle-stimulating hormone n. A glycoprotein hormone of the anterior pituitary gland that stimulates the Graafian follicles of the ovary and assists in follicular maturation and in the secretion of estradiol. It also stimulates the epithelium of the seminiferous tubules and assists in inducing spermatogenesis.

fol·lic·u·lar (fə-lĭk′yə-lər) adj. **1.** Relating to, having, or resembling a follicle or follicles. **2.** Affecting or growing out of a follicle or follicles.

follicular cyst n. A cyst caused by the blockage of a duct of a follicle, especially a graafian follicle, which fills with fluid.

follicular phase n. Period during which the ovarian follicle develops during the menstrual cycle.

follicular stigma n. The point where the Graafian follicle is about to rupture on the surface of the ovary.

fol·lic·u·li·tis (fə-lĭk′yə-lī′tĭs) n. Inflammation of a follicle, especially of a hair follicle.

fol·lic·u·lus (fə-lĭk′yə-ləs) n., pl. **-li** (-lī′). Follicle.

fol·li·tro·pin (fŏl′ĭ-trō′pĭn) n. See **follicle-stimulating hormone**.

fol·low·ing bougie (fŏl′ō-ĭng) n. A flexible tapered bougie with a screw tip that is attached to the tailing end of a filiform bougie, allowing the progressive dilation of a passage.

fo·men·ta·tion (fō′mən-tā′shən, -mĕn-) n. **1.** A substance or material used as a warm, moist medicinal compress. **2.** The therapeutic application of warmth and moisture, as to relieve pain.

fo·mes (fō′mēz) n., pl. **fom·i·tes** (fŏm′ĭ-tēz′, fō′mī-). Fomite.

fo·mite (fō′mīt′) n. An inanimate object or substance, such as clothing, furniture, or soap, that is capable of transmitting infectious organisms from one person to another.

fon·ta·nel or **fon·ta·nelle** (fŏn′tə-nĕl′) n. Any of the soft membranous gaps between the incompletely formed cranial bones of a fetus or an infant.

fon·tic·u·lus (fŏn-tĭk′yə-ləs) n., pl. **fon·tic·u·li** (-lī′). Fontanel.

food (fōōd) n. Material, usually of plant or animal origin, that contains essential body nutrients, such as carbohydrates, fats, proteins, vitamins, or minerals, and is ingested and assimilated by an organism to produce energy, stimulate growth, and maintain life.

food poisoning n. **1.** Bacterial food poisoning. **2.** Poisoning caused by ingesting substances, such as certain mushrooms, that contain natural toxins.

foot (fōōt) n., pl. **feet** (fēt). **1.** The lower extremity of the vertebrate leg that is in direct contact with the ground in standing or walking. **2.** A unit of length in the U.S. Customary and British Imperial systems equal to 12 inches (30.48 cm).

foot-and-mouth disease n. An acute, highly contagious degenerative viral disease of cattle and other cloven-hoofed animals, characterized by fever and the eruption of vesicles around the mouth and hoofs.

foot-drop n. Paralysis or weakness of the dorsiflexor muscles of the foot and ankle, resulting in dragging of the foot and toes.

foot·ling presentation (fōōt′lĭng) n. Breech presentation of the fetus during birth in which the feet are the presenting part.

foot presentation n. See **footling presentation**.

fo·ra·men (fə-rā′mən) n., pl. **-ra·mens** or **-ram·i·na** (-răm′ə-nə). An aperture or perforation through a bone or a membranous structure. — **fo·ram′i·nal** (-răm′ə-nəl), **fo·ram′i·nous** (-nəs) adj.

foramen mag·num (măg′nəm) n. See **great foramen**.

force (fôrs) n. External energy that produces a change in the motion of an object; energy, strength, or active power.

forced alimentation n. See **forced feeding** (sense 1).

forced beat n. **1.** A premature beat believed to be precipitated by the preceding normal beat to which it is coupled. **2.** An extrasystole caused by artificial stimulation of the heart.

forced feeding n. **1.** Administration of liquid food through a nasal tube passed into the stomach. **2.** Forcing a person to eat more food than desired. — **force′-feed′** v.

force-feed (fôrs′fēd′) v. **-fed** (-fĕd′), **-feed·ing**, **-feeds**. To compel to take food or nourishment, especially to supply nourishment through a nasal tube passed into the stomach of someone unable or unwilling to eat.

for·ceps (fôr′səps, -sĕps) n., pl. **forceps**. **1.** An instrument resembling a pair of pincers or tongs, used for grasping, manipulating, or extracting, especially in surgery. **2.** Either of two bands of white fibers composing the radiation of the corpus callosum to the cerebrum.

forceps delivery n. The birth of a child assisted by extraction with a forceps designed to grasp the head.

for·ci·pres·sure (fôr′sə-prĕsh′ər) n. A method of

arresting hemorrhage by compressing a blood vessel with forceps.

Fordyce's spots *n.* A condition marked by the presence of small yellowish-white granules on the inner surface and border of the lips.

fore·arm (fôr′ärm′) *n.* The part of the arm between the wrist and the elbow.

fore·brain (fôr′brān′) *n.* The prosencephalon.

fore·fin·ger (fôr′fĭng′gər) *n.* See **index finger**.

fore·head (fôr′ĭd, -hĕd′) *n.* The part of the face between the eyebrows, the normal hairline, and the temples.

for·eign body (fôr′ĭn) *n.* An object or entity in the tissues or cavities of the body that has been introduced from outside.

fore·milk (fôr′mĭlk′) *n.* See **colostrum**.

fo·ren·sic medicine (fə-rĕn′sĭk, -zĭk) *n.* The branch of medicine that interprets or establishes the facts in civil or criminal law cases.

fore·play (fôr′plā′) *n.* Sexual stimulation preceding intercourse.

fore·skin (fôr′skĭn′) *n.* The loose fold of skin that covers the glans of the penis.

fore·wa·ters (fôr′wô′tərz) *n.* The amniotic fluid between the presenting part, usually the head, and the intact fetal membranes.

For·mad's kidney (fôr′mădz) *n.* An enlarged and deformed kidney sometimes seen in chronic alcoholism.

for·mal·de·hyde (fôr-măl′də-hīd′) *n.* A colorless, gaseous compound that is the simplest aldehyde, used for embalming fluids and in aqueous solution as a preservative and disinfectant.

for·ma·lin (fôr′mə-lĭn) *n.* An aqueous solution of formaldehyde that is 37 percent by weight.

formalin pigment *n.* A pigment formed in blood-rich tissues that come in contact with aqueous solutions of formaldehyde that have acidic pH values.

for·ma·tion (fôr-mā′shən) *n.* **1.** The act or process of forming something or of taking form. **2.** Something formed.

for·mi·ca·tion (fôr′mĭ-kā′shən) *n.* An abnormal sensation as of insects running over or into the skin, associated with cocaine intoxication or disease of the spinal cord and peripheral nerves.

for·mu·la (fôr′myə-lə) *n., pl.* **-las** or **-lae** (-lē′). **1.** A symbolic representation of the chemical composition or of the chemical composition and structure of a compound. **2.** The chemical compound so represented. **3.** A prescription of ingredients in fixed proportion; a recipe. **4.** A liquid food for infants, containing most of the nutrients in human milk.

for·ni·ca·tion (fôr′nĭ-kā′shən) *n.* Sexual intercourse between partners who are not married to each other.

for·nix (fôr′nĭks) *n., pl.* **-ni·ces** (-nĭ-sēz′). **1.** An arch-shaped structure, especially the arch-shaped roof of an anatomical space. **2.** The compact bundle of white fiber by which the hippocampus of each cerebral hemisphere projects to the opposite hippocampus and to the septum, the anterior nu-

cleus of the thalamus, and the mamillary body.

Fort Bragg fever (fôrt brăg′) *n.* See **pretibial fever**.

for·ward heart failure (fôr′wərd) *n.* Congestive heart failure resulting from inadequate cardiac output, characterized by weakness, fatigue, and the retention of sodium and water.

fos·car·net (fŏs-kär′nĭt) *n.* A pyrophosphate analogue used to treat herpes simplex infections.

fos·sa (fŏs′ə) *n., pl.* **fos·sae** (fŏs′ē′). A small longitudinal cavity or depression, as in a bone.

fos·sette (fŏ-sĕt′) *n.* **1.** A small depression; a dimple. **2.** A small deep ulcer of the cornea.

fos·su·la (fŏs′ə-lə, -yə-lə) *n., pl.* **-lae** (-lē′). A small fossa.

Fos·ter frame (fô′stər) *n.* A reversible bed similar to a Stryker frame.

Foth·er·gill's disease (fŏth′ər-gĭlz′) *n.* See **trigeminal neuralgia**.

Fothergill's operation *n.* See **Manchester operation**.

fou·lage (foō-läzh′) *n.* A form of massage in which the muscles are kneaded and pressed.

foun·da·tion (foun-dā′shən) *n.* The basis on which something stands or is supported; a base.

fourth cranial nerve *n.* See **trochlear nerve**.

fourth disease *n.* A mild exanthematous disease of childhood resembling scarlatina.

fourth heart sound *n.* The heart sound that occurs in late diastole and corresponds with atrial contraction.

fo·ve·a (fō′vē-ə) *n., pl.* **-ve·ae** (-vē-ē′). **1.** A small pit or cuplike depression in a bone or an organ. **2.** The fovea centralis.

fovea cen·tra·lis (sĕn-trā′lĭs) *n.* A depression in the center of the macula of the retina, the area of the most acute vision, where only cones are present and where blood vessels are lacking.

fo·ve·a·tion (fō′vē-ā′shən) *n.* **1.** The state of being pitted or scarred, as occurs in smallpox, chickenpox, or vaccinia. **2.** Any of the pits formed under such conditions.

Fow·ler's position (fou′lərz) *n.* An inclined position obtained by raising the head of the bed to promote better dependent drainage after an abdominal operation.

Fox-Fordyce disease (fŏks′-) *n.* A rare chronic eruption of dry papules and distended ruptured apocrine glands, with intense pruritis and follicular hyperkeratosis of the nipples, armpits, and pubic and chest regions.

fox·glove (fŏks′glŭv′) *n.* Any of several herbs of the genus *Digitalis*, having a long cluster of large, tubular, pinkish-purple flowers and leaves that are the source of the drug digitalis.

frac·ture (frăk′chər) *n.* **1.** The act or process of breaking. **2.** A break, rupture, or crack, especially in bone or cartilage. —*v.* To cause to break.

frag·ile X-chromosome (frăj′əl ĕks′) *n.* An X-chromosome with a fragile site near the end of the long arm, resulting in the appearance of an almost detached fragment.

fragile X syndrome *n.* An inherited disorder causing mental retardation, enlarged testes, and facial abnormalities in males and mild mental retardation in females.

fra·gil·i·ty (frə-jĭl′ĭ-tē) *n.* The quality or state of being easily broken or destroyed.

fragility test *n.* A test to measure the resistance of red blood cells to hemolysis in hypotonic saline solutions; in thalassemia, sickle cell anemia, and obstructive jaundice, red-blood-cell fragility is usually reduced.

frag·ment (frăg′mənt) *n.* **1.** A small part broken off or detached. **2.** An incomplete or isolated portion; a bit. — *v.* -ment·ed, -ment·ing, -ments. To break or separate into fragments.

fram·be·sia (frăm-bē′zhə, -zhē-ə) *n.* See yaws.

frame (frām) *n.* Something composed of parts fitted and joined together.

Fran·ci·sel·la (frăn′sĭ-sĕl′ə) *n.* A genus of nonmotile, gram-negative, rod-shaped or coccoid aerobic bacteria, some species of which cause disease in humans.

fran·ci·um (frăn′sē-əm) *n.* An unstable radioactive element with atomic number 87 of the alkali metals.

fra·ter·nal (frə-tûr′nəl) *adj.* **1.** Of or relating to brothers. **2.** Of, relating to, or being a twin developed from two separately fertilized ova.

fra·ter·nal twins (frə-tûr′nəl) *pl.n.* Twins derived from two separately fertilized ova and having different genetic makeup. They may be of the same or opposite sex.

Fra·zier-Spil·ler operation (frā′zhər-spĭl′ər) *n.* A subtemporal trigeminal rhizotomy.

freck·le (frĕk′əl) *n.* A small brownish spot on the skin, often turning darker or increasing in number upon exposure to the sun.

Fre·det-Ramstedt operation (frə-dā′-) *n.* See **pyloromyotomy.**

free association *n.* A psychoanalytic technique in which a patient verbalizes the passing contents of his or her mind without reservation.

free flap *n.* An island flap in which the donor vessels are severed and the flap is transported as a free object to the recipient site, where it is revascularized by connecting its supplying vessels to vessels.

free gingiva *n.* The portion of the gum that surrounds the tooth but is not directly attached to the tooth surface.

free graft *n.* A graft cut free from its attachments and transplanted to another site.

free macrophage *n.* An actively motile macrophage typically found in sites of inflammation.

free radical *n.* An uncharged atom or group of atoms having at least one unpaired electron, which makes it highly reactive.

freeze (frēz) *v.* **froze** (frōz), **fro·zen** (frō′zən), **freez·ing, freez·es. 1.** To pass from the liquid to the solid state by loss of heat. **2.** To make or become congealed, stiffened, or hardened by exposure to cold.

freeze-drying *n.* See **lyophilization.**

Frei test (frī) *n.* A skin test for lymphogranuloma venereum, using antigen prepared from chlamyd-iae grown in the yolk sac of a chick embryo,

Frej·ka pillow splint (frā′kə) *n.* A pillow splint used for abduction and flexion of the femurs in treating congenital hip dysplasia or dislocation in infants.

frem·i·tus (frĕm′ĭ-təs) *n., pl.* **fremitus.** A palpable vibration, as felt by the hand placed on the chest during coughing or speaking.

fre·nec·to·my (frə-nĕk′tə-mē) *n.* Surgical excision of a frenum.

fre·no·plas·ty (frē′nə-plăs′tē) *n.* Surgical correction of an abnormally attached frenum.

fre·not·o·my (frə-nŏt′ə-mē) *n.* Surgical incision of a frenum, especially of the tongue.

fren·u·lum (frĕn′yə-ləm) *n., pl.* **-la** (-lə). A small frenum.

fre·num (frē′nəm) *n., pl.* **-nums** or **-na** (-nə). **1.** A membranous fold of skin or mucous membrane that supports or restricts the movement of a part or organ, such as the band of tissue that connects the tongue to the floor of the mouth. **2.** An anatomical structure resembling such a fold.

fre·quen·cy distribution (frē′kwən-sē) *n.* A set of intervals, usually adjacent and of equal width, into which the range of a statistical distribution is divided, each associated with the number of measurements in that interval.

fresh frozen plasma *n.* Blood plasma frozen within 6 hours of collection, used in treating hypovolemia and coagulation-factor deficiency.

Freud·i·an (froi′dē-ən) *adj.* Relating to or being in accordance with the psychoanalytic doctrines of Sigmund Freud, who theorized that the symptoms of hysterical patients represent unresolved infantile psychosexual conflicts.

Frey's irritation hairs (frīz) *pl.n.* Short hairs of varying degrees of stiffness, embedded at right angles into the end of a light wooden handle and used for determining the presence and sensitivity of pressure points of the skin.

FRF *abbr.* follicle-stimulating hormone-releasing factor

fric·tion (frĭk′shən) *n.* **1.** The rubbing of one object or surface against another. **2.** A physical force that resists the relative motion or tendency to such motion of two bodies in contact.

friction rub *n.* See **friction sound.**

friction sound *n.* The sound heard on auscultation caused by the rubbing together of two opposing serous surfaces that are roughened by an inflammatory exudate.

Fried·länd·er's bacillus (frēd′lĕn′dərz) *n.* The pathogenic bacterium *Klebsiella pneumoniae* that often causes pneumonia.

Friedländer's pneumonia *n.* A severe form of lobar pneumonia caused by infection with Friedländer's bacillus and characterized by swelling of the affected lobe.

Fried·reich's ataxia (frēd′rīks, -rīкнs) *n.* See **hereditary spinal ataxia.**

Friedreich's sign *n.* An indication of adherent pericardium in which previously distended neck veins collapse with each diastole of the heart.

frig·id (frĭj′ĭd) *adj.* **1.** Extremely cold. **2.** Persistently averse to sexual intercourse.

fri·gid·i·ty (frĭ-gĭd′ĭ-tē) *n.* The state of marked or abnormal sexual indifference.

frôle·ment (frōl-män′) *n.* **1.** A succession of slow, brushing movements in massage, done with the palm of the hand. **2.** A rustling sound sometimes heard during auscultation in pericardial disease.

fron·tal (frŭn′tl) *adj.* **1.** Of, relating to, directed toward, or situated at the front. **2.** Of or relating to the forehead or frontal bone. **3.** Of or relating to the coronal plane.

frontal bone *n.* A cranial bone consisting of a vertical portion corresponding to the forehead and a horizontal portion that forms the roofs of the orbital and nasal cavities.

frontal lobe *n.* The largest portion of each cerebral hemisphere, anterior to the central sulcus.

fron·to·an·te·ri·or position (frŭn′tō-ăn-tēr′ē-ər) *n.* A cephalic presentation of the fetus with the forehead directed toward either the right or left front quarter of the mother's pelvis.

fron·to·pos·te·ri·or position (frŭn′tō-pō-stēr′-ē-ər, -pō-) *n.* A cephalic presentation of the fetus with the forehead directed toward either the right or left rear quarter of the mother's pelvis.

fron·to·trans·verse position (frŭn′tō-trăns-vûrs′, -trănz-, -trăns′vûrs′, -trănz′-) *n.* A cephalic presentation of the fetus with the forehead directed toward either the right or left iliac fossa of the mother's pelvis.

frost·bite (frôst′bīt′) *n.* Injury or destruction of skin and underlying tissue, most often that of the nose, ears, fingers, or toes, resulting from prolonged exposure to freezing or subfreezing temperatures.

Frost-Lang operation (-lăng′) *n.* Insertion of a spherical prosthesis after the enucleation of the eyeball.

Frost suture *n.* An intermarginal suture between the eyelids to protect the cornea.

frot·tage (frô-täzh′) *n.* **1.** Massage; rubbing. **2.** The act of rubbing against the body of another person, as in a crowd, to attain sexual gratification.

fro·zen section (frō′zən) *n.* A thin slice of tissue cut from a frozen specimen, often used for rapid microscopic diagnosis.

fruc·tose (frŭk′tōs, frōōk′-) *n.* A very sweet sugar occurring in many fruits and honey and used as a preservative in food and as an intravenous nutrient.

fruc·to·se·mi·a (frŭk′tō-sē′mē-ə, frōōk′-) *n.* The presence of fructose in the blood.

fruc·to·su·ria (frŭk′tō-sōōr′ē-ə, -syōōr′-, frōōk′-) *n.* The presence of fructose in the urine.

fruit sugar *n.* See **fructose.**

frus·tra·tion (frŭ-strā′shən) *n.* **1.** The condition that results when an impulse or an action is thwarted by external or internal forces. **2.** The blocking or thwarting of an impulse, purpose, or action.

FSH *abbr.* follicle-stimulating hormone

ft. or **ft** *abbr.* **1.** foot **2.** *Latin.* fiat, fiant (let there de done; let there be made)

fuch·sin (fyōōk′sĭn) or **fuch·sine** (-sĭn, -sēn′) *n.* Any of various red to purple-red rosanilin dyes used as bacterial and histological stains.

fuch·sin·o·phil (fyōōk-sĭn′ə-fĭl′) *adj.* Staining readily with fuchsin. — *n.* A cell or tissue that stains readily with fuchsin. — **fuch·sin′o·phil′ic** *adj.*

fu·co·si·do·sis (fyōō-kō′sĭ-dō′sĭs) *n.* An inherited metabolic storage disease caused by a deficiency of alpha-fucosidase and the accumulation of fucose-containing glycolipids. Clinical symptoms include progressive neurologic deterioration, spasticity, tremor, and mild skeletal changes.

fugue (fyōōg) *n.* A pathological amnesiac condition that may persist for several months and usually results from severe mental stress, in which one is apparently conscious of one's actions but has no recollection of them after returning to a normal state.

ful·gu·ra·tion (fōōl′gyə-rā′shən, -gə-, fŭl′-) *n.* The destruction of tissue, usually malignant tumors, by means of a high-frequency electric current applied with a needlelike electrode.

full denture *n.* See **complete denture.**

full-thickness flap *n.* A surgical flap consisting of the full thickness of the mucosa and submucosa or skin and subcutaneous tissues.

full-thickness graft *n.* A skin graft including the full thickness of the skin and subcutaneous tissue.

ful·mi·nant (fōōl′mə-nənt, fŭl′-) *adj.* Occurring suddenly, rapidly, and with great severity or intensity, usually of pain.

fu·mi·gant (fyōō′mĭ-gənt) *n.* A chemical compound used in its gaseous state as a pesticide or disinfectant.

fu·mi·gate (fyōō′mĭ-gāt′) *v.* **-gat·ed, -gat·ing, -gates.** To subject to smoke or fumes, usually in order to exterminate pests or disinfect. — **fu′mi·ga′tion** *n.*

func·tion (fŭngk′shən) *n.* **1.** The special action or physiological property of an organ or a body part. **2.** Something closely related to another thing and dependent on it for its existence, value, or significance, such as growth resulting from nutrition. **3.** The general properties of a substance, depending on its chemical character and relation to other substances, according to which it may be grouped, for example, among acids, bases, alcohols, or esters. **4.** A particular reactive grouping in a molecule.

func·tion·al (fŭngk′shə-nəl) *adj.* **1.** Of or relating to a function. **2.** Affecting the physiological function but not the structure.

functional blindness *n.* Loss of vision related to conversion hysteria.

functional disorder *n.* A physical disorder in which the symptoms have no known or detectable organic basis but are believed to be the result of psychological factors such as emotional conflicts or stress.

functional murmur *n.* A cardiac murmur not associated with a heart lesion.

functional neurosurgery *n.* The surgical destruction or chronic excitation of a part of the brain as treatment of a physiological or psychological disorder.

functional occlusion *n.* **1.** Tooth contact occurring within the functional range of the surfaces of opposing teeth. **2.** Occlusion that occurs during biting and chewing.

functional residual capacity *n.* The volume of gas remaining in the lungs at the end of a normal expiration.

functional splint *n.* See **dynamic splint.**

fun·dec·to·my (fŭn-dĕk′tə-mē) *n.* See **fundusectomy.**

fun·do·pli·ca·tion (fŭn′dō-plĭ-kā′shən) *n.* The surgical procedure of tucking or folding the fundus of the stomach around the esophagus to prevent reflux, used in the repair of a hiatal hernia.

fun·dus (fŭn′dəs) *n., pl.* **-di** (-dī′). The bottom of or part farthest from the opening of a sac or hollow organ. — **fun′dic** *adj.*

fun·du·sec·to·my (fŭn′də-sĕk′tə-mē) *n.* Surgical excision of the fundus of an organ, as of uterus.

fundus gland *n.* See **gastric gland.**

fundus of stomach *n.* The portion of the stomach that lies above the cardiac notch.

fun·gal (fŭng′gəl) or **fun·gous** (-gəs) *adj.* **1.** Of, relating to, resembling, or characteristic of a fungus. **2.** Caused by a fungus.

fun·ge·mi·a (fŭn-jē′mē-ə, fŭng-gē′-) *n.* The presence of fungi in the blood.

fun·gi·cide (fŭn′jĭ-sīd′, fŭng′gĭ-) *n.* A chemical substance that destroys or inhibits the growth of fungi. — **fun′gi·cid′al** (-sīd′l) *adj.*

fun·gi·form papilla (fŭn′jə-fôrm′, fŭng′gə-) *n.* Any of numerous minute mushroomlike elevations on the back of the tongue. The epithelium of many of these papillae have taste buds.

fun·gus (fŭng′gəs) *n., pl.* **fun·gus·es** or **fun·gi** (fŭn′jī, fŭng′gī). Any of numerous eukaryotic organisms of the kingdom Fungi, which lack chlorophyll and vascular tissue and range in form from a single cell to a body mass of branched filamentous hyphae that often produce specialized fruiting bodies; they include the yeasts, molds, smuts, and mushrooms.

fungus ball *n.* **1.** A compact mass of fungal mycelium and cellular debris produced by bacterial and mycotic infectious agents and residing within a lung cavity. **2.** See **aspergilloma** (sense 2).

fu·nic souffle or **funicular souffle** (fyoō′nĭk) *n.* See **fetal souffle.**

funicular graft *n.* A nerve graft in which each funiculus is approximated and sutured separately.

fu·nic·u·li·tis (fyoō-nĭk′yə-lī′tĭs, fə-) *n.* **1.** Inflam-

mation of a funiculus, especially of the spermatic cord. **2.** Inflammation of the portion of a spinal nerve root that lies in the intervertebral canal.

fu·nic·u·lo·pexy (fyoō-nĭk′yə-lō-pĕk′sē, fə-) *n.* The suturing of the spermatic cord to surrounding tissue to correct an undescended testicle.

fu·nic·u·lus (fyoō-nĭk′yə-ləs, fə-) or **fu·ni·cle** (fyoō′nĭ-kəl) *n., pl.* **-li** (-lī′) or **-cles. 1.** A slender cordlike strand or band, especially a bundle of nerve fibers in a nerve trunk. **2.** Any of three major divisions of white matter in the spinal cord, consisting of fasciculi. **3.** The umbilical cord. — **fu·nic′u·lar** (-lər) *adj.*

fu·nis (fyoō′nĭs) *n.* **1.** See **umbilical cord. 2.** A cordlike structure.

fun·nel breast (fŭn′əl) *n.* See **funnel chest.**

funnel chest *n.* A hollow at the lower part of the chest caused by a backward displacement of the xiphoid cartilage.

fun·ny bone (fŭn′ē) *n.* A point on the elbow where the ulnar nerve runs close to the surface and produces a sharp tingling sensation if knocked against the bone.

FUO *abbr.* fever of unknown origin

fur·ca·tion (fûr-kā′shən) *n.* A forking, or a forklike part or branch.

fu·ror ep·i·lep·ti·cus (fyoōr′ôr′ ĕp′ə-lĕp′tĭ-kəs, fyoōr′ər) *n.* The sudden unprovoked attacks of intense anger and violence to which persons with psychomotor epilepsy are occasionally subject.

fur·row (fûr′ō, fûr′ō) *n.* **1.** A rut, groove, or narrow depression. **2.** A deep wrinkle in the skin, as on the forehead.

fu·run·cle (fyoōr′ŭng′kəl) *n.* See **boil.** — **fu·run′·cu·lar** (fyoō-rŭng′kyə-lər), **fu·run′cu·lous** (-ləs) *adj.*

fu·run·cu·loid (fyoō-rŭng′kyə-loid′) *adj.* Resembling a boil.

fu·run·cu·lo·sis (fyoō-rŭng′kyə-lō′sĭs) *n.* A skin condition characterized by the development of recurring boils.

fused kidney *n.* A single anomalous organ produced by congenital fusion of the embryonic kidneys.

fu·sion (fyoō′zhən) *n.* **1.** The act or procedure of liquefying or melting by the application of heat. **2.** The merging of different elements into a union, as of vertebrae. **3.** The mechanism by which both eyes are able to blend slightly different images from each eye into a single image.

fusion beat *n.* The atrial or ventricular complex in an electrocardiogram when either the atria or the ventricles are activated by two simultaneously invading impulses.

fu·so·spi·ro·chet·al gingivitis (fyoō′zō-spī′rə-kēt′l) *n.* See **trench mouth.**

G

g *abbr.* gram

G *abbr.* glucose; guanine

GABA-al·pha (jē′ā-bē′ā-ăl′fə) *n.* A cell receptor that inhibits brain cells from responding to neuronal messages.

gad·o·lin·i·um (găd′l-ĭn′ē-əm) *n.* A malleable, ductile metallic rare-earth element with atomic number 64, used in improving the ferromagnetic characteristics of iron, cerium, and related alloys.

gag (găg) *v.* **gagged, gag·ging, gags.** **1.** To choke, retch, or undergo a regurgitative spasm. **2.** To prevent from talking. — *n.* An instrument adjusted between the teeth to keep the mouth from closing during operations in the mouth or throat.

gag reflex *n.* Retching or gagging caused by the contact of a foreign body with the mucous membrane of the throat.

gait (gāt) *n.* A particular way or manner of walking.

gal. *abbr.* gallon

ga·lac·to·cele (gə-lăk′tə-sēl′) *n.* A retention cyst caused by occlusion of a milk duct.

gal·ac·toph·o·rous duct (găl′ək-tŏf′ə-rəs) *n.* See **lactiferous duct.**

ga·lac·to·poi·e·sis (gə-lăk′tə-poi-ē′sĭs) *n.* Production and secretion of milk by the mammary glands. — **ga·lac′to·poi·et′ic** (-ĕt′ĭk) *adj.*

ga·lac·tor·rhe·a (gə-lăk′tə-rē′ə) *n.* **1.** A continued discharge of milk from the breasts between intervals of nursing or after weaning. **2.** Excessive flow of milk during lactation.

ga·lac·tose (gə-lăk′tōs′) *n.* A monosaccharide commonly occurring in lactose and in certain pectins, gums, and mucilages.

ga·lac·to·se·mia (gə-lăk′tə-sē′mē-ə) *n.* An inherited metabolic disorder characterized by the deficiency of an enzyme that is necessary for the metabolism of galactose. The disorder results in elevated levels of galactose in the blood and, if untreated, can lead to mental retardation and eye and liver abnormalities. — **ga·lac′to·se′mic** *adj.*

galactose tolerance test *n.* A liver function test based on the ability of the liver to convert galactose to glycogen, in which the rate of excretion of galactose following ingestion or intravenous injection of a known amount is measured.

ga·lac·to·side (gə-lăk′tə-sīd′) *n.* Any of a group of glycosides that yield galactose on hydrolysis and exist in alpha and beta forms.

ga·lac·to·sis (găl′ək-tō′sĭs) *n.* The formation of milk by the mammary glands.

ga·lac·to·su·ri·a (gə-lăk′tə-sŏŏr′ē-ə, -syŏŏr′-, -shŏŏr′-) *n.* The excretion of galactose in the urine.

ga·lac·to·ther·a·py (gə-lăk′tō-thĕr′ə-pē) *n.* **1.** The treatment of disease by means of an exclusive

or nearly exclusive milk diet. **2.** Medicinal treatment of a nursing infant by giving to the mother a drug that is excreted in part with her milk.

gal·ba·num (găl′bə-nəm, gôl′-) *n.* A bitter, aromatic gum resin extracted from an Asiatic plant (*Ferula galbaniflua*) or any of several related plants, used medicinally as a counterirritant.

ga·le·a (gā′lē-ə) *n., pl.* **-le·ae** (-lē-ē′). **1.** An anatomical structure shaped like a helmet. **2.** The aponeurosis connecting the occipitofrontal muscle to form the epicranium. **3.** A type of bandage for covering the head.

gall (gôl) *n.* See **bile** (sense 1).

gall (gôl) *n.* A skin sore caused by friction and abrasion. — *v.* **galled, gall·ing, galls.** To become irritated, chafed, or sore.

gallbladder or **gall bladder** *n.* A small, pear-shaped muscular sac, located under the right lobe of the liver, in which bile secreted by the liver is stored until needed by the body for digestion.

gall duct *n.* **1.** See **bile duct. 2.** See **common bile duct.**

gal·li·um (găl′ē-əm) *n.* A rare metallic element with atomic number 31 that is liquid near room temperature and is found as a trace element in coal, bauxite, and other minerals.

gal·lon (găl′ən) *n.* A unit of volume in the U.S. Customary System, used in liquid measure, equal to 4 quarts, 231 cubic inches, or 8.3389 pounds of distilled water (3.7853 liters).

gal·lop (găl′əp) *n.* A triple cadence to the heart sounds at rates of 100 beats per minute or more due to an abnormal third or fourth heart sound being heard in addition to the first and second sounds; usually indicative of heart disease.

gallop rhythm *n.* See **gallop.**

gall·stone (gôl′stōn′) *n.* A concretion in the gallbladder or in a bile duct, composed chiefly of cholesterol, calcium salts, and bile pigments.

gal·van·ic skin response (găl-văn′ĭk) *n.* A measure of electrical resistance as a reflection of changes in emotional arousal, taken by attaching electrodes to any part of the skin and recording changes in moment-to-moment perspiration and related activity of the autonomic nervous system.

Gam·bi·an trypanosomiasis (găm′bē-ən) *n.* A type of African trypanosomiasis caused by *Trypanosoma brucei gambiense,* and transmitted by tsetse flies, characterized by erythematous patches and local edemas, cramps, tremors, and paresthesia, enlargement of the lymph glands, spleen, and liver, emaciation, and in later stages lethargy deepening to coma before death.

gam·ete (găm′ēt′, gə-mēt′) *n.* A reproductive cell having the haploid number of chromosomes, especially a mature sperm or egg capable of fusing with a gamete of the opposite sex to produce the fertilized egg.

ga·me·to·cyte (gə-mē′tə-sīt′) *n.* A cell from which gametes develop by meiotic division, especially a spermatocyte or an oocyte.

ga·me·to·gen·e·sis (gə-mē′tə-jĕn′ĭ-sĭs) *n.* The formation and development of gametes. **— ga·me′to·gen′ic, gam′e·tog′e·nous** (găm′ĭ-tŏj′-ə-nəs) *adj.*

gam·ma (găm′ə) *adj.* Relating to or characterizing a polypeptide chain that is one of five types of heavy chains present in immunoglobins.

gam·ma-a·mi·no·bu·tyr·ic acid (găm′ə-ə-mē′nō-byōō-tēr′ĭk, -ăm′ə-nō-) *n.* An amino acid that occurs in the central nervous system and is associated with the transmission of inhibitory nerve impulses.

gam·ma angle (găm′ə) *n.* The angle formed between the line joining the fixation point to the center of the eye and the optic axis.

gamma globulin *n.* A protein fraction of blood serum containing numerous antibodies, used in the prevention and treatment of certain diseases, such as measles, poliomyelitis, and hepatitis.

gam·mop·a·thy (gă-mŏp′ə-thē) *n.* An abnormal condition marked by a disturbance of immunoglobulin synthesis.

gam·o·gen·e·sis (găm′ə-jĕn′ĭ-sĭs) *n.* Sexual reproduction.

gan·ci·clo·vir (găn-sī′klō-vēr) *n.* An antiviral agent used in the treatment of opportunistic cytomegalovirus infections.

gan·gli·ec·to·my (găng′glē-ĕk′tə-mē) *n.* See **ganglionectomy.**

gan·gli·o·blast (găng′glē-ō-blăst′) *n.* An embryonic cell giving rise to ganglion cells.

gan·gli·o·cyte (găng′glē-ō-sīt′) *n.* See **ganglion cell.**

gan·gli·o·cy·to·ma (găng′glē-ō-sī-tō′mə) *n.* See **ganglioneuroma.**

gan·gli·o·gli·o·ma (găng′glē-ō-glē-ō′mə, -glī-) *n.* See **central ganglioneuroma.**

gan·gli·ol·y·sis (găng′glē-ŏl′ĭ-sĭs) *n.* The dissolution or breaking up of a ganglion.

gan·gli·o·ma (găng′glē-ō′mə) *n.* See **ganglioneuroma.**

gan·gli·on (găng′glē-ən) *n., pl.* **-gli·ons** or **-gli·a** (-glē-ə). **1.** A group of nerve cells forming a nerve center, especially one located outside the brain or spinal cord. **2.** A benign tumorlike fibrous cyst containing mucopolysaccharide-rich fluid, usually attached to a tendon sheath in the hand, wrist, or foot. **— gan′gli·al** *adj.*

ganglion cell *n.* A neuron having its cell body outside the central nervous system.

gan·gli·on·ec·to·my (găng′glē-ə-nĕk′tə-mē) *n.* Excision of a ganglion.

gan·gli·o·neu·ro·ma (găng′glē-ō-nōō-rō′mə, -nyōō-) *n.* A benign neoplasm composed of mature ganglionic neurons scattered singly or in clumps within a relatively abundant and dense stroma of neurofibrils and collagenous fibers.

gan·gli·on·ic (găng′glē-ŏn′ĭk) *adj.* Relating to a ganglion; ganglial.

ganglionic blocking agent *n.* A substance that blocks nerve impulses in autonomic ganglia.

gan·gli·on·i·tis (găng′glē-ə-nī′tĭs) *n.* Inflammation of a ganglion.

gan·gli·on·os·to·my (găng′glē-ə-nŏs′tə-mē) *n.* The surgical formation of an opening into a ganglion.

gan·gli·o·side (găng′glē-ə-sīd′) *n.* Any of a group of glycosphingolipids chemically similar to the cerebrosides but containing one or more sialic acid residues, found principally in the surface membrane of nerve cells and in the spleen.

gan·gli·o·si·do·sis (găng′glē-ō-sī-dō′sĭs) *n.* Any of a group of diseases characterized by the abnormal accumulation of gangliosides within the nervous system.

gan·grene (găng′grēn, găng-grēn′) *n.* Death and decay of body tissue, often occurring in a limb, caused by insufficient blood supply and usually following injury or disease. **— gan′gre·nous** (găng′grə-nəs) *adj.*

gangrenous stomatitis *n.* Stomatitis characterized by necrosis of the oral tissue.

Gan·ser's syndrome (găn′zərz, gän′-) *n.* A pseudo-psychotic condition typically occurring in persons feigning insanity and characterized by wrong but related answers to questions.

gap (găp) *n.* **1.** An opening in a structure or surface; a cleft or breach. **2.** An interval or discontinuity in any series or sequence.

gap 1 *n.* In the somatic cell cycle, the gap that follows mitosis and is followed by synthesis for the next cycle.

gap 2 *n.* In the somatic cell cycle, a pause between the completion of synthesis and the onset of cell division.

gap phenomenon *n.* A short period in the cycle of atrioventricular or intraventricular conduction during which an impulse, which at other times would be blocked in transit, is allowed to pass.

Gard·ner's syndrome (gärd′nərz) *n.* An inherited syndrome characterized by the development of multiple tumors, including osteomas of the skull, epidermoid cysts, and fibromas before 10 years of age, and of multiple polyposis predisposing to carcinoma of the colon.

gar·gle (gär′gəl) *v.* **-gled, -gling, -gles.** To force exhaled air through a liquid held in the back of the mouth, with the head tilted back, in order to cleanse or medicate the mouth or throat. **—** *n.* A medicated fluid used for gargling.

gar·goyl·ism (gär′goil′ĭz′əm) *n.* A condition characterized by coarsened facial surface and distorted features and associated with Hurler's syndrome and Hunter's syndrome.

Gärt·ner's bacillus (gĕrt′nərz) *n.* A gram-negative, motile, rod-shaped bacterium *Salmonella enteritidis* that causes gastroenteritis in humans.

gas (găs) *n., pl.* **gas·es** or **gas·ses. 1.** The state of matter distinguished from the solid and liquid states by relatively low density and viscosity, relatively great expansion and contraction with changes in pressure and temperature, the ability to diffuse readily, and the spontaneous tendency to become distributed uniformly throughout any container. **2.** A substance in the gaseous state. **3.** A gaseous asphyxiant, irritant, or poison. **4.** A gaseous anesthetic, such as nitrous oxide. **5.** Flatulence. **6.** Flatus. — *v.* **gassed, gas·sing, gas·es** or **gas·ses. 1.** To treat chemically with gas. **2.** To overcome, disable, or kill with poisonous fumes. **3.** To give off gas.

gas abscess *n.* An abscess containing gas caused by a gas-forming microorganisms.

gas bacillus *n.* An anaerobic, gram-negative, motile bacterium *Clostridium perfringens* that causes gas gangrene in humans.

gas chromatography *n.* Chromatography in which the moving phase is a mixture of gases or vapors, which separate during their differential adsorption by a stationary phase.

gas·e·ous (găs′ē-əs, găsh′əs) *adj.* **1.** Of, relating to, or existing as a gas. **2.** Full of or containing gas; gassy. — **gas′e·ous·ness** *n.*

gas gangrene *n.* A form of gangrene occurring in a wound infected with anaerobic bacteria, especially *Clostridium perfringens* and *C. novyi,* and characterized by the presence of gas in the affected tissue and constitutional septic symptoms.

gash (găsh) *v.* **gashed, gash·ing, gash·es.** To make a long, deep cut in; slash deeply. — *n.* **1.** A long, deep cut. **2.** A deep flesh wound.

gas·trad·e·ni·tis (găs-străd′n-ī′tĭs) *n.* Inflammation of the glands of the stomach.

gas·tral·gi·a (gă-străl′jē-ə, -jə) *n.* See **gastrodynia.**

gas·trec·ta·sis (gă-strĕk′tə-sĭs) or **gas·trec·ta·si·a** (găs′trĭk-tā′zē-ə, -zhə) *n.* Dilation of the stomach.

gas·trec·to·my (gă-strĕk′tə-mē) *n.* Excision of a part or all of the stomach.

gas·tric (găs′trĭk) *adj.* Of, relating to, or associated with the stomach.

gastric analysis *n.* The determination of the pH and acid output of the contents of the stomach.

gastric bypass *n.* A surgical prcedure used for treatment of morbid obesity, consisting of the severeance of the upper stomach, anastomosis of the upper pouch of the stomach to the jejunum, and closure of the distal part of the stomach.

gastric calculus *n.* See **gastrolith.**

gastric digestion *n.* The part of digestion, chiefly of proteins, carried on in the stomach by the enzymes of the gastric juices.

gastric feeding *n.* The administration of food directly into the stomach by a tube inserted either through the nasopharynx and esophagus or directly through the abdominal wall.

gastric gland *n.* Any of the branched tubular glands in the mucosa of the fundus and body of the stomach, containing parietal cells and zymogenic cells.

gastric indigestion *n.* Indigestion occurring in the stomach.

gastric juice *n.* The colorless, watery, acidic diges-

tive fluid that is secreted by various glands in the mucous membrane of the stomach and consists chiefly of hydrochloric acid, pepsin, rennin, and mucin.

gastric secretin *n.* Gastrin.

gastric stapling *n.* The partitioning of the stomach by rows of staples in the treatment of morbid obesity.

gastric ulcer *n.* An ulcer occurring in the mucous membrane of the stomach.

gas·trin (găs′trĭn) *n.* Any of the hormones that are secreted in the pyloric-antral mucosa of the stomach and stimulate secretion of gastric juice by the parietal cells of the gastric glands.

gas·tri·no·ma (găs′trə-nō′mə) *n., pl.* -**mas** or -**ma·ta** (-mə-tə). A gastrin-secreting tumor associated with Zollinger–Ellison syndrome.

gas·tri·tis (gă-strī′tĭs) *n.* Chronic or acute inflammation of the stomach, especially of the mucous membrane of the stomach.

gastritis cys·ti·ca pol·y·po·sa (sĭs′tĭ-kə pŏl′ə-pō′sə, -zə) *n.* Large fixed mucosal polyps arising in the stomach proximal to an old gastroenterostomy.

gas·tro·a·nas·to·mo·sis (găs′trō-ə-năs′tə-mō′sĭs) *n.* Anastomosis of the cardiac and the antral segments of the stomach.

gas·tro·cele (găs′trə-sēl′) *n.* **1.** The cavity of the gastrula of an embryo. **2.** Hernia of a portion of the stomach.

gas·troc·ne·mi·us (găs′trŏk-nē′mē-əs, găs′trə-) *n., pl.* -**mi·i** (-mē-ī′). A muscle with its origin from the lateral and medial condyles of the femur, with insertion by the Achilles tendon into the lower half of the posterior surface of the calcaneus, and whose action causes plantar flexion of the foot.

gastrocolic reflex *n.* A mass movement of the contents of the colon that sometimes occurs immediately following the entrance of food into the stomach.

gas·tro·co·li·tis (găs′trō-kə-lī′tĭs) *n.* Inflammation of the stomach and the colon.

gas·tro·co·los·to·my (găs′trō-kə-lŏs′tə-mē) *n.* The surgical formation of a communication between the stomach and the colon.

gas·tro·du·o·de·ni·tis (găs′trō-dōō′ō-də-nī′tĭs, -dyōō′-, -dŏō-ŏd′n-ī′-, -dyōō-) *n.* Inflammation of the stomach and the duodenum.

gas·tro·du·o·de·nos·co·py (găs′trō-dōō′ə-də-nŏs′kə-pē, -dyōō′-, -dŏō-ŏd′n-ŏs′-, -dyōō-) *n.* Visualization of the interior of the stomach and the duodenum by a gastroscope.

gas·tro·du·o·de·nos·to·my (găs′trō-dōō′ə-də-nŏs′tə-mē, -dyōō′-, -dŏō-ŏd′n-ŏs′-, -dyōō-) *n.* The surgical formation of a communication between the stomach and the duodenum.

gas·tro·dyn·i·a (găs′trō-dĭn′ē-ə) *n.* Pain in the stomach; a stomach ache.

gas·tro·en·ter·i·tis (găs′trō-ĕn′tə-rī′tĭs) *n.* Inflammation of the mucous membrane of the stomach and intestines.

gas·tro·en·ter·o·co·li·tis (găs′trō-ĕn′tə-rō-kō-lī′tĭs, -kə-) *n.* Inflammation of the stomach, small intestines, and colon.

gas·tro·en·ter·ol·o·gy (găs′trō-ĕn′tə-rŏl′ə-jē) *n.* The medical specialty concerned with the function and disorders of the stomach, intestines, and related organs of the gastrointestinal tract. — **gas·tro·en′ter·o·log′ic** (-ə-lŏj′ĭk), **gas′tro·en′ter·o·log′i·cal** *adj.*

gas·tro·en·ter·op·a·thy (găs′trō-ĕn′tə-rŏp′ə-thē) *n.* A disorder of the stomach and intestines.

gas·tro·en·ter·o·plas·ty (găs′trō-ĕn′tə-rō-plăs′-tē) *n.* Surgical repair of defects in the stomach and the intestine.

gas·tro·en·ter·op·to·sis (găs′trō-ĕn′tə-rŏp-tō′-sĭs) *n.* Downward displacement of the stomach and a portion of the intestine.

gas·tro·en·ter·os·to·my (găs′trō-ĕn′tə-rŏs′tə-mē) *n.* The surgical formation of a new opening between the stomach and the intestine, either anterior or posterior to the mesocolon.

gas·tro·en·ter·ot·o·my (găs′trō-ĕn′tə-rŏt′ə-mē) *n.* Incision into the stomach and the intestine.

gas·tro·e·soph·a·gi·tis (găs′trō-ĭ-sŏf′ə-jī′tĭs) *n.* Inflammation of the stomach and the esophagus.

gas·tro·e·soph·a·gos·to·my (găs′trō-ĭ-sŏf′ə-gŏs′tə-mē) *n.* The surgical formation of a new opening between the esophagus and the stomach.

gas·tro·gas·tros·to·my (găs′trō-gă-strŏs′tə-mē) *n.* See **gastroanastomosis**.

gas·tro·ga·vage (găs′trō-gə-väzh′) *n.* See **gavage** (sense 1).

gas·tro·il·e·ac reflex (găs′trō-ĭl′ē-ăk′) *n.* Opening of the ileocolic valve as food enters the stomach.

gas·tro·il·e·i·tis (găs′trō-ĭl′ē-ī′tĭs) *n.* Inflammation of the stomach and the ileum.

gas·tro·il·e·os·to·my (găs′trō-ĭl′ē-ŏs′tə-mē) *n.* The surgical formation of a direct communication between the stomach and the ileum.

gas·tro·in·tes·ti·nal (găs′trō-ĭn-tĕs′tə-nəl) *adj.* Relating to the stomach and the intestines.

gastrointestinal tract *n.* The part of the digestive system consisting of the stomach, and intestines.

gas·tro·je·ju·nos·to·my (găs′trō-jə-jōō′nŏs′tə-mē, -jē′jōō-) *n.* The surgical formation of a direct communication between the stomach and the jejunum.

gas·tro·lith (găs′trə-lĭth′) *n.* A pathological concretion formed in the stomach.

gas·tro·li·thi·a·sis (găs′trō-lĭ-thī′ə-sĭs) *n.* Presence of one or more gastroliths in the stomach.

gas·trol·y·sis (gă-strŏl′ĭ-sĭs) *n.* Surgical division of perigastric adhesions.

gas·tro·ma·la·ci·a (găs′trō-mə-lā′shē-ə, -shə) *n.* Softening of the walls of the stomach.

gas·tro·meg·a·ly (găs′trō-mĕg′ə-lē) *n.* Enlargement of the abdomen or the stomach.

gas·tro·myx·or·rhe·a (găs′trō-mĭk′sə-rē′ə) *n.* Excessive secretion of mucus in the stomach.

gas·tro·pa·ral·y·sis (găs′trō-pə-rāl′ĭ-sĭs) *n.* Paralysis of the muscular coat of the stomach.

gas·tro·pa·re·sis (găs′trō-pə-rē′sĭs, -pār′ĭ-sĭs) *n.* Mild gastroparalysis.

gas·trop·a·thy (gă-strŏp′ə-thē) *n.* Any disease of the stomach.

gas·tro·pex·y (găs′trə-pĕk′sē) *n.* Surgical attachment of the stomach to the abdominal wall or to the diaphragm.

gas·tro·plas·ty (găs′trə-plăs′tē) *n.* Surgical repair of a defect in the stomach or lower esophagus.

gas·tro·pli·ca·tion (găs′trō-plī-kā′shən) *n.* A surgical procedure for reducing of the size of the stomach by suturing a fold in the stomach wall.

gas·trop·to·sis (găs′trŏp-tō′sĭs) *n.* Downward displacement of the stomach.

gas·tror·rha·gi·a (găs′trə-rā′jē-ə, -jə) *n.* Hemorrhage from the stomach.

gas·tror·rha·phy (gă-strôr′ə-fē) *n.* **1.** Suture of a stomach perforation. **2.** See **gastroplication**.

gas·tror·rhe·a (găs′trə-rē′ə) *n.* Excessive secretion of gastric juice or mucus by the stomach.

gas·tros·chi·sis (gă-strŏs′kĭ-sĭs) *n.* A congenital fissure in the abdominal wall usually accompanied by protrusion of the viscera.

gas·tro·scope (găs′trə-skōp′) *n.* An endoscope for examining the inner surface of the stomach. — **gas′tro·scop′ic** (-skŏp′ĭk) *adj.* — **gas·tros′co·py** (-kə-pē) *n.*

gas·tro·spasm (găs′trə-spăz′əm) *n.* Spasmodic contraction of the walls of the stomach.

gas·tro·stax·is (găs′trō-stăk′sĭs) *n.* Oozing of blood from the mucous membrane of the stomach.

gas·tro·ste·no·sis (găs′trō-stə-nō′sĭs) *n.* Diminution in size of the cavity of the stomach.

gas·tros·to·la·vage (gă-strŏs′tō-lä-väzh′) *n.* Washing out of the stomach through a gastric fistula.

gas·tros·to·my (gă-strŏs′tə-mē) *n.* Surgical construction of a permanent opening from the external surface of the abdominal wall into the stomach, usually for inserting a feeding tube.

gas·trot·o·my (gă-strŏt′ə-mē) *n.* Incision into the stomach.

gas·tro·to·nom·e·try (găs′trō-tō-nŏm′ĭ-trē) *n.* The measurement of intragastric pressure.

gas·tru·la (găs′trə-lə) *n., pl.* **-las** or **-lae** (-lē′). An embryo at the stage following the blastula, consisting of a hollow, two-layered sac of ectoderm and endoderm surrounding a gastrocele.

gas·tru·la·tion (găs′trə-lā′shən) *n.* Transformation of the blastula into the gastrula.

Gau·cher's disease (gō-shāz′) *n.* A rare familial disorder of fat metabolism caused by a genetic enzyme deficiency and characterized by enlargement of the liver and spleen, lymphadenopathy, and bone destruction.

gaunt·let bandage (gônt′lĭt, -gänt′-) *n.* A figure-of-8 bandage covering the hand and fingers.

gauze (gôz) *n.* A bleached cotton cloth of plain weave, used for dressings, bandages, and absorbent sponges.

ga·vage (gə-väzh′) *n.* **1.** Introduction of nutritive material into the stomach by means of a tube. **2.** The therapeutic use of a high-potency diet.

gay (gā) *adj.* Relating to a homosexual or the lifestyle thereof. — *n.* A homosexual, especially male.

gaze (gāz) *n.* The act of looking steadily in one direction for a period of time. — **gaze** *v.*

G cell *n.* An enteroendocrine cell that secretes gastrin, found primarily in the gastric glands of the pyloric cavity mucosa of the stomach.

gel·a·tin or **gel·a·tine** (jĕl′ə-tn) *n.* A derived protein formed from the collagen of animal tissues by boiling.

ge·lat·i·nous (jə-lăt′n-əs) *adj.* **1.** Of, relating to, or containing gelatin. **2.** Resembling gelatin; viscous.

ge·lo·sis (jĕ-lō′sĭs) *n.* An extremely firm mass in a tissue, especially in a muscle, with a consistency resembling that of frozen tissue.

gem·el·lip·a·ra (jĕm′ə-lĭp′ər-ə) *n.* A woman who has given birth to twins.

gen·der (jĕn′dər) *n.* **1.** The sex of an individual, male or female, based on reproductive anatomy. **2.** Sexual identity, especially in relation to society or culture.

gender identity *n.* A person's sense of being male or female, resulting from a combination of genetic and environmental influences.

gender role *n.* The pattern of masculine or feminine behavior of an individual as defined by a particular culture and largely as determined by a child's upbringing.

gene (jēn) *n.* A hereditary unit that occupies a specific location on a chromosome, determines a particular characteristic in an organism by directing the formation of a specific protein, and is capable of self-replication at each cell division.

ge·ne·al·o·gy (jē′nē-ŏl′ə-jē, -ăl′-, jĕn′ē-) *n.* **1.** A record or table of the descent of a person, family, or group from an ancestor or ancestors; a family tree. **2.** The study or investigation of ancestry and family histories.

gene amplification *n.* A cellular process characterized by the production of multiple copies of a particular gene or genes to amplify the phenotype that the gene confers on the cell.

gene augmentation therapy *n.* A procedure for correcting metabolic deficiencies caused by a missing or defective gene by having a healthy gene produce the necessary product without actually substituting that gene for the flawed or absent gene in the DNA.

gene dosage compensation *n.* The putative mechanism that adjusts the X-linked phenotypes of males and females to compensate for the haploid state in males and the diploid state in females.

gene mapping *n.* The determination of the sequence of genes and their relative distances from one another on a specific chromosome.

gene pool *n.* The collective genetic information contained within a population of sexually reproducing organisms.

general-adaptation syndrome *n.* The nonspecific reactions of organisms to injury or stress,

grouped into alarm, resistance, and exhaustion stages.

general anesthesia *n.* Loss of the ability to perceive pain associated with loss of consciousness, produced by intravenous or inhalation anesthetic agents.

general anesthetic *n.* An agent that produces loss of sensation and loss of consciousness.

general duty nurse *n.* A nurse who does not specialize in a particular area of practice but is available for any duty.

general immunity *n.* Immunity that protects the body as a whole.

gen·er·al·ist (jĕn′ər-ə-lĭst) *n.* A physician whose practice is not oriented in a specific medical specialty but instead covers a variety of medical problems.

gen·er·al·i·za·tion (jĕn′ər-ə-lĭ-zā′shən) *n.* **1.** The act or an instance of generalizing. **2.** A principle, a statement, or an idea having general application.

gen·er·al·ize (jĕn′ər-ə-līz′) *v.* **-ized, -iz·ing, -iz·es.** **1.** To render indefinite or unspecific. **2.** To infer from many particulars. **3.** To draw inferences or a general conclusion from. **4.** To make generally or universally applicable.

gen·er·al·ized (jĕn′ər-ə-līzd′) *adj.* **1.** Involving an entire organ, as when an epileptic seizure involves all parts of the brain. **2.** Not specifically adapted to a particular environment or function; not specialized. **3.** Generally prevalent.

generalized anaphylaxis *n.* The immediate anaphylactic response of a sensitized person following inoculation with an antigen.

generalized vaccinia *n.* A skin eruption following vaccination for smallpox, seen most commonly in people with previously traumatized skin.

generalized xanthelasma *n.* Xanthoma planum of the neck, trunk, extremities, and eyelids in persons with normal plasma lipid levels.

general paresis *n.* A brain disease occurring as a late consequence of syphilis, characterized by dementia, muscular weakness, and paralysis.

general practitioner *n.* A physician whose practice consists of providing ongoing care covering a variety of medical problems in patients of all ages, often including referral to appropriate specialists. — **general practice** *n.*

gen·er·a·tion (jĕn′ə-rā′shən) *n.* **1.** All of the offspring that are at the same stage of descent from a common ancestor. **2.** The average interval of time between the birth of parents and the birth of their offspring. **3.** A group of individuals born and living about the same time. **4.** The act or process of generating; origination, production, or procreation.

ge·ner·ic (jə-nĕr′ĭk) *adj.* **1.** Of or relating to a genus. **2.** Relating to or descriptive of an entire group or class; general. **3.** Not having a trademark or brand name. — *n.* A drug sold without a brand name or trademark.

gen·e·sis (jĕn′ĭ-sĭs) *n., pl.* **-ses** (-sēz′). The coming into being of something; the origin.

gene-splicing *n.* The process in which fragments of DNA from one or more different organisms are combined to form recombinant DNA and are made to function within the cells of a host organism.

gene therapy *n.* A technique for the treatment of genetic disease, such as enzyme deficiencies, in which a gene that is absent or defective is replaced by a healthy gene.

ge·net·ic (jə-nĕt′ĭk) or **ge·net·i·cal** (-ĭ-kəl) *adj.* **1.** Of or relating to genetics or genes. **2.** Affecting or affected by genes, as a disorder or deficiency. **3.** Of, relating to, or influenced by the origin or development of something; ontogenic.

genetic amplification *n.* A process for increasing specific DNA sequences, especially used to increase the proportion of plasmid DNA to that of bacterial DNA.

genetic association *n.* The occurrence together in a population, more often than can be readily explained by chance, of two or more traits of which at least one is known to be genetic.

genetic code *n.* The sequence of nucleotides that is the basis of heredity in the DNA molecule of a chromosome and that specifies the amino acid sequence in the synthesis of proteins.

genetic counseling *n.* The counseling of prospective parents on the probabilities and dangers of inherited diseases occurring in their offspring and on the diagnosis and treatment of such diseases.

genetic disease *n.* A disease caused by the absence of a gene or by the substances produced by a defective gene.

genetic female *n.* **1.** A person with a normal female karyotype, including two X-chromosomes. **2.** A person whose cell nuclei contain Barr bodies, which are normally present in females and absent in males.

genetic fitness *n.* The reproductive success of a genotype, usually measured as the number of offspring produced by an individual that survive to reproductive age relative to the average for the population.

ge·net·i·cist (jə-nĕt′ĭ-sĭst) *n.* A specialist in genetics.

genetic lethal *n.* A disorder that prevents effective reproduction by those affected, such as Klinefelter syndrome.

genetic male *n.* **1.** A person having one X-chromosome and one Y-chromosome, the normal male karyotype. **2.** A person whose cell nuclei do not contain Barr bodies.

genetic map *n.* A graphic representation of the arrangement of genes or mutable sites on a chromosome.

genetic marker *n.* A gene phenotypically associated with a particular, easily identified trait and used to identify an individual or cell carrying that gene. Genetic markers associated with certain diseases can often be detected in the blood serum, where their presence is used to determine whether one is at high risk for developing a disease.

ge·net·ics (jə-nĕt′ĭks) *n.* The branch of biology

that deals with heredity, especially the mechanisms of hereditary transmission and the variation of inherited characteristics among similar or related organisms.

ge·nic·u·lum (jə-nĭk′yə-ləm) *n., pl.* **-la** (-lə). **1.** A small kneelike anatomical structure. **2.** A sharp bend in an organ.

ge·ni·o·plas·ty (jē′nē-ō-plăs′tē, jə-nī′ə-) *n.* See **mentoplasty.**

gen·i·tal (jĕn′ĭ-tl) *adj.* **1.** Of or relating to biological reproduction. **2.** Of or relating to the genitalia. **3.** Of or relating to the stage of psychosexual development in psychoanalytic theory during which the genitals become the focus of sexual gratification. — *n.* A reproductive organ, especially one of the external sex organs.

genital cord *n.* One of a pair of mesenchymal ridges bulging into the caudal part of the celom of a embryo containing the primordium of the uterine ligaments and walls in the female and the site of fusion with the urinary bladder in the male.

genital herpes *n.* A highly contagious, sexually transmitted viral infection caused by herpesvirus type two and characterized by painful lesions in the genital and anal regions.

gen·i·ta·li·a (jĕn′ĭ-tā′lē-ə, -tāl′yə) *pl.n.* The reproductive organs, especially the external sex organs; the genitals.

gen·i·tal·i·ty (jĕn′ĭ-tăl′ĭ-tē) *n.* **1.** In psychoanalytic theory, the genital components of sexuality. **2.** The capacity to experience erotic sensation in the genitalia.

genital organ *n.* Any of the organs of reproduction or generation, including, in the female, the vulva, clitoris, ovaries, uterine tubes, uterus, and vagina, and in the male, the penis, scrotum, testes, epididymides, deferent ducts, seminal vesicles, prostate, and bulbourethral glands.

genital phase *n.* In psychoanalytic theory, the final stage of psychosexual development, reached in puberty, when erotic interest and activity are focused on a sexual partner.

gen·i·tals (jĕn′ĭ-tlz) *pl.n.* Genitalia.

genital tract *n.* The genital passages of the urogenital system.

genital wart *n.* A pointed papilloma typically found on the skin or mucous membranes of the anus and external genitalia, caused by a virus transmitted mainly through sexual contact.

gen·i·to·u·ri·nar·y (jĕn′ĭ-tō-yŏŏr′ə-nĕr′ē) *adj.* Of or relating to the genital and urinary organs or their functions.

genitourinary system *n.* See **urogenital system.**

gen·o·cop·y (jĕn′ə-kŏp′ē) *n.* A trait that is a phenotypic copy of a genetic trait but is caused by a mechanism other than genotype expression.

ge·nome (jē′nōm′) or **ge·nom** (-nōm) *n.* A complete haploid set of chromosomes with its associated genes. — **ge·nom′ic** (-nŏm′ĭk) *adj.*

gen·o·type (jĕn′ə-tīp′, jē′nə-) *n.* **1.** The genetic constitution of an organism or a group of organisms. **2.** A group or class of organisms having the same genetic constitution. — gen′o·typ′i·cal (-tĭp′ĭ-kəl) adj.

gen·ta·mi·cin or gen·ta·my·cin (jĕn′tə-mī′sĭn) n. A broad-spectrum antibiotic derived from an actinomycete and used to treat various infections.

gen·tian·o·phil (jĕn′shə-nō-fĭl′) or gen·tian·o·phile (-fīl′, -fĭl′) adj. Staining readily with gentian violet. — gen′tian·o·phil′ic adj. — gen′tian·oph′i·lous (jĕn′shə-nŏf′ə-ləs) adj.

ge·nu (jē′nōō, jĕn′yōō) n., pl. gen·u·a (jĕn′yōō-ə). 1. Knee. 2. An anatomical structure resembling the angular shape of a flexed knee.

genu re·cur·va·tum (rē′kûr-vā′təm) n. The backward curvature of the knee; hyperextension of the knee.

ge·nus (jē′nəs) n., pl. gen·er·a (jĕn′ər-ə). A taxonomic category ranking below a family and generally consisting of a group of species exhibiting similar characteristics; the genus name is used, either alone or followed by a Latin adjective or epithet, to form the name of a species.

genu val·gum (văl′gəm) n. Knock-knee.

ge·ode (jē′ōd′) n. A cystlike space with or without an epithelial lining, usually observed in subarticular bone in arthritic disorders.

ge·o·graph·i·cal tongue (jē′ə-grăf′ĭ-kəl) n. A chronic inflamation of the tongue characterized by distinct somewhat circular groupings of lesions bounded by a white band; the groupings may vary in shape and position.

ge·oph·a·gy (jē-ŏf′ə-jē) or ge·oph·a·gism (-jĭz′əm) or ge·o·pha·gia (jē′ə-fā′jə) n. The eating of earthy substances, such as clay, practiced among various peoples as a custom or for dietary or subsistence reasons. — ge·oph′a·gist n.

ger·i·at·ric (jĕr′ē-ăt′rĭk) adj. 1. Of or relating to geriatrics. 2. Of or relating to the aged or to characteristics of the aging process. — n. An aged person.

ger·i·at·rics (jĕr′ē-ăt′rĭks) n. The branch of medicine that deals with the diagnosis and treatment of diseases and problems specific to the aged.

germ (jûrm) n. 1. A small mass of protoplasm or cells from which a new organism or one of its parts may develop. 2. A microorganism, especially a pathogen.

ger·ma·ni·um (jər-mā′nē-əm) n. A brittle crystalline gray-white metalloid element with atomic number 32, widely used as a semiconductor.

Ger·man measles (jûr′mən) n. See rubella.

German measles virus n. See rubella virus.

germ cell n. An ovum or a sperm cell or one of their developmental precursors.

ger·mi·nal disk (jûr′mə-nəl) n. See embryonic disk.

germinal epithelium n. See surface epithelium.

ger·mi·no·ma (jûr′mə-nō′mə) n. A neoplasm derived from germ tissue of the testes or ovum.

germ layer n. Any of the three primary cellular layers, the ectoderm, endoderm, or mesoderm, into which most animal embryos differentiate and from which the organs and tissues of the body develop through further differentiation.

germ line n. Cells from which gametes are derived.

germ plasm n. 1. The cytoplasm of a germ cell, especially that part containing the chromosomes. 2. Germ cells as distinguished from other body cells. 3. Hereditary material; genes.

germ theory n. The doctrine holding that infectious diseases are caused by the activity of microorganisms within the body.

ger·o·der·ma (jĕr′ō-dûr′mə) n. Thinning of the skin accompanied by the loss of elasticity and subcutaneous fat, as in the aged.

ger·o·mor·phism (jĕr′ō-môr′fĭz′əm) n. Premature senility.

ger·on·tol·o·gy (jĕr′ən-tŏl′ə-jē) n. The scientific study of the biological, psychological, and sociological phenomena associated with old age and aging. — ger′on·tol′o·gist n.

ges·ta·gen (jĕs′tə-jən, -jĕn′) n. A substance, such as a steroid hormone, that affects the uterus in a manner similar to progesterone.

ge·stalt·ism (gə-shtäl′tĭz′əm, -shtôl′-, -stäl′-, -stôl′-) n. The school or theory of psychology that emphasizes the wholeness and organized structure of every psychological, physiological, and behavioral experience, maintaining that experiences are not reducible and thus cannot be derived from a simple summation of perceptual elements such as sensation and response.

Ge·stalt psychology (gə-shtält′, -shtôlt′, -stält′, -stôlt′) n. See gestaltism.

gestalt therapy n. Psychotherapy with individuals or groups that emphasizes treatment of the person as a whole, including a person's biological components and their organic functioning, perceptual configuration, and interrelationships with the external world.

ges·ta·tion (jĕ-stā′shən) n. The period of development in the uterus from conception until birth; pregnancy.

ges·ta·tion·al edema (jĕ-stā′shə-nəl) n. The occurrence of a generalized and excessive accumulation of fluid in the tissues due to the influence of pregnancy.

ges·to·sis (jĕ-stō′sĭs) n., pl. ges·to·ses (jĕ-stō′sēz). A toxemic disorder of pregnancy.

GFR abbr. glomerular filtration rate

GH abbr. growth hormone

ghost cell n. 1. A dead cell in which the outline remains visible, but whose nucleus and cytoplasmic structures are not stainable. 2. A red blood cell after loss of its hemoglobin.

ghost corpuscle n. See achromocyte.

GI abbr. gastrointestinal

gi·ant axonal neuropathy (jī′ənt) n. A generalized disorder of neurofilaments characterized by progressive peripheral neural degeneration during childhood.

giant cell n. An unusually large cell, especially a large multinucleated, phagocytic cell.

giant cell carcinoma n. A malignant epithelial neoplasm characterized by large undifferentiated cells.

giant cell fibroma *n.* A form of irritation fibroma, occurring most frequently on the gingiva of young adults, composed of fibroblasts with large stellate or multiple nuclei.

giant cell sarcoma *n.* A malignant giant cell tumor of bone.

giant cell tumor of the tendon sheath *n.* A nodule, possibly inflammatory, that usually develops from the flexor sheath of the fingers and thumb and is composed of fibrous tissue, lipid- and hemosiderin-containing macrophages, and giant cells.

gi·ant·ism (jī′ən-tĭz′əm) *n.* **1.** The quality or condition of being a giant. **2.** See **gigantism** (sense 2).

Gi·ar·di·a (jē-är′dē-ə) *n.* A genus of flagellated, usually nonpathogenic protozoa that are intestinal parasites in humans and most domestic animals.

gi·ar·di·a·sis (jē′är-dī′ə-sĭs) *n.* Intestinal infection with the protozoan *Giardia lamblia.*

gib·bos·i·ty (gĭ-bŏs′ĭ-tē) *n.* **1.** The condition of being gibbous. **2.** A rounded hump or protuberance.

gib·bus (gĭb′əs) *n.* The hump of a deformed spine.

Gib·son murmur (gĭb′sən) *n.* The typical continuous rumbling murmur associated with patent ductus arteriosus.

gi·gan·tism (jī-găn′tĭz′əm) *n.* **1.** The quality or state of being gigantic; abnormally large size. **2.** Excessive growth of the body or any of its parts, especially as a result of oversecretion of the growth hormone by the pituitary gland.

Gilles de la Tour·ette's disease or **Gilles de la Tour·ette's syndrome** (zhēl də lä tōō-rĕts′) *n.* See **Tourette's syndrome.**

gill slit *n.* One of several rudimentary invaginations in the surface of the embryo, present during development of all air-breathing vertebrates and corresponding to the functional gill slits of aquatic species.

gin·gi·va (jĭn′jə-və, jĭn-jī′-) *n., pl.* **-vae** (-vē′). See **gum.** — **gin′gi·val** (jĭn′jə-vəl, jĭn-jī′-) *adj.*

gingival massage *n.* Stimulation of the gingiva by rubbing or rhythmic pressure.

gin·gi·vec·to·my (jĭn′jə-vĕk′tə-mē) *n.* Surgical removal of gum tissue.

gin·gi·vi·tis (jĭn′jə-vī′tĭs) *n.* Inflammation of the gums, characterized by redness and swelling.

gin·gi·vo·glos·si·tis (jĭn′jə-vō-glŏ-sī′tĭs) *n.* Inflammation of the tongue and the gums.

gin·gi·vo·plas·ty (jĭn′jə-vō-plăs′tē) *n.* The surgical reshaping and recontouring of gum tissue for cosmetic, physiological, or functional purposes.

gir·dle (gûr′dl) *n.* **1.** Something that encircles like a belt. **2.** An elasticized, flexible undergarment worn over the waist and hips. **3.** The pelvic or pectoral girdle.

girdle anesthesia *n.* Anesthesia distributed as a band encircling the abdomen.

girdle sensation *n.* See **zonesthesia.**

git·a·lin (jĭt′l-ĭn, jĭ-tä′lĭn, -tăl′ĭn) *n.* **1.** A crystalline glycoside obtained from digitalis. **2.** An amorphous mixture of the glycosides obtained from digitalis.

gla·bel·la (glə-bĕl′ə) *n., pl.* **-bel·lae** (-bĕl′ē). **1.** The smooth area between the eyebrows just above the nose. **2.** The most forward projecting point of the forehead in the midline of the supraorbital ridges.

glad·i·o·lus (glăd′ē-ō′ləs) *n., pl.* **-lus·es** or **-li** (-lī). The large middle section of the sternum.

gland (glănd) *n.* **1.** A cell, a group of cells, or an organ that produces a secretion for use elsewhere in the body or in a body cavity or for elimination from the body. **2.** Any of various organs, such as lymph nodes, that resemble true glands but perform a nonsecretory function.

glan·di·lem·ma (glăn′də-lĕm′ə) *n.* The capsule of a gland.

gland of Moll *n.* See **ciliary gland.**

glan·du·lar (glăn′jə-lər) *adj.* **1.** Of, relating to, affecting, or resembling a gland or its secretion. **2.** Functioning as a gland. **3.** Having glands. **4.** Resulting from the abnormal function of a gland or glands.

glandular epithelium *n.* Epithelium made up of cells that produce secretions.

glan·dule (glăn′jōōl) *n.* A small gland.

glans (glănz) *n., pl.* **glan·des** (glăn′dēz). **1.** A conical vascular body forming the distal end of the penis. **2.** A conical vascular body forming the distal end of the clitoris.

Glanz·mann's thrombasthenia (glănz′menz, glänts′mänz′) *n.* An inherited hemorrhagic disorder characterized by normal or prolonged bleeding time, normal coagulation time but defective clot retraction, and normal platelet count but morphologic or functional abnormality of platelets.

glass (glăs) *n.* **1.** Any of a large class of materials with highly variable mechanical and optical properties that solidify from the molten state without crystallization, are generally hard, brittle, and transparent or translucent, and are considered to be supercooled liquids rather than true solids. **2.** Something usually made of glass, such as a window, or mirror, or drinking vessel. **3.** **glasses.** A pair of lenses mounted in a light frame, used to correct faulty vision or protect the eyes.

glass eye *n.* **1.** An artificial eye fashioned of glass. **2.** An eye whose iris is whitish, pale, or colorless.

glass·es (glăs′ĭz) *n.* See **spectacles.**

glau·co·ma (glou-kō′mə, glô-) *n.* Any of a group of eye diseases marked by abnormally high intraocular fluid pressure, damaged optic disk, hardening of the eyeball, and partial to complete vision loss. — **glau·co′ma·tous** (-kō′mə-təs) *adj.*

glaucomatous cataract *n.* A nuclear opacity usually seen in absolute glaucoma.

glaucomatous halo *n.* **1.** A yellowish ring surrounding the optic disk, indicating atrophy of the choroid in glaucoma. **2.** A ring or circle of illumination seen around lights, caused by corneal edema in glaucoma.

gleet (glēt) *n.* **1.** Inflammation of the urethra resulting from chronic gonorrhea and marked by a mucopurulent discharge. **2.** The discharge characteristic of this inflammation. — **gleet′y** *adj.*

Glenn's operation (glĕnz) *n.* Surgical anastomosis between the superior vena cava and the right main pulmonary artery to increase pulmonary blood flow as a correction for tricuspid atresia.

gli·a (glē′ə, glī′ə) *n.* See **neuroglia.**

gli·a·din (glī′ə-dĭn) *n.* Any of a class of simple proteins separable from wheat and rye glutens.

glid·ing joint (glī′dĭng) *n.* See **plane joint.**

gli·o·blast (glē′ə-blăst′, glī′-) *n.* An early neural cell developing from the early ependymal cell of the neural tube.

gli·o·blas·to·ma (glē′ō-blă-stō′mə, glī′-) *n.* A glioma consisting chiefly of undifferentiated anaplastic cells frequently arranged radially about an irregular focus of necrosis; it grows rapidly and invades extensively, occurring most frequently in the cerebrum of adults.

glioblastoma mul·ti·for·me (mŭl′tə-fôr′mē) *n.* A virulent type of brain cancer that is fatal in almost all cases.

gli·o·ma (glē-ō′mə, glī-) *n., pl.* **-mas** or **-ma·ta** (-mə-tə). A tumor originating in the neuroglia of the brain or spinal cord. — **gli·om′a·tous** (-ŏm′-ə-təs, -ō′mə-) *adj.*

gli·o·ma·to·sis (glē-ō′mə-tō′sĭs, glī-) *n.* Neoplastic growth of neuroglial cells in the brain or spinal cord, especially such a growth of relatively large size or having multiple foci.

gli·o·neu·ro·ma (glē′ō-nŏŏ-rō′mə, -nyŏŏ-, glī′-) *n.* A ganglioneuroma derived from neurons, containing many glial cells and fibers in the matrix.

gli·o·sar·co·ma (glē′ō-sär-kō′mə, glī′-) *n.* A glioma consisting of immature, undifferentiated, pleomorphic, spindle-shaped cells with relatively large, hyperchromatic nuclei and poorly formed fibrillary processes.

gli·o·sis (glē-ō′sĭs, glī-) *n.* Excessive proliferation of the neuroglia.

glip·i·zide (glĭp′ĭ-zīd′) *n.* An oral sulfonylurea having hypoglycemic activity and used therapeutically as an antidiabetic.

glob·al (glō′bəl) *adj.* **1.** Having the shape of a globe; spherical. **2.** Of or involving the entire earth; worldwide. **3.** Comprehensive; total. **4.** Of or relating to the eyeball. — **glob′al·ly** *adv.*

glo·bin (glō′bĭn) *n.* The protein that is a constituent of hemoglobin.

glo·bo·side (glō′bə-sīd′) *n.* A glycosphingolipid, especially a ceramide tetrasaccharide, occurring in the kidneys, red blood cells, blood serum, liver, and spleen and accumulating in tissues in a form of gangliosidosis.

glob·ule (glŏb′yōōl) *n.* A small spherical body, as a drop of liquid. — **glob′u·lar** (-yə-lər) *adj.*

glob·u·lin (glŏb′yə-lĭn) *n.* Any of a family of proteins that can be precipitated from plasma and may be further fractionated by separation methods into many subgroups that differ with respect to associated lipids or carbohydrates.

glob·u·li·nu·ri·a (glŏb′yə-lə-nŏŏr′ē-ə, -nyŏŏr′-) *n.* Excretion of globulin in the urine.

glo·bus (glō′bəs) *n., pl.* **-bi** (-bī′). **1.** A round or spherical body. **2.** Any of the brown bodies sometimes found in the granulomatous lesions of leprosy.

glo·mec·to·my (glō-mĕk′tə-mē) *n.* Surgical excision of a glomus tumor.

glom·er·ule (glŏm′ə-rōōl′, glŏm′yə-) *n.* A glomerulus. — **glo·mer′u·late** (glō-mĕr′yə-lĭt) *adj.*

glo·mer·u·li·tis (glō-mĕr′yə-lī′tĭs) *n.* Inflammation of a glomerulus, especially of the renal glomeruli, as in glomerulonephritis.

glo·mer·u·lo·ne·phri·tis (glō-mĕr′yə-lō-nə-frī′-tĭs) *n.* Renal disease characterized by bilateral inflammatory changes in glomeruli that are not the result of infection of the kidneys.

glo·mer·u·lop·a·thy (glō-mĕr′yə-lŏp′ə-thē) *n.* Disease of the renal glomeruli.

glo·mer·u·lo·scle·ro·sis (glō-mĕr′yə-lō-sklə-rō′-sĭs) *n.* Hyaline deposits or scarring within the renal glomeruli, a degenerative process occurring in renal arteriosclerosis or diabetes.

glo·mer·u·lus (glō-mĕr′yə-ləs) *n., pl.* **-li** (-lī′). **1.** A small cluster or intertwined mass, as of blood vessels or nerve fibers. **2.** A tuft of capillaries situated within a Bowman's capsule at the end of a renal tubule in the vertebrate kidney that filters waste products from the blood and thus initiates urine formation. **3.** The twisted secretory portion of a sweat gland. **4.** A nerve ending consisting of a cluster of dendritic ramifications and axon terminals surrounded by a glial sheath.

glo·mus (glō′məs) *n., pl.* **glom·er·a** (glŏm′ər-ə). **1.** A small globular body. **2.** A small body surrounded by many nerve fibers, consisting of an anastomosis between fine arterioles and veins and functioning as a regulation mechanism in the flow of blood, control of temperature, and conservation of heat in a particular organ or part.

glomus tumor *n.* A painful tumor composed of specialized pericytes usually arranged in single encapsulated nodular masses that occur almost exclusively in the skin.

glos·sa (glô′sə) *n., pl.* **glos·sas** or **glos·sae** (glô′sē). The tongue.

glos·sal (glô′səl) *adj.* Of or relating to the tongue.

glos·sec·to·my (glô-sĕk′tə-mē) *n.* Surgical excision or amputation of the tongue.

glos·si·tis (glô-sī′tĭs) *n.* Inflammation of the tongue. — **glos·sit′ic** (-sĭt′ĭk) *adj.*

glos·so·dyn·i·a (glôs′ō-dĭn′ē-ə) *n.* A burning or painful sensation in the tongue.

glos·so·la·li·a (glô′sə-lā′lē-ə) *n.* Fabricated and nonmeaningful speech, especially such speech associated with a trance state or certain schizophrenic syndromes.

glos·sop·a·thy (glō-sŏp′ə-thē) *n.* A disease of the tongue.

glos·so·pha·ryn·ge·al (glŏs′ō-fə-rĭn′jē-əl, -jəl, -făr′ən-jē′əl) *adj.* Relating to the tongue and the pharynx.

glossopharyngeal breathing *n.* Respiration unaided by the primary muscles of respiration, the air being forced into the lungs by use of the tongue and muscles of the pharynx.

glossopharyngeal nerve *n.* Either of a pair of nerves that emerge from the rostral end of the medulla, pass through the jugular foramen, and supply sensation to the pharynx and the back third of tongue.

glos·so·plas·ty (glŏ′sə-plăs′tē) *n.* Reparative or plastic surgery of the tongue.

glos·sor·rha·phy (glŏ-sôr′ə-fē) *n.* Suture of a wound of the tongue.

glos·sot·o·my (glŏ-sŏt′ə-mē) *n.* Surgical incision of the tongue.

glot·tis (glŏt′ĭs) *n., pl.* **glot·tis·es** or **glot·ti·des** (glŏt′ĭ-dēz′). The vocal apparatus of the larynx, consisting of the true vocal cords and the narrow opening between them.

glot·ti·tis (glŏ-tī′tĭs) *n.* Inflammation of the glottic portion of the larynx.

glove anesthesia (glŭv) *n.* Loss of sensation in an area that would be covered by a glove.

Glu *abbr.* glutamic acid; glutamine

glu·ca·gon (glōō′kə-gŏn′) *n.* A polypeptide hormone secreted by the alpha cells of the islets of Langerhans of the pancreas that initiates a rise in blood sugar levels by stimulating the breakdown of glycogen by the liver.

glu·ca·go·no·ma (glōō′kə-gŏ-nō′mə) *n.* A glucagon-secreting tumor, usually derived from pancreatic islet cells.

glu·can (glōō′kăn′, -kən) *n.* A polysaccharide, such as cellulose, that is a polymer of glucose.

glu·co·cor·ti·coid (glōō′kō-kôr′tĭ-koid′) *n.* Any of a group of steroid hormones, such as cortisone, that are produced by the adrenal cortex, are involved in carbohydrate, protein, and fat metabolism, and have anti-inflammatory properties. — **glu′co·cor′ti·coid′** *adj.*

glu·co·fu·ra·nose (glōō′kō-fyŏŏr′ə-nōs′) *n.* A cyclic glucose in which an oxygen atom links carbons located at particular positions in the ring.

glu·co·gen·e·sis (glōō′kō-jĕn′ĭ-sĭs) *n.* The formation of glucose through the breakdown of glycogen. — **glu′co·gen′ic** *adj.*

glu·co·ne·o·gen·e·sis (glōō′kō-nē′ə-jĕn′ĭ-sĭs) *n.* The formation of glucose, especially by the liver, from noncarbohydrate sources, such as amino acids and the glycerol portion of fats.

glu·co·pro·tein (glōō′kō-prō′tēn′, -tē-ĭn) *n.* A glycoprotein containing glucose as carbohydrate.

glu·co·san (glōō′kə-săn′) *n.* **1.** A polysaccharide yielding glucose upon hydrolysis. **2.** Any of several anhydrides of glucose.

glu·cose (glōō′kōs′) *n.* A monosaccharide sugar that is the principal circulating sugar in the blood and the major energy source of the body; it occurs widely in most plant and animal tissue.

glucose-6-phosphate *n.* An essential intermediate formed from glucose and ATP during the metabolism of glucose.

glucose tolerance test *n.* A test for evaluating the body's capability to metabolize glucose based

upon the ability of the liver to absorb and store excess glucose as glycogen.

glucose transport maximum *n.* The maximal rate of reabsorption of glucose from the glomerular filtrate.

glu·co·side (glōō′kə-sīd′) *n.* A glycoside, the sugar component of which is glucose. — **glu′co·sid′ic** (-sĭd′ĭk) *adj.*

glu·co·su·ri·a (glōō′kə-sŏŏr′ē-ə, -shŏŏr′-) *n.* Excretion of glucose in the urine, especially in elevated quantities.

glu·co·syl·cer·a·mide (glōō′kə-sĭl-sə-răm′ĭd′, -sĕr′ə-mīd′) *n.* A glycolipid containing a fatty acid, glucose, and sphingosine.

glu·cu·ron·ic acid (glōō′kyə-rŏn′ĭk) *n.* The uronic acid of glucose that conjugates various substances in the liver to detoxicate or inactivate them.

glu·cu·ro·nide (glōō-kyŏŏr′ə-nīd′) *n.* Any of various derivatives of glucuronic acid that often combine with toxic organic compounds and are excreted.

glu·tam·ic acid (glōō-tăm′ĭk) *n.* A nonessential amino acid occurring widely in plant and animal tissue and having a salt, sodium glutamate, that is used as a flavor-intensifying seasoning.

glu·ta·mine (glōō′tə-mēn′) *n.* A nonessential amino acid that occurs widely in proteins and blood and other tissue, and is metabolized to yield urinary ammonia.

glu·tar·ic acid (glōō-tăr′ĭk) *n.* An acid formed during the catabolism of tryptophan.

glu·ta·thi·one (glōō′tə-thī′ōn′) *n.* A tripeptide of the amino acids glycine, cystine, and glutamic acid occurring widely in plant and animal tissues and forming reduced and oxidized forms important in biological oxidation-reduction reactions.

glu·te·al (glōō′tē-əl, glōō-tē′-) *adj.* Relating to the buttocks.

gluteal fold *n.* A prominent fold on the back of the upper thigh that marks the upper limit of the thigh from the lower limit of the buttock.

glu·ten (glōōt′n) *n.* A mixture of insoluble plant proteins occurring in cereal grains, chiefly corn and wheat, used as a flour substitute.

glu·teth·i·mide (glōō-tĕth′ə-mīd′) *n.* A nonbarbiturate sedative and hypnotic drug.

glu·te·us (glōō′tē-əs, glōō-tē′-) *n., pl.* **glu·te·i** (glōō′tē-ī′, glōō-tē′ī′). Any of three large muscles of each buttock, especially gluteus maximus, that extend, abduct, and rotate the thigh.

glu·ti·nous (glōōt′n-əs) *adj.* Adhesive; sticky. — **glu′ti·nous·ness, glu′ti·nos′i·ty** (-ŏs′ĭ-tē) *n.*

Gly *abbr.* glycine

gly·can (glī′kăn′, -kən) *n.* See **polysaccharide**.

gly·ce·mi·a (glī-sē′mē-ə) *n.* The presence of glucose in the blood.

glyc·er·ide (glĭs′ə-rīd′) *n.* A natural or synthetic ester of glycerol and fatty acids.

glyc·er·in or **glyc·er·ine** (glĭs′ər-ĭn) *n.* Glycerol or a preparation of glycerol.

glyc·er·ol (glĭs′ə-rôl′, -rōl′) *n.* A sweet syrupy fluid used as a solvent, a skin emollient, and as a vehicle and sweetening agent; it is also used by injection or in suppository form for constipation and orally to reduce ocular tension.

gly·cine (glī'sēn', -sĭn) *n.* A nonessential amino acid derived from the alkaline hydrolysis of gelatin and used as a nutrient and dietary supplement, also used in biochemical research and in the treatment of certain myopathies.

gly·co·ca·lyx (glī'kō-kā'lĭks, -kăl'ĭks) *n.* An outer filamentous coating of carbohydrate-rich molecules on the surface of certain cells.

gly·co·cho·lic acid (glī'kō-kō'lĭk) *n.* A crystalline acid occurring in bile and formed through the conjugation of cholic acid and glycine.

gly·co·gen (glī'kə-jən) *n.* A polysaccharide that is the main form of carbohydrate storage in animals and occurs primarily in the liver and muscle tissue; it is readily converted to glucose as needed by the body to satisfy its energy needs. — **gly'co·gen'ic** (-jĕn'ĭk) *adj.*

gly·co·gen·e·sis (glī'kə-jĕn'ĭ-sĭs) *n.* The formation or synthesis of glycogen. — **gly'co·ge·net'ic** (-jə-nĕt'ĭk) *adj.*

glycogen granule *n.* A granule of glycogen occurring in a cell as an alpha or a beta granule.

gly·co·ge·nol·y·sis (glī'kə-jə-nŏl'ĭ-sĭs) *n.* The hydrolysis of glycogen to glucose. — **gly'co·gen·o·lyt'ic** (-jĕn'ə-lĭt'ĭk) *adj.*

gly·co·ge·no·sis (glī'kə-jə-nō'sĭs) *n.* Any of various inheritable diseases caused by enzyme deficiencies and characterized by the abnormal accumulation of glycogen in tissue.

glycogen storage disease *n.* See **glycogenosis.**

gly·col·ic acid (glī-kŏl'ĭk) *n.* A colorless crystalline compound found in sugar beets, cane sugar, and unripe grapes that is used in pharmaceuticals, pesticides, adhesives, and plasticizers.

gly·co·lip·id (glī'kə-lĭp'ĭd) *n.* A lipid, such as a cerebroside, that contains a carbohydrate groups.

gly·col·y·sis (glī-kŏl'ə-sĭs) *n.* The ATP-generating metabolic process that occurs in nearly all living cells by which carbohydrates and sugars, typically glucose, are converted in a series of steps to pyruvic acid. — **gly'co·lyt'ic** (glī'kə-lĭt'ĭk) *adj.*

gly·co·ne·o·gen·e·sis (glī'kə-nē'ə-jĕn'ĭ-sĭs) *n.* See **gluconeogenesis.**

gly·co·pe·ni·a (glī'kə-pē'nē-ə) *n.* A deficiency of any or all sugars in an organ or a tissue.

gly·co·pep·tide (glī'kō-pĕp'tīd') *n.* Glycoprotein.

gly·co·phil·i·a (glī'kə-fĭl'ē-ə) *n.* A condition in which one tends to develop hyperglycemia after ingesting even a small amount of glucose.

gly·co·pro·tein (glī'kō-prō'tēn', -tē-ĭn) *n.* Any of a group of conjugated proteins that contain a carbohydrate as the nonprotein component.

gly·co·pty·a·lism (glī'kō-tī'ə-lĭz'əm) *n.* See **glycosialia.**

gly·cor·rha·chi·a (glī'kə-rā'kē-ə, -răk'ē-ə) *n.* The presence of sugar in the cerebrospinal fluid.

gly·cor·rhe·a (glī'kə-rē'ə) *n.* Discharge of sugar from the body, especially in large quantities.

gly·co·si·a·li·a (glī'kō-sī-ā'lē-ə, -ăl'ē-ə) *n.* The presence of sugar in the saliva.

gly·co·side (glī'kə-sīd') *n.* Any of a group of organic compounds, occurring abundantly in plants, that yield a sugar and one or more nonsugar substances on hydrolysis. — **gly'co·sid'ic** (-sĭd'ĭk) *adj.*

gly·co·su·ri·a (glī'kə-sŏŏr'ē-ə, -shŏŏr'-) *n.* **1.** See **glucosuria. 2.** Excretion of carbohydrates in the urine. — **gly'co·su'ric** *adj.*

gly·co·syl (glī'kə-sĭl') *n.* A univalent radical resulting from detachment of a hydroxyl group (OH) from a cyclic glucose.

gly·co·sy·lat·ed hemoglobin (glī-kō'sə-lā'tĭd) *n.* Any of four hemoglobin fractions that together account for less than 4 percent of the total hemoglobin in the blood.

gm. *abbr.* gram

GMP (jē'ĕm-pē') *n.* A nucleotide composed of guanine, ribose, and one phosphate group that is formed during protein synthesis.

gnat (năt) *n.* Any of various small, biting, two-winged flies, such as a biting midge or black fly.

gnath·o·plas·ty (năth'ə-plăs'tē) *n.* Reparative surgery of the jaw.

gno·si·a (nō'sē-ə, -zē-ə) *n.* The perceptive faculty enabling one to recognize the form and the nature of persons and things.

GnRH *abbr.* gonadotropin-releasing hormone

gob·let cell (gŏb'lĭt) *n.* A mucus-secreting epithelial cell that distends with mucin before secretion and collapses to a goblet shape after secretion.

goi·ter (goi'tər) *n.* A noncancerous enlargement of the thyroid gland, visible as a swelling at the front of the neck, that is often associated with iodine deficiency. — **goi'trous** (-trəs) *adj.*

gold (gōld) *n.* A soft, yellow, corrosion-resistant element with atomic number 79 that is the most malleable and ductile metal. Gold is generally alloyed to increase its strength.

Gold·blatt phenomenon (gōld'blăt') *n.* Hypertension occurring as a result of the partial occlusion of a renal artery.

Gold·stein's toe sign (gōld'stīnz) *n.* Increased space between the big toe and its neighbor, seen in Down syndrome and occasionally cretinism.

Golgi apparatus *n.* See **Golgi complex.**

Golgi complex *n.* A complex of parallel, flattened saccules, vesicles, and vacuoles that lies adjacent to the nucleus of a cell and is concerned with the formation of secretions within the cell.

gom·pho·sis (gŏm-fō'sĭs) *n., pl.* **-ses** (-sēz). A type of immovable articulation, as of a tooth inserted into its bony socket.

go·nad (gō'năd') *n.* An organ that produces gametes, especially a testis or an ovary. — **go·nad'-al** (gō-năd'l), **go·nad'ic** *adj.*

go·nad·ec·to·my (gō'nə-dĕk'tə-mē) *n.* Surgical excision of an ovary or a testis.

gon·a·dop·a·thy (gŏn'ə-dŏp'ə-thē) *n.* A disease affecting the gonads.

go·nad·o·troph (gō-năd'ə-trŏf', -trŏf', gŏn'ə-dō-) *n.* A cell of the anterior lobe of the pituitary gland that affects certain cells of the ovary or the testis.

go·nad·o·trop·ic hormone (gō-năd'ə-trŏp'ĭk, -trō'pĭk) *n.* See **gonadotropin.**

go·nad·o·tro·pin (gō-năd′ə-trō′pĭn, -trŏp′ĭn) or **go·nad·o·tro·phin** (-trō′fĭn) *n.* A hormone that stimulates the growth and activity of the gonads, especially any of several pituitary hormones that stimulate the function of the ovaries and testes.

gonadotropin-releasing hormone *n.* A hormone produced by the hypothalamus that stimulates the anterior pituitary gland to begin secreting luteinizing hormone and follicle-stimulating hormone.

gon·an·gi·ec·to·my (gŏn′ăn-jē-ĕk′tə-mē) *n.* See **vasectomy.**

gon·ar·throt·o·my (gŏn′är-thrŏt′ə-mē) *n.* Incision into the knee joint.

Go·nin operation (gō-năn′, gô-) *n.* Treatment of retinal detachment by closure of the break in the retina through cauterization.

go·ni·o·punc·ture (gō′nē-ə-pŭngk′chər) *n.* An operation for congenital glaucoma in which a puncture is made in the filtration angle of the anterior chamber of the eye.

go·ni·o·scope (gō′nē-ə-skōp′) *n.* An ophthalmoscope used to examine the angle of the anterior chamber of the eye.

go·ni·os·co·py (gō′nē-ŏs′kə-pē) *n.* Examination of the angle of the anterior chamber of the eye with a gonioscope or with a contact prism lens.

go·ni·ot·o·my (gō′nē-ŏt′ə-mē) *n.* Surgical opening of the vascular structure encircling the cornea by way of the angle of the anterior chamber of the eye to treat congenital glaucoma.

gonococcal conjunctivitis *n.* Severe conjunctivitis caused by gonococci and marked by intense swelling of the conjunctiva and eyelids and by a profuse purulent discharge.

gon·o·coc·ce·mi·a (gŏn′ə-kŏk-sē′mē-ə) *n.* The presence of gonococci in the circulating blood.

gon·o·coc·cus (gŏn′ə-kŏk′əs) *n., pl.* **-coc·ci** (-kŏk′sī′, -kŏk′ī′). The bacterium *Neisseria gonorrhoeae,* which is the causative agent of gonorrhea. — **gon′o·coc′cal** *adj.*

gon·or·rhe·a (gŏn′ə-rē′ə) *n.* A sexually transmitted disease caused by gonococci that affects the mucous membrane chiefly of the genital and urinary tracts and is characterized by an acute purulent discharge and painful or difficult urination, though women often have no symptoms. — **gon′or·rhe′al, gon′or·rhe′ic** *adj.*

gonorrheal ophthalmia *n.* Acute purulent conjunctivitis due to gonococcal infection.

Good·pas·ture′s syndrome (gŏod′păs′chərz) *n.* Glomerulonephritis associated with circulating antibodies against basement-membrane antigens; it may be preceded by hemoptysis.

goose bumps *pl.n.* Momentary roughness of the skin caused by erection of the papillae in response to cold or fear.

gor·get (gôr′jĭt) *n.* A surgical director or guide with a wide groove for use in lithotomy.

Gor·man′s syndrome (gôr′mənz) *n.* A disorder characterized by hemangiomatosis of the skeletal system with or without involvement of the over-

lying skin and resulting in osteolysis and fibrous replacement of bone.

go·se·rel·in (gō′sə-rĕl′ĭn) *n.* A synthetic peptide analogue of gonadotropin-releasing hormone used to treat prostate cancer, endometriosis, and advanced breast cancer.

gouge (gouj) *n.* A strong curved chisel used in bone surgery.

Gou·ley′s catheter (gōo′lēz) *n.* A solid, curved steel instrument grooved on its inferior surface so that it can be passed over a guide inserted through a urethral stricture.

goun·dou (gōon′dōo) *n.* A disease characterized by exostoses of the nasal processes of the maxillary bones, causing swelling on each side of the nose; believed to be a result of yaws.

gout (gout) *n.* An inherited disorder of uric-acid metabolism marked by painful inflammation of the joints, especially of the feet and hands, and arthritic attacks resulting from elevated levels of uric acid in the blood and deposition of urate crystals around the joints. — **gout′y** *adj.*

G.P. or **GP** *abbr.* general practitioner

gr or **gr.** *abbr.* grain; gram

Graaf·i·an follicle or **Graaf·i·an follicle** (grä′fē-ən, gräf′ē-) *n.* A mature ovarian follicle in which the oocyte attains its full size and the surrounding follicular cells are permeated by one or more fluid-filled cavities.

grac·i·lis muscle (grăs′ə-lĭs) *n.* A muscle with its origin in the pubic ramus near the symphysis and insertion to the shaft of the tibia, and whose action adducts the thigh, flexes the knee, and rotates the leg medially.

grad. *abbr. Latin.* gradatim (gradually)

grad·u·at·ed tenotomy (grăj′ōo-ā′tĭd) *n.* Partial incisions of the tendon of an eye muscle to correct a slight degree of strabismus.

Grae·fe′s operation (grā′fəz) *n.* **1.** The removal of cataract by a limbal incision with capsulotomy and iridectomy. **2.** Iridectomy for the treatment of glaucoma.

Graefe′s sign or **von Graefe′s sign** (vŏn) *n.* An indication of Graves′ disease in which the upper eyelid does not evenly follow the downward movement of the eyeball, but instead lags or moves jerkily.

graft (grăft) *v.* **graft·ed, graft·ing, grafts.** To transplant or implant tissue surgically into a body part to replace a damaged part or compensate for a defect. — *n.* **1.** Material, especially living tissue or an organ, surgically attached to or inserted into a body part to replace a damaged part or compensate for a defect. **2.** The procedure of implanting or transplanting such material.

graft-versus-host disease *n.* A type of incompatibility reaction of transplanted cells against host tissues that have an antigen different from that of the donor.

Gra·ham Steell′s murmur (grā′əm stēlz′) *n.* An early diastolic murmur caused by pulmonary insufficiency secondary to pulmonary hypertension, as in mitral stenosis.

grain (grān) *n.* **1.** A small, dry, one-seeded fruit of a cereal grass, having the fruit and the seed walls united. **2.** The fruits of cereal grasses especially after having been harvested. **3.** A small discrete particulate or crystalline mass. **4.** A unit of weight in the U.S. Customary System, an avoirdupois unit equal to 0.002285 ounce (0.065 gram).

gram (grăm) *n.* A metric unit of mass equal to 15.432 grains, one thousandth (10^{-3}) of a kilogram, or 0.035 ounce.

gram·i·ci·din (grăm′ĭ-sīd′n) *n.* An antibiotic produced by the soil bacterium *Bacillus brevis* and used to treat infections caused by certain grampositive bacteria.

gram-negative or **Gram-negative** *adj.* Of, relating to, or being a bacterium that does not retain the violet stain used in Gram's method.

gram-positive or **Gram-pos·i·tive** (grăm′pŏz′ĭ-tĭv) *adj.* Of, relating to, or being a bacterium that retains the violet stain used in Gram's method.

Gram's stain (grămz) *n.* A method of staining technique used to classify bacteria in which a bacterial specimen is first stained with crystal violet, then treated with an iodine solution, decolorized with alcohol, and counterstained with safranine. Gram-positive bacteria retain the violet stain; gram-negative bacteria do not.

grand mal (grän′ mäl′, gränd′ măl′) *n.* A severe form of epilepsy characterized by seizures involving spasms and loss of consciousness.

grand mal epilepsy *n.* See **grand mal**.

grand mal seizure *n.* A sudden attack or convulsion characterized by generalized muscle spasms and loss of consciousness, recurrent in grand mal.

gran·u·lar endoplasmic reticulum (grăn′yə-lər) *n.* Endoplasmic reticulum in which the cisternae are studded with ribosomes, associated with the synthesis of proteins.

granular layer *n.* **1.** The deeper of the two layers of the cortex of the cerebellum, containing many granule cells whose dendrites synapse with incoming highly branched nerve fibers, but whose axons form numerous synapses with the dendrites of Purkinje cells, basket cells, and stellate cells. **2.** A layer of somewhat flattened cells containing keratin granules, lying just above the prickle cell layer of the epidermis. **3.** The layer of small cells that forms the wall of an ovarian follicle.

granular leukoblast *n.* See **promyelocyte**.

granular leukocyte *n.* A white blood cell having granules in its cytoplasm.

gran·u·la·tion (grăn′yə-lā′shən) *n.* **1.** The process of forming grains or granules. **2.** The state or appearance of having grains or granules. **3.** Small, fleshy, beadlike protuberances, consisting of outgrowths of new capillaries, on the surface of a wound that is healing. **4.** The formation of these protuberances.

granulation tissue *n.* See **granulation** (sense 3).

gran·ule (grăn′yōōl) *n.* **1.** A small grain or pellet; a particle. **2.** A cellular or cytoplasmic particle, es-

pecially one that stains readily. **3.** A very small pill, usually coated with gelatin or sugar.

granule cell *n.* One of the small neurons of the cortex of the cerebellum and cerebrum.

gran·u·lo·cyte (grăn′yə-lō-sīt′) *n.* Any of a group of white blood cells having granules in the cytoplasm. — **gran′u·lo·cyt′ic** (-sĭt′ĭk) *adj.*

granulocytic leukemia *n.* Leukemia characterized by proliferation of myeloid tissue in areas such as bone marrow and the spleen and by the abnormal increase of granulocytes, myelocytes, and myeloblasts in tissues and in blood.

granulocytic series *n.* The cells in various stages of granulopoietic development in the bone marrow.

gran·u·lo·cy·to·pe·ni·a (grăn′yə-lō-sī′tə-pē′nē-ə) *n.* A condition marked by an abnormally low number of granular white blood cells.

gran·u·lo·cy·to·poi·e·sis (grăn′yə-lō-sī′tə-poi-ē′sĭs) *n.* See **granulopoiesis**. — **gran′u·lo·cy′to·poi·et′ic** (-ĕt′ĭk) *adj.*

gran·u·lo·cy·to·sis (grăn′yə-lō-sī-tō′sĭs) *n.* A condition characterized by an abnormally large number of granulocytes in the blood or tissues.

gran·u·lo·ma (grăn′yə-lō′mə) *n.*, *pl.* **-mas** or **-ma·ta** (-mə-tə). A mass of inflamed granulation tissue, usually associated with ulcerated infections. — **gran′u·lo′ma·tous** (-mə-təs) *adj.*

granuloma in·gui·na·le (ĭng′gwə-nä′lē) *n.* See **donovanosis**.

granuloma mul·ti·for·me (mŭl′tə-fôr′mē) *n.* A chronic granulomatous annular eruption of the skin on the upper body in older adults, usually seen in central Africa.

granulomatous colitis *n.* Colitis characterized by granulomas.

granulomatous inflammation *n.* A form of proliferative inflammation characterized by the formation of granulomas.

granuloma trop·i·cum (trŏp′ĭ-kəm) *n.* See **yaws**.

gran·u·lo·mere (grăn′yə-lō-mêr′) *n.* The central part of a blood platelet.

gran·u·lo·pe·ni·a (grăn′yə-lō-pē′nē-ə) *n.* See **granulocytopenia**.

gran·u·lo·poi·e·sis (grăn′yə-lō-poi-ē′sĭs) *n.* The formation of granulocytes. — **gran′u·lo·poi·et′ic** (-ĕt′ĭk) *adj.*

gran·u·lo·sa cell (grăn′yə-lō′sə) *n.* A cell lining the vesicular ovarian follicle that becomes a luteal cell after ovulation.

granulosa cell tumor *n.* A benign or malignant tumor of the ovary developing from the granular layer of the Graafian follicle and frequently secreting estrogen.

gran·u·lo·sis (grăn′yə-lō′sĭs) *n.* The formation of a mass of granules.

grat·tage (gră-täzh′, grə-) *n.* Scraping or brushing an ulcer or surface that has granulations in order to stimulate the healing process.

grave (grāv) *adj.* Serious or dangerous, as a symptom or disease.

grav·el (grăv′əl) *n.* Sandlike concretions of uric acid, calcium oxalate, and mineral salts formed in the passages of the biliary and urinary tracts.

Graves' disease (grāvz) n. A condition usually caused by excessive production of thyroid hormone and characterized by an enlarged thyroid gland, protrusion of the eyeballs, a rapid heartbeat, and nervous excitability.

grav·id (grăv′ĭd) adj. Carrying eggs or developing young. — **gra·vid′i·ty** (grə-vĭd′ĭ-tē) n.

grav·i·da (grăv′ĭ-də) n., pl. **-das** or **-dae** (-dē′). A pregnant woman.

gravid uterus n. The condition of the uterus in pregnancy.

grav·i·ta·tion·al ulcer (grăv′ĭ-tā′shə-nəl) n. A chronic ulcer of the leg that is slow to heal because of the dependent position of the extremity and the incompetence of the valves of the varicosed veins.

gray hepatization (grā) n. The second stage of hepatization of lung tissue in pneumonia, when the yellowish-gray exudate is beginning to degenerate before breaking down.

gray matter n. Brownish-gray nerve tissue, especially of the brain and spinal cord, composed of nerve cell bodies and their dendrites and some supportive tissue.

gray substance n. See **gray matter**.

great·er omentum (grā′tər) n. A peritoneal fold passing from the greater curvature of the stomach to the transverse colon, hanging like an apron in front of the intestines.

greater trochanter n. A strong process overhanging the root of the neck of the femur, giving attachment to the middle and least gluteal muscles as well as other muscles that control thigh movement.

greater vestibular gland n. Either of two compound tubuloalveolar mucus-secreting glands situated in the lateral walls on each side of the vestibule of the vagina.

great foramen n. The large orifice in the base of the skull through which the spinal cord passes to the cranial cavity and becomes continuous with the medulla oblongata.

great saphenous vein n. A vein formed by the union of the dorsal vein of the big toe and the dorsal venous arch of the foot and emptying into the femoral vein in the region of the upper thigh.

Green·field's disease (grēn′fēldz′) n. The late-infantile form of metachromatic leukodystrophy.

green soap n. A translucent, yellowish-green soft or liquid soap made chiefly from vegetable oils and used in the treatment of skin disorders.

green·stick fracture (grēn′stĭk′) n. A fracture in which one side of the bone is broken and the other side is bent.

Greig's syndrome (grēgz) n. See **ocular hypertelorism**.

grenz rays (grĕnts) pl.n. Very soft x-rays, closely allied to ultraviolet rays in their wavelength and in their biological action upon tissues.

grief (grēf) n. Deep mental anguish, as that arising from bereavement.

gripe (grīp) v. **griped**, **grip·ing**, **gripes**. To have sharp pains in the bowels. — n. **1. gripes**. Sharp,

spasmodic pains in the bowels. **2.** A firm grasp.

grippe or **grip** (grĭp) n. See **influenza**.

gris·e·o·ful·vin (grĭz′ē-ə-fŭl′vĭn) n. An antibiotic administered orally for the treatment of fungal infections of the skin, hair, and nails.

groin (groin) n. The crease or hollow at the junction of the inner part of each thigh with the trunk, together with the adjacent region and often including the external genitals.

groove (grōōv) n. A rut, groove, or narrow depression or channel in a surface.

ground substance n. **1.** The amorphous intercellular material in which the cells and fibers of connective tissue are embedded, composed of proteoglycans, plasma constituents, metabolites, water, and ions. **2.** See **hyaloplasm**.

group A streptococcus (grōōp) n. A common but very virulent type of streptococcus that kills the tissue it infects and produces toxins that trigger a form of shock that affects vital organs.

group practice n. The practice of medicine by a group of physicians, each of whom is usually confined to some special field but all of whom share a common facility.

group therapy n. A form of psychotherapy that involves sessions guided by a therapist and attended by several clients who confront their personal problems together.

grow (grō) v. **grew** (grōō), **grown** (grōn), **grow·ing**, **grows**. **1.** To increase in size by a natural process. **2.** To develop and reach maturity. **3.** To be capable of growth; thrive.

growing pains pl.n. Pains in the limbs and joints of children or adolescents, frequently occurring at night and often attributed to rapid growth but arising from various unrelated causes.

growth (grōth) n. **1.** The process of growing. **2.** Full development; maturity. **3.** An increase, as in size, number, value, or strength. **4.** Something that grows or has grown. **5.** An abnormal mass of tissue growing in or on a living organism.

growth factor n. A substance that affects the growth of an organism.

growth hormone n. See **somatotropin**.

growth line n. Any of various dense transverse lines observed in radiographs of long bones, representing bone regrowth after temporary cessation of longitudinal growth.

growth rate n. Absolute or relative growth increase, expressed in units of time.

GSR abbr. galvanic skin response

GTP (jē′tē-pē′) n. Guanosine triphosphate; a nucleotide similar to ATP, composed of guanine, ribose, and three phosphate groups, and necessary for the synthesis of proteins.

gtt. abbr. Latin. guttae (drops)

GU abbr. genitourinary

guai·a·col (gwī′ə-kôl′, -kōl′) n. A yellowish, oily, aromatic substance used chiefly as an expectorant, a local anesthetic, and an antiseptic.

gua·nine (gwä′nēn′) n. A purine base that is an essential constituent of both RNA and DNA.

guanine ribonucleotide *n.* See **GMP**.
gua·no·sine (gwä′nə-sēn′, -sĭn) *n.* A nucleoside consisting of guanine and ribose.
guanosine triphosphate *n.* GTP.
gua·nyl·ic acid (gwä-nĭl′ĭk) *n.* See **GMP**.
guard (gärd) *v.* **guard·ed, guard·ing, guards. 1.** To protect from harm by or as if by watching over. **2.** To furnish a device or object with a protective piece. **3.** To take precautions. —*n.* **1.** A device attached to a knife to prevent too deep an incision. **2.** A padded covering worn to protect a body part from injury.
guard·ed (gär′dĭd) *adj.* Watched over; supervised, as of the condition of a patient.
guarding *n.* A spasm of muscles that minimizes the motion or agitation of sites affected by injury or disease.
gu·ber·nac·u·lum (gōō′bər-năk′yə-ləm) *n., pl.* **-la** (-lə). A fibrous cord connecting two structures.
guide (gīd) *n.* A device or instrument by which something is led into its proper course, such as a grooved director or a catheter guide.
Guil·lain–Bar·ré syndrome (gē-yăn′bə-rā′, gē-yăn′-) *n.* See **acute idiopathic polyneuritis**.
guil·lo·tine (gĭl′ə-tēn′, gē′ə-) *n.* An instrument in the shape of a metal ring with a sliding knifeblade running through it, used in cutting off an enlarged tonsil.
guin·ea worm (gĭn′ē) *n.* A long, threadlike nematode worm *(Dracunculus medinensis)* of tropical Asia and Africa that is a subcutaneous parasite of humans and other mammals and causes ulcerative lesions on the legs and feet.
gul·let (gŭl′ĭt) *n.* **1.** The esophagus. **2.** The throat.
gum (gŭm) *n.* The firm connective tissue covered by mucous membrane that envelops the alveolar arches of the jaw and surrounds the bases of the teeth. —*v.* **gummed, gum·ming, gums.** To chew food with toothless gums.
gum line *n.* The position of the margin of the gingiva in relation to teeth in the dental arch.
gum·ma (gŭm′ə) *n., pl.* **gum·mas** (gŭm′əz) or **gum·ma·ta** (gŭm′ə-tə). A small, rubbery granuloma with a necrotic center and an inflamed, fibrous capsule. It is characteristic of an advanced stage of syphilis. —**gum′ma·tous** *adj.*
gum resection *n.* See **gingivectomy**.
Gunn's dot (gŭnz) *n.* Any of the minute glistening white or yellowish nonpathogenic spots usually occurring on the posterior part of a fundus.
Gunn's sign *n.* An indication of arteriolar sclerosis observed ophthalmoscopically, in which the underlying vein at arteriovenous crossings is compressed.
Günz·berg's test (günts′bərgz, -bĕrks′) *n.* A test for detecting hydrochloric acid using indicators that produce a bright red color in the presence of the acid.

gur·ney (gûr′nē) *n., pl.* **-neys.** A metal stretcher with wheeled legs, used for transporting patients.
gus·ta·tion (gŭ-stā′shən) *n.* The act or faculty of tasting.
gus·ta·to·ry (gŭs′tə-tôr′ē) or **gus·ta·tive** (-tə-tĭv) *adj.* Of or relating to the sense of taste.
gustatory cell *n.* See **taste cell**.
gut (gŭt) *n.* **1.** The alimentary canal or a portion thereof, especially the intestine or stomach. **2.** The embryonic digestive tube, consisting of the foregut, the midgut, and the hindgut. **3. guts.** The bowels; entrails; viscera. **4.** A thin, tough cord made from the intestines of animals, usually sheep, used as suture material in surgery.
Guth·rie test (gŭth′rē) *n.* A bacterial inhibition assay for measuring serum phenylalanine, used to detect phenylketonuria in the newborn.
gut·ta (gŭt′ə) *n., pl.* **gut·tae** (gŭt′ē′). A drop, as of liquid medicine.
guttat. *abbr. Latin.* guttatim (drop by drop)
GYN *abbr.* gynecology
gy·nan·dro·mor·phism (jī-năn′drə-môr′fĭz′əm, gī-, jī-) *n.* The occurrence of both male and female characteristics in an organism.
gy·nan·dro·mor·phous (jī-năn′drə-môr′fəs, gī-, jī-) *adj.* Having both male and female characteristics.
gy·ne·cog·ra·phy (gī′nĭ-kŏg′rə-fē, jĭn′ĭ-, jī′nĭ-) *n.* See **hysterosalpingography**.
gyn·e·coid (jĭn′ĭ-koid′, gī′nĭ-, jī′-) *adj.* Characteristic of a woman.
gynecoid pelvis *n.* The normal female pelvis.
gy·ne·col·o·gist (gī′nĭ-kŏl′ə-jĭst, jĭn′ĭ-, jī′nĭ-) *n.* A physician specializing in gynecology.
gy·ne·col·o·gy (gī′nĭ-kŏl′ə-jē, jĭn′ĭ-, jī′nĭ-) *n.* The branch of medicine dealing with the administration of health care to women, especially the diagnosis and treatment of disorders affecting the female reproductive organs. —**gy′ne·co·log′i·cal** (-kə-lŏj′ĭ-kəl), **gy′ne·co·log′ic** *adj.*
gyn·e·co·mas·ti·a (jĭn′ĭ-kō-măs′tē-ə, gī′nĭ-, jī′-) *n.* Abnormal enlargement of the male mammary glands, sometimes to the point of secreting milk.
gyn·e·pho·bi·a (jĭn′ĭ-fō′bē-ə, gī′nĭ-, jī′-) *n.* An abnormal or irrational fear of women.
gy·no·plas·tics (jĭn′ə-plăs′tĭks, gī′nə-, jī′-) or **gyn·o·plas·ty** (jĭn′ə-plăs′tē, gī′nə-, jī′-) *n.* Reparative or reconstructive surgery of the female reproductive organs.
gy·rate (jī′rāt′) *v.* **-rat·ed, -rat·ing, -rates. 1.** To revolve around a fixed point or axis. **2.** To revolve in or as if in a circle or spiral. —*adj.* In rings; coiled or convoluted. —**gy·ra′tion** *n.*
gy·rec·to·my (jī-rĕk′tə-mē) *n.* Surgical excision of a cerebral gyrus.
gy·rus (jī′rəs) *n., pl.* **-ri** (-rī′). Any of the prominent, rounded, elevated convolutions on the surfaces of the cerebral hemispheres.

H

haar·schei·be tumor (här'shī'bə) *n.* Hamartoma of the hair disk.

hab·it-forming (hăb'ĭt) *adj.* Capable of leading to physiological or psychological dependence.

ha·bit·u·al abortion (hə-bĭch'o͞o-əl) *n.* Three or more consecutive spontaneous abortions occurring at about the same stage of pregnancy.

ha·bit·u·ate (hə-bĭch'o͞o-āt') *v.* **-at·ed, -at·ing, -ates. 1.** To accustom by frequent repetition or prolonged exposure. **2.** To cause physiological or psychological habituation, as to a drug. **3.** To experience psychological habituation.

ha·bit·u·a·tion (hə-bĭch'o͞o-ā'shən) *n.* **1.** The process of habituating or the state of being habituated. **2.** Physiological tolerance to a drug resulting from repeated use. **3.** Psychological dependence on a drug.

hab·i·tus (hăb'ĭ-təs) *n., pl.* **habitus.** The physical and constitutional characteristics of an individual, especially as related to the tendency to develop a certain disease.

Hae·moph·i·lus or **He·moph·i·lus** (hē-mŏf'ə-ləs) *n.* A genus of aerobic to facultatively anaerobic parasitic bacteria of the family Brucellaceae that contain minute, gram-negative, rod-shaped cells.

haf·ni·um (hăf'nē-əm) *n.* A metallic element with atomic number 72.

hair (hâr) *n.* **1.** Any of the cylindrical, keratinized, often pigmented filaments characteristically growing from the epidermis of a mammal. **2.** A growth of such filaments, as that covering the scalp of a human. **3.** One of the fine hairlike processes of a sensory cell.

hair cell *n.* A cell with hairlike processes, especially one of the sensory epithelial cells present in the spiral organ.

hair follicle *n.* A deep narrow pit that is formed by the tubular invagination of the epidermis and corium and encloses the root of the hair.

hair·line (hâr'līn') *n.* The outline of the growth of hair on the head, especially across the front.

hairline fracture *n.* A fracture in which the fragments do not separate because the line of break is so fine, often occurs in the skull.

hair root *n.* The part of a hair embedded in the hair follicle.

hair·y cell (hâr'ē) *n.* White blood cells having multiple processes and characteristically present in hairy cell leukemia, where they replace bone marrow.

hairy cell leukemia *n.* A form of lymphocytic leukemia, usually originating with B cells, that is characterized by splenomegaly and the presence of cells with a ciliated appearance in the spleen, bone marrow, liver, and blood.

hairy heart *n.* See **fibrinous pericarditis.**

hairy mole *n.* A nevus covered with a growth of hair.

ha·la·tion (hā-lā'shən) *n.* Blurring of the visual image due to glare from strong illumination.

hal·az·e·pam (hă-lăz'ə-păm') *n.* A benzodiazepine used in the management of anxiety disorders and for short-term relief of symptoms of anxiety.

hal·cin·o·nide (hăl-sĭn'ə-nīd') *n.* An anti-inflammatory corticosteroid used in topical preparations.

Hal·dane effect (hôl'dān') *n.* The promotion of carbon dioxide dissociation by the oxygenation of hemoglobin.

half and half nail *n.* Division of the nail by a transverse line into a proximal dull white part and a distal pink or brown part. It is seen in uremia.

half-life *n.* **1.** The time required for half the quantity of a drug or other substance deposited in a living organism to be metabolized or eliminated by normal biological processes. **2.** The time required for the radioactivity of material taken in by or administered to a living organism to be reduced to half its initial value by a combination of biological elimination processes and radioactive decay.

half·way house (hăf'wā') *n.* A rehabilitation facility for people, such as mental patients or substance abusers, who no longer require the complete facilities of a hospital or other institution but who are not yet prepared to return to their communities.

hal·i·to·sis (hăl'ĭ-tō'sĭs) *n.* The condition of having foul-smelling breath; bad breath.

hal·i·tus (hăl'ĭ-təs) *n.* An exhalation, as of a breath or vapor.

Hal·lion's test (äl-yôNz') *n.* A test of collateral circulation in cases of aneurysm, in which the main artery and vein of a limb are compressed; the veins of the hand or foot swell up if the collateral circulation is unimpeded.

hal·lu·ci·na·tion (hə-lo͞o'sə-nā'shən) *n.* **1.** False or distorted perception of objects or events with a compelling sense of their reality, usually resulting from a mental disorder or as a response to a drug. **2.** The objects or events so perceived. — **hal·lu'·ci·nate'** *v.* — **hal·lu'ci·na'tion·al, hal·lu'ci·na'·tive** *adj.*

hal·lu·ci·no·gen (hə-lo͞o'sə-nə-jən) *n.* A substance that induces hallucination. — **hal·lu'cin·o·gen'ic** (-jĕn'ĭk) *adj.*

hal·lu·ci·no·sis (hə-lo͞o'sə-nō'sĭs) *n.* Abnormal condition or mental state marked by hallucination.

hal·lux (hăl'əks) *n., pl.* **hal·lu·ces** (hăl'yə-sēz', hăl'ə-). The innermost or first digit of the human foot; the big toe.

hallux val·gus (văl′gəs) *n.* Deviation of the tip or main axis of the big toe toward the outer side of the foot.

hal·o·gen (hăl′ə-jən) *n.* Any of a group of five chemically related nonmetallic elements: fluorine, chlorine, bromine, iodine, and astatine.

hal·o·per·i·dol (hăl′ō-pĕr′ĭ-dôl′, -dōl′) *n.* A tranquilizer used especially in the treatment of psychotic disorders, including schizophrenia.

ha·lo sign (hā′lō) *n.* A radiologic indication of a dead or dying fetus in which the subcutaneous fat layer is elevated over the fetal skull.

hal·o·thane (hăl′ə-thān′) *n.* A colorless, nonflammable liquid widely used as an inhalation anesthetic that takes effect rapidly and can be rapidly counteracted.

Hal·stead–Rei·tan battery (hôl′stĕd′rī′tăn′) *n.* An array of neuropsychological tests used to determine the effects of brain damage on behavior.

Hal·sted's operation (hôl′stədz, -stĕdz′) *n.* **1.** An operation for the radical correction of inguinal hernia. **2.** See **radical mastectomy.**

Halsted's suture *n.* A suture through the subcuticular fascia, used for exact skin approximation.

ham·ar·to·ma (hăm′är-tō′mə) *n., pl.* **-mas** or **-ma·ta** (-mə-tə) A benign tumorlike formation resulting from faulty tissue development in an organ.

ha·mate bone (hā′māt′) *n.* A bone on the medial side of the carpus, articulating with the fourth and fifth metacarpal, triquetrum, lunate, and capitate bones.

ham·mer (hăm′ər) *n.* See **malleus.**

hammer finger *n.* See **baseball finger.**

ham·mer·toe or **ham·mer toe** (hăm′ər-tō′) *n.* A toe, usually the second, that is permanently flexed downward, resulting in a clawlike shape.

ham·string (hăm′strĭng′) *n.* **1.** Any of the tendons at the rear hollow of the human knee. **2.** Or **hamstrings.** The hamstring muscle.

hamstring muscle *n.* Any of the three muscles constituting the back of the upper leg that flex the knee joint, adduct the leg, and extend the thigh.

hand (hănd) *n.* The terminal part of the human arm located below the forearm, used for grasping and holding and consisting of the wrist, palm, four fingers, and an opposable thumb.

hand·ed (hăn′dĭd) *adj.* Relating to dexterity, preference, or size with respect to a hand or hands.

hand·ed·ness (hăn′dĭd-nĭs) *n.* A preference for using one hand as opposed to the other.

hand-foot-and-mouth disease *n.* An exanthematous eruption of the toes, palms, soles, and fingers with often painful blistering and ulceration of the buccal mucous membrane, tongue, and soft palate, caused by a Coxsackie virus.

hand·i·cap (hăn′dē-kăp′) *n.* A physical or mental disability.

Hand–Schüller–Christian disease (hănd′-) *n.* A progressive disease beginning in childhood that is characterized by protruding eyeballs, diabetes insipidus, and the softening and ultimate destruction of bone tissue, especially the skull, and caused by abnormal cholesterol metabolism.

hang·man's fracture (hăng′mən) *n.* A fracture or dislocation fracture of the cervical vertebrae near the base of the skull.

hang·nail (hăng′nāl′) *n.* A small piece of dead skin at the side or the base of a fingernail that is partly detached from the rest of the skin.

Han·sen's bacillus (hăn′sənz) *n.* An aerobic, nonmotile, gram-positive bacterium *Mycobacterium leprae* that causes leprosy in humans.

Han·sen's disease (hăn′sənz) *n.* See **leprosy.**

han·ta·vi·rus (hăn′tə-vī′rəs) *n.* A type of virus carried by rodents causing severe respiratory infections in humans and, in some cases, hemorrhaging, kidney disease, and death.

hap·loid (hăp′loid′) *adj.* Having the same number of sets of chromosomes as a germ cell, or half the diploid number of a somatic cell. The haploid number (23 in humans) is the normal chromosome complement of germ cells.

hap·lo·scope (hăp′lə-skōp′) *n.* An instrument for presenting separate views to each eye so that they may be seen as one integrated view. **— hap′lo·scop′ic** (-skŏp′ĭk) *adj.*

hap·lo·type (hăp′lə-tīp′) *n.* **1.** The set of alleles that determine different antigens but are closely linked on one chromosome and inherited as a unit, providing a distinctive genetic pattern that can be used in settling paternity disputes and in histocompatibility testing for organ transplants. **2.** The antigenic phenotype determined by closely linked genes inherited as a unit from one parent.

hap·ten (hăp′tən) *n.* A substance that is capable of reacting with a specific antibody but cannot induce the formation of antibodies unless bound to a carrier protein or other molecule.

hap·tics (hăp′tĭks) *n.* The science that deals with the sense of touch.

hap·to·glo·bin (hăp′tə-glō′bĭn) *n.* A plasma protein that is a normal constituent of blood serum and functions in the binding of free hemoglobin in the bloodstream.

Ha·ra·da's syndrome (hə-rä′dəz) *n.* A syndrome of unknown cause, usually occurring in young adults, marked by bilateral fundal edema; inflammation of the choroid, ciliary body, and iris of the eye; and retinal detachment as well as temporary or permanent loss of hearing and visual acuity, and graying and loss of the hair.

hard·en·ing of the arteries (här′dn-ĭng) *n.* Arteriosclerosis.

hard palate *n.* The anterior part of the palate, consisting of the bony palate covered above by the mucous membrane of the floor of the nose, and below by the mucous membrane and periosteum of the roof of the mouth.

hard pulse *n.* A pulse that strikes forcibly against the tip of the finger and is difficult to compress, indicating hypertension.

hard tubercle *n.* A nonnecrotic tubercle.

Har·dy–Rand–Ritter test (här′dē-rănd′-) *n.* A test for color-vision deficiency similar to the Ishihara test.

hare·lip (hâr′lĭp′) *n.* See **cleft lip.**

Har·ris' line (hăr′ĭ-sīz) *n.* See **growth line**.

Hart·mann's operation (härt′mənz) *n.* Resection of the rectosigmoid colon, with closure of the rectal stump and colostomy.

Hart·nup disease (härt′nəp) *n.* A congenital metabolic disorder characterized by aminoaciduria, a pellagralike, light-sensitive skin rash, and temporary cerebellar ataxia.

Ha·shi·mo·to's disease (häsh′ĭ-mō′tōz, hä′shē-) *n.* An autoimmune diease of the thyroid gland, resulting in diffuse goiter, infiltration of the thyroid gland with lymphocytes, and hypothyroidism.

Has·sall's concentric corpuscle (hăs′ôlz, -əlz) *n.* See **thymic corpuscle**.

has·si·um (hä′sē-əm) *n.* An artifically produced radioactive element with atomic number 108.

haus·tra·tion (hô-strā′shən) *n.* **1.** The formation of a haustrum. **2.** A haustrum.

haus·trum (hô′strəm) *n., pl.* **haus·tra** (hô′strə). Any of a series of saccules or pouches, especially one of the sacculations of the colon.

HAV *abbr.* hepatitis A virus

Hav·er·hill fever (hăv′rəl, hā′vər-əl) *n.* An infection by *Streptobacillus moniliformis* marked by initial chills and high fever gradually subsiding and followed by arthritis usually in the larger joints and spine, and by a rash occurring over the joints and on the surfaces of the extremities.

ha·ver·sian canal (hə-vûr′zhən) *n.* Any of various canals in compact bone through which blood vessels, nerve fibers, and lymphatics pass.

hay fever *n.* An allergic condition affecting the mucous membranes of the upper respiratory tract and the eyes, usually characterized by nasal discharge, sneezing, and itchy, watery eyes and usually caused by an abnormal sensitivity to airborne pollen.

Hb *abbr.* hemoglobin

Hb F *n.* A form of hemoglobulin present in high concentrations in the fetal stage of development but normally diminishing to a low concentration in children and adults except in certain anemias, leukemias, and hemoglobin disorders.

HCS *abbr.* human chorionic somatomammotropic hormone

Hct *abbr.* hematocrit

h.d. *abbr. Latin.* hora decubitus (before sleep, at bedtime)

HDL *abbr.* high-density lipoprotein

HDRV *abbr.* human diploid cell rabies vaccine

head (hĕd) *n.* **1.** The uppermost or forwardmost part of the human body, containing the brain and the eyes, ears, nose, mouth, and jaws. **2.** The tip of an abscess, a boil, or a pimple, in which pus forms. **3.** The proximal end of a long bone. **4.** The end of a muscle that is attached to the less movable part of the skeleton.

head·ache (hĕd′āk′) *n.* A pain in the head.

head cap *n.* See **acrosomal cap**.

head cold *n.* A common cold mainly affecting the mucous membranes of the nasal passages, characterized by congestion and sneezing.

head-dropping test *n.* A test used in the diagnosis of disease of the extrapyramidal system in which the head of a person in supine position is lifted by the examiner with one hand and allowed to fall into the other.

heal (hēl) *v.* **healed, heal·ing, heals. 1.** To restore to health or soundness; cure. **2.** To become well; return to sound health.

healing by first intention *n.* Healing by fibrous adhesion, without suppuration or formation of granulation tissue.

health (hĕlth) *n.* **1.** The overall condition of an organism at a given time. **2.** Soundness, especially of body or mind; freedom from disease or abnormality.

health care or **healthcare** *n.* The prevention, treatment, and management of illness and the preservation of mental and physical well-being through the services offered by the medical and allied health professions.

health·ful (hĕlth′fəl) *adj.* **1.** Conducive to good health; salutary. **2.** Healthy. — **health′ful·ly** *adv.* — **health′ful·ness** *n.*

health insurance *n.* Insurance against expenses incurred through illness of the insured.

health maintenance organization *n.* An HMO.

health·y (hĕl′thē) *adj.* **-i·er, -i·est. 1.** Possessing good health. **2.** Conducive to good health; healthful. **3.** Indicative of sound, rational thinking or frame of mind. — **health′i·ly** *adv.* — **health′i·ness** *n.*

hear (hēr) *v.* **heard** (hûrd), **hear·ing, hears.** To perceive (sound) by the ear.

hear·ing (hēr′ĭng) *n.* The sense by which sound is perceived; the capacity to hear.

hearing aid *n.* A small electronic apparatus that amplifies sound and is worn in or behind the ear to compensate for impaired hearing.

hearing dog *n.* A dog trained to assist a deaf or hearing-impaired person by signaling the occurrence of certain sounds, such as a doorbell.

hearing-impaired *adj.* **1.** Having a diminished or defective sense of hearing, but not deaf; hard of hearing. **2.** Completely incapable of hearing; deaf. — *n.* Persons who are deficient in hearing or are deaf.

hearing impairment *n.* A reduction or defect in the ability to perceive sound.

heart (härt) *n.* The four-chambered, muscular organ that pumps blood received from the veins into the arteries, thereby maintaining the flow of blood through the entire circulatory system.

heart attack *n.* Acute myocardial infarction typically resulting from an occlusion or obstruction of a coronary artery and characterized by sudden, severe pain in the chest that often radiates to the shoulder, arm, or jaw.

heart·beat (härt′bēt′) *n.* A single complete pulsation of the heart.

heart block *n.* A condition in which faulty transmission of the impulses that control the heartbeat results in a lack of coordination in the contraction of the atria and ventricles of the heart.

heart·burn (härt′bûrn′) *n.* A burning sensation, usually centered in the mid chest near the sternum, caused by the reflux of acidic stomach fluids that enter the lower end of the esophagus.

heart disease *n.* A structural or functional abnormality of the heart, or of the blood vessels supplying the heart, that impairs its normal functioning.

heart failure *n.* **1.** A condition marked by weakness, edema, and shortness of breath that is caused by the inability of the heart to maintain adequate blood circulation in the peripheral tissues and the lungs. **2.** The resulting clinical syndrome, consisting of shortness of breath, pitting edema, enlarged tender liver, engorged neck veins, and pulmonary rales.

heart-lung machine *n.* An apparatus through which blood is temporarily diverted, especially during heart surgery, to oxygenate it and pump it throughout the body until the heart and lungs are able to return to normal functioning.

heart massage *n.* See **cardiac massage.**

heart rate *n.* The number of heartbeats per unit of time, usually expressed as beats per minute.

heart sac *n.* See **pericardium.**

heart sound *n.* Any of the sounds heard on auscultation over the heart.

heat (hēt) *n.* **1.** A form of energy associated with the motion of atoms or molecules and capable of being transmitted through solid and fluid media by conduction, through fluid media by convection, and through empty space by radiation. **2.** The sensation or perception of such energy as warmth or hotness. **3.** An abnormally high bodily temperature, as from a fever. **4.** Estrus.

heat cramps *pl.n.* Painful muscle spasms following hard work in intense heat, caused by loss of salt and water from profuse sweating.

heat exhaustion *n.* A condition caused by exposure to heat, marked by prostration, weakness, and collapse, resulting from dehydration.

heat lamp *n.* A lamp that emits infrared light and produces heat, used to apply topical heat to the skin for therapeutic purposes.

heat prostration *n.* See **heat exhaustion.**

heat rash *n.* An inflammatory skin condition caused by obstruction of the ducts of the sweat glands, due to exposure to high heat and humidity and marked by eruption of small, red papules and an itching or prickling sensation.

heat stroke *n.* A severe condition caused by impairment of the body's temperature-regulating abilities, resulting from prolonged exposure to excessive heat and characterized by cessation of sweating, severe headache, high fever, hot dry skin, and in serious cases, collapse and coma.

heav·y eye (hĕv′ē) *n.* The affected eye in severe uniocular myopia.

heavy-ion treatment *n.* A cancer treatment method in which cancer cells are bombarded with the positively-charged nuclei of ions of carbon, neon, and other elements in order to kill the cells.

he·be·phre·ni·a (hē′bə-frē′nē-ə, -frĕn′ē-ə) *n.* A type of schizophrenia, usually starting at puberty, marked by foolish mannerisms, senseless laughter, delusions, hallucinations, and regressive behavior. — **he′be·phren′ic** (-frĕn′ĭk, -frē′nĭk) *adj.*

heb·e·tude (hĕb′ĭ-tood′, -tyood′) *n.* Dullness of mind; mental lethargy. — **heb′e·tu′di·nous** (-tood′n-əs, -tyood′-) *adj.*

he·bi·at·rics (hē′bē-ăt′rĭks) *n.* See **adolescent medicine.**

hed·ro·cele (hĕd′rə-sēl′) *n.* Prolapse of the intestine through the anus.

heel (hēl) *n.* **1.** The rounded posterior portion of the human foot under and behind the ankle. **2.** A similar anatomical part, such as the fleshy rounded base of the human palm.

heel bone *n.* See **calcaneus.**

heel tendon *n.* See **Achilles tendon.**

Heg·glin's anomaly (hĕg′lĭnz) *n.* A hereditary disorder characterized by the presence of basophilic structures in most granulocytes, faulty maturation of platelets, and thrombocytopenia.

height (hīt) *n.* **1.** The distance from the base of something to the top. **2.** Stature, especially of the human body.

Heim·lich maneuver (hīm′lĭk′, -lĸн′) *n.* An emergency technique used to eject an object, such as food, from the trachea of a choking person. The technique employs a firm upward thrust just below the rib cage to force air from the lungs up through the trachea.

he·li·en·ceph·a·li·tis (hē′lē-ĕn-sĕf′ə-lī′tĭs) *n.* Inflammation of the brain following sunstroke.

he·li·um (hē′lē-əm) *n.* An inert gaseous element found in natural gas and with atomic number 2.

he·lix (hē′lĭks) *n., pl.* **-lix·es** or **hel·i·ces** (hĕl′ĭ-sēz′, hē′lĭ-). **1.** A spiral form or structure. **2.** The folded rim of skin and cartilage around most of the outer ear.

hel·minth (hĕl′mĭnth′) *n.* A worm, especially a parasitic roundworm or tapeworm.

hel·min·thi·a·sis (hĕl′mĭn-thī′ə-sĭs) *n., pl.* **-ses** (-sēz′). A disease caused by infestation with parasitic worms.

hel·min·tho·ma (hĕl′mĭn-thō′mə) *n., pl.* **-mas** or **-ma·ta** (-mə-tə). A tumor of granulomatous tissue caused by a parasitic worm.

he·lo·ma (hē-lō′mə) *n., pl.* **-mas** or **-ma·ta** (-mə-tə). See **corn.**

he·lot·o·my (hē-lŏt′ə-mē) *n.* Treatment of a corn or corns by surgery.

help·er T cell (hĕl′pər) *n.* Any of the T cells that, when stimulated by a specific antigen, release lymphokines that promote the activation and function of B cells and killer cells.

he·mad·sorp·tion (hē′măd-sôrp′shən, -zôrp′-) *n.* The adherence of an agent or a substance to the surface of a red blood cell.

he·mag·glu·ti·na·tion (hē′mə-glōot′n-ā′shən) *n.* The agglutination of red blood cells, which may be caused by a specific antibody either for red blood cell antigens or for antigens that coat red blood cells or by viruses or other microbes.

hemagglutination inhibition test *n.* A test to determine the amount of a specific antigen in a blood serum sample, in which the sample is incubated with antibody, and antigen-coated red blood cells are added; the amount of antigen can be deteimined by the percentage of red blood cells that do not agglutinate.

he·mag·glu·ti·nin (hē'mə-gloŏt'n-ĭn) n. A substance, such as an antibody, that causes agglutination of red blood cells.

he·ma·gogue (hē'mə-gôg') n. 1. An agent that promotes the flow of blood. 2. See emmenagogue. — he'ma·gog'ic (-gŏj'ĭk) adj.

he·mal·um (hē-măl'əm) n. A solution of hematoxylin and alum used as a nuclear stain in histology, especially with eosin as a counterstain.

he·mam·e·bi·a·sis (hē'măm-ə-bī'ə-sĭs) n. An infection of red blood cells with ameboid forms of parasites, as in malaria.

he·ma·nal·y·sis (hē'mə-năl'ĭ-sĭs) n. Analysis of the blood, especially by chemical methods.

he·man·gi·ec·ta·sis (hē'măn-jē-ĕk'tə-sĭs) n. Dilation of the blood vessels.

he·man·gi·o·blast (hĭ-măn'jē-ō-blăst') n. A primitive embryonic cell of mesodermal origin that produces cells giving rise to vascular endothelium, reticuloendothelial elements, and blood-forming cells of all types.

he·man·gi·o·ma (hĭ-măn'jē-ō'mə) n., pl. -mas or -ma·ta (-mə-tə). A congenital benign skin lesion consisting of dense, usually elevated masses of dilated blood vessels.

he·man·gi·o·sar·co·ma (hĭ-măn'jē-ō-sär-kō'mə) n. A rare malignant neoplasm characterized by rapidly proliferating anaplastic cells derived from blood vessels and lining blood-filled spaces.

he·ma·pher·e·sis (hē'mə-fĕr'ə-sĭs, hĕm'ə-) n. See apheresis.

he·ma·tem·e·sis (hē'mə-tĕm'ĭ-sĭs, hĕm'ə-, hē'mə-tə-mē'sĭs) n. The vomiting of blood.

he·mat·en·ceph·a·lon (hē'mə-tĕn-sĕf'ə-lŏn') n. See cerebral hemorrhage.

he·ma·ti·dro·sis (hē'mə-tĭ-drō'sĭs, hĕm'ə-) n. The excretion of blood or blood pigment in the sweat.

he·ma·to·blast (hē'mə-tə-blăst', hĭ-măt'ə-) n. An immature undifferentiated blood cell. — he'ma·to·blas'tic adj.

he·mat·o·crit (hĭ-măt'ə-krĭt') n. The percentage by volume of packed red blood cells in a given sample of blood after centrifugation.

he·ma·to·cy·tu·ri·a (hē'mə-tō-sī-toŏr'ē-ə, -tyoŏr'-, hĭ-măt'ō-) n. The presence of red blood cells in the urine.

he·ma·to·gen·e·sis (hē'mə-tə-jĕn'ĭ-sĭs, hĭ-măt'ə-) or he·mo·gen·e·sis (hē'mə-) n. See hematopoiesis. — he'ma·to·gen'ic (-jĕn'ĭk), he'ma·to·ge·net'ic (-jə-nĕt'ĭk) adj.

he·ma·to·his·ton (hē'mə-tō-hĭs'tŏn', hĭ-măt'ə-) n. See globin.

he·ma·toi·din (hē'mə-toid'n) n. A ironless pigment derived from hemoglobin and formed within tissues, chemically similar to bilirubin.

he·ma·tol·o·gist (hē'mə-tŏl'ə-jĭst) n. A physician specializing in hematology.

he·ma·tol·o·gy (hē'mə-tŏl'ə-jē) n. The science dealing with the medical study of the blood and blood-producing organs. — he'ma·to·log'ic (-tə-lŏj'ĭk), he'ma·to·log'i·cal adj.

he·ma·to·ma (hē'mə-tō'mə) n., pl. -mas or -ma·ta (-mə-tə). A localized swelling filled with blood resulting from a break in a blood vessel.

he·ma·to·me·tra (hē'mə-tō-mē'trə, hĭ-măt'ə-) n. A collection or retention of blood in the uterine cavity.

he·ma·to·my·e·li·a (hē'mə-tō-mī-ē'lē-ə, hĭ-măt'ə-) n. Hemorrhage into the substance of the spinal cord, usually caused by trauma.

he·ma·to·poi·e·sis (hē'mə-tō-poi-ē'sĭs, hĭ-măt'ə-) or he·mo·poi·e·sis (hē'mə-poi-ē'-sĭs) n. The formation of blood or blood cells in the body. — he'-ma·to·poi·et'ic (-ĕt'ĭk) adj.

hematopoietic gland n. An organ involved in the formation of blood or blood cells, such as the spleen.

hematopoietic system n. The blood-making organs, principally the bone marrow and lymph nodes.

he·ma·to·sal·pinx (hē'mə-tō-săl'pĭngks, hĭ-măt'ə-) n. A collection of blood in a tube, as in a fallopian tube, where it is often associated with a tubal pregnancy.

he·ma·to·tox·in (hē'mə-tō-tŏk'sĭn, hĭ-măt'ə-) n. See hemotoxin.

he·ma·tox·y·lin (hē'mə-tŏk'sə-lĭn) n. A yellow or red crystalline compound used in histological dyes and as an indicator.

hematoxylin-eosin stain n. A widely used, two-stage stain for cells in which hematoxylin is followed by a counterstain of red eosin so that the nuclei stain a deep blue-black and the cytoplasm stains pink.

he·ma·tu·ri·a (hē'mə-toŏr'ē-ə, -tyoŏr'-) n. The presence of blood in urine. — he'ma·tu'ric adj.

heme (hēm) n. The deep red, oxygen-carrying, nonprotein, ferrous component of hemoglobin.

hem·i·al·gi·a (hĕm'ē-ăl'jē-ə, -jə) n. Pain affecting one half of the body.

hem·i·an·es·the·sia (hĕm'ē-ăn'ĭs-thē'zhə) n. Loss of tactile sensibility on one side of the body.

hem·i·a·nop·si·a (hĕm'ē-ə-nŏp'sē-ə) or hem·i·a·no·pi·a (-nŏ'pē-ə) n. Loss of vision in one half of the visual field of one or both eyes.

hem·i·ar·thro·plas·ty (hĕm'ē-är'thrə-plăs'tē) n. Arthroplasty in which one joint surface is replaced with an artificial material, usually metal.

hem·i·a·tax·i·a (hĕm'ē-ə-tăk'sē-ə) n. Ataxia affecting one side of the body.

hem·i·at·ro·phy (hĕm'ē-ăt'rə-fē) n. Atrophy of one side of a body part or organ.

hem·i·ceph·a·lal·gia (hĕm'ē-sĕf'ə-lăl'jə, -jē-ə) n. Headache affecting one side of the head, characteristic of migraine.

he·mic murmur (hē'mĭk) n. A cardiac or vascular murmur heard in anemic persons who have no valvular lesion.

hem·i·co·lec·to·my (hĕm'ē-kə-lĕk'tə-mē) n. Surgical removal of the right or left side of the colon.

hem·i·des·mo·some (hĕm′ĭ-dĕz′mə-sōm′, dĕs′-) *n.* Any of the specialized structures representing half desmosomes that occur on the basal surface of certain stratified squamous epithelial cells.

hem·i·di·a·pho·re·sis (hĕm′ē-dī′ə-fə-rē′sĭs, -dī-ăf′ə-) *n.* Sweating on one side of the body.

hem·i·dys·tro·phy (hĕm′ĭ-dĭs′trə-fē) *n.* Underdevelopment of one side of the body.

hem·i·ec·tro·me·li·a (hĕm′ē-ĕk′trō-mē′lē-ə) *n.* Defective development of the limbs on one side of the body.

hem·i·ep·i·lep·sy (hĕm′ē-ĕp′ə-lĕp′sē) *n.* Epilepsy in which the convulsive movements are confined to one side of the body.

hem·i·gas·trec·to·my (hĕm′ĭ-gă-strĕk′tə-mē) *n.* Surgical excision of the distal half of the stomach.

hem·i·glos·sec·to·my (hĕm′ĭ-glô-sĕk′tə-mē) *n.* Surgical removal of one half of the tongue.

hem·i·gna·thi·a (hĕm′ĭ-nā′thē-ə, -năth′ē-ə) *n.* Defective development of one side of the mandible.

hem·i·hyp·es·the·sia (hĕm′ĭ-hī′pĭs-thē′zhə) *n.* Diminished sensibility on one side of the body.

hem·i·lam·i·nec·to·my (hĕm′ĭ-lăm′ə-nĕk′tə-mē) *n.* Surgical removal of a portion of a vertebral lamina.

hem·i·lar·yn·gec·to·my (hĕm′ĭ-lăr′ən-jĕk′tə-mē) *n.* Surgical excision of one side of the larynx.

hem·i·op·ic pupillary reaction (hĕm′ē-ŏp′ĭk, -ō′-pĭk) *n.* See **Wernicke's reaction.**

hem·i·par·a·ple·gia (hĕm′ĭ-păr′ə-plē′jə, -jē-ə) *n.* Paralysis of one leg.

hem·i·pa·re·sis (hĕm′ē-pə-rē′sĭs, -păr′ĭ-sĭs) *n.* Slight paralysis or weakness affecting one side of the body.

hem·i·ple·gia (hĕm′ĭ-plē′jə, -jē-ə) *n.* Paralysis affecting only one side of the body. — **hem′i·ple′gic** (-plē′jĭk) *adj.*

hemiplegic gait *n.* The walk of hemiplegics, characterized by swinging the affected leg in a half circle.

hem·i·sphere (hĕm′ĭ-sfêr′) *n.* **1.** A half of a symmetrical spherical structure as divided by a plane of symmetry. **2.** Either of the lateral halves of the cerebrum; a cerebral hemisphere. — **hem′i·spher′ic** (-sfêr′ĭk, -sfêr′-), **hem′i·spher′i·cal** *adj.*

hem·i·tho·rax (hĕm′ĭ-thôr′ăks′) *n.* One side of the chest.

he·mo·blast (hē′mə-blăst′) *n.* See **hemocytoblast.**

he·mo·ca·ther·e·sis (hē′mō-kă-thĕr′ĭ-sĭs, -thĕr′-, -kăth′ə-rē′-) *n.* Destruction of blood cells, especially of red blood cells. — **he′mo·cath′e·ret′ic** (-kăth′ə-rĕt′ĭk) *adj.*

he·moc·cult test (hē′mə-kŭlt′) *n.* A qualitative test for hidden blood in the stool, based upon detecting the peroxidase activity of hemoglobin.

he·mo·chro·ma·to·sis (hē′mə-krō′mə-tō′sĭs) *n.* A hereditary disorder of iron metabolism characterized by excessive accumulation of iron in the body tissues, diabetes mellitus, liver dysfunction, and a bronze pigmentation of the skin.

he·moc·la·sis (hē-mŏk′lə-sĭs) *n.* The rupture, hemolysis, or destruction of red blood cells. — **he′mo·clas′tic** (hē′mə-klăs′tĭk) *adj.*

he·mo·con·cen·tra·tion (hē′mō-kŏn′sən-trā′-shən) *n.* A decrease in the volume of plasma resulting in an increase in the concentration of red blood cells in the circulating blood.

he·mo·cyte (hē′mə-sīt′) *n.* A cellular component or formed element of the blood.

he·mo·cy·to·blast (hē′mə-sī′tə-blăst′) *n.* A stem cell derived from the embryonic mesenchyme and believed to have the capability of developing into any of the various types of blood cells.

he·mo·cy·to·ca·ther·e·sis (hē′mə-sī′tō-kă-thĕr′ĭ-sĭs, -thĕr′-, -kăth′ə-rē′-) *n.* The destruction of red blood cells, as by hemolysis.

he·mo·cy·tol·y·sis (hē′mō-sī-tŏl′ĭ-sĭs) *n.* The dissolution of blood cells.

he·mo·cy·to·trip·sis (hē′mō-sī′tə-trĭp′sĭs) *n.* The fragmentation or disintegration of blood cells by means of mechanical trauma.

he·mo·di·ag·no·sis (hē′mō-dī′əg-nō′sĭs) *n.* Diagnosis by examination of the blood.

he·mo·di·al·y·sis (hē′mō-dī-ăl′ĭ-sĭs) *n.* A procedure for removing metabolic waste products or toxic substances from the blood by dialysis.

he·mo·di·a·lyz·er (hē′mō-dī′ə-lī′zər) *n.* A machine for performing hemodialysis in acute or chronic renal failure that removes toxic substances from the blood by exposure to dialyzing fluid across a semipermeable membrane.

he·mo·en·do·the·li·al placenta (hē′mō-ĕn′dō-thē′lē-əl) *n.* A placenta in which the trophoblast becomes so attenuated that maternal blood is separated from fetal blood only by the endothelium of the chorionic capillaries.

he·mo·fil·tra·tion (hē′mō-fĭl-trā′shən) *n.* A process similar to hemodialysis, by which blood is dialyzed using ultrafiltration and simultaneous reinfusion of physiologic saline solution.

he·mo·glo·bin (hē′mə-glō′bĭn) *n.* The red iron-containing respiratory protein of red blood cells that transports oxygen as oxyhemoglobin from the lungs to the tissues, where the oxygen is readily released and the oxyhemoglobin becomes hemoglobin.

hemoglobin A *n.* Normal adult hemoglobin, made up of two alpha chains and two beta chains.

hemoglobin C *n.* An abnormal hemoglobin in which lysine has been substituted for glutamic acid.

hemoglobin disease *n.* Any of several inherited diseases characterized by the presence of various abnormal hemoglobin molecules in the blood.

he·mo·glo·bi·ne·mi·a (hē′mə-glō′bə-nē′mē-ə) *n.* The presence of free hemoglobin in the blood plasma.

hemoglobin H *n.* An abnormal hemoglobin that is not effective in oxygen transport and is associated with a thalassemialike syndrome.

hemoglobin M *n.* A group of abnormal hemoglobins in which a single amino acid substitution favors the formation of methemoglobin and is thus associated with methemoglobinemia.

he·mo·glo·bi·nol·y·sis (hē′mə-glō′bə-nŏl′ĭ-sĭs)

n. The destruction or chemical splitting of hemoglobin.

he·mo·glo·bi·nop·a·thy (hē′mə-glō′bə-nŏp′-ə-thē) *n.* A disorder caused by or associated with the presence of abnormal hemoglobins in the blood.

hemoglobin S *n.* An abnormal hemoglobin that becomes less soluble under decreasing oxygen concentrations and that polymerizes into crystals that distort the red blood cells into a sickle shape.

he·mo·glo·bi·nu·ri·a (hē′mə-glō′bə-nŏŏ′ē-ə, -nyŏŏr′-) *n.* The presence of free hemoglobin in the urine. — **he′mo·glo′bi·nu′ric** *adj.*

he·mo·gram (hē′mə-grăm′) *n.* A record of the findings from an examination of the blood, especially with reference to the numbers, proportions, and morphological features of its elements.

he·mo·his·ti·o·blast (hē′mō-hĭs′tē-ə-blăst′) *n.* A primitive mesenchymal cell believed to be capable of developing into a histiocyte or into any of the various types of blood cells, including monocytes.

he·mo·lith (hē′mə-lĭth′) *n.* A concretion in the wall of a blood vessel.

he·mo·lymph (hē′mə-lĭmf′) *n.* The blood and lymph considered as a circulating tissue.

he·mol·y·sate (hĭ-mŏl′ĭ-sāt′) *n.* The product resulting from the lysis of red blood cells.

he·mol·y·sin (hĭ-mŏl′ĭ-sĭn, hē′mə-lī′-) *n.* An agent or a substance, such as an antibody or a bacterial toxin, that causes the destruction of red blood cells, thereby liberating hemoglobin.

he·mo·ly·sin·o·gen (hē′mə-lī-sĭn′ə-jən, hĭ-mŏl′ĭ-sĭn′ə-jən) *n.* The antigenic material in red blood cells that stimulates the formation of hemolysin.

he·mol·y·sis (hĭ-mŏl′ĭ-sĭs, hē′mə-lī′sĭs) or **he·ma·tol·y·sis** (hē′mə-tŏl′ĭ-sĭs) *n.* The destruction or dissolution of red blood cells, with subsequent release of hemoglobin.

he·mo·lyt·ic (hē′mə-lĭt′ĭk) *adj.* Destructive to red blood cells; hematolytic.

hemolytic anemia *n.* Anemia resulting from the abnormal destruction of red blood cells, as in response to certain toxic or infectious agents and in certain inherited blood disorders.

hemolytic disease of the newborn *n.* See **erythroblastosis fetalis.**

hemolytic jaundice *n.* Jaundice resulting from the lysis of red blood cells and the consequent increased production of bilirubin, as in response to toxic or infectious agents or in immune disorders.

hemolytic uremic syndrome *n.* A syndrome in which hemolytic anemia and thrombocytopenia occur with acute renal failure, characterized in children by gastrointestinal bleeding, scanty urine that contains red blood cells, and microangiopathic hemolytic anemia; in adults it is associated with complications of pregnancy following delivery, oral contraceptive use, or infection.

he·mo·lyze (hē′mə-līz′) *v.* **-lyzed, -lyz·ing, -lyz·es.** To undergo or cause to undergo hemolysis.

he·mo·me·di·as·ti·num (hē′mō-mē′dē-ə-stī′nəm) *n.* Blood in the mediastinum.

he·mop·a·thy (hē-mŏp′ə-thē) *n.* Any of various abnormal conditions or diseases of the blood or blood-forming tissues.

he·mo·per·fu·sion (hē′mō-pər-fyŏŏ′zhən) *n.* The passage of blood through columns of adsorptive material, such as activated charcoal, to remove toxic substances from the blood.

he·mo·per·i·car·di·um (hē′mō-pĕr′ĭ-kär′dē-əm) *n.* Blood in the pericardial sac.

he·mo·per·i·to·ne·um (hē′mō-pĕr′ĭ-tn-ē′əm) *n.* Blood in the peritoneal cavity.

he·mo·pex·in (hē′mō-pĕk′sĭn) *n.* A serum protein that is part of the beta-globulin fraction and functions in binding heme and porphyrins.

he·mo·phil·i·a (hē′mə-fĭl′ē-ə, -fēl′yə) *n.* Any of several hereditary blood-coagulation disorders, manifested almost exclusively in males, in which the blood fails to clot normally because of a deficiency or an abnormality of one of the clotting factors.

hemophilia A *n.* Hemophilia due to deficiency of factor VIII, characterized by prolonged clotting time, decreased formation of thromboplastin, and diminished conversion of prothrombin.

hemophilia B *n.* A clotting disorder of the blood resembling hemophilia A, caused by the hereditary deficiency of factor IX.

he·mo·phil·i·ac (hē′mə-fĭl′ē-ăk′, -fēl′ē-) *n.* A person who is affected with hemophilia.

he·mo·pho·bi·a (hē′mə-fō′bē-ə) *n.* An abnormal fear of blood.

he·mo·pho·re·sis (hē′mō-fə-rē′sĭs) *n.* Blood convection or irrigation of the tissues.

he·mo·pleu·ro·pneu·mo·nia syndrome (hē′mō-plŏŏr′ō-nŏŏ-mōn′yə, -nyŏŏ-) *n.* A respiratory syndrome that, in cases of puncture wounds to the chest, indicates pneumonia together with blood in the pleural cavity and that is characterized by fever, spitting of blood, shortness of breath, and moderate tachycardia.

he·mo·pre·cip·i·tin (hē′mō-prĭ-sĭp′ĭ-tĭn) *n.* An antibody that combines with and precipitates soluble antigenic material from red blood cells.

he·mo·pro·tein (hē′mə-prō′tēn′, -tē-ĭn) *n.* A conjugated protein containing a metal-porphyrin compound as the prosthetic group.

he·mop·ty·sis (hĭ-mŏp′tĭ-sĭs) *n.* The spitting of blood derived from the lungs or from the bronchial tubes.

hem·or·rhage (hĕm′ər-ĭj) *n.* An escape of blood from the blood vessels, especially when excessive. — **hem′or·rhage** *v.* — **hem′or·rhag′ic** (hĕm′ə-răj′ĭk) *adj.*

hemorrhagic colitis *n.* Abdominal cramps and bloody diarrhea, without fever, attributed to infection by a strain of *Escherichia coli.*

hemorrhagic disease of the newborn *n.* A syndrome characterized by spontaneous internal or external bleeding accompanied by hypoprothrombinemia and markedly elevated bleeding and clotting times, usually occurring between the third and sixth day after birth.

hemorrhagic endovasculitis *n.* Endothelial and medial hyperplasia of placental blood vessels with thrombosis, fragmentation, and diapedesis of red blood cells resulting in stillbirth or fetal developmental disorders.

hemorrhagic fever *n.* A syndrome that occurs in perhaps 20 percent to 40 percent of infections by arboviruses of the hemorrhagic fever group, characterized by high fever, scattered petechiae, bleeding from the gastrointestinal tract and other organs, hypotension, and shock.

hemorrhagic fever with renal syndrome *n.* See **epidemic hemorrhagic fever.**

hemorrhagic measles *n.* See **black measles.**

hemorrhagic plague *n.* The hemorrhagic form of bubonic plague.

hemorrhagic rickets *n.* Bone changes occurring in infantile scurvy, marked by subperiosteal hemorrhage and deficient bone tissue formation.

hemorrhagic shock *n.* Hypovolemic shock resulting from acute hemorrhage and characterized by hypotension, tachycardia, oliguria, and by pale, cold, and clammy skin.

hem·or·rhag·in (hĕm′ə-răj′ĭn, -rā′jĭn) *n.* Any of a group of toxins found in certain venoms and plant poisons that cause degeneration and lysis of endothelial cells in capillaries and small vessels, thereby producing numerous small hemorrhages in the tissues.

hem·or·rhoid (hĕm′ə-roid′) *n.* **1.** An itching or painful mass of dilated veins in swollen anal tissue. **2.** *or* **hemorrhoids.** The pathological condition in which such painful masses occur.

hem·or·rhoi·dal (hĕm′ə-roid′l) *adj.* **1.** Of or relating to hemorrhoids. **2.** Relating to certain arteries and veins supplying the rectal and anal regions.

hem·or·rhoid·ec·to·my (hĕm′ə-rci-dĕk′tə-mē) *n.* Surgical removal of hemorrhoids.

he·mo·sal·pinx (hē′mō-săl′pĭngks) *n.* See **hematosalpinx.**

he·mo·sid·er·in (hē′mō-sĭd′ər-ĭn) *n.* An iron-containing insoluble protein produced by phagocytic digestion of hematin and found as granules in most tissues, especially in the liver.

he·mo·sper·mia (hē′mə-spûr′mē-ə) *n.* The presence of blood in the seminal fluid.

he·mo·sta·sis (hē′mə-stā′sĭs, hē-mŏs′stə-) *n.* **1.** The stoppage of bleeding or hemorrhage. **2.** The stoppage of blood flow through a blood vessel or body part. **3.** The stagnation of blood.

he·mo·stat (hē′mə-stăt′) *n.* **1.** An agent, such as a chemical, that stops bleeding. **2.** An instrument for arresting hemorrhage by compression of the bleeding vessel.

he·mo·stat·ic forceps (hē′mə-stăt′ĭk) *n.* A forceps with a catch for locking the blades, used for seizing the end of a blood vessel to control hemorrhage.

he·mo·ther·a·py (hē′mə-thĕr′ə-pē) or **he·mo·ther·a·peu·tics** (-thĕr′ə-pyōō′tĭks) *n.* The treatment of disease by the use of blood or blood derivatives, as in transfusion.

he·mo·tho·rax (hē′mə-thôr′ăks′) *n.* Blood in the pleural cavity.

he·mo·tox·in (hē′mə-tŏk′sĭn) *n.* A substance, especially one produced by a bacterium, that destroys red blood cells.

he·mo·troph (hē′mə-trŏf′, -trôf′) *n.* The nutritive materials supplied to the embryo through the placenta from the maternal bloodstream.

Hen·der·so·nu·la to·ru·loi·de·a (hĕn′dər-sə-nyōō′lə tôr′yə-loi′dē-ə) *n.* A species of black yeast capable of producing infections of the toenails as well as of the skin of the feet.

Hen·le's loop (hĕn′lēz) *n.* See **nephronic loop.**

He·noch–Schönlein purpura (hā′nŏk-, -nôkʜ-) *n.* A form of nonthrombocytopenic purpura occurring most commonly in boys and associated with pain or swelling of the joints, colic, vomiting of blood, passage of bloody stools, and sometimes inflammation of the kidneys.

HEPA *abbr.* high-efficiency particulate arresting, used of air purification filters designed to remove allergens and other respiratory irritants.

hep·a·rin (hĕp′ər-ĭn) *n.* A complex organic acid found especially in lung and liver tissue that functions to prevent platelet agglutination and blood clotting, and is used in the form of its sodium salt to treat thrombosis. — **hep′a·rin′i·za′tion** (-ə-rĭn′ĭ-zā′shən) *n.* — **hep′a·rin·ize′** (-ər-ə-nīz′) *v.*

hep·a·tal·gi·a (hĕp′ə-tăl′jē-ə, -jə) *n.* Pain in the liver.

hep·a·ta·tro·phi·a (hĕp′ə-tə-trō′fē-ə) or **hep·a·tat·ro·phy** (hĕp′ə-tăt′rə-fē) *n.* Liver atrophy.

hep·a·tec·to·my (hĕp′ə-tĕk′tə-mē) *n.* Excision of liver tissue.

he·pa·tic (hĭ-păt′ĭk) *adj.* **1.** Of, relating to, or resembling the liver. **2.** Acting on or occurring in the liver. — *n.* A drug that acts on the liver.

hepatic artery *n.* **1.** An artery with its origin in the celiac artery, with branches to the right gastric, gastroduodenal, and proper hepatic arteries. **2.** An artery with its origin in the common hepatic artery, and with branches to the right and left hepatic arteries.

hepatic duct *n.* **1.** Left hepatic duct. **2.** Right hepatic duct.

he·pat·i·co·do·chot·o·my (hĭ-păt′ĭ-kō-dō-kŏt′ə-mē) *n.* Incision into the common bile duct and the hepatic duct.

he·pat·i·co·du·o·de·nos·to·my (hĭ-păt′ĭ-kō-dōō′ə-də-nŏs′tə-mē, -dyōō′-, -dōō-ŏd′n-ŏs′-, -dyōō-) *n.* Surgical formation of a communication between a hepatic duct and the duodenum.

he·pat·i·co·en·ter·os·to·my (hĭ-păt′ĭ-kō-ĕn′tə-rŏs′tə-mē) *n.* Surgical formation of a communication between a hepatic duct and the intestine.

he·pat·i·co·gas·tros·to·my (hĭ-păt′ĭ-kō-gă-strŏs′tə-mē) *n.* Surgical formation of a communication between a hepatic duct and the stomach.

he·pat·i·co·li·thot·o·my (hĭ-păt′ĭ-kō-lĭ-thŏt′ə-mē) *n.* Surgical removal of one or more calculi from a hepatic duct.

he·pat·i·co·lith·o·trip·sy (hĭ-păt′ĭ-kō-lĭth′ə-trĭp′sē) *n.* The crushing of a biliary calculus in a hepatic duct.

he·pat·i·cos·to·my (hǐ-pǎt′ǐ-kǒs′tə-mē) *n.* The surgical formation of an opening into a hepatic duct.

he·pat·i·cot·o·my (hǐ-pǎt′ǐ-kǒt′ə-mē) *n.* Incision into a hepatic duct.

hepatic vein *n.* Any of the veins that collect blood from the central veins of the liver and terminate in three large veins opening into the inferior vena cava below the diaphragm and in several small veins entering the lower vena cava.

hep·a·ti·tis (hěp′ə-tī′tĭs) *n., pl.* **-ti·tis·es** (-tĭt′ĭ-dēz′). Inflammation of the liver, caused by infectious or toxic agents and characterized by jaundice, fever, liver enlargement, and abdominal pain.

hepatitis A *n.* A form of hepatitis caused by an RNA virus that does not persist in the blood serum and is transmitted by ingestion of infected food and water. The disease has a shorter incubation period and generally milder symptoms than hepatitis B.

hepatitis-associated antigen *n.* See **Australia antigen.**

hepatitis B *n.* A form of hepatitis caused by a DNA virus that persists in the blood serum and is transmitted by infected blood or blood derivatives, or by contaminated needles or other instruments. The disease has a long incubation period and symptoms that may become severe or chronic, causing serious damage to the liver.

hepatitis B core antigen *n.* A core protein antigen of the hepatitis B virus found in the Dane particle and also in hepatocyte nuclei in hepatitis B infections.

hepatitis B e antigen *n.* A core protein antigen of the hepatitis B virus that is distinct from both the surface antigen and the core antigen.

hepatitis B surface antigen *n.* An antigen of the small spherical and filamentous forms of hepatitis B antibodies that is also present on the Dane particle.

hepatitis B vaccine *n.* A vaccine prepared from the inactivated surface antigen of the virus causing hepatitis B, which is obtained from the plasma of human carriers of the virus or by genetic engineering, used to immunize against hepatitis B.

hep·a·ti·za·tion (hěp′ə-tĭ-zā′shən) *n.* The conversion of a loose tissue into a firm mass like the substance of the liver, especially such a conversion of lung tissue in pneumonia.

hep·a·to·blas·to·ma (hěp′ə-tō-blă-stō′mə) *n.* A malignant neoplasm occurring in young children, primarily in the liver, composed of tissue resembling embryonic hepatic epithelium.

he·pat·o·cele (hǐ-pǎt′ə-sēl′, hěp′ə-tō-) *n.* Hernial protrusion of part of the liver through the abdominal wall or through the diaphragm.

hep·a·to·cho·lan·gi·o·je·ju·nos·to·my (hěp′ə-tō-kō-lǎn′jē-ō-jə-jōo′nŏs′tə-mē, -jē′jōo-) *n.* Surgical union of the hepatic duct to the jejunum.

hep·a·to·cho·lan·gi·os·to·my (hěp′ə-tō-kō-lǎn′jē-ŏs′tə-mē) *n.* The surgical formation of an opening into the common bile duct to establish drainage.

hep·a·to·cho·lan·gi·tis (hěp′ə-tō-kō′lăn-jī′tĭs) *n.* Inflammation of the liver and bile ducts.

hep·a·to·cyte (hěp′ə-tə-sīt′, hǐ-pǎt′ə-) *n.* A parenchymal liver cell.

hep·a·to·dyn·i·a (hěp′ə-tō-dĭn′ē-ə) *n.* See **hepatalgia.**

hep·a·tog·ra·phy (hěp′ə-tŏg′rə-fē) *n.* Radiographic examination of the liver.

hep·a·to·jug·u·lar reflux (hěp′ə-tō-jŭg′yə-lər, hǐ-pǎt′ə-) *n.* An elevation of venous pressure, visible in the jugular veins and measurable in the veins of the arm, that is produced in active or impending congestive heart failure by firm pressure with the flat hand over the abdomen.

hep·a·to·lith (hěp′ə-tə-lĭth′) *n.* A concretion in the liver.

hep·a·to·li·thec·to·my (hěp′ə-tō-lə-thĕk′tə-mē) *n.* Surgical removal of a calculus from the liver.

hep·a·to·li·thi·a·sis (hěp′ə-tō-lə-thī′ə-sĭs) *n.* The presence of calculi in the liver.

hep·a·tol·o·gy (hěp′ə-tŏl′ə-jē) *n.* The branch of medical science concerned with the liver and its diseases.

hep·a·tol·y·sin (hěp′ə-tŏl′ĭ-sĭn) *n.* A cytolysin that destroys parenchymal liver cells.

hep·a·to·ma (hěp′ə-tō′mə) *n., pl.* **-mas** or **-ma·ta** (-mə-tə). A usually malignant tumor occurring in the liver.

hep·a·to·ma·la·ci·a (hěp′ə-tō-mə-lā′shē-ə, -shə) *n.* Softening of the liver.

hep·a·to·meg·a·ly (hěp′ə-tə-měg′ə-lē, hǐ-pǎt′ə-) *n.* Abnormal enlargement of the liver.

hep·a·to·mel·a·no·sis (hěp′ə-tō-měl′ə-nō′sĭs) *n.* Deep pigmentation of the liver.

hep·a·top·a·thy (hěp′ə-tŏp′ə-thē) *n.* A disease or disorder of the liver. — **hep·a·to·path·ic** (hěp′ə-tō-păth′ĭk, hǐ-pǎt′ō-) *adj.*

hep·a·to·pex·y (hěp′ə-tə-pěk′sē) *n.* Surgical anchoring of the liver to the abdominal wall.

hep·a·to·re·nal (hěp′ə-tō-rē′nəl) *adj.* Relating to the liver and the kidney.

hepatorenal syndrome *n.* A condition in which acute renal failure occurs with disease of the liver or biliary tract.

hep·a·tor·rha·phy (hěp′ə-tôr′ə-fē) *n.* Suture of a wound of the liver.

hep·a·tos·co·py (hěp′ə-tŏs′kə-pē) *n.* Examination of the liver.

hep·a·to·sple·ni·tis (hěp′ə-tō-splĭ-nī′tĭs) *n.* Inflammation of the liver and the spleen.

hep·a·to·sple·nog·ra·phy (hěp′ə-tō-splĭ-nŏg′rə-fē) *n.* Radiographic visualization of the liver and the spleen following the injection of a contrast medium.

hep·a·to·sple·no·meg·a·ly (hěp′ə-tō-splē′nō-měg′ə-lē, -splěn′ō-) *n.* Enlargement of the liver and the spleen.

hep·a·to·sple·nop·a·thy (hěp′ə-tō-splĭ-nŏp′ə-thē) *n.* A disease of the liver and spleen.

hep·a·to·tom·y (hěp′ə-tŏt′ə-mē) *n.* Incision into the liver.

hep·a·to·tox·in (hěp′ə-tō-tŏk′sĭn, hǐ-pǎt′ō-) *n.* A

toxin that is destructive to parenchymal cells of the liver.

hep·tose (hĕp′tōs′, -tōz′) *n.* A monosaccharide containing seven carbon atoms in a molecule.

herb·al·ist (ûr′bə-lĭst, hûr′-) *n.* **1.** One who grows, collects, or specializes in the use of herbs, especially medicinal herbs. **2.** See **herb doctor.**

herb doctor *n.* One who practices healing with herbs.

Her·bert's operation (hûr′bərts) *n.* An operation for creating a filtering cicatrix in glaucoma by cutting and displacing, without removing, a wedge-shaped scleral flap.

he·red·i·tar·y (hə-rĕd′ĭ-tĕr′ē) *adj.* Transmitted or capable of being transmitted genetically from parent to offspring.

hereditary cerebellar ataxia *n.* A disease of later childhood and early adult life characterized by ataxic gait, hesitating and explosive speech, nystagmus, and sometimes optic neuritis.

hereditary hypertrophic neuropathy *n.* An inherited chronic sensorimotor multiple neuropathy characterized by the progressive swelling and mucoid degeneration of peripheral nerves.

hereditary spinal ataxia *n.* Sclerosis of posterior and lateral columns of the spinal cord, occurring in children and marked by ataxia in the lower extremities spreading to the upper extremities and followed by paralysis and contractures.

he·red·i·ty (hə-rĕd′ĭ-tē) *n.* **1.** The genetic transmission of characteristics from parent to offspring. **2.** One's genetic constitution.

her·i·ta·bil·i·ty (hĕr′ĭ-tə-bĭl′ĭ-tē) *n.* **1.** The quality of being heritable. **2.** The proportion of phenotypic variance that can be attributed to variance in genotypes.

her·i·ta·ble (hĕr′ĭ-tə-bəl) *adj.* **1.** Capable of being passed from one generation to another; hereditary. **2.** Capable of inheriting or taking by inheritance. — **her′i·ta·bly** *adv.*

her·maph·ro·dite (hər-măf′rə-dīt′) *n.* A person having the reproductive organs and many of the secondary sex characteristics of both sexes. — **her·maph′ro·dit′ic** (-dĭt′ĭk) *adj.*

her·maph·ro·dit·ism (hər-măf′rə-dī-tĭz′əm) *n.* The presence of both ovarian and testicular tissue in a person.

her·met·ic (hər-mĕt′ĭk) or **her·met·i·cal** (-ĭ-kəl) *adj.* Completely sealed, especially against the escape or entry of air. — **her·met′i·cal·ly** *adv.*

her·ni·a (hûr′nē-ə) *n., pl.* **-ni·as.** The protrusion of an organ or other bodily structure through the wall that normally contains it. — **her′ni·al** *adj.*

hernial sac *n.* The peritoneal envelope of a hernia.

her·ni·ate (hûr′nē-āt′) *v.* **-at·ed, -at·ing, -ates.** To protrude through an abnormal bodily opening. — **her′ni·a′tion** *n.*

herniated *adj.* Of or relating to a bodily structure that has protruded through an abnormal opening in the wall that contains it.

herniated disk *n.* The protrusion of a degenerated or fragmented intervertebral disk into the intervertebral foramen, compressing the nerve root.

her·ni·o·plas·ty (hûr′nē-ə-plăs′tē) *n.* Surgical correction of a hernia.

her·ni·or·rha·phy (hûr′nē-ôr′ə-fē) *n.* Surgical correction of a hernia by suturing.

her·ni·ot·o·my (hûr′nē-ŏt′ə-mē) *n.* The surgical correction of a hernia by cutting through a band of tissue that constricts it.

her·o·in (hĕr′ō-ĭn) *n.* A white, odorless, bitter crystalline compound that is derived from morphine and is a highly addictive narcotic.

her·pan·gi·na (hûr′păn-jī′nə, hûr-păn′jə-) *n.* A mild disease of children caused by a coxsackievirus and marked by fever, dysphagia, and vesicopapular lesions of the mucous membranes of the throat.

her·pes (hûr′pēz) *n.* Any of several viral diseases causing the eruption of small blisterlike vesicles on the skin or mucous membranes, especially herpes simplex or herpes zoster. — **her·pet′ic** (hər-pĕt′ĭk) *adj.*

herpes sim·plex (sĭm′plĕks′) *n.* **1.** A recurrent viral disease caused by herpesvirus type one, and marked by the eruption of fluid-containing vesicles on the mouth, lips, or face; cold sore; fever blister. **2.** A recurrent viral disease caused by herpesvirus type two, and marked by the eruption of fluid-containing vesicles on the genitals.

herpes simplex virus *n.* See **herpesvirus.**

her·pes·vi·rus (hûr′pēz-vī′rəs) *n.* Either of two types of DNA-containing animal viruses of the genus *Herpesvirus,* herpesvirus type one or herpesvirus type two, which form characteristic inclusion bodies within the nuclei of host cells.

herpes zoster *n.* See **shingles.**

her·sage (ĕr-säzh′) *n.* Surgical separation of the individual fibers of a nerve trunk.

Herx·hei·mer's reaction (hûrks′hī′mərz, hĕrks′-) *n.* An inflammatory reaction in syphilitic tissues induced in certain cases by treatment with mercury, antibiotics, or other drugs.

hes·i·tan·cy (hĕz′ĭ-tən-sē) *n.* An involuntary delay or inability in starting the urinary stream.

het·er·es·the·sia (hĕt′ər-ĭs-thē′zhə) *n.* A variation in the degree of the sensory response to a cutaneous stimulus as the stimulus crosses different areas on the surface of the skin.

het·er·o·ag·glu·ti·nin (hĕt′ə-rō-ə-glōōt′n-ĭn) *n.* A hemagglutinin that agglutinates red blood cells in one or more species other than the species from which it was derived.

het·er·o·an·ti·bod·y (hĕt′ə-rō-ăn′tĭ-bŏd′ē) *n.* An antibody specific for antigens originating in species other than that of the antibody producer.

het·er·o·an·ti·se·rum (hĕt′ə-rō-ăn′tĭ-sēr′əm) *n.* An antiserum developed in one animal species against antigens or cells of another species.

het·er·o·chro·ma·tin (hĕt′ə-rō-krō′mə-tĭn) *n.* The part of the chromonema that is coiled and condensed during interphase, thus stains readily.

het·er·o·chro·mic uveitis (hĕt′ə-rō-krō′mĭk) *n.* Pigmentary changes in the iris with inflammation of the anterior uvea.

het·er·o·chro·mo·some (hĕt′ə-rō-krō′mə-sōm′)

n. **1.** A chromosome composed primarily of heterochromatin. **2.** See allosome.

het·er·o·cy·to·tro·pic antibody *n.* A cytotropic antibody similar in activity to a homocytotropic antibody but having an affinity for cells of a different species rather than for cells of the same or a closely related species.

het·er·o·er·o·tism (hĕt′ə-rō-ĕr′ə-tĭz′əm) *n.* See alloerotism. — **het′er·o·e·rot′ic** (-ĭ-rŏt′ĭk) *adj.*

het·er·o·gam·ete (hĕt′ə-rō-găm′ēt′, -gə-mēt′) *n.* Either of two conjugating gametes that differ in structure or behavior, such as the small motile male spermatozoon and the larger nonmotile female ovum.

het·er·og·a·my (hĕt′ə-rŏg′ə-mē) *n.* The state or condition in which conjugating gametes are dissimilar in structure and size as well as in function.

het·er·o·ge·ne·ous (hĕt′ər-ə-jē′nē-əs, -jēn′yəs) *adj.* Composed of parts having dissimilar characteristics or properties.

het·er·o·gen·e·sis (hĕt′ə-rō-jĕn′ĭ-sĭs) *n.* The production of offspring unlike the parents.

het·er·o·ge·net·ic antigen (hĕt′ə-rō-jə-nĕt′ĭk) *n.* An antigen occurring in several different phylogenetically unrelated species.

het·er·o·ge·nous vaccine (hĕt′ə-rŏj′ə-nəs) *n.* Vaccine prepared from microorganisms obtained from a source other than the person who is to be vaccinated.

het·er·o·graft (hĕt′ə-rō-grăft′) *n.* A type of tissue graft in which the donor and recipient are of different species.

het·er·o·ki·ne·sis (hĕt′ə-rō-kə-nē′sĭs, -kī-) *n.* Differential distribution of X-chromosomes and Y-chromosomes during meiotic cell division.

het·er·ol·o·gous graft (hĕt′ə-rŏl′ə-gəs) *n.* See heterograft.

heterologous stimulus *n.* A stimulus that acts upon any part of the sensory apparatus or a nerve tract.

heterologous tumor *n.* A tumor composed of a tissue unlike that from which it develops.

het·er·ol·o·gy (hĕt′ə-rŏl′ə-jē) *n.* Lack of correspondence between bodily parts, as in structure, arrangement, or development, arising from differences in origin.

het·er·ol·y·sis (hĕt′ə-rŏl′ĭ-sĭs, -ə-rō-lī′sĭs) *n., pl.* **-ses** (-sēz′). Dissolution or digestion of cells or protein components from one species by a lytic agent from a different species. — **het′er·o·lyt′ic** (-ə-rō-lĭt′ĭk) *adj.*

het·er·o·met·ric autoregulation (hĕt′ə-rō-mĕt′rĭk) *n.* Autoregulation of the strength of ventricular contraction that occurs in direct relation to the end-diastolic fiber length.

het·er·o·mor·pho·sis (hĕt′ə-rō-môr′fə-sĭs, -môr-fō′sĭs) *n.* **1.** The development of one tissue from a tissue of another kind or type. **2.** The embryonic development of a tissue or an organ inappropriate to its site.

het·er·op·a·thy (hĕt′ə-rŏp′ə-thē) *n.* Abnormal sensitivity to stimuli.

het·er·oph·a·gy (hĕt′ə-rŏf′ə-jē) *n.* Digestion within a cell of a substance taken in by phagocytosis from the cell's environment.

het·er·o·pha·sia (hĕt′ə-rō-fā′zhə, -zē-ə) *n.* See heterolalia.

het·er·o·phe·mi·a (hĕt′ə-rō-fē′mē-ə) *n.* See heterolalia.

het·er·o·pho·ni·a (hĕt′ə-rō-fō′nē-ə) *n.* **1.** The change of voice at puberty. **2.** An abnormality in the voice sounds.

het·er·o·pho·ri·a (hĕt′ə-rō-fôr′ē-ə) *n.* A tendency of the eyes to deviate from the parallel.

het·er·oph·thal·mus (hĕt′ə-rŏf-thăl′məs, -ŏp-) *n.* A difference in the appearance of the two eyes, as in the color or direction of the visual axes.

het·er·o·phy·i·a·sis (hĕt′ə-rō-fī-ī′ə-sĭs) *n.* Infection with trematodes of the genus *Heterophyes*.

het·er·o·pla·sia (hĕt′ə-rō-plā′zhə, -zhē-ə) *n.* **1.** The development of cytologic and histologic elements that are not normal for the organ or part in which they occur. **2.** Malposition of tissue or a part that is otherwise normal.

het·er·o·plas·tic graft (hĕt′ə-rō-plăs′tĭk) *n.* See heterograft.

het·er·o·plas·ty (hĕt′ər-ə-plăs′tē) *n.* The surgical grafting of tissue obtained from one person or species to another.

het·er·o·pyk·no·sis (hĕt′ə-rō-pĭk-nō′sĭs) *n.* A state of variable density between chromosomes of different cells or between individual chromosomes. — **het′er·o·pyk·not′ic** (-nŏt′ĭk) *adj.*

het·er·o·sex·u·al (hĕt′ə-rō-sĕk′shōō-əl) *adj.* Sexually oriented to persons of the opposite sex. — *n.* A heterosexual person.

het·er·o·sex·u·al·i·ty (hĕt′ə-rō-sĕk′shōō-ăl′ĭ-tē) *n.* Erotic attraction, predisposition, or sexual behavior between persons of the opposite sex.

het·er·o·tax·i·a (hĕt′ə-rō-tăk′sē-ə) *n.* Abnormal arrangement of organs or parts of the body in relation to one another.

het·er·o·to·ni·a (hĕt′ə-rō-tō′nē-ə) *n.* A state of abnormality or variation in tension or tone.

het·er·o·to·pi·a (hĕt′ər-ə-tō′pē-ə) or **het·er·ot·o·py** (hĕt′ə-rŏt′ə-pē) *n.* **1.** Displacement of an organ or other body part to an abnormal location. **2.** Displacement of gray matter, usually into the deep cerebral white matter. — **het′er·o·top′ic** (-tŏp′ĭk) *adj.*

het·er·o·trans·plant (hĕt′ə-rō-trăns′plănt′) *n.* See heterograft.

het·er·o·trans·plan·ta·tion (hĕt′ə-rō-trăns′plăn-tā′shən) *n.* The transplantation of a heterograft.

het·er·o·tri·cho·sis (hĕt′ə-rō-trĭ-kō′sĭs) *n.* Hair growth of variegated color.

het·er·o·tro·pi·a (hĕt′ə-rō-trō′pē-ə) *n.* See strabismus.

heterotypical chromosome *n.* See allosome.

het·er·o·zy·gote (hĕt′ə-rō-zī′gōt′) *n.* An organism that has different alleles at a particular gene locus on homologous chromosomes.

hex·a·dac·ty·ly (hĕk′sə-dăk′tə-lē) or **hex·a·dac·tyl·ism** (-lĭz′əm) *n.* The presence of six digits on one or both hands or feet.

hex·os·a·min·i·dase (hĕk′sō-sə-mĭn′ĭ-dās′, -dāz′)

n. Any of at least four enzymes, each of which is the catalyst for the removal of hexose residues from gangliosides; deficiencies of these enzymes can cause certain metabolic disorders.

hex·ose (hĕk′sōs′) *n.* Any of various simple sugars, such as glucose and fructose, that have six carbon atoms per molecule.

hex·yl·caine hydrochloride (hĕk′səl-kān′) *n.* A local anesthetic agent used for surface application, infiltration, or nerve block.

hex·yl·re·sor·ci·nol (hĕk′səl-rĭ-zôr′sə-nôl′, -nōl′) *n.* A yellowish-white crystalline phenol used as an antiseptic and anthelmintic.

Hey·er–Pu·denz valve (hā′ər-pyoō′dĕnz′) *n.* A valve used in the shunting procedure to relieve hydrocephaly, in which cerebrospinal fluid drains from a ventricular catheter to the right atrium of the heart.

HGH *abbr.* human growth hormone

hi·a·tal hernia (hī-ā′təl) *n.* A hernia in which part of the stomach protrudes through the esophageal opening of the diaphragm.

hi·a·tus (hī-ā′təs) *n., pl.* **hiatus** or **-tus·es. 1.** An aperture or fissure in an organ or a body part. **2.** A foramen.

Hib *abbr.* Haemophilus influenza type b conjugate vaccine

hic·cup or **hic·cough** (hĭk′əp) *n.* A spasm of the diaphragm causing sudden inhalation that is interrupted by a spasmodic closure of the glottis, producing the characteristic noise. — **hic′cup,** **hic′cough** *v.*

hi·drad·e·ni·tis (hī-drăd′n-ī′tĭs, hī-) *n.* Inflammation of the sweat glands.

hi·drad·e·no·ma (hī-drăd′n-ō′mə, hī-) *n.* A benign tumor derived from epithelial cells of sweat glands.

hi·dro·poi·e·sis (hī′drō-poi-ē′sĭs) *n.* The formation of sweat.

hi·dros·che·sis (hī-drŏs′kĭ-sĭs, hī-) *n.* The suppression of sweating.

hi·dro·sis (hī-drō′sĭs, hī-) *n., pl.* **-ses** (-sēz). **1.** The formation and excretion of sweat. **2.** Sweat, especially in excessive or abnormal amounts. — **hi·drot′ic** (-drŏt′ĭk) *adj.*

high blood pressure *n.* Hypertension.

high calorie diet *n.* A diet containing more than 4,000 calories per day.

high-density lipoprotein *n.* A complex of lipids and proteins that functions as a transporter of cholesterol in the blood and which, in high concentrations, is associated with a decreased risk of atherosclerosis and coronary heart disease.

high enema *n.* An enema instilled high up into the colon.

high-energy phosphate bond *n.* A phosphate linkage present in certain intermediates of carbohydrate metabolism the stored energy of which is used in metabolic processes, transferred, or stored.

high-pressure oxygen *n.* See **hyperbaric oxygen.**

Hill operation (hĭl) *n.* A surgical procedure to prevent esophageal reflux.

Hill's sign (hĭlz) *n.* An indication of aortic insufficiency in which systolic blood pressure is higher in the legs than in the arms.

hi·lum (hī′ləm) *n., pl.* **-la** (-lə). A depression or slit-like opening through which nerves, ducts, or blood vessels enter and leave in an organ or a gland. — **hi′lar** (-lər) *adj.*

hi·lus cell (hī′ləs) *n.* A cell in the hilum of the ovary that produces androgens and thus is functionally analogous to an interstitial cell.

hind·brain (hīnd′brān′) *n.* See **rhombencephalon.**

hind·gut (hīnd′gŭt′) *n.* **1.** The large intestine, rectum, and anal canal. **2.** The caudal or terminal part of the embryonic gut.

hinged flap *n.* A turnover flap transferred by lifting it over on its pedicle as though the pedicle was a hinge.

hinge joint (hĭnj) *n.* A uniaxial joint in which a broad, transversely cylindrical convexity on one bone fits into a corresponding concavity on the other, allowing motion in one plane only, as in the elbow.

hip (hĭp) *n.* **1.** The lateral prominence of the pelvis from the waist to the thigh. **2.** The hip joint.

hip·bone (hĭp′bōn′) *n.* Either of two large flat bones formed by the fusion of ilium, ischium, and pubis (in the adult), constituting the lateral half of the pelvis and articulating with its fellow, with the sacrum, and with the femur.

hip joint *n.* The ball-and-socket joint formed by the head of the femur and the cup-shaped cavity of the hipbone.

Hip·pel's disease (hĭp′əlz) *n.* See **Lindau's disease.**

hip·po·cam·pus (hĭp′ə-kăm′pəs) *n., pl* **-pi** (-pī′). The complex, internally convoluted structure that forms the medial margin of the cortical mantle of the cerebral hemisphere, is composed of two gyri with their white matter, and forms part of the limbic system. — **hip′po·cam′pal** (-pəl) *adj.*

Hip·poc·ra·tes (hĭ-pŏk′rə-tēz′) Called "the Father of Medicine." 460?–377? B.C. Greek physician who laid the foundations of scientific medicine by freeing medical study from philosophical speculation and superstition.

hippocratic nail *n.* The coarse curved nail of a clubbed finger.

Hirsch·o·witz syndrome (hûr′shə-wĭts′) *n.* A skin condition in which acanthosis nigricans occurs in association with hypovitaminosis.

hir·sut·ism (hûr′soō-tĭz′əm, hĭr′-, hər-soō′-) *n.* The presence of excessive body and facial hair, especially in women.

hir·u·din (hĭr-ōōd′n, hĭr′ə-dən, -yə-) *n.* A substance extracted from the salivary glands of leeches and used as an anticoagulant.

His *abbr.* histidine

His bundle electrogram (hĭs) *n.* An electrogram recorded from the atrioventricular trunk during cardiac catheterization.

His's line (hĭs′ĭz) *n.* An imaginary line extending from the tip of the anterior nasal spine to the hindmost point on the posterior margin of the foramen magnum, dividing the face into an upper and a lower part.

His·ta·log test (hĭs′tə-lôg′) *n.* A test for measuring maximal production of gastric acidity or anacidity using betazole hydrochloride.

his·ta·mine (hĭs′tə-mēn′, -mĭn) *n.* A physiologically active depressor amine found in plant and animal tissue, derived from histidine by decarboxylation and released from cells in the immune system as part of an allergic reaction. It is a powerful stimulant of gastric secretion, constrictor of bronchial smooth muscle, and vasodilator. — **his′ta·min′ic** (-mĭn′ĭk) *adj.*

his·ta·mi·ne·mi·a (hĭs′tə-mə-nē′mē-ə, hĭ-stăm′ə-) *n.* The presence of histamine in the blood.

histamine test *n.* A test for measuring maximal production of gastric acidity or anacidity.

his·ta·mi·nu·ri·a (hĭs′tə-mə-nŏŏr′ē-ə, -nyŏŏr′-) *n.* The excretion of histamine in the urine.

his·ti·dine (hĭs′tĭ-dēn′, -dĭn) *n.* An essential amino acid important for tissue growth and repair.

his·ti·di·ne·mi·a (hĭs′tĭ-də-nē′mē-ə) *n.* A hereditary disorder characterized by an elevated histidine level, excretion of histidine in urine due to deficient enzyme activity, and often manifested by mild mental retardation.

his·ti·di·nu·ri·a (hĭs′tĭ-də-nŏŏr′ē-ə, -nyŏŏr′-) *n.* The excretion of excessive histidine in the urine.

his·ti·o·blast (hĭs′tē-ə-blăst′) *n.* A tissue-forming cell.

his·ti·o·cyte (hĭs′tē-ə-sīt′) *n.* A relatively inactive, immobile macrophage found in normal connective tissue. — **his′ti·o·cyt′ic** (-sĭt′ĭk) *adj.*

his·ti·o·cy·to·sis (hĭs′tē-ō′sī-tō′sĭs) *n., pl.* **-ses** (-sēz). Abnormal multiplication of histiocytes.

his·to·blast (hĭs′tə-blăst′) *n.* See **histioblast.**

his·to·com·pat·i·bil·i·ty (hĭs′tō-kəm-păt′ə-bĭl′-ĭ-tē) *n.* A state or condition in which the absence of immunologic interference permits tissue grafting or blood transfusion without rejection.

histocompatibility antigen *n.* Any of various antigens on the surface of cell membranes that serve to identify a cell as self or nonself, thus determining whether a tissue graft or transfusion will be accepted by a recipient.

histocompatibility gene *n.* A gene that is part of the major histocompatibility complex and is responsible for the production of a histocompatibility antigen.

his·to·cyte (hĭs′tə-sīt′) *n.* See **histiocyte.**

his·to·cy·to·sis (hĭs′tō-sī-tō′sĭs) *n.* See **histiocytosis.**

his·to·dif·fer·en·ti·a·tion (hĭs′tō-dĭf′ə-rĕn′shē-ā′shən) *n.* The morphologic appearance of tissue characteristics during embryonic development.

his·to·gen·e·sis (hĭs′tō-jĕn′ĭ-sĭs) *n.* The formation and development of the tissues of the body. — **his′to·ge·net′ic** (-jə-nĕt′ĭk), **his′to·gen′ic** (-jĕn′-ĭk) *adj.*

his·toid tumor (hĭs′toid′) *n.* A type of connective tumor that is composed of a single type of differentiated tissue.

his·to·in·com·pat·i·bil·i·ty (hĭs′tō-ĭn′kəm-păt′ə-

bĭl′ĭ-tē) *n.* A state of immunologic dissimilarity of tissues sufficient to cause rejection of transplanted tissue.

histologic accommodation *n.* Change in the shape of cells to meet altered physical conditions, such as the flattening of cuboidal cells in cysts as a result of pressure.

his·tol·o·gy (hĭ-stŏl′ə-jē) *n.* The science concerned with the minute structure of tissues and organs in relation to their function. — **his′to·log′i·cal** (hĭs′-tə-lŏj′ĭ-kəl), **his′to·log′ic** *adj.* — **his·tol′o·gist** *n.*

his·tol·y·sis (hĭ-stŏl′ĭ-sĭs) *n.* The breakdown and disintegration of tissue. — **his′to·lyt′ic** (hĭs′tə-lĭt′ĭk) *adj.*

his·to·ma (hĭ-stō′mə) *n., pl.* **-mas** or **-ma·ta** (-mə-tə). A benign tumor having cytologic and histologic elements closely similar to those of normal tissue from which the tumor cells are derived.

his·tone (hĭs′tōn′) *n.* Any of several small simple proteins that are most commonly found in association with the DNA in chromatin and contain a high proportion of basic amino acids.

his·to·nu·ri·a (hĭs′tō-nŏŏr′ē-ə, -nyŏŏr′-) *n.* The excretion of histone in the urine.

his·to·path·o·gen·e·sis (hĭs′tō-păth′ə-jĕn′ĭ-sĭs) *n.* The development of tissue in relation to disease.

his·to·pa·thol·o·gy (hĭs′tō-pə-thŏl′ə-jē, -pă-) *n.* The science concerned with the cytologic and histologic structure of abnormal or diseased tissue.

his·to·phys·i·ol·o·gy (hĭs′tō-fĭz′ē-ŏl′ə-jē) *n.* The microscopic study of tissues in relation to their functions.

his·to·plas·min (hĭs′tə-plăz′mĭn) *n.* An antigenic extract of *Histoplasma capsulatum,* used in immunological tests for histoplasmosis.

his·to·plas·mo·sis (hĭs′tō-plăz-mō′sĭs) *n., pl.* **-ses** (-sēz). An infectious disease caused by the inhalation of spores of *Histoplasma capsulatum,* most often asymptomatic but occasionally producing acute pneumonia or an influenzalike illness and spreading to other organs and body systems.

his·tor·rhex·is (hĭs′tə-rĕk′sĭs) *n.* Breakdown of tissue by a process other than infection.

his·to·tome (hĭs′tə-tōm′) *n.* See **microtome.**

his·tot·o·my (hĭ-stŏt′ə-mē) *n.* See **microtomy.**

HI test *n.* See **hemagglutination inhibition test.**

HIV (āch′ī-vē′) *n.* Human immunodeficiency virus; a cytopathic retrovirus that is the cause of AIDS; HTLV-III.

hives (hīvz) *pl.n.* (*used with a sing. or pl. verb*) See **urticaria.**

HLA *abbr.* human leukocyte antigen

HLA complex *n.* See **major histocompatibility complex.**

HLA typing (āch′ĕl-ā′) *n.* A method for determining compatibility for bone marrow transplantation using the tissue of unrelated donors and recipients.

HMO (āch′ĕm-ō′) *n.* A corporation financed by insurance premiums whose member physicians and professional staff provide curative and preventive medicine within certain financial, geographic, and professional limits to enrolled volunteer members and their families.

hnRNA (āch'ĕn-är'ĕn-ā') *n.* Heterogeneous nuclear RNA; any of the various extrachromosomal molecules of RNA found in the nucleus, especially those transcribed from DNA rather than other RNA, and the proteins produced from such RNA molecules.

hoarse (hôrs) *adj.* **hoars·er, hoars·est. 1.** Rough or grating in sound, as of a voice. **2.** Having or characterized by a husky, grating voice.

Hodg·kin's disease (hŏj'kĭnz) *n.* A malignant, progressive, sometimes fatal disease of unknown etiology, marked by enlargement of the lymph nodes, spleen, and liver and often accompanied by anemia and fever.

Hodg·son's disease (hŏj'sənz) *n.* Dilation of the aortic arch associated with insufficiency of the aortic valve.

Hoff·mann's reflex (hôf'mənz) *n.* See **Hoffmann's sign.**

Hoffmann's sign *n.* **1.** Severe pain in the trigeminal nerve in response to mild mechanical stimulation, characteristic of latent tetany. **2.** Flexion of the terminal phalanx of the thumb and of the second and third phalanges of other fingers when one of the middle fingertips is flicked.

Hof·meis·ter's operation (hôf'mī'stərz) *n.* Partial gastrectomy with closure of a portion of the lesser curvature of the stomach and anastomosis of the remainder to the jejunum.

ho·lis·tic medicine (hō-lĭs'tĭk) *n.* An approach to medical care that emphasizes the study of all aspects of a person's health, including psychological, social, and economic influences on health status.

Hol·len·horst plaques (hŏl'ən-hôrst') *pl.n.* Glittering orange-yellow atheromatous emboli in the retinal arterioles containing cholesterin crystals, indicative of cardiovascular disease.

hollow back *n.* See **lordosis.**

Holmes—Adie syndrome *n.* A syndrome of unknown etiology and pathology characterized by tonic pupillary reactions with tendon reflexes possibly absent or diminished.

hol·mi·um (hōl'mē-əm) *n.* A soft malleable rare-earth element with atomic number 67.

hol·o·crine gland (hŏl'ə-krĭn, -krīn', -krēn', hō'lə-) *n.* A gland whose secretion consists of its own disintegrated secretory cells along with its secretory product.

hol·o·en·zyme (hŏl'ō-ĕn'zīm', hō'lō-) *n.* An active, complex enzyme consisting of an apoenzyme and a coenzyme.

ho·log·raph·y (hō-lŏg'rə-fē) *n.* A method of producing a three-dimensional image of an object by recording on a photographic plate or film the pattern of interference formed by a split laser beam and then illuminating the pattern either with a laser or with ordinary light.

hol·o·pros·en·ceph·a·ly (hŏl'ō-prŏs'ĕn-sĕf'ə-lē, hō'lō-) *n.* Failure of the forebrain to divide into hemispheres or lobes causing insufficient development of facial characteristics such as the nose, lips, and palate and in severe cases, cyclopia.

hol·o·ra·chis·chi·sis (hŏl'ō-rə-kĭs'kĭ-sĭs, hō'lō-) *n.* A form of spina bifida in which the entire spinal column is open.

Ho·mans' sign (hō'mănz') *n.* An indication of incipient or established thrombosis in the leg veins in which slight pain occurs at the back of the knee or calf when, with the knee bent, the ankle is slowly and gently dorsiflexed.

ho·me·o·met·ric autoregulation (hō'mē-ə-mĕt'-rĭk) *n.* Autoregulation of the strength of ventricular contraction by mechanisms or agents that do not depend upon change in the end-diastolic fiber length.

ho·me·op·a·thy (hō'mē-ŏp'ə-thē) *n.* A system for treating disease based on the administration of minute doses of a drug that in massive amounts produces symptoms in healthy individuals similar to those of the disease itself. — **ho'me·o·path'ic** (-ə-păth'ĭk) *adj.* — **ho'me·o·path', ho'-me·op'a·thist** *n.*

ho·me·o·pla·sia (hō'mē-ə-plā'zhə, -zhē-ə) *n.* **1.** The growth of new tissue having the same form and properties as normal tissue. **2.** The tissue formed in this manner. — **homeoplastic** *adj.*

ho·me·o·sta·sis (hō'mē-ō-stā'sĭs) *n.* **1.** The ability or tendency of an organism or a cell to maintain internal equilibrium by adjusting its physiological processes. **2.** The processes used to maintain such bodily equilibrium. — **ho'me·o·stat'ic** (-stăt'ĭk) *adj.*

ho·me·o·ther·a·py (hō'mē-ō-thĕr'ə-pē) or **ho·me·o·ther·a·peu·tics** (-thĕr'ə-pyōō'tĭks) *n.* The treatment or prevention of disease using homeopathic principles. — **ho'me·o·ther'a·peu'tic** *adj.*

ho·mo·cys·te·ine (hō'mə-sĭs'tə-ēn', -ĭn, -tē-) *n.* An amino acid that is a homologue of cysteine, is produced by the demethylation of methionine, and forms a complex with serine that metabolizes to produce cysteine and homoserine.

ho·mo·cys·tine (hō'mə-sĭs'tēn') *n.* An amino acid resulting from the oxidation of homocysteine and excreted in the urine in homocystinuria.

ho·mo·cys·ti·ne·mi·a (hō'mə-sĭs'tə-nē'mē-ə) *n.* The presence of an excess of homocystine in the blood plasma.

ho·mo·cys·ti·nu·ri·a (hō'mə-sĭs'tə-nŏŏr'ē-ə, -nyŏŏr'-) *n.* An inherited metabolic disorder caused by a deficiency of an enzyme important in the metabolism of homocysteine and characterized by the excretion of homocystine in the urine, mental retardation, dislocation of the crystalline lens of the eye, sparse blond hair, and cardiovascular and skeletal deformities.

ho·mo·cy·to·trop·ic antibody (hō'mō-sī'tə-trŏp'ĭk, -trō'pĭk) *n.* An antibody that has an affinity especially for mast cells of the same or a closely related species, combines with a specific antigen, and triggers the release of mediators of anaphylaxis from the cells to which it is attached.

ho·mog·a·my (hō-mŏg'ə-mē) *n.* Reproduction within a group that perpetuates qualities or traits that distinguish the group from a larger group of which it is part.

ho·mo·gen·e·sis (hō'mə-jĕn'ĭ-sĭs) *n*. Reproduction in which the offspring are similar to the parents.

ho·mog·e·nous (hə-mŏj'ə-nəs, hō-) *adj*. Of or exhibiting homogeny.

ho·mo·gen·ti·su·ri·a (hō'mō-jĕn'tĭ-sŏor'ē-ə) *n*. See **alkaptonuria**.

ho·mog·e·ny (hə-mŏj'ə-nē, hō-) *n*. Similarity of structure between organs or parts, possibly of dissimilar function, that are related by common descent.

ho·mo·graft (hō'mə-grăft', hŏm'ə-) *n*. See **allograft**.

ho·mol·o·gous (hə-mŏl'ə-gəs, hō-) *adj*. **1.** Corresponding or similar in position, value, structure, or function. **2.** Similar in structure and evolutionary origin, though not necessarily in function, as the flippers of a seal and the hands of a human. **3.** Relating to the correspondence between an antigen and the antibody produced in response to it. **4.** Having the same morphology and linear sequence of gene loci as another chromosome.

homologous chromosome *n*. Either member of a single pair of chromosomes.

homologous graft *n*. See **allograft**.

homologous stimulus *n*. A stimulus that acts only on the nerve endings in a special sense organ.

homologous tumor *n*. A tumor composed of the same type of tissue as that from which it develops.

ho·mo·logue or **hom·o·log** (hŏm'ə-lôg', hō'mə-) *n*. Something homologous; a homologous organ or part.

ho·mol·y·sin (hō-mŏl'ĭ-sĭn) *n*. A sensitizing, hemolytic antibody formed as the result of stimulation by an antigen derived from an animal of the same species.

ho·mol·y·sis (hō-mŏl'ĭ-sĭs) *n*. **1.** Lysis of a cell by extracts of the same type of tissue. **2.** Lysis of red blood cells by homolysin and complement.

ho·mo·plas·tic graft (hō'mə-plăs'tĭk, hŏm'ə-) *n*. See **allograft**.

ho·mo·plas·ty (hō'mə-plăs'-tē) *n*. Surgical repair using grafts from an individual of the same species.

ho·mo·ser·ine (hō'mə-sĕr'ēn') *n*. An amino acid formed when methionine is converted to cysteine.

ho·mo·sex·u·al (hō'mə-sĕk'shŏo-əl, -mō-) *adj*. Of, relating to, or having a sexual orientation to persons of the same sex. — *n*. A homosexual person; a gay man or a lesbian.

ho·mo·sex·u·al·i·ty (hō'mə-sĕk'shŏo-ăl'ĭ-tē, -mō-) *n*. **1.** Sexual orientation to persons of the same sex. **2.** Sexual activity with another of the same sex.

homosexual panic *n*. An acute, severe attack of anxiety based on unconscious conflicts regarding homosexuality.

ho·mo·top·ic (hō'mə-tŏp'ĭk) *adj*. Relating to or occurring in the same or corresponding place or part of the body.

ho·mo·type (hō'mə-tīp', hŏm'ə-) *n*. A part or organ that has the same structure or function as another, especially to a corresponding one on the opposite side of the body. — **ho'mo·typ'ic** (-tĭp'-ĭk), **ho'mo·typ'i·cal** *adj*.

ho·mo·zy·gos·i·ty (hō'mō-zī-gŏs'ĭ-tē, hŏm'ō-) *n*. The condition of having identical genes at one or more loci in homologous chromosome segments.

ho·mo·zy·gote (hō'mō-zī'gōt', -mə-, hŏm'ə-) *n*. An organism that has the same alleles at a particular gene locus on homologous chromosomes.

hon·ey·comb lung (hŭn'ē-kōm') *n*. The radiological and gross appearance of the lungs resulting from diffuse fibrosis and cystic dilation of bronchioles.

Hong Kong influenza (hŏng'kŏng') *n*. Influenza caused by a serotype of influenza virus type A; it was first identified in Hong Kong during the 1968 epidemic.

hoof-and-mouth disease *n*. See **foot-and-mouth disease**.

Hooke's law (hŏoks) *n*. The principle that the stress applied to stretch or compress a body is proportional to the strain or to the change in length thus produced, so long as the limit of elasticity of the body is not exceeded.

hook·worm (hŏok'wûrm') *n*. Any of numerous small parasitic nematode worms of the family Ancylostomatidae, having hooked mouthparts with which they fasten themselves to the intestinal walls of various hosts, including humans.

hookworm disease *n*. A disease, such as ancylostomiasis, resulting from infestation with hookworms and usually marked by abdominal discomfort, diarrhea, and anemia.

Hoo·ver's sign (hŏo'vərz) *n*. **1.** An indication of compensatory movement in legs whether normal or paralyzed; missing in hysteric paralysis. **2.** An indication of a change in the contour of the diaphragm as a result of empyema or other intrathoracic conditions in which there is a modification in the movement of the costal margins of the diaphragm during respiration.

hor. decub. *abbr*. *Latin*. hora decubitus (before sleep, at bedtime)

hore·hound (hôr'hound') *n*. **1.** An aromatic Eurasian plant (*Marrubium vulgare*) the leaves of which yield a bitter extract used in flavoring and as a cough remedy. **2.** A candy or preparation flavored with this extract.

horizontal plane *n*. A plane crossing the body at right angles to the coronal and sagittal planes.

hor·mone (hôr'mōn') *n*. A substance, usually a peptide or steroid, produced by one tissue and conveyed by the bloodstream to another to effect physiological activity, such as growth or metabolism. — **hor·mon'al** (-mō'nəl), **hor·mon'ic** (-mŏn'ĭk) *adj*.

hormone-replacement therapy *n*. The therapeutic administration of estrogen and perhaps other hormones to postmenopausal women to reduce the occurrence of hot flashes and to prevent osteoporosis and coronary disease.

hor·mo·no·gen·e·sis (hôr-mō'nə-jĕn'ĭ-sĭs) *n.* The formation of hormones. — **hor·mo'no·gen'ic** *adj.*

hor·mo·no·poi·e·sis (hôr-mō'nə-poi-ē'sĭs) *n.* The production of hormones. — **hor·mo'no·poi·et'ic** (-poi-ĕt'ĭk) *adj.*

Hor·ner's syndrome (hôr'nərz) *n.* A syndrome caused by a lesion in the sympathetic nervous system, especially the cervical chain or central pathways, that is characterized by drooping of the upper eyelid, pupillary contraction, absence of sweating, and receding of the eyeball into its orbit.

Horner–Trantas dot *n.* Any of the small, white, calcareouslike cellular infiltrates occurring on the edge of the conjunctiva in vernal conjunctivitis.

horny layer *n.* See **stratum corneum.**

ho·rop·ter (hô-rŏp'tər) *n.* The sum of all points in space whose images form at corresponding points on the plane of the retina.

hor·rip·i·la·tion (hō-rĭp'ə-lā'shən, hŏ-) *n.* The bristling of the body hair, as from fear or cold; goose bumps.

hor. som. *abbr. Latin.* hora somni (before sleep, at bedtime)

Hor·te·ga cell (ôr-tā'gə) *n.* See **microglia.**

hos·pice (hŏs'pĭs) *n.* A program or facility that provides palliative care and attends to the emotional, spiritual, social, and financial needs of terminally ill patients at an inpatient facility or at the patient's home.

hos·pi·tal (hŏs'pĭ-tl, -pĭt'l) *n.* An institution that provides medical, surgical, or psychiatric care and treatment for the sick or the injured.

hos·pi·tal·i·za·tion (hŏs'pĭ-tl-ĭ-zā'shən) *n.* **1.** The act of placing a person in a hospital as a patient. **2.** The condition of being hospitalized. **3.** Insurance that fully or partially covers a patient's hospital expenses.

hospital record *n.* The medical record for a patient generated during a period of hospitalization, usually including written accounts of consultants' opinions as well as nurses' observations and treatments.

host (hōst) *n.* **1.** The animal or plant on which or in which a parasitic organism lives. **2.** The recipient of a transplanted tissue or organ.

hot flash *n.* A sudden, brief sensation of heat, often over the entire body, caused by a transient dilation of the blood vessels of the skin and experienced by some women during menopause.

hot flush *n.* See **hot flash.**

hot spot *n.* A region in a gene in which there is a high rate of mutation.

hour·glass contraction (our'glăs') *n.* Constriction of the middle portion of a hollow organ, such as the stomach or the uterus.

hourglass murmur *n.* A murmur in which there are two areas of maximum loudness, one preceding and the other following a softer midpoint. Its graph resembles an hourglass.

hourglass stomach *n.* A condition in which there is an abnormal constriction of the stomach wall

dividing it into two cavities, cardiac and pyloric.

house call *n.* A professional visit made to a home, especially by a physician.

house·maid's knee (hous'mādz') *n.* Swelling and inflammation of the bursa in front of the patella just beneath the skin, caused by trauma, such as that caused by excessive kneeling.

house officer *n.* An intern or resident employed by a hospital to provide service to patients during the period he or she is receiving training in a medical specialty.

house physician *n.* **1.** A physician, especially an intern or a resident who cares for hospitalized patients under the supervision of the surgical and medical staff of a hospital. **2.** A physician employed by a hotel or another establishment.

house staff *n.* The physicians and surgeons in specialty training at a hospital who care for the patients under the direction and responsibility of the attending staff.

How·ell–Jol·ly body (hou'əl-zhô-lē') *n.* A spherical granule occasionally observed in the stroma of a circulating red blood cell, especially after a splenectomy.

How·ship's lacuna (hou'shĭps) *n.* Any of the tiny depressions, pits, or irregular grooves in bone that is being resorbed by osteoclasts.

HPL *abbr.* human placental lactogen

HPV *abbr.* human papilloma virus

HR *abbr.* heart rate

HTLV (āch'tē-ĕl-vē') *n.* Human T-cell lymphotropic virus; any of a group of lymphotropic retroviruses that have a selective affinity for the helper/inducer cell subset of T lymphocytes and are associated with adult T-cell leukemia and lymphoma. One type, HTLV-III, causes AIDS.

HTLV-I *n.* Human T-cell lymphotropic virus type I; a retrovirus that causes diseases similar to multiple sclerosis.

HTLV-III *n.* Human T-cell lymphotropic virus type III; HIV.

hu·man antihemophilic factor (hyōō'mən) *n.* A lyophilized concentrate of factor VIII, obtained from fresh normal human plasma and used as a hemostatic agent in hemophilia.

human chorionic gonadotropin *n.* See **chorionic gonadotropin.**

human chorionic so·ma·to·mam·mo·trop·ic hormone (sō'mə-tə-măm'ə-trŏp'ĭk, -trō'pĭk, sə-măt'ə-) or **human chorionic so·ma·to·mam·mo·tro·pin** (-măm'ə-trō'pĭn, -mə-mŏt'rə-pĭn) *n.* See **human placental lactogen.**

human diploid cell rabies vaccine *n.* Rabies vaccine composed of inactive virus prepared from fixed rabies virus cultured on human diploid cells.

human gamma globulin *n.* A preparation of the proteins of human plasma containing the antibodies of normal adults.

Human Genome Project *n.* An international research effort to map and identify the role of all genes in the human genome.

human growth hormone *n.* See **somatotropin.**

human immunodeficiency virus *n.* HIV.

human insulin *n.* A protein that has the normal structure of insulin produced by the human pancreas but that is prepared by recombinant DNA techniques and by semisynthetic processes.

human leukocyte antigen *n.* A gene product of the major histocompatibility complex; these antigens have been shown to strongly influence human allotransplantation, transfusions in refractory patients, and certain disease associations.

human menopausal gonadotropin *n.* An injectable preparation obtained from the urine of menopausal women with effects similar to those of follicle-stimulating hormone; it mimics the effects of luteinizing hormone and is used with chorionic gonadotropin to induce ovulation.

human papilloma virus *n.* A DNA virus of the genus *Papillomavirus,* certain types of which cause cutaneous and genital warts in humans, including condyloma acuminatum. Other types are associated with severe cervical intraepithelial neoplasia and with anogenital and laryngeal carcinomas.

human placental lactogen *n.* A hormone originating from the placenta whose biological activity weakly mimics that of human pituitary growth hormone and prolactin.

human plasma protein fraction *n.* A sterile solution of selected proteins removed by fractionation from the blood plasma of adult human donors and used to augment blood volume.

human T-cell leukemia virus *n.* See **HTLV.**

hu·mer·al (hyōō′mər-əl) *adj.* **1.** Of, relating to, or located in the region of the humerus or the shoulder. **2.** Relating to or being a body part analogous to the humerus.

hu·mer·us (hyōō′mər-əs) *n., pl.* **-mer·i** (-mə-rī′). The long bone of the arm or forelimb, extending from the shoulder to the elbow.

hu·mor (hyōō′mər) *n.* **1.** A body fluid, such as blood, lymph, or bile. **2.** Aqueous humor. **3.** Vitreous humor. **4.** A person's characteristic disposition or temperament.

hu·mor·al (hyōō′mər-əl) *adj.* **1.** Relating to body fluids, especially serum. **2.** Relating to or arising from any of the bodily humors.

humoral immunity *n.* The component of the immune response involving the transformation of B-lymphocytes into plasma cells that produce and secrete antibodies to a specific antigen.

hump·back (hŭmp′băk′) or **hunch·back** (hŭnch′-) *n.* See **kyphosis.**

hunch·back (hŭnch′băk′) *n.*

hun·ger (hŭng′gər) *n.* **1.** A strong desire or need for food. **2.** The discomfort, weakness, or pain caused by a prolonged lack of food. **3.** A strong desire or craving, as for affection.

hunger contractions *pl.n.* Strong contractions of the stomach associated with hunger pains.

hunger pain *n.* Pain or discomfort in the epigastrium associated with hunger.

Hun·ner's ulcer (hŭn′ərz) *n.* A focal lesion involving all layers of the bladder wall in chronic interstitial cystitis.

Hunter's syndrome *n.* A metabolic deficiency syndrome caused by an inability to break down mucopolysaccharides and characterized by lack of a specific sulfatase, urinary excretion of an ester of heparin, and the presence of mucopolysaccharides in connective tissue.

Hun·ting·ton's chorea (hŭn′tĭng-tənz) *n.* A chronic disorder marked by choreic movements in the face and extremities, accompanied by a progressive loss of mental faculties.

Hunt's syndrome (hŭnts) *n.* **1.** A tremor beginning in one extremity and gradually increasing in intensity until it involves other parts of the body. **2.** Facial paralysis, otalgia, and herpes zoster resulting from viral infection of the facial nerve and geniculate ganglion. **3.** A form of juvenile paralysis associated with primary atrophy of the pallidal system.

Hur·ler's syndrome (hûr′lərz) *n.* A hereditary defect in mucopolysaccharide metabolism characterized by abnormal development of skeletal cartilage and bone, corneal clouding, enlarged liver and spleen, mental retardation, hearing loss, and a coarsened facial surface.

Hürth·le cell (hûr′tl, hürt′lə) *n.* A thyroid follicular cell that is enlarged and has acidophilic cytoplasm, especially present in adenomas.

Hürthle cell tumor *n.* A benign or malignant tumor of the thyroid gland.

Hutch·in·son–Gil·ford syndrome or **Hutch·in·son-Gil·ford disease** (hŭch′ĭn-sən-gĭl′fərd) *n.* See **progeria.**

hy·a·lin (hī′ə-lĭn) or **hy·a·line** (-lĭn, -lĭn′) *n.* **1.** The uniform matrix of hyaline cartilage. **2.** A translucent product of some types of tissue degeneration.

hyaline cartilage *n.* Semitransparent opalescent cartilage forming most of the fetal skeleton and consisting of cells that synthesize a collagen-protein matrix; in the adult, it is found in the trachea, larynx, and joint surfaces.

hyaline degeneration *n.* Any of several degenerative processes that affect various cells and tissues, resulting in the formation of rounded masses or broad bands of homogeneous acidophilic substances that have a glassy appearance.

hyaline membrane *n.* The thin, clear basement membrane between the inner fibrous layer of a hair follicle and its outer root sheath.

hyaline membrane disease *n.* See **respiratory distress syndrome.**

hy·a·lin·i·za·tion (hī′ə-lĭn′ĭ-zā′shən) *n.* The formation of hyalin. — **hy′a·lin·ized** (hī′ə-lə-nīzd) *adj.*

hy·a·li·nu·ri·a (hī′ə-lə-nŏŏr′ē-ə, -nyŏŏr′-) *n.* The excretion of hyalin or casts of hyaline material in the urine.

hy·a·li·tis (hī′ə-lī′tĭs) *n.* Inflammation of the vitreous humor of the eye in which the inflammatory changes extend into the avascular vitreous from adjacent structures.

hy·al·o·gen (hī-ăl′ə-jən) *n.* Any of various insoluble substances related to mucoids occurring in structures such as cartilage, vitreous humor, and hydatid cysts and yielding sugars on hydrolysis.

hyaloid body *n.* See **vitreous body.**

hy·a·lo·plasm (hī′ə-lō-plăz′əm) *n.* The clear, fluid portion of cytoplasm as distinguished from the granular and netlike components.

hy·al·o·some (hī-ăl′ə-sōm′) *n.* An oval or round structure within a cell nucleus that stains faintly but otherwise resembles a nucleolus.

H–Y antigen *n.* An antigen factor, dependent on the Y-chromosome, responsible for differentiating the human embryo into the male phenotype by inducing the embryonic gonad to develop into a testis.

hy·brid·o·ma (hī′brī-dō′mə) *n.* A cell hybrid produced in vitro by the fusion of an antibody-producing lymphocyte and a myeloma tumor cell. It proliferates into clones that produce a continuous supply of a specific antibody.

hy·da·tid (hī′də-tĭd) *n.* **1.** A hydatid cyst. **2.** The encysted larva of *Echinococcus granulosus.* **3.** An abnormal vascular structure that is usually filled with fluid.

hydatid cyst *n.* A cyst formed as a result of infestation by larvae of the tapeworm *Echinococcus granulosus.*

hydatid disease *n.* An infection, usually of the liver or lungs, with the larvae of an *Echinococcus* tapeworm and characterized by the formation of hydatid cysts.

hydatid fremitus *n.* See **hydatid thrill.**

hy·da·tid·i·form mole (hī′də-tĭd′ə-fôrm′) *n.* A vesicular or polycystic placental mass resulting from the proliferation of the trophoblast and the hydropic degeneration and avascularity of the chorionic villi, usually indicative of an abnormal pregnancy.

hydatid thrill *n.* The trembling or vibratory sensation felt by the hand when examining a hydatid cyst.

hy·dra·gogue (hī′drə-gôg′) *n.* Any of a class of cathartics that aid in the removal of edematous fluids and thus promote the discharge of watery fluid from the bowels.

hy·dral·a·zine (hī-drăl′ə-zēn′) *n.* A crystalline compound whose hydrochloride form is used in the treatment of hypertension.

hy·dram·ni·on (hī-drăm′nē-ən, -ŏn′) *n.* The presence of an excessive amount of amniotic fluid.

hy·dran·en·ceph·a·ly (hī′drăn-ən-sĕf′ə-lē) *n.* The congenital absence of the cerebral hemispheres in which the space in the cranium that they normally occupy is filled with fluid.

hy·drar·gyr·i·a (hī′drär-jĭr′ē-ə, -jĭ′rē-ə) or **hy·drar·gy·rism** (hī-drär′jə-rĭz′əm) *n.* See **mercury poisoning.**

hy·drar·thro·sis (hī′drär-thrō′sĭs) *n.* An effusion of serous fluid into a joint cavity. — **hy′drar·thro′di·al** (-thrō′dē-əl) *adj.*

hy·drate (hī′drāt′) *v.* **-drat·ed, -drat·ing, -drates.** **1.** To rehydrate. **2.** To supply water to a person or thing in order to restore or maintain fluid balance.

hy·dra·tion (hī-drā′shən) *n.* **1.** The addition of water to a chemical molecule without hydrolysis. **2.** The process of providing an adequate amount of liquid to bodily tissues.

hy·dre·mi·a (hī-drē′mē-ə) *n.* An increase in blood volume because of excessive plasma or water with or without a reduction in the concentration of blood proteins.

hy·dro·a (hī-drō′ə) *n.* A vesicular or bullous eruption, especially of the skin.

hy·dro·car·bon (hī′drə-kär′bən) *n.* Any of numerous organic compounds, such as benzene and methane, that contain only carbon and hydrogen.

hy·dro·cele (hī′drə-sēl′) *n.* A pathological accumulation of serous fluid in a bodily cavity, especially in the scrotal pouch.

hy·dro·ce·lec·to·my (hī′drə-sĭ-lĕk′tə-mē) *n.* Surgical excision of a hydrocele.

hy·dro·ceph·a·lus (hī′drō-sĕf′ə-ləs) or **hy·dro·ceph·a·ly** (-lē) *n.* A usually congenital condition in which an abnormal accumulation of fluid in the cerebral ventricles causes enlargement of the skull and compression of the brain, destroying much of the neural tissue. — **hy′dro·ce·phal′ic** (-sə-făl′ĭk), **hy′dro·ceph′a·loid′**

hy·dro·chlo·ride (hī′drə-klôr′īd′) *n.* A compound resulting or regarded as resulting from the reaction of hydrochloric acid with an organic base.

hy·dro·cho·le·cys·tis (hī′drō-kō′lĭ-sĭs′tĭs) *n.* The effusion of serous fluid into the gallbladder.

hy·dro·col·po·cele (hī′drō-kŏl′pə-sēl′) *n.* The accumulation of watery or mucoid fluid in the vagina.

hy·dro·cor·ti·sone (hī′drə-kôr′tĭ-sōn′, -zōn′) *n.* **1.** A steroid hormone, produced by the adrenal cortex, that regulates carbohydrate metabolism and maintains blood pressure. **2.** A preparation of this hormone obtained from natural sources or produced synthetically and used to treat inflammatory conditions and adrenal failure.

hy·dro·cyst (hī′drə-sĭst′) *n.* A cyst having clear watery contents.

hy·dro·gel (hī′drə-jĕl′) *n.* A colloidal gel in which the particles are dispersed in water.

hy·dro·gen (hī′drə-jən) *n.* A colorless, highly flammable gaseous element, with atomic number 1, the most abundant in the universe, found in water and nearly all organic compounds, used in the hydrogenation of organic materials.

hy·dro·gen·a·tion (hī′drə-jə-nā′shən, hī-drŏj′ə-) *n.* The addition of hydrogen to a compound, especially to an unsaturated fat or fatty acid so as to solidify it.

hydrogen chloride *n.* A colorless, fuming, corrosive, very soluble, suffocating gas that forms hydrochloric acid in solution.

hydrogen peroxide *n.* A colorless, heavy, strongly oxidizing liquid capable of reacting explosively with combustibles and used principally in aqueous solution as a mild antiseptic, an oxidizing agent, and a laboratory reagent.

hy·drol·y·sis (hī-drŏl′ĭ-sĭs) *n.* Decomposition of a chemical compound by reaction with water, such as the dissociation of a dissolved salt or the catalytic conversion of starch to glucose. — **hy·dro·lyt'ic** (-drə-lĭt'ĭk) *adj.*

hy·dro·me·nin·go·cele (hī'drō-mə-nĭng'gə-sēl') *n.* A fluid-filled protrusion of the meninges of the brain or spinal cord through a defect in the skull or vertebral column.

hy·dro·me·tra (hī'drō-mē'trə) *n.* The accumulation of thin mucus or other watery fluid in the uterus.

hy·dro·mor·phone hydrochloride (hī'drō-môr'fōn') *n.* A synthetic derivative of morphine used as a respiratory sedative and analgesic that is more potent than morphine.

hy·dro·my·e·li·a (hī'drō-mī-ē'lē-ə) *n.* A dilation of the central canal of the spinal cord caused by an increase of fluid.

hy·dro·my·e·lo·cele (hī'drō-mī'ə-lō-sēl') *n.* The protrusion through a spina bifida of a saclike portion of the spinal cord containing cerebrospinal fluid.

hy·dro·ne·phro·sis (hī'drō-nə-frō'sĭs) *n.* The dilation of the pelvis and calices of one or both kidneys because of the accumulation of urine resulting from obstruction to urine outflow. — **hy'dro·ne·phrot'ic** (-frŏt'ĭk) *adj.*

hy·dro·per·i·car·di·tis (hī'drō-pĕr'ĭ-kär-dī'tĭs) *n.* Pericarditis accompanied by with an effusion of serous fluid into the pericardial cavity.

hy·dro·per·i·car·di·um (hī'drō-pĕr'ĭ-kär'dē-əm) *n.* The noninflammatory accumulation of watery fluid in the pericardial cavity.

hy·dro·per·i·to·ne·um (hī'drō-pĕr'ĭ-tn-ē'əm) *n.* See ascites.

hy·dro·phil·i·a (hī'drə-fĭl'ē-ə) *n.* **1.** A tendency of the blood and tissues to absorb fluid. **2.** The ability to combine with or attract water.

hy·dro·phil·ic (hī'drə-fĭl'ĭk) *adj.* Having an affinity for water; readily absorbing or dissolving in water.

hy·dro·pho·bi·a (hī'drə-fō'bē-ə) *n.* **1.** An abnormal fear of water. **2.** Rabies.

hy·dro·pho·bic (hī'drə-fō'bĭk, -fŏb'ĭk) *adj.* **1.** Repelling, tending not to combine with, or incapable of dissolving in water. **2.** Of or exhibiting hydrophobia.

hy·dro·pneu·ma·to·sis (hī'drō-nōō'mə-tō'sĭs, -nyōō'-) *n.* The presence of gas and liquid in the tissues.

hy·dro·pneu·mo·go·ny (hī'drō-nōō-mō'gə-nē, -nyōō-) *n.* The injection of air into a joint to determine the amount of effusion.

hy·dro·pneu·mo·per·i·car·di·um (hī'drō-nōō'-mō-pĕr'ĭ-kär'dē-əm) *n.* The accumulation of serous fluid and gas in the pericardial sac.

hy·dro·pneu·mo·per·i·to·ne·um (hī'drō-nōō'-mō-pĕr'ĭ-tn-ē'əm, -nyōō'-) *n.* The accumulation of serous fluid and gas in the peritoneal cavity.

hy·dro·pneu·mo·tho·rax (hī'drō-nōō'mō-thôr'ăks', -nyōō'-) *n.* The accumulation of serous fluid and gas in the pleural cavity.

hy·drops (hī'drŏps') *n.* The excessive accumulation of serous fluid in tissues or cavities of the body as in ascites, anasarca, and edema.

hy·dror·rhe·a (hī'drə-rē'ə) *n.* A profuse watery discharge from any part of the body, such as the nose.

hydrorrhea grav·i·dar·um (grăv'ĭ-dâr'əm) *n.* The discharge of a watery fluid from the vagina during pregnancy.

hy·dro·sal·pinx (hī'drō-săl'pĭngks) *n.* The accumulation of serous fluid in the fallopian tube.

hy·dro·sar·co·cele (hī'drō-sär'kə-sēl') *n.* A chronic swelling of the testis accompanied by a hydrocele.

hy·dro·stat·ic (hī'drə-stăt'ĭk) or **hy·dro·stat·i·cal** (-ĭ-kəl) *adj.* Of or relating to fluids at rest or under pressure.

hy·dro·tax·is (hī'drə-tăk'sĭs) *n.* Movement of a cell or an organism in response to moisture.

hy·dro·ther·a·py (hī'drə-thĕr'ə-pē) *n.* External use of water in the medical treatment of certain diseases.

hy·dro·tho·rax (hī'drə-thôr'ăks') *n.* Accumulation of serous fluid in one or both pleural cavities.

hy·dro·tu·ba·tion (hī'drō-tōō-bā'shən, -tyōō-) *n.* The injection of liquid medication or saline solution through the cervix into the uterine cavity and fallopian tubes for therapeutic purposes.

hy·dro·u·re·ter (hī'drō-yōō-rē'tər, -yōōr'ĭ-tər) *n.* The distention of the ureter with urine due to blockage.

hy·dro·var·i·um (hī'drō-vâr'ē-əm) *n.* The accumulation of fluid in the ovary.

hy·drox·ide (hī-drŏk'sīd') *n.* A chemical compound containing the hydroxyl (OH) group, especially a compound that releases a hydroxyl group when dissolved.

hy·drox·y·ky·nu·re·ni·nu·ri·a (hī-drŏk'sē-kī-nōōr'ə-nĭ-nōōr'ē-ə, -nyōōr'ə-nĭ-nyōōr'-) *n.* An inherited abnormality in tryptophan metabolism believed to be due to a defect in a liver enzyme and characterized by mild mental retardation, migrainelike headaches, and urinary excretion of excessive amounts of certain metabolites of tryptophan.

hy·drox·y·phen·yl·u·ri·a (hī-drŏk'sē-fĕn'ə-lōōr'ē-ə, -lyōōr'-, fē'nə-) *n.* The presence of tyrosine and phenylalanine in the urine as a result of a deficiency of ascorbic acid.

hy·drox·y·zine (hī-drŏk'sĭ-zēn') *n.* A mild sedative and minor tranquilizer used in the treatment of psychological neuroses.

hy·giene (hī'jēn') *n.* **1.** The science that deals with the promotion and preservation of health. **2.** Conditions and practices that serve to promote or preserve health, as in personal hygiene. — **hy·gien'ist** (hī-jē'nĭst, hī'jē'-, hī-jēn'ĭst) *n.*

hy·gi·en·ic (hī'jē-ĕn'ĭk, hī-jēn'-) *adj.* **1.** Of or relating to hygiene. **2.** Tending to promote or preserve health. **3.** Sanitary.

hy·gi·en·ics (hī'jē-ĕn'ĭks, hī-jēn'-, -jē'nĭks) *n.* See hygiene.

hy·gro·ma (hī-grō'mə) *n., pl.* **-mas** or **-ma·ta** (-mə-tə). A cystic swelling containing a serous fluid.

hy·men (hī′mən) *n.* A membranous fold of tissue that partly or completely occludes the external vaginal orifice. — **hy′men·al** *adj.*

hy·men·ec·to·my (hī′mə-něk′tə-mē) *n.* Surgical excision of the hymen.

hy·o·glos·sus muscle (hī′ō-glŏs′əs) or **hyoglossal muscle** *n.* A muscle with its origin from the hyoid bone, with insertion to the side of the tongue, and whose action retracts and pulls down the side of the tongue.

hy·oid arch (hī′oid′) *n.* The second postoral arch in the branchial arch series.

hyoid bone *n.* A U-shaped bone at the base of the tongue that supports the muscles of the tongue.

hyp·a·cu·sis (hĭp′ə-kōō′sĭs, -kyōō′-, hī′pə-) or **hy·po·a·cu·sis** (hī′pō-ə-) *n.* An hearing impairment associated with a deficiency in the peripheral neurosensory or conductive organs of hearing.

hyp·al·ge·si·a (hĭp′ăl-jē′zē-ə, -zhə, hī′păl-) or **hy·po·al·ge·si·a** (hī′pō-ăl-) *n.* Diminished sensitivity to pain. — **hyp′al·ge′sic** (-sĭk, -zĭk) *adj.*

hyp·am·ni·os (hĭ-păm′nē-ŏs′, hī-) *n.* The presence of an abnormally small amount of amniotic fluid.

hyp·an·a·ki·ne·sis (hĭ-păn′ə-kə-nē′sĭs, -kĭ-, hī-) *n.* A diminishing of normal gastric or intestinal movements.

hy·per·a·cid·i·ty (hī′pər-ə-sĭd′ĭ-tē) *n.* Abnormally high acidity, as of the stomach.

hy·per·ac·tive (hī′pər-ăk′tĭv) *adj.* **1.** Highly or excessively active, as of a gland. **2.** Having behavior characterized by constant overactivity. **3.** Afflicted with attention deficit disorder.

hy·per·ac·tiv·i·ty (hī′pər-ăk-tĭv′ĭ-tē) *n.* A general restlessness or excess of movement, such as that in children with minimal brain dysfunction or hyperkinesis.

hy·per·ad·e·no·sis (hī′pər-ăd′n-ō′sĭs) *n.* Enlargement of glands, especially of the lymph glands.

hy·per·ad·i·po·sis (hī′pər-ăd′ə-pō′sĭs) *n.* Excessive accumulation of body fat; extreme adiposis.

hy·per·a·dre·no·cor·ti·cal·ism (hī′pər-ə-drē′nō-kôr′tĭ-kə-lĭz′əm) *n.* Excessive secretion of adrenocortical hormones, especially cortisol.

hy·per·al·ge·si·a (hī′pər-ăl-jē′zē-ə, -zhə) *n.* Extreme sensitivity to pain. — **hy′per·al·ge′sic** (-sĭk, -zĭk) *adj.*

hy·per·al·i·men·ta·tion (hī′pər-ăl′ə-měn-tā′-shən) *n.* **1.** The administration or consumption of nutrients beyond normal requirements. **2.** The administration of nutrients by intravenous feeding, especially to persons who cannot take in food through the alimentary tract.

hy·per·bar·ic chamber (hī′pər-băr′ĭk) *n.* A compartment capable of high-pressure oxygenation, used to treat decompression sickness and anaerobic infections.

hyperbaric oxygen *n.* Oxygen at a pressure greater than one atmosphere.

hy·per·bar·ism (hī′pər-băr′ĭz′əm) *n.* Disturbances to the body resulting from the pressure of ambient gases at greater than normal atmospheric pressure.

hy·per·bil·i·ru·bi·ne·mi·a (hī′pər-bĭl′ĭ-rōō′bə-

nē′mē-ə) *n.* An abnormally high concentration of bilirubin in the blood.

hy·per·cal·ce·mi·a (hī′pər-kăl-sē′mē-ə) *n.* An abnormally high concentration of calcium in the blood.

hy·per·cal·ci·u·ri·a (hī′pər-kăl′sē-yŏŏr′ē-ə) *n.* The excretion of abnormally high concentrations of calcium in the urine.

hy·per·cap·ni·a (hī′pər-kăp′nē-ə) *n.* An increased concentration of carbon dioxide in the blood.

hy·per·chlo·re·mi·a (hī′pər-klôr-ē′mē-ə) *n.* An abnormally large amount of chloride ions in the blood.

hy·per·chlor·hy·dri·a (hī′pər-klôr-hī′drē-ə) *n.* The presence of an abnormal amount of hydrochloric acid in the stomach.

hy·per·cho·les·ter·ol·e·mia (hī′pər-kə-lĕs′tər-ə-lē′mē-ə) or **hy·per·cho·les·ter·e·mi·a** (-kə-lĕs′tə-rē′mē-ə) *n.* **1.** An abnormally high concentration of cholesterol in the blood. **2.** A familial disorder characterized by an abnormally high concentration of cholesterol in the blood.

hy·per·cho·li·a (hī′pər-kō′lē-ə) *n.* A condition in which an abnormally large amount of bile is formed in the liver.

hy·per·chro·ma·tism (hī′pər-krō′mə-tĭz′əm) *n.* Excessive formation of skin pigment. — **hy′per·chro·mat′ic** (-krə-măt′ĭk) *adj.*

hy·per·chro·mi·a (hī′pər-krō′mē-ə) *n.* See **hyperchromatism**.

hy·per·cy·to·sis (hī′pər-sī-tō′sĭs) *n.* An abnormal increase in the number of cells in the blood or the tissues, especially of white blood cells.

hy·per·dac·ty·ly (hī′pər-dăk′tə-lē) See **polydactyly**.

hy·per·e·che·ma (hī′pər-ĭ-kē′mə) *n.* The auditory magnification or exaggeration of a sound.

hy·per·em·e·sis (hī′pər-ĕm′ĭ-sĭs) *n.* Excessive vomiting. — **hy′per·e·met′ic** (-ĭ-mĕt′ĭk) *adj.*

hy·per·e·mi·a (hī′pər-ē′mē-ə) *n.* An increase in the quantity of blood flow to a body part; engorgement. — **hy′per·e′mic** (-mĭk) *adj.*

hy·per·e·o·sin·o·phil·ic syndrome (hī′pər-ē′ə-sĭn′ə-fĭl′ĭk) *n.* A syndrome in which the concentration of eosinophils increases in peripheral blood with later infiltration into bone marrow, heart, and other organ systems; it is accompanied by nocturnal sweating, coughing, anorexia and weight loss, itching and various skin lesions.

hy·per·es·the·sia or **hy·per·aes·the·sia** (hī′pər-ĭs-thē′zhə) *n.* An abnormal or pathological increase in sensitivity to sensory stimuli, as of the skin to touch or the ear to sound. — **hy′per·es·thet′ic** (-thĕt′ĭk) *adj.*

hy·per·ex·ten·sion (hī′pər-ĭk-stĕn′shən) *n.* Extension of a joint beyond its normal range of motion. — **hy′per·ex·tend′** (-ĭk-stĕnd′) *v.*

hyperextension-hyperflexion injury *n.* Violence to the body causing the unsupported head to rapidly hyperextend and hyperflex the neck, as in whiplash injury.

hy·per·fi·brin·o·ge·ne·mi·a (hī′pər-fī-brĭn′ə-jə-nē′mē-ə) *n.* An increased level of fibrinogen in the blood.

hy·per·flex·ion (hī′pər-flĕk′shən) *n.* Flexion of a limb or part beyond its normal range. — **hy′per·flex′** *v.*

hy·per·gal·ac·to·sis (hī′pər-găl′ək-tō′sĭs) *n.* The excessive secretion of milk.

hy·per·gam·ma·glob·u·li·ne·mi·a (hī′pər-găm′-ə-glŏb′yə-lə-nē′mē-ə) *n.* An increased concentration of gamma globulins in plasma, such as in chronic infectious diseases.

hy·per·gen·e·sis (hī′pər-jĕn′ĭ-sĭs) *n.* Excessive development or redundancy of parts or organs of the body. — **hy′per·ge·net′ic** (-jə-nĕt′ĭk) *adj.*

hy·per·glob·u·li·ne·mi·a (hī′pər-glŏb′yə-lə-nē′mē-ə) *n.* A condition characterized by abnormally large amounts of globulins in the blood.

hy·per·gly·ce·mi·a (hī′pər-glī-sē′mē-ə) *n.* The presence of an abnormally high concentration of glucose in the blood. — **hy′per·gly·ce′mic** (-mĭk) *adj.*

hy·per·glyc·er·i·de·mi·a (hī′pər-glĭs′ə-rĭ-dē′mē-ə) *n.* A condition characterized by an elevated concentration of glycerides in the blood, usually present within chylomicrons.

hy·per·gly·ci·ne·mi·a (hī′pər-glī′sə-nē′mē-ə) *n.* A hereditary disorder marked by an elevated concentration of glycine in the blood.

hy·per·gly·ci·nu·ri·a (hī′pər-glī′sə-noŏr′ē-ə, -nyoŏr′-) *n.* An abnormally high level of glycine in the urine.

hy·per·gly·co·su·ri·a (hī′pər-glī′kə-soŏr′ē-ə, -shoŏr′-) *n.* The persistent excretion of unusually large amounts of glucose in the urine.

hy·per·go·nad·ism (hī′pər-gō′năd-ĭz′əm, -gŏn′ə-dĭz′əm) *n.* A condition marked by excessive secretion of gonadal hormones, with precocious sexual development.

hy·per·he·mo·glo·bi·ne·mi·a (hī′pər-hē′mə-glō′bə-nē′mē-ə) *n.* A condition marked by an unusually large amount of hemoglobin in the circulating blood.

hy·per·hy·dra·tion (hī′pər-hī-drā′shən) *n.* Excess water content of the body.

hy·per·in·fec·tion (hī′pər-ĭn-fĕk′shən) *n.* Infection by very large numbers of organisms as a result of immunologic deficiency.

hy·per·in·su·lin·ism (hī′pər-ĭn′sə-lə-nĭz′əm) *n.* A condition marked by excessive secretion of insulin by the islets of Langerhans, resulting in hypoglycemia; the symptoms are similar to those of insulin shock, though more chronic in character.

hy·per·ka·le·mi·a (hī′pər-kə-lē′mē-ə) *n.* An abnormally high concentration of potassium ions in the blood.

hy·per·ka·le·mic periodic paralysis (hī′pər-kə-lē′mĭk) *n.* An inherited form of periodic paralysis in which the serum potassium level is elevated during attacks. Onset occurs in infancy, attacks are frequent but relatively mild, and myotonia is often present.

hy·per·ker·a·to·sis (hī′pər-kĕr′ə-tō′sĭs) *n., pl.* **-ses** (-sēz). Hypertrophy of the cornea or the horny layer of the skin. — **hy′per·ker′a·tot′ic** (-tŏt′ĭk) *adj.*

hy·per·ke·to·ne·mi·a (hī′pər-kē′tə-nē′mē-ə) *n.* The presence of elevated concentrations of ketone bodies in the blood.

hy·per·ke·to·nu·ri·a (hī′pər-kē′tə-noŏr′ē-ə, -nyoŏr′-) *n.* Increased urinary excretion of ketonic compounds.

hy·per·ki·net·ic syndrome (hī′pər-kə-nĕt′ĭk) *n.* A childhood or adolescent disorder characterized by excessive activity, emotional instability, significantly reduced attention span, and an absence of shyness and fear; it occasionally develops in persons with brain injury, mental defect, or epilepsy.

hy·per·lac·ta·tion (hī′pər-lăk-tā′shən) *n.* Continuance of lactation beyond the normal period.

hy·per·leu·ko·cy·to·sis (hī′pər-loŏ′kə-sī-tō′sĭs) *n.* An unusually large increase in the number and proportion of white blood cells in the blood or the tissues.

hy·per·lip·o·pro·tein·e·mi·a (hī′pər-lĭp′ō-prō′-tē-nē′mē-ə, -tē-ə-nē′-, -lĭ′pō-) *n.* A condition marked by an abnormally high level of lipoproteins in the blood.

hy·per·li·po·sis (hī′pər-lĭ-pō′sĭs) *n.* **1.** An extreme accumulation of fat in the body. **2.** An extreme degree of fatty degeneration.

hy·per·lu·cent lung (hī′pər-loŏ′sənt) *n.* The radiographic finding that one lung is less dense than the other normal lung, as from infection or a bronchial foreign body.

hy·per·ly·si·ne·mi·a (hī′pər-lī′sə-nē′mē-ə) *n.* A hereditary disorder marked by an abnormal increase of lysine in the blood and associated with mental retardation, convulsions, and anemia.

hy·per·men·or·rhe·a (hī′pər-mĕn′ə-rē′ə) *n.* Excessively prolonged or profuse menstrual flow.

hy·per·me·tab·o·lism (hī′pər-mĭ-tăb′ə-lĭz′əm) *n.* An abnormal increase in metabolic rate, as in thyrotoxicosis.

hy·per·me·tro·pi·a (hī′pər-mĭ-trō′pē-ə) *n.* See **hyperopia.**

hy·perm·ne·sia (hī′pərm-nē′zhə) *n.* Exceptionally exact or vivid memory, especially as associated with certain mental illnesses.

hy·per·na·tre·mi·a (hī′pər-nə-trē′mē-ə) *n.* An abnormally high concentration of sodium ions in the blood.

hy·per·o·pi·a (hī′pə-rō′pē-ə) *n.* An abnormal condition of the eye in which vision is better for distant objects than for near objects. — **hy′per·ope′** (hī′pə-rōp′) *n.* — **hy′per·o′pic** (-ō′pĭk, -ŏp′ĭk) *adj.*

hyperopic astigmatism *n.* Astigmatism in which one meridian is hyperopic while the one at a right angle to it is without refractive error.

hy·per·o·rex·i·a (hī′pə-rō-rĕk′sē-ə) *n.* See **bulimia.**

hy·per·os·mi·a (hī′pər-ŏz′mē-ə) *n.* An exaggerated or abnormally acute sense of smell.

hy·per·os·to·sis (hī′pər-ŏ-stō′sĭs) *n., pl.* **-ses** (-sēz). **1.** Excessive or abnormal thickening or growth of bone tissue. **2.** See **exostosis.** — **hy′per·os·tot′ic** (-ŏ-stŏt′ĭk) *adj.*

hy·per·o·var·i·an·ism (hī′pər-ō-vâr′ē-ə-nĭz′əm) *n.* A condition of sexual precocity in girls due to premature development of the ovaries accompanied by the secretion of ovarian hormones.

hy·per·ox·i·a (hī′pər-ŏk′sē-ə) *n.* **1.** An excess of oxygen in tissues and organs. **2.** A higher than normal oxygen tension, such as that produced by breathing air or oxygen at greater than atmospheric pressures.

hy·per·par·a·thy·roid·ism (hī′pər-păr′ə-thī′roi-dĭz′əm) *n.* An increase in the secretory activity of the parathyroid glands, causing resorption of calcified bone, elevated serum calcium, decreased serum phosphorus, and increased excretion of both calcium and phosphorus.

hy·per·per·i·stal·sis (hī′pər-pĕr′ĭ-stôl′sĭs, -stăl′-) *n.* A condition marked by excessive rapidity of the passage of food through the stomach and intestine.

hy·per·pha·lan·gism (hī′pər-fə-lăn′jĭz′əm, -fā-) *n.* The presence of a supernumerary phalanx or phalanges in a finger or toe.

hy·per·phen·yl·al·a·ni·ne·mi·a (hī′pər-fĕn′əl-ăl′ə-nə-nē′mē-ə, -fē′nəl-) *n.* Abnormally high blood levels of phenylalanine, which may or may not be associated with elevated tyrosine levels, observed especially in newborn infants.

hy·per·pho·ne·sis (hī′pər-fō-nē′sĭs) *n.* A noticeable increase in the perceived sound in auscultation or percussion.

hy·per·phos·pha·te·mi·a (hī′pər-fŏs′fə-tē′mē-ə) *n.* An abnormally high concentration of phosphates in the blood.

hy·per·phos·pha·tu·ri·a (hī′pər-fŏs′fə-tŏŏr′ē-ə, -tyŏŏr′-) *n.* An increased excretion of phosphates in the urine.

hy·per·pig·men·ta·tion (hī′pər-pĭg′mən-tā′shən) *n.* The presence of excess pigment in a tissue or body part.

hy·per·pi·tu·i·ta·rism (hī′pər-pĭ-tōō′ĭ-tə-rĭz′əm, -tyōō′-) *n.* **1.** Pathologically excessive production of anterior pituitary hormones, especially somatotropin. **2.** The condition resulting from an excess of pituitary hormones, characterized by gigantism in children and acromegaly in adults. — **hy′per·pi·tu′i·tar′y** (-tēr′ē) *adj.*

hy·per·pla·sia (hī′pər-plā′zhə) *n.* An abnormal increase in the number of cells in a tissue or organ, excluding tumor formation, whereby the bulk of the part or organ is increased. — **hy′per·plas′tic** (-plăs′tĭk) *adj.*

hyperplastic polyp *n.* A benign small sessile polyp of the large bowel with lengthening and cystic dilation of mucosal glands.

hy·perp·ne·a (hī′pərp-nē′ə, hī′pər-nē′ə) *n.* Abnormally deep and rapid breathing. — **hy′perp·ne′ic** (-ĭk) *adj.*

hy·per·pro·li·ne·mi·a (hī′pər-prō′lə-nē′mē-ə) *n.* A hereditary metabolic disorder characterized by elevated proline concentrations in the blood and

by urinary excretion of proline, hydroxyproline, and glycine.

hy·per·pro·tein·e·mi·a (hī′pər-prō′tē-nē′mē-ə, -tē-ə-nē′-) *n.* An abnormally high concentration of protein in the blood.

hy·per·py·rex·i·a (hī′pər-pī-rĕk′sē-ə) *n.* Abnormally high fever. — **hy′per·py·rex′i·al, hy′per·py·ret′ic** (-rĕt′ĭk) *adj.*

hy·per·sal·i·va·tion (hī′pər-săl′ə-vā′shən) *n.* See **ptyalism.**

hy·per·sar·co·si·ne·mi·a (hī′pər-sär′kə-sə-nē′-mē-ə) *n.* See **sarcosinemia.**

hy·per·se·cre·tion (hī′pər-sĭ-krē′shən) *n.* The excessive production of any bodily secretion.

hypersecretory *adj.* Of or relating to excessive production of a bodily secretion.

hy·per·sen·si·tive (hī′pər-sĕn′sĭ-tĭv) *adj.* Responding excessively to the stimulus of a foreign agent, such as an allergen; abnormally sensitive. — **hy′per·sen′si·tive·ness, hy′per·sen′si·tiv′i·ty** (-tĭv′ĭ-tē) *n.*

hy·per·sen·si·ti·za·tion (hī′pər-sĕn′sĭ-tĭ-zā′shən) *n.* The act of inducing hypersensitiveness.

hy·per·som·ni·a (hī′pər-sŏm′nē-ə) *n.* A condition in which one sleeps for an excessively long time but is normal in the waking intervals.

hy·per·splen·ism (hī′pər-splĕn′ĭz′əm, splē′nĭz′-əm) *n.* A condition in which the hemolytic action of the spleen is greatly increased.

hy·per·sthe·nu·ri·a (hī′pər-sthē-nŏŏr′ē-ə, -nyŏŏr′-) *n.* Excretion of urine of unusually high specific gravity and concentration of solutes, resulting usually from loss or deprivation of water.

hy·per·ten·sion (hī′pər-tĕn′shən) *n.* **1.** Persistent high blood pressure. **2.** Arterial disease marked by chronic high blood pressure.

hy·per·ten·sive (hī′pər-tĕn′sĭv) *adj.* **1.** Of or characterized by abnormally increased blood pressure. **2.** Causing an increase in blood pressure. — *n.* A person having or susceptible to high blood pressure.

hypertensive retinopathy *n.* A retinal condition occurring in accelerated hypertension and characterized by arteriolar constriction, flame-shaped hemorrhages, cotton-wool patches, progressive severity of star-shaped edematous spot at the macula, and papilledema.

hy·per·ther·mi·a (hī′pər-thûr′mē-ə) *n.* Extremely high fever or body temperature, especially when therapeutically induced. — **hy′per·ther′mal** *adj.*

hy·per·throm·bi·ne·mi·a (hī′pər-thrŏm′bə-nē′-mē-ə) *n.* An abnormal increase of thrombin in the blood, frequently resulting in a tendency to intravascular coagulation.

hy·per·thy·mism (hī′pər-thī′mĭz′əm) *n.* Excessive activity of the thymus gland. — **hy′per·thy′mic** *adj.*

hy·per·thy·roid·ism (hī′pər-thī′roi-dĭz′əm) *n.* **1.** Pathologically excessive production of thyroid hormones. **2.** The condition resulting from excessive activity of the thyroid gland, characterized by increased basal metabolism. — **hy′per·thy′-roid** *adj.*

hy·per·to·ni·a (hī′pər-tō′nē-ə) *n*. Extreme tension of the muscles or arteries.

hy·per·ton·ic (hī′pər-tŏn′ĭk) *adj*. Having extreme muscular or arterial tension; spastic. — **hy′per·to·nic′i·ty** (-tə-nĭs′ĭ-tē, -tō-) *n*.

hy·per·tri·cho·sis (hī′pər-trĭ-kō′sĭs) *n*. Growth of hair in excess of the normal.

hy·per·tri·glyc·er·i·de·mi·a (hī′pər-trī-glĭs′ər-ĭ-dē′mē-ə) *n*. An elevated triglyceride concentration in the blood.

hypertrophic hy·per·se·cre·to·ry gastropathy (sī-krē′tə-rē) *n*. Nodular thickenings of the gastric mucosa with acid hypersecretion and frequently with peptic ulceration that is not associated with a gastrin-secreting tumor.

hypertrophic rhinitis *n*. Chronic rhinitis with permanent thickening of the mucous membrane.

hy·per·tro·phy (hī-pûr′trə-fē) *n*. A nontumorous enlargement of an organ or a tissue as a result of an increase in the size rather than the number of constituent cells. — *v*. **-phied, -phy·ing, -phies.** To grow or cause to grow abnormally large. — **hy′per·tro′phic** (-trō′fĭk, -trŏf′ĭk) *adj*.

hy·per·u·ri·ce·mi·a (hī′pər-yŏŏr′ĭ-sē′mē-ə) *n*. An abnormally high concentration of uric acid in the blood, associated with gout. — **hy′per·u′ri·ce′mic** *adj*.

hy·per·ven·ti·late (hī′pər-vĕn′tl-āt′) *v*. **-lat·ed, -lat·ing, -lates.** **1.** To breathe abnormally fast or deeply so as to effect hyperventilation. **2.** To breathe in this manner as from excitement or anxiety.

hy·per·ven·ti·la·tion (hī′pər-vĕn′tl-ā′shən) *n*. Abnormally fast or deep respiration resulting in the loss of carbon dioxide from the blood, thereby causing a fall in blood pressure, tingling of the extremities, and sometimes fainting. — **hy′per·ven′ti·late′** *v*.

hy·per·vi·ta·min·o·sis (hī′pər-vī′tə-mə-nō′sĭs) *n*. Any of various abnormal conditions caused by excessive intake of a vitamin.

hy·per·vo·le·mi·a (hī′′pər-vŏ-lē′mē-ə) *n*. An abnormally increased volume of circulating blood. — **hy′per·vo·le′mic** *adj*.

hy·phe·mi·a (hī-fē′mē-ə) *n*. See **oligemia.**

hyp·nes·the·sia (hĭp′nĭs-thē′zhə) *n*. See **drowsiness.**

hyp·no·a·nal·y·sis (hĭp′nō-ə-năl′ĭ-sĭs) *n*. The use of hypnosis in conjunction with psychoanalytic techniques.

hyp·no·gen·e·sis (hĭp′nō-jĕn′ĭ-sĭs) *n*. The process of inducing or entering sleep or a hypnotic state. — **hyp′no·ge·net′ic** (-jə-nĕt′ĭk), **hyp′no·gen′ic, hyp′nog′e·nous** (hĭp-nŏj′ə-nəs) *adj*.

hyp·no·pho·bi·a (hĭp′nə-fō′bē-ə) *n*. An abnormal fear of falling asleep. — **hyp′no·pho′bic** *adj*.

hyp·no·sis (hĭp-nō′sĭs) *n*., *pl*. **-ses** (-sēz). **1.** A trancelike state resembling somnambulism, usually induced by another person, in which the subject may experience forgotten or suppressed memories, hallucinations, and heightened suggestibility. **2.** A sleeplike state or condition. **3.** Hypnotism.

hyp·no·ther·a·py (hĭp′nō-thĕr′ə-pē) *n*. **1.** Therapy based on or using hypnosis, especially for treatment of chronic pain. **2.** Treatment of disease by inducing prolonged sleep.

hyp·not·ic (hĭp-nŏt′ĭk) *adj*. **1.** Of or relating to hypnotism or hypnosis. **2.** Inducing or tending to induce sleep; soporific. — *n*. An agent that causes sleep; a soporific.

hyp·no·tism (hĭp′nə-tĭz′əm) *n*. **1.** The theory or practice of inducing hypnosis. **2.** The act of inducing hypnosis. — **hyp′no·tist** *n*.

hyp·no·tize (hĭp′nə-tīz′) *v*. **-tized, -tiz·ing, -tiz·es.** To put a person into a state of hypnosis. — **hyp′no·tiz′a·bil′i·ty** *n*. — **hyp′no·tiz′a·ble** *adj*. — **hyp′no·ti·za′tion** (-tĭ-zā′shən) *n*.

hy·po (hī′pō) *n*. **1.** A hypodermic syringe. **2.** A hypodermic injection.

hy·po·ad·re·nal·ism (hī′pō-ə-drē′nə-lĭz′əm, -drĕn′ə-) *n*. Reduced adrenocortical function.

hy·po·al·bu·mi·ne·mi·a (hī′pō-ăl-byōō′mə-nē′mē-ə) or **hyp·al·bu·mi·ne·mi·a** (hĭp′ăl-, hī′păl-) *n*. An abnormally low concentration of albumin in the blood.

hy·po·al·i·men·ta·tion (hī′pō-ăl′ə-mĕn-tā′shən) *n*. A condition of insufficient nourishment.

hy·po·al·ler·gen·ic (hī′pō-ăl′ər-jĕn′ĭk) *adj*. Having a decreased tendency to provoke an allergic reaction.

hy·po·bar·ism (hī′pə-băr′ĭz′əm) *n*. Dysbarism resulting from greater gas pressure within the body than in the surrounding medium, so that gas in body cavities expands and gases in body fluids bubble out of solution.

hy·po·blast (hī′pə-blăst′) *n*. See **endoderm.** — **hy′po·blas′tic** *adj*.

hy·po·cal·ce·mi·a (hī′pō-kăl-sē′mē-ə) *n*. Abnormally low levels of calcium in the blood. — **hy′po·cal·ce′mic** *adj*.

hy·po·cap·ni·a (hī′pō-kăp′nē-ə) *n*. A deficient level of carbon dioxide in the blood.

hy·po·chlo·re·mi·a (hī′pō-klôr-ē′mē-ə) *n*. An abnormally low concentration of chloride ions in the blood. — **hy′po·chlo·re′mic** *adj*.

hy·po·chlor·hy·dri·a (hī′pō-klôr-hī′drē-ə) *n*. An abnormally small amount of hydrochloric acid in the stomach.

hy·po·chlor·u·ri·a (hī′pō-klôr-yŏŏr′ē-ə) *n*. The excretion of abnormally small quantities of chloride ions in the urine.

hy·po·cho·les·ter·ol·e·mi·a (hī′pō-kə-lĕs′tər-ə-lē′mē-ə) *n*. Abnormally small amounts of cholesterol in the blood.

hy·po·chon·dri·a (hī′pə-kŏn′drē-ə) *n*. The persistent neurotic conviction that one is or is likely to become ill, often involving experiences of real pain when illness is neither present nor likely.

hy·po·chon·dri·ac (hī′pə-kŏn′drē-ăk′) *n*. A person afflicted with hypochondria. — *adj*. **1.** Relating to or afflicted with hypochondria. **2.** Relating to or located in the left or right hypochondrium. — **hy′po·chon·dri′a·cal** (-kŏn-drī′ə-kəl) *adj*.

hy·po·chon·dri·um (hī′pə-kŏn′drē-əm) *n*., *pl*. **-dri·a** (-drē-ə). The upper lateral region of the abdomen on either side of the epigastrium and below the lower ribs.

hy·po·chon·dro·pla·sia (hī′pō-kŏn′drō-plā′zhə, -zhē-ə) *n.* A form of congenital dwarfism similar to but milder than achondroplasia, not familial and not evident until mid-childhood, in which the skull and facial features are normal.

hy·po·cy·the·mi·a (hī′pō-sī-thē′mē-ə) *n.* Abnormally low numbers of red and white blood cells and other formed elements of the circulating blood, as in aplastic anemia.

hy·po·dac·ty·ly (hī′pō-dăk′tə-lē) *n.* The condition of having fewer than five digits on a hand or foot.

hy·po·der·mic (hī′pə-dûr′mĭk) *adj.* **1.** Of or relating to the layer just beneath the epidermis. **2.** Relating to the hypodermis. **3.** Injected beneath the skin. — *n.* **1.** A hypodermic injection. **2.** A hypodermic needle. **3.** A hypodermic syringe. — **hy′-po·der′mi·cal·ly** *adv.*

hypodermic injection *n.* A subcutaneous, intracutaneous, intramuscular, or intravenous injection by means of a hypodermic syringe and needle.

hypodermic needle *n.* **1.** A hollow needle used with a hypodermic syringe. **2.** A hypodermic syringe including the needle.

hypodermic syringe *n.* A small syringe with a calibrated barrel, plunger, and tip, used with a hypodermic needle for hypodermic injections and for aspiration.

hy·po·der·mis (hī′pə-dûr′mĭs) or **hy·po·derm** (hī′pə-dûrm′) *n.* A loose fibrous envelope beneath the skin, containing the cutaneous vessels and nerves.

hy·po·der·moc·ly·sis (hī′pə-dûr-mŏk′lĭ-sĭs) *n.* Subcutaneous injection of a saline or other solution.

hy·po·er·gi·a (hī′pō-ûr′jē-ə) or **hy·po·er·gy** (hī′-pō-ûr′jē) *n.* See **hyposensitivity.**

hy·po·es·the·sia (hī′pō-ĭs-thē′zhə) or **hy·pes·the·sia** (hī′pĭs-) *n.* Partial loss of sensitivity to sensory stimuli; diminished sensation. — **hy′pes·the′sic** (-thē′sĭk, -zĭk), **hy′pes·thet′ic** (-thět′ĭk) *adj.*

hy·po·func·tion (hī′pō-fŭngk′shən) *n.* Diminished, abnormally low, or inadequate functioning.

hy·po·ga·lac·ti·a (hī′pō-gə-lăk′tē-ə, -shē-ə) *n.* Abnormally low milk secretion.

hy·po·gam·ma·glob·u·li·ne·mi·a (hī′pō-găm′ə-glŏb′yə-lə-nē′mē-ə) *n.* **1.** Decreased quantity of the gamma fraction of serum globulin. **2.** A decreased quantity of immunoglobulins.

hy·po·gas·tri·um (hī′pə-găs′trē-əm) *n., pl.* **-tri·a** (-trē-ə). See **pubic region.** — **hy′po·gas′tric** *adj.*

hy·po·geu·si·a (hī′pə-gyōō′zē-ə, -zhə, -jōō′-) *n.* Impairment of the sense of taste.

hy·po·glos·sal nerve (hī′pə-glŏ′səl) *n.* Either of a pair of nerves that arise from the medulla, and supply the intrinsic and extrinsic muscles of the tongue.

hy·po·gly·ce·mi·a (hī′pō-glī-sē′mē-ə) *n.* An abnormally low concentration of glucose in the blood.

hy·po·gly·ce·mic (hī′pō-glī-sē′mĭk) *adj.* **1.** Of or

relating to hypoglycemia. **2.** Lowering the concentration of glucose in the blood. Used of a drug.

hy·po·go·nad·ism (hī′pō-gō′năd-ĭz′əm, -gŏn′ə-dĭz′əm) *n.* Inadequate functioning of the testes or ovaries as manifested by deficiencies in gametogenesis or the secretion of gonadal hormones.

hy·po·hi·dro·sis (hī′pō-hī-drō′sĭs, -hī-) or **hyp·hi·dro·sis** (hĭp′hī-drō′sĭs, -hī-, hĭp′-) *n.* Diminished perspiration. — **hy′po·hi·drot′ic** (-drŏt′ĭk) *adj.*

hy·po·ka·le·mi·a (hī′pō-kə-lē′mē-ə) *n.* An abnormally low concentration of potassium ions in the blood.

hy·po·ka·le·mic periodic paralysis (hī′pō-kə-lē′-mĭk) *n.* An inherited form of periodic paralysis in which the serum potassium level is low during attacks. Onset usually occurs between the ages of 7 and 21 years; attacks may occur with exposure to cold or ingestion of a high-carbohydrate meal or alcohol, and may cause respiratory paralysis.

hy·po·men·or·rhe·a (hī′pō-měn′ə-rē′ə) *n.* A diminution of the flow or a shortening of the duration of menstruation.

hy·po·me·tab·o·lism (hī′pō-mĭ-tăb′ə-lĭz′əm) *n.* An abnormal decrease in metabolic rate.

hy·pom·ne·sia (hī′pŏm-nē′zhə) *n.* Impaired memory.

hy·po·na·tre·mi·a (hī′pō-nə-trē′mē-ə) *n.* An abnormally low concentration of sodium ions in the blood.

hy·po·nych·i·um (hī′pō-nĭk′ē-əm) *n.* The epithelium of the nail bed, especially its posterior part in the region of the lunula. — **hy′po·nych′i·al** *adj.*

hy·po·pan·cre·a·tism (hī′pō-păng′krē-ə-tĭz′əm, păn′-) *n.* A condition of diminished secretory activity of the pancreas.

hy·po·par·a·thy·roid·ism (hī′pō-păr′ə-thī′roi-dĭz′əm) *n.* A condition due to diminution or absence of the secretion of the parathyroid hormones; parathyroid insufficiency.

hy·po·pha·lan·gism (hī′pō-fə-lăn′jĭz′əm) *n.* Congenital absence of one or more of the phalanges of a finger or toe.

hy·po·phos·pha·te·mi·a (hī′pō-fŏs′fə-tē′mē-ə) *n.* Abnormally low concentrations of phosphates in the blood.

hy·po·phos·pha·tu·ri·a (hī′pō-fŏs′fə-tŏŏr′ē-ə, -tyŏŏr′-) *n.* Abnormally low urinary excretion of phosphates.

hy·poph·y·sec·to·my (hī-pŏf′ĭ-sĕk′tə-mē) *n.* Surgical excision or destruction of the pituitary gland.

hy·poph·y·sis (hī-pŏf′ĭ-sĭs) *n., pl.* **-ses** (-sēz′). See **pituitary gland.**

hy·poph·y·si·tis (hī-pŏf′ĭ-sī′tĭs) *n.* Inflammation of the pituitary gland.

hy·po·pi·tu·i·ta·rism (hī′pō-pĭ-tōō′ĭ-tə-rĭz′əm, -tyōō′-) *n.* **1.** Deficient or diminished production of pituitary hormones. **2.** The condition resulting from a deficiency in pituitary hormone, especially growth hormone, characterized by dwarfism in children and various hormonal deficiencies. — **hy′po·pi·tu′i·tar′y** (-tĕr′ē) *adj.*

hy·po·pla·sia (hī′pō-plā′zhə, -zhē-ə) *n.* **1.** Incomplete or arrested development of an organ or a part. **2.** Atrophy due to destruction of some of the elements of a tissue or an organ. — **hy′po·plas′tic** (-plăs′tĭk) *adj.*

hypoplastic anemia *n.* Progressive nonregenerative anemia resulting from greatly depressed, inadequately functioning bone marrow that may lead to aplastic anemia.

hy·pop·ne·a (hī-pŏp′nē-ə, hī′pō-nē′ə) *n.* Abnormally slow or shallow breathing. — **hy′pop·ne′ic** *adj.*

hy·po·po·tas·se·mi·a (hī′pō-pə-tă-sē′mē-ə) *n.* See **hypokalemia.**

hy·po·pro·tein·e·mi·a (hī′pō-prō′tē-nē′mē-ə, -tē-ə-nē′-) *n.* Abnormally small amounts of total protein in the blood.

hy·po·py·on (hī-pō′pē-ŏn′) *n.* The presence of pus or a puslike fluid in the anterior chamber of the eye.

hy·po·sal·i·va·tion (hī′pō-săl′ə-vā′shən) *n.* Abnormally reduced salivation.

hy·po·sen·si·tiv·i·ty (hī′pō-sĕn′sĭ-tĭv′ĭ-tē) *n.* Less than normal sensitivity to a foreign agent, such as an allergen, in which the response is unusually delayed or lessened in degree. — **hy′po·sen′si·tive** *adj.*

hy·po·sen·si·tize (hī′pō-sĕn′sĭ-tīz′) *n.* **-tized, -tiz·ing, -tiz·es.** To make less sensitive, as to an allergen; desensitize.

hy·po·spa·di·as (hī′pō-spā′dē-əs) or **hy·po·spa·di·a** (-dē-ə) *n.* **1.** A developmental anomaly of the urethra in which part of the urethral canal is open on the undersurface of the penis or on the perineum. **2.** A similar anomaly in which the urethra opens into the vagina.

hy·pos·the·nu·ri·a (hī-pŏs′thə-nŏŏr′ē-ə, -nyŏŏr′-) *n.* Excretion of urine of low specific gravity due to an inability of the tubules of the kidneys to produce concentrated urine.

hy·po·tel·or·ism (hī′pō-tĕl′ə-rĭz′əm) *n.* Abnormal closeness of the eyes.

hy·po·ten·sion (hī′pə-tĕn′shən) *n.* **1.** Abnormally low arterial blood pressure. **2.** Reduced pressure or tension of any kind, as of intraocular fluids.

hy·po·ten·sive (hī′pə-tĕn′sĭv) *adj.* **1.** Of or characterized by low blood pressure. **2.** Causing a reduction in blood pressure.

hy·po·thal·a·mus (hī′pō-thăl′ə-məs) *n.* The part of the brain that lies below the thalamus, functioning to regulate bodily temperature, certain metabolic processes, and other autonomic activities. — **hy′po·tha·lam′ic** (-thə-lăm′ĭk) *adj.*

hy·po·the·nar (hī′pō-thē′när′, -nər, hī-pŏth′ə-) *n.* The fleshy mass at the medial side of the palm. — *adj.* Of or relating to this part.

hy·po·ther·mi·a (hī′pə-thûr′mē-ə) *n.* Abnormally low body temperature. — **hy′po·ther′mic** (-mĭk) *adj.*

hy·po·throm·bi·ne·mi·a (hī′pō-thrŏm′bə-nē′mē -ə) *n.* Abnormally low levels of thrombin in the blood, resulting in a tendency to bleed without clotting.

hy·po·thy·mi·a (hī′pō-thī′mē-ə) *n.* A state of diminished emotional response; despondency or depression.

hy·po·thy·mism (hī′pō-thī′mĭz′əm) *n.* Reduced or inadequate functioning of the thymus.

hy·po·thy·roid·ism (hī′pō-thī′roi-dĭz′əm) *n.* **1.** Insufficient production of thyroid hormones. **2.** A pathological condition resulting from thyroid insufficiency, which may lead to cretinism or myxedema.

hy·po·to·ni·a (hī′pō-tō′nē-ə) *n.* **1.** Reduced tension or pressure, as of the intraocular fluid in the eyeball. **2.** Relaxation of the arteries. **3.** Loss of muscle tone, resulting in stretching of the muscles beyond their normal limits.

hy·po·tri·cho·sis (hī′pō-trĭ-kō′sĭs) *n.* A less than normal amount of hair on the head or body.

hy·pot·ro·phy (hī-pŏt′rə-fē) *n.* Progressive degeneration of an organ or tissue caused by loss of cells.

hy·po·u·ri·ce·mi·a (hī′pō-yŏŏr′ĭ-sē′mē-ə) *n.* Abnormally reduced blood concentration of uric acid.

hy·po·u·ri·cu·ri·a (hī′pō-yŏŏr′ĭ-kyŏŏr′ē-ə) *n.* Abnormally small amounts of uric acid in the urine.

hy·po·ven·ti·la·tion (hī′pə-vĕn′tl-ā′shən) *n.* Reduced or deficient ventilation of the lungs, resulting in reduced aeration of blood in the lungs and an increased level of carbon dioxide in the blood.

hy·po·vi·ta·min·o·sis (hī′pō-vī′tə-mə-nō′sĭs) *n.* Insufficiency of one or more essential vitamins.

hy·po·vo·le·mi·a (hī′′pō-vō-lē′mē-ə) *n.* See **oligemia.** — **hy′po·vo·le′mic** *adj.*

hypovolemic shock *n.* Shock caused by a reduction in the volume of blood, as from hemorrhage or dehydration.

hy·po·xan·thine (hī′pō-zăn′thēn′) *n.* A purine present in muscle and other tissues, formed during uric acid synthesis.

hy·pox·e·mi·a (hī′pŏk-sē′mē-ə) *n.* Insufficient oxygenation of arterial blood. — **hy′pox·e′mic** *adj.*

hy·pox·i·a (hī-pŏk′sē-ə, hī-) *n.* Deficient levels of oxygen in blood or tissue. — **hy·pox′ic** *adj.*

hypoxic hypoxia *n.* Hypoxia resulting from defective oxygenation in the lungs, as is caused by low oxygen tension, abnormal pulmonary function, or a right-to-left shunt in the heart.

hys·ter·ec·to·my (hĭs′tə-rĕk′tə-mē) *n.* Surgical removal of part or all of the uterus.

hys·ter·eu·ry·sis (hĭs′tər-yŏŏr′ĭ-sĭs) *n.* Dilation of the lower segment and cervical canal of the uterus.

hys·ter·i·a (hĭ-stĕr′ē-ə, -stĕr′-) *n.* **1.** A neurosis characterized by the presentation of a physical ailment without an organic cause, sleepwalking, amnesia, episodes of hallucinations, and other mental and behavioral aberrations. **2.** Excessive or uncontrollable emotion, such as fear or panic. — **hys·ter′i·cal** (hĭ-stĕr′ĭ-kəl) *adj.*

hysterical personality *n.* A personality disorder characterized by immaturity, dependence, self-centeredness, and vanity, with a craving for attention, activity, or excitement, and behavior that is markedly unstable or manipulative.

hys·ter·o·cele (hĭs′tə-rō-sēl′) *n.* **1.** An abdominal or perineal hernia containing part or all of the uterus. **2.** Protrusion of uterine contents into a weakened, bulging area of the uterine wall.

hys·ter·o·clei·sis (hĭs′tə-rō-klī′sĭs) *n., pl.* **-ses** (-sēz′). Surgical occlusion of the uterus.

hys·ter·o·ep·i·lep·sy (hĭs′tə-rō-ĕp′ə-lĕp′sē) *n.* Hysteria accompanied by convulsions resembling epileptic seizures.

hys·ter·o·gram (hĭs′tə-rō-grăm′) *n.* **1.** An x-ray of the uterus, usually using contrast media. **2.** A graphic record of the strength of uterine contractions during labor.

hys·ter·o·graph (hĭs′tə-rō-grăf′) *n.* An apparatus for recording the strength of uterine contractions during labor.

hys·ter·og·ra·phy (hĭs′tə-rŏg′rə-fē) *n.* **1.** Radiography of a uterine cavity filled with contrast medium. **2.** The procedure of recording uterine contractions during labor.

hys·ter·o·my·o·ma (hĭs′tə-rō-mī-ō′mə) *n.* A myoma of the uterus.

hys·ter·o·my·o·mec·to·my (hĭs′tə-rō-mī′ə-mĕk′tə-mē) *n.* Surgical removal of a uterine myoma.

hys·ter·o·my·ot·o·my (hĭs′tə-rō-mī-ŏt′ə-mē) *n.* Surgical incision into the uterine muscles.

hys·ter·o·o·o·pho·rec·to·my (hĭs′tə-rō-ō′ə-fə-rĕk′tə-mē) *n.* Surgical removal of the uterus and ovaries.

hys·ter·op·a·thy (hĭs′tə-rŏp′ə-thē) *n.* A disease or disorder of the uterus. **— hys′ter·o·path′ic** (-rō-păth′ĭk) *adj.*

hys·ter·o·pex·y (hĭs′tə-rō-pĕk′sē) *n.* Surgical fixation of a misplaced or overly movable uterus.

hys·ter·o·plas·ty (hĭs′tə-rō-plăs′tē) *n.* See **uteroplasty**.

hys·ter·or·rha·phy (hĭs′tə-rôr′ə-fē) *n.* Repair of a torn or lacerated uterus by suturing.

hys·ter·or·rhex·is (hĭs′tə-rō-rĕk′sĭs) *n.* Rupture of the uterus.

hys·ter·o·sal·pin·gec·to·my (hĭs′tə-rō-săl′pĭn-jĕk′tə-mē) *n.* Surgical removal of the uterus and one or both oviducts.

hys·ter·o·sal·pin·gog·ra·phy (hĭs′tə-rō-săl′pĭng-gŏg′rə-fē) *n.* Radiography of the uterus and oviducts after the injection of radiopaque material.

hys·ter·o·sal·pin·go·o·o·pho·rec·to·my (hĭs′tə-rō-săl-pĭng′gō-ō′ə-fə-rĕk′tə-mē) *n.* Surgical excision of the uterus, oviducts, and ovaries.

hys·ter·o·sal·pin·gos·to·my (hĭs′tə-rō-săl′pĭng-gŏs′tə-mē, -pĭn-) *n.* Surgical restoration of a connection between the uterus and an occluded fallopian tube.

hys·ter·o·scope (hĭs′tə-rō-skōp′) *n.* An endoscope used in direct visual examination of the uterine cavity.

hys·ter·os·co·py (hĭs′tə-rŏs′kə-pē) *n.* Visual inspection of the uterine cavity with an endoscope.

hys·ter·ot·o·my (hĭs′tə-rŏt′ə-mē) *n.* Surgical incision of the uterus.

hys·ter·o·tra·che·lec·to·my (hĭs′tə-rō-trā′kə-lĕk′tə-mē, -trăk′ə-) *n.* Surgical removal of the uterine cervix.

hys·ter·o·tra·che·lo·plas·ty (hĭs′tə-rō-trā′kə-lō-plăs′tē, -trăk′ə-) *n.* Surgical repair of the uterine cervix.

hys·ter·o·tra·che·lor·rha·phy (hĭs′tə-rō-trā′kə-lôr′ə-fē, -trăk′ə-) *n.* Repair of a lacerated uterine cervix by suturing.

hys·ter·o·tra·che·lot·o·my (hĭs′tə-rō-trā′kə-lŏt′ə-mē, -trăk′ə-) *n.* Surgical incision of the uterine cervix.

hys·ter·o·tu·bog·ra·phy (hĭs′tə-rō-tōō-bŏg′rə-fē, -tyōō-) *n.* See **hysterosalpingography**.

~ ~ ~ ~ ~ ~ I ~ ~ ~ ~ ~ ~

I 131 uptake test *n.* A test of thyroid function in which ¹³¹I-iodide is given orally and 24 hours later the amount present in the thyroid gland is measured and compared with normal levels.

i·at·ro·gen·ic (ī-ăt′rə-jĕn′ĭk) *adj.* Induced in a patient by a physician's activity, manner, or therapy. Used especially of an infection or other complication of treatment.

iatrogenic transmission *n.* Transmission of infectious agents due to a medical procedure.

IBD *abbr.* inflammatory bowel disease

i·bo·ga·ine (ĭ-bō′gə-ēn′, -ĭn) *n.* A white powdery substance that can act as a stimulant, hallucinogen, or memory stimulant, or as a selective dopamine blocker that stems the craving for heroin and cocaine without causing dependency.

i·bu·pro·fen (ī′byōō-prō′fən) *n.* A nonsteroidal anti-inflammatory medication used especially in the treatment of arthritis and commonly taken for its analgesic and antipyretic properties.

ice bag *n.* See **ice pack**.

I cell *n.* See **inclusion cell**.

ice pack *n.* A folded sac filled with crushed ice and applied to sore or swollen parts of the body to reduce pain and inflammation.

i·chor (ī′kôr′, ī′kər) *n.* A watery, acrid discharge from a wound or ulcer. **— i′chor·ous** (ī′kər-əs) *adj.*

ich·thy·ism (ĭk′thē-ĭz′əm) *n.* See **ichthyotoxism**.

ich·thy·o·sis (ĭk′thē-ō′sĭs) *n.* A congenital, often hereditary skin disease characterized by dry, thickened, scaly skin.

ich·thy·o·tox·ism (ĭk′thē-ō-tŏk′sĭz′əm) *n.* Poisoning by a toxic substance derived from fish.

ic·ter·us (ĭk′tər-əs) *n.* See **jaundice.**

ic·tus (ĭk′təs) *n., pl.* **ictus** or **-tus·es.** A sudden attack, stroke, or seizure.

ICU *abbr.* intensive care unit

id (ĭd) *n.* In psychoanalytic theory, the division of the psyche that is unconscious and serves as the source of instinctual impulses and demands for immediate satisfaction of primitive needs.

IDD *abbr.* insulin-dependent diabetes

i·de·a (ī-dē′ə) *n.* A thought or conception that exists in the mind as a product of mental activity.

idea of reference *n.* The belief that other people's statements or acts have special reference to oneself when in fact they do not.

i·de·a·tion (ī′dē-ā′shən) *n.* The formation of ideas or mental images. — **i′de·ate′** *v.*

i·dée fixe (ē-dā fēks′) *n., pl.* **i·dées fixes** (ē-dā fēks′). A fixed idea; an obsession.

i·den·ti·cal (ī-dĕn′tĭ-kəl) *adj.* **1.** Exactly equal and alike. **2.** Of or relating to a twin or twins developed from the same fertilized ovum and having the same genetic makeup and closely similar appearance; monozygotic.

identical twins *pl.n.* Twins derived from the same fertilized ovum that at an early stage of development becomes separated into independently growing cell aggregations, giving rise to two individuals of the same sex, identical genetic makeup, and closely similar appearance.

i·den·ti·fi·ca·tion (ī-dĕn′tə-fĭ-kā′shən) *n.* **1.** A person's association with the qualities, characteristics, or views of another person or group. **2.** An unconscious process by which a person transfers the response appropriate to a particular person or group to a different person or group.

i·den·ti·ty (ī-dĕn′tĭ-tē) *n.* **1.** The set of behavioral or personal characteristics by which an individual is recognizable as a member of a group. **2.** The distinct personality of an individual.

identity crisis *n.* A psychosocial state or condition of disorientation and role confusion occurring especially in adolescents as a result of conflicting pressures and expectations.

identity disorder *n.* A disorder occurring in late adolescence and characterized by feelings of uncertainty and distress due to issues such as long-term goals, sexuality, morality, and religion.

id·i·o·ag·glu·ti·nin (ĭd′ē-ō-ə-glōōt′n-ĭn) *n.* An agglutinin that occurs in the blood of a person or animal without injection of a stimulating antigen or without passive transfer of antibodies.

id·i·o·gram (ĭd′ē-ə-grăm′) *n.* A diagrammatic representation of chromosome morphology characteristic of a species or a population.

id·i·o·het·er·ol·y·sin (ĭd′ē-ō-hĕt′ə-rŏl′ĭ-sĭn, -rō-lī′sĭn) *n.* An idiolysin in the blood of an animal of one species, but capable of combining with the red blood cells of another species, thereby causing hemolysis when complement is present.

id·i·ol·y·sin (ĭd′ē-ŏl′ĭ-sĭn, ĭd′ē-ō-lī′sĭn) *n.* A lysin that occurs in the blood of a person or an animal without the injection of a stimulating antigen or the passive transfer of antibodies.

id·i·o·path·ic (ĭd′ē-ə-păth′ĭk, ĭd′ē-ō-) *adj.* **1.** Of or relating to a disease having no known cause. **2.** Of or relating to a disease that is not the result of any other disease. — **id′i·o·path′i·cal·ly** *adv.*

idiopathic pulmonary hemosiderosis *n.* Repeated attacks of difficulty in breathing and hemoptysis leading to the deposition of abnormal amounts of hemosiderin in the lungs.

id·i·op·a·thy (ĭd′ē-ŏp′ə-thē) *n.* **1.** A disease of unknown origin or cause. **2.** A primary disease arising with no apparent external cause.

id·i·o·syn·cra·sy (ĭd′ē-ō-sĭng′krə-sē) *n.* **1.** A structural or behavioral characteristic peculiar to an individual or a group. **2.** A physiological or temperamental peculiarity. **3.** An unusual individual reaction to food or a drug. — **id′i·o·syn·crat′ic** (-sĭn-krăt′ĭk) *adj.*

id·i·ot (ĭd′ē-ət) *n.* A person of profound mental retardation having a mental age below three years. The term is no longer in use and is considered offensive.

idiot savant (ĭd′ē-ət să-vänt′) *n., pl.* **idiot savants.** A mentally retarded person who exhibits genius in a highly specialized area, such as mathematics.

id·i·o·type (ĭd′ē-ə-tīp′) *n.* A determinant that confers on an immunoglobulin molecule an antigenic individuality that is analogous to the individuality of the molecule's antibody activity.

id·i·o·ven·tric·u·lar rhythm (ĭd′ē-ō-vĕn-trĭk′yə-lər) *n.* A slow independent cardiac rhythm under control of an ectopic ventricular center.

i·dox·u·ri·dine (ī′dŏks-yōōr′ĭ-dēn′) *n.* A pyrimidine analogue with both antiviral and anticancer effects and used locally in the eye for the treatment of keratitis from herpes simplex or vaccinia.

IFN *abbr.* interferon

Ig *abbr.* immunoglobulin

IgA *abbr.* immunoglobulin A

IgD *abbr.* immunoglobulin D

IgE *abbr.* immunoglobulin E

IgG *abbr.* immunoglobulin G

IgM *abbr.* immunoglobulin M

ig·ni·punc·ture (ĭg′nə-pŭngk′chər) *n.* Surgical closing of retinal break in retinal separation by cauterizing the site of the break with a hot needle.

IH *abbr.* infectious hepatitis

IL-1 *abbr.* interleukin-1

IL-2 *abbr.* interleukin-2

Ile *abbr.* isoleucine; isoleucyl

il·e·al (ĭl′ē-əl) *adj.* Of or relating to the ileum.

il·e·ec·to·my (ĭl′ē-ĕk′tə-mē) *n.* Surgical removal of the ileum.

il·e·i·tis (ĭl′ē-ī′tĭs) *n.* Inflammation of the ileum.

il·e·o·ce·cos·to·my (ĭl′ē-ō-sē-kŏs′tə-mē) *n.* Surgical construction of an opening between the ileum and cecum.

il·e·o·co·li·tis (ĭl′ē-ō-kə-lī′tĭs) *n.* Inflammation of the mucous membrane of the ileum and colon.

il·e·o·co·los·to·my (ĭl′ē-ō-kə-lŏs′tə-mē) *n.* Surgical construction of an opening between the ileum and colon.

il·e·o·cys·to·plas·ty (ĭl′ē-ō-sĭs′tə-plăs′tē) *n.* Surgical reconstruction of the bladder involving the use of an isolated intestinal segment to augment bladder capacity.

il·e·o·il·e·os·to·my (ĭl′ē-ō-ĭl′ē-ŏs′tə-mē) *n.* Surgical construction of an opening between two segments of the ileum.

il·e·o·je·ju·ni·tis (ĭl′ē-ō-jə-jōō′nī′tĭs, -jē′jōō-, -jĕj′-ōō-) *n.* A chronic inflammatory condition involving the jejunum and parts or most of the ileum.

il·e·o·pex·y (ĭl′ē-ō-pĕk′sē) *n.* Surgical fixation of the ileum.

il·e·o·proc·tos·to·my (ĭl′ē-ō-prŏk-tŏs′tə-mē) *n.* Surgical construction of an opening between the ileum and the rectum.

il·e·or·rha·phy (ĭl′ē-ôr′ə-fē) *n.* The suturing of the ileum.

il·e·o·sig·moid·os·to·my (ĭl′ē-ō-sĭg′moi-dŏs′-tə-mē) *n.* Surgical construction of an opening between the ileum and the sigmoid colon.

il·e·os·to·my (ĭl′ē-ŏs′tə-mē) *n.* **1.** Surgical construction of an artificial excretory opening through the abdominal wall into the ileum. **2.** The opening created by such a procedure.

il·e·ot·o·my (ĭl′ē-ŏt′ə-mē) *n.* An incision into the ileum.

il·e·um (ĭl′ē-əm) *n., pl.* **-e·a** (-ē-ə). The third and terminal portion of the small intestine, extending from the jejunum to the cecum.

il·e·us (ĭl′ē-əs) *n.* Intestinal obstruction causing severe colicky pain, vomiting, constipation, and often fever and dehydration.

il·i·ac bone (ĭl′ē-ăk′) *n.* The broad flaring portion of the hipbone, distinct at birth but later becoming fused with the ischium and the pubis to form the acetabulum and the ala.

iliac region *n.* See **inguinal region**.

il·i·um (ĭl′ē-əm) *n., pl.* **-i·a** (-ē-ə). The uppermost and widest of the three bones constituting either of the lateral halves of the pelvis.

ill·ness (ĭl′nĭs) *n.* Disease of body or mind; poor health; sickness.

il·lu·sion (ĭ-lōō′zhən) *n.* **1.** An erroneous perception or belief. **2.** The condition of being deceived by a false perception or belief. **3.** Something, such as a fantastic plan or desire, that causes an erroneous belief or perception. — **il·lu′sion·al, il·lu′-sion·ar′y** (-zhə-nĕr′ē) *adj.*

IM *abbr.* internal medicine; intramuscular (as for injection site)

im·age (ĭm′ĭj) *n.* **1.** An optically formed duplicate, counterpart, or other representative reproduction of an object. **2.** A mental picture of something. — *v.* **-aged, -ag·ing, -ag·es. 1.** To make or produce a likeness of. **2.** To picture something mentally; imagine. **3.** To visualize something, as by magnetic resonance imaging.

im·age·ry (ĭm′ĭj-rē) *n.* **1.** A set of mental pictures or images. **2.** A technique in behavior therapy in which the patient is conditioned to use pleasant fantasies to counteract the unpleasant feelings associated with anxiety.

im·ag·ing (ĭm′ĭ-jĭng) *n.* **1.** Visualization of internal body organs, tissues, or cavities using specialized instruments and techniques, such as radiology and ultrasonography, for diagnostic purposes. **2.** The use of mental images to influence bodily processes and to control pain, or to achieve a goal one has visualized or imagined.

i·ma·go (ĭ-mā′gō, ĭ-mä′-) *n., pl.* **-goes** or **-gi·nes** (-gə-nēz′). **1.** An often idealized image of a person, usually a parent, formed in childhood and persisting unconsciously into adulthood. **2.** See **archetype** (sense 2).

im·bal·ance (ĭm-băl′əns) *n.* **1.** A lack of balance, as in distribution or functioning. **2.** Lack of equality in some aspect of binocular vision, as in strabismus or heterophobia.

im·be·cile (ĭm′bə-sĭl, -səl) *n.* A person of moderate to severe mental retardation having a mental age of three to seven years. The term is no longer in use and is considered offensive.

im·bi·bi·tion (ĭm′bə-bĭsh′ən) *n.* Absorption of fluid by a solid or colloid that results in swelling.

im·id·az·ole (ĭm′ĭ-dăz′ōl′) *n.* An organic crystalline base that is an inhibitor of histamine.

im·i·no·gly·ci·nu·ri·a (ĭm′ə-nō-glī′sə-nōōr′ē-ə, -nyōōr′-) *n.* A benign inborn error of amino acid transport, causing glycine, proline, and hydroxyproline to be excreted in the urine.

im·ma·ture (ĭm′ə-tyŏŏr′, -tŏŏr′, -chŏŏr′) *adj.* Not fully grown or developed.

im·me·di·ate auscultation (ĭ-mē′dē-ĭt) *n.* The direct application of an examiner's ear to the surface of a patient's body in order to listen to the internal sounds of the body.

immediate flap *n.* See **direct flap**.

immediate percussion *n.* Percussion performed directly with the finger or a plexor, without the intervention of another finger or pleximeter.

immediate reaction *n.* An allergic or immune response that begins within a few minutes to about an hour after exposure to a sensitizing antigen.

immediate transfusion *n.* See **direct transfusion**.

im·mis·ci·ble (ĭ-mĭs′ə-bəl) *adj.* Incapable of being mixed or blended, as oil and water.

im·mo·bile (ĭ-mō′bəl, -bēl′, -bĭl′) *adj.* **1.** Immovable; fixed. **2.** Not moving; motionless. — **im′mo·bil′i·ty** (-bĭl′-ĭ-tē) *n.*

im·mo·bi·lize (ĭ-mō′bə-līz′) *v.* **-lized, -liz·ing, -liz·es. 1.** To render immobile. **2.** To fix the position of a joint or fractured limb, as with a splint or cast. — **im·mo′bi·li·za′tion** (-lĭ-zā′shən) *n.*

im·mo·tile cilia syndrome (ĭ-mōt′l, ĭ-mō′tĭl′) *n.* An inherited syndrome characterized by the inability of cilia to beat effectively and by recurrent sinopulmonary infections.

im·mov·a·ble joint (ĭ-mōō′və-bəl) *n.* A union of two bones by fibrous tissue, such as a syndesmosis or gomphosis, in which there is no joint cavity and little motion is possible.

im·mune (ĭ-myōōn′) *adj.* **1.** Of, relating to, or having immunity to infection by a specific pathogen. **2.** Relating to the mechanism of sensitization whereby reactivity is altered by previous contact with an antigen, so that the involved tissues respond quickly upon subsequent contact.

immune adsorption *n.* **1.** Removal of antibody from antiserum by specific antigen, with aggregation and separation of the antigen-antibody complex by centrifugation or filtration. **2.** Similar removal of antigen by a specific antiserum.

immune complex *n.* Any of various complexes of an antigen and an antibody in the blood, to which complement may also be fixed, and which may form a precipitate.

immune complex disease *n.* A disease caused by the deposition of antigen-antibody or antigen-antibody-complement complexes on cell surfaces, resulting in chronic or acute inflammation, which may be manifested by vasculitis, endocarditis, neuritis, or glomerulonephritis.

immune deficiency *n.* See **immunodeficiency**.

immune electron microscopy *n.* The use of an electron microscope to examine viral specimens bound to specific antibody.

immune fetal hydrops *n.* Edema and ascites in a fetus, due to erythroblastosis fetalis.

immune reaction *n.* The reaction resulting from the recognition and binding of an antigen by its specific antibody or by a previously sensitized lymphocyte.

immune response *n.* An integrated bodily response to an antigen, especially one mediated by lymphocytes and involving recognition of antigens by specific antibodies or previously sensitized lymphocytes.

immune response gene *n.* A gene in the major histocompatibility complex that controls a cell's immune response to specific antigens.

immune serum *n.* See **antiserum**.

immune serum globulin *n.* A sterile solution of globulins from pooled human blood containing antibodies normally present in the blood of adults, used as a passive immunizing agent against rubella, measles, and hepatitis A and as treatment for hypogammaglobulinemia.

immune surveillance *n.* See **immunological surveillance**.

immune system *n.* The integrated body system of organs, tissues, cells, and cell products, such as antibodies, that differentiates self from nonself and neutralizes potentially pathogenic organisms or substances.

im·mu·ni·ty (ĭ-myoo′nĭ-tē) *n.* **1.** The quality or condition of being immune. **2.** Inherited, acquired, or induced resistance to infection by a specific pathogen.

im·mu·nize (ĭm′yə-nīz′) *v.* -nized, -niz·ing, -niz·es. **1.** To render immune. **2.** To produce immunity in, as by inoculation. — **im′mu·ni·za′tion** (-nĭ-zā′shən) *n.*

im·mu·no·as·say (ĭm′yə-nō-ăs′ā, ĭ-myoo′-) *n.* A laboratory or clinical technique that makes use of the specific binding between an antigen and its homologous antibody in order to identify and quantify a substance in a sample.

im·mu·no·chem·i·cal assay (ĭm′yə-nō-kĕm′ĭ-kəl) *n.* See **immunoassay**.

im·mu·no·chem·is·try (ĭm′yə nō kĕm′ĭ strē, ĭ myoo′-) *n.* The chemistry of immunologic phenomena, as of antigen-antibody reactions.

im·mu·no·com·pe·tent (ĭm′yə-nō-kŏm′pĭ-tənt, ĭ-myoo′-) *adj.* Having the normal bodily capacity to develop an immune response following exposure to an antigen. — **im′mu·no·com′pe·tence** *n.*

im·mu·no·com·pro·mised (ĭm′yə-nō-kŏm′prə-mīzd, ĭ-myoo′-) *adj.* Incapable of developing a normal immune response, usually as a result of disease, malnutrition, or immunosuppressive therapy.

im·mu·no·con·glu·ti·nin (ĭm′yə-nō-kŏn-gloot′-n-ĭn, ĭ-myoo′-) *n.* An autoantibodylike immunoglobulin formed by animals against their own complement after injection of complement-containing complexes or of sensitized bacteria.

im·mu·no·de·fi·cien·cy (ĭm′yə-nō-dĭ-fĭsh′ən-sē, ĭ-myoo′-) *n.* A disorder or deficiency of the normal immune response, resulting from a defect in the immune mechanism or the effects of a disease.

immunodeficiency syndrome *n.* A syndrome associated with an immunological deficiency or disorder and characterized primarily by an increased susceptibility to infection.

im·mu·no·dif·fu·sion (ĭm′yə-nō-dĭ-fyoo′zhən, ĭ-myoo′-) *n.* A technique for studying antigen-antibody reactions by observing precipitates formed by the combination of antigens and antibodies that have been placed in a gel.

im·mu·no·e·lec·tro·pho·re·sis (ĭm′yə-nō-ĭ-lĕk′trə-fə-rē′sĭs, ĭ-myoo′-) *n.* The separation and identification of proteins based on differences in their mobility through a liquid or gel in response to changes in an electric field, and in their reactivity with antibodies.

im·mu·no·en·hance·ment (ĭm′yə-nō-ĕn-hăns′mənt, ĭ-myoo′-) *n.* The potentiating effect of immunoenhancers such as specific antibodies in establishing or in delaying rejection of a tumor allograft.

im·mu·no·en·hanc·er (ĭm′yə-nō-ĕn-hăn′sər, ĭ-myoo′-) *n.* A substance that increases an immune response.

im·mu·no·gen (ĭm′yə-nə-jən, -jĕn′, ĭ-myoo′-) *n.* See **antigen**.

im·mu·no·ge·nic·i·ty (ĭm′yə-nō-jə-nĭs′ĭ-tē) *n.* See **antigenicity**.

im·mu·no·glob·u·lin (ĭm′yə-nō-glŏb′yə-lĭn, ĭ-myoo′-) *n.* Any of a group of glycoproteins secreted by plasma cells that function as antibodies in the immune response by binding with specific antigens.

immunoglobulin A *n.* The class of antibodies produced predominantly against ingested antigens, found in body secretions such as saliva or sweat, and functioning to prevent attachment of viruses and bacteria to epithelial surfaces.

immunoglobulin D *n.* The class of antibodies found only on the surface of B cells, possibly functioning as antigen receptors to initiate differentiation of B cells into plasma cells.

immunoglobulin E *n.* The class of antibodies produced in the lungs, skin, and mucous membranes and responsible for allergic reactions.

immunoglobulin G *n.* The most abundant class of antibodies, found in blood serum and lymph and active against bacteria, viruses, fungi, and foreign particles; it activates the complement system.

immunoglobulin M *n.* The class of antibodies found in circulating body fluids and being the first antibodies to appear in response to an initial exposure to an antigen.

im·mu·no·his·to·chem·is·try (ĭm′yə-nō-hĭs′tō-kĕm′ĭ-strē, ĭ-myōō′-) *n.* Microscopic localization of specific antigens in tissues by staining with antibodies labeled with fluorescent or pigmented material.

immunological mechanism *n.* The collection of cells, chiefly lymphocytes and cells of the reticuloendothelial system, that function in establishing active acquired immunity.

immunological paralysis *n.* Lack of specific antibody production after exposure to large doses of an antigen.

immunological surveillance *n.* A theory holding that malignant cells are recognized as such and removed by the immune system.

immunological tolerance *n.* Acquired specific failure of the immunological mechanism to respond to a given antigen, induced by exposure to the antigen.

immunologic pregnancy test *n.* Any of various pregnancy tests to detect increased human chorionic gonadotropin in the blood or urine by immunologic techniques such as radioimmunoassay.

im·mu·nol·o·gist (ĭm′yə-nŏl′ə-jĭst) *n.* A specialist in immunology.

im·mu·nol·o·gy (ĭm′yə-nŏl′ə-jē) *n.* The branch of biomedicine concerned with the structure and function of the immune system, innate and acquired immunity, and laboratory techniques involving the interaction of antigens with specific antibodies. — **im′mu·no·log′ic** (-nə-lŏj′ĭk), **im′-mu·no·log′i·cal** *adj.*

im·mu·no·per·ox·i·dase technique (ĭm′yə-nō-pə-rŏk′sĭ-dās′, -dāz′, ĭ-myōō′nō-) *n.* An enzymatic antigen detection technique that uses horseradish peroxidase to label antibody-antigen complexes in tissues, used to demonstrate hormones, tissue-specific antigens, structural proteins, microorganisms, and viruses.

im·mu·no·po·ten·ti·a·tion (ĭm′yə-nō-pə-tĕn′-shē-ā′shən, ĭ-myōō′-) *n.* Enhancement of the immune response by increasing the speed and extent of its development and prolonging its duration.

im·mu·no·pre·cip·i·ta·tion (ĭm′yə-nō-prĭ-sĭp′ĭ-tā′shən, ĭ-myōō′-) *n.* The precipitation of sensitized antigen as the result of the interaction of antigen with a specific antibody in solution.

im·mu·no·pro·lif·er·a·tive disorder (ĭm′yə-nō-prə-lĭf′ə-rā′tĭv, ĭ-myōō′-) *n.* A disorder characterized by the production of an abnormally high number of antibody-producing cells, especially those associated with autoallergic disturbances and gamma-globulin abnormalities.

im·mu·no·re·ac·tion (ĭm′yə-nō-rē-ăk′shən, ĭ-myōō′-) *n.* See **immune reaction**. — **im′mu·no·re·ac′tive** (-tĭv) *adj.* — **im′mu·no·re·ac·tiv′i·ty** *n.*

im·mu·no·sor·bent (ĭm′yə-nō-sôr′bənt, -zôr′-, ĭ-myōō′-) *n.* An antibody used to remove specific antigen, or an antigen used to remove specific antibody, from solution or suspension.

im·mu·no·sup·pres·sion (ĭm′yə-nō-sə-prĕsh′ən, ĭ-myōō′-) *n.* Suppression of the immune response in order to prevent the rejection of grafts or transplants or control autoimmune diseases. — **im′-mu·no·sup·pres′sive** *adj.*

im·mu·no·ther·a·py (ĭm′yə-nō-thĕr′ə-pē, ĭ-myōō′-) *n.* Treatment of disease by inducing, enhancing, or suppressing an immune response.

im·mu·no·trans·fu·sion (ĭm′yə-nō-trăns-fyōō′-zhən, ĭ-myōō′-) *n.* A transfusion of blood from a donor who has been immunized by injections of an antigen prepared from microorganisms isolated the recipient; the recipient then gains passive immunity from the donor's antibodies.

im·pact·ed (ĭm-păk′tĭd) *adj.* **1.** Wedged together at the broken ends. Used of a fractured bone. **2.** Placed in the alveolus in a manner prohibiting eruption into a normal position. Used of a tooth. **3.** Wedged or packed in, so as to fill or block an organ or a passage.

impacted fetus *n.* A fetus that has become wedged and is incapable of spontaneous advance or recession.

impacted fracture *n.* A bone fracture in which one of the fragments is firmly driven into another fragment.

im·pair·ment (ĭm-pâr′mənt) *n.* Weakening, damage, or deterioration, especially as a result of injury or disease. — **im·pair′** *v.*

im·ped·i·ment (ĭm-pĕd′ə-mənt) *n.* **1.** Something that impedes. **2.** An organic defect preventing clear articulation of speech.

im·per·fo·rate anus (ĭm-pûr′fər-ĭt) *n.* See **anal atresia**.

im·per·fo·ra·tion (ĭm-pûr′fə-rā′shən) *n.* The condition of being abnormally occluded or closed.

im·per·me·a·ble (ĭm-pûr′mē-ə-bəl) *adj.* Impossible to permeate; not permitting passage.

im·pe·ti·go (ĭm′pĭ-tī′gō) *n., pl.* **-gos.** A contagious skin infection caused by staphylococcal or streptococcal bacteria and characterized by the eruption of pustules that form crusts, usually on the face; it most commonly occurs in children.

im·plant (ĭm-plănt′) *v.* **-plant·ed, -plant·ing, -plants.** **1.** To insert or embed an object or a device surgically. **2.** To graft or insert a tissue within the body. **3.** To become attached to and embedded in the uterine lining. Used of a fertilized egg. — *n.* (ĭm′plănt′). Something implanted, especially a surgically implanted tissue or device.

im·plan·ta·tion (ĭm′plăn-tā′shən) *n.* **1.** The act or an instance of implanting. **2.** The condition of being implanted. **3.** The process by which a fertilized egg implants in the uterine lining.

implanted suture *n.* A suture created by passing a pin through each lip of a wound, parallel to the line of incision, and then looping the pins together with stitches.

im·plo·sion (ĭm-plō′zhən) *n.* A type of behavior therapy in which the patient is repeatedly subjected to extreme anxiety-arousing stimuli in an attempt to extinguish anxious feelings and behavior and replace them with more appropriate responses.

im·po·tence (ĭm′pə-təns) or **im·po·ten·cy** (-tən-sē) *n.* The quality or condition of being impotent.

im·po·tent (ĭm′pə-tənt) *adj.* **1.** Incapable of sexual intercourse, often because of an inability to achieve or sustain an erection. **2.** Sterile. Used of males.

im·preg·nate (ĭm-prĕg′nāt) *v.* **-nat·ed, -nat·ing, -nates. 1.** To make pregnant; inseminate. **2.** To fertilize an ovum. **3.** To fill throughout; saturate. — **im′preg·na′tion** *n.* — **im·preg′na′tor** *n.*

im·pres·sion (ĭm-prĕsh′ən) *n.* **1.** An effect, a feeling, or an image retained as a consequence of experience. **2.** A mark or indentation made by the pressure of one organ on the surface of another.

im·print·ing (ĭm′prĭn′tĭng) *n.* A learning process occurring early in life in which a specific behavior pattern is established through association with a parent or other role model.

im·pulse (ĭm′pŭls′) *n.* **1.** A sudden pushing or driving force. **2.** A sudden wish or urge that prompts an unpremeditated act or feeling. **3.** The electrochemical transmission of a signal along a nerve fiber that produces an excitatory or inhibitory response at a target tissue, such as a muscle or another nerve.

im·pul·sion (ĭm-pŭl′shən) *n.* An urge to perform certain actions without regard for internal or social constraints, as occurs in young children and in adults with certain psychological disorders.

im·pul·sive (ĭm-pŭl′sĭv) *adj.* **1.** Inclined to act on impulse rather than thought. **2.** Motivated by or resulting from impulse. — **im·pul′sive·ness, im′pul·siv′i·ty** *n.*

impulsive obsession *n.* An obsession accompanied by action; it sometimes becomes a mania.

in·ac·ti·vat·ed poliovirus vaccine (ĭn-ăk′tə-vā-təd) *n.* See **poliovirus vaccine** (sense 1).

in·ac·tive repressor (ĭn-ăk′tĭv) *n.* See **aporepressor.**

in·ad·e·quate personality (ĭn-ăd′ĭ-kwĭt) *n.* A personality disturbance characterized by an inability to cope with the social, emotional, occupational, and intellectual demands of life.

inadequate stimulus *n.* A stimulus too weak to evoke a response.

in·an·i·mate (ĭn-ăn′ə-mĭt) *adj.* Not having the qualities associated with active, living organisms; not animate. — **in·an′i·mate·ness** *n.*

in·a·ni·tion (ĭn′ə-nĭsh′ən) *n.* Exhaustion, as from lack of nourishment or vitality.

in·ar·tic·u·late (ĭn′är-tĭk′yə-lĭt) *adj.* **1.** Uttered without the use of normal words or syllables; incomprehensible as speech or language. **2.** Unable to speak; speechless. **3.** Unable to speak with clarity or eloquence. **4.** Not having joints or segments. — **in′ar·tic′u·late·ness, in′ar·tic′u·la·cy** (-lə-sē) *n.*

in·born (ĭn′bôrn′) *adj.* **1.** Possessed by an organism at birth. **2.** Inherited or hereditary.

inborn error of metabolism *n.* Any of a group of congenital disorders caused by an inherited defect in a single specific enzyme that results in a characteristic disruption or abnormality in a specific metabolic pathway.

in·bred (ĭn′brĕd′) *adj.* **1.** Produced by inbreeding. **2.** Fixed in the character or disposition as if inherited; deep-seated.

in·breed·ing (ĭn′brē′dĭng) *n.* See **homogamy.**

in·cest (ĭn′sĕst′) *n.* **1.** Sexual relations between persons who are so closely related that their marriage is illegal or forbidden by custom. **2.** The statutory crime of sexual relations with such a near relative.

in·cise (ĭn-sīz′) *v.* **-cised, -cis·ing, -cis·es.** To cut into with a sharp instrument.

incised wound *n.* A wound characterized by a clean cut, as by a sharp instrument.

in·ci·sion (ĭn-sĭzh′ən) *n.* **1.** A cut into a body tissue or organ, especially one made during surgery. **2.** The scar resulting from such a cut.

in·ci·sion·al hernia (ĭn-sĭzh′ə-nəl) *n.* A hernia occurring through a surgical incision or scar.

incision biopsy *n.* Excision of only a part of a lesion for gross and microscopic examination.

in·ci·sor (ĭn-sī′zər) *n.* Any of the four teeth adapted for cutting or gnawing, having a chisel-shaped crown and a single conical root and located in the front part of both jaws in both deciduous and permanent dentitions.

in·ci·sure (ĭn-sī′zhər) *n.* An indentation at the edge of a structure; a notch. — **in·ci′su·ral** *adj.*

in·cli·na·tion (ĭn′klə-nā′shən) *n.* **1.** A deviation or the degree of deviation from the horizontal or vertical; a slant. **2.** A tendency toward a certain condition or character: **3.** A characteristic disposition to do, prefer, or favor one thing rather than another; a propensity.

in·clu·sion body (ĭn-kloō′zhən) *n.* An abnormal structure in a cell nucleus or cytoplasm having characteristic staining properties and associated especially with certain viral infections, such as rabies and smallpox.

inclusion cell *n.* A cultured skin fibroblast containing membrane-bound inclusions.

inclusion conjunctivitis *n.* A form of conjunctivitis caused by *Chlamydia trachomatis* and often affecting newborn infants but also contracted by adults in swimming pools or from sexual intimacy, characterized by enlarged papilla on the inner eyelids and purulent discharge.

in·com·pat·i·ble (ĭn′kəm-păt′ə-bəl) *adj.* **1.** Producing an undesirable effect when used in combination with a particular substance, as a medicine in combination with alcohol. **2.** Not suitable for combination or administration because of immunological differences, as blood types. — in′com·pat·i·bil′i·ty (ĭn′kəm-păt′ə-bĭl′ĭ-tē) *n.*

in·com·pe·tence (ĭn-kŏm′pĭ-təns) or in·com·pe·ten·cy (-tən-sē) *n.* **1.** The quality of being incompetent or incapable of performing a function, as the failure of the cardiac valves to close properly. **2.** The condition of being not legally qualified, as to stand trial. **3.** The inability to distinguish right from wrong or to manage one's affairs.

in·com·pe·tent (ĭn-kŏm′pĭ-tənt) *adj.* **1.** Not qualified in legal terms. **2.** Inadequate for or unsuited to a particular purpose or application. **3.** Incapable of proper functioning, as a heart valve.

incompetent cervix *n.* A defect in the muscular ring at the isthmus of the uterus, allowing premature dilation of the cervix during pregnancy.

in·com·plete abortion (ĭn′kəm-plēt′) *n.* Abortion in which all of the products of conception are not expelled from the uterus.

incomplete antibody *n.* See **serum agglutinin.**

incomplete antigen *n.* See **hapten.**

incomplete dominance *n.* A heterozygous condition in which both alleles at a gene locus are partially expressed, often producing an intermediate phenotype.

incomplete fistula *n.* See **blind fistula.**

incomplete foot presentation *n.* Breech presentation of the fetus during birth in which a single foot is the presenting part.

incomplete fracture *n.* A fracture in which the line of fracture does not include the entire bone.

in·con·ti·nence (ĭn-kŏn′tə-nəns) *n.* **1.** The inability to control excretory functions. **2.** Lack of restraint in sexual relations; immoderation.

in·con·ti·nent (ĭn-kŏn′tə-nənt) *adj.* **1.** Lacking normal voluntary control of excretory functions. **2.** Lacking sexual restraint; unchaste.

in·co·or·di·na·tion (ĭn′kō-ôr′dn-ā′shən) *n.* See **ataxia.**

in·cre·tion (ĭn-krē′shən) *n.* **1.** The process of internal secretion characteristic of endocrine glands. **2.** The product of this process; a hormone.

in·crust·a·tion (ĭn′krŭ-stā′shən) *n.* **1.** The formation of a crust or a scab. **2.** A coating of hardened exudate or other material on a body or body part; a scale or scab.

in·cu·bate (ĭn′kyə-bāt′, ĭng′-) *v.* -bat·ed, -bat·ing, -bates. To maintain eggs, organisms, or living tissue at optimal environmental conditions for growth and development.

in·cu·ba·tion (ĭn′kyə-bā′shən, ĭng′-) *n.* **1.** The act of incubating or the state of being incubated. **2.** The maintenance of controlled environmental conditions for the purpose of favoring the growth or development of microbial or tissue cultures. **3.** The maintenance of an infant, especially a premature infant, in an environment of controlled temperature, humidity, and oxygen concentration in order to provide optimal conditions for growth and development. **4.** The development of an infection from the time the pathogen enters the body until signs or symptoms first appear.

incubation period *n.* See **latent period** (sense 2).

in·cu·ba·tor (ĭn′kyə-bā′tər, ĭng′-) *n.* **1.** An apparatus in which environmental conditions, such as temperature and humidity, can be controlled, often used for growing bacterial cultures. **2.** An apparatus for maintaining an infant, especially a premature infant, in an environment of controlled temperature, humidity, and oxygen concentration.

in·cu·bus (ĭn′kyə-bəs, ĭng′-) *n., pl.* -bus·es or -bi (-bī′). A nightmare.

in·cu·dec·to·my (ĭng′kyə-dĕk′tə-mē) *n.* Surgical removal of the incus.

in·cur·a·ble (ĭn-kyoor′ə-bəl) *adj.* Being such that a cure is impossible; not curable.

in·cur·va·tion (ĭn′kûr-vā′shən) *n.* An inward curvature.

in·cus (ĭng′kəs) *n., pl.* in·cu·des (ĭng-kyōō′dēz). The middle of the three ossicles in the middle ear, located between the malleus and the stapes.

in d. *abbr. Latin.* in dies (daily)

in·dane·di·one (ĭn′dān-dī′ōn′) *n.* Any of a class of rapidly acting, orally administered anticoagulants.

in·dap·a·mide (ĭn-dăp′ə-mīd′) *n.* A loop diuretic used to treat edema associated with congestive heart failure, hepatic cirrhosis, and renal disease.

in·den·ta·tion (ĭn′dĕn-tā′shən) *n.* A notch, pit, or depression.

in·dex (ĭn′dĕks′) *n., pl.* -dex·es or -di·ces (-dĭ-sēz′). **1.** A guide, standard, indicator, symbol, or number indicating the relation of one part or thing to another in respect to size, capacity, or function. **2.** A guide, usually made of plaster, used to reposition teeth, casts, or parts. **3.** The index finger. — in′dex′ *v.*

index case *n.* See **proband.**

index finger *n.* The finger next to the thumb.

in·di·ca·tion (ĭn′dĭ-kā′shən) *n.* **1.** Something that points to or suggests the proper treatment of a disease, as that demanded by its cause or symptoms. **2.** Something indicated as necessary or expedient, as in the treatment of a disease or the administration of a drug.

in·di·ca·tor (ĭn′dĭ-kā′tər) *n.* **1.** One that indicates, especially a pointer or an index. **2.** Any of various substances, such as litmus or phenolphthalein, that indicate the presence, absence, or concentration of another substance or the degree of reaction between two or more substances by means of a characteristic change, especially in color.

in·di·ges·tion (ĭn′dĭ-jĕs′chən, -dī-) *n.* **1.** The inability to digest or a difficulty in properly digesting food in the alimentary tract. **2.** Abdominal discomfort or illness resulting from this inability or difficulty.

in·din·a·vir (ĭn-dĭn′-ə-vîr) *n.* A protease-inhibiting drug usually used in combination to suppress the production of HIV.

in·di·rect fracture (ĭn′dĭ-rĕkt′, -dĭ-) *n.* A fracture, especially of the skull, that occurs at a point other than the point of impact or injury.

indirect hemagglutination test *n.* See **passive hemagglutination.**

indirect ophthalmoscope *n.* An instrument designed to visualize the interior of the eye, with the instrument at arm's length from the subject's eye and the observer viewing an inverted image through a convex lens located between the instrument and the subject's eye.

indirect reacting bilirubin *n.* Serum bilirubin that has not been conjugated with glucuronic acid in the liver.

indirect transfusion *n.* Transfusion of blood previously obtained from a donor.

indirect vision *n.* See **peripheral vision.**

in·dis·pose (ĭn′dĭ-spōz′) *v.* **-posed, -pos·ing, -pos·es.** To cause to be or feel ill; sicken.

in·di·um (ĭn′dē-əm) *n.* A soft, malleable, metallic element with atomic number 49 and found primarily in ores of zinc.

in·di·vid·u·a·tion (ĭn′də-vĭj′ōō-ā′shən) *n.* **1.** The act or process of becoming distinct or individual, especially the process by which social individuals become differentiated one from the other. **2.** In Jungian psychology, the gradual integration and unification of the self through the resolution of successive layers of psychological conflict. **3.** The formation of distinct organs or structures through the interaction of adjacent tissues in an embryo.

individuation field *n.* The region within which an organizer influences the rearrangement of primordial tissues so that a complete embryo is formed.

in·dole (ĭn′dōl) *n.* **1.** A white crystalline compound obtained from coal tar or various plants and found in the intestines and feces as a product of the bacterial decomposition of tryptophan. **2.** Any of various derivatives of this compound.

in·do·lent bubo (ĭn′də-lənt) *n.* An indurated enlargement of an inguinal node.

in·do·meth·a·cin (ĭn′dō-mĕth′ə-sĭn) *n.* A nonsteroidal anti-inflammatory, antipyretic, and analgesic drug used especially in the treatment of some forms of arthritis.

in·do·pro·fen (ĭn′dō-prō′fən) *n.* A nonsteroidal anti-inflammatory agent with analgesic and antipyretic properties.

in·dox·yl (ĭn-dŏk′səl) *n.* A product of intestinal bacterial degradation of indoleacetic acid, excreted in the urine.

in·duce (ĭn-dōōs′, -dyōōs′) *v.* **-duced, -duc·ing, -duc·es. 1.** To bring about or stimulate the occurrence of something, such as labor. **2.** To initiate or increase the production of an enzyme or other protein at the level of genetic transcription.

in·duced abortion (ĭn-dōōst′, -dyōōst′) *n.* Abortion caused intentionally by the administration of drugs or by mechanical means.

induced enzyme *n.* An enzyme that is produced by the cell only in response to the accumulation or addition of a particular substance.

induced hypotension *n.* Deliberate acute reduction of arterial blood pressure to reduce surgical blood loss, either by pharmacologic means during anesthesia and surgery or by presurgical withdrawal of blood which is returned to the circulation postsurgically.

induced radioactivity *n.* See **artificial radioactivity.**

in·duc·er (ĭn-dōō′sər, -dyōō′-) *n.* **1.** One that induces, especially a molecule that is usually a substrate of a specific enzyme pathway and combines with an active repressor produced by a regulator gene to deactivate the repressor. **2.** A part or structure in an embryo that influences the differentiation of another part.

in·duc·i·ble enzyme (ĭn-dōō′sə-bəl, -dyōō′-) *n.* An enzyme normally present in minute quantities within a cell, but whose concentration increases dramatically when a substrate is added.

in·duc·tion (ĭn-dŭk′shən) *n.* **1.** The process of initiating or increasing the production of an enzyme or other protein at the level of genetic transcription. **2.** The period from the first administration of anesthesia to the establishment of a depth of anesthesia adequate for surgery. **3.** The change in form or shape caused by the action of one tissue of an embryo on adjacent tissues or parts, as by the diffusion of hormones or chemicals. **4.** A modification imposed upon the offspring by the action of environment on the germ cells of one or both parents.

induction period *n.* The interval between an initial injection of an antigen and the appearance of demonstrable antibodies in the blood.

in·duc·tor (ĭn-dŭk′tər) *n.* See **evocator.**

in·du·ra·tion (ĭn′də-rā′shən, -dyə-) *n.* **1.** The hardening of a normally soft tissue or organ, especially the skin, because of inflammation, infiltration of a neoplasm, or an accumulation of blood. **2.** A focus or region of abnormally hardened tissue.

in·dus·tri·al disease (ĭn-dŭs′trē-əl) *n.* **1.** A pathological condition resulting from exposure to a toxin discharged by a business or industry into the environment. **2.** An occupational disease.

in·dwell·ing catheter (ĭn′dwĕl′ĭng) *n.* A catheter that remains in place in the bladder.

in·e·bri·a·tion (ĭn-ē′brē-ā′shən) *n.* The condition of being intoxicated, as with alcohol.

in·ert (ĭn-ûrt′) *adj.* **1.** Sluggish in action or motion; lethargic. **2.** Having no pharmacologic or therapeutic action.

in·er·tia (ĭ-nûr′shə) *n.* Resistance or disinclination to motion, action, or change.

in ex·tre·mis (ĭn ĕk-strē′mĭs) *adv.* At the point of death.

in·fan·cy (ĭn′fən-sē) *n.* **1.** The earliest period of childhood, especially before the ability to walk has been acquired. **2.** The state of being an infant.

in·fant (ĭn′fənt) *n.* A child in the earliest period of life, especially before he or she has acquired the ability to walk.

in·fan·ti·cide (ĭn-făn′tĭ-sīd′) *n.* **1.** The act of killing an infant. **2.** The practice of killing infants.

in·fan·tile (ĭn′fən-tīl′, -tĭl) *adj.* **1.** Of or relating to infants or infancy. **2.** Displaying or suggesting a lack of maturity; extremely childish.

infantile autism *n.* A severe disorder of childhood characterized by withdrawal, preoccupation with fantasy, language impairment, and abnormal behavior, such as ritualistic acts and excessive object attachment.

infantile fibrosarcoma *n.* A rapidly growing but infrequently metastasizing fibrosarcoma that usually appears on the extremities in the first year of life.

infantile paralysis *n.* See **poliomyelitis.**

infantile sexuality *n.* In psychoanalytic theory, the overlapping oral, anal, and phallic phases of psychosexual development that occur during the first five years of life.

in·fan·til·ism (ĭn′fən-tl-ĭz′əm, ĭn-făn′tl-) *n.* **1.** A state of arrested development in an adult, characterized by retention of infantile mentality, accompanied by stunted growth and sexual immaturity, and often by dwarfism. **2.** Extreme immaturity, as in behavior or character.

infant mortality rate *n.* The ratio of the number of deaths in the first year of life to the number of live births occurring in the same population during the same period of time.

in·farct (ĭn′färkt′, ĭn-färkt′) *n.* An area of tissue that undergoes necrosis as a result of obstruction of local blood supply, as by a thrombus or an embolus. — **in·farct′ed** *adj.*

in·farc·tion (ĭn-färk′shən) *n.* **1.** The formation or development of an infarct. **2.** An infarct.

in·fect (ĭn-fĕkt′) *v.* **-fect·ed, -fect·ing, -fects. 1.** To contaminate with a pathogenic microorganism or agent. **2.** To communicate a pathogen or disease to another organism. **3.** To invade and produce infection in an organ or body part.

in·fect·ed abortion (ĭn-fĕk′tĭd) *n.* Abortion complicated by infection of the genital tract.

in·fec·tion (ĭn-fĕk′shən) *n.* **1.** Invasion by and multiplication of pathogenic microorganisms in a bodily part or tissue, which may produce subsequent tissue injury and progress to overt disease through a variety of cellular or toxic mechanisms. **2.** An instance of being infected. **3.** An agent or a contaminated substance responsible for one's becoming infected. **4.** The pathological state resulting from having been infected. **5.** An infectious disease.

infection-exhaustion psychosis *n.* A psychosis that occurs following an acute infection, shock, or chronic intoxication.

infection immunity *n.* Relative immunity to severe infection by a particular pathogen as a result of a chronic low-grade infection induced earlier by the same pathogen.

in·fec·tious (ĭn-fĕk′shəs) *adj.* **1.** Capable of causing infection. **2.** Caused by or capable of being transmitted by infection. **3.** Caused by a pathogenic microorganism or agent. — **in·fec′tious·ness** *n.*

infectious disease *n.* A disease resulting from the

presence and activity of a pathogenic microbial agent.

infectious hepatitis *n.* See **hepatitis A.**

infectious mononucleosis *n.* A common, acute, infectious disease, usually affecting young people, caused by Epstein-Barr virus and characterized by fever, swollen lymph nodes, sore throat, and lymphocyte abnormalities.

infectious papilloma virus *n.* See **human papilloma virus.**

infectious polyneuritis *n.* See **acute idiopathic polyneuritis.**

infectious warts virus *n.* See **human papilloma virus.**

in·fec·tive (ĭn-fĕk′tĭv) *adj.* Capable of producing infection; infectious. — **in·fec′tive·ness, in′fec·tiv′i·ty** *n.*

in·fe·ri·or (ĭn-fēr′ē-ər) *adj.* **1.** Low or lower in order, degree, or value. **2.** Situated below or directed downward. **3.** In human anatomy, situated nearer the soles of the feet in relation to a specific reference point. — **in·fe′ri·or′i·ty** (-ôr′ĭ-tē) *n.*

in·fe·ri·or·i·ty complex (ĭn-fēr′ē-ôr′ĭ-tē) *n.* A persistent sense of inadequacy or a tendency to self-diminishment, sometimes resulting in excessive aggressiveness through overcompensation.

inferior limb *n.* See **lower extremity.**

inferior vena cava *n.* A large vein formed by the union of the two common iliac veins that receives blood from the lower limbs and the pelvic and abdominal viscera and empties into the right atrium of the heart.

in·fer·tile (ĭn-fûr′tl) *adj.* Incapable of producing offspring; sterile.

in·fer·til·i·ty (ĭn′fər-tĭl′ĭ-tē) *n.* **1.** Absent or diminished fertility. **2.** The persistent inability to conceive a child.

in·fest (ĭn-fĕst′) *v.* **-fest·ed, -fest·ing, -fests.** To live as a parasite in or on tissues or organs or on the skin and its appendages. — **in′fes·ta′tion** *n.*

in·fil·trate (ĭn-fĭl′trāt′, ĭn′fĭl′-) *v.* **-trat·ed, -trat·ing, -trates. 1.** To cause a liquid to permeate a substance by passing through its interstices or pores. **2.** To permeate a porous substance with a liquid or gas. — *n.* An abnormal substance that accumulates gradually in cells or body tissues.

in·fil·tra·tion (ĭn′fĭl-trā′shən) *n.* **1.** The act or process of infiltrating. **2.** The state of being infiltrated. **3.** The gas, fluid, or dissolved matter that has entered a substance, cell, or tissue. — **in·fil′tra·tive** (-trə-tĭv) *adj.*

infiltration anesthesia *n.* See **local anesthesia.**

in·firm (ĭn-fûrm′) *adj.* Weak in body, especially from old age or disease; feeble.

in·fir·ma·ry (ĭn-fûr′mə-rē) *n.* A place for the care of the infirm, sick, or injured, especially a small hospital or clinic in an institution or school.

in·fir·mi·ty (ĭn-fûr′mĭ-tē) *n.* **1.** A bodily ailment or weakness, especially one brought on by old age. **2.** A condition or disease producing weakness. **3.** A failing or defect in a person's character.

in·flam·ma·tion (ĭn′flə-mā′shən) *n.* A localized protective reaction of tissue to irritation, injury, or infection, characterized by pain, redness, swelling, and sometimes loss of function.

in·flam·ma·to·ry (ĭn-flăm′ə-tôr′ē) *adj.* Characterized or caused by inflammation.

inflammatory bowel disease *n.* Any of several incurable and debilitating diseases of the gastrointestinal tract marked by inflammation and obstruction of one or several parts of the intestine.

in·flec·tion (ĭn-flĕk′shən) *n.* An inward bending.

in·flu·en·za (ĭn′flōō-ĕn′zə) *n.* An acute contagious viral infection, commonly occuring in epidemics or pandemics, characterized by inflammation of the respiratory tract and by sudden onset, fever, chills, muscular pain, headache, and severe prostration. — **in′flu·en′zal** *adj.*

influenza A *n.* Influenza caused by infection with a strain of influenza virus type A.

influenza B *n.* Influenza caused by infection with influenza virus type B.

influenza C *n.* Influenza caused by infection with a strain of influenza virus type C.

influenzal pneumonia *n.* **1.** Pneumonia complicating influenza. **2.** Pneumonia due to *Haemophilus influenzae.*

influenza virus *n.* Any of three viruses of the genus *Influenzavirus* that cause influenza and influenzalike infections.

influenza virus type A *n.* A myxovirus of the genus *Influenzavirus,* antigenically varying from influenza virus type B and influenza virus type C, that causes acute respiratory illness in humans.

Influenza virus type B *n.* A myxovirus of the genus *Influenzavirus,* antigenically varying from influenza virus type A and influenza virus type C, that causes various respiratory illnesses in humans.

Influenza virus type C *n.* A myxovirus of the genus *Influenzavirus,* antigenically varying from influenza virus type A and influenza virus type B, that causes respiratory illness in humans.

influenza virus vaccine *n.* A vaccine containing several strains of influenza virus prepared in chick embryos and used to immunize against influenza; because of their antigenic variation, the influenza viruses in the vaccine are regularly changed to include the most recently isolated strains.

in·formed consent (ĭn-fôrmd′) *n.* Consent by a patient to a surgical or medical procedure or participation in a clinical study after achieving an understanding of the relevant medical facts and the risks involved.

in·frac·tion (ĭn-frăk′shən) *n.* A bone fracture, especially one without displacement.

in·fra·nod·al extrasystole (ĭn′frə-nōd′l) *n.* See **ventricular extrasystole.**

in·fun·dib·u·lec·to·my (ĭn′fən-dĭb′yə-lĕk′tə-mē) *n.* Excision of the conus arteriosus, especially of hypertrophied myocardium encroaching on the ventricular outflow tract.

in·fun·dib·u·lum (ĭn′fən-dĭb′yə-ləm) *n.,* pl. **-la** (-lə). **1.** A funnel or funnel-shaped structure or passage. **2.** The infundibulum of the fallopian tube. **3.** The expanding portion of a calix as it opens into the pelvis of the kidney. **4.** A termina-

tion of a bronchiole in the alveolus. **5.** Termination of the cochlear canal beneath the cupola. **6.** The funnel-shaped, unpaired prominence of the base of the hypothalamus behind the optic chiasm, enclosing the infundibular recess of the third ventricle and continuous below with the stalk of the pituitary gland. — **in′fun·dib′u·lar** (-lər), **in′fun·dib′u·late′** (-lāt′, -lĭt) *adj.*

in·fuse (ĭn-fyōōz′) *v.* **-fused, -fus·ing, -fus·es.** To introduce a solution into the body through a vein for therapeutic purposes.

in·fu·sion (ĭn-fyōō′zhən) *n.* **1.** The process of steeping a substance in water to extract its soluble principles. **2.** A medicinal preparation from such a process. **3.** Introduction of a solution into the body through a vein for therapeutic purposes. **4.** The solution so introduced.

infusion-aspiration drainage *n.* The continuous infusion of antibiotics into a cavity while fluid is being drained from the cavity.

in·gest (ĭn-jĕst′) *v.* **-gest·ed, -gest·ing, -gests.** To take into the body by the mouth for digestion or absorption.

in·ges·ta (ĭn-jĕs′tə) *pl.n.* Ingested matter, especially food taken into the body through the mouth.

in·ges·tion (ĭn-jĕs′chən) *n.* **1.** The act of taking food and drink into the body by the mouth. **2.** The taking in of particles by a phagocytic cell. — **in·gest′** (-jĕst′) *v.* — **in·ges′tive** (-jĕs′tĭv) *adj.*

in·grown hair (ĭn′grōn′) *n.* A hair that grows at an abnormal angle and turns back into the skin, causing the formation of a pustule or papule.

ingrown nail *n.* A toenail, one edge of which has grown abnormally into the nail fold.

in·growth (ĭn′grōth′) *n.* Something that grows inward or into a part of the body.

in·gui·nal (ĭng′gwə-nəl) *adj.* **1.** Of or located in the groin. **2.** Relating to the left or right inguinal region of the abdomen.

inguinal canal *n.* The oblique passage through the lower abdominal wall, transmitting the spermatic cord in the male and the round ligament in the female.

inguinal hernia *n.* A hernia into the inguinal canal.

inguinal region *n.* The lower lateral region of the abdomen on either side of the pubic region.

in·ha·lant (ĭn-hā′lənt) *adj.* Used in or for inhaling. — *n.* Something that is inhaled, especially a drug that is delivered to the respiratory passages by a nebulizer or an aerosol container.

in·ha·la·tion (ĭn′hə-lā′shən) *n.* **1.** The act or an instance of inhaling. **2.** A solution of a drug or a combination of drugs administered to the respiratory passages as a nebulized mist.

inhalation anesthesia *n.* General anesthesia resulting from breathing of anesthetic gases or vapors.

inhalation therapy *n.* The therapeutic use of gases or of aerosols by inhalation.

in·ha·la·tor (ĭn′hə-lā′tər) *n.* **1.** See **respirator** (sense 1). **2.** See **inhaler.**

in·hale (ĭn-hāl′) *v.* **-haled, -hal·ing, -hales. 1.** To breathe in; inspire. **2.** To draw something such as smoke or a medicinal mist into the lungs by breathing; inspire.

in·hal·er (ĭn-hā′lər) *n*. A device that produces a vapor to ease breathing or is used to medicate by inhalation, especially a small nasal applicator containing a volatile medicament.

in·her·it (ĭn-hĕr′ĭt) *v*. **-it·ed, -it·ing, -its**. To receive a trait from one's parents by genetic transmission.

in·her·it·a·ble (ĭn-hĕr′ĭ-tə-bəl) *adj*. Capable of being inherited. — **in·her′it·a·bil′i·ty** *n*.

in·her·i·tance (ĭn-hĕr′ĭ-təns) *n*. **1.** The process of genetic transmission of traits from parents to offspring. **2.** A characteristic so inherited. **3.** The sum of characteristics genetically transmitted from parents to offspring.

inherited character *n*. A single attribute of an animal or plant transmitted from generation to generation in accordance with genetic principles.

in·hib·it (ĭn-hĭb′ĭt) *v*. **-it·ed, -it·ing, -its**. **1.** To hold back; restrain. **2.** To suppress or restrain a behavioral process, an impulse, or a desire consciously or unconsciously. **3.** To decrease, limit, or block the action or function of something in the body, as an enzyme or organ. — **in·hib′i·to′ry** (-tôr′ē) *adj*.

in·hi·bi·tion (ĭn′hə-bĭsh′ən, ĭn′ə-) *n*. **1.** The act of inhibiting or the state of being inhibited. **2.** Something that restrains, blocks, or suppresses. **3.** The conscious or unconscious restraint of a behavioral process, a desire, or an impulse. **4.** Any of a variety of processes associated with the gradual attenuation, masking, and extinction of a previously conditioned response. **5.** The condition in which or the process by which a reaction is inhibited. **6.** The condition in which or the process by which an enzyme is inhibited.

inhibitory nerve *n*. A nerve conveying impulses that diminish functional activity in a part.

in·i·ti·a·tion (ĭ-nĭsh′ē-ā′shən) *n*. **1.** The act or an instance of initiating. **2.** The condition of being initiated. **3.** The first stage of tumor induction by a carcinogen in which cells are altered so that they are likely to form a tumor upon subsequent exposure to a promoting agent.

initiation factor *n*. Any of several soluble proteins involved in the initiation of protein synthesis and released from the ribosome as it progresses into chain elongation.

in·ject (ĭn-jĕkt′) *v*. **-ject·ed, -ject·ing, -jects**. **1.** To introduce a substance, such as a drug or vaccine, into a body part. **2.** To treat a patient by means of injection.

in·ject·a·ble (ĭn-jĕk′tə-bəl) *adj*. Capable of being injected. Used of a drug. — *n*. A drug or medicine that can be injected.

in·jec·tion (ĭn-jĕk′shən) *n*. **1.** The act of injecting a substance into a tissue, vessel, canal, or organ. **2.** Something that is injected, especially a dose of liquid medicine injected into the body. **3.** Congestion or hyperemia.

in·ju·ry (ĭn′jə-rē) *n*. **1.** Damage, harm, or loss, as

from trauma. **2.** A particular form of hurt, damage, or loss.

in·lay (ĭn′lā′, ĭn-lā′) *n*. **1.** A solid filling, as of gold or porcelain, fitted to a cavity in a tooth and cemented into place. **2.** A graft of bone, skin, or other tissue. **3.** An orthomechanical device inserted into a shoe.

inlay graft *n*. A skin graft wrapped raw side out around a stent of dental compound and inserted into a prepared surgical pocket.

in·let (ĭn′lĕt′, -lĭt) *n*. A passage leading into a cavity.

in·nate (ĭ-nāt′, ĭn′āt′) *adj*. Possessed at birth; inborn. — **in·nate′ness** *n*.

innate immunity *n*. Immunity that occurs naturally as a result of a person's genetic constitution or physiology and does not arise from a previous infection or vaccination.

in·ner cell mass (ĭn′ər) *n*. The mass at the embryonic pole of the blastocyst concerned with the formation of the body of the embryo.

inner ear *n*. The portion of the ear located within the temporal bone that is involved in both hearing and balance and includes the semicircular canals, vestibule, and cochlea.

in·ner·vate (ĭ-nûr′vāt′, ĭn′ər-) *v*. **-vat·ed, -vat·ing, -vates**. **1.** To supply an organ or a body part with nerves. **2.** To stimulate a nerve, muscle, or body part to action. — **in′ner·va′tion·al** (-vā′shə-nəl) *adj*.

in·ner·va·tion (ĭn′ər-vā′shən) *n*. **1.** The arrangement or distribution of nerves to an organ or body part. **2.** The amount or degree of stimulation of a muscle or organ by nerves. — **in′ner·va′tion·al** (-vā′shə-nəl) *adj*.

in·no·cent murmur (ĭn′ə-sənt) *n*. See **functional murmur**.

innominate artery *n*. An artery with its origin in the arch of the aorta and with branches to the right subclavian and the right common carotid arteries.

innominate bone *n*. See **hipbone**.

in·nu·tri·tion (ĭn′nōō-trĭsh′ən, -nyōō-) *n*. Poor nourishment; lack of good nutrition.

in·oc·u·la·ble (ĭ-nŏk′yə-lə-bəl) *adj*. **1.** Transmissible by inoculation. **2.** Susceptible to a disease transmitted by inoculation. **3.** That can be used in an inoculation. — **in·oc′u·la·bil′i·ty** *n*.

in·oc·u·lant (ĭ-nŏk′yə-lənt) *n*. See **inoculum**.

in·oc·u·late (ĭ-nŏk′yə-lāt′) *v*. **-lat·ed, -lat·ing, -lates**. **1.** To introduce a serum, a vaccine, or an antigenic substance into the body, especially to produce or boost immunity to a specific disease. **2.** To implant microorganisms or infectious material into or on a culture medium. **3.** To communicate a disease to a living organism by transferring its causative agent into the organism. — **in·oc′u·la′tive** *adj*.

in·oc·u·la·tion (ĭ-nŏk′yə-lā′shən) *n*. The act or an instance of inoculating, especially the introduction of an antigenic substance or vaccine into the body to produce immunity to a specific disease.

in·oc·u·lum (ĭ-nŏk′yə-ləm) *n*., *pl*. **-lums** or **-la** (-lə).

The microorganisms or other material used in an inoculation.

in·op·er·a·ble (ĭn-ŏp'ər-ə-bəl, -ŏp'rə-) adj. Unsuitable for a surgical procedure. — **in·op'er·a·bil'i·ty** n.

in·or·gan·ic (ĭn'ôr-găn'ĭk) n. **1.** Not formed by or involving organic life or the products of organic life. **2.** Not composed of organic matter. — **in'or·gan'i·cal·ly** adv.

inorganic compound n. A compound that does not contain hydrocarbon groups.

in·os·co·py (ĭ-nŏs'kə-pē) n. Microscopic examination of biological materials after dissecting or chemically digesting the fibrillary elements and strands of fibrin.

in·os·cu·late (ĭn-ŏs'kyə-lāt') v. **-lat·ed, -lat·ing, -lates. 1.** To unite parts such as blood vessels, nerve fibers, or ducts by small openings. **2.** To unite so as to be continuous; blend.

in·o·se·mi·a (ĭn'ō-sē'mē-ə) n. See **fibremia.**

in·pa·tient (ĭn'pā'shənt) n. A patient who is admitted to a hospital or clinic for treatment that requires at least one overnight stay.

in·quest (ĭn'kwĕst') n. **1.** A legal inquiry into the cause of violent or mysterious death. **2.** The finding based on such an inquiry.

in·sane (ĭn-sān') adj. Of, exhibiting, or afflicted with insanity.

in·san·i·ty (ĭn-săn'ĭ-tē) n. **1.** Persistent mental disorder or derangement. **2.** Unsoundness of mind sufficient in the judgment of a civil court to render a person unfit to maintain a contractual or other legal relationship or to warrant commitment to a mental health facility. **3.** In most criminal jurisdictions, a degree of mental malfunctioning sufficient to relieve the accused of legal responsibility for the act committed.

in·sec·ti·cide (ĭn-sĕk'tĭ-sīd') n. A chemical substance that kills insects. — **in·sec'ti·cid'al** (-sīd'l) adj.

in·se·cure (ĭn'sĭ-kyŏŏr') adj. **1.** Lacking emotional stability; not well-adjusted. **2.** Lacking self-confidence; plagued by anxiety. — **in'se·cu'ri·ty** (-kyŏŏr'ĭ-tē) n.

in·sem·i·nate (ĭn-sĕm'ə-nāt') v. **-nat·ed, -nat·ing, -nates.** To introduce or inject semen into a female's reproductive tract. — **in·sem'i·na'tion** n.

in·se·nes·cence (ĭn'sĭ-nĕs'əns) n. The process of becoming old; senescence.

in·sen·si·ble (ĭn-sĕn'sə-bəl) adj. **1.** Having lost consciousness, especially temporarily; unconscious. **2.** Lacking physical sensation or the power to react, as to pain or cold; numb.

insensible perspiration n. Perspiration that evaporates before it is perceived as moisture on the skin.

in·ser·tion (ĭn-sûr'shən) n. The point or mode of attachment of a skeletal muscle to the bone or other body part that it moves.

in·sid·i·ous (ĭn-sĭd'ē-əs) adj. Of or being a disease that progresses with few or no symptoms to indicate its gravity. — **in·sid'i·ous·ly** adv. — **in·sid'i·ous·ness** n.

in·sight (ĭn'sīt') n. Understanding, especially self-understanding of the motives and reasons behind one's actions. — **in'sight·ful** (ĭn'sīt'fəl, ĭn-sīt'-) adj.

in si·tu (ĭn sī'tōō) adj. **1.** In the original position. **2.** Confined to the site of origin. — **in situ** adv.

in·som·ni·a (ĭn-sŏm'nē-ə) n. Chronic inability to fall asleep or remain asleep for an adequate length of time.

in·som·ni·ac (ĭn-sŏm'nē-ăk') n. One who suffers from insomnia.

in·sorp·tion (ĭn-sôrp'shən) n. Movement of substances from the intestinal tract into the blood.

in·sper·sion (ĭn-spûr'shən, -zhən) n. The act of sprinkling with a fluid or a powder.

in·spi·ra·tion (ĭn'spə-rā'shən) n. The inhalation of air into the lungs.

in·spi·ra·to·ry (ĭn-spīr'ə-tôr'ē) adj. Of, relating to, or used for the drawing in of air.

inspiratory capacity n. The volume of air that can be inhaled after normal inspiration.

inspiratory stridor n. A crowing sound during the inspiratory phase of respiration during general anesthesia due to relaxation of the laryngeal muscles that maintain vocal cord abduction.

in·spire (ĭn-spīr') v. **-spired, -spir·ing, -spires.** To inhale.

inspired gas n. A gas that has been inhaled; specifically, an inhaled gas after it has been humidified at body temperature.

in·spis·sate (ĭn-spĭs'āt', ĭn'spĭ-sāt') v. **-sat·ed, -sat·ing, -sates.** To undergo thickening or cause to thicken, as by evaporation or the absorption of fluid. — **in'spis·sa'tion** n. — **in·spis'sa'tor** n.

in·step (ĭn'stĕp') n. The arched middle part of the human foot between the toes and the ankle.

in·still (ĭn-stĭl') v. **-stilled, -still·ing, -stills.** To add drop by drop. — **in'stil·la'tion** (ĭn'stə-lā'shən) n.

in·stinct (ĭn'stĭngkt') n. **1.** An inborn pattern of behavior that is characteristic of a species and is often a response to specific environmental stimuli. **2.** A powerful motivation or impulse. — **in·stinc'tive, in·stinc'tu·al** (ĭn-stĭngk'chōō-əl) adj.

in·sti·tu·tion·al·ize (ĭn'stĭ-tōō'shə-nə-līz', -tyōō'-) v. **-ized, -iz·ing, -iz·es.** To place a person in the care of an institution, especially one providing care for the disabled or mentally ill. — **in'sti·tu'tion·al·i·za'tion** (-shə-nə-lĭ-zā'shən) n.

in·stru·ment (ĭn'strə-mənt) n. A tool or implement, as for surgery.

in·stru·men·tar·i·um (ĭn'strə-mən-târ'ē-əm, -mĕn-) n., pl. **-i·a** (-ē-ə). A collection of instruments and other equipment for a surgical operation or for a medical procedure.

in·suf·fi·cien·cy (ĭn'sə-fĭsh'ən-sē) n. **1.** Inability of a bodily part or an organ to function normally. **2.** Moral or mental incompetence.

in·suf·fi·cient (ĭn'sə-fĭsh'ənt) adj. **1.** Not sufficient; inadequate. **2.** Incapable of proper functioning; incompetent.

in·suf·flate (ĭn'sə-flāt', ĭn-sŭf'lāt') v. **-flat·ed, -flat·ing, -flates. 1.** To blow into, especially to fill the lungs of an asphyxiated person with air, or to blow a medicated vapor, powder, or anesthetic into the lungs, or into any cavity or orifice of the body. **2.** To treat by blowing a medicated powder, gas, or vapor into a bodily cavity. — **in′suf·fla′tor** *n.*

in·suf·fla·tion anesthesia (ĭn′sə-flā′shən) *n.* The maintenance of inhalation anesthesia by delivery of anesthetic gases or vapors directly to a person's airway.

in·su·la (ĭn′sə-lə, ĭns′yə-) *n., pl.* **in·su·lae** (-lē′). **1.** A circumscribed body or patch on the skin. **2.** An oval region of the cerebral cortex that is involved in processing both physical actions and mental imaging.

in·su·lin (ĭn′sə-lĭn) *n.* **1.** A polypeptide hormone that is secreted by the islets of Langerhans, helps regulate the metabolism of carbohydrates and fats, especially the conversion of glucose to glycogen, and promotes protein synthesis and the formation and storage of neutral lipids. **2.** Any of various pharmaceutical preparations containing this hormone that are derived from the pancreas of certain animals or produced through genetic engineering and are used parenterally in the treatment of insulin-dependent diabetes mellitus.

insulin-dependent diabetes *n.* See **diabetes mellitus** (sense 1).

in·su·li·ne·mi·a (ĭn′sə-lə-nē′mē-ə) *n.* An abnormally large concentration of insulin in the blood.

in·su·lin·like activity (ĭn′sə-lĭn-līk′) *n.* A measure of the substances, usually in plasma, that exert biological effects similar to those of insulin in various bioassays.

in·su·lin·o·gen·e·sis (ĭn′sə-lĭn′ə-jĕn′ĭ-sĭs) *n.* Production of insulin by the islets of Langerhans. — **in′su·lin′o·gen′ic, in′su·lo·gen′ic** (ĭn′sə-lō-gĕn′ĭk) *adj.*

in·su·li·no·ma (ĭn′sə-lə-nō′mə) *n., pl.* **-mas** or **-ma·ta** (-mə-tə). An islet cell adenoma that secretes insulin.

insulin pump *n.* A portable device for people with diabetes that injects insulin at programmed intervals in order to regulate blood sugar levels.

insulin resistance *n.* A state of diminished effectiveness of insulin in lowering the levels of blood sugar, usually resulting from insulin binding by antibodies, and associated with conditions such as obesity, ketoacidosis, and infection.

insulin shock *n.* Acute hypoglycemia usually resulting from an overdose of insulin and characterized by sweating, trembling, dizziness, and, if left untreated, convulsions and coma.

in·su·lo·ma (ĭn′sə-lō′mə) *n., pl.* **-mas** or **-ma·ta** (-mə-tə). See **insulinoma**.

in·sus·cep·ti·bil·i·ty (ĭn′sə-sĕp′tə-bĭl′ĭ-tē) *n.* The state or condition of not being susceptible to a disease or infection. — **in′sus·cep′ti·ble** *adj.*

int. cib. *abbr. Latin.* inter cibos (between meals)

in·te·gra·tion (ĭn′tĭ-grā′shən) *n.* **1.** The organization of the psychological or social traits and tendencies of a personality into a harmonious whole. **2.** A physiological increase or building up, as by accretion or anabolism. **3.** A recombination

event in which a genetic element is inserted.

in·teg·ri·ty (ĭn-tĕg′rĭ-tē) *n.* The state of being unimpaired; soundness or wholeness.

in·teg·u·ment (ĭn-tĕg′yŏo-mənt) *n.* **1.** The enveloping membrane of the body, including the dermis, epidermis, hairs, nails, and sebaceous, mammary, and sweat glands. **2.** The membrane, capsule, skin, or other covering of any body or part. — **in·teg′u·men′ta·ry** (-mĕn′tə-rē, -mĕn′-trē) *adj.*

in·tel·lec·tu·al·ize (ĭn′tl-ĕk′chŏo-ə-līz′) *v.* **-ized, -iz·ing, -iz·es. 1.** To furnish a rational structure or meaning for. **2.** To engage in excessive intellectual reasoning as an unconscious defense against the emotional stress associated with painful personal fears or problems.

in·tel·li·gence (ĭn-tĕl′ə-jəns) *n.* **1.** The capacity to acquire and apply knowledge, especially toward a purposeful goal. **2.** A person's relative standing on two quantitative indices, namely measured intelligence, as expressed by an intelligence quotient, and effectiveness of adaptive behavior.

intelligence quotient *n.* An index of measured intelligence expressed as the ratio of tested mental age to chronological age, multiplied by 100.

in·ten·sive care (ĭn-tĕn′sĭv) *n.* Continuous and closely monitored health care that is provided to critically ill patients.

intensive care unit *n.* A specialized section of a hospital containing the equipment, medical and nursing staff, and monitoring devices necessary to provide intensive care.

in·ten·tion (ĭn-tĕn′shən) *n.* **1.** An aim that guides action; an objective. **2.** The process by which a wound heals. — **in·ten′tion·al** *adj.*

intention tremor *n.* A tremor that occurs when a voluntary movement is made.

in·ter·brain (ĭn′tər-brān′) *n.* See **diencephalon**.

in·ter·ca·lat·ed disk (ĭn-tûr′kə-lā′tĭd) *n.* An undulating double membrane separating adjacent cells in cardiac muscle fibers.

in·ter·cel·lu·lar canaliculus (ĭn′tər-sĕl′yə-lər) *n.* Any of various fine channels between adjoining secretory cells.

in·ter·cil·i·um (ĭn′tər-sĭl′ē-əm) *n.* Glabella.

in·ter·cos·tal (ĭn′tər-kŏs′təl) *adj.* Located or occurring between the ribs.

intercostal membrane *n.* Any of the membranous layers between the ribs.

intercostal nerve *n.* Any of the ventral branches of the thoracic nerves.

intercostal space *n.* The interval between each rib.

in·ter·course (ĭn′tər-kôrs′) *n.* **1.** Dealings or communications between persons or groups. **2.** Sexual intercourse.

in·ter·cri·co·thy·rot·o·my (ĭn′tər-krī′kō-thī-rŏt′ə-mē) *n.* See **cricothyrotomy**.

in·ter·cus·pa·tion (ĭn′tər-kŭ-spā′shən) *n.* The interlocking of the cusps of opposing teeth.

in·ter·dig·it (ĭn′tər-dĭj′ĭt) *n.* The area of the hand or foot between any two adjacent fingers or toes.

in·ter·dis·ci·pli·nar·y (ĭn′tər-dĭs′ə-plə-nĕr′ē) *adj.* Of or involving two or more medical or scientific disciplines that are usually considered distinct.

in·ter·face (ĭn′tər-fās′) *n.* A surface forming a common boundary between adjacent regions or bodies.

in·ter·fer·ence (ĭn′tər-fēr′əns) *n.* **1.** The condition in which infection of a cell by one virus prevents superinfection by another virus. **2.** The condition in which superinfection by a second virus prevents effects that would result from infection by either virus alone, even though both viruses persist.

in·ter·fer·on (ĭn′tər-fēr′ŏn′) *n.* Any of a group of glycoproteins that are produced by different cell types in response to various stimuli and that block viral replication in newly infected cells and, in some cases, modulate specific cellular functions such as growth and differentiation.

in·ter·ki·ne·sis (ĭn′tər-kə-nē′sĭs, -kī-) *n.* See **interphase**.

in·ter·lam·i·nar jelly (ĭn′tər-lăm′ə-nər) *n.* The gelatinous material between ectoderm and endoderm that serves as the substrate on which mesenchymal cells migrate.

in·ter·leu·kin (ĭn′tər-lōō′kĭn) *n.* Any of a class of lymphokines that act to stimulate, regulate, or modulate lymphocytes such as T cells.

interleukin-1 *n.* Any of a group of cytokines, released by macrophages and other cells, that induce the production of interleukin-2 by helper T cells and stimulate the inflammatory response.

interleukin-2 *n.* A lymphokine that is released by helper T cells in response to an antigen and interleukin-1 and stimulates the proliferation of helper T cells. It has been used experimentally to treat cancer.

in·ter·lo·bi·tis (ĭn′tər-lō-bī′tĭs) *n.* Inflammation of the pleura separating two pulmonary lobes.

intermediate host *n.* A host in which a parasite goes through its larval or developmental stages.

in·ter·me·din (ĭn′tər-mēd′n) *n.* See **melanocyte-stimulating hormone**.

in·ter·mit·tent (ĭn′tər-mĭt′nt) *adj.* **1.** Stopping and starting at intervals. **2.** Marked by intervals of complete quietude between two periods of activity. — **in′ter·mit′tence** *n.*

intermittent acute porphyria *n.* Porphyria caused by overproduction of ALA, with greatly increased urinary excretion of it and of porphobilinogen, due to a deficiency of porphobilinogen deaminase. It is characterized by intermittent acute attacks of hypertension, abdominal colic, psychosis, and neuropathy.

intermittent claudication *n.* A condition caused by ischemia of the leg muscles due to sclerosis and narrowing of the arteries, characterized by attacks of lameness and pain and brought on by walking.

intermittent mandatory ventilation *n.* Mechanical application of positive pressure at a determined frequency to the airway to increase tidal volume.

intermittent positive pressure ventilation *n.* See **controlled mechanical ventilation**.

intermuscular septum *n.* Any of the aponeurotic sheets separating various muscles of the extremities, including the anterior and posterior crural septa, the lateral and medial femoral septa, and the lateral and medial humeral septa.

in·tern or **in·terne** (ĭn′tûrn′) *n.* An advanced student or recent graduate who assists in the medical or surgical care of hospital patients and who resides within the institution. — *v.* **-terned, -terning, -terns.** To train or serve as an intern. — **in′tern·ship′** *n.*

in·ter·nal (ĭn-tûr′nəl) *adj.* **1.** Located, acting, or effective within the body. **2.** Relating to or located within the limits or surface; inner.

internal ear *n.* See **inner ear**.

internal fixation *n.* The stabilization of fractured bony parts by direct fixation to one another with surgical wires, screws, pins, or plates.

internal hemorrhage *n.* Bleeding into organs or cavities of the body.

internal hemorrhoids *pl.n.* Hemorrhoids occurring beneath the mucous membrane of the anal sphincter.

in·ter·nal·ize (ĭn-tûr′nə-līz′) *v.* **-ized, -iz·ing, -iz·es.** **1.** To make internal, personal, or subjective. **2.** To take in and adopt as an integral part of one's attitudes or beliefs. — **in·ter′nal·i·za′tion** (-nə-lĭ-zā′shən) *n.*

internal medicine *n.* The branch of medicine that deals with the diagnosis and nonsurgical treatment of diseases affecting the internal organs of the body, especially in adults.

internal oblique muscle *n.* The oblique muscle that forms the middle layer in the lateral and ventral abdominal wall.

internal respiration *n.* See **tissue respiration**.

internal secretion *n.* A secretion that is produced by an endocrine gland and discharged directly into the bloodstream; a hormone.

internal traction *n.* A pulling force created by using one of the cranial bones, above the point of fracture, for anchorage.

internal version *n.* Version of a fetus performed with one hand inside the uterus.

in·ter·neu·ron (ĭn′tər-nōōr′ŏn′, -nyōōr′-) *n.* A nerve cell found entirely within the central nervous system that acts as a link between sensory neurons and motor neurons. — **in′ter·neu′ro·nal** (-nōōr′ə-nəl, -nyōōr′-, -nōō-rō′-, -nyōō-) *adj.*

in·ter·nist (ĭn-tûr′nĭst) *n.* A physician specializing in internal medicine.

in·ter·nod·al segment (ĭn′tər-nōd′l) *n.* The portion of a myelinated nerve fiber between two successive nodes.

in·ter·o·cep·tor (ĭn′tər-ō-sĕp′tər) *n.* A specialized sensory nerve receptor that receives and responds to stimuli originating from within the body. — **in′ter·o·cep′tive** *adj.*

in·ter·phase (ĭn′tər-fāz′) *n.* The stage of a cell between two successive mitotic or meiotic divisions.

in·ter·pleu·ral space (ĭn′tər-plōōr′əl) *n.* See **mediastinum** (sense 2).

in·ter·po·lat·ed extrasystole (ĭn-tûr′pə-lā′tĭd) *n.*

A ventricular contraction that occurs between two normal heartbeats.

in·ter·pre·ta·tion (ĭn-tûr′prĭ-tā′shən) *n.* **1.** The act or process of explaining the meaning of something. **2.** A psychotherapist's explanation of the meaning of a patient's remarks, dreams, memories, experiences, and behavior.

in·ter·space (ĭn′tər-spās′) *n.* A space between two things; an interval. — **in′ter·space′** *v.* — **in′ter·spa′tial** (-spā′shəl) *adj.*

in·ter·stice (ĭn-tûr′stĭs) *n., pl.* **-stic·es** (-stĭ-sēz′, -sĭz). A small area, space, or hole in the substance of an organ or tissue.

in·ter·sti·tial (ĭn′tər-stĭsh′əl) *adj.* Relating to or situated in the small, narrow spaces between tissues or parts of an organ.

interstitial cell *n.* A cell occurring between the germ cells of the gonads and believed to furnish the male sex hormone.

interstitial cystitis *n.* A chronic inflammatory condition of unknown cause involving the mucosa and muscular tissue of the bladder and resulting in reduced bladder capacity.

interstitial disease *n.* A disease that chiefly affects the connective-tissue framework of an organ.

interstitial fluid *n.* The fluid in spaces between the tissue cells, constituting about 16 percent of the weight of the body.

interstitial gastritis *n.* Inflammation of the stomach involving the submucous and muscle coats.

interstitial growth *n.* Growth originating in a number of different centers within a structure or an area, characteristic of tissues formed of nonrigid materials.

interstitial tissue *n.* See **connective tissue.**

in·ter·sti·ti·um (ĭn′tər-stĭsh′ē-əm) *n.* An interstice.

in·ter·tri·go (ĭn′tər-trī′gō′) *n.* Dermatitis occurring between folds or juxtaposed surfaces of the skin and caused by moisture, warmth, and the overgrowth of resident microorganisms.

in·ter·val (ĭn′tər-vəl) *n.* **1.** A space between two objects, points, or units. **2.** The amount of time between two specified instants, events, or states.

interval phase *n.* Ovulation.

in·ter·ven·tion (ĭn′tər-vĕn′shən) *n.* Interference so as to modify a process or situation. — **in′ter·vene′** (ĭn′tər-vēn′) *v.*

in·ter·ven·tric·u·lar foramen (ĭn′tər-vĕn-trĭk′-yə-lər) *n.* The short, often slitlike passage that connects the third ventricle of the diencephalon with the lateral ventricle in the cerebral hemisphere.

interventricular septum *n.* The wall between the ventricles of the heart.

in·ter·ver·te·bral (ĭn′tər-vûr′tə-brəl, -vûr-tē′-) *adj.* Located between vertebrae.

intervertebral disk *n.* Any of the disks between the bodies of adjacent vertebrae.

intervertebral foramen *n.* Any of the openings into the vertebral canal bounded by the pedicles of adjacent vertebra, the vertebral bodies, and the articular processes.

in·ter·vil·lous lacuna (ĭn′tər-vĭl′əs) *n.* One of the spaces in the placenta that contain maternal blood and into which the chorionic villi project.

intervillous space *n.* Any of the spaces between placental villi containing maternal blood.

in·tes·ti·nal (ĭn-tĕs′tə-nəl) *adj.* Of, relating to, or constituting the intestine.

intestinal anastomosis *n.* See **enteroenterostomy.**

intestinal atresia *n.* Congenital absence or closure of the lumen of the small intestine involving the ileum, jejunum, or duodenum.

intestinal digestion *n.* The part of digestion carried on in the intestine and affecting all food, including starches, fats, and proteins.

intestinal fistula *n.* A tract leading from the lumen of the bowel to the exterior.

intestinal gland *n.* Any of the tubular glands in the mucous membrane of the intestines.

intestinal villus *n.* Any of the many projections of the mucous membrane of the intestine that serve as sites of absorption and are leaf-shaped in the duodenum and become shorter, more finger-shaped, and sparser in the ileum.

in·tes·tine (ĭn-tĕs′tĭn) *n.* The portion of the alimentary canal extending from the stomach to the anus and consisting of two segments, the small intestine and the large intestine.

in·ti·ma (ĭn′tə-mə) *n., pl.* **-mas** or **-mae** (-mē′). The tunica intima. — **in′ti·mal** *adj.*

in·tol·er·ance (ĭn-tŏl′ər-əns) *n.* Extreme sensitivity or allergy to a drug, food, or other substance.

in·tor·sion (ĭn-tôr′shən) *n.* The inward rotation of a limb or an organ.

in·tor·tor (ĭn-tôr′tər) *n.* A muscle that turns a part medially.

in·tox·i·cate (ĭn-tŏk′sĭ-kāt′) *v.* **-cat·ed, -cat·ing, -cates.** To stupefy or excite, as by the action of a chemical substance such as alcohol.

in·tox·i·ca·tion (ĭn-tŏk′sĭ-kā′shən) *n.* **1.** The pathological state produced by a drug, serum, alcohol, or any toxic substance; poisoning. **2.** Acute alcoholism. **3.** A state of mental excitement.

in·tra-a·or·tic balloon device (ĭn′trə-ā-ôr′tĭk) *n.* An inflatable balloon placed into the descending aorta to assist the heart in pumping blood; the balloon is inflated between contractions, increasing blood pressure and perfusion of the blood to the organs, and deflated during contractions, thus reducing the amount of work the heart must accomplish.

intra-aortic balloon pump *n.* The pump connected to an intra-aortic balloon device.

in·tra·car·di·ac catheter (ĭn′trə-kär′dē-ăk′) *n.* See **cardiac catheter.**

in·tra·cath·e·ter (ĭn′trə-kăth′ĭ-tər) *n.* A plastic tube, usually attached to a puncturing needle, inserted into a blood vessel for infusion, injection, or pressure monitoring.

in·tra·cel·lu·lar (ĭn′trə-sĕl′yə-lər) *adj.* Occurring or situated within a cell or cells.

in·tra·cel·lu·lar canaliculus (ĭn′trə-sĕl′yə-lər) *n.* A fine canal formed by invagination of a cell membrane into the cytoplasm of a cell.

intracellular fluid *n.* The fluid within the tissue

cells, constituting about 30 percent to 40 percent of the body weight.

in·tra·cra·ni·al hemorrhage (ĭn'trə-krā'nē-əl) n. The escape of blood within the cranium due to the loss of integrity of vascular channels and frequently leading to formation of a hematoma.

intracranial pressure n. Pressure within the cranial cavity.

in·trac·ta·ble (ĭn-trăk'tə-bəl) adj. **1.** Difficult to manage or govern; stubborn. **2.** Difficult to alleviate, remedy, or cure. — **in·trac'ta·bil'i·ty, in·trac'ta·ble·ness** n.

in·tra·cu·ta·ne·ous reaction (ĭn'trə-kyōō-tā'-nē-əs) n. A skin reaction following the intracutaneous injection of an antigen to which one has been sensitized, as in the tuberculin test.

in·tra·der·mal reaction (ĭn'trə-dûr'məl) n. See **intracutaneous reaction**.

intradermal test n. A test for hypersensitivity or allergy in which a small amount of the suspected allergen is injected into the skin.

in·tra·lob·u·lar duct (ĭn'trə-lŏb'yə-lər) n. One of the ducts contained within a lobule of a gland.

in·tra·mus·cu·lar (ĭn'trə-mŭs'kyə-lər) adj. Within a muscle.

in·tra·na·sal anesthesia (ĭn'trə-nā'zəl) n. **1.** Insufflation anesthesia in which an inhalation anesthetic is added to inhaled air as it passes through the nose or nasopharynx. **2.** Anesthesia of nasal passages by topical application of a local anesthetic solution to nasal mucosa.

in·tra·oc·u·lar pressure (ĭn'trə-ŏk'yə-lər) n. The pressure of the intraocular fluid within the eye.

intraocular tension n. The pressure within the eyeball, measured by the resistance of the tunics of the eye to indentation.

in·tra·o·ral anesthesia (ĭn'trə-ôr'əl) n. **1.** Insufflation anesthesia in which an inhalation anesthetic is added to inhaled air passing through the mouth. **2.** Regional anesthesia of the mouth and associated structures by topical application of local anesthetic solutions to oral mucosa.

in·tra·par·tum hemorrhage (ĭn'trə-pär'təm) n. Hemorrhage occurring in the course of normal labor and delivery.

in·tra·u·ter·ine (ĭn'trə-yōō'tər-ĭn, -tə-rīn') adj. Within the uterus.

intrauterine contraceptive n. An intrauterine device.

intrauterine device n. A birth control device, such as a plastic or metallic loop, ring, or spiral, that is inserted into the uterus to prevent implantation of a fertilized egg in the uterine lining.

in·trav·a·sa·tion (ĭn-trăv'ə-sā'shən) n. Entry of foreign matter into a blood vessel.

in·tra·ve·nous (ĭn'trə-vē'nəs) adj. Within or administered into a vein. — **in'tra·ve'nous·ly** adv.

in·tra·ve·nous anesthesia (ĭn'trə-vē'nəs) n. General anesthesia in which venipuncture is used as a means of injecting central nervous system depressants into the bloodstream.

intravenous anesthetic n. An agent that produces

anesthesia when injected into the bloodstream via venipuncture.

intravenous drip n. The continuous introduction of a solution intravenously, a drop at a time.

intravenous urography n. X-ray examination of kidneys, ureters, and bladder following the injection of a contrast agent into a vein.

in·tra·ven·tric·u·lar conduction (ĭn'trə-vĕn-trĭk'yə-lər) n. The conduction of the cardiac impulse through the ventricular muscle tissue, represented by the QRS complex in an electrocardiogram.

in·trin·sic (ĭn-trĭn'zĭk, -sĭk) adj. **1.** Of or relating to the essential nature of a thing; inherent. **2.** Situated within or belonging solely to the organ or body part on which it acts. Used of certain nerves and muscles.

intrinsic factor n. A relatively small mucoprotein secreted by the parietal cells of gastric glands and required for adequate absorption of vitamin B_{12} for production of red blood cells.

intrinsic reflex n. A reflex muscular contraction elicited by the application of a stimulus, usually stretching, to the muscle.

in·tro·duc·er (ĭn'trə-dōō'sər, -dyōō'-) n. An instrument or stylet used to insert a catheter, an endotracheal tube, or similar flexible device into the body.

in·tro·flec·tion or **in·tro·flex·ion** (ĭn'trə-flĕk'-shən) n. A bending inward.

in·tro·i·tus (ĭn-trō'ĭ-təs) n., pl. **introitus**. The entrance into a canal or hollow organ, such as the vagina.

in·tro·jec·tion (ĭn'trə-jĕk'shən) n. The process of incorporating the characteristics of a person or object unconsciously into one's psyche, often as a defense mechanism. — **in'tro·ject'** v.

in·tro·mis·sion (ĭn'trə-mĭsh'ən) n. The act or process of intromitting. — **in'tro·mis'sive** (-mĭs'ĭv) adj.

in·tro·mit (ĭn'trə-mĭt') v. **-mit·ted, -mit·ting, -mits**. To cause or permit to enter; introduce or admit.

in·tron (ĭn'trŏn) n. A segment of a gene situated between exons that does not function in coding for protein synthesis.

in·tro·spec·tion (ĭn'trə-spĕk'shən) n. Contemplation of one's own thoughts, feelings, and sensations; self-examination. — **in'tro·spect'** v. — **in'-tro·spec'tion·al** adj. — **in'tro·spec'tive** (-tĭv) adj.

in·tro·sus·cep·tion (ĭn'trō-sə-sĕp'shən) n. See **intussusception**.

in·tro·ver·sion (ĭn'trə-vûr'zhən, -shən) n. **1.** The act or process of introverting or the condition of being introverted. **2.** The direction or tendency to direct one's thoughts and feelings toward oneself. — **in'tro·ver'sive** (-vûr'sĭv) adj.

in·tro·vert (ĭn'trə-vûrt', ĭn'trə-vûrt') v. **-vert·ed, -vert·ing, -verts**. **1.** To turn or direct inward. **2.** To concentrate one's interests upon oneself. **3.** To turn a tubular organ or part inward upon itself. — n. (ĭn'trə-vûrt'). **1.** One whose thoughts and feelings are directed toward oneself. **2.** An anatomical structure that is capable of being introverted.

in·tu·bate (ĭn′tōō-bāt′, -tyōō-) *v.* **-bat·ed, -bat·ing, -bates.** To insert a tube into a hollow organ or body passage. — **in′tu·ba′tion** *n.* — **in′tu·ba′tion·al** *adj.*

in·tu·i·tive stage (ĭn-tōō′ĭ-tĭv, -tyōō′-) *n.* A stage of development, usually between 4 and 7 years of age, in which thought processes are determined by the prominent aspects of stimuli to which one is exposed, rather than by logical thought.

in·tu·mesce (ĭn′tōō-mĕs′, -tyōō-) *v.* **-mesced, -mesc·ing, -mesc·es.** **1.** To swell or expand; enlarge. **2.** To bubble up, especially from the effect of heating.

in·tu·mes·cence (ĭn′tōō-mĕs′əns, -tyōō-) *n.* **1.** The act or process of swelling or the condition of being swollen. **2.** A swollen organ or body part. — **in′tu·mes′cent** *adj.*

in·tus·sus·cept (ĭn′tə-sə-sĕpt′) *v.* **-cept·ed, -cept·ing, -cepts.** To take within, as in telescoping one part of the intestine into another; invaginate.

in·tus·sus·cep·tion (ĭn′tə-sə-sĕp′shən) *n.* **1.** Invagination, especially an infolding of one part of the intestine into another. **2.** Assimilation of new substances into the existing components of living tissue.

in·u·lin clearance (ĭn′yə-lĭn) *n.* A method for determining the rate of filtration in the renal glomeruli, since inulin, a fructose polysaccharide found in plants, is completely filterable through them and is neither excreted nor reabsorbed by the renal tubules.

in·unc·tion (ĭn-ŭngk′shən) *n.* The process of applying and rubbing in an ointment.

in u·ter·o (ĭn yōō′tə-rō) *adv.* — *adj.* In the uterus.

in·vag·i·nate (ĭn-văj′ə-nāt′) *v.* **-nat·ed, -nat·ing, -nates.** To infold or become infolded so as to form a hollow space within a previously solid structure, as in the formation of a gastrula from a blastula.

in·vag·i·na·tion (ĭn-văj′ə-nā′shən) *n.* **1.** The act or process of invaginating or the condition of being invaginated. **2.** An invaginated organ or part. **3.** The infolding of a portion of the outer layer of a blastula in the formation of a gastrula.

in·va·lid (ĭn′və-lĭd) *n.* One who is incapacitated by a chronic illness or disability. — *adj.* Incapacitated by illness or injury.

in·va·sive (ĭn-vā′sĭv) *adj.* **1.** Marked by the tendency to spread, especially into healthy tissue, as a tumor. **2.** Of or relating to a medical procedure in which a part of the body is entered, as by puncture or surgical incision. — **in·va′sive·ness** *n.*

in·ver·sion (ĭn-vûr′zhən, -shən) *n.* **1.** The act of inverting or the state of being inverted. **2.** The taking on of the gender role of the opposite sex. **3.** Homosexuality. Used in psychology. **4.** A chromosomal defect in which a segment of the chromosome breaks off and reattaches in the reverse direction.

in·vert (ĭn-vûrt′) *v.* **-vert·ed, -vert·ing, -verts. 1.** To turn inside out or upside down. **2.** To reverse

the position, order, or condition of. **3.** To subject to inversion. — *n.* (ĭn′vûrt′). **1.** Something inverted. **2.** One who takes on the gender role of the opposite sex. **3.** A homosexual. Used in psychology.

in·ver·tase (ĭn-vûr′tās, ĭn′vər-tās, -tāz′) *n.* An enzyme that catalyzes the hydrolysis of sucrose into glucose and fructose.

in·ver·tin (ĭn-vûr′tn), *n.* See **invertase**.

in·ver·tor (ĭn-vûr′tər) *n.* A muscle that turns a body part such as the foot inward.

in·vert sugar (ĭn′vûrt) *n.* A mixture of equal parts of glucose and fructose resulting from the hydrolysis of sucrose, found naturally in fruits and honey, and produced artificially for use in the food industry.

in·vet·er·ate (ĭn-vĕt′ər-ĭt) *adj.* **1.** Firmly and long established; deep-rooted. **2.** Persisting in an ingrained habit; habitual. — **in·vet′er·a·cy** (-ər-ə-sē), **in·vet′er·ate·ness** *n.*

in·vis·ca·tion (ĭn′vĭ-skā′shən) *n.* **1.** Smearing with mucilaginous matter. **2.** The mixing of food with the buccal secretions during chewing.

in vi·tro (ĭn vē′trō) *adj.* In an artificial environment outside a living organism.

in vitro fertilization *n.* Fertilization of an egg outside the body of a female animal or human by the addition of sperm, as a means of producing a zygote either for laboratory analysis or for implantation into a uterus.

in vi·vo (vē′vō) *adj.* Within a living organism.

in vivo fertilization *n.* Fertilization of a ripe egg within the uterus of a fertile donor female, rather than in an artificial medium, for subsequent nonsurgical transfer to an infertile recipient.

in·vol·un·tar·y (ĭn-vŏl′ən-tĕr′ē) *adj.* **1.** Not subject to control of the volition. **2.** Acting or done without or against one's will.

involuntary muscle *n.* Any of the muscles, which are all smooth except for the heart muscles, not under control of the will.

in·vo·lu·tion (ĭn′və-lōō′shən) *n.* **1.** A decrease in size of an organ, as of the uterus following childbirth. **2.** The ingrowth and curling inward of a group of cells, as in the formation of a gastrula from a blastula. **3.** A progressive decline or degeneration of normal physiological functioning occurring as a result of the aging process. — **in′vo·lu′tion·al** *adj.*

involutional psychosis *n.* A mental disturbance occurring during menopause or later life, characterized chiefly by depression.

i·o·dine (ī′ə-dīn′, -dĭn, -dēn′) *n.* **1.** A poisonous halogen element with atomic number 53 and forming compounds used as germicides, antiseptics, and food supplements, with radioactive isotopes used in thyroid disease diagnosis and therapy. **2.** A liquid containing iodine dissolved in ethyl alcohol, used as an antiseptic.

io·dip·a·mide (ī′ə-dĭp′ə-mīd′) *n.* A radiopaque contrast medium used for diagnostic tests for the biliary system.

i·o·do·chlor·hy·drox·y·quin (ī-ō′də-klôr′hī-drŏk′sĭ-kwĭn′) or **i·o·do·chlor·o·hy·drox·y·quin·o·line** (-klôr′ō-hī′drŏk′sĭ-kwĭn′ə-lēn′, -lĭn) *n.* A compound used topically as a local antibacterial agent and in the treatment of a wide range of dermatoses, intravaginally in the treatment of *Trichomonas vaginalis* vaginitis, and internally in the treatment of mild or asymptomatic intestinal amebiasis.

io·do·hip·pu·rate sodium (ī-ō′də-hĭp′yə-rāt′) *n.* A radiopaque compound administered intravenously and orally, especially when tagged with ¹³¹I, for diagnostic applications such as retrograde urography and renography.

io·do·meth·a·mate sodium (ī-ō′də-mĕth′ə-māt′) *n.* An organic iodine radiopaque compound used in intravenous urography and retrograde pyelography.

i·o·dom·e·try (ī′ō-dŏm′ĭ-trē) *n.* An analytical technique involving titrations in which the sudden appearance or disappearance of iodine marks the end point. — **i·o′do·met′ric** (ī-ō′də-mĕt′rĭk) *adj.*

i·o·do·phil·i·a (ī-ō′də-fĭl′ē-ə) *n.* An affinity for iodine, as manifested by some white blood cells in certain conditions.

i·o·dop·sin (ī′ə-dŏp′sĭn) *n.* A violet, light-sensitive visual pigment found in the cones of the retina.

i·o·do·py·ra·cet (ī-ō′də-pī′rə-sĕt′) *n.* A radiopaque contrast medium used intravenously in urography and also used to determine renal plasma flow and renal tubular excretory mass.

i·o·do·thy·ro·nine (ī-ō′dō-thī′rə-nēn′, -nĭn) *n.* Any of the iodinated derivatives of thyronine.

i·o·du·ria (ī′ə-dŏor′ē-ə, -dyŏor′-) *n.* The excretion of iodine in the urine.

i·on (ī′ən, ī′ŏn′) *n.* An atom or a group of atoms that has acquired a net electric charge by gaining or losing one or more electrons.

i·on·ic (ī-ŏn′ĭk) *adj.* Of, containing, or involving an ion or ions.

i·on·i·za·tion (ī′ə-nĭ-zā′shən) *n.* The formation of or separation into ions by heat, electrical discharge, radiation, or chemical reaction; electrolytic dissociation.

i·on·ize (ī′ə-nīz′) *v.* **-ized, -iz·ing, -iz·es.** To dissociate atoms or molecules into electrically charged atoms or radicals; to separate into ions. — **i′on·iz′er** *n.*

ionizing radiation *n.* High-energy radiation capable of producing ionization in substances through which it passes.

i·o·pam·i·dol (ī′ə-păm′ĭ-dôl′) *n.* A diagnostic radiopaque medium used in myelography, urography, and ventriculography.

i·ox·ag·late (ī′ŏks-ăg′lāt′) *n.* A diagnostic radiopaque medium used in angiography, aortography, and urography.

ip·e·cac (ĭp′ĭ-kăk′) *n.* A medicinal preparation made from the dried roots and rhizomes of the shrub *Cephaelis ipecacuanha* that is used to induce vomiting.

ip·ra·tro·pi·um (ĭp′rə-trō′pē-əm) *n.* A synthetic compound, chemically related to atropine, that is

used as an inhalant in the treatment of bronchospasm.

IPV *abbr.* inactivated poliovirus vaccine

IQ or **I.Q.** *abbr.* intelligence quotient

ir·i·dec·to·my (ĭr′ĭ-dĕk′tə-mē, ĭ′rĭ-) *n.* Surgical removal of part of the iris of the eye.

ir·i·de·re·mi·a (ĭr′ĭ-də-rē′mē-ə, ĭ′rĭ-) *n.* An iris so rudimentary that it appears to be absent.

i·rid·e·sis (ĭ-rĭd′ĭ-sĭs, ī′rĭ-dē′sĭs) *n.* Ligature of a portion of the iris brought out through an incision in the cornea.

i·rid·ic (ĭ-rĭd′ĭk, ī-rĭd′-) *adj.* Of or relating to the iris of the eye.

i·rid·i·um (ĭ-rĭd′ē-əm) *n.* A hard, brittle, corrosion-resistant metallic element with atomic number 77 and used principally to harden platinum.

ir·i·do·a·vul·sion (ĭr′ĭ-dō-ə-vŭl′shən, ĭ′rĭ-dō-) *n.* A tearing away of the iris.

ir·i·do·cele (ĭr′ĭ-dō-sēl′, ī-rĭd′ə-, ĭ-rĭd′ə-) *n.* Protrusion of a portion of the iris through a corneal defect.

ir·i·do·cho·roid·i·tis (ĭr′ĭ-dō-kôr′oi-dī′tĭs, ĭ′rĭ-) *n.* Inflammation of both the iris and choroid.

ir·i·do·cy·clec·to·my (ĭr′ĭ-dō-sī-klĕk′tə-mē, -sī-klĕk′-, ĭ′rĭ-) *n.* Removal of the iris and the ciliary body.

ir·i·do·cy·cli·tis (ĭr′ĭ-dō-sī-klī′tĭs, -sī-, ĭ′rĭ-) *n.* Inflammation of the iris and the ciliary body.

ir·i·do·cys·tec·to·my (ĭr′ĭ-dō-sĭ-stĕk′tə-mē, ĭ′rĭ-) *n.* The surgical creation of an artificial pupil in which the border of the iris and a portion of the capsule of the lens are drawn out through an incision in the cornea and cut off.

ir·i·dod·e·sis (ĭr′ĭ-dŏd′ĭ-sĭs, ĭ′rĭ-) *n.* See **iridesis.**

ir·i·do·di·al·y·sis (ĭr′ĭ-dō-dī-ăl′ĭ-sĭs, ĭ′rĭ-) *n.* Separation of the iris from its ciliary attachment.

ir·i·do·di·as·ta·sis (ĭr′ĭ-dō-dī-ăs′tə-sĭs, ĭ′rĭ-) *n.* A defect of the peripheral border of the iris with an intact pupil.

ir·i·don·co·sis (ĭr′ĭ-dŏng-kō′sĭs, ĭ′rĭ-) *n.* Thickening of the iris.

ir·i·don·cus (ĭr′ĭ-dŏng′kəs, ĭ′rĭ-) *n.* A tumefaction of the iris.

ir·i·do·pa·ral·y·sis (ĭr′ĭ-dō-pə-răl′ĭ-sĭs, ĭ′rĭ-) *n.* See **iridoplegia.**

ir·i·do·ple·gi·a (ĭr′ĭ-dō-plē′jē-ə, -jə, ĭ′rĭ-) *n.* Paralysis of the sphincter of the iris.

ir·i·dop·to·sis (ĭr′ĭ-dŏp-tō′sĭs, ĭ′rĭ-) *n.* Prolapse of the iris.

ir·i·dor·rhex·is (ĭr′ĭ-dō-rĕk′sĭs, ĭ′rĭ-) *n.* The tearing away of the iris from its peripheral attachment.

ir·i·do·scle·rot·o·my (ĭr′ĭ-dō-sklə-rŏt′ə-mē, ĭ′rĭ-) *n.* Surgical incision of the sclera and the iris.

ir·i·dot·a·sis (ĭr′ĭ-dŏt′ə-sĭs, ĭ′rĭ-) *n.* The surgical stretching of the iris in glaucoma treatment.

ir·i·dot·o·my (ĭr'ĭ-dŏt'ə-mē, ĭr'ĭ-) n. Surgical incision of the iris to form an artificial pupil.

i·ris (ī'rĭs) n., pl. **i·ris·es** or **i·ri·des** (ī'rĭ-dēz', ĭr'ĭ-). The round pigmented contractile membrane of the eye that is perforated in the center by the pupil, forms the front part of the vascular tunic, and is attached on the margin to the ciliary body. It contains a double layer of pigmented retinal epithelium that gives rise to the sphincter and dilator muscles of the pupil that regulate the amount of light entering the eye. **—i'ri·dal** (ī'rĭ-dl, ĭr'ĭ-), **i·rid'i·al** (ī-rĭd'ē-əl, ĭ-rĭd'-), **i·rid'i·an** adj.

i·ri·tis (ī-rī'tĭs) n. Inflammation of the iris.

i·rit·o·my (ī-rĭt'ə-mē) n. See **iridotomy**.

i·ron (ī'ərn) n. **1.** A lustrous, malleable, ductile, magnetic or magnetizable metallic element having atomic number 26 and occurring abundantly in ores such as hematite and magnetite and used alloyed in a wide range of important structural materials. **2.** A medication containing iron and taken as a dietary supplement.

iron deficiency anemia n. A form of hypochromic microcytic anemia due to the dietary lack of iron or to a loss of iron from chronic bleeding.

iron lung n. See **Drinker respirator**.

iron-storage disease n. Any of various diseases characterized by the storage of excess iron in the parenchyma of many organs, as in idiopathic hemochromatosis or transfusion hemosiderosis.

i·rot·o·my (ī-rŏt'ə-mē) n. See **iridotomy**.

ir·ra·di·ate (ĭ-rā'dē-āt') v. **-at·ed, -at·ing, -ates. 1.** To expose to radiation, as for diagnostic or therapeutic purposes. **2.** To treat with radiation. **3.** To apply radiation to a structure or organism.

ir·ra·di·a·tion (ĭ-rā'dē-ā'shən) n. **1.** Exposure or subjection to the action of radiation for diagnostic or therapeutic purposes. **2.** Medical treatment by exposure to radiation. **3.** The spread of a nervous impulse beyond the usual path of conduction.

ir·re·duc·i·ble (ĭr'ĭ-dōō'sə-bəl, -dyōō'-) adj. Impossible to reduce to a desired, simpler, or smaller form or amount; not reducible. **— ir're·duc'i·bil'i·ty, ir're·duc'i·ble·ness** n. **— ir're·duc'i·bly** adv.

ir·reg·u·lar (ĭ-rĕg'yə-lər) adj. **1.** Not straight, uniform, or symmetrical, as of facial features. **2.** Of uneven rate, occurrence, or duration, such as a heartbeat. **3.** Deviating from a type; atypical.

irregular astigmatism n. Astigmatism in which different parts of the same meridian have different degrees of curvature.

ir·ri·gate (ĭr'ĭ-gāt') v. **-gat·ed, -gat·ing, -gates.** To wash out a cavity or wound with a fluid.

ir·ri·ta·bil·i·ty (ĭr'ĭ-tə-bĭl'ĭ-tē) n. **1.** The capacity to respond to stimuli. **2.** Abnormal or excessive sensitivity to stimuli of an organism, organ, or body part.

ir·ri·ta·ble (ĭr'ĭ-tə-bəl) adj. **1.** Capable of reacting to a stimulus. **2.** Abnormally sensitive to a stimulus.

irritable colon n. Chronic disordered motility in

the intestines often accompanied by colicky pains and diarrhea.

ir·ri·ta·tion (ĭr'ĭ-tā'shən) n. **1.** Extreme incipient inflammatory reaction of the body tissues to an injury. **2.** The normal response of a nerve or muscle to a stimulus. **3.** The evocation of a reaction in the body tissues by the application of a stimulus.

irritation fibroma n. Slow-growing fibrous nodules on the oral mucosa, resulting from irritation caused by cheek biting or objects such as dentures and fillings.

Ir·vine–Gass syndrome (ûr'vīn'-găs') n. A syndrome of the eye characterized by macular edema and loss of vision following cataract surgery.

is·aux·e·sis (ī'sôg-zē'sĭs, -sŏk-sē'-) n. Growth of parts at the same rate as growth of the whole.

is·che·mi·a (ĭ-skē'mē-ə) n. A decrease in the blood supply to a bodily organ, tissue, or part caused by constriction or obstruction of the blood vessels. **— i·sche'mic** adj.

ischemic hypoxia n. Tissue hypoxia resulting from slower circulation through the tissues so that oxygen tension in capillary blood is less than normal, even though the saturation, content, and tension in arterial blood are normal.

ischial bone n. See **ischium**.

is·chi·al·gi·a (ĭs'kē-ăl'jē-ə, -jə) n. Pain occurring in the ischium.

is·chi·o·dyn·i·a (ĭs'kē-ō-dĭn'ē-ə) n. See **ischialgia**.

is·chi·o·ni·tis (ĭs'kē-ə-nī'tĭs) n. Inflammation of the ischium.

is·chi·um (ĭs'kē-əm) n., pl. **-chi·a** (-kē-ə). The lowest of the three major bones that constitute each half of the pelvis, distinct at birth but later becoming fused with the ilium and pubis. **— is'chi·ad'ic** (-ăd'ĭk) adj. **— is'chi·al** (-əl) adj. **— is'chi·at'ic** (-ăt'ĭk) adj.

is·chu·ri·a (ĭs-kyōōr'ē-ə) n. Retention or suppression of urine.

Ish·i·ha·ra test (ĭsh'ĭ-hä'rə) n. A test for color-vision deficiency employing a series of plates on which numbers or letters are printed in dots of primary colors surrounded by dots of other colors; the figures are discernable by people with normal color vision.

is·land (ī'lənd) n. An isolated tissue or group of cells that is separated from the surrounding tissues by a groove or is marked by a difference in structure or function.

island flap n. A surgical flap in which the pedicle consists solely of the supplying blood vessels.

islands of Langerhans n. See **islets of Langerhans**.

is·let (ī'lĭt) n. A small island.

islet cell n. One of the endocrine cells making up the islets of Langerhans.

islets of Langerhans pl.n. Irregular clusters of endocrine cells scattered throughout the tissue of the pancreas that secrete insulin and glucagon.

i·so·ag·glu·ti·na·tion (ī'sō-ə-glōōt'n-ā'shən) n. The agglutination of the red blood cells of an individual by antibodies in the serum of another individual of the same species.

i·so·ag·glu·ti·nin (ī'sō-ə-glōōt'n-ĭn) n. An isoantibody normally present in the serum of one person that causes the agglutination of the red blood cells of another person.

i·so·ag·glu·tin·o·gen (ī′sō-ăg′lōō-tǐn′ə-jən) *n.* An isoantigen that on exposure to its corresponding isoantibody causes agglutination of the red blood cells to which it is attached.

i·so·an·ti·bod·y (ī′sō-ăn′tǐ-bŏd′ē) *n.* An antibody produced by or derived from the same species as the antigen with which it reacts.

i·so·an·ti·gen (ī′sō-ăn′tǐ-jən) *n.* A protein or other antigenic substance present in only some members of a species and therefore able to stimulate antibody production in members that lack it.

i·so·cap·ni·a (ī′sə-kăp′nē-ə) *n.* A state in which the arterial carbon dioxide pressure remains constant or unchanged.

i·so·chro·mo·some (ī′sə-krō′mə-sōm′) *n.* A chromosomal aberration that arises as a result of transverse rather than longitudinal division of the centromere during meiosis; two daughter chromosomes are formed, each lacking one chromosome arm but with the other doubled.

i·so·cit·rate dehydrogenase (ī′sə-sǐt′rāt′) *n.* Either of two enzymes that catalyze the oxidative decarboxylation of isocitrate during the Krebs cycle.

i·so·co·ri·a (ī′sō-kôr′ē-ə) *n.* Equality in the size of the two pupils.

i·so·cor·tex (ī′sō-kôr′tĕks′) *n.* The larger part of the cerebral cortex, distinguished from the allocortex by having a larger number of nerve cells arranged in six layers.

i·so·cy·tol·y·sin (ī′sō-sī-tŏl′ǐ-sǐn) *n.* A cytolysin that reacts with the cells of certain people, but not with the cells of the person that formed it.

i·so·dac·tyl·ism (ī′sō-dăk′tə-lǐz′əm) *n.* A condition in which each of the fingers or toes is approximately equal in length.

i·so·en·zyme (ī′sō-ĕn′zīm′) *n.* See **isozyme.** — **i′·so·en·zy′mic** (-zī′mǐk, -zīm′ǐk) *adj.*

i·so·er·y·th·rol·y·sis (ī′sō-ĕr′ə-thrŏl′ǐ-sǐs) *n.* The destruction of red blood cells by isoantibodies.

i·so·flu·rane (ī′sō-flŏor′ān′) *n.* A halogenated ether with potent anesthetic action.

i·sog·a·my (ī-sŏg′ə-mē) *n.* Conjugation between two gametes of equal size and structure, or between two individual cells alike in all respects. — **i·sog′a·mous** *adj.*

i·so·ge·ne·ic (ī′sō-jə-nē′ǐk) or **i·so·gen·ic** (-jĕn′ǐk) *adj.* Relating to a group of individuals or to a strain of animals genetically alike with respect to specified gene pairs.

isogeneic graft *n.* See **syngraft.**

isogeneic homograft *n.* See **syngraft.**

i·so·gen·e·sis (ī′sō-jĕn′ĭ-sǐs) *n.* Similarity in development.

i·so·graft (ī′sə-grăft′) *n.* See **syngraft.**

i·so·he·mag·glu·ti·na·tion (ī′sō-hē′mə-glŏot′n-ā′shən) *n.* See **isoagglutination.**

iso·he·mag·glu·ti·nin (ī′sō-hē′mə-glŏot′n-ĭn) *n.* See **isoagglutinin.**

i·so·he·mo·ly·sin (ī′sō-hǐ-mŏl′ǐ-sǐn, -hē′mə-lī′-)

n. An isolysin that reacts with red blood cells.

i·so·he·mol·y·sis (ī′sō-hǐ-mŏl′ǐ-sǐs, -hē′mə-lī′sǐs) *n.* A form of isolysis in which there is dissolution of red blood cells as a result of the reaction between an isolysin and a specific antigen in or on the cells.

i·so·i·co·ni·a (ī′sō-ī-kō′nē-ə) *n.* A condition in which the two retinal images are of equal size. — **i′so·i·con′ic** (-kŏn′ĭk) *adj.*

i·so·im·mu·ni·za·tion (ī′sō-ĭm′yə-nǐ-zā′shən) *n.* The development of specific antibodies as a result of antigenic stimulation using material derived from the red blood cells of another individual of the same species.

i·so·ki·net·ic exercise (ī′sō-kə-nĕt′ĭk, -kī-) *n.* Exercise performed with a specialized apparatus that provides variable resistance to a movement, so that no matter how much effort is exerted, the movement takes place at a constant speed. Such exercise is used to test and improve muscular strength and endurance, especially after injury.

i·so·late (ī′sə-lāt′) *v.* **-lat·ed, -lat·ing, -lates. 1.** To set apart or cut off from others. **2.** To place in quarantine. **3.** To separate a pure strain from a mixed bacterial or fungal culture. **4.** To separate experiences or memories from the emotions relating to them. — *n.* (-lǐt, -lāt′). A bacterial or fungal strain that has been isolated. — **i′so·la′tor** *n.*

i·so·la·tion (ī′sə-lā′shən) *n.* The act of isolating or the state of being isolated.

i·so·leu·cine (ī′sə-lōō′sēn′) *n.* An essential amino acid that is isomeric with leucine.

isologous graft *n.* See **syngraft.**

i·sol·y·sin (ī-sŏl′ǐ-sǐn, ī′sə-lī′sǐn) *n.* An antibody that combines with, sensitizes, and causes complement-fixation and the dissolution of the cells that contain the specific isoantigen.

i·sol·y·sis (ī-sŏl′ǐ-sǐs) *n.* Lysis or dissolution of cells as a result of the reaction between an isolysin and a specific antigen in or on the cells. — **i′so·lyt′ic** (ī′sə-lǐt′ĭk) *adj.*

i·so·mer (ī′sə-mər) *n.* Any of two or more substances that are composed of the same elements in the same proportions but differ in properties because of differences in the arrangement of atoms. — **i′so·mer′ic** (-mĕr′ĭk) *adj.*

i·so·met·ric (ī′sə-mĕt′rĭk) *adj.* Of or involving muscular contraction against resistance in which the length of the muscle remains the same.

isometric exercise *n.* Exercise performed by the exertion of effort against a resistance that strengthens and tones the muscle without changing the length of the muscle fibers.

isometric period of cardiac cycle *n.* The period in the cardiac cycle, extending from the closing of the atrioventricular valves to the opening of the semilunar valves, in which the muscle fibers do not shorten although the cardiac muscle is excited and the pressure in the ventricles rises.

isometrics *n.* Isometric exercise.

isometric scale *n.* A radiopaque strip of metal calibrated in centimeters, placed between the buttocks of a person to be x-rayed, used to measure anteroposterior diameters of the pelvis.

i·so·me·tro·pi·a (ī'sō-mĭ-trō'pē-ə) *n.* Equality of refraction in both eyes.

i·so·ni·a·zid (ī'sə-nī'ə-zĭd) *n.* A crystalline antibacterial compound used in the treatment of tuberculosis.

i·sop·a·thy (ī-sŏp'ə-thē) *n.* **1.** The treatment of disease by means of the causal agent or a product of the same disease. **2.** The treatment of a diseased organ by an extract of a similar organ from a healthy animal.

i·soph·a·gy (ī-sŏf'ə-jē) *n.* Autolysis.

i·so·pho·ri·a (ī'sə-fōr'ē-ə) *n.* A state of equality in the tension of the vertical muscles of each eye.

i·so·pre·cip·i·tin (ī'sō-prĭ-sĭp'ĭ-tĭn) *n.* An antibody that combines with and precipitates soluble antigenic material in the plasma or serum of another member, but not all members, of the same species.

i·sop·ter (ī-sŏp'tər) *n.* A curve of equal retinal sensitivity in the visual field designated by a fraction, the numerator being the diameter of the white test object, and the denominator being the testing distance.

i·sor·rhe·a (ī'sə-rē'ə) *n.* A state of physiological equilibrium between the intake and output of water and solutes.

i·so·to·ni·a (ī'sə-tō'nē-ə) *n.* A condition of tonic equality, in which the tension or osmotic pressure in two substances or solutions is the same.

i·so·ton·ic (ī'sə-tŏn'ĭk) *adj.* **1.** Of equal tension. **2.** Isosmotic. **3.** Having the same concentration of solutes as the blood. **4.** Of or involving muscular contraction in which the muscle remains under relatively constant tension while its length changes. — **i'so·ton·ic'i·ty** (-tə-nĭs'ĭ-tē) *n.*

isotonic exercise *n.* Exercise in which isotonic muscular contraction is used to strengthen muscles and improve joint mobility.

i·so·tope (ī'sə-tōp') *n.* One of two or more atoms having the same atomic number but different mass numbers. — **i'so·top'ic** (-tŏp'ĭk) *adj.*

i·so·tre·tin·o·in (ī'sō-trĭ-tĭn'ō-ĭn, -tĭn'oin) *n.* A chemical compound that inhibits the secretion of sebum and is used in the treatment of severe forms of acne.

i·so·trop·ic (ī'sə-trŏp'ĭk, -trō'pĭk) *adj.* Identical in all directions; invariant with respect to direction. — **i·sot'ro·py** (ī-sŏt'rə-pē), **i·sot'ro·pism** (-pĭz'-əm) *n.*

i·so·type (ī'sə-tīp') *n.* An antigenic marker that occurs in all members of a subclass of an immunoglobulin class. — **i·so·typ'ic** (-tīp'ĭk) *adj.*

i·so·zyme (ī'sə-zīm') *n.* Any of a group of enzymes that are similar in catalytic properties but are differentiated by variations in physical properties.

is·sue (ĭsh'ōō) *n.* **1.** A discharge, as of blood or pus. **2.** A lesion, a wound, or an ulcer producing such a discharge.

isth·mec·to·my (ĭs-měk'tə-mē, ĭsth-) *n.* Surgical excision of the midportion of the thyroid.

isth·mus (ĭs'məs) *n., pl.* **-mus·es** or **-mi** (-mī'). A constriction or narrow passage connecting two larger parts of an organ or other anatomical structure.

itch (ĭch) *n.* **1.** An irritating skin sensation causing a desire to scratch. **2.** Any of various skin disorders, such as scabies, marked by intense irritation and itching. — *v.* **itched, itch·ing, itch·es.** To feel, have, or produce an itch.

itch mite *n.* A parasitic mite *(Sarcoptes scabiei)* that burrows into the skin and causes scabies.

i·ter (ī'tər) *n.* A passage leading from one anatomical part to another.

IU *abbr.* international unit

IUD *abbr.* intrauterine device

IV *abbr.* intravenous; intravenously; intraventricular

Ix·o·des (ĭk-sō'dēz') *n.* A genus of hard-bodied ticks, many species of which are parasitic on humans and animals.

ix·o·di·a·sis (ĭk'sō-dī'ə-sĭs) *n.* **1.** Skin lesions caused by the bites of certain ticks. **2.** A disease, such as Rocky Mountain fever, that is transmitted by ticks.

~ ~ ~ ~ ~ ~ **J** ~ ~ ~ ~ ~ ~

Ja·bou·lay's method (zhä-bōō-lāz') *n.* A surgical method of linking arteries by splitting the cut ends a short distance and suturing the flaps together with the inner coats touching each other.

jack·et (jăk'ĭt) *n.* A fixed bandage applied around the body to immobilize the spine.

jack·so·ni·an epilepsy (jăk-sō'nē-ən) *n.* A form of focal epilepsy in which a seizure progresses from the distal to the proximal muscles of a limb.

jac·ti·ta·tion (jăk'tĭ-tā'shən) *n.* Extreme restlessness or tossing in bed.

Ja·das·sohn—Le·wan·dow·sky syndrome (yä'-däs-zōn-lěv'ən-dŏv'skē, -lā'vän-dôf'skē) *n.* See **pachyonychia congenita.**

Jae·ger's test types (yā'gərz, yěg'ərz) *pl.n.* Printed letters of different sizes used for testing the acuity of near vision.

Ja·kob—Creutz·feldt disease (yä'kôp-) *n.* See **Creutzfeldt—Jakob disease.**

Jan·sky—Biel·schow·sky disease (jăn'skē-, yän'-) *n.* The early juvenile type of cerebral sphingolipidosis.

Ja·nus green B (jā'nəs) *n.* A basic dye used as a histological stain.

Jap·a·nese B encephalitis virus (jăp′ə-nēz′, -nēs′) *n.* A mosquito-borne virus of the genus *Flavivirus* capable of causing fever and sometimes encephalitis.

jar·gon (jär′gən) *n.* **1.** Nonsensical, incoherent, or meaningless talk. **2.** The specialized or technical language of a trade, profession, or similar group.

Ja·risch–Herxheimer reaction (yä′rĭsh-) *n.* See **Herxheimer's reaction.**

jaun·dice (jôn′dĭs, jän′-) *n.* Yellowish discoloration of the whites of the eyes, skin, and mucous membranes due to deposition of bile salts, occurring as a symptom of diseases, such as hepatitis, that affect the processing of bile.

jaundice of the newborn *n.* **1.** A mild temporary jaundice in newborns caused mainly by functional immaturity of the liver. **2.** A severe, sometimes fatal form of jaundice in newborns, caused by several conditions, including congenital blockage of the common bile duct, erythroblastosis fetalis, congenital syphilitic cirrhosis of the liver, and septic pylephlebitis.

jaw (jô) *n.* **1.** Either of two bony structures that form the framework of the mouth and hold the teeth. **2.** The mandible or maxilla or the part of the face covering these bones. —**jaw′less** *adj.*

jaw·bone (jô′bōn′) *n.* The maxilla or, especially, the mandible.

jaw reflex *n.* A spasmodic contraction of the temporal muscles following a downward tap on the loosely hanging mandible; it is seen in lesions of the corticospinal tract.

jaw-winking syndrome *n.* An increase in the width of the eyelids that occurs during chewing, sometimes with a rhythmic raising of the upper lid when the mouth is open and its subsequent drooping when the mouth is closed.

je·ju·nal (jə-jōō′nəl) *adj.* Relating to the jejunum.

je·ju·nec·to·my (jə-jōō′něk′tə-mē, jē′jōō-, jĕj′ōō-) *n.* Surgical excision of all or a part of the jejunum.

je·ju·ni·tis (jə-jōō′nī′tĭs, jē′jōō-, jĕj′ōō-) *n.* Inflammation of the jejunum.

je·ju·no·co·los·to·my (jə-jōō′nō-kə-lŏs′tə-mē, jĕj′ōō-) *n.* The surgical creation of an opening or passage between the jejunum and the colon.

je·ju·no·il·e·al bypass (jə-jōō′nō-ĭl′ē-əl, jĕj′ōō-) *n.* Anastomosis of the upper jejunum to the terminal ileum for treating morbid obesity.

jejunoileal shunt *n.* See **jejunoileal bypass.**

je·ju·no·il·e·i·tis (jə-jōō′nō-ĭl′ē-ī′tĭs, jĕj′ōō-) *n.* Inflammation of the jejunum and the ileum.

je·ju·no·il·e·os·to·my (jə-jōō′nō-ĭl′ē-ŏs′tə-mē, jĕj′ōō-) *n.* The surgical creation of an opening or passage between the jejunum and the ileum.

je·ju·no·je·ju·nos·to·my (jə-jōō′nō-jə-jōō′nŏs′-tə-mē, jĕj′ōō-nō-jĕj′ōō-) *n.* The surgical creation of an opening or passage between two portions of jejunum.

je·ju·no·plas·ty (jə-jōō′nə-plăs′tē) *n.* A corrective surgical procedure on the jejunum.

je·ju·nos·to·my (jə-jōō′nŏs′tə-mē, jē′jōō-, jĕj′ōō-) *n.* The surgical creation of an opening from the

abdominal wall into the jejunum, usually with a stoma on the abdominal wall.

je·ju·not·o·my (jə-jōō′nŏt′ə-mē, jē′jōō-, jĕj′ōō-) *n.* Surgical incision into the jejunum.

je·ju·num (jə-jōō′nəm) *n.*, *pl* **-na** (-nə). The section of the small intestine between the duodenum and the ileum.

jel·ly (jĕl′ē) *n.* A semisolid resilient substance usually containing some form of gelatin in solution.

jerk (jûrk) *v.* **jerked, jerk·ing, jerks.** To make spasmodic motions. —*n.* **1.** A sudden reflexive or spasmodic muscular movement. **2.** See **deep reflex. 3. jerks.** Involuntary convulsive twitching often resulting from excitement. Often used with *the.*

jet injection *n.* The injection of a liquid drug by means of a device that uses high pressure to force the liquid to penetrate the skin or mucous membrane without the use of a needle.

jet lag or **jetlag** *n.* A temporary disruption of circadian rhythm caused by high-speed travel across several time zones typically in a jet aircraft, resulting in fatigue and other symptoms.

jim-jams (jĭm′jămz′) *pl.n.* **1.** The jitters. **2.** Delirium tremens.

Jo·cas·ta complex (jō-kăs′tə) *n.* In psychoanalytic theory, a mother's libidinous fixation on a son.

jock itch *n.* See **tinea cruris.**

Jof·froy's sign (zhô-frwäz′) *n.* **1.** An indication of exophthalmic goiter in which the facial muscles remain immobile when the eyeballs are rolled upward. **2.** An indication of the early stages of brain disease in which a person is unable to mentally compute simple mathematical calculations.

john·ny (jŏn′ē) *n.* A loose short-sleeved gown opening in the back, worn by patients undergoing medical treatment or examination.

joint (joint) *n.* A point of articulation between two or more bones, especially such a connection that allows motion.

Jou·bert's syndrome (zhōo-bĕrz′) *n.* A syndrome of neurological disorders caused by agenesis of the vermis of the brain and marked by attacks of tachypnea or prolonged apnea, abnormal eye movements, ataxia, and mental retardation.

jowl¹ (joul) *n.* **1.** The jaw, especially the lower jaw. **2.** The cheek.

jowl² (joul) *n.* The flesh under the lower jaw, especially when plump or flaccid.

J point *n.* The point marking the end of the QRS complex and the beginning of the S-T segment in an electrocardiogram.

ju·gal bone (jōo′gəl) *n.* See **zygomatic bone.**

jug·u·lar (jŭg′yə-lər) *adj.* Of, relating to, or located in the region of the neck or throat. —*n.* A jugular vein.

jugular pulse *n.* The pulse in the right internal jugular vein at the root of the neck.

jugular vein *n.* Any of the three veins located in the jugular region: anterior jugular vein, external jugular vein, and internal jugular vein.

ju·gum (jōo′gəm) *n.*, *pl.* **-gums** or **-ga** (-gə). **1.** A ridge or furrow connecting two structures. **2.** A type of forceps.

juice (jōōs) *n.* **1.** A fluid naturally contained in plant or animal tissue. **2.** A bodily secretion, especially that secreted by the glands of the stomach and intestines.

jump flap *n.* A distant flap transferred in stages via an intermediate carrier, as an abdominal flap that is first attached to the wrist so that the wrist can be brought to the face at a later stage.

junc·tion (jŭngk′shən) *n.* **1.** The act or process of joining or the condition of being joined. **2.** A place where two things join or meet, especially a place where two things come together and one terminates. **3.** A transition layer or boundary between two different materials or between physically different regions in a single material. — **junc′tion·al** *adj.*

junctional epithelium *n.* A circular arrangement of epithelial cells occurring at the base of the gingival crevice and attached to both the tooth and the subepithelial connective tissue.

junc·tu·ra (jŭngk-tŏōr′ə, -tyŏōr′-, -chŏōr′-) *n., pl.* **-tu·rae** (-tŏōr′ē, -tyŏōr′-, -chŏōr′-). A juncture; junction.

Jung·i·an (yŏōng′ē-ən) *adj.* **1.** Of, relating to, or characteristic of Carl Gustav Jung or his theories of psychology. **2.** Maintaining Jung's psychological theories, especially those that stress the contribution of racial and cultural inheritance to the psychology of the individual.

jun·gle fever (jŭng′gəl) *n.* See **malaria**.

ju·ve·nile cell (jōō′və-nīl′, -nəl) *n.* See **metamyelocyte**.

juvenile diabetes *n.* Insulin-dependent diabetes.

juvenile-onset diabetes *n.* Insulin-dependent diabetes.

juvenile palmo-plantar fibromatosis *n.* Fibromatosis that occurs in children as a single poorly demarcated nodule on the palm of the hand or sole of the foot.

juvenile papillomatosis *n.* A form of fibrocystic disease of the breast in young women, with florid and sclerosing adenosis that microscopically may suggest carcinoma.

juvenile polyp *n.* A smoothly rounded, mucosal benign growth of the large intestine, which may be multiple and cause rectal bleeding, especially in the first decade of life.

juvenile retinoschisis *n.* A hereditary condition of retinal degeneration occurring in children under the age of 10 and characterized by cyst development within the nerve-fiber layer of the retina, often with macular involvement.

jux·ta·glo·mer·u·lar cell (jŭk′stə-glō-mĕr′yə-lər) *n.* A cell occurring in the kidney and producing renin.

juxtaglomerular granule *n.* Any of the stainable osmophilic secretory granules present in juxtaglomerular cells, resembling zymogen granules.

jux·ta·po·si·tion (jŭk′stə-pə-zĭsh′ən) *n.* The state of being placed or situated side by side.

~ ~ ~ ~ ~ ~ **K** ~ ~ ~ ~ ~

K *abbr.* Kelvin

ka·la·a·zar (kä′lə-ə-zär′) *n.* See **visceral leishmaniasis**.

ka·le·mi·a (kä-lē′mē-ə) *n.* The presence of potassium in the blood.

ka·li·o·pe·ni·a (kā′lē-ō-pē′nē-ə, kăl′ē-) *n.* A low potassium concentration in the blood. — **ka′li·o·pe′nic** (-pē′nĭk) *adj.*

kal·lak (kăl′ăk) *n.* A pustular dermatitis, occurring especially among the Eskimos.

kal·u·re·sis (kăl′yōō-rē′sĭs, kăl′-) or **ka·li·u·re·sis** (kā′lē-yōō-rē′sĭs, kăl′ē-) *n.* The excretion of increased amounts of potassium in the urine. — **kal′u·ret′ic** (-rĕt′ĭk) *adj.*

kan·a·my·cin (kăn′ə-mī′sĭn) *n.* A water-soluble broad-spectrum antibiotic obtained from the soil bacterium *Streptomyces kanamyceticus*.

Kan·ner's syndrome (kăn′ərz) *n.* See **infantile autism**.

ka·o·lin·o·sis (kā′ə-lə-nō′sĭs) *n.* Pneumoconiosis caused by the inhalation of clay dust.

Ka·po·si's sarcoma (kə-pō′sēz, kăp′ə-) *n.* A cancer characterized by bluish-red nodules on the skin, usually on the lower extremities, that is endemic to equatorial Africa and often occurs in people with AIDS.

kap·pa (kăp′ə) *adj.* Relating to or characterizing a polypeptide chain that is one of two types of light chains present in immunoglobins.

kappa angle *n.* The angle between the pupillary axis and the visual axis.

Kar·ta·ge·ner's syndrome (kär′tə-gā′nərz, kär-tä′gə-nərz) *n.* A syndrome of disorders in which complete transposition of the viscera is associated with bronchiectasis and chronic sinusitis.

kar·y·o·cyte (kăr′ē-ə-sīt′) *n.* An immature normoblast.

kar·y·og·a·my (kăr′ē-ŏg′ə-mē) *n.* The coming together and fusing of cell nuclei, as in fertilization. — **kar′y·o·gam′ic** (-ə-găm′ĭk) *adj.*

kar·y·o·gen·e·sis (kăr′ē-ə-jĕn′ĭ-sĭs) *n.* Formation of a cell nucleus. — **kar′y·o·gen′ic** (-jĕn′ĭk) *adj.*

kar·y·o·ki·ne·sis (kăr′ē-ō-kə-nē′sĭs) *n.* See **mitosis** (sense 1). — **kar′y·o·ki·net′ic** (-nĕt′ĭk) *adj.*

kar·y·o·lymph (kăr′ē-ə-lĭmf′) *n.* The colorless, liquid component of the cell nucleus.

kar·y·ol·y·sis (kăr′ē-ŏl′ĭ-sĭs) *n.* The dissolution of the nucleus of a cell by swelling or necrosis with

the loss of its affinity for staining with basic dyes.
— **kar′y·o·lyt′ic** (-ə-lĭt′ĭk) *adj.*

kar·y·on (kăr′ē-ŏn′) *n.* See **nucleus** (sense 1).

kar·y·o·plasm (kăr′ē-ə-plăz′əm) *n.* See **nucleoplasm**.

kar·y·o·plast (kăr′ē-ə-plăst′) *n.* A cell nucleus surrounded by a narrow band of cytoplasm and a plasma membrane.

kar·y·o·pyk·no·sis (kăr′ē-ō-pĭk-nō′sĭs) *n.* The shrinkage of the nucleus of a cell with the condensation of the chromatin into structureless masses, as in superficial or cornified cells of stratified squamous epithelium.

kar·y·o·some (kăr′ē-ə-sōm′) *n.* An aggregation of chromatin in the nucleus of a cell not undergoing mitosis.

kar·y·o·type (kăr′ē-ə-tīp′) *n.* **1.** The characterization of the chromosomal complement of an individual or a species, including number, form, and size of the chromosomes. **2.** A photomicrograph of chromosomes arranged according to a standard classification. — *v.* **-typed, -typ·ing, -types.** To classify and array the chromosome complement of an organism or a species according to the arrangement, number, size, shape, or other characteristics of the chromosomes.

Ka·sai operation (kä-sī′) *n.* See **portoenterostomy.**

Kay·ser–Flei·scher ring (kī′zər-flī′shər) *n.* A greenish-yellow pigmented ring encircling the cornea just within the corneoscleral margin.

kcal *abbr.* kilocalorie

Kel·ly′s operation (kĕl′ēz) *n.* **1.** Surgical correction of retroversion of the uterus by plication of the uterosacral ligaments. **2.** Surgical correction of stress-related urinary incontinence by placing sutures beneath the bladder neck.

ke·loid or **che·loid** (kē′loid′) *n.* A red, raised formation of fibrous scar tissue caused by excess tissue growth following trauma or surgical incision.

ke·loi·do·sis (kē′loi-dō′sĭs) *n.* The presence of multiple keloids.

ke·lo·plas·ty (kē′lə-plăs′tē) *n.* The surgical removal of a scar or keloid.

Kel·vin (kĕl′vĭn) *adj.* Of or relating to a temperature scale in which absolute zero equals −273° on the Celsius scale. The freezing point of water is 273°K; the boiling point of water is 373°K.

Ken·ny′s treatment (kĕn′ēz) *n.* Sister Kenney's treatment.

ker·a·tec·to·my (kĕr′ə-tĕk′tə-mē) *n.* Surgical excision of a portion of the cornea.

ker·a·tin (kĕr′ə-tĭn) *n.* A tough, insoluble, sulfur-containing protein that is the chief structural constituent of hair, nails, and other horny tissues.

ker·a·tin·i·za·tion (kĕr′ə-tn-ĭ-zā′shən) *n.* The conversion of squamous epithelial cells into a keratinized, horny material, such as hair or nails.

ke·rat·i·no·cyte (kə-răt′n-ə-sīt′, kĕr′ə-tĭn′ə-) *n.* An epidermal cell that produces keratin.

ke·rat·i·no·some (kə-răt′n-ə-sōm′, kĕr′ə-tĭn′ə-) *n.* A membrane-bound granule located in the up-

per layers of the stratum spinosum of certain stratified squamous epithelia.

keratin pearl *n.* A focus of central keratinization within concentric layers of abnormal squamous cells, occurring in squamous cell carcinoma.

ker·a·ti·tis (kĕr′ə-tī′tĭs) *n., pl.* **-tit·i·des** (-tĭt′ĭ-dēz′). Inflammation of the cornea.

keratitis sic·ca (sĭk′ə) *n.* Inflammation of the conjunctiva and cornea of the eye associated with decreased tears.

ker·a·to·ac·an·tho·ma (kĕr′ə-tō-ăk′ən-thō′mə) *n.* A rapidly growing skin tumor having a central keratin mass and usually occurring on exposed areas, invading the dermis but remaining localized and usually healing spontaneously.

ker·a·to·cele (kĕr′ə-tō-sēl′) *n.* A herniation of the posterior basement membrane of the cornea through a defect in the outer layer of the cornea.

ker·a·to·con·junc·ti·vi·tis (kĕr′ə-tō-kən-jŭngk′-tə-vī′tĭs) *n.* Inflammation of the cornea and conjunctiva resulting from a hypersensitivity reaction to an endogenous toxin.

ker·a·to·co·nus (kĕr′ə-tō-kō′nəs) *n.* A conical protrusion of the center of the cornea caused by noninflammatory thinning of the stroma; it usually affects both eyes.

ker·a·to·cyte (kĕr′ə-tō-sīt′) *n.* A fibroblastic stromal cell of the cornea.

ker·a·to·der·ma (kĕr′ə-tō-dûr′mə) *n.* **1.** A horny growth or covering, especially of the skin. **2.** A generalized thickening of the horny layer of the epidermis.

ker·a·to·ep·i·the·li·o·plas·ty (kĕr′ə-tō-ĕp′ə-thē′lē-ō-plăs′tē) *n.* Keratoplasty in which corneal epithelium is transplanted with minimal supporting tissue.

ker·a·tog·e·nous membrane (kĕr′ə-tŏj′ə-nəs) *n.* See **nail bed.**

ker·a·to·hy·a·lin (kĕr′ə-tō-hī′ə-lĭn) *n.* A colorless translucent protein present in the granules of the stratum granulosum of the epidermis.

ker·a·toid exanthema (kĕr′ə-toid) *n.* A symptom occurring in the secondary stage of yaws and consisting of patches of fine, light-colored scales scattered irregularly over the limbs and trunk.

ker·a·to·lep·tyn·sis (kĕr′ə-tō-lĕp-tĭn′sĭs) *n.* Cosmetic surgery to remove the corneal surface and cover the area with bulbar conjunctiva.

ker·a·tol·y·sis (kĕr′ə-tŏl′ĭ-sĭs) *n.* **1.** The separation or loosening of the horny layer of the epidermis. **2.** A skin disease marked by periodic epidermal shedding. — **ker′a·to·lyt′ic** (-tō-lĭt′ĭk) *adj.*

ker·a·to·ma (kĕr′ə-tō′mə) *n.* **1.** See **callosity. 2.** A horny tumor.

ker·a·to·ma·la·ci·a (kĕr′ə-tō-mə-lā′shē-ə, -shə) *n.* A condition, usually occurring in children with vitamin A deficiency, characterized by corneal softening, ulceration, and perforation.

ker·a·tom·e·ter (kĕr′ə-tŏm′ĭ-tər) *n.* An instrument for measuring the curvature of the anterior surface of the cornea. — **ker′a·tom′e·try** *adj.*

ker·a·to·mi·leu·sis (kĕr′ə-tō-mə-lōō′sĭs) *n.* A procedure to correct refraction of the cornea by removing a deep corneal lamella, freezing it, reshaping its curvature, and reattaching it.

ker·a·top·a·thy (kĕr′ə-tŏp′ə-thē) *n.* A noninflammatory disease of the cornea.

ker·a·to·pha·ki·a (kĕr′ə-tō-fā′kē-ə) *n.* Keratoplasty in which corneal tissue from a donor is frozen, reshaped, and transplanted into the corneal stroma of the recipient to modify refractive error.

ker·a·to·plas·ty (kĕr′ə-tō-plăs′tē) *n.* Surgical replacement of a portion of the cornea with corneal tissue having the same size and shape.

ker·a·to·pros·the·sis (kĕr′ə-tō-prŏs-thē′sĭs) *n.* An acrylic plastic replacement for the central area of an opacified cornea.

ker·a·to·rhex·is or **ker·a·tor·rhex·is** (kĕr′ə-tō-rĕk′sĭs) *n.* Rupture of the cornea due to trauma or a perforating ulcer.

ker·a·to·scle·ri·tis (kĕr′ə-tō-sklə-rī′tĭs) *n.* Inflammation of the cornea and the sclera.

ker·a·to·scope (kĕr′ə-tō-skōp′) *n.* An instrument marked with lines or circles for use in examining the curvature of the cornea.

ker·a·tos·co·py (kĕr′ə-tŏs′kə-pē) *n.* Examination of the anterior surface of the cornea to determine the character and amount of astigmatism.

ker·a·to·sis (kĕr′ə-tō′sĭs) *n., pl.* **-ses** (-sēz). Excessive growth of horny tissue of the skin. — **ker′a·tot′ic** (-tŏt′ĭk) *adj.*

ker·a·to·tome (kĕr′ə-tō-tōm′) or **ker·a·tome** (kĕr′ə-tōm′) *n.* A knife used for surgical incisions of the cornea.

ker·a·tot·o·my (kĕr′ə-tŏt′ə-mē) *n.* Surgical incision of the cornea.

ke·ri·on (kĕr′ē-ŏn′) *n.* Fungal infection of the hair follicles accompanied by secondary bacterial infection and marked by raised, usually pus-filled and spongy lesions.

ker·nic·ter·us (kûr-nĭk′tər-əs) *n.* A severe form of jaundice of the newborn, characterized by very high levels of unconjugated bilirubin in the blood and by yellow staining and degenerative lesions in the cerebral gray matter.

Ker·nig's sign (kûr′nĭgz) *n.* An indication of meningitis in which complete extension of the leg on the thigh is impossible when the individual lies on the back and flexes the thigh at a right angle to the axis of the trunk.

ke·ta·mine (kē′tə-mēn′) *n.* A general anesthetic given intravenously or intramuscularly in the form of its hydrochloride that produces analgesia with little relaxation of the skeletal muscles.

ke·to·ac·i·do·sis (kē′tō-ăs′ĭ-dō′sĭs) *n.* Acidosis caused by the increased production of ketone bodies, as in diabetic acidosis.

ke·to·ac·i·du·ri·a (kē′tō-ăs′ĭ-dŏŏr′ē-ə, -dyŏŏr′-) *n.* The presence in the urine of excessive amounts of compounds containing a ketone and carboxyl group.

ke·to·co·na·zole (kē′tō-kō′nə-zōl′) *n.* A broad-spectrum antifungal agent used to treat systemic and topical fungal infections.

ke·to·gen·e·sis (kē′tō-jĕn′ĭ-sĭs) *n.* The formation

of ketone bodies, as occurs in diabetes mellitus. — **ke′to·gen′ic** *adj.*

ketogenic diet *n.* A high-fat, low-carbohydrate diet that includes normal amounts of protein.

ke·tole (kē′tōl′) *n.* See **indole**.

ke·tone (kē′tōn′) *n.* Any of a class of organic compounds having a carbonyl group linked to a carbon atom in each of two hydrocarbon radicals.

ketone body *n.* A ketone-containing substance that is an intermediate of fatty acid metabolism, tends to accumulate in the blood, and is excreted in the urine of persons affected by starvation or uncontrolled diabetes mellitus.

ke·to·ne·mi·a (kē′tə-nē′mē-ə) *n.* The presence of detectable concentrations of ketone bodies in the plasma.

ke·to·nu·ri·a (kē′tə-nŏŏr′ē-ə, -nyŏŏr′-) *n.* The presence of an excessive concentration of ketone bodies in the urine.

ke·to·sis (kē-tō′sĭs) *n., pl.* **-ses** (-sēz). A pathological increase in the production of ketone bodies, as in uncontrolled diabetes mellitus.

key-in-lock maneuver *n.* A method by which obstetrical forceps are used to rotate the fetal head.

kg *abbr.* kilogram

kibe (kīb) *n.* A chapped or inflamed area on the skin, especially on the heel, resulting from exposure to cold.

kid·ney (kĭd′nē) *n., pl.* **-neys**. Either of a pair of organs in the dorsal region of the abdominal cavity, functioning to maintain proper water and electrolyte balance, regulate acid-base concentration, and filter the blood of metabolic wastes, which are then excreted as urine.

kidney stone *n.* A small hard mass in the kidney that forms from deposits chiefly of phosphates and urates.

Kier·nan's space (kēr′nənz) *n.* Interlobular space in the liver.

kill·er cell (kĭl′ər) *n.* A large, differentiated T cell that attacks and lyses target cells bearing specific antigens.

killer T cell *n.* See **killer cell**.

kil·o·cal·o·rie (kĭl′ə-kăl′ə-rē) *n.* See **calorie** (sense 2).

kil·o·gram (kĭl′ə-grăm′) *n.* The base unit of mass in the International System, equal to 1,000 grams (2.2046 pounds).

Kim·mel·stiel–Wilson disease (kĭm′əl-stēl′-) *n.* Nephrotic syndrome and hypertension in diabetics associated with diabetic glomerulosclerosis.

kin·an·es·the·sia (kĭn′ăn-ĭs-thē′zhə) *n.* A disturbance of deep nerve sensitivity characterized by an inability to perceive either direction or extent of movement.

ki·nase (kī′nās′, -nāz′, kĭn′ās′, -āz′) *n.* **1.** An enzyme that catalyzes the conversion of a proenzyme to an active enzyme. **2.** Any of various enzymes that catalyze the transfer of a phosphate group from a donor, such as ADP or ATP, to an acceptor.

kin·e·sal·gi·a (kĭn′ĭ-săl′jē-ə, -jə) or **ki·ne·si·al·**

gi·a (kĭ-nē′sē-ăl′jē-ə, -jə) *n.* Pain caused by muscular movement.

ki·ne·sia (kə-nē′zhə, kī-) *n.* See **motion sickness**.

ki·ne·si·at·rics (kə-nē′sē-ăt′rĭks, -zē-) *n.* See **kinesitherapy**.

ki·ne·si·ol·o·gy (kə-nē′sē-ŏl′ə-jē, -zē-, kī-) *n.* The study of muscular movement, especially the mechanics of human motion. — **kin′e·sim′e·ter** (kĭn′ĭ-sĭm′ĭ-tər, kī′nĭ-) *n.*

ki·ne·sis (kə-nē′sĭs, kī-) *n., pl.* **-ses** (-sēz′). Motion or physical movement, especially that induced by stimulation.

kin·es·the·sia (kĭn′ĭs-thē′zhə, kī′nĭs-) *n.* **1.** The sense that detects bodily position, weight, or movement of the muscles, tendons, and joints. **2.** The sensation of moving in space. — **kin′es·thet′ic** (-thĕt′ĭk) *adj.*

kin·es·the·si·om·e·ter (kĭn′ĭs-thē′zē-ŏm′ĭ-tər, kī′nĭs-) *n.* An instrument for determining the degree of muscular sensation in response to movement, weight, and position.

kinesthetic sense *n.* See **myesthesia**.

ki·net·ic (kə-nĕt′ĭk, kī-) *adj.* Of, relating to, or produced by motion.

ki·net·ics (kə-nĕt′ĭks, kī-) *n.* The branch of mechanics concerned with the effects of forces on the motion of a body or system of bodies, especially of forces that do not originate within the system itself.

ki·net·o·car·di·o·gram (kə-nĕt′ō-kär′dē-ə-grăm′, -nē′tō-, kī-) *n.* A graphic recording of the vibrations of the chest wall produced by cardiac activity. — **ki·net′o·car′di·o·graph′** (-grăf′) *adj.*

ki·net·o·chore (kə-nĕt′ə-kôr′, -nē′tə-, kī-) *n.* See **centromere**.

ki·nin (kī′nĭn) *n.* Any of various structurally related polypeptides that act locally to induce vasodilation and contraction of smooth muscle.

kink·y-hair disease (kĭng′kē-hâr′) *n.* A congenital metabolic defect manifested by short, sparse, poorly pigmented kinky hair and associated with failure to thrive, physical and mental retardation, and progressive deterioration of the brain.

kiss·ing disease (kĭs′ĭng) *n.* Infectious mononucleosis.

kiss of life *n.* Mouth-to-mouth resuscitation.

Kleb·si·el·la (klĕb′zē-ĕl′ə) *n.* A genus of bacteria of the family Enterobacteriaceae containing gram-negative, nonmotile, frequently encapsulated rods arranged singly, in pairs, or in short chains; some species are human pathogens.

klep·to·ma·ni·a (klĕp′tə-mā′nē-ə, -mān′yə) *n.* An obsessive impulse to steal regardless of economic need. — **klep′to·ma′ni·ac′** (-nē-ăk′) *adj.*

Kline·fel·ter's syndrome (klīn′fĕl′tərz) *n.* A chromosomal anomaly in males characterized by the presence of two X-chromosomes and one Y-chromosome, causing reduced testicular size, seminiferous tubule dysgenesis, and infertility.

Klip·pel–Feil syndrome (klĭ-pĕl′fīl′, -fēl′) *n.* A congenital syndrome of anatomical defects characterized by a short neck, extensive fusion of the cervical vertebrae, and abnormalities of the brain stem and cerebellum.

Klump·ke's paralysis (klŭmp′kēz) *n.* Brachial plexus injury, often due to birth trauma, resulting in atrophic paralysis of the forearm and small muscles of the hand.

knee (nē) *n.* **1.** The joint between the thigh and the lower leg, formed by the articulation of the femur and the tibia and covered anteriorly by the patella. **2.** The region of the leg that encloses and supports this joint.

knee·cap (nē′kăp′) *n.* See **patella** (sense 1).

knee-chest position *n.* A prone position in which the patient rests on the knees and upper part of the chest, assumed for gynecologic or rectal examination.

knee-elbow position *n.* A prone position in which the patient rests on the knees and elbows, assumed for rectal or gynecologic examination or operation.

knee jerk *n.* See **patellar reflex**.

knee-jerk reflex *n.* See **patellar reflex**.

knee joint *n.* A compound condylar joint consisting of the joint between the condyles of the femur and the condyles of the tibia, and the articulation between the femur and the patella.

knee presentation *n.* Breech presentation of the fetus during birth in which a knee is the presenting part.

knee reflex *n.* See **patellar reflex**.

knit·ting (nĭt′ĭng) *n.* The physiological process by which the fragments of a broken bone are united or the edges of a wound are closed.

knock-knee (nŏk′nē′) *n.* A deformity of the legs in which the knees are abnormally close together and the ankles are spread widely apart.

knot (nŏt) *n.* A protuberant growth or swelling in a tissue, as of a gland or ganglion.

knuck·le (nŭk′əl) *n.* **1.** The prominence of the dorsal aspect of a joint of a finger, especially of one of the joints connecting the fingers to the hand. **2.** A rounded protuberance formed by the bones in a joint. **3.** A loop of intestine, as in a hernia.

Köb·ner's phenomenon (kœb′nərz) *n.* An isomorphic cutaneous reaction occurring in response to trauma and affecting previously uninvolved sites of patients with psoriasis, lichen planus, and flat wart.

Koch's bacillus (kôks, kôKHs) *n.* **1.** See **tubercle bacillus**. **2.** The gram-negative bacterium (*Vibrio cholerae*) that produces a soluble exotoxin believed to be the cause of Asiatic cholera.

Koch–Weeks bacillus (-wēkz′) *n.* A gram-negative, rod-shaped, parasitic bacterium (*Haemophilus aegyptius*) that causes acute conjunctivitis.

Kock pouch (kôk) *n.* An ileostomy with a reservoir and valved opening surgically created from doubled loops of ileum.

Kon·do·le·on operation (kŏn′dō-lē′ŏn, kôn′dō-lē′ŏn) *n.* Excision of strips of subcutaneous connective tissue for the relief of elephantiasis.

Ko·rot·koff sounds (kə-rŏt′kôf, kô-) *pl.n.* The

sounds heard over an artery when blood pressure is determined by the auscultatory method.

Ko·rot·koff's test (kə-rŏt′kôfs, kô-) *n.* A test of collateral circulation in cases of aneurysm, in which the artery is compressed above the aneurysm.

Kor·sa·koff's syndrome (kôr′sə-kôfs′) *n.* A syndrome characterized by confusion and severe impairment of memory for which the patient compensates by confabulation.

Kras·ke's operation (krăs′kēz, krä′skəz) *n.* Removal of the coccyx and excision of the left wing of the sacrum to afford approach for resection of the rectum in cases of cancer or stenosis.

krau·ro·sis vul·vae (krô-rō′sĭs vŭl′vē) *n.* Atrophy and shrinkage of the skin of the vagina and vulva often accompanied by a chronic inflammatory reaction in the deeper tissues.

Krebs cycle (krĕbz) *n.* A series of enzymatic reactions in aerobic organisms involving oxidative metabolism of acetyl units and producing high-energy phosphate compounds, which serve as the main source of cellular energy.

Kru·ken·berg's tumor (krōō′kĭn-bûrgz′) *n.* A malignant tumor of the ovary that usually occurs bilaterally and in association with mucous carcinoma of the stomach.

kryp·ton (krĭp′tŏn′) *n.* A largely inert gaseous element with atomic number 36.

Kufs disease (kŭfs, kōōfs) *n.* The adult type of cerebral sphingolipidosis.

Kupf·fer cell (kŏŏp′fər) *n.* Macrophages lining the walls of the hepatic sinusoids.

ku·ru (kŏŏr′ōō) *n.* A progressive, fatal form of spongiform encephalopathy, probably caused by a slow-acting virus, that is endemic to certain peoples of New Guinea and is thought to be transmitted through cannibalism.

Kuss·maul–Kien respiration (kōōs′moul-kēn′) *n.* See **Kussmaul respiration.**

Kussmaul respiration *n.* Deep, rapid respiration characteristic of diabetic acidosis or other conditions causing acidosis.

Kuss·maul's coma (kōōs′moulz) *n.* See **diabetic coma.**

Kussmaul's sign *n.* An indication of cardiac tamponade in which an increase in venous distention and pressure occurs during inspiration.

Kveim antigen (kvām) *n.* A saline suspension of human sarcoid tissue prepared from the spleen of a person with active sarcoidosis.

Kveim test *n.* An intradermal test for the detection of sarcoidosis, performed by injecting Kveim antigen and examining skin biopsies after three and six weeks.

kwa·shi·or·kor (kwä′shē-ôr′kôr′) *n.* A severe malnutrition of infants and young children caused by deficiency in the quality and quantity of protein in the diet and characterized by anemia, edema, pot belly, changes in skin and hair pigmentation, hypoalbuminemia, and bulky stools containing undigested food.

ky·ma·tism (kī′mə-tĭz′əm) *n.* See **myokymia.**

ky·mo·graph (kī′mə-grăf′) *n.* An instrument for recording variations in pressure, as of the blood, or in tension, as of a muscle, by means of a pen or stylus that marks a rotating drum. — **ky′mo·graph′ic** *adj.* — **ky′mo·gram′** (-grăm′) *n.* — **ky·mog′ra·phy** (-mŏg′rə-fē) *n.*

ky·phos (kī′fŏs′) *n.* The convex part of the back produced by kyphosis; the hump.

ky·pho·sco·li·o·sis (kī′fō-skō′lē-ō′sĭs, skŏl′ē-) *n.* A condition in which the spinal disorders of kyphosis and scoliosis occur together.

ky·pho·sis (kī-fō′sĭs) *n.* Abnormal rearward curvature of the spine, resulting in protuberance of the upper back. — **ky·phot′ic** (-fŏt′ĭk) *adj.*

L

L or **l** *abbr.* liter

la·bet·a·lol hydrochloride (lə-bĕt′ə-lôl′, -lōl′) *n.* An alpha-adrenergic and beta-adrenergic blocking agent that is used in the treatment of hypertension.

la·bi·al (lā′bē-əl) *adj.* Of or relating to the lips or labia.

labial splint *n.* An appliance made to conform to the outer aspect of the dental arch and used in the management of jaw and facial injuries.

labia ma·jo·ra (mə-jôr′ə) *pl.n.* The two outer rounded folds of adipose tissue that lie on either side of the vaginal opening and form the external lateral boundaries of the vulva.

labia mi·no·ra (mə-nôr′ə) *pl.n.* The two thin inner folds of skin within the vestibule of the vagina enclosed within the cleft of the labia majora.

labia o·ris (ôr′ĭs) *pl.n.* The lips of the mouth.

la·bi·o·plas·ty (lā′bē-ə-plăs′tē) *n.* Plastic surgery on a lip.

la·bi·um (lā′bē-əm) *n., pl* **-bi·a** (-bē-ə). **1.** A lip or lip-shaped anatomical structure. **2.** Any of four folds of tissue of the female external genitalia.

la·bor (lā′bər) *n.* The physical efforts of expulsion of the fetus and the placenta from the uterus during parturition. — *v.* **-bored, -bor·ing, -bors.** To undergo the efforts of childbirth.

lab·o·ra·to·ry diagnosis (lăb′rə-tôr′ē) *n.* Diagnosis based on the results of laboratory studies, including chemical, microscopic, bacteriologic, or biopsy studies.

labor pains *pl.n.* Rhythmical uterine contractions

that, under normal conditions, increase in intensity, frequency, and duration, and culminate in vaginal delivery of the infant.

lab·ro·cyte (lăb′rə-sīt′) n. See **mast cell.**

la·brum (lā′brəm) n., pl. **-bra** (-brə). A lip-shaped anatomical edge, rim, or structure.

lab·y·rinth (lăb′ə-rĭnth′) n. **1.** A group of complex interconnecting anatomical cavities. **2.** See **inner ear.**

lab·y·rin·thec·to·my (lăb′ə-rĭn-thĕk′tə-mē) n. Surgical excision of the labyrinth of the ear.

lab·y·rin·thine fluid (lăb′ə-rĭn′thĭn, -thēn′) n. The fluid separating the osseous and the membranous labyrinths of the inner ear.

lab·y·rin·thi·tis (lăb′ə-rĭn-thī′tĭs) n. Inflammation of the inner ear, sometimes accompanied by vertigo.

lab·y·rin·thot·o·my (lăb′ə-rĭn-thŏt′ə-mē) n. Incision into the labyrinth of the ear.

lac·er·ate (lăs′ə-rāt′) v. **-at·ed, -at·ing, -ates.** To rip, cut, or tear. — adj. (-rĭt, -rāt′). **1.** Torn; mangled. **2.** Wounded.

lacerated wound n. A wound caused by laceration.

lac·er·a·tion (lăs′ə-rā′shən) n. **1.** A jagged wound or cut. **2.** The process or act of tearing tissue.

lach·ry·ma·tor or **lach·ri·ma·tor** (lăk′rə-mā′tər) n. A tear-producing agent.

lac·ri·mal or **lach·ry·mal** (lăk′rə-məl) adj. **1.** Of or relating to tears. **2.** Of, relating to, or constituting the glands that produce tears.

lacrimal bone n. A thin irregularly rectangular plate forming part of the medial wall of the eye socket behind the frontal process of the maxilla.

lacrimal canal n. See **lacrimal duct.**

lacrimal caruncle n. A small reddish body at the medial angle of the eye, containing modified sebaceous and sweat glands.

lacrimal duct n. A curved canal beginning at the lacrimal point in the margin of each eyelid near the medial commissure, and running transversely to empty with the duct from the other eye into the lacrimal sac.

lacrimal gland n. An almond-shaped gland that secretes tears into ducts that empty onto the surface of the conjunctiva of the eye.

lacrimal sac n. The upper portion of the nasolacrimal duct into which the lacrimal ducts empty.

lac·ri·ma·tion or **lach·ry·ma·tion** (lăk′rə-mā′-shən) n. The secretion of tears, especially in excess.

lac·ri·mot·o·my (lăk′rə-mŏt′ə-mē) n. Incision of the lacrimal duct or sac.

La Crosse encephalitis (lə krôs′) n. An often fatal infection of the brain caused by a virus occasionally present in the bloodstream of birds and transmitted to humans by the mosquito *Aedes triseriatus.*

lac·tal·bu·min (lăk′tăl-byōō′mĭn) n. The albumin contained in milk and obtained from whey.

lac·tate (lăk′tāt′) v. **-tat·ed, -tat·ing, -tates.** To secrete or produce milk.

lactated Ringer's injection n. A sterile solution of calcium chloride, potassium chloride, sodium chloride, and sodium lactate in water, given intravenously as a systemic alkalizer and as a fluid and electrolyte replenisher.

lactated Ringer's solution n. A solution containing sodium chloride, potassium chloride, calcium chloride, and sodium lactate in distilled water, used for the same purposes as Ringer's solution.

lac·ta·tion (lăk-tā′shən) n. **1.** The secretion or formation of milk by the mammary glands. **2.** The period during which the mammary glands secrete milk. — **lac·ta′tion·al** adj.

lac·te·al (lăk′tē-əl) adj. **1.** Of, relating to, or resembling milk. **2.** Of or relating to a lacteal. — n. Any of numerous minute lymphatic vessels that convey chyle from the intestine to the thoracic duct.

lactic acid n. A syrupy, water-soluble liquid existing in three isomeric forms: one produced in muscle tissue and blood as a result of the anaerobic metabolism of glucose and glycogen, a second, present in sour milk, molasses, various fruits, and wines as a result of fermentation, and a third, produced through bacterial fermentation, is used in foods and beverages as a flavoring and preservative and in pharmaceuticals.

lac·tif·er·ous duct (lăk-tĭf′ər-əs) n. Any of the ducts that drain the lobes of the mammary gland at the nipple.

lac·to·ba·cil·lus (lăk′tō-bə-sĭl′əs) n. Any of various rod-shaped, nonmotile, aerobic bacteria of the genus *Lactobacillus* that ferment lactic acid from sugars and are the causative agents in the souring of milk.

lac·to·cele (lăk′tə-sēl′) n. See **galactocele.**

lac·to·fla·vin (lăk′tə-flā′vĭn, lăk′tə-flā′-) n. See **riboflavin.**

lac·to·gen·e·sis (lăk′tə-jĕn′ĭ-sĭs) n. The production of milk by the mammary glands.

lac·to·gen·ic (lăk′tə-jĕn′ĭk) adj. Inducing lactation.

lactogenic hormone n. See **prolactin.**

lac·to·glob·u·lin (lăk′tō-glŏb′yə-lĭn) n. The globulin present in milk, comprising from 50 to 60 percent of bovine whey protein.

lac·to·pro·tein (lăk′tō-prō′tēn′, -tē-ən) n. A protein normally present in milk.

lac·tose (lăk′tōs′) n. **1.** A disaccharide that is found in milk and hydrolyzes to yield glucose and galactose. **2.** A white crystalline substance obtained from whey and used in infant foods and pharmaceuticals as a diluent and excipient.

lac·to·ther·a·py (lăk′tō-thĕr′ə-pē) n. See **galactotherapy** (sense 2).

lac·to·tro·pin (lăk′tō-trō′pĭn) n. See **prolactin.**

la·cu·na (lə-kyōō′nə) n., pl. **-nas** or **-nae** (-nē). **1.** An anatomical cavity, space, or depression, especially in a bone. **2.** An abnormal space between the strata or between the cellular elements of the epidermis. — **la·cu′nal** adj.

la·cu·nar amnesia (lə-kyōō′nər) n. A condition in which memory is partially lost or the memory of isolated events is lost.

la·cu·nule (lə-kyōō'nyōōl') *n.* A very small lacuna.

lad·der splint (lăd'ər) *n.* A flexible splint consisting of two stout parallel wires with finer cross wires.

la·e·trile (lā'ĭ-trĭl', -trəl) *n.* A drug derived from amygdalin and purported to have antineoplastic properties.

lag·ging (lăg'ĭng) *n.* Retarded or diminished movement of the affected side of the chest in pulmonary tuberculosis.

lag·oph·thal·mi·a (lăg'ŏf-thăl'mē-ə) or **lag·oph·thal·mos** (-mŏs') *n.* A condition in which it is difficult or impossible to close the eyelids completely. — **lag'oph·thal'mic** (lăg'ŏf-thăl'mĭk) *adj.*

La·grange's operation (lə-grănʒ'zhīz) *n.* A combined iridectomy and sclerectomy performed in glaucoma for the purpose of forming a filtering cicatrix.

lake (lāk) *n.* A small collection of fluid.

lal·ling (lăl'ĭng) *n.* A form of stammering in which the speech is almost unintelligible.

lal·o·che·zi·a (lăl'ō-kē'zē-ə) *n.* Emotional relief gained by using indecent or vulgar language.

lal·o·ple·gi·a (lăl'ō-plē'jē-ə, -jə) *n.* Paralysis of the muscles involved in speech.

La·maze method (lə-mäz') *n.* A method of childbirth in which the expectant mother is prepared psychologically and physically to give birth without the use of pain-relieving drugs.

lamb·da (lăm'də) *n.* The craniometric point at the junction of the sagittal and lambdoid sutures. — *adj.* Relating to or characterizing a polypeptide chain that is one of two types of light chains present in immunoglobins.

Lam·bert–Eaton syndrome (lăm'bərt-) *n.* Progressive proximal muscle weakness in persons with carcinoma, in the absence of dermatomyositis or polymyositis.

Lam·bri·nu·di operation (lăm'brə-nōō'dē, -nyōō'-) *n.* A triple arthrodesis done to prevent foot drop.

LAMB syndrome (lăm) *n.* A syndrome of dermatological disorders characterized by the simultaneous appearance of lentigines, atrial and mucocutaneous myxomas, and blue nevi.

lame (lām) *adj.* **lam·er, lam·est. 1.** Disabled so that movement, especially walking, is difficult or impossible. **2.** Marked by pain or rigidity. — *v.* **lamed, lam·ing, lames.** To cause to become lame.

la·mel·la (lə-mĕl'ə) *n., pl.* **-mel·las** or **-mel·lae** (-mĕl'-ē'). **1.** A thin scale, plate, or layer of bone or tissue. **2.** A medicated gelatin disk, used instead of a solution for application to the conjunctiva.

lamellar bone *n.* A bone in which the tubular lamellae are formed, which are characterized by parallel spirally arranged collagen fibers.

la·mel·late (lə-mĕl'āt', lăm'ə-lāt') *adj.* **1.** Having, composed of, or arranged in lamellae. **2.** Resembling a lamella. — **lam'el·la'ted** *adj.* — **lam'el·la'tion** *n.*

la·mel·li·po·di·um (lə-mĕl'ə-pō'dē-əm) *n., pl.* **-di·a** (-dē-ə). A sheetlike cytoplasmic extension produced by migrating polymorphonuclear white blood cells that permits movement along a substrate.

lam·i·na (lăm'ə-nə) *n., pl.* **-nas** or **-nae** (-nē'). **1.** A thin plate, sheet, or layer. **2.** A thin layer of bone, membrane, or other tissue. — **lam'i·nar, lam'i·nal** *adj.*

lam·i·na·gram (lăm'ə-nə-grăm') *n.* An x-ray image taken by a laminagraph.

lam·i·na·graph (lăm'ə-nə-grăf') *n.* An x-ray machine that uses a technique in which tissues above and below the level of a suspected lesion are blurred out to emphasize a specific area.

lam·i·nag·ra·phy (lăm'ə-năg'rə-fē) *n.* See **tomography.**

lam·i·nat·ed clot (lăm'ə-nā'tĭd) *n.* A clot formed in a succession of layers, as occurs in the natural course of an aneurysm.

laminated epithelium *n.* See **stratified epithelium.**

lam·i·nec·to·my (lăm'ə-nĕk'tə-mē) *n.* Surgical excision of a vertebral lamina.

lam·i·not·o·my (lăm'ə-nŏt'ə-mē) *n.* Surgical division of one or more vertebral laminae.

lamp (lămp) *n.* A device that generates light, heat, or therapeutic radiation.

lance (lăns) *n.* See **lancet.** — *v.* **lanced, lanc·ing, lanc·es.** To make a surgical incision in, as with a lancet.

lan·cet (lăn'sĭt) *n.* A surgical knife with a short, wide, pointed double-edged blade, used especially for making punctures and small incisions.

Lan·dry's paralysis (lăn'drēz, län-drēz') *n.* See **acute ascending paralysis.**

Land·ström's muscle (länd'strœmz') *n.* Microscopic muscle fibers that are located in the fascia behind and about the eyeball, and draw the eyeball forward and the lids backward, resisting the pull of the four orbital muscles.

Lang·er·hans cell (läng'ər-häns') *n.* **1.** Any of the dendritic cells of the interstitial spaces of the mammalian epidermis that appear rod- or racket-shaped histologically; they are similar to melanocytes but lack the ability to oxidize phenols.

Langerhans granule *n.* A membrane-bound granule having a characteristic platelike arrangement of particles, first observed in Langerhans cells of the epidermis.

lan·o·lin (lăn'ə-lĭn) *n.* A fatty substance obtained from wool and used in soaps, cosmetics, and ointments.

lan·tha·nide (lăn'thə-nīd') *n.* Any of the abundant elements with atomic numbers 57 through 71, which closely resemble one another chemically.

lan·tha·num (lăn'thə-nəm) *n.* A soft malleable metallic rare-earth element with atomic number 57.

la·nu·gi·nous (lə-nōō'jə-nəs, -nyōō'-) or **la·nu·gi·nose** (-nōs') *adj.* Covered with soft, short hair; downy. — **la·nu'gi·nous·ness** *n.*

la·nu·go (lə-nōō'gō, -nyōō'-) *n., pl.* **-gos.** The fine, soft hair that grows on a fetus and is present on a newborn child.

lanugo hair *n.* See **lanugo.**

lap·a·ror·rha·phy (lăp′ə-rôr′ə-fē) *n.* See **celiorrha·phy.**

lap·a·ro·scope (lăp′ər-ə-skōp′) *n.* A slender, tubular endoscope inserted through an incision in the abdominal wall to examine or perform minor surgery in the abdominal or pelvic cavities.

lap·a·ros·co·py (lăp′ə-rŏs′kə-pē) *n.* **1.** Examination of the interior of the abdomen by a laparoscope; peritoneoscopy. **2.** A surgical procedure using laparoscopy.

lap·a·rot·o·my (lăp′ə-rŏt′ə-mē) *n.* **1.** Surgical incision into the abdominal cavity through the loin or flank. **2.** See **celiotomy.**

laparotomy pad *n.* A pad made from several layers of gauze folded into a rectangular shape and used especially as a sponge for packing off the viscera in abdominal operations.

large calorie *n.* See **calorie** (sense 2).

large intestine *n.* The portion of the intestine that extends from the ileum to the anus, forming an arch around the convolutions of the small intestine and including the cecum, colon, rectum, and anal canal.

lar·va (lär′və) *n., pl.* **-vas** or **-vae** (-vē). The newly hatched, wingless, often wormlike form of many insects before metamorphosis. — **lar′val** *adj.*

larva cur·rens (kûr′ənz) *n.* Creeping eruption caused by rapidly moving larvae of *Strongyloides stercoralis,* typically extending from the anal area down the upper thighs.

la·ryn·ge·al (lə-rĭn′jē-əl, -jəl, lăr′ən-jē′əl) or **la·ryn·gal** (lə-rĭng′gəl) *adj.* Of, relating to, affecting, or near the larynx.

laryngeal papillomatosis *n.* A condition characterized by multiple squamous cell papillomas of the larynx, seen most commonly in young children, usually due to infection by the human papilloma virus transmitted at birth from the maternal genital warts. Recurrences are common, with remission after several years.

laryngeal stenosis *n.* Narrowing or stricture of the larynx.

laryngeal syncope *n.* A paroxysmal neurosis characterized by unusual sensations in the throat and attacks of coughing, followed by a brief period of unconsciousness.

lar·yn·gec·to·my (lăr′ən-jĕk′tə-mē) *n.* Surgical removal of part or all of the larynx.

lar·yn·gis·mus (lăr′ĭn-jĭz′məs) *n.* Spasmodic narrowing or closure of the opening between the vocal cords.

laryngismus stri·du·lus (strī′jə-ləs, strĭj′ə-) *n.* A spasmodic closure of the glottis, lasting a few seconds, followed by noisy inspiration.

lar·yn·gi·tis (lăr′ĭn-jī′tĭs) *n.* Inflammation of the larynx. — **lar′yn·git′ic** (-jĭt′ĭk) *adj.*

la·ryn·go·cele (lə-rĭng′gə-sēl′) *n.* An air sac connected to the larynx through the ventricle, often bulging outward into the tissue of the neck, especially during coughing.

la·ryn·go·fis·sure (lə-rĭng′gō-fĭsh′ər) *n.* Surgical opening of the larynx, usually through the midline of the thyroid cartilage.

la·ryn·go·pa·ral·y·sis (lə-rĭng′gō-pə-răl′ĭ-sĭs) *n.* Paralysis of the laryngeal muscles.

lar·yn·gop·a·thy (lăr′ĭng-gŏp′ə-thē) *n.* A disease of the larynx.

la·ryn·go·phar·yn·gec·to·my (lə-rĭng′gō-făr′ĭn-jĕk′tə-mē) *n.* Surgical resection or excision of the larynx and the pharynx.

la·ryn·go·phar·yn·gi·tis (lə-rĭng′gō-făr′ĭn-jī′tĭs) *n.* Inflammation of the larynx and the pharynx.

la·ryn·go·phar·ynx (lə-rĭng′gō-făr′ĭngks) *n.* The part of the pharynx lying below the aperture of the larynx and behind the larynx, extending to the esophagus at the level of the cricoid cartilage.

lar·yn·goph·o·ny (lăr′ĭn-gŏf′ə-nē) *n.* The voice sounds heard in auscultation of the larynx.

la·ryn·go·plas·ty (lə-rĭng′gə-plăs′tē) *n.* Reparative or plastic surgery of the larynx.

la·ryn·go·scope (lə-rĭng′gə-skōp′, -rĭn′jə-) *n.* A tubular endoscope that is inserted into the larynx through the mouth and used for examining the interior of the larynx. — **la·ryn′go·scop′ic** (-skōp′ĭk), **la·ryn′go·scop′i·cal** *adj.*

lar·yn·gos·co·py (lăr′ĭn-gŏs′kə-pē) *n.* Examination of the larynx by means of a laryngoscope.

la·ryn·go·spasm (lə-rĭng′gə-spăz′əm) *n.* Spasmodic closure of the larynx.

la·ryn·go·ste·no·sis (lə-rĭng′gō-stə-nō′sĭs) *n.* Stricture or narrowing of the larynx.

lar·yn·gos·to·my (lăr′ĭn-gŏs′tə-mē) *n.* Surgical creation of a permanent opening into the larynx.

lar·yn·got·o·my (lăr′ĭn-gŏt′ə-mē) *n.* See **laryngofissure.**

la·ryn·go·tra·che·i·tis (lə-rĭng′gō-trā′kē-ī′tĭs) *n.* Inflammation of the larynx and the trachea.

la·ryn·go·tra·che·o·bron·chi·tis (lə-rĭng′gō-trā′kē-ō-brŏn-kī′tĭs, -brŏng-) *n.* An acute respiratory infection of the larynx, trachea, and bronchi.

la·ryn·go·tra·che·ot·o·my (lə-rĭng′gō-trā′kē-ŏt′ə-mē) *n.* Surgical incision of the larynx and trachea.

lar·ynx (lăr′ĭngks) *n., pl.* **lar·ynx·es** or **la·ryn·ges** (lə-rĭn′jēz). The part of the respiratory tract between the pharynx and the trachea, having walls of cartilage and muscle and containing the vocal cords enveloped in folds of mucous membrane.

La·sægue's sign (lə-sĕgz′, lä-) *n.* An indication of lumbar root or sciatic nerve irritation in which dorsiflexion of the ankle when the hip is flexed causes pain or muscle spasm in the posterior thigh.

lase (lāz) *v.* **lased, las·ing, las·es.** To cut, divide, or dissolve a substance with a laser.

la·ser (lā′zər) *n.* Any of several devices that convert incident electromagnetic radiation to highly amplified and coherent ultraviolet, visible, or infrared radiation; lasers are used in surgery to cut and dissolve tissue.

Las·sa fever or **Las·sa hemorrhagic fever** (läs′ə, lä′sə) *n.* A highly fatal form of epidemic hemorrhagic fever caused by Lassa virus and characterized by high fever, sore throat, severe muscle aches, skin rash with hemorrhages, headache, abdominal pain, vomiting, and diarrhea.

Lassa virus *n.* A virus of the genus *Arenavirus* that causes Lassa fever.

las·si·tude (lăs′ĭ-tōōd′, -tyōōd′) *n.* A state or feeling of weariness, diminished energy, or listlessness.

la·tah (lä′tə) *n.* A nervous disorder characterized by an exaggerated physical response to being startled or to unexpected suggestion.

la·ten·cy (lāt′n-sē) *n.* **1.** The state of being latent. **2.** Latency phase.

latency period *n.* See **latency phase.**

latency phase *n.* In psychoanalytic theory, the stage in psychosexual development, extending from about age 5 to age 12, when overt sexual interest is repressed or sublimated and the person focuses on skills and activities with members of his or her own sex.

la·tent (lāt′nt) *adj.* **1.** Present or potential but not evident or active. **2.** In a dormant or hidden stage, as an infection. **3.** Undeveloped but capable of normal growth under the proper conditions. **4.** Present in the unconscious mind but not consciously expressed.

latent content *n.* The hidden meaning of a dream, fantasy, or thought that can be revealed through interpretation or in psychoanalysis.

latent diabetes *n.* A mild form of diabetes mellitus in which a person displays no overt symptoms, but has abnormal responses to various diagnostic tests, as for glucose tolerance or fasting blood glucose concentration.

latent homosexuality *n.* A sexual tendency toward members of the same sex that is not consciously recognized or not expressed overtly.

latent learning *n.* Learning that is not the result of determined effort and is not evident at the time it occurs, but remains subconscous or latent until a need for it arises.

latent period *n.* **1.** The period elapsing between the application of a stimulus and the obvious response, such as the contraction of a muscle. **2.** The interval between exposure to an infectious organism or a carcinogen and the clinical appearance of disease.

latent reflex *n.* A reflex considered normal but usually appearing only with a pathological condition that makes its manifestation more likely.

latent schizophrenia *n.* A condition characterized by symptoms of schizophrenia but lacking a psychotic schizophrenic episode. The condition may indicate a preexisting susceptibility for the full development of schizophrenia.

late-onset diabetes *n.* See **diabetes mellitus**

lat·er·al (lăt′ər-əl) *adj.* **1.** Relating to or situated at or on the side. **2.** Situated or extending away from the median plane of the body. **3.** Relating to the left or right lateral region of the abdomen. — *n.* A lateral part, position, or appendage. — **lat′er·al·ly** *adv.*

lateral hermaphroditism *n.* Hermaphroditism in which a testis is present on one side of the body and an ovary on the other.

lat·er·al·i·ty (lăt′ə-răl′ĭ-tē) *n.* Preferential use of members of one side of the body in voluntary motor movements over those on the other side.

lat·er·al·i·za·tion (lăt′ər-ə-lī-zā′shən) *n.* Localization of function attributed to either the right or left side of the brain.

lateral recumbent position *n.* See **Sims′ position.**

lateral region *n.* The region of the abdomen lying on either side of the umbilical region and between the hypochondriac and inguinal regions.

lat·er·o·duc·tion (lăt′ə-rō-dŭk′shən) *n.* Movement to one side, as of an eye.

lat·er·o·flex·ion (lăt′ə-rō-flĕk′shən) *n.* A bending or curvature to one side.

lat·er·o·tor·sion (lăt′ə-rō-tôr′shən) *n.* A twisting to one side, especially the turning of the eyeball to the left or right on its anteroposterior axis.

lat·er·o·tru·sion (lăt′ə-rō-trōō′zhən) *n.* The outward thrust given by the muscles of chewing to the rotating mandibular condyle during movement of the mandible.

lat·er·o·ver·sion (lăt′ə-rō-vûr′zhən, -shən) *n.* A turning to one side, as of the uterus.

late systole *n.* See **prediastole.**

la·tex (lā′tĕks′) *n.* An emulsion of rubber or plastic globules in water. — **la′tex′** *adj.*

latex agglutination test *n.* A passive agglutination test in which antigen is adsorbed onto latex particles.

la·tis·si·mus dor·si (lă-tĭs′ə-məs dôr′sī) *n.* A muscle with origin from the spinous processes of the lower thoracic and lumbar vertebrae, the sacrum, and the iliac crest, with insertion into the humerus, and whose action adducts the arm, rotates it medially, and extends it.

laugh·ing gas (lăf′ĭng) *n.* Nitrous oxide, especially as used as an anesthetic.

Lau·rence–Moon syndrome (lôr′əns-mōōn′) *n.* An inherited syndrome believed to be caused by recessive mutations of two genes on the same chromosome and marked by mental retardation, pigmentary retinopathy, hypogenitalism, and spastic paraplegia.

lav·age (lăv′ĭj, lä-väzh′) *n.* A washing, especially of a hollow organ such as the stomach or lower bowel, with repeated injections of water.

law (lô) *n.* **1.** A formulation describing a relationship observed to be invariable between or among phenomena for all cases in which the specified conditions are met. **2.** A generalization based on consistent experience or results.

law of referred pain *n.* The principle that pain arises only from irritation of nerves that are sensitive to those stimuli that produce pain when applied to the surface of the body.

law of the heart *n.* The principle that the energy released by the heart when it contracts is a function of the length of its muscle fibers at the end of diastole.

law·ren·ci·um (lô-rĕn′sē-əm, lō-) *n.* A radioactive synthetic element that is produced from californium and has atomic number 103.

lax·a·tive (lăk′sə-tĭv) *n.* A food or drug that stimulates evacuation of the bowels. — *adj.* Stimulating evacuation of the bowels.

lay·er (lā′ər) *n.* A single thickness of a material covering a surface or forming an overlying part or segment. — *v.* **-ered, -er·ing, -ers.** To divide or form into layers.

LBT *abbr.* lupus band test

LCAT deficiency *abbr.* lecithin cholesterol acyltransferase deficiency — *n.* A rare inherited condition due to very low lecithin cholesterol acyltransferase activity, marked by corneal opacities, anemia, proteinuria, and the accumulation of unesterfied cholesterol in plasma and tissues.

LDL *abbr.* low-density lipoprotein

L-dopa *n.* A form of dopa used to treat Parkinson's disease.

L dose *n.* Any of a group of terms indicating the relative activity, potency, or combining effect of the diphtheria toxin with an antitoxin.

LE *abbr.* left eye; lupus erythematosus

lead (lēd) *n.* **1.** Any of the conductors designed to detect changes in electrical potential when situated in or on the body and connected to an instrument that registers and records these changes, such as an electrocardiograph. **2.** A record made from the current supplied by such a conductor.

lead (lĕd) *n.* A soft ductile dense metallic element that has poisonous salts; is extracted chiefly from galena; used in pipes, solder, bullets, paints, and antiknock compounds; and has atomic number 82.

lead line (lĕd) *n.* An irregular dark deposit in the gums occurring in lead poisoning.

lead poisoning (lĕd) *n.* Acute or chronic poisoning by lead or any of its salts, with the acute form causing severe gastroenteritis and encephalopathy and the chronic form causing anemia and damage to the gastrointestinal tract and nervous system.

Lear complex (lēr) *n.* In psychoanalytic theory, a father's libidinous fixation on a daughter.

learned helplessness *n.* A laboratory model of depression in which exposure to a series of unforeseen adverse situations gives rise to a sense of helplessness or an inability to cope with or devise ways to escape such situations.

learn·ing (lûr′nĭng) *n.* **1.** The act, process, or experience of gaining knowledge or skill. **2.** Behavioral modification especially through experience or conditioning.

learning disability *n.* A disorder in one or more of the basic cognitive and psychological processes involved in using language or performing mathematical calculations, affecting persons of normal intelligence and not due to emotional disturbance or impairment of sight or hearing. — **learn′ing·dis·a′bled** *adj.*

leath·er·bot·tle stomach (lĕth′ər-bŏt′l) *n.* Marked thickening and rigidity of the stomach wall, with reduced capacity of the lumen.

Le·ber's hereditary optic atrophy (lā′bərz, -bĕrz) *n.* The degeneration of the optic nerve and papillomacular bundle with resulting rapid loss of central vision, occurring most often in males.

LE cell *abbr.* lupus erythematosus cell

LE cell test *n.* See **lupus erythematosus cell test.**

lec·i·thin (lĕs′ə-thĭn) *n.* Any of a group of phospholipids that are found in nervous tissue, especially myelin sheaths and egg yolk, and in the plasma membranes of cells and are used as emulsifiers in a wide range of commercial products, including foods.

lec·i·tho·blast (lĕs′ə-thō-blăst′) *n.* One of the cells proliferating to form the yolk-sac endoderm.

lec·tin (lĕk′tĭn) *n.* Any of several plant glycoproteins that bind to specific carbohydrate groups on the plasma membrane of cells, used to stimulate lymphocyte proliferation and agglutinate red blood cells.

leech (lēch) *n.* Any of various chiefly aquatic bloodsucking or carnivorous annelid worms of the class Hirudinea, one species *(Hirudo medicinalis)* was formerly used by physicians to bleed patients. — *v.* **leeched, leech·ing, leech·es.** To bleed with leeches.

LE factor (ĕl′ē′) *n.* Any of the antinuclear immunoglobulins in the plasma of persons with disseminated lupus erythematosus.

Le·Fort II fracture (lə-fôr′) *n.* See **pyramidal fracture.**

left atrioventricular valve *n.* See **mitral valve.**

left brachiocephalic vein *n.* A vein that receives the left vertebral, internal thoracic, superior intercostal, inferior thyroid, and other veins.

left brain *n.* The cerebral hemisphere to the left of the corpus callosum, controlling the right side of the body.

left heart *n.* The left atrium and left ventricle.

left hepatic duct *n.* The duct that drains bile from the left half of the liver.

left-to-right shunt *n.* **1.** A diversion of blood from the left side of the heart to the right, as through a septal defect. **2.** A diversion of blood from the systemic circulation to the pulmonary circulation, as through a patent ductus arteriosus.

left ventricle *n.* The chamber on the left side of the heart that receives arterial blood from the left atrium and contracts to force it into the aorta.

left ventricular failure *n.* Congestive heart failure manifested by signs of pulmonary congestion and edema.

leg (lĕg) *n.* **1.** One of the two lower limbs of the human body, especially the part between the knee and the foot. **2.** A supporting part resembling a leg in shape or function.

le·gal blindness (lē′gəl) *n.* Visual acuity of less than ⁶⁄₆₀ or 20/200 using Snellen's test types, or visual field restriction to 20 degrees or less.

legal medicine *n.* See **forensic medicine.**

Le·gion·el·la (lē′jə-nĕl′ə) *n.* A genus of gramnegative bacilli that includes the species *(L. pneumophila)* that causes Legionnaires' disease.

Le·gion·naires' disease (lē′jə-nârz′) *n.* An acute, sometimes fatal respiratory disease caused by a bacterium of the genus *Legionella*, especially *L.*

pneumophila, and characterized by severe pneumonia, headache, and a dry cough.

lei·o·my·o·fi·bro·ma (lī′ō-mī′ō-fī-brō′mə) *n.* See **fibroleiomyoma.**

lei·o·my·o·ma (lī′ō-mī-ō′mə) *n.* A benign tumor derived from smooth muscle, occurring most often in the uterus.

Leish·man·i·a (lēsh-măn′ē-ə, -mā′nē-ə) *n.* A genus of flagellate protozoa, several species of which cause leishmaniasis; all species are indistinguishable morphologically but may be separated by their serological reactions and by their clinical manifestations of leishmaniasis.

leish·man·i·a·sis (lēsh′mə-nī′ə-sĭs) *n.* **1.** An infection caused by any of the flagellate protozoans of the genus *Leishmania,* transmitted to humans and animals by bloodsucking sand flies. **2.** A disease, such as kala-azar or any of various ulcerative skin diseases, caused by flagellate protozoans of the genus *Leishmania.*

Le·jeune syndrome (lə-zhœn′) *n.* See **cri-du-chat syndrome.**

Lem·bert suture (län-bĕr′) *n.* A continuous or interrupted suture for intestinal surgery that produces serosal apposition and includes the collagenous submucosal layer without entering the lumen of the intestine.

lem·mo·blast (lĕm′ō-blăst′) *n.* A cell developing from the neural crest in an embryo, capable of forming a cell of the neurilemma sheath.

lem·mo·cyte (lĕm′ō-sīt′) *n.* Any of the cells of the neurilemma.

lem·nis·cus (lĕm-nĭs′kəs) *n., pl.* **-nis·ci** (-nĭs′ī′, -nĭs′kī′, -nĭs′kē). A bundle of nerve fibers ascending from sensory nuclei in the spinal cord and the rhombencephalon to the thalamus.

Len·nox–Gas·taut syndrome (lĕn′əks-gä-stō′, -gä-) or **Len·nox syndrome** *n.* A generalized myoclonic astatic epilepsy that occurs in children as a result of various cerebral afflictions such as perinatal hypoxia, cerebral hemorrhage, encephalitis, and maldevelopment or metabolic disorders of the brain; it is marked by mental retardation and generalized tonic seizures or akinetic attacks.

lens (lĕnz) *n., pl.* **lens·es. 1.** A ground or molded piece of glass, plastic, or other transparent material with opposite surfaces either or both of which are curved, by means of which light rays are refracted so that they converge or diverge to form an image. **2.** A transparent, biconvex body of the eye between the iris and the vitreous humor that focuses light rays entering through the pupil to form an image on the retina. — **lensed** *adj.*

lens·ec·to·my (lĕn-zĕk′tə-mē) *n.* Surgical removal of the lens, usually done by puncture incision through the ciliary disk during vitrectomy.

lens stars *pl.n.* Congenital cataracts with opacities along the suture lines of the lens of the eye.

len·tic·u·lar astigmatism (lĕn-tĭk′yə-lər) *n.* Astigmatism due to a defect in the curvature, position, or index of refraction of the lens.

len·tic·u·lus (lĕn-tĭk′yə-ləs) *n., pl.* **-li** (-lī′). An intraocular lens of inert plastic placed in the ante-

rior chamber of the eye or behind the iris or clipped to the iris after cataract extraction.

len·ti·go (lĕn-tī′gō) *n., pl.* **-tig·i·nes** (-tĭj′ə-nēz′). A small, flat, pigmented spot on the skin.

len·ti·vi·rus (lĕn′tə-vī′rəs) *n.* See **slow virus.**

lep·er (lĕp′ər) *n.* One who has leprosy.

lep·o·thrix (lĕp′ə-thrĭks′) *n.* See **trichomycosis axillaris.**

lep·re·chaun·ism (lĕp′rĭ-kŏn′ĭz′əm) *n.* A rare genetic disorder characterized by mental and physical retardation, emaciation, endocrine disorders, hirsutism, and facial features dominated by large wide-set eyes and large low-set ears.

lep·rid (lĕp′rĭd) *n.* A skin lesion characteristic of leprosy.

lep·ro·ma (lĕ-prō′mə) *n., pl.* **-mas** or **-ma·ta** (-mə-tə). A circumscribed, discrete nodular skin lesion characteristic of leprosy.

lep·ro·ma·tous leprosy (lĕ-prō′mə-təs, -prŏm′ə-) *n.* A form of leprosy yielding a negative lepromin test that is contagious until treated and is characterized by lepromas, macular lesions having ill-defined borders, and, in advanced cases, nerve involvement and destructive lesions of the face, mouth, throat, and larynx.

lep·ro·min (lĕp′rə-mĭn) *n.* An extract of human tissue infected with *Mycobacterium leprae* and used in skin tests to classify the stage of leprosy.

lepromin test *n.* A nondiagnostic test to evaluate leprosy using an intradermal injection of a lepromin; the test classifies the stage and type of leprosy based on the lepromin reaction.

lep·ro·sar·i·um (lĕp′rə-sâr′ē-əm) *n., pl.* **-i·ums** or **-i·a** (-ē-ə). A hospital for the treatment of leprosy.

lep·ro·sy (lĕp′rə-sē) *n.* A chronic, mildly contagious granulomatous disease of tropical and subtropical regions, caused by the bacillus *Mycobacterium leprae,* marked by ulcers of skin, bone, and viscera and leading to loss of sensation, paralysis, gangrene, and deformation. It occurs in two principal types: lepromatous and tuberculoid. — **lep′rous** (lĕp′rəs), **lep·rot′ic** (lĕ-prŏt′ĭk) *adj.*

lep·to·ceph·a·ly (lĕp′tə-sĕf′ə-lē) *n.* A malformation marked by an abnormally small cranium.

lep·to·cyte (lĕp′tə-sīt′) *n.* An abnormally thin or flattened red blood cell having a central rounded pigmented area, a middle pigmentless zone, and a pigmented edge.

lep·to·cy·to·sis (lĕp′tō-sī-tō′sĭs) *n.* The presence of leptocytes in the blood.

lep·to·me·nin·ges (lĕp′tō-mə-nĭn′jēz) *n.* The pia mater and arachnoid considered together as one unit enveloping the brain and spinal cord. — **lep′to·me·nin′ge·al** (-jē-əl) *adj.*

lep·to·men·in·gi·tis (lĕp′tō-mĕn′ĭn-jī′tĭs) *n.* Inflammation of the leptomeninges.

Lep·to·spi·ra (lĕp′tō-spī′rə) *n.* A genus of aerobic spirochetes of the order Spirochaetales, consisting of thin, tightly coiled cells, many species of which cause leptospirosis.

lep·to·spi·ro·sis (lĕp′tō-spī-rō′sĭs) *n.* Any of a

group of infectious diseases that are caused by spirochetes of the genus *Leptospira*, are characterized by jaundice and fever, and are transmitted to humans by contact with the urine of infected animals.

lep·to·tene (lĕp′tə-tēn′) *n.* The early stage of prophase in meiosis in which the replicated chromosomes contract and become visible as long filaments well separated from one another.

Le·ri's sign (lā-rēz′) *n.* An indication of hemiplegia in which the voluntary flexion of the elbow is impossible when the wrist on the paralyzed side is passively flexed.

Leri–Weill syndrome (-vĕl′) *n.* See **dyschondrosteosis**.

Ler·moy·ez syndrome (lĕr-mwä-yā′) *n.* A hearing disorder in which the degree of deafness increases until a sudden attack of dizziness occurs, after which hearing improves.

les·bi·an (lĕz′bēən) *n.* A gay or homosexual woman. — *adj.* Of, relating to, or being a lesbian.

les·bi·an·ism (lĕz′bē-ə-nĭz′əm) *n.* Sexual orientation of women to other women.

Lesch–Ny·han syndrome (lĕsh′nī′ən) *n.* A sex-linked metabolic disorder in males, associated with an enzyme deficiency and characterized by hyperuricemia and uric acid urolithiasis, mental retardation, spastic cerebral palsy, and self-mutilation of fingers and lips by biting.

le·sion (lē′zhən) *n.* **1.** A wound or an injury. **2.** A localized pathological change in a bodily organ or tissue. **3.** An infected or diseased patch of skin.

less·er omentum (lĕs′ər) *n.* A peritoneal fold passing from the margins of the portal fissure to the lesser curvature of the stomach and to the upper border of the duodenum.

lesser trochanter *n.* A pyramidal process that projects from the shaft of the femur at the junction of the shaft and the neck.

lesser vestibular gland *pl.n.* Any of the small branched tubular mucous glands opening on the surface of the vestibule between the orifices of the vagina and urethra.

le·thal (lē′thəl) *adj.* **1.** Capable of causing death. **2.** Of, relating to, or causing death.

lethal factor *n.* A gene mutation or chromosomal structural change that when expressed causes death before sexual maturity.

lethal gene *n.* A gene whose expression results in the death of the organism.

lethal mutation *n.* A mutant trait that leads to a phenotype incapable of effective reproduction.

leth·ar·gy (lĕth′ər-jē) *n.* **1.** A state of sluggishness, inactivity, and apathy. **2.** A state of unconsciousness resembling deep sleep.

Leu *abbr.* leucine

leu·cine (lōō′sēn′) *n.* An essential amino acid derived from the hydrolysis of protein by pancreatic enzymes during digestion and necessary for optimal growth in infants and children and for the maintenance of nitrogen balance in adults.

leu·ka·phe·re·sis (lōō′kə-fə-rē′sĭs) *n.* The removal of a quantity of white blood cells from the blood

of a donor with the remaining portions of the blood retransfused into the donor.

leu·ke·mi·a (lōō-kē′mē-ə) *n.* Any of various acute or chronic neoplastic diseases of the bone marrow in which unrestrained proliferation of white blood cells occurs, usually accompanied by anemia, impaired blood clotting, and enlargement of the lymph nodes, liver, and spleen. — **leu·ke′mic** *adj.*

leukemic retinopathy *n.* A condition of the retina occurring in all types of leukemia and characterized by the presence of a yellow-orange fundus, engorgement and tortuosity of retinal veins, scattered hemorrhages, and edema of the retina and optic disk.

leu·ke·mid (lōō-kē′mĭd) *n.* Any of various nonspecific cutaneous lesions that are associated with leukemia but are not localized accumulations of leukemic cells.

leu·ke·mo·gen·e·sis (lōō-kē′mə-jĕn′ĭ-sĭs) *n.* Induction, development, and progression of a leukemic disease.

leu·ke·moid reaction (lōō-kē′moid′) *n.* A moderate, advanced, or sometimes extreme degree of leukocytosis that is similar or possibly identical to that occurring in various forms of leukemia but is due to some other cause.

leu·ko·ag·glu·ti·nin (lōō′kō-ə-glōōt′n-ĭn) *n.* An antibody that agglutinates white blood cells.

leu·ko·blast (lōō′kə-blăst′) *n.* An immature white blood cell formed during the transition from hemocytoblast to promyelocyte. — **leu′ko·blas′-tic** *adj.*

leu·ko·blas·to·sis (lōō′kō-blă-stō′sĭs) *n.* The abnormal proliferation of immature white blood cells, especially in granulocytic and lymphocytic leukemia.

leu·ko·ci·din (lōō′kə-sīd′n, lōō-kō′sĭ-dn) *n.* A heat-labile substance, made by certain species of *Staphylococcus* and *Streptococcus* bacteria, that can destroy or lyse white blood cells.

leu·ko·cyte or **leu·co·cyte** (lōō′kə-sīt′) *n.* See **white blood cell.** — **leu′ko·cyt′ic** (-sĭt′ĭk) *adj.*

leu·ko·cy·to·blast (lōō′kə-sī′tə-blăst′) *n.* A white blood cell precursor.

leu·ko·cy·to·gen·e·sis (lōō′kə-sī′tə-jĕn′ĭ-sĭs) *n.* Formation and development of white blood cells.

leu·ko·cy·tol·y·sin (lōō′kə-sī-tŏl′ĭ-sĭn) *n.* A substance that destroys or lyses white blood cells.

leu·ko·cy·tol·y·sis (lōō′kə-sī-tŏl′ĭ-sĭs) *n.* The destruction or lysis of white blood cells. — **leu′ko·cy′to·lyt′ic** (-sī′tə-lĭt′ĭk) *adj.*

leu·ko·cy·to·ma (lōō′kə-sī′tə-tō′mə) *n.* A fairly well circumscribed, nodular, dense accumulation of white blood cells.

leu·ko·cy·to·pe·ni·a (lōō′kə-sī′tə-pē′nē-ə) *n.* See **leukopenia.**

leu·ko·cy·to·pla·ni·a (lōō′kə-sī′tə-plā′nē-ə) *n.* The movement of white blood cells from blood vessels, through serous membranes, or in tissues.

leu·ko·cy·to·poi·e·sis (lōō′kə-sī′tə-poi-ē′sĭs) *n.* See **leukopoiesis.**

leu·ko·cy·to·sis or **leu·co·cy·to·sis** (lōō′kə-sī-tō′-

sĭs) *n., pl.* **-ses** (-sēz). An abnormally large increase in the number of white blood cells in the blood, often occurring during an acute infection or inflammation. — **leu′ko·cy·tot′ic** (-tŏt′ĭk) *adj.*

leu·ko·cy·to·tax·i·a (lōō′kə-sī′tə-tăk′sē-ə) *n.* **1.** The active ameboid movement of white blood cells, especially of neutrophilic granulocytes, toward or away from certain microorganisms or certain substances formed in inflamed tissue. **2.** The property of attracting or repelling white blood cells. — **leu′ko·cy′to·tac′tic** (-tăk′tĭk) *adj.*

leu·ko·cy·to·tox·in (lōō′kə-sī′tə-tŏk′sĭn) *n.* A substance that causes degeneration and necrosis of white blood cells.

leu·ko·cy·tu·ri·a (lōō′kə-sī-tōōr′ē-ə, -tyōōr′-) *n.* The presence of white blood cells in the urine.

leu·ko·der·ma or **leu·co·der·ma** (lōō′kə-dûr′mə) *n.* Partial or total loss of skin pigmentation, often occurring in patches.

leu·ko·dys·tro·phy (lōō′kō-dĭs′trə-fē) *n.* Degeneration of the white matter of the brain characterized by demyelination and glial reaction, probably related to defects of lipid metabolism.

leu·ko·e·de·ma (lōō′kō-ĭ-dē′mə) *n.* A benign abnormality of the buccal mucosa characterized by a filmy, opalescent-to-whitish gray, wrinkled epithelium similar to that seen in leukoplakia.

leu·ko·en·ceph·a·li·tis (lōō′kō-ĕn-sĕf′ə-lī′tĭs) *n.* Inflammation of the white matter of the brain.

leu·ko·e·ryth·ro·blas·to·sis (lōō′kō-ĭ-rĭth′rō-blă-stō′sĭs) *n.* An anemic condition resulting from space-occupying lesions in the bone marrow and characterized by the presence of immature granular white blood cells and nucleated red blood cells in the blood.

leu·ko·ko·ri·a (lōō′kō-kôr′ē-ə) *n.* A condition characterized by a reflective white mass within the eye that gives the appearance of white pupil.

leu·ko·lym·pho·sar·co·ma (lōō′kō-lĭm′fō-sär-kō′mə) *n.* See **leukosarcoma**.

leu·kol·y·sin (lōō-kŏl′ĭ-sĭn) *n.* See **leukocytolysin**.

leu·ko·ma (lōō-kō′mə) *n., pl.* **-mas** or **-ma·ta** (-mə-tə). A dense white opacity of the cornea. — **leu·kom′a·tous** (lōō-kŏm′ə-təs) *adj.*

leu·ko·my·e·lop·a·thy (lōō′kō-mī′ə-lŏp′ə-thē) *n.* Any of various diseases involving the white substance of the spinal cord.

leu·kon (lōō′kŏn′) *n.* The total mass of circulating white blood cells, their precursors, and the leukopoietic cells from which they arise.

leu·ko·nych·i·a (lōō′kō-nĭk′ē-ə) *n.* The occurrence of white spots or patches under the nails due to the presence of air bubbles between the nail and its bed.

leu·ko·pe·de·sis (lōō′kō-pĭ-dē′sĭs) *n.* The movement of white blood cells through the walls of capillaries and into the tissues.

leu·ko·pe·ni·a or **leu·co·pe·ni·a** (lōō′kə-pē′nē-ə) *n.* An abnormally low number of white blood cells in the blood. — **leu′ko·pe′nic** *adj.*

leu·ko·pla·ki·a (lōō′kə-plā′kē-ə) *n.* An abnormal condition characterized by white spots or patches on mucous membranes, especially of the mouth and vulva.

leu·ko·pla·sia (lōō′kə-plā′zhə, -zhē-ə, -zē-ə) *n.* See **leukoplakia**.

leu·ko·poi·e·sis (lōō′kō-poi-ē′sĭs) *n.* The formation and development of the various types of white blood cells. — **leu′ko·poi·et′ic** (-ĕt′ĭk) *adj.*

leu·ko·sar·co·ma (lōō′kō-sär-kō′mə) *n.* A type of lymphoma characterized by large numbers of abnormal lymphocyte precursors in the blood.

leu·ko·sis (lōō-kō′sĭs) *n.* The abnormal proliferation of one or more of the leukopoietic tissues.

leu·ko·tax·i·a (lōō′kə-tăk′sē-ə) *n.* See **leukocytotaxia** (sense 1). — **leu′ko·tac′tic** (-tăk′tĭk) *adj.*

leu·ko·tax·ine (lōō′kə-tăk′sēn′, -sĭn) *n.* A crystalline nitrogenous material produced in injured, acutely degenerating tissue and found in inflammatory exudates that acts to increase capillary permeability and white blood cell migration.

leu·ko·tax·is (lōō′kə-tăk′sĭs) *n.* See **leukocytotaxia** (sense 1).

leu·kot·o·my or **leu·cot·o·my** (lōō-kŏt′ə-mē) *n.* A prefrontal lobotomy.

leu·ko·trich·i·a (lōō′kə-trĭk′ē-ə) *n.* Whiteness of the hair.

leu·pro·lide acetate (lōō′prō-līd′) *n.* A synthetic polypeptide analog of naturally occurring gonadotropin-releasing hormone used in the treatment of advanced prostate cancer.

le·va·tor (lə-vā′tər) *n., pl.* **lev·a·to·res** (lĕv′ə-tôr′ēz). **1.** A surgical instrument for lifting the depressed fragments of a fractured skull. **2.** A muscle that raises a body part.

lev·el (lĕv′əl) *n.* **1.** Relative position or rank on a graded scale, such as mental or emotional development. **2.** A relative degree, as of intensity or concentration.

Le·vin tube (lə-vĭn′) *n.* A tube that is inserted through the nose into the upper alimentary canal and is used to facilitate intestinal decompression.

le·vo·bu·no·lol hydrochloride (lē′vō-byōō′nə-lôl′) *n.* A beta-blocker used primarily as an eyedrop in the treatment of chronic open-angle glaucoma and ocular hypertension.

le·vo·car·di·a (lē′və-kär′dē-ə) *n.* Situs inversus of the viscera but with normal positioning of the heart on the left, usually associated with congenital cardiac lesions.

le·vo·do·pa (lē′və-dō′pə) *n.* See **L-dopa**.

le·vo·duc·tion (lē′və-dŭk′shən) *n.* The rotation of one or both eyes to the left.

Lev's syndrome (lĕvz) *n.* A condition in which bundle-branch block occurs but the myocardium and coronary arteries are normal and in which there is fibrosis or calcification of the membranous septum, the muscular septum, and the mitral and aortic rings of the heart.

lev·u·lose (lĕv′yə-lōs′, -lōz′) *n.* See **fructose**.

Ley·dig cell (lī′dĭg, -dĭкʜ) *n.* See **interstitial cell**.

LH *abbr.* luteinizing hormone

Lher·mitte–Du·clos disease (lâr′mĭt-dōō-klō′, -dyōō-, lĕr-mĕt′-dü-klō′) *n.* A disease occurring chiefly in adults characterized by abnormal development and enlargement of the cerebellum and an increase in intracranial pressure.

Lher·mitte's sign (lăr´mĭts, lĕr-mēts´) *n.* An indication of multiple sclerosis and of disorders of the cervical cord, especially compression, in which sudden electriclike shocks extend down the spine when the head is flexed.

LHRH *abbr.* luteinizing hormone releasing hormone

li·bi·do (lĭ-bē´dō, -bī´-) *n., pl.* **-dos. 1.** The psychic and emotional energy associated with instinctual biological drives. **2.** Sexual desire. **3.** Manifestation of the sexual drive.

Lib·ri·um (lĭb´rē-əm) A trademark used for preparations of chlordiazepoxide hydrochloride.

li·chen (lī´kən) *n.* Any of various skin diseases characterized by patchy eruptions of small, firm papules.

li·chen·i·fi·ca·tion (lī-kĕn´ə-fĭ-kā´shən, lī´kə-nə-) *n.* Thickening of the skin with hyperkeratosis caused by chronic inflammation resulting from prolonged scratching or irritation.

lichen myx·e·de·ma·to·sus (mĭk´sĭ-dē´mə-tō´səs) *n.* A skin condition characterized by the widespread eruption of papules or plaques of mucinous edema caused by the deposition of acid mucopolysaccharides in the skin.

lichen nit·i·dus (nĭt´ĭ-dəs) *n.* A skin condition characterized by minute, asymptomatic, whitish or pinkish, flat-topped skin papules that may occur in conjunction with lichen planus.

li·chen·oid keratosis (lī´kə-noid´) *n.* A solitary benign skin papule or plaque having microscopic features resembling lichen planus.

lichen pla·nus (plā´nəs) *n.* A skin condition characterized by the eruption of flat-topped, shiny, violaceous papules on flexor surfaces, male genitalia, and the mucosa of the oral cavity.

lichen sim·plex (sĭm´plĕks´) *n.* A skin condition characterized by small, intensely pruritic papules.

li·do·caine (lī´də-kān´) *n.* A synthetic amide used chiefly in the form of its hydrochloride as a local anesthetic and antiarrhythmic agent.

Lie·ber·kühn's crypt (lē´bər-kyōonz´, -künz´) *n.* See **intestinal gland.**

li·en (lī´ən, -ĕn´) *n.* The spleen.

lien mo·bi·lis (mō´bə-lĭs) *n.* See **floating spleen.**

lienteric diarrhea *n.* Diarrhea in which undigested food appears in the stools.

li·en·ter·y (lī´ən-tĕr´ē) *n.* The passage of undigested or partially digested food in the stool. — **li´en·ter´ic** (lī´ən-tĕr´ĭk) *adj.*

life (līf) *n., pl.* **lives** (līvz). **1.** The property or quality that distinguishes living organisms from dead organisms and inanimate matter, manifested in functions such as metabolism, growth, reproduction, and response to stimuli or adaptation to the environment originating from within the organism. **2.** The characteristic state or condition of a living organism.

life cycle *n.* **1.** The course of developmental changes through which an organism passes from its inception as a fertilized zygote to the mature state in which another zygote may be produced. **2.** A

progression through a series of differing stages of development.

life expectancy *n.* The number of years that one is expected to live as determined by statistics.

life instinct *n.* In psychoanalytic theory, the instinct of self-preservation and sexual procreation; the basic urge toward preservation of the species.

life science *n.* Any of several branches of science, such as biology, medicine, anthropology, or ecology, that deal with living organisms and their organization, life processes, and relationships to each other and their environment.

life span *n.* **1.** A lifetime. **2.** The average or maximum length of time an organism, a material, or an object can be expected to survive or last.

life-support system *n.* Medical equipment that augments or substitutes for an essential bodily function, such as respiration or excretion, enabling a patient who otherwise might not survive to live.

life·time (līf´tīm´) *n.* **1.** The period of time during which an individual is alive. **2.** The period of time during which property, an object, a process, or a phenomenon exists or functions.

lig·a·ment (lĭg´ə-mənt) *n.* **1.** A band or sheet of tough fibrous tissue connecting two or more bones, cartilages, or other structures, or serving as support for fasciae or muscles. **2.** A fold of peritoneum supporting any of the abdominal viscera. **3.** The cordlike remains of a fetal vessel or other structure that has lost its original lumen. — **lig´a·men´tal** (-mĕn´tl), **lig´a·men´ta·ry** (-mĕn´tə-rē, -mĕn´trē), **lig´a·men´tous** *adj.*

lig·a·men·to·pex·is (lĭg´ə-mĕn´tə-pĕk´sĭs) or **lig·a·men·to·pex·y** (-mĕn´tə-pĕk´sē) *n.* A shortening of a ligament of the uterus.

li·gase (lī´gās´, -gāz´) *n.* Any of a class of enzymes, including the carboxylases, that catalyze the linkage of two molecules, generally using ATP as the energy donor.

li·gate (lī´gāt´) *v.* **-gat·ed, -gat·ing, -gates.** To tie or bind with a ligature.

li·ga·tion (lī-gā´shən) *n.* **1.** The act of binding or of applying a ligature. **2.** The state of being bound. **3.** Something that binds; a ligature.

lig·a·ture (lĭg´ə-chŏŏr´, -chər) *n.* **1.** The act of tying or binding. **2.** A thread, wire, or cord used in surgery to close vessels or tie off ducts.

light (līt) *n.* **1.** Electromagnetic radiation that stimulates the retina and is perceived as the sensation of vision.

light adaptation *n.* The adjustment of the eye under increased illumination, in which the sensitivity to light is reduced.

light-adapted eye *n.* An eye that has been exposed to light of relatively high intensity and has undergone adjustments of photochemical change and constriction of the pupil.

light·en·ing (līt´n-ĭng) *n.* The sensation of decreased abdominal distention during the latter weeks of pregnancy following the descent of the fetal head into the pelvic inlet.

light reflex *n.* **1.** Contraction of the pupil of the eye in response to an increase in light. **2.** A circular red light reflected from the retina of the eye, as observed in retinoscopy. **3.** See **cone of light**.

light treatment *n.* See **phototherapy**.

limb (lǐm) *n.* **1.** One of the paired jointed extremities of the body; an arm or a leg. **2.** A segment of such a jointed structure.

limb bud *n.* A mesenchymal outgrowth covered with ectoderm on the flank of an embryo that gives rise to a limb.

lim·bic system (lǐm′bǐk) *n.* A group of deep brain structures that includes the hippocampus, amygdala, and connecting structures, associated with olfaction, emotion, motivation, behavior, and various autonomic functions.

limb lead (lēd) *n.* **1.** Any of the three standard leads used in electrocardiography, having one electrode attached to the chest and another to a limb. **2.** A unipolar lead in which one electrode is placed on a limb. **3.** A record obtained from such leads.

lim·bus (lǐm′bəs) *n., pl.* **-bi** (-bī′). An edge, border, or fringe of an anatomical part.

li·men (lī′mən) *n., pl.* **li·mens** or **lim·i·na** (lǐm′ə-nə). **1.** The threshold of a physiological or psychological response. **2.** The external opening of a canal; an entrance. — **lim′i·nal** (lǐm′ə-nəl) *adj.*

limp (lǐmp) *n.* An irregular, jerky, or awkward gait; a claudication. — *v.* **limped, limp·ing, limps.** To walk lamely, especially with irregularity, as if favoring one leg.

lim·u·lus·ly·sate test (lǐm′yə-ləs-lī′sāt′) *n.* A test for the rapid detection of gram-negative bacterial meningitis.

lin·co·my·cin (lǐng′kə-mī′sǐn) *n.* An antibiotic derived from cultures of the bacterium *Streptomyces lincolnensis*, used in the treatment of certain penicillin-resistant infections.

lin·dane (lǐn′dān) *n.* A white crystalline powder used topically in the treatment of scabies and pediculosis.

Lin·dau's disease (lǐn′douz′) *n.* A hereditary disease marked by hemangiomas of the retina, the cerebellum and occasionally the spinal cord, and sometimes associated with cysts or hamartomas of kidney, adrenal glands, or other organs.

line (līn) *n.* **1.** A crease in the skin, especially on the face; a wrinkle. **2.** In anatomy, a long narrow mark, strip, or streak distinguished from adjacent tissue by color, texture, or elevation. **3.** A real or imaginary mark positioned in relation to fixed points of reference. **4.** A border, boundary, or demarcation. **5.** A contour or an outline. **6.** Ancestry or lineage. **7.** A series of persons, especially from one family, who succeed each other.

lin·e·a (lǐn′ē-ə) *n., pl.* **-e·ae** (-ē-ē′). A line.

linea al·ba (ǎl′bə) *n.* A fibrous band that runs vertically along the center of the anterior abdominal wall and receives the attachments of the oblique and transverse abdominal muscles.

linea ni·gra (nī′grə, nǐg′rə) *n.* The linea alba in pregnancy, which then becomes pigmented.

lin·e·ar accelerator (lǐn′ē-ər) *n.* A device that produces high energy photons (x-rays) on charged particles for use in radiation therapy.

linear atrophy *n.* Stretch marks.

linear fracture *n.* A fracture that runs parallel to the long axis of a bone.

line of fixation *n.* An imaginary line joining the optical point of fixation with the fovea and passing through the nodal point.

lin·gua (lǐng′gwə) *n., pl.* **-guae** (-gwē′). **1.** The tongue. **2.** A tonguelike anatomical structure.

lin·gual (lǐng′gwəl) *n.* **1.** Of or relating to the tongue or any tonguelike part; glossal. **2.** Next to or toward the tongue.

lingual papilla *n.* Any of the papillae on the tongue.

lingua ni·gra (nī′grə, nǐg′rə) *n.* Black tongue.

lin·gu·lec·to·my (lǐng′gyə-lěk′tə-mē) *n.* **1.** Surgical excision of the lingular portion of the left upper lobe of the lung. **2.** See **glossectomy**.

lin·i·ment (lǐn′ə-mənt) *n.* A liquid preparation rubbed into the skin or gums as a counterirritant, rubefacient, anodyne, or cleansing agent.

li·ni·tis (lǐ-nī′tǐs, lī-) *n.* Inflammation of cellular tissue, especially of the perivascular tissue of the stomach.

linitis plas·ti·ca (plǎs′tǐ-kə) *n.* Thickening and fibrous proliferation in the wall of the stomach caused by the infiltration of scirrhous carcinoma.

link·age (lǐng′kǐj) *n.* An association between two or more genes such that the traits they control tend to be inherited together.

link·er (lǐng′kər) *n.* A fragment of synthetic DNA containing a restriction site that may be used for splicing of genes.

lin·o·le·ic acid (lǐn′ə-lē′ǐk) *n.* An unsaturated fatty acid considered essential to the human diet and an important component of drying oils, such as linseed oil.

lip (lǐp) *n.* **1.** Either of two fleshy folds that surround the opening of the mouth. **2.** A liplike structure bounding or encircling a bodily cavity or groove.

lip·ase (lǐp′ās′, lī′pās′) *n.* Any of a group of fat-splitting or lipolytic enzymes that cleave a fatty acid residue from the glycerol residue in a neutral fat or a phospholipid.

lip·ec·to·my (lǐ-pěk′tə-mē, lī-) *n.* Surgical excision of subcutaneous fatty tissue.

lip·e·de·ma (lǐp′ǐ-dē′mə) *n.* Chronic swelling, usually of the lower extremities, caused by the widespread, even distribution of subcutaneous fat and fluid.

li·pe·mi·a (lǐ-pē′mē-ə) *n.* An excess of fat or lipids in the blood.

lipemia ret·i·na·lis (rět′n-ā′lǐs) *n.* A creamy appearance of the retinal blood vessels when the lipids of the blood are over five percent.

lip·id (lǐp′ǐd, lī′pǐd) or **lip·ide** (lǐp′ǐd′, lī′pǐd′) *n.* Any of a group of organic compounds, including the fats, oils, waxes, sterols, and triglycerides, that are insoluble in water but soluble in common organic solvents, are oily to the touch, and together with carbohydrates and proteins constitute the principal structural material of living cells. — **lip·id'ic** adj.

lip·i·do·sis (lĭp'ĭ-dō'sĭs) n., pl. **-ses** (-sēz). An inborn or acquired disorder of the lipid metabolism.

lipid proteinosis n. An inherited lipid metabolism disorder characterized by deposits of a protein-lipid complex on the labial mucosa and sublingual and faucial areas, and by papillomatous eyelid lesions.

lip·o·ar·thri·tis (lĭp'ō-är-thrī'tĭs) n. Inflammation of the periarticular fatty tissues of the knee.

lip·o·at·ro·phy (lĭp'ō-ăt'rə-fē) n. The loss of subcutaneous fat.

lip·o·blast (lĭp'ə-blăst') n. An embryonic fat cell.

lip·o·blas·to·ma (lĭp'ō-blă-stō'mə) n. **1.** See **liposarcoma**. **2.** A tumor, usually occurring in infants, composed of embryonal fat cells separated into distinct lobules.

lip·o·blas·to·ma·to·sis (lĭp'ō-blă-stō'mə-tō'sĭs) n. A diffuse form of lipoblastoma that infiltrates locally but does not metastasize.

lip·o·crit (lĭp'ə-krĭt') n. A procedure for separating and volumetrically analyzing the amount of lipid in the blood or other body fluid.

lip·o·cyte (lĭp'ə-sīt') n. A fat-storing stellate cell of the liver.

lip·o·der·moid (lĭp'ō-dûr'moid') n. A congenital, yellowish-white, fatty, benign tumor located beneath the conjunctiva of the eye.

lip·o·e·de·ma (lĭp'ō-ĭ-dē'mə) n. Edema of subcutaneous fat, which causes painful swellings, especially of the legs in women.

lip·o·fi·bro·ma (lĭp'ō-fī-brō'mə) n. A benign neoplasm of fibrous connective tissue, with conspicuous numbers of adipose cells.

lip·o·fus·cin (lĭp'ō-fŭs'ĭn, -fyōō'sĭn) n. Brown pigment granules representing lipid-containing residues of lysosomal digestion.

lip·o·gen·e·sis (lĭp'ə-jĕn'ĭ-sĭs) n. **1.** Production of fat, either fatty degeneration or fatty infiltration. **2.** The normal deposition of fat or the conversion of carbohydrate or protein to fat. — **lip'o·gen'ic** (-jĕn'ĭk), **li·pog'e·nous** (lĭ-pŏj'ə-nəs) adj.

lip·oi·do·sis (lĭp'oi-dō'sĭs) n. Lipidosis.

li·pol·y·sis (lĭ-pŏl'ĭ-sĭs, lī-) n., pl **-ses** (-sēz'). The hydrolysis of lipids. — **lip'o·lyt'ic** (lĭp'ə-lĭt'ĭk, lī'-pə-) adj.

li·po·ma (lĭ-pō'mə, lī-) n., pl. **-mas** or **-ma·ta** (-mətə). A benign tumor composed chiefly of fat cells.

lipoma sar·co·ma·to·des (sär-kō'mə-tō'dēz) n. Liposarcoma.

li·po·ma·to·sis (lĭ-pō'mə-tō'sĭs) n. See **adiposis**.

lip·o·me·nin·go·cele (lĭp'ō-mə-nĭng'gə-sēl') n. An intraspinal lipoma associated with a spina bifida.

lip·o·mu·co·pol·y·sac·cha·ri·do·sis (lĭp'ō-myōō'kō-pŏl'ē-săk'ə-rĭ-dō'sĭs) n. See **mucolipidosis I**.

lip·o·pe·ni·a (lĭp'ə-pē'nē-ə) n. An abnormally small amount or a deficiency of lipids in the body.

lip·o·phage (lĭp'ə-fāj') n. A cell that ingests fat.

li·poph·a·gy (lĭ-pŏf'ə-jē, lĭp'ə-fā'jē) n. The ingestion of fat by a lipophage.

lip·o·phil (lĭp'ə-fĭl') n. A substance having an affinity for, tending to combine with, or capable of dissolving in lipids. — **lip'o·phil'ic** adj. & n.

lip·o·pol·y·sac·cha·ride (lĭp'ō-pŏl'ē-săk'ə-rīd', lī'pō-) n. Any of a group of polysaccharides in which a lipid constitutes a portion of the molecule.

lip·o·pro·tein (lĭp'ō-prō'tēn', -tē-ĭn, lī'pō-) n. Any of a group of conjugated proteins in which at least one of the components is a lipid. Lipoproteins, classified according to their densities and chemical qualities, are the principal means by which lipids are transported in the blood.

lip·o·sar·co·ma (lĭp'ō-sär-kō'mə) n. A malignant tumor consisting chiefly of immature, anaplastic lipoblasts of varying sizes, including giant forms, with bizarre nuclei and vacuoles of varying sizes in the cytoplasm, usually in association with a rich network of capillaries.

li·po·sis (lĭ-pō'sĭs) n. **1.** See **adiposis**. **2.** Fatty infiltration of tissue, with neutral fats being present in the cells.

lip·o·some (lĭp'ə-sōm', lī'pə-) n. An artificial microscopic vesicle consisting of an aqueous core enclosed in one or more phospholipid layers, used to convey vaccines, drugs, enzymes, or other substances to target cells or organs.

lip·o·suc·tion·ing (lĭp'ō-sŭk'shə-nĭng, lī'pō-) or **lip·o·suc·tion** (-sŭk'shən) n. A usually cosmetic surgical procedure in which excess subcutaneous fat is removed from a specific area of the body, such as the thighs or abdomen, by means of suction.

li·pot·ro·phy (lĭ-pŏt'rə-fē) n. An increase of fat in the body.

lip·o·tro·pin (lĭp'ə-trō'pĭn, lī'pə-) n. A hormone produced by the anterior pituitary gland that promotes the use of fat by the body and is a precursor to the endorphins.

lip·ping (lĭp'ĭng) n. The formation of a liplike structure, as at the articular end of a bone in osteoarthritis.

lip reflex n. A pouting movement of the lips in young infants occurring in response to tapping near the angle of the mouth.

li·pu·ri·a (lĭ-pōōr'ē-ə, -pyōōr'-) n. Excretion of fat in the urine. — **li·pu'ric** adj.

liq·ue·fac·tion (lĭk'wə-făk'shən) n. **1.** The process of liquefying. **2.** The state of being liquefied.

liq·ue·fac·tive necrosis (lĭk'wə-făk'tĭv) n. Necrosis characterized by a circumscribed lesion that consists of the fluid remains of tissue that had become necrotic and that was digested by enzymes.

liq·uid (lĭk'wĭd) n. **1.** The state of matter in which a substance exhibits a characteristic readiness to flow, little or no tendency to disperse, and relatively high incompressibility. **2.** Matter or a specific body of matter in this state. — adj. **1.** Of or being a liquid. **2.** Having been liquefied, especially melted by heating or condensed by cooling. **3.**

Flowing readily; fluid. — **liq′uid·ly** *adv.* — **liq′uid·ness** *n.*

lisp (lĭsp) *n.* A speech defect or mannerism characterized by mispronunciation of the sounds (s) and (z) as (th) and (*th*). — *v.* lisped, lisp·ing, lisps. To speak with a lisp.

lis·sen·ce·pha·li·a (lĭs′ĕn-sə-fā′lē-ə, -fāl′yə) or **lis·sen·ceph·a·ly** (-sĕf′ə-lē) *n.* See **agyria**. — **lis′sen·ce·phal′ic** (-sə-fāl′ĭk) *adj.*

Lis·te·ri·a (lĭ-stēr′ē-ə) *n.* A genus of aerobic bacteria containing small, coccoid, gram-positive rods that tend to form chains. They are found in the feces of humans and other animals, on vegetation, and in silage.

lis·ter·ism (lĭs′tə-rĭz′əm) *n.* See **Lister's method**.

Lis·ter's method (lĭs′tərz) *n.* Antiseptic surgery, as first advocated by English surgeon Joseph Lister.

Lis·ting's law (lĭs′tĭngz) *n.* The principle that when the eye turns from looking at one object and fixes upon another, it revolves about an axis perpendicular to a plane cutting both the former and the present lines of vision.

li·ter (lē′tər) *n.* A unit of volume equal to 1000 cubic centimeters or or 1 cubic decimeter (1.0567 quarts).

li·thec·to·my (lĭ-thĕk′tə-mē) *n.* See **lithotomy**.

li·thi·a·sis (lĭ-thī′ə-sĭs) *n.*, *pl.* -ses (-sēz′). The formation of calculi of any kind, especially biliary or urinary calculi.

lith·i·um (lĭth′ē-əm) *n.* A soft, highly reactive metallic element with atomic number 3, the salts of which are used for the treatment of psychiatric disorders such as bipolar disorder.

lithium car·bon·ate (kär′bə-nāt′) *n.* An agent used in the treatment of depression and bipolar disorder.

lith·o·clast (lĭth′ə-klăst′) *n.* See **lithotrite**.

lith·o·di·al·y·sis (lĭth′ō-dī-ăl′ĭ-sĭs) *n.* The fragmentation or dissolution of a calculus.

lith·o·gen·e·sis (lĭth′ə-jĕn′ĭ-sĭs) *n.* The formation of calculi.

li·thol·a·pax·y (lĭ-thŏl′ə-păk′sē, lĭth′ə-lə-) *n.* See **lithotripsy**.

li·thol·y·sis (lĭ-thŏl′ĭ-sĭs) *n.* The dissolution of urinary calculi.

lith·o·lyt·ic (lĭth′ə-lĭt′ĭk) *n.* An agent that dissolves calculi. — **lith′o·lyt′ic** *adj.*

lith·o·ne·phri·tis (lĭth′ō-nə-frī′tĭs) *n.* Inflammation of the kidney due to irritation by calculi.

lith·o·scope (lĭth′ə-skōp′) *n.* See **cystoscope**.

li·thot·o·my (lĭ-thŏt′ə-mē) *n.* Surgical removal of a calculus, especially from the urinary tract.

lith·o·trip·sy (lĭth′ə-trĭp′sē) *n.* The procedure of crushing a stone in the urinary bladder or urethra.

lith·o·trip·ter (lĭth′ə-trĭp′tər) *n.* A device that pulverizes kidney stones by passing shock waves through a water-filled tub in which the patient sits.

lith·o·trip·tic (lĭth′ə-trĭp′tĭk) *n.* An agent that effects the dissolution of a calculus. — **lith′o·trip′tic** *adj.*

lith·o·trip·tos·co·py (lĭth′ə-trĭp-tŏs′kə-pē) *n.* The

crushing of a stone in the bladder while viewing directly through a cystoscope.

lith·o·trite (lĭth′ə-trīt′) *n.* An instrument used to crush a stone in the bladder or urethra.

li·thot·ri·ty (lĭ-thŏt′rĭ-tē) *n.* See **lithotripsy**.

lith·u·re·sis (lĭth′yōō-rē′sĭs) *n.* The passage of small calculi in the urine.

lit·mus (lĭt′məs) *n.* A water-soluble blue powder derived from certain lichens that changes to red with increasing acidity and to blue with increasing basicity.

litmus paper *n.* Paper that is impregnated with litmus and used as a pH or acid-base indicator.

litmus test *n.* A test for chemical acidity or basicity using litmus paper.

Lit·ten's phenomenon (lĭt′nz) *n.* See **diaphragm phenomenon**.

lit·ter (lĭt′ər) *n.* A flat supporting framework, such as a piece of canvas stretched between parallel shafts, for carrying a disabled or dead person; a stretcher.

Lit·tle Leagu·er's elbow (lĭt′l lē′gərz) *n.* Epicondylitis of the elbow at the origin of the flexor muscles of the forearm due to throwing; usually seen in children or adolescents.

live (lĭv) *adj.* **1.** Having life; alive. **2.** Capable of replicating in a host's cells. **3.** Containing living microorganisms or active virus, as a vaccine.

li·ve·do (lĭ-vē′dō) *n.* A bluish skin discoloration.

liv·er (lĭv′ər) *n.* The largest gland of the body comprising four lobes and lying beneath the diaphragm in the upper right portion of the abdominal cavity; it secretes bile and is active in the formation of certain blood proteins and in the metabolism of carbohydrates, fats, and proteins.

liver spot *n.* A benign, localized brownish patch on the skin, often occurring in old age and in people with sun-damaged skin.

live vaccine *n.* A vaccine prepared from living attenuated microorganisms or from viruses that have been attenuated but retain the ability to act as antigens and stimulate an immune response.

liv·id (lĭv′ĭd) *adj.* Having a black-and-blue or a leaden or ashy-gray color, as in discoloration from a contusion, congestion, or cyanosis. — **li·vid′i·ty, liv′id·ness** *n.*

liv·ing will (lĭv′ĭng) *n.* A will in which the signer requests not to be kept alive by medical life-support systems in the event of a terminal illness.

li·vor (lī′vôr, -vər) *n.* The livid discoloration of the skin on the dependent parts of a body after death.

load (lōd) *n.* A departure from normal body content, as of water, salt, or heat. A positive load is a quantity in excess of the normal; a negative load is a deficit.

load·ing (lō′dĭng) *n.* The administration of a substance for the purpose of testing metabolic function.

Loa loa (lō′ə lō′ə) *n.* A threadlike worm, a species of the family Onchocercidae indigenous to the western part of equatorial Africa. It is the causative agent of loiasis.

lo·bar pneumonia (lō′bər, -bär′) *n.* Pneumonia

affecting one or more lobes of the lung, commonly due to infection by *Streptococcus pneumoniae.*

lo·bate (lō′bāt′) *adj.* **1.** Divided into lobes. **2.** Lobe-shaped. — **lo′bate′ly** *adv.*

lobe (lōb) *n.* **1.** A rounded projection, especially a rounded, projecting anatomical part, such as the lobe of the ear. **2.** A subdivision of a body organ or part bounded by fissures, connective tissue, or other structural boundaries.

lo·bec·to·my (lō-bĕk′tə-mē) *n.* Excision of a lobe of an organ or a gland.

lo·bi·tis (lō-bī′tĭs) *n.* Inflammation of a lobe.

lo·bot·o·my (lə-bŏt′ə-mē, lō-) *n.* **1.** Incision into a lobe. **2.** The division of one or more nerve tracts in a lobe of the cerebrum.

lob·ster-claw deformity (lŏb′stər-clô′) *n.* A deformity of a hand or foot in which the middle digits are missing or fused.

lob·ule (lŏb′yōōl) *n.* **1.** A small lobe. **2.** A section or subdivision of a lobe. — **lob′u·lar** (-yə-lər), **lob′-u·lose′** (-yə-lōs′) *adj.*

lo·cal (lō′kəl) *adj.* Affecting or confined to a limited part; not general or systemic.

local anaphylaxis *n.* The immediate, temporary, localized anaphylactic response of a sensitized person following injection of an antigen into the skin.

local anesthesia *n.* Regional anesthesia produced by direct infiltration of local anesthetic solution into the surgical site.

local anesthetic *n.* An agent that, when applied directly to mucous membranes or when injected about the nerves, produces loss of sensation by inhibiting nerve excitation or conduction.

local death *n.* Death of a part of the body or of a tissue by necrosis.

local flap *n.* A surgical flap that is transferred to an adjacent area.

local immunity *n.* Natural or acquired immunity to an infectious agent limited to a particular organ or tissue.

lo·cal·i·za·tion (lō′kə-lĭ-zā′shən) *n.* **1.** Limitation to a specific area. **2.** The reference of a sensation to its point of origin. **3.** The determination of the location of a pathological process.

lo·cal·ized nodular tenosynovitis (lō′kə-līzd′) *n.* See **giant cell tumor of tendon sheath.**

local reaction *n.* See **focal reaction.**

lo·ca·tor (lō′kā′tər) *n.* An instrument or apparatus for finding a foreign object in tissue.

lo·chi·a (lō′kē-ə, lŏk′ē-ə) *pl.n.* The normal uterine discharge of blood, tissue, and mucus from the vagina after childbirth. — **lo′chi·al** *adj.*

locked knee *n.* A knee joint disorder that prevents the leg from being fully extended, usually resulting from damage to the semilunar cartilage.

lock·jaw (lŏk′jô′) *n.* **1.** See **tetanus** (sense 1). **2.** See **trismus.**

loc·ule (lŏk′yōōl) or **loc·u·lus** (-yə-ləs) *n.* A small cavity or compartment within an organ or a part of an animal.

lo·cus (lō′kəs) *n., pl.* **-ci** (-sī′, -kē, -kī′). **1.** A place;

site. **2.** The position that a given gene occupies on a chromosome.

locus of control *n.* A theoretical construct designed to assess a person's perceived control over his or her own behavior.

Loeb's deciduoma (lōbz) *n.* A mass of decidual tissue produced in the uterus in the absence of a fertilized ovum by means of mechanical or hormonal stimulation.

lo·fen·ta·nil (lō-fĕn′tə-nĭl) *n.* A potent, long lasting narcotic and analgesic that is chemically related to fentanyl.

log·ag·no·sia (lŏg′ăg-nō′zhə) *n.* See **aphasia.**

log·am·ne·sia (lŏg′ăm-nē′zhə) *n.* See **aphasia.**

log·a·pha·sia (lŏg′ə-fā′zhə) *n.* Aphasia of articulation.

log·as·the·ni·a (lŏg′ăs-thē′nē-ə) *n.* See **aphasia.**

log·o·ple·gi·a (lŏg′ə-plē′jē-ə, -jə) *n.* Paralysis of the organs of speech.

log·or·rhe·a (lŏg′ə-rē′ə) *n.* Excessive use of words.

lo·i·a·sis (lō-ī′ə-sĭs) *n.* A chronic disease caused by infestation of the subcutaneous tissue with the worm *Loa loa* and characterized by hyperemia, exudation of fluid, and a creeping sensation in the tissues with intense itching.

loin (loin) *n.* The part of the body on either side of the spinal column between the ribs and the pelvis.

long-acting thyroid stimulator *n.* A substance that is found in the blood of hyperthyroid patients, exerts a prolonged stimulatory effect on the thyroid gland, and is associated in plasma with the insulinlike growth factor.

long axis *n.* A line parallel to an object lengthwise, as in the body the imaginary line that runs vertically through the head down to the space between the feet.

long bone *n.* One of the elongated bones of the extremities, consisting of a tubular shaft, which is composed of compact bone surrounding a central marrow-filled cavity, and two expanded portions that usually serve as articulation points.

lon·gev·i·ty (lŏn-jĕv′ĭ-tē) *n.* Duration of an individual life beyond the norm for the species.

lon·gi·tu·di·nal (lŏn′jĭ-tōōd′n-əl, -tyōōd′-) *n.* Running in the direction of the long axis of the body or any of its parts.

longitudinal fracture *n.* A fracture that follows the long axis of the bone.

long-term memory *n.* The phase of the memory process considered the permanent storehouse of retained information.

loos·en·ing of association (lōō′sə-nĭng) *n.* A manifestation of a severe thought disorder characterized by the lack of an obvious connection between one thought or phrase and the next.

Lo·rain–Lé·vi syndrome (lə-rān′lā-vē′, lô-răn′-) *n.* See **pituitary dwarfism.**

lor·do·sco·li·o·sis (lôr′dō-skō′lē-ō′sĭs, -skŏl′ē-) *n.* Combined backward and lateral curvature of the spine.

lor·do·sis (lôr-dō′sĭs) *n.* An abnormal forward curvature of the spine in the lumbar region. — **lor·dot′ic** (-dŏt′ĭk) *adj.*

lo·tion (lō′shən) *n.* A medicated preparation consisting of a liquid suspension or dispersion intended for external application.

Lou Geh·rig's disease (lōō′ gĕr′ĭgz) *n.* See **amyotrophic lateral sclerosis.**

loupe (lōōp) *n.* A small magnifying lens.

louse (lous) *n., pl.* **lice** (līs). Any of numerous small, flat-bodied, wingless biting or sucking insects of the orders Mallophaga or Anoplura, many of which are external parasites on various animals, including humans.

lo·va·stat·in (lō′və-stăt′n) *n.* A cholesterol-lowering agent isolated from a strain of *Aspergillus terreus.*

low calorie diet *n.* A diet of 1,200 calories or less per day.

low-density lipoprotein *n.* A complex of lipids and proteins that functions as a transporter of cholesterol in the blood, and which, in high concentrations, is associated with an increased risk of atherosclerosis and coronary heart disease.

low·er airway (lō′ər) *n.* The portion of the respiratory tract that extends from the subglottis through the terminal bronchioles.

lower extremity *n.* The hip, thigh, leg, ankle, or foot.

lower motor neuron *n.* A motor neuron whose cell body is located in the brainstem or in the anterior horn of the spinal cord and whose axon innervates skeletal muscle fibers.

lox·os·ce·lism (lŏk-sŏs′ə-līz′əm) *n.* A condition produced by the bite of the brown recluse spider, *Loxosceles reclusus,* of North America. It is characterized by a gangrenous slough at the site of bite, nausea, malaise, fever, hemolysis, and thrombocytopenia.

loz·enge (lŏz′ĭnj) *n.* A small, medicated candy intended to be dissolved slowly in the mouth to lubricate and soothe irritated tissues of the throat.

LPN or **L.P.N.** *abbr.* licensed practical nurse

LRH *abbr.* luteinizing hormone-releasing hormone

LSD (ĕl′ĕs-dē′) *n.* Lysergic acid diethylamide; a crystalline compound derived from lysergic acid and used as a powerful hallucinogenic drug.

LTH *abbr.* luteotropic hormone

LTM *abbr.* long term memory

lu·cid·i·ty (lōō-sĭd′ĭ-tē) *n.* Clarity, especially mental clarity.

lu·es (lōō′ēz) *n., pl.* **lues.** Syphilis. — **lu·et′ic** (-ĕt′-ĭk) *adj.*

lu·lib·er·in (lōō-lĭb′ər-ĭn) *n.* See **gonadotropin-releasing hormone.**

lum·ba·go (lŭm-bā′gō) *n.* A painful condition of the lower back, as one resulting from muscle strain or a slipped disk.

lum·bar (lŭm′bər, -bär′) *adj.* Of, near, or situated in the part of the back and sides between the lowest ribs and the pelvis.

lumbar nerve *n.* Any of five nerves on either side that emerge from the lumbar portion of the spinal cord, the first four of which enter into formation of the lumbar plexus, and the fourth and fifth into that of the sacral plexus.

lumbar puncture *n.* Puncture into the subarachnoid space of the lumbar region for diagnostic or therapeutic purposes.

lumbar rheumatism *n.* See **lumbago.**

lumbar rib *n.* A rib articulating with the transverse process of the first lumbar vertebra; occurring only occasionally.

lum·bo·co·los·to·my (lŭm′bō-kə-lŏs′tə-mē) *n.* The formation of a permanent opening into the colon through an incision in the lumbar region.

lum·bri·cide (lŭm′brĭ-sīd′) *n.* An agent that kills intestinal worms.

lum·bri·co·sis (lŭm′brĭ-kō′sĭs) *n.* Infestation with intestinal worms.

lu·men (lōō′mən) *n., pl.* **lumens** or **-mi·na** (-mə-nə). The inner open space or cavity of a tubular organ, as of a blood vessel or an intestine. **lu′men·al, lu′min·al** *adj.*

lu·mi·nes·cence (lōō′mə-nĕs′əns) *n.* **1.** The emission of light that does not derive energy from the temperature of the emitting body, as in fluorescence, phosphorescence, and bioluminescence. **2.** The light so emitted.

lu·mi·no·phore (lōō′mə-nə-fôr′) *n.* An atom or atomic grouping that when present in an organic compound increases the ability of the compound to luminesce.

lump·ec·to·my (lŭm-pĕk′tə-mē) *n.* See **tylectomy.**

lunate bone *n.* The second of three bones forming the proximal row of bones in the wrist between the scaphoid and triquetrum bones and articulating with the radius, scaphoid, triquetrum, hamate, and capitate bones.

lung (lŭng) *n.* Either of the two saclike organs of respiration, occupying the cavity of the thorax, in which aeration of the blood takes place. The right lung is slightly larger than the left, and is divided into three lobes, while the left has two lobes.

lu·nu·la (lōōn′yə-lə) *n., pl.* **-lae** (-lē′). A small crescent-shaped structure or marking, especially the white area at the base of a fingernail that resembles a half-moon.

lu·poid hepatitis (lōō′poid′) *n.* A form of active chronic hepatitis characterized by jaundice with liver cell damage and positive lupus erythematosus cell tests, but without physical manifestations of systemic lupus erythematosus.

lu·pus (lōō′pəs) *n.* Any of several diseases, especially systemic lupus erythematosus, that principally affect the skin and joints but often also involve other systems of the body.

lupus er·y·the·ma·to·sus (ĕr′ə-thē′mə-tō′səs, -thĕm′ə-) *n.* **1.** A chronic disease of unknown origin characterized by the appearance of red, scaly lesions or patches on the face and upper portion of the trunk. **2.** Systemic lupus erythematosus.

lupus erythematosus cell *n.* A polymorphonuclear white blood cell that has ingested another cell's nuclear material that has been denatured by a substance in the blood and bodily fluids of those with systemic lupus erythematosus.

lupus erythematosus cell test *n.* A test for systemic lupus erythematosus in which characteristic lupus erythematosus cells are formed by incubation of blood or bone marrow of an affected person or by the action of an affected person's serum on normal white blood cells.

lupus nephritis *n.* Glomerulonephritis that occurs with systemic lupus erythematosus and is characterized by hematuria progressing to renal failure.

lupus vul·gar·is (vŭl-găr′ĭs) *n.* Cutaneous tuberculosis with characteristic reddish-brown ulcerating nodular lesions on the face, particularly about the nose and ears.

lu·te·al cell (lo͞o′tē-əl) *n.* See lutein cell.

luteal phase *n.* The portion of the menstrual cycle that begins with the formation of the corpus luteum and ends with the start of the menstrual flow, usually 14 days in length.

lu·te·in (lo͞o′tē-ĭn, -tēn′) *n.* **1.** A yellow carotenoid pigment that was first isolated in corpus luteum and is also in body fat, egg yolk, and green plants. **2.** A dried preparation of corpus luteum.

lutein cell *n.* A cell of the ovary's corpus luteum.

lu·te·in·i·za·tion (lo͞o′tē-ə-nĭ-zā′shən) *n.* The transformation of the mature ovarian follicle into a corpus luteum after ovulation. — **lu′te·in·ize** (lo͞o′tē-ə-nīz′) *v.*

luteinizing hormone-releasing hormone *n.* See gonadotropin-releasing hormone.

Lu·tem·bach·er's syndrome (lo͞o′təm-băk′ərz, -bä′kərz) *n.* A congenital cardiac abnormality consisting of mitral stenosis, an enlarged right atrium, and a defect of the interatrial septum of the heart.

lu·te·o·hor·mone (lo͞o′tē-ō-hôr′mōn′) *n.* See progesterone (sense 1).

lu·te·o·ma (lo͞o′tē-ō′mə) *n.,* *pl.* **-mas** or **-ma·ta** (-mə-tə). An ovarian tumor of granulosa- or theca-cell origin in which luteinization has occurred.

lu·te·o·tro·pin (lo͞o′tē-ə-trō′pĭn) *n.* See prolactin.

lu·te·ti·um or **lu·te·ci·um** (lo͞o-tē′shē-əm) *n.* A rare-earth element with atomic number 71.

lux·ate (lŭk′sāt′) *v.* **-at·ed, -at·ing, -ates.** To put out of joint; dislocate. — **lux·a′tion** *n.*

LVN or **L.V.N.** *abbr.* licensed vocational nurse

ly·co·pene (lī′kə-pēn′) *n.* The red pigment of the tomato that is considered chemically to be the parent substance from which all natural carotenoid pigments are derived.

ly·co·per·do·no·sis (lī′kə-pûr′də-nō′sĭs) *n.* A respiratory disease caused by inhaling the spores of the puffballs *Lycoperdon pyriforme* and *L. bovista.*

ly·ing-in (lī′ĭng-ĭn′) *n.,* *pl.* **ly·ings-in** (lī′ĭngz-) or **ly·ing-ins.** The confinement of a woman in childbirth.

Lyme arthritis (līm) *n.* Arthritis associated with Lyme disease.

Lyme disease *n.* An inflammatory disease caused by the spirochete *Borrelia burgdorferi,* transmitted by ticks, and characterized by a rash followed by flulike symptoms including fever, joint pain, and headache; if untreated, it can result in chronic arthritis and nerve and heart dysfunction.

lymph (lĭmf) *n.* A clear, watery fluid derived from body tissues that contains white blood cells and circulates throughout the lymphatic system, returning to the venous bloodstream through the thoracic duct. Lymph acts to remove bacteria and certain proteins from the tissues, transport fat from the small intestine, and supply mature lymphocytes to the blood.

lym·phad·e·nec·to·my (lĭm-făd′n-ĕk′tə-mē) *n.* Surgical excision of one or more lymph nodes.

lym·phad·e·ni·tis (lĭm-făd′n-ī′tĭs, lĭm′fə-də-nī′-) *n.* Inflammation of one or more lymph nodes.

lym·phad·e·nog·ra·phy (lĭm-făd′n-ŏg′rə-fē) *n.* Radiography of an enlarged lymph node following the injection of a radiopaque substance into the node.

lym·phad·e·nop·a·thy (lĭm-făd′n-ŏp′ə-thē, lĭm′-fə-dn-) *n.* A chronic, abnormal enlargement of the lymph nodes, usually associated with disease.

lym·phad·e·no·sis (lĭm-făd′n-ō′sĭs) *n.* The basic underlying proliferative process that results in enlargement of lymph nodes.

lym·phan·gi·al (lĭm-făn′jē-əl) *adj.* Of or relating to a lymphatic vessel.

lym·phan·gi·ec·ta·sis (lĭm-făn′jē-ĕk′tə-sĭs) or **lym·phan·gi·ec·ta·si·a** (lĭm-făn′jē-ĭk-tā′zē-ə, -zhə) *n.* Dilation of the lymphatic vessels. — **lym·phan′gi·ec·tat′ic** (-ĭk-tăt′ĭk) *adj.*

lym·phan·gi·ec·to·my (lĭm-făn′jē-ĕk′tə-mē) *n.* Surgical excision of a lymphatic vessel.

lym·phan·gi·o·en·do·the·li·o·ma (lĭm-făn′jē-ō-ĕn′dō-thē′lē-ō′mə) *n.* A tumor consisting of irregular groups of endothelial cells with aggregates of tubate structures thought to be derived from lymphatic vessels.

lym·phan·gi·og·ra·phy (lĭm-făn′jē-ŏg′rə-fē) *n.* Radiography of the lymph nodes and lymphatic vessels following the injection of a radiopaque substance. — **lym·phan′gi·o·gram′** (-ə-grăm′) *n.*

lym·phan·gi·ol·o·gy (lĭm-făn′jē-ŏl′ə-jē) *n.* The branch of medical science concerned with the lymphatic system.

lym·phan·gi·o·ma (lĭm-făn′jē-ō′mə) *n.* A benign tumorlike mass of lymphatic vessels or channels that vary in size, are frequently greatly dilated, and are lined with normal endothelial cells.

lym·phan·gi·o·phle·bi·tis (lĭm-făn′jē-ō-flĭ-bī′tĭs) *n.* Inflammation of lymphatic vessels and veins.

lym·phan·gi·o·plas·ty (lĭm-făn′jē-ə-plăs′tē) *n.* Surgical alteration of lymphatic vessels.

lym·phan·gi·o·sar·co·ma (lĭm-făn′jē-ō-sär-kō′mə) *n.* An angiosarcoma in which the tumor cells originate from the endothelial cells of lymphatic vessels.

lym·phan·gi·ot·o·my (lĭm-făn′jē-ŏt′ə-mē) *n.* Surgical incision of lymphatic vessels.

lym·phan·gi·tis (lĭm′făn-jī′tĭs) or **lym·phan·gi·i·tis** (lĭm-făn′jē-ī′tĭs) *n.* Inflammation of the lymphatic vessels.

lym·pha·phe·re·sis (lĭm′fə-fə-rē′sĭs) *n.* See lymphocytapheresis.

lym·phat·ic (lĭm-făt′ĭk) *adj.* Of or relating to

lymph, a lymph node, or a lymphatic vessel. — *n.* A lymphatic vessel.

lymphatic duct *n.* Either of the two terminal lymph vessels that convey lymph to the bloodstream.

lym·phat·i·cos·to·my (lĭm-făt′ĭ-kŏs′tə-mē) *n.* Surgical construction of an opening into a lymphatic duct.

lymphatic system *n.* The interconnected system of spaces and vessels between body tissues and organs by which lymph circulates the body.

lymphatic tissue *n.* Tissue consisting of a three-dimensional network of reticular fibers and cells, the meshes of which are occupied by lymphocytes.

lymphatic vessel *n.* Any of the vascular channels that transport lymph throughout the lymphatic system and freely anastomose with one another.

lym·pha·ti·tis (lĭm′fə-tī′tĭs) *n.* Inflammation of the lymphatic vessels or lymph nodes.

lym·pha·tol·y·sis (lĭm′fə-tŏl′ĭ-sĭs) *n.* The destruction or dissolution of lymphatic vessels or lymphoid tissue. — **lym′pha·to·lyt′ic** (-tə-lĭt′ĭk) *adj.*

lym·phec·ta·si·a (lĭm′fĭk-tā′zē-ə, -zhə) *n.* See **lymphangiectasis.**

lym·phe·de·ma (lĭm′fĭ-dē′mə) *n.* Swelling, especially in subcutaneous tissues, as a result of obstruction of lymphatic vessels or lymph nodes, with accumulation of large amounts of lymph in the affected region.

lym·phe·mi·a (lĭm-fē′mē-ə) *n.* The presence of unusually large numbers of lymphocytes or their precursors in the blood.

lymph gland *n.* See **lymph node.**

lymph node *n.* Any of the small, oval or round bodies, located along the lymphatic vessels, that supply lymphocytes to the bloodstream and remove bacteria and foreign particles from the lymph.

lymph node permeability factor *n.* A substance released by stimulated or damaged lymphocytes that increases capillary permeability and the accumulation of mononuclear cells.

lym·pho·blast (lĭm′fə-blăst′) *n.* An immature cell that gives rise to a lymphocyte. — **lym′pho·blas′-tic** *adj.*

lymphoblastic lymphoma *n.* A diffuse malignant lymphoma occurring in children, composed of T-lymphocytes that have convoluted nuclei.

lym·pho·blas·to·ma (lĭm′fō-blă-stō′mə) *n.* A form of malignant lymphoma composed chiefly of lymphoblasts.

lym·pho·blas·to·sis (lĭm′fō-blă-stō′sĭs) *n.* The presence of lymphoblasts in the peripheral blood.

lym·pho·cy·ta·phe·re·sis (lĭm′fō-sī′tə-fə-rē′sĭs) *n.* Separation and removal of lymphocytes from donated blood, with the remainder of the blood retransfused into the donor.

lym·pho·cyte (lĭm′fə-sīt′) *n.* Any of the nearly colorless cells formed in lymphoid tissue, as in the lymph nodes, spleen, thymus, and tonsils, constituting between 22 and 28 percent of all white blood cells in the blood of a normal adult human.

They function in the development of immunity and include two specific types, B cells and T cells. — **lym′pho·cyt′ic** (-sĭt′ĭk) *adj.*

lym·pho·cy·the·mi·a (lĭm′fō-sī-thē′mē-ə) *n.* See **lymphocytosis.**

lymphocytic choriomeningitis virus *n.* A virus of the genus *Arenavirus* that causes lymphocytic choriomeningitis.

lymphocytic leukemia *n.* Leukemia characterized by the proliferation and enlargement of lymphoid tissue in various sites and by increased numbers of lymphocytic cells in the blood and in various tissues and organs.

lymphocytic leukocytosis *n.* See **lymphocytosis.**

lymphocytic series *n.* The cells at various states of lymphopoietic development in lymphoid tissue.

lym·pho·cy·to·ma (lĭm′fō-sī-tō′mə) *n., pl.* **-mas** or **-ma·ta** (-mə-tə). **1.** A circumscribed nodule or mass of mature lymphocytes, having the appearance of a neoplasm. **2.** A malignant lymphoma whose cells closely resemble mature lymphocytes.

lym·pho·cy·to·pe·ni·a (lĭm′fō-sī′tə-pē′nē-ə) *n.* See **lymphopenia.**

lym·pho·cy·to·poi·e·sis (lĭm′fō-sī′tə-poi-ē′sĭs) *n.* Formation of lymphocytes.

lym·pho·cy·to·sis (lĭm′fō-sī-tō′sĭs) *n.* A condition marked by an abnormal increase in the number of lymphocytes in the bloodstream, usually resulting from infection or inflammation. — **lym′-pho·cy·tot′ic** (-tŏt′ĭk) *adj.*

lym·pho·ep·i·the·li·o·ma (lĭm′fō-ĕp′ə-thē′lē-ō′mə) *n.* A poorly differentiated squamous cell carcinoma involving lymphoid tissue in the region of the tonsils and the nasopharynx.

lym·pho·gen·e·sis (lĭm′fə-jĕn′ĭ-sĭs) *n.* Lymph production.

lym·pho·gran·u·lo·ma (lĭm′fō-grăn′yə-lō′mə) *n.* Any of several unrelated diseases in which the pathological processes result in the formation of granulomas or granulomalike lesions, especially in various groups of lymph nodes which then become conspicuously enlarged.

lym·phog·ra·phy (lĭm-fŏg′rə-fē) *n.* See **lymphangiography.**

lym·phoid (lĭm′foid′) *adj.* Of or relating to lymph or the lymphatic tissue where lymphocytes are formed.

lym·phoid·ec·to·my (lĭm′foi-dĕk′tə-mē) *n.* Surgical excision of lymphoid tissue.

lym·phoi·do·cyte (lĭm-foi′də-sīt′) *n.* See **hemocytoblast.**

lymphoid series *n.* See **lymphocytic series.**

lymphoid tissue *n.* See **lymphatic tissue.**

lym·pho·kine (lĭm′fə-kīn′) *n.* Any of various soluble substances, released by sensitized lymphocytes on contact with specific antigens, that help effect cellular immunity by stimulating activity of monocytes and macrophages.

lym·pho·ki·ne·sis (lĭm′fō-kə-nē′sĭs) *n.* **1.** The circulation of lymph in the lymphatic vessels and through the lymph nodes. **2.** The movement of lymph in the semicircular canals.

lym·phol·o·gy (lǐm-fŏl′ə-jē) *n.* See **lymphangiol·ogy.**

lym·pho·ma (lǐm-fō′mə) *n., pl.* **-mas** or **-ma·ta** (-mə-tə). Any of various usually malignant neoplasms of lymphatic and reticuloendothelial tissues that occur as circumscribed solid tumors composed of cells that resemble lymphocytes, plasma cells, or histiocytes. — **lym·pho′ma·toid′, lym·pho′ma·tous** (-təs) *adj.*

lym·pho·ma·to·sis (lǐm-fō′mə-tō′sǐs) *n., pl.* **-ses** (-sēz). Any of various conditions characterized by the occurrence of multiple, widely distributed lymphomas in the body.

lym·pho·myx·o·ma (lǐm′fō-mǐk-sō′mə) *n.* A soft nonmalignant tumor containing lymphoid tissue in a matrix of loose areolar connective tissue.

lym·phop·a·thy (lǐm-fŏp′ə-thē) *n.* A disease of the lymphatic vessels or lymph nodes.

lym·pho·pe·ni·a (lǐm′fə-pē′nē-ə) *n.* A reduction in the number of lymphocytes in the blood.

lym·pho·plas·ma·phe·re·sis (lǐm′fō-plǎz′mə-fə-rē′sǐs) *n.* Separation and removal of lymphocytes and plasma from donated blood that is then retransfused into the donor.

lym·pho·poi·e·sis (lǐm′fō-poi-ē′sǐs) *n.* The formation of lymphocytes. — **lym′pho·poi·et′ic** (-ět′ǐk) *adj.*

lym·phor·rhe·a (lǐm′fə-rē′ə) *n.* An escape of lymph from ruptured, torn, or cut lymph vessels.

lym·pho·sar·co·ma (lǐm′fō-sär-kō′mə) *n.* A diffuse malignant lymphoma.

lym·pho·sar·co·ma·to·sis (lǐm′fō-sär-kō′mə-tō′-sǐs) *n.* A condition characterized by the presence of multiple, widely distributed lymphosarcomas in the body.

lym·pho·tax·is (lǐm′fə-tǎk′sǐs) *n.* The property of attracting or repelling lymphocytes.

lym·pho·tox·ic·i·ty (lǐm′fō-tŏk-sǐs′ǐ-tē) *n.* The potential of an antibody in the serum of an allograft recipient to react directly with the lymphocytes or other cells of an allograft donor to produce a hyperacute type of graft rejection.

lym·pho·tox·in (lǐm′fə-tŏk′sǐn) *n.* A lymphokine that is toxic to certain susceptible target cells.

lymph vessel *n.* A lymphatic vessel.

Ly·on·i·za·tion (lī′ə-nī-zā′shən) *n.* The phenomenon in which heterozygous females do not phenotypically express their X-linked recessive genotype or do so only randomly.

ly·oph·i·li·za·tion (lī-ŏf′ə-lī-zā′shən) *n.* The process of isolating a solid substance from solution by freezing the solution and vaporizing the ice away under vacuum conditions. — **ly·oph′i·lize′** (-līz′) *v.*

ly·pres·sin (lī-prĕs′ǐn) *n.* An antidiuretic and vasopressor substance obtained from the pituitary glands of swine.

Lys *abbr.* lysine

ly·sate (lī′sāt′) *n.* The cellular debris and fluid produced by lysis.

lyse (līs, līz) or **lyze** (līz) *v.* **lysed** or **lyzed, lys·ing** or **lyz·ing, lys·es** or **lyz·es.** To undergo or cause to undergo lysis.

ly·ser·gic acid (lī-sûr′jĭk, lī-) *n.* A crystalline alkaloid derived from ergot and used in medical research as a psychotomimetic agent.

ly·sin (lī′sĭn) *n.* **1.** An antibody that is capable of causing the destruction or dissolution of red blood cells, bacteria, or other cellular elements. **2.** A substance that causes lysis.

ly·sine (lī′sēn′, -sĭn) *n.* An essential amino acid derived from the hydrolysis of proteins and required by the body for optimum growth.

ly·si·ne·mi·a (lī′sə-nē′mē-ə) *n.* Increased concentration of lysine in the blood, associated with mental and physical retardation.

ly·sin·o·gen (lī-sĭn′ə-jən, -jĕn′) *n.* An antigen that stimulates the formation of a specific lysin.

ly·si·nu·ri·a (lī′sə-noŏr′ē-ə, -nyoŏr′-) *n.* The presence of lysine in the urine.

ly·sis (lī′sĭs) *n., pl.* **-ses** (-sēz). **1.** The gradual subsiding of the symptoms of an acute disease. **2.** The dissolution or destruction of cells, such as blood cells or bacteria, as by the action of a specific lysin.

ly·so·gen (lī′sə-jən) *n.* An agent capable of inducing lysis.

ly·so·gen·e·sis (lī′sə-jĕn′ĭ-sĭs) *n.* The production of lysins.

ly·so·gen·ic (lī′sə-jĕn′ĭk) *adj.* Causing or having the power to cause lysis.

ly·so·ge·nic·i·ty (lī′sə-jə-nĭs′ĭ-tē) *n.* The property of being lysogenic.

ly·sog·e·nize (lī-sŏj′ĭ-nīz′) *v.* **-nized, -niz·ing, -niz·es.** To make lysogenic. — **ly·sog′e·ni·za′tion** (-nī-zā′shən) *n.*

lysosomal disease *n.* A disease caused by the inadequate functioning of a lysosomal enzyme and usually characterized by an excess or an absence of storage of a vital cellular component.

ly·so·some (lī′sə-sōm′) *n.* A membrane-bound organelle in the cytoplasm of most cells containing various hydrolytic enzymes that function in intracellular digestion. — **ly·so·so′mal** *adj.*

ly·so·zyme (lī′sə-zīm′) *n.* An enzyme occurring naturally in egg white, human tears, saliva, and other body fluids, capable of destroying the cell walls of certain bacteria and thereby acting as a mild antiseptic.

lyt·ic cocktail (lĭt′ĭk) *n.* A mixture of drugs injected intravenously to produce sedation, analgesia, amnesia, hypotension, hypothermia, and blockade of the functions of the sympathetic and parasympathetic nervous systems during surgical anesthesia.

~ ~ ~ ~ ~ ~ M ~ ~ ~ ~ ~ ~

μ *The symbol for* micro-.

μμ. *The symbol for* micromicro-.

μg *abbr.* microgram

μm *abbr.* micrometer; micron

m *abbr.* meter

mμ *abbr.* millimicron

MA or **M.A.** *abbr.* mental age

Mace or **MACE** (mās) An alternate trademark used for Chemical Mace, an aerosol used to immobilize an attacker temporarily.

mac·er·a·tion (măs′ə-rā′shən) *n.* **1.** Softening by soaking in a liquid. **2.** Softening of tissues after death by autolysis, especially of a stillborn fetus.

ma·chin·er·y murmur (mə-shē′nə-rē, -shēn′rē) *n.* See **Gibson murmur.**

mac·ren·ceph·a·ly (măk′rĕn-sĕf′ə-lē) *n.* Hypertrophy of the brain.

mac·ro·bi·ot·ics (măk′rō-bī-ŏt′ĭks) *n.* The theory or practice of promoting well-being and longevity, principally by a diet consisting chiefly of whole grains and beans. — **mac′ro·bi·ot′ic** *adj.*

mac·ro·ceph·a·ly (măk′rō-sĕf′ə-lē) or **mac·ro·ce·pha·li·a** (-sə-fā′lē-ə, -fāl′yə) *n.* Abnormal largeness of the head. — **mac′ro·ce·phal′ic** (-sə-fāl′ĭk), **mac′ro·ceph′a·lous** *adj.*

mac·ro·cry·o·glob·u·li·ne·mi·a (măk′rō-krī′ō-glŏb′yə-lə-nē′mē-ə) *n.* The presence in the peripheral blood of a type of hemagglutinin that agglutinates red blood cells at cold temperatures.

mac·ro·cyte (măk′rə-sīt′) *n.* An abnormally large red blood cell, especially one associated with pernicious anemia. — **mac′ro·cyt′ic** (-sĭt′ĭk) *adj.*

mac·ro·cy·the·mi·a (măk′rō-sī-thē′mē-ə) *n.* The presence of unusually large numbers of macrocytes in the blood.

ma·crog·li·a (mă-krŏg′lē-ə) *n.* See **astrocyte.**

mac·ro·glob·u·lin (măk′rō-glŏb′yə-lĭn) *n.* A plasma globulin of high molecular weight.

mac·ro·mon·o·cyte (măk′rō-mŏn′ə-sīt′) *n.* An unusually large monocyte.

mac·ro·my·e·lo·blast (măk′rō-mī′ə-lə-blăst′) *n.* An abnormally large myeloblast.

mac·ro·nor·mo·blast (măk′rō-nôr′mə-blăst′) *n.* A large normoblast.

mac·ro·phage (măk′rə-fāj′) *n.* Any of the large phagocytic cells of the reticuloendothelial system. — **mac′ro·phag′ic** (-făj′ĭk) *adj.*

mac·ro·scop·ic (măk′rə-skŏp′ĭk) or **mac·ro·scop·i·cal** (-ĭ-kəl) *adj.* **1.** Large enough to be perceived or examined by the unaided eye. **2.** Relating to observations made by the unaided eye.

ma·cros·co·py (mă-krŏs′kə-pē) *n.* Examination with the naked eye.

mac·ro·so·mi·a (măk′rə-sō′mē-ə) *n.* Abnormally large size of the body.

mac·u·la (măk′yə-lə) *n., pl.* **-las** or **-lae** (-lē′). **1.**

Also **mac·ule** (-yōōl′) A spot, stain, or blemish, especially an area of discoloration on the skin caused by excess or lack of pigment. **2.** A small area distinguishable from the surrounding tissue. **3.** The macula lutea. — **mac′u·lar** *adj.*

macula lu·te·a (lōō′tē-ə) *n., pl.* **maculae lu·te·ae** (lōō′tē-ē′). A minute yellowish area containing the fovea centralis located near the center of the retina where visual perception is most acute.

macular area *n.* The portion of the retina used for central vision.

macular degeneration *n.* Degeneration of the macula lutea, characterized by spots of pigmentation and causing a reduction or loss of central vision.

macula ret·i·nae (rĕt′n-ē′) *n.* See **macula lutea.**

mad (măd) *adj.* **1.** Angry; resentful. **2.** Suffering from a disorder of the mind; insane. **3.** Affected by rabies; rabid.

Ma·de·lung′s disease (măd′ə-lŭngz′, mä′də-lōōngz) *n.* The symmetrical deposition of fatty tissue on the upper part of the back, shoulders, and neck.

Mad Hatter syndrome *n.* A complex of disorders caused by chronic mercury poisoning, includes stomatitis, diarrhea, ataxia, tremor, sensorineural impairment, and emotional instability.

mad·ness (măd′nĭs) *n.* The quality or condition of being insane.

mad·u·ro·my·co·sis (măd′ə-rō-mī-kō′sĭs, măd′yə-) *n.* A form of mycetoma caused by a varied group of fungi and characterized by formation of swellings and sinuses that discharge oily pus.

mag·got (măg′ət) *n.* The legless, soft-bodied, wormlike larva of any of various flies of the order Diptera, often found in decaying matter.

mag·ic bullet (măj′ĭk) *n.* A drug, therapy, or preventive therapy that cures or prevents a disease.

mag·ne·si·um (măg-nē′zē-əm, -zhəm) *n.* A light, naturally occurring metallic element with atomic number 12, found in muscle, bone, and body fluids, and essential for the activity of many enzymes.

magnesium salicylate *n.* A sodium-free salicylate derivative with anti-inflammatory, analgesic, and antipyretic actions, used for relief of mild to moderate pain.

magnesium sulfate *n.* A colorless, crystalline compound used as a cathartic and applied locally as an anti-inflammatory agent.

mag·net·ic resonance (măg-nĕt′ĭk) *n.* The phenomenon of absorption of certain frequencies of radio and microwave radiation by atoms placed in a magnetic field. The pattern of absorption reveals molecular structure.

magnetic resonance imaging *n.* The use of a nuclear magnetic resonance spectrometer to produce electronic images of specific atoms and molecular structures in solids, especially human cells, tissues, and organs.

mag·ne·to·en·ceph·a·log·ra·phy (măg-nē′tō-ĕn-sĕf′ə-lŏg′rə-fē) *n.* An imaging technique used to detect electro-magnetic and metabolic shifts occurring in the brain during trauma such as during migraine attacks.

mag·ni·fi·ca·tion (măg′nə-fĭ-kā′shən) *n.* **1.** The act of magnifying or the state of being magnified. **2.** The process of enlarging the size of something, as an optical image. **3.** Something that has been magnified; an enlarged representation, image, or model.

mag·ni·fy (măg′nə-fī′) *v.* **-fied, -fy·ing, -fies.** To increase the apparent size of, especially by means of a lens.

main·stream·ing (mān′strē′mĭng) *n.* The process of integrating physically or intellectually disadvantaged students into regular school classes. — **main′stream′** *v.*

main·te·nance (mān′tə-nəns) *n.* The extent to which a patient continues good health practices without supervision, incorporating them into his or her lifestyle.

maintenance drug therapy *n.* In chemotherapy, the systematic reduction of the dosage of a drug to a level that protects against against exacerbation of the condition.

ma·jor histocompatibility complex (mā′jər) *n.* A chromosomal segment that codes for cell-surface histocompatibility antigens and is the principal determinant of tissue type and transplant compatibility.

mal (măl, mäl) *n.* A disease or disorder.

mal·ab·sorp·tion (măl′əb-sôrp′shən, -zôrp′-) *n.* Defective or inadequate absorption of nutrients from the intestinal tract.

malabsorption syndrome *n.* A nutritional syndrome caused by any of various disorders in which there is ineffective absorption of nutrients from the gastrointestinal tract, characterized by diverse conditions such as diarrhea, weakness, edema, lassitude, weight loss, poor appetite, protuberant abdomen, pallor, bleeding tendencies, paresthesias, and muscle cramps.

ma·la·ci·a (mə-lā′shē-ə, -shə) *n.* A softening or loss of consistency in any of the organs or tissues.

mal·a·co·sis (măl′ə-kō′sĭs) *n.* See **malacia**.

mal·ad·just·ed (măl′ə-jŭs′tĭd) *adj.* Inadequately adjusted to the demands or stresses of daily living.

mal·a·dy (măl′ə-dē) *n.* A disease, a disorder, or an ailment.

mal·aise (mă-lāz′, -lĕz′) *n.* A vague feeling of bodily discomfort, as at the beginning of an illness.

mal·a·lign·ment (măl′ə-līn′mənt) *n.* Displacement of a tooth or teeth from a normal position in the dental arch.

ma·lar (mā′lər, -lär′) *adj.* Of or relating to the cheekbone or the cheek. — *n.* The cheekbone.

malar bone *n.* See **zygomatic bone**.

ma·lar·i·a (mə-lâr′ē-ə) *n.* An infectious disease characterized by cycles of chills, fever, and sweating, caused by the parasitic infection of red blood cells by a protozoan of the genus *Plasmodium*, which is transmitted by the bite of an infected female anopheles mosquito. — **ma·lar′i·al, ma·lar′i·an, ma·lar′i·ous** *adj.*

malar process *n.* See **zygomatic process of maxilla**.

mal·as·sim·i·la·tion (măl′ə-sĭm′ə-lā′shən) *n.* Incomplete or imperfect assimilation of nutrients by the body.

mal·ate (măl′āt′, mā′lāt′) *n.* A salt or ester of malic acid.

malate dehydrogenase *n.* An enzyme that catalyzes, through NAD or NADP, dehydrogenation or decarboxylation of malate.

mal de mer (măl′ də mâr′) *n.* See **seasickness**.

male (māl) *adj.* Of, relating to, or designating the sex that has organs to produce spermatozoa for fertilizing ova. — *n.* **1.** A member of the sex that begets young by fertilizing ova. **2.** A man or boy.

ma·le·ic acid (mə-lē′ĭk) *n.* A colorless crystalline dibasic acid that is used as an oil and fat preservative.

mal·for·ma·tion (măl′fôr-mā′shən) *n.* Abnormal or anomalous formation or structure; deformity.

mal·formed (măl-fôrmd′) *adj.* Abnormally or faultily formed.

mal·func·tion (măl-fŭngk′shən) *v.* **-tioned, -tion·ing, -tions. 1.** To fail to function. **2.** To function improperly. — *n.* **1.** Failure to function. **2.** Faulty or abnormal functioning.

mal·ic acid (măl′ĭk, mā′lĭk) *n.* A colorless crystalline intermediate in the Krebs cycle that occurs naturally in apples and other fruits.

ma·lig·nan·cy (mə-lĭg′nən-sē) *n.* **1.** The state or quality of being malignant. **2.** A malignant tumor.

ma·lig·nant (mə-lĭg′nənt) *adj.* **1.** Threatening to life, as a disease; virulent. **2.** Tending to metastasize; cancerous. Used of a tumor.

malignant bubo *n.* The bubo associated with bubonic plague.

malignant hypertension *n.* Severe hypertension that runs a rapid course, causing necrosis of arteriolar walls and hemorrhagic lesions.

malignant lentigo *n.* A precancerous brown or black lesion of the skin, often of older persons, that appears on areas that are exposed to the sun, is irregular in shape, and is slow growing.

malignant lymphoma *n.* See **lymphoma**.

malignant melanoma *n.* See **melanoma**.

malignant nephrosclerosis *n.* Nephrosclerosis occurring in malignant hypertension.

malignant tumor *n.* A tumor that invades surrounding tissues, is usually capable of producing metastases, may recur after attempted removal, and may cause death unless adequately treated.

ma·lin·ger (mə-lĭng′gər) *v.* **-gered, -ger·ing, -gers.** To feign illness or other incapacity in order to avoid duty or work. — **ma·lin′ger·er** *n.*

mal·le·o·lus (mə-lē′ə-ləs) *n., pl.* **mal·le·o·li** (-lī′). A rounded bony prominence, such as on either side of the ankle joint. — **mal·le′o·lar** (-lər) *adj.*

mal·le·ot·o·my (măl′ē-ŏt′ə-mē) *n.* **1.** Surgical division of the malleus. **2.** Surgical division of the ligaments holding the malleoli of the ankle in apposition.

mallet finger *n.* See **baseball finger**.

mal·le·us (măl′ē-əs) *n., pl.* **mal·le·i** (măl′ē-ī′). The hammer-shaped bone that is the outermost of the three auditory ossicles and articulates with the body of the incus.

Mal·lo·ry—Weiss lesion (măl′ə-rē-wīs′) *n.* Laceration of the gastric cardia, as seen in Mallory-Weiss syndrome.

Mallory—Weiss syndrome *n.* A disorder of the lower end of the esophagus caused by severe retching and vomiting and characterized by laceration associated with bleeding, or by penetration into the mediastinum.

Mallory—Weiss tear *n.* See **Mallory—Weiss lesion**.

mal·nour·ished (măl-nûr′ĭsht, -nûr′-) *adj.* Affected by improper nutrition or an insufficient diet.

mal·nour·ish·ment (măl-nûr′ĭsh-mənt, -nûr′-) *n.* Malnutrition.

mal·nu·tri·tion (măl′nōō-trĭsh′ən, -nyōō-) *n.* Poor nutrition because of an insufficient or poorly balanced diet or faulty digestion or utilization of foods.

mal·oc·clu·sion (măl′ə-klōō′zhən) *n.* Faulty contact between the upper and lower teeth when the jaw is closed.

mal·po·si·tion (măl′pə-zĭsh′ən) *n.* See **dystopia**.

mal·prac·tice (măl-prăk′tĭs) *n.* Improper or negligent treatment of a patient, as by a physician, resulting in injury, damage, or loss.

mal·pres·en·ta·tion (măl′prĕz-ən-tā′shən, -prē′-zən-) *n.* Presentation of a part of a fetus other than the back of the head during parturition.

MALT (môlt) *n.* Mucosal-associated lymphoid tissue; a rare type of lymphoma of the stomach that may be associated with infection by the bacteria *Helicobacter pylori*.

mal·tase (môl′tās′, -tāz′) *n.* An enzyme that catalyzes the hydrolysis of maltose to glucose.

mal·tose (môl′tōs′, -tōz′) *n.* A white crystalline sugar formed during the digestion of starch.

ma·mil·la (mă-mĭl′ə) *n., pl.* **-mil·lae** (-mĭl′ē). **1.** A small rounded elevation resembling the female breast. **2.** See **nipple**.

mam·il·lar·y (măm′ə-lĕr′ē) *adj.* Relating to or shaped like a nipple.

mamillary duct *n.* See **lactiferous duct**.

mam·ma (măm′ə) *n., pl.* **mam·mae** (măm′ē). An organ of female mammals that contains milk-producing glands; a mammary gland.

mam·ma·plas·ty or **mam·mo·plas·ty** (măm′ə-plăs′tē) *n.* Reconstructive or cosmetic plastic surgery to alter the size or shape of the breast.

mam·ma·ry (măm′ə-rē) *adj.* Of or relating to a breast or mamma.

mammary duct *n.* See **lactiferous duct**.

mammary gland *n.* Either of the two milk-producing apocrine glands typically occurring in

female mammals, that consist of lobes containing clusters of alveoli with a system of ducts to convey the milk to an external nipple and that begin secreting milk when young are born; mamma.

mam·mec·to·my (mă-mĕk′tə-mē) *n.* See **mastectomy**.

mam·mil·la (mă-mĭl′ə) *n.* **1.** A nipple. **2.** A nipple-shaped protuberance.

mam·mil·la·plas·ty (mă-mĭl′ə-plăs′tē) *n.* Plastic surgery of the nipple and the areola.

mam·mil·li·tis (măm′ə-lī′tĭs) *n.* Inflammation of the nipple.

mam·mo·gram (măm′ə-grăm′) *n.* An x-ray image of the breast produced by mammography.

mam·mog·ra·phy (mă-mŏg′rə-fē) *n.* Radiographic examination of the breasts for diagnostic purposes, as for the early detection of malignancies.

mam·mot·o·my (mă-mŏt′ə-mē) *n.* See **mastotomy**.

man·aged care (măn′ĭjd) *n.* Any arrangement for health care in which an organization, such as an HMO, another type of doctor-hospital network, or an insurance company, acts as intermediate between the person seeking care and the physician.

Man·ches·ter operation (măn′chĕs′tər, -chĭ-stər) *n.* A vaginal operation for prolapsed uterus consisting of cervical amputation and parametrial fixation of the cervical ligaments of the uterus.

man·del·ic acid (măn-dĕl′ĭk) *n.* An acid that has both antibacterial and bacteriostatic properties, used in treating urinary tract infections.

man·di·ble (măn′də-bəl) *n.* A U-shaped bone forming the lower jaw, articulating with the temporal bone on either side; jawbone; lower jawbone. — **man·dib′u·lar** (-dĭb′yə-lər) *adj.*

mandibular joint *n.* The joint between the head of the mandible and the mandibular fossa and articular tubercle of the temporal bone.

man·drel or **man·dril** (măn′drəl) *n.* **1.** A shaft on which a working tool is mounted, as in a dental drill. **2.** See **mandrin**.

man·drin (măn′drĭn) *n.* A stiff wire or stylet inserted into a soft catheter to give it shape and firmness while passing through a hollow tubular structure.

ma·neu·ver (mə-nōō′vər, -nyōō′-) *n.* A movement or procedure involving skill and dexterity. — *v.* **-vered, -ver·ing, -vers.** To manipulate into a desired position.

man·ga·nese (măng′gə-nēz′, -nēs′) *n.* A brittle metallic element with atomic number 25, found in certain ores and in trace amounts in body tissues.

mange (mānj) *n.* Any of several chronic skin diseases of animals, sometimes humans, caused by parasitic mites and characterized by skin lesions, itching, and loss of hair. — **mang′y** (măn′jē) *adj.*

ma·ni·a (mā′nē-ə, măn′yə) *n.* A manifestation of manic-depressive illness, characterized by profuse and rapidly changing ideas, exaggerated gaiety, and excessive physical activity.

ma·ni·ac (mā′nē-ăk′) *n.* An insane person. — *adj.*

ma·ni·a·cal (mə-nī′ə-kəl) or **ma·ni·ac** (mā′nē-ăk′) *adj.* Suggestive of or afflicted with insanity.

man·ic (măn′ĭk) *adj.* Relating to, affected by, or resembling mania.

manic-depressive *adj.* Of, relating to, or affected by bipolar disorder. — *n.* A person afflicted with bipolar disorder.

manic-depressive illness *n.* See **bipolar disorder.**

man·i·fes·ta·tion (măn′ə-fĕ-stā′shən) *n.* An indication of the existence, reality, or presence of something, especially an illness.

man·i·fest content (măn′ə-fĕst′) *n.* The content of a dream, fantasy, or thought as it is remembered and reported in psychoanalysis.

man·i·fest·ing carrier (măn′ə-fĕs′tĭng) *n.* See **manifesting heterozygote.**

ma·nip·u·la·tion (mə-nĭp′yə-lā′shən) *n.* **1.** The act or practice of manipulating. **2.** The state of being manipulated.

man·ner·ism (măn′ə-rĭz′əm) *n.* A distinctive behavioral trait; an idiosyncrasy.

man·ni·tol (măn′ĭ-tôl′, -tōl′) *n.* A white, crystalline, water-soluble, slightly sweet alcohol, used as a dietary supplement and dietetic sweetener and in medical tests of renal function.

man·nose (măn′ōs′) *n.* A monosaccharide obtained from various plants by the oxidation of mannitol.

man·no·si·do·sis (măn′ə-sĭ-dō′sĭs) *n.* An inherited disorder caused by the deficiency of an enzyme necessary for the metabolism of mannose and characterized by mental retardation, kyphosis, and an enlarged tongue.

ma·nom·e·ter (mă-nŏm′ĭ-tər) *n.* **1.** An instrument used for measuring the pressure of liquids and gases. **2.** A sphygmomanometer. — **man′o·met′ric** (măn′ə-mĕt′rĭk), **man′o·met′ri·cal** *adj.* — **ma·nom′e·try** *n.*

man. pr. *n.* — *abbr. Latin.* mane primo (early morning, first thing in the morning)

Man·son·el·la (măn′sə-nĕl′ə) *n.* A genus of filarial worms that are found chiefly in Central and South America and cause mansonelliasis.

man·so·nel·li·a·sis (măn′sə-nĕl-ī′ə-sĭs) *n.* Infection with a species of filarial worms of the genus *Mansonella,* the adult worms live in the serous cavities, especially the peritoneal cavity, in mesenteric and perivisceral adipose tissue, and in the skin.

man·tle (măn′tl) *n.* **1.** A covering layer of tissue. **2.** See **pallium.**

mantle radiotherapy *n.* The use of radiotherapy with protection of uninvolved radiosensitive structures or organs.

Man·toux test (măn′tōō′) *n.* A tuberculin test in which a small amount of tuberculin is injected under the skin.

man·u·al ventilation (măn′yōō-əl) *n.* A method of assisted or controlled ventilation in which the hands are used to generate airway pressures.

ma·nu·bri·um (mə-nōō′brē-əm, -nyōō′-) *n., pl.* **-bri·a** (-brē-ə). **1.** The upper segment of the sternum with which the clavicle and the first two pairs of ribs articulate. **2.** See **episternum. 3.** The portion of the malleus embedded in the tympanic membrane and extending down, in and back from the neck of the malleus.

ma·nus (mā′nəs, măn′əs) *n., pl.* **manus. 1.** The distal part of the arm, including the carpus, metacarpus, and digits. **2.** The hand.

man·y-tailed bandage (mĕn′ē-tāld′) *n.* A large oblong cloth, applied to the thorax or abdomen, with ends that are cut into narrow strips that are tied or overlapped and pinned.

map (măp) *n.* A genetic map. — *v.* **mapped, map·ping, maps.** To locate a gene or DNA sequence in a specific region of a chromosome in relation to known genes or DNA sequences.

ma·ple syr·up urine disease (mā′pəl sĭr′əp, sûr′-) *n.* A hereditary metabolic disorder due to a deficiency of decarboxylase that leads to high concentrations of leucine, isoleucine, and valine in the blood and urine, characterized by urine with a maple syrup odor, mental retardation, and seizures.

map·ping function (măp′ĭng) *n.* A mathematical formula that relates distances on a gene map to recombination frequencies.

ma·pro·ti·line (mə-prōt′l-ēn′) *n.* A tricyclic antidepressant used in the treatment of depressive illnesses and for the relief of anxiety.

Ma·ra·ñon′s sign (mär′ən-yōnz′, mä′rä-nyônz′) *n.* An indication of Graves' disease in which a vasomotor reaction occurs after the skin over the throat is stimulated.

ma·ras·mus (mə-răz′məs) *n.* Chronic wasting of body tissues, especially in young children, commonly due to prolonged dietary deficiency of protein and calories. — **ma·ras′mic** *adj.*

Mar·burg virus disease (mär′bûrg′) *n.* An often fatal infection of humans by the Marburg virus, characterized by severe fever, diarrhea, a maculopapular rash, and hemorrhaging.

march fracture *n.* A fatigue fracture occurring in a metatarsal bone of the foot.

Mar·chia·fa·va–Bi·gna·mi disease (mär′kyə-fä′və-bĭ-nyä′mē, -bē-) *n.* Degeneration of the corpus callosum, characterized by mental deterioration, dementia, and convulsions, and occurring predominately in chronic alcoholics.

Mar·cus Gunn phenomenon or **Mar·cus Gunn syndrome** (mär′kəs gŭn′) *n.* See **jaw-winking syndrome.**

Mar·cus Gunn's sign (mär′kəs gŭnz′) *n.* See **Gunn's sign.**

Mar·fan syndrome (mär′făn) *n.* A hereditary disorder principally affecting connective tissues, manifested in varying degrees by excessive bone elongation and joint flexibility and by abnormalities of the eye and cardiovascular system.

mar·gin (mär′jĭn) *n.* **1.** A border or edge, as of an organ. **2.** A limit in a condition or process, beyond or below which something is no longer possible or acceptable.

mar·gin·al (mär′jə-nəl) *adj.* **1.** Of, relating to, located at, or constituting a margin, a border, or an edge. **2.** Barely within a lower standard or limit of quality. **3.** Relating to or located at the fringe of consciousness. — **mar·gin·al´i·ty** (-jə-năl´ĭ-tē) n.

mar·gin·a·tion (mär´jə-nā´shən) n. The adhesion of white blood cells to the endothelial cells of blood vessels at the site of an injury during the early phases of inflammation.

mar·gi·no·plas·ty (mär´jə-nō-plăs´tē) n. Plastic surgery of the tarsal border of an eyelid.

mar·i·jua·na or **mar·i·hua·na** (măr´ə-wä´nə) n. **1.** The cannabis plant. **2.** A preparation made from the dried flowers and leaves of the cannabis plant, usually smoked or eaten to induce euphoria.

mark (märk) n. **1.** A spot or line on a surface, visible through difference in color or elevation from that of the surrounding area. **2.** A distinctive trait or property. — v. **marked, mark·ing, marks. 1.** To make a visible trace or impression on, as with a spot, line, or dent. **2.** To form, make, or depict by making a mark. **3.** To distinguish or characterize.

mark·er (mär´kər) n. **1.** A physiological substance, such as human chorionic gonadotropin or alpha-fetoprotein, that when present in abnormal amounts in the serum may indicate the presence of disease, as that caused by a malignancy. **2.** A genetic marker.

marker trait n. A trait that may be of little importance in itself but which facilitates the detection or understanding of a particular disease.

Ma·ro·teaux–La·my syndrome (mär´ə-tō´lä-mē´, mä-rô-) n. An inherited defect in mucopolysaccharide metabolism characterized by retarded growth, lumbar kyphosis, sternal protrusion, knock-knee, and usually enlargement of the liver and spleen.

mar·row (măr´ō) n. **1.** Bone marrow. **2.** The spinal cord.

mar·su·pi·al·i·za·tion (mär-sōō´pē-ə-lĭ-zā´shən) n. Surgical alteration of a cyst or similar enclosed cavity by making an incision in the cyst or enclosed cavity and suturing the flaps to the adjacent tissue, thereby creating a pouch.

mas·cu·line (măs´kyə-lĭn) n. **1.** Of or relating to men or boys; male. **2.** Suggestive or characteristic of a man. — **mas´cu·line·ness** n.

mas·cu·lin·i·ty (măs´kyə-lĭn´ĭ-tē) n. **1.** The quality or condition of being masculine. **2.** Something traditionally considered to be characteristic of a male.

mas·cu·lin·ize (măs´kyə-lə-nīz´) v. **-ized, -iz·ing, -iz·es. 1.** To give a masculine appearance or character to. **2.** To cause a female to assume masculine characteristics, as through hormonal imbalance or male hormone therapy. — **mas´cu·lin·i·za´tion** (-lə-nĭ-zā´shən) n.

MASH abbr. Mobile Army Surgical Hospital

mask (măsk) n. **1.** A covering for the nose and mouth that is used for inhaling oxygen or an anesthetic. **2.** A covering worn over the nose and mouth, as by a surgeon or dentist, to prevent infection. **3.** A facial bandage. **4.** Something, often a trait, that disguises or conceals. **5.** Any of various conditions producing alteration or discoloration of the skin of the face. **6.** An expressionless appearance of the face seen in certain diseases, such as Parkinsonism. — v. **masked, mask·ing, masks. 1.** To cover with a protective mask. **2.** To cover in order to conceal or protect.

mask·ing (măs´kĭng) n. **1.** The concealment or screening of one sensory process or sensation by another. **2.** An opaque covering used to camouflage the metal parts of a prosthesis.

mask of pregnancy n. See **chloasma.**

mas·och·ism (măs´ə-kĭz´əm) n. **1.** The act or an instance of deriving sexual gratification from being physically or emotionally abused. **2.** A psychological disorder in which sexual gratification is derived from being physically or emotionally abused. **3.** The act or an instance of deriving pleasure from being offended, dominated, or mistreated. **4.** The tendency to seek such mistreatment. — **mas´och·ist** n. — **mas´och·is´tic** adj.

masochistic personality n. A personality disorder characterized by the exploitation or infliction of pain on others or oneself so as to gain personal satisfaction or pleasure.

mass (măs) n. **1.** The physical volume or bulk of a solid body. **2.** The measure of the quantity of matter that a body or an object contains. The mass of the body is not dependent on gravity and therefore is different from but proportional to its weight. **3.** A thick, pasty pharmacological mixture containing drugs from which pills are formed.

mas·sage (mə-säzh´ -säj´) n. The rubbing or kneading of parts of the body for therapeutic purposes. — v. **-saged, -sag·ing, -sag·es. 1.** To give a massage to. **2.** To treat by means of a massage.

mas·se·ter muscle (mə-sē´tər) n. A muscle with origin from the inferior border and medial surface of the zygomatic arch, with insertion into the lateral surface of the ramus and coronoid process of the mandible, and whose action closes the jaw in chewing. — **mas´se·ter´ic** (măs´ĭ-tĕr´ĭk) adj.

mass hysteria n. **1.** Spontaneous, en masse development of identical physical or emotional symptoms among a group of individuals, as in a classroom of schoolchildren. **2.** A socially contagious frenzy of irrational behavior in a group of people as a reaction to an event.

mas·so·ther·a·py (măs´ō-thĕr´ə-pē) n. The therapeutic use of massage.

mass peristalsis n. Brief, forcible peristaltic movements that move the contents through long segments of the large intestine, such as from the ascending colon to the transverse colon.

mas·tad·e·no·ma (măs´tă-dn-ō´mə) n. A benign tumor of the breast.

mast cell n. A cell found in connective tissue that contains basophilic granules and releases substances such as heparin and histamine in response to injury or inflammation of bodily tissues.

mas·tec·to·my (mă-stĕk´tə-mē) n. Surgical removal of all or part of a breast, sometimes including excision of the underlying pectoral muscles and regional lymph nodes, usually performed as a treatment for cancer.

mas·ter gland (măs′tər) *n.* See **pituitary gland.**

Mas·ter's two-step exercise test (măs′tərz) *n.* See **two-step exercise test.**

mas·ti·cate (măs′tĭ-kāt′) *v.* **-cat·ed, -cat·ing, -cates.** To chew food. — **mas′ti·ca′tion** *n.*

mas·ti·ca·to·ry (măs′tĭ-kə-tôr′ē) *adj.* **1.** Of, relating to, or used in mastication. **2.** Adapted for chewing. — *n.* A medicinal substance chewed to increase salivation.

masticatory system *n.* The organs and structures primarily functioning in mastication, including the jaws and jaw muscles, teeth, temporomandibular joints, tongue, lips, cheeks, and oral mucosa.

mas·ti·tis (mă-stī′tĭs) *n.* Inflammation of the breast.

mas·to·cyte (măs′tə-sīt′) *n.* See **mast cell.**

mas·to·cy·to·ma (măs′tō-sī-tō′mə) *n., pl.* **-mas** or **-ma·ta** (-mə-tə). An accumulation or nodule of mast cells that resembles a tumor.

mas·to·dyn·i·a (măs′tə-dĭn′ē-ə) *n.* Pain in the breast.

mas·toid (măs′toid′) *n.* The mastoid process. — *adj.* **1.** Of or relating to the mastoid process, antrum, or cells. **2.** Shaped like a breast or nipple.

mastoid bone *n.* See **mastoid process** (sense 1).

mas·toid·ec·to·my (măs′toi-dĕk′tə-mē) *n.* Surgical removal of mastoid cells or part or all of the mastoid process.

mas·toi·de·o·cen·te·sis (măs-toi′dē-ō-sĕn-tē′sĭs) *n.* Surgical puncture of the mastoid cells and the mastoid antrum.

mas·toid·i·tis (măs′toi-dī′tĭs) *n.* Inflammation of the mastoid process and mastoid cells.

mas·toid·ot·o·my (măs′toi-dŏt′ə-mē) *n.* Surgical incision into the subperiosteum or the mastoid process of the temporal bone.

mastoid part *n.* The portion of the petrous part of the temporal bone bearing the mastoid process.

mastoid process *n.* **1.** A conical protuberance of the posterior portion of the temporal bone that is situated behind the ear and serves as a site of muscle attachment. **2.** The part of the first pharyngeal arch in the embryo, developing into the upper jaw in the embryo.

mas·to·plas·ty (măs′tə-plăs′tē) *n.* Plastic surgery of the breast.

mas·tot·o·my (mă-stŏt′ə-mē) *n.* Surgical incision of the breast.

mas·tur·bate (măs′tər-bāt′) *v.* **-bat·ed, -bat·ing, -bates.** To perform an act of masturbation.

mas·tur·ba·tion (măs′tər-bā′shən) *n.* Excitation of one's own or another's genital organs, usually to orgasm, by manual contact or means other than sexual intercourse.

Mat·as operation (măt′əs) *n.* See **aneurysmoplasty** (sense 1).

match·ing (măch′ĭng) *n.* The process of comparing a study group and a comparison group in an epidemiological study with respect to extraneous or confounding factors such as age, sex, or breed.

mate (māt) *v.* **mat·ed, mat·ing, mates. 1.** To be paired for reproducing; breed. **2.** To copulate.

ma·ter·nal (mə-tûr′nəl) *adj.* **1.** Relating to or characteristic of a mother. **2.** Inherited from one's mother.

maternal dystocia *n.* A difficult delivery caused by an abnormality in the mother.

maternal placenta *n.* The part of the placenta derived from uterine tissue.

ma·ter·ni·ty (mə-tûr′nĭ-tē) *n.* **1.** The state of being a mother; motherhood. **2.** The feelings or characteristics associated with being a mother. **3.** A maternity ward. — *adj.* Relating to pregnancy, childbirth, or the first months of motherhood.

maternity ward *n.* The department of a hospital that provides care for women during pregnancy and childbirth as well as for newborn infants.

mat·ri·cide (măt′rĭ-sīd′) *n.* The act of killing one's mother. — **mat′ri·cid′al** (-sīd′l) *adj.*

ma·trix (mā′trĭks) *n., pl.* **ma·trix·es** or **ma·tri·ces** (mā′trĭ-sēz′, măt′rĭ-). **1.** A surrounding substance within which something else originates, develops, or is contained. **2.** The formative cells or tissue of a fingernail, toenail, or tooth. **3.** See **ground substance.**

mat·ter (măt′ər) *n.* **1.** A specific type of substance. **2.** Discharge or waste, such as pus or feces, from a living organism.

mat·tress suture (măt′rĭs) *n.* A suture made with a double stitch that forms a loop about the tissue on both sides of a wound and produces eversion of the edges.

mat·u·rate (măch′ə-rāt′) *v.* **-ra·ted, -rat·ing, -rates. 1.** To mature, ripen, or develop. **2.** To suppurate.

mat·u·ra·tion (măch′ə-rā′shən) *n.* **1.** The process of becoming mature. **2.** Production or discharge of pus. **3.** The processes by which gametes are formed, including the meiotic reduction of chromosomes in a germ cell from a diploid to a haploid number. **4.** The final differentiation processes in biological systems, such as the attainment of full functional capacity by a cell, a tissue, or an organ. — **mat′u·ra′tion·al** *adj.*

maturation arrest *n.* The cessation of complete differentiation of cells at an immature stage.

maturation division *n.* Either of the two successive cell divisions of meiosis, with only one duplication of the chromosomes, that results in the formation of haploid gametes.

ma·ture (mə-tyŏor′, -tŏor′, -chŏor′) *adj.* **1.** Having reached full natural growth or development. **2.** Of, relating to, or characteristic of full development, either mental or physical. — *v.* **-tured, -tur·ing, -tures.** To evolve toward or reach full development.

mature-onset diabetes *n.* Non-insulin-dependent diabetes mellitus.

ma·tu·ri·ty (mə-tyŏor′ĭ-tē, -tŏor′-, -chŏor′-) *n.* **1.** The state or quality of being fully grown or developed. **2.** The state or quality of being mature.

Mau·rer's dot (mou′rərz) *n.* Any of the fine granular precipitates or irregular cytoplasmic particles usually present in red blood cells infected with the trophozoites of *Plasmodium falciparum*.

Mau·riac's syndrome (môr′ē-äks′, môr-yäks′) *n.* Dwarfism accompanied by obesity and enlargement of the liver and spleen in children with poorly controlled diabetes mellitus.

Mau·ri·ceau's maneuver (mô-rē-sōz′) *n.* A method of delivering the head in an assisted breech delivery in which the infant's body is supported by the right forearm while traction is made upon the shoulders by the left hand.

max·il·la (măk-sĭl′ə) *n., pl.* **max·il·las** or **max·il·lae** (măk-sĭl′ē). Either of a pair of irregularly shaped bones of the skull, fusing in the midline, supporting the upper teeth, and forming part of the eye sockets, hard palate, and nasal cavity; upper jaw.

max·il·lar·y (măk′sə-lĕr′ē) *adj.* Of or relating to a jaw or jawbone, especially the upper one. —*n.* A maxillary bone; a jawbone.

maxillary artery *n.* An artery with origin in the external carotid artery and with branches to the tonsils, pharynx, jaw, and other deep facial structures; internal maxillary artery.

maxillary bone *n.* Maxilla.

max·il·lot·o·my (măk′sə-lŏt′ə-mē) *n.* Surgical sectioning of the maxilla to allow movement of all or a part of the maxilla into the desired position.

max·i·mal permissible dose (măk′sə-məl) *n.* The largest dose of radiation one may be exposed to without experiencing harmful effects.

max·i·mum breathing capacity (măk′sə-məm) *n.* The volume of gas that can be breathed in 15 seconds when a person is breathing as deeply and as quickly as possible.

maximum velocity *n.* **1.** The maximum rate of an enzymatic reaction that can be achieved by progressively increasing the substrate concentration. **2.** The maximum initial rate of shortening of a myocardial fiber that can be obtained under zero load. Used to evaluate the fiber's contractility.

maximum voluntary ventilation *n.* See **maximum breathing capacity.**

May·er's reflex (mī′ərz) *n.* See **basal joint reflex.**

Ma·yo–Rob·son's position (mā′ō-rŏb′sənz) *n.* A supine position with a thick pad under the loins to elevate the lumbocostal region, used in operations on the gallbladder.

Ma·yo's operation (mā′ōz) *n.* An operation for the radical correction of umbilical hernia.

Mb *abbr.* myoglobin

M band *n.* See **M line.**

MBC *abbr.* maximum breathing capacity

MCAT *abbr.* Medical College Admissions Test

Mc·Bur·ney's point (mək-bûr′nēz) *n.* A point above the anterior superior spine of the ilium, located on a straight line joining that process and the umbilicus, where pressure of the finger elicits tenderness in acute appendicitis.

Mc·Mur·ray test (mək-mûr′ē, -mûr′ē) *n.* A test for injury to meniscal structures of the knee in which the lower leg is rotated while the leg is extended; pain and a cracking in the knee indicates injury.

Mc·Vay's operation (mĭk-vāz′) *n.* Surgical repair

of femoral hernias by suture of the transverse muscle of the abdomen and its associated fasciae to the pectineal ligament.

MD *abbr.* Also **M.D.** *Latin.* Medicinae Doctor (Doctor of Medicine); muscular dystrophy

ME *abbr.* medical examiner

Mead·ows's syndrome (mĕd′ōz) *n.* Disease of the myocardium developing during pregnancy or the puerperium.

mean cell hemoglobin (mēn) *n.* The hemoglobin content of the average red blood cell, calculated from the hemoglobin therein and the red cell count in red blood cell indices.

mean cell hemoglobin concentration *n.* The average mean hemoglobin concentration in a given volume of packed red blood cells.

mean cell volume *n.* The average volume of red cells in red blood cell indices, calculated from the hematocrit and the red blood cell count.

mea·sles (mē′zəlz) *n.* **1.** An acute, contagious viral disease, usually occurring in childhood and characterized by eruption of red spots on the skin, fever, and catarrhal symptoms. **2.** Black measles. **3.** Any of several other diseases, especially German measles, that cause similar but milder symptoms.

measles, mumps, rubella vaccine *n.* A vaccine containing live attenuated measles, mumps, and rubella viruses in an aqueous suspension.

measles virus *n.* An RNA virus of the genus *Morbillivirus* that causes measles in humans.

measles virus vaccine *n.* A vaccine containing live attenuated strains of measles virus prepared in chick embryo cell cultures.

meas·ure (mězh′ər) *n.* **1.** A reference standard used for the quantitative comparison of properties. **2.** A unit specified by a scale, such as a degree, or by variable conditions, such as room temperature. **3.** A system of measurement, such as the metric system. **4.** An evaluation or a basis of comparison. **5.** A measured quantity. —*v.* **-ured, -ur·ing, -ures. 1.** To ascertain the dimensions, quantity, or capacity of. **2.** To mark off or apportion, usually with reference to a given unit of measurement.

me·at·o·plas·ty (mē-ăt′ə-plăs′tē) *n.* Reparative or reconstructive surgery of a meatus or canal.

me·a·tor·rha·phy (mē′ə-tôr′ə-fē) *n.* Suture of the wound made by performing a meatotomy.

me·a·tos·co·py (mē′ə-tŏs′kə-pē) *n.* The inspection of a meatus, especially of the urethra.

me·a·tot·o·my (mē′ə-tŏt′ə-mē) *n.* A surgical incision made to enlarge a meatus, as of the urethra or ureter.

me·a·tus (mē-ā′təs) *n., pl.* **-tus·es** or **meatus.** A body opening or passage, especially the external opening of a canal.

me·chan·i·cal (mĭ-kăn′ĭ-kəl) *adj.* **1.** Operated or produced by a mechanism or machine. **2.** Relating to or produced by physical forces.

mechanical alternation *n.* A disorder in which contractions of the heart are regular in time but are alternately stronger and weaker.

mechanical ventilation *n.* A mode of assisted or controlled ventilation using mechanical devices that cycle automatically to generate airway pressure.

mech·a·nism (mĕk′ə-nĭz′əm) *n.* **1.** A machine or mechanical appliance. **2.** A system of parts that operate or interact like those of a machine. **3.** The involuntary and consistent response of an organism to a given stimulus. **4.** A usually unconscious mental and emotional pattern that dominates behavior in a given situation or environment. **5.** The sequence of steps in a chemical reaction.

mech·a·no·re·cep·tor (mĕk′ə-nō-rĭ-sĕp′tər) *n.* A specialized sensory end organ that responds to mechanical stimuli such as tension, pressure, or displacement.

mech·a·no·ther·a·py (mĕk′ə-nō-thĕr′ə-pē) *n.* Medical treatment by mechanical methods, such as massage. — **mech′a·no·ther′a·pist** *n.*

Meck·el's cartilage (mĕk′əlz) *n.* See **mandibular cartilage.**

Meck·el syndrome (mĕk′əl) *n.* A hereditary malformation syndrome marked by sloping forehead, cleft palate, ocular anomalies, and polydactyly and resulting in death during the perinatal period.

mec·li·zine (mĕk′lĭ-zēn′) *n.* An antihistaminic used in the prevention and treatment of nausea and motion sickness.

me·co·ni·um (mĭ-kō′nē-əm) *n.* **1.** A dark green fecal material that accumulates in the fetal intestines and is discharged at or near the time of birth. **2.** See **opium.**

meconium aspiration *n.* Aspiration of amniotic fluid contaminated with meconium by a fetus in hypoxic distress.

meconium ileus *n.* Intestinal obstruction in a newborn child following the thickening of meconium resulting from a lack of trypsin; it is associated with cystic fibrosis of the pancreas.

med (mĕd) *adj.* Of or relating to medicine or things medical.

med·e·vac (mĕd′ĭ-văk′) *n.* **1.** Air transport of persons to a place where they can receive medical or surgical care; medical evacuation. **2.** A helicopter or other aircraft used for such transport. — *v.* **-vaced, -vac·ing, -vacs.** To transport a patient to a place where medical care is available.

me·di·a (mē′dē-ə) *n.* The tunica media.

me·di·al (mē′dē-əl) *adj.* Relating to, situated in, or extending toward the middle.

me·di·an (mē′dē-ən) *adj.* **1.** Relating to, located in, or extending toward the middle. **2.** Of, relating to, or situated in or near the plane that divides a bilaterally symmetrical animal into right and left halves. — *n.* A median point, plane, line, or part.

median artery *n.* An artery arising in the anterior interosseous artery and distributed with the median nerve to the palm, and with anastomoses to branches of the superficial palmar arch.

median line *n.* **1.** Anterior median line. **2.** Posterior median line.

median plane *n.* A vertical plane along the midline of the body dividing the body into right and left halves.

median rhinoscopy *n.* Examination of the roof of the nasal cavity and openings of the posterior ethmoid cells and sphenoidal sinus using a long-bladed nasal speculum or a nasopharyngoscope.

median vein *n.* An intermediate vein.

mediastinal vein *n.* Any of several small veins from the mediastinum emptying into brachiocephalic vein or the superior vena cava.

me·di·as·ti·ni·tis (mē′dē-ăs′tə-nī′tĭs) *n.* Inflammation of the cellular tissue of the mediastinum.

me·di·as·ti·nog·ra·phy (mē′dē-ăs′tə-nŏg′rə-fē) *n.* Radiography of the mediastinum.

me·di·as·tin·o·scope (mē′dē-ăs-tĭn′ə-skōp′) *n.* An endoscope inserted through an incision above the sternum to examine the mediastinum.

me·di·as·ti·nos·co·py (mē′dē-ăs′tə-nŏs′kə-pē) *n.* Exploration of the mediastinum through a suprasternal incision.

me·di·as·ti·not·o·my (mē′dē-ăs′tə-nŏt′ə-mē) *n.* Incision into the mediastinum.

me·di·as·ti·num (mē′dē-ə-stī′nəm) *n., pl.* **-na** (-nə). **1.** A septum between two parts of an organ or a cavity. **2.** The region between the pleural sacs, containing the heart and all of the thoracic viscera except the lungs. — **me′di·as·ti′nal** (-nəl) *adj.*

me·di·ate auscultation (mē′dē-āt′) *n.* The use of a stethoscope to examine the internal sounds of a body.

mediate percussion *n.* Percussion effected by the intervention of a finger or a pleximeter between the striking finger or plexor and the part percussed.

med·ic (mĕd′ĭk) *n.* **1.** A member of a military medical corps. **2.** A physician or surgeon. **3.** A medical student or intern.

Med·i·caid or **med·i·caid** (mĕd′ĭ-kād′) *n.* A program in the United States, jointly funded by the states and the federal government, that reimburses hospitals and physicians for providing care to qualifying people who cannot finance their own medical expenses.

med·i·cal (mĕd′ĭ-kəl) *adj.* **1.** Of or relating to the study or practice of medicine. **2.** Requiring treatment by medicine. — *n.* A thorough physical examination.

medical diathermy *n.* Diathermy in which the tissues are warmed but not destroyed.

medical examiner *n.* **1.** A physician officially authorized by a governmental unit to ascertain causes of deaths, especially those not occurring under natural circumstances. **2.** A physician who examines employees of a particular firm or applicants for life insurance.

medical jurisprudence *n.* See **forensic medicine.**

medical law *n.* The branch of law that deals with the application of medical knowledge to legal problems.

medical record *n.* A chronological written account of a patient's examination and treatment that includes the patient's medical history and complaints, the physician's physical findings, the results of diagnostic tests and procedures, and medications and therapeutic procedures.

medical tran·scrip·tion·ist (trăn-skrĭp′shə-nĭst) *n.* A person who transcribes a physician's medical reports concerning a patient's health care.

Med·i·care or **med·i·care** (mĕd′ĭ-kâr′) *n.* A program under the U.S. Social Security Administration that reimburses hospitals and physicians for medical care provided to qualifying people over 65 years of age.

med·i·cate (mĕd′ĭ-kāt′) *v.* **-cat·ed, -cat·ing, -cates.** **1.** To treat by medicine. **2.** To tincture or permeate with a medicinal substance.

med·i·ca·tion (mĕd′ĭ-kā′shən) *n.* **1.** A medicine; a medicament. **2.** The act or process of treating with medicine. **3.** Administration of medicine.

med·i·cine (mĕd′ĭ-sĭn) *n.* **1.** The science of diagnosing, treating, or preventing disease and other damage to the body or mind. **2.** The branch of this science encompassing treatment by drugs, diet, exercise, and other nonsurgical means. **3.** The practice of medicine. **4.** An agent, such as a drug, used to treat disease or injury.

med·i·co (mĕd′ĭ-kō′) *n.* **1.** A physician. **2.** A medical student.

med·i·co·chi·rur·gi·cal (mĕd′ĭ-kō-kī-rûr′jĭ-kəl) *adj.* Relating to medicine and surgery.

med·i·co·le·gal (mĕd′ĭ-kō-lē′gəl) *adj.* Of, relating to, or concerned with medicine and law.

Med·i·ter·ra·ne·an exanthematous fever (mĕd′-ĭ-tə-rā′nē-ən) *n.* A disease occurring sporadically in the Mediterranean littoral marked by severe chills with abrupt temperature rise, tonsillitis, joint pains, diarrhea, vomiting, and a rash of elevated nonconfluent macules beginning on the thighs and spreading to the entire body.

Mediterranean fever *n.* See **brucellosis.**

me·di·um (mē′dē-əm) *n., pl.* **-di·ums** or **-di·a** (-dē-ə). **1.** Something, such as an intermediate course of action, that occupies a position or represents a condition midway between extremes. **2.** An intervening substance through which something else is transmitted or carried on. **3.** The substance in which a specific organism lives and thrives. **4.** A culture medium. **5.** A filtering substance, such as filter paper. — *adj.* Occurring or being between two degrees, amounts, or quantities; intermediate.

MEDLARS *abbr.* Medical Literature Analysis and Retrieval System (computerized index system of the U. S. National Library of Medicine)

MEDLINE (mĕd′līn′) *n.* A system providing telephone linkage between a number of medical libraries in the United States and MEDLARS for rapid retrieval of medical bibliographies.

me·dul·la (mĭ-dŭl′ə) *n., pl.* **-dul·las** or **-dul·lae** (-dŭl′ē). The inner core of certain organs or body structures, such as the marrow of bone. — **me·dul′lar, med·ul·lar′y** (mĕd′l-ĕr′ē, mə-dŭl′ə-rē) *adj.*

medulla ob·lon·ga·ta (ŏb′lŏng-gä′tə, -gä′tə) *n., pl.* **-ga·tas** or **-ga·tae** (-gä′tē, -gä′tē). The lower-

most portion of the human brain, continuous with the spinal cord and responsible for the control of respiration, circulation, and certain other bodily functions.

medullary membrane *n.* See **endosteum.**

medullary sheath *n.* See **myelin sheath.**

medullated fiber *n.* See **myelinated fiber.**

med·ul·lec·to·my (mĕd′l-ĕk′tə-mē) *n.* Surgical removal of a medullary substance or part.

med·ul·li·za·tion (mĕd′l-ĭ-zā′shən) *n.* Replacement of bone tissue by marrow, as in osteitis.

med·ul·lo·blas·to·ma (mĕd′l-ō-blă-stō′mə, mĭ-dŭl′ō-) *n.* A glioma consisting of neoplastic cells that resemble the undifferentiated cells of the primitive medullary tube.

Me·du·sa head (mĭ-dōō′sə, -zə, -dyōō′-) *n.* Dilated cutaneous veins radiating from the umbilicus.

mef·e·nam·ic acid (mĕf′ə-năm′ĭk) *n.* A crystalline compound used as an anti-inflammatory drug and as an analgesic.

meg·a·co·lon (mĕg′ə-kō′lən) *n.* Extreme dilation and hypertrophy of the colon.

meg·a·cys·tic syndrome (mĕg′ə-sĭs′tĭk) *n.* A syndrome characterized by a large thin-walled bladder, regurgitation of the urine into the ureters, and dilated ureters.

meg·a·kar·y·o·blast (mĕg′ə-kăr′ē-ə-blăst′) *n.* The precursor of a megakaryocyte.

meg·a·kar·y·o·cyte (mĕg′ə-kăr′ē-ə-sīt′) *n.* A large bone marrow cell with a lobulate nucleus that gives rise to blood platelets.

meg·a·lo·blast (mĕg′ə-lō-blăst′) *n.* An abnormally large nucleated red blood cell found especially in pernicious anemia or in certain vitamin deficiencies. — **meg′a·lo·blas′tic** *adj.*

megaloblastic anemia *n.* Anemia in which there is a predominant number of megaloblasts and relatively few normoblasts among the hyperplastic erythroid cells in the bone marrow, as in pernicious anemia.

meg·a·lo·cys·tis (mĕg′ə-lō-sĭs′tĭs) *n.* An abnormally enlarged or distended bladder.

meg·a·lo·cyte (mĕg′ə-lō-sīt′) *n.* A large nonnucleated red blood cell.

meg·a·lo·en·ceph·a·ly (mĕg′ə-lō-ĕn-sĕf′ə-lē) *n.* Abnormal largeness of the brain. — **meg′a·lo·en′ce·phal′ic** (-ĕn′sə-făl′ĭk) *adj.*

meg·a·lo·kar·y·o·cyte (mĕg′ə-lō-kăr′ē-ə-sīt′) *n.* See **megakaryocyte.**

meg·a·lo·ma·ni·a (mĕg′ə-lō-mā′nē-ə, -mān′yə) *n.* A psychopathological condition in which delusional fantasies of wealth, power, or omnipotence predominate. — **meg′a·lo·ma′ni·ac′** *n.* — **meg′a·lo·ma·ni′a·cal** (-mə-nī′ə-kəl), **meg′a·lo·man′ic** (-măn′ĭk) *adj.*

meg·a·vi·ta·min (mĕg′ə-vī′tə-mĭn) *n.* A dose of a vitamin greatly exceeding the amount required to maintain health.

meibomian cyst *n.* See **chalazion.**

mei·bo·mi·an gland (mī-bō′mē-ən) *n.* Any of the branched modified sebaceous glands situated in the tarsus of the eyelid, the secretions of which prevent the eyelids from sticking together.

mei·bo·mi·tis (mī′bō-mī′tĭs) or **mei·bo·mi·a·ni·tis** (mĭ-bō′mē-ə-nī′tĭs) *n.* Inflammation of the Meibomian glands.

mei·o·sis (mī-ō′sĭs) *n., pl.* **-ses** (-sēz′). The special process of cell division in sexually reproducing organisms that results in the formation of gametes, consisting of two nuclear divisions in rapid succession that in turn result in the formation of four gametocytes, each containing half the number of chromosomes found in somatic cells. — **mei·ot′ic** (-ŏt′ĭk) *adj.* — **mei·ot′i·cal·ly** *adv.*

meit·ner·i·um (mīt-nûr′ē-əm) *n.* An artificially produced roadioactive element with atomic number 109.

me·lag·ra (mĕ-lăg′rə) *n.* Rheumatic or muscular pains in the arms or legs.

mel·an·cho·li·a (mĕl′ən-kō′lē-ə) *n.* A mental disorder marked by depression, apathy, and withdrawal. — **mel′an·cho′li·ac** (-lē-ăk′) *adj. & n.*

mel·an·chol·y (mĕl′ən-kŏl′ē) *n.* **1.** Sadness or depression of the spirits; gloom. **2.** Melancholia.

mel·a·nin (mĕl′ə-nĭn) *n.* Any of a group of naturally occurring dark pigments composed of granules of highly irregular polymers that usually contain nitrogen or sulfur atoms, especially the pigment found in skin and hair.

mel·a·nism (mĕl′ə-nĭz′əm) *n.* **1.** See **melanosis. 2.** Dark coloration of the skin or hair because of a high concentration of melanin.

mel·a·no·blast (mĕl′ə-nō-blăst′, mə-lăn′ə-) *n.* A precursor cell of a melanocyte or melanophore. — **mel′a·no·blas′tic** *n.*

mel·a·no·cyte (mĕl′ə-nō-sīt′) *n.* An epidermal cell capable of synthesizing melanin. — **mel′a·no·cyt′ic** (-sĭt′ĭk) *adj.*

melanocyte-stimulating hormone *n.* A pituitary hormone that regulates skin color by stimulating melanin synthesis in melanocytes and melanin granule dispersal in melanophores.

mel·a·no·cy·to·ma (mĕl′ə-nō-sī-tō′mə) *n.* **1.** A benign neoplasm composed of melanocytes. **2.** A usually benign, deeply pigmented melanoma of the optic disk.

mel·a·no·der·ma (mĕl′ə-nō-dûr′mə) *n.* An abnormal darkening of the skin caused by deposition of excess melanin or of metallic substances.

me·lan·o·gen (mĕ-lăn′ə-jən, -jĕn′, mĕl′ə-nō-jĕn′) *n.* A colorless precursor of melanin.

mel·a·no·gen·e·sis (mĕl′ə-nō-jĕn′ĭ-sĭs) *n.* The formation of melanin by living cells.

mel·a·no·ma (mĕl′ə-nō′mə) *n., pl.* **-mas** or **-ma·ta** (-mə-tə). A dark-pigmented, malignant, often widely metastasizing tumor arising from a melanocyte and occurring most commonly in the skin.

mel·a·no·phage (mĕl′ə-nə-fāj′, mə-lăn′ə-) *n.* A histiocyte that contains phagocytized melanin.

mel·a·no·phore (mĕl′ə-nə-fôr′, mə-lăn′ə-) *n.* A pigment cell that contains melanin.

mel·a·no·sis (mĕl′ə-nō′sĭs) *n.* Abnormally dark pigmentation of the skin or other tissues, resulting from a disorder of pigment metabolism. — **mel′a·not′ic** (-nŏt′ĭk) *adj.*

mel·a·no·some (mĕl′ə-nō-sōm′, mə-lăn′ə-) *n.* Any

of the usually oval pigment granules produced by melanocytes.

mel·a·no·troph (mĕl′ə-nō-trŏf′, -trōf′) *n.* A cell of the pituitary gland that produces melanocyte-stimulating hormone.

me·las·ma (mə-lăz′mə) *n.* **1.** A patchy or generalized dark pigmentation of the skin. **2.** See **chloasma.**

mel·a·to·nin (mĕl′ə-tō′nĭn) *n.* A hormone derived from serotonin, produced by the pineal gland, and believed to influence estrus in mammals.

me·le·na (mə-lē′nə) *n.* The passage of black tarry stools containing blood that has been acted on by the intestinal juices.

Me·le·ney′s gangrene (mə-lē′nēz) *n.* A form of gangrene of the skin and subcutaneous tissues, usually following an operation, caused by a synergistic interaction between microaerophilic nonhemolytic streptococci and aerobic hemolytic staphylococci.

Meleney's ulcer *n.* See **Meleney's gangrene.**

mel·o·plas·ty (mĕl′ə-plăs′tē) *n.* Reparative or plastic surgery of the cheek.

mem·ber (mĕm′bər) *n.* A part or an organ of the body, especially a limb.

mem·brane (mĕm′brān′) *n.* **1.** A thin pliable layer of tissue covering surfaces, enveloping a part, lining a cavity, or separating or connecting structures or organs. **2.** Cell membrane. **3.** A thin sheet of natural or synthetic material that is permeable to substances in solution.

membrane potential *n.* The potential inside a cell membrane measured relative to the fluid just outside; it is negative under resting conditions and becomes positive during an action potential.

mem·bra·nous (mĕm′brə-nəs) *adj.* **1.** Relating to, made of, or similar to a membrane. **2.** Characterized by the formation of a membrane or a layer similar to a membrane.

membranous labyrinth *n.* The fluid-filled membranous sacs of the inner ear that are associated with the senses of hearing and balance.

membranous ossification *n.* The development of bone tissue within connective tissue.

membranous rhinitis *n.* Chronic inflammation of the nasal mucous membrane with a fibrinous or pseudomembranous exudate.

mem·o·ry (mĕm′ə-rē) *n.* **1.** The mental faculty of retaining and recalling past experience based on the mental processes of learning, retention, recall, and recognition. **2.** Persistent modification of behavior resulting from experience. **3.** The ability of the immune system to produce a specific secondary response to an antigen that has been previously encountered.

men·ac·me (mĕ-năk′mē) *n.* The period of a woman's life in which menstrual activity occurs.

men·a·di·one (mĕn′ə-dī′ōn′) *n.* A synthetic vitamin K derivative occurring as a yellow crystalline powder and used as a vitamin K supplement.

men·a·quin·one (mĕn′ə-kwĭn′ōn′, -kwī′nōn′) *n.* See **vitamin K₂.**

me·nar·che (mə-när′kē) *n.* The first menstrual period, usually occurring during puberty. — **me·nar′che·al** *adj.*

Mendel–Bechterew reflex *n.* See **Bechterew–Mendel reflex.**

men·de·le·vi·um (měn′də-lē′vē-əm) *n.* A synthetic radioactive element with atomic number 101.

men·de·li·an inheritance (měn-dē′lē-ən, -dēl′yən) *n.* Inheritance that conforms to Mendel's laws.

Men·del·ism (měn′dl-ĭz′əm) or **Men·de·li·an·ism** (měn-dē′lē-ə-nĭz′əm) *n.* The theoretical principles of heredity formulated by Gregor Mendel; Mendel's laws.

Mé·nière's disease (mān-yârz′) *n.* A pathological condition of the inner ear characterized by dizziness, ringing in the ears, and progressive loss of hearing.

me·nin·ge·or·rha·phy (mə-nĭn′jē-ôr′ə-fē) *n.* Suture of the cranial or spinal meninges.

me·nin·gi·o·ma (mə-nĭn′jē-ō′mə) *n., pl.* **-mas** or **-ma·ta** (-mə-tə). A slow-growing tumor of the meninges occurring primarily in adults and often creating pressure and damaging the brain and adjacent tissues.

me·nin·gism (mə-nĭn′jĭz′əm, měn′ĭn-) *n.* A condition of irritation of the brain or spinal cord meninges in which the symptoms resemble those of meningitis but without inflammation, often occurring in children.

meningitic streak *n.* A line of redness following the drawing of the fingernail or of a pencil point across the skin, especially in cases of meningitis.

men·in·gi·tis (měn′ĭn-jī′tĭs) *n., pl.* **men·in·git·i·des** (-jĭt′ĭ-dēz′). Inflammation of the meninges of the brain and the spinal cord, most often caused by a bacterial or viral infection and characterized by fever, vomiting, intense headache, and stiff neck. — **men′in·git′ic** (-jĭt′ĭk) *adj.*

meningococcal meningitis *n.* An acute infectious disease affecting children and young adults characterized by inflammation of the meninges of the brain and spinal cord, headache, vomiting, convulsions, stiff neck, light sensitivity, and purpuric eruptions, and caused by the meningococcus, *Neisseria meningitidis.*

me·nin·go·coc·ce·mi·a (mə-nĭng′gō-kŏk-sē′mē-əs) *n.* The presence of the meningococci in the blood.

me·nin·go·coc·cus (mə-nĭng′gə-kŏk′əs, -nĭn′jə-) *n., pl.* **-coc·ci** (-kŏk′sī, -kī). A bacterium *(Neisseria meningitidis)* that causes cerebrospinal meningitis. — **me·nin′go·coc′cal** (-kŏk′əl), **me·nin′go·coc′cic** (-kŏk′sĭk)

me·nin·go·en·ceph·a·li·tis (mə-nĭng′gō-ĕn-sĕf′ə-lī′tĭs) *n.* Inflammation of the brain and its membranes.

me·nin·go·en·ceph·a·lo·cele (ĕn-sĕf′ə-lō-sēl′) *n.* Protrusion of the meninges and brain through a congenital defect in the cranium.

me·nin·go·my·e·li·tis (mə-nĭng′gō-mī′ə-lī′tĭs) *n.* Inflammation of the spinal cord and its enveloping arachnoid and pia mater, and, less commonly, dura mater.

me·nin·go·my·e·lo·cele (mə-nĭng′gō-mī′ə-lə-sēl′) *n.* Protrusion of the spinal membranes and cord through a defect in the vertebral column.

men·in·go·sis (měn′ĭng-gō′sĭs) *n.* The membranous union of bones, as in the skull of a newborn.

me·ninx (mē′nĭngks) *n., pl.* **me·nin·ges** (mə-nĭn′jēz). A membrane, especially one of the three membranes enclosing the brain and spinal cord.

men·is·cec·to·my (měn′ĭ-sĕk′tə-mē) *n.* Surgical excision of a meniscus, usually from the knee joint.

men·is·ci·tis (měn′ĭ-sī′tĭs) *n.* Inflammation of a fibrocartilaginous meniscus.

me·nis·co·cyte (mə-nĭs′kə-sīt′) *n.* See **sickle cell.**

me·nis·cus (mə-nĭs′kəs) *n., pl.* **-nis·cus·es** or **-nis·ci** (-nĭs′ī, -kī, -kē). **1.** A crescent-shaped body. **2.** A disk of cartilage that acts as a cushion between the ends of bones that meet in a joint. — **me·nis′cal** (-kəl), **me·nis′cate** (-kāt′), **me·nis′coid** (-koid′), **men′is·coi′dal** (měn′ĭs-koid′l) *adj.*

men·o·pause (měn′ə-pôz′) *n.* The period marked by the natural and permanent cessation of menstruation, occurring usually between the ages of 45 and 55. — **men′o·paus′al** *adj.*

me·nos·che·sis (mə-nŏs′kĭ-sĭs, měn′ə-skē′sĭs) *n.* Suppression of menstruation.

men·ses (měn′sēz) *n.* The monthly flow of blood and cellular debris from the uterus that begins at puberty and ceases at menopause.

men·stru·al (měn′strōō-əl) or **men·stru·ous** (-əs) *adj.* Of or relating to menstruation.

menstrual cycle *n.* The recurring cycle of physiological changes in the uterus and ovaries that occur from the beginning of one menstrual period through the beginning of the next.

menstrual period *n.* See **menses.**

men·stru·ate (měn′strōō-āt′) *v.* **-at·ed**, **-at·ing**, **-ates**. To undergo menstruation.

men·stru·a·tion (měn′strōō-ā′shən) *n.* The process or an instance of discharging the menses.

men·tal¹ (měn′tl) *adj.* **1.** Of or relating to the mind; intellectual. **2.** Of, relating to, or affected by a disorder of the mind. **3.** Intended for treatment of people affected with disorders of the mind.

mental² *adj.* Of or relating to the chin.

mental age *n.* A measure of mental development as determined by intelligence tests, generally restricted to children and expressed as the age at which that level is typically attained.

mental deficiency *n.* See **mental retardation.**

mental disease *n.* See **mental illness.**

mental disorder *n.* See **mental illness.**

mental illness *n.* Any of various disorders characterized chiefly by abnormal behavior or an inability to function socially, including diseases of the mind and personality and certain diseases of the brain.

mental image *n.* A mental picture of something not real or present produced by memory or imagination.

men·tal·i·ty (mĕn-tăl'ĭ-tē) *n.* The sum of a person's intellectual capabilities or endowment.

mental retardation *n.* Subnormal intellectual development or functioning that is the result of congenital causes, brain injury, or disease and is characterized by any of various deficiencies, ranging from impaired learning ability to social and vocational inadequacy.

men·thol (mĕn'thôl') *n.* A white crystalline organic compound obtained from peppermint oil or synthesized and used as a mild topical anesthetic and as a mint flavoring.

men·to·plas·ty (mĕn'tə-plăs'tē) *n.* Surgical alteration of the size or shape of the chin.

me·phi·tis (mə-fī'tĭs) *n.* An offensive smell.

me·piv·a·caine hy·dro·chlo·ride (mə-pĭv'ə-kān') *n.* A local anesthetic agent similar in action to lidocaine.

mep·ro·bam·ate (mĕp'rō-băm'āt', mĕ-prō'bə-) *n.* A bitter white powder used as a tranquilizer, a muscle relaxant, and an anticonvulsant.

mEq or **meq** *abbr.* milliequivalent

me·ral·gi·a (mə-răl'jē-ə, -jə) *n.* Pain in the thigh.

mer·bro·min (mər-brō'mĭn) *n.* A green crystalline compound that forms a red aqueous solution, used as a germicide and an antiseptic.

mer·cap·to·pu·rine (mər-kăp'tō-pyŏor'ēn) *n.* A purine analogue that acts as an antimetabolite by interfering with purine synthesis, used primarily in the treatment of acute leukemia.

Mer·cu·ro·chrome (mər-kyŏor'ə-krōm') A trademark used for a solution of merbromin.

mer·cu·ry (mûr'kyə-rē) *n.* A silvery-white poisonous metallic element with atomic number 80, liquid at room temperature and used in dental amalgams, thermometers, and batteries, and sometimes in pharmaceuticals.

mercury poisoning *n.* Poisoning caused by mercury or a compound containing mercury, with the acute form characterized by stomach ulcers and renal tubule toxicity and the chronic form affecting the central nervous system and causing emotional instability.

mer·cy killing (mûr'sē) *n.* Euthanasia.

mer·o·crine gland (mĕr'ə-krĭn, -krīn', -krēn') *n.* A gland whose secretory cells produce and discharge a secretion but are not destroyed or damaged during the process.

me·rog·o·ny (mə-rŏg'ə-nē) *n.* Incomplete development of an ovum.

mer·o·me·li·a (mĕr'ō-mē'lē-ə) *n.* Congenital absence of part of a limb.

me·ro·pi·a (mə-rō'pē-ə) *n.* Partial blindness.

me·ros·mi·a (mə-rŏz'mē-ə) *n.* A partial loss of the sense of smell leading to an inability to perceive certain odors.

me·rot·o·my (mə-rŏt'ə-mē) *n.* Division into parts, especially of a cell.

mer·o·zo·ite (mĕr'ə-zō'īt) *n.* A protozoan cell that arises from the schizogony of a parent sporozoan and may enter either the asexual or sexual phase of the life cycle.

mer·o·zy·gote (mĕr'ə-zī'gōt') *n.* An incomplete bacterial zygote containing only a fragment of the genome from one of its parent cells.

Merz·bach·er–Pelizaeus disease (mûrts'băk'ər-, mĕrts'bäкн'ər) *n.* A familial degenerative disease of the brain marked by progressive sclerosis of white substance of the frontal lobes, mental deficiency, and vasomotor disorders.

me·sal·a·mine (mə-săl'ə-mēn') *n.* A salicylate used as an anti-inflammatory gastrointestinal agent for the treatment of ulcerative colitis, proctosigmoiditis, and proctitis.

mes·an·gi·um (mĕs-ăn'jē-əm) *n.* The central part of the renal glomerulus between capillaries. — **mes·an'gi·al** *adj.*

mes·a·or·ti·tis (mĕs'ā-ôr-tī'tĭs) *n.* Inflammation of the middle layer of the aorta.

mes·en·ceph·a·lon (mĕz'ĕn-sĕf'ə-lŏn', mĕs'-) *n.* The portion of the vertebrate brain that develops from the middle section of the embryonic brain.

mes·en·ceph·a·lot·o·my (mĕz'ĕn-sĕf'ə-lŏt'ə-mē, mĕs'-) *n.* Surgical sectioning of any structure in the mesencephalon, especially of the pain-conducting tracts for the relief of unbearable pain.

mes·en·chyme (mĕz'ən-kīm', mĕs'-) *n.* The part of the embryonic mesoderm, consisting of loosely packed, unspecialized cells set in a gelatinous ground substance, from which connective tissue, bone, cartilage, and the circulatory and lymphatic systems develop. — **mes·en'chy·mal** (mĕz-ĕng'kə-məl, mĕs-, mĕz'ən-kī'məl, mĕs'-) *adj.*

mes·en·chy·mo·ma (mĕz'ən-kī-mō'mə, -kə-, mĕs'-) *n., pl.* **-mas** or **-ma·ta** (-mə-tə). A neoplasm containing a mixture of cells resembling those of the mesenchyme and its derivatives other than fibrous tissue.

mesenteric artery *n.* **1.** An artery with its origin in the aorta, with branches to the left colic, sigmoid, and superior rectal arteries. **2.** An artery with its origin in the aorta, with branches to the inferior pancreaticoduodenal, jejunal, ileal, ileocolic, appendicular, right colic, and middle colic arteries.

mes·en·ter·i·o·pex·y (mĕz'ən-tĕr'ē-ə-pĕk'sē, mĕs'-) *n.* Surgical fixation of a torn or incised mesentery.

mes·en·ter·i·or·rha·phy (mĕz'ən-tĕr'ē-ôr'ə-fē, mĕs'-) *n.* Suture of the mesentery.

mes·en·ter·i·pli·ca·tion (mĕz'ən-tĕr'ə-plĭ-kā'shən, mĕs'-) *n.* Surgical reduction of a mesentery by making one or more tucks in it.

mes·en·te·ri·um (mĕz'ən-tĕr'ē-əm, mĕs'-) *n., pl.* **-te·ri·a** (-tĕr'ē-ə). Mesentery.

mes·en·ter·y (mĕz'ən-tĕr'ē, mĕs'-) *n.* **1.** A double layer of peritoneum attached to the abdominal wall and enclosing in its fold certain organs of the abdominal viscera. **2.** A fold of the peritoneum that connects the intestines to the dorsal abdominal wall, especially such a fold that envelops the jejunum and ileum. — **mes'en·ter'ic** *adj.*

mes·mer·ism (mĕz'mə-rĭz'əm, mĕs'-) *n.* **1.** A strong or spellbinding appeal. **2.** Hypnotism.

mes·o·blast (mĕz'ə-blăst', mĕs'-) *n.* The middle germinal layer of an early embryo, consisting of undifferentiated cells destined to become the mesoderm. — **mes'o·blas'tic** *adj.*

mes·o·blas·te·ma (mĕz'ə-blă-stē'mə, mĕs'-) *n.* The cells that collectively constitute the early undifferentiated mesoderm. — **mes'o·blas·te'mic** (-stē'mĭk) *adj.*

mes·o·car·di·a (mĕz'ə-kär'dē-ə, mĕs'-) *n.* An atypical central position of the heart in the chest, as in the embryo.

mes·o·car·di·um (mĕz'ə-kär'dē-əm, mĕs'-) *n., pl.* **-di·a** (-dē-ə). Either of the two layers of the embryonic mesentery supporting the embryonic heart in the pericardial cavity.

mes·o·ca·val shunt (mĕz'ə-kā'vəl, mĕs'-) *n.* Anastomosis or graft anastomosis of the side of the superior mesenteric vein to the proximal end of the divided inferior vena cava for control of portal hypertension.

mes·o·co·lon (mĕz'ə-kō'lən, mĕs'-) *n.* The peritoneal fold attaching the colon to the posterior abdominal wall. — **mes'o·col'ic** (-kŏl'ĭk, -kō'lĭk) *adj.*

mes·o·col·o·pex·y (mĕz'ə-kŏl'ə-pĕk'sē, -kō'lə-) *n.* The surgical shortening of the mesocolon to suspend it or fix it in place.

mes·o·co·lo·pli·ca·tion (mĕz'ō-kō'lə-plĭ-kā'-shən, mĕs'-) *n.* See **mesocolopexy.**

mes·o·derm (mĕz'ə-dûrm', mĕs'-) *n.* The middle embryonic germ layer, lying between the ectoderm and the endoderm, from which connective tissue, muscle, bone, and the urogenital and circulatory systems develop. — **mes'o·der'mic** *adj.*

mes·o·lym·pho·cyte (mĕz'ə-lĭm'fə-sīt', mĕs'-) *n.* A mononuclear white blood cell of medium size, believed to be a lymphocyte, having a deeply staining nucleus that is relatively smaller than that in most lymphocytes.

mes·o·me·li·a (mĕz'ə-mē'lē-ə, mĕs'-) *n.* A condition in which the forearms and lower legs are abnormally short. — **mes'o·mel'ic** (-mĕl'ĭk) *adj.*

mes·o·mere (mĕz'ə-mêr', mĕs'-) *n.* **1.** A blastomere of intermediate size, larger than a micromere but smaller than a macromere. **2.** The middle zone of the mesoderm of a chordate vertebrate embryo, from which excretory tissue develops.

mes·o·morph (mĕz'ə-môrf', mĕs'-) *n.* A person having a robust, muscular body build in which tissues derived from the embryonic mesodermal layer predominate. — **mes'o·mor'phic** *adj.* — **mes'o·mor'phism, mes'o·mor'phy** *n.*

mes·o·neph·ros (mĕz'ə-nĕf'rəs, -rŏs', mĕs'-) *n., pl.* **-neph·roi** (-nĕf'roi'). The second of the three excretory organs that develop in a vertebrate embryo, replaced by the metanephros in humans and higher vertebrates. — **mes'o·neph'ric** *adj.*

mes·o·pex·y (mĕz'ə-pĕk'sē, mĕs'-) *n.* See **mesenteriopexy.**

mes·o·sig·moi·do·pex·y (mĕz'ō-sĭg-moi'də-pĕk'-sē, mĕs'-) *n.* The surgical fixation of the mesentery of the sigmoid flexure.

mes·o·the·li·o·ma (mĕz'ə-thē'lē-ō'mə, mĕs'-) *n., pl.* **-mas** or **-ma·ta** (-mə-tə). A rare neoplasm derived from cells lining the pleura and peritoneum and growing as a thick sheet composed of spindle cells or fibrous tissue covering the viscera.

mes·sen·ger RNA (mĕs'ən-jər) *n.* mRNA.

mes·tra·nol (mĕs'trə-nôl', -nōl') *n.* A synthetic estrogen used in combination with a progestin in oral contraceptive preparations.

Met *abbr.* methionine

me·tab·a·sis (mĭ-tăb'ə-sĭs) *n.* A change in the symptoms, course, or treatment of a disease.

met·a·bi·o·sis (mĕt'ə-bī-ō'sĭs) *n.* Dependence of one organism on another for the preparation of an environment in which it can live.

met·a·bi·sul·fite test (mĕt'ə-bī-sŭl'fīt') *n.* A test for sickle-cell hemoglobin in which red blood cells are deoxygenated by the addition of sodium metabisulfite and the cells containing the defective hemoglobin assume a sickle shape.

met·a·bol·ic (mĕt'ə-bŏl'ĭk) *adj.* Of, relating to, or resulting from metabolism.

metabolic acidosis *n.* Decreased pH and bicarbonate concentration of the body fluids caused either by the accumulation of excess acids stronger than carbonic acid or by abnormal losses of bicarbonate from the body.

metabolic alkalosis *n.* An increase in the alkalinity of body fluids due to an increase in alkali intake or a decrease in acidity, as from vomiting.

metabolic equivalent *n.* The energy expended while resting, usually calculated as the energy used to burn 3 to 4 milliliters of oxygen per kilogram of body weight per minute.

me·tab·o·lism (mĭ-tăb'ə-lĭz'əm) *n.* **1.** The physical and chemical processes occurring within a living cell or organism that are necessary for the maintenance of life. In metabolism some substances are broken down to yield energy for vital processes while other substances, necessary for life, are synthesized. **2.** The functioning of a specific substance, such as water, within the living body.

me·tab·o·lite (mĭ-tăb'ə-līt') *n.* **1.** A substance produced by metabolism. **2.** A substance necessary for or taking part in a metabolic process.

me·tab·o·lize (mĭ-tăb'ə-līz') *v.* **-lized, -liz·ing, -liz·es.** **1.** To subject to metabolism. **2.** To produce by metabolism. **3.** To undergo change by metabolism.

met·a·car·pal (mĕt'ə-kär'pəl) *adj.* Of or relating to the metacarpus. — *n.* Any of the five long bones that form the metacarpus and articulate with the bones of the distal row of the carpus and with the five proximal phalanges. — **met'a·car'pal·ly** *adv.*

met·a·car·pec·to·my (mĕt'ə-kär-pĕk'tə-mē) *n.* Surgical excision of one or all of the metacarpals of the hand.

met·a·car·pus (mĕt'ə-kär'pəs) *n., pl.* **-pi** (-pī). The part of the human hand that includes the five bones between the fingers and the wrist.

met·a·cen·tric chromosome (mĕt'ə-sĕn'trĭk) *n.* A chromosome with a centrally placed centromere that divides the chromosome into two arms of approximately equal length.

met·a·chro·ma·si·a (mĕt′ə-krō-mā′zē-ə, -zhə) *n.* The characteristic of a cell or tissue component of taking on a color different from that of the dye with which it is stained.

met·a·chro·ma·tic stain (mĕt′ə-krō-măt′ĭk) *n.* A stain that has the ability to produce different colors in various histological or cytological structures.

met·a·chro·ma·tism (mĕt′ə-krō′mə-tĭz′əm) *n.* Metachromasia.

met·a·gen·e·sis (mĕt′ə-jĕn′ĭ-sĭs) *n.* See **alternation of generations.**

me·tal fume fever (mĕt′l) *n.* An occupational disease caused by inhalation of particles and fumes of metallic oxides and characterized by malaria-like symptoms.

met·a·mor·pho·sis (mĕt′ə-môr′fə-sĭs) *n., pl.* **-ses** (-sēz′). **1.** A marked change in appearance, character, condition, or function. **2.** A usually degenerative pathological change in the structure of a particular body tissue. — **met·a·mor·phot′ic** (-môr-fŏt′ĭk) *adj.*

met·a·my·el·o·cyte (mĕt′ə-mī′ə-lə-sīt′) *n.* A transitional form of myelocyte having a nuclear construction intermediate between the mature myelocyte and the two-lobed granular white blood cell.

met·a·phase (mĕt′ə-fāz′) *n.* The stage of mitosis and meiosis, following prophase and preceding anaphase, during which the chromosomes align along the metaphase plate.

metaphase plate *n.* An imaginary plane perpendicular to the spindle fibers of a dividing cell, along which chromosomes align during metaphase.

me·taph·y·sis (mĭ-tăf′ĭ-sĭs) *n., pl.* **-ses** (-sēz′). The zone of growth between the epiphysis and diaphysis during development of a bone. — **met′a·phys′i·al** (mĕt′ə-fĭz′ē-əl, mĭ-tăf′ĭ-zē′əl, -sē′-) *adj.*

met·a·pla·sia (mĕt′ə-plā′zhə, -zhē-ə) *n.* **1.** Normal transformation of tissue from one type to another, as in the ossification of cartilage to form bone. **2.** Transformation of cells from a normal to an abnormal state.

met·a·plas·tic anemia (mĕt′ə-plăs′tĭk) *n.* Pernicious anemia in which the various elements in the blood change into multisegmented, unusually large neutrophiles, immature myeloid cells, and distorted platelets.

metaplastic polyp *n.* See **hyperplastic polyp.**

met·a·pro·ter·e·nol sulfate (mĕt′ə-prō-tĕr′-ə-nôl) *n.* A bronchodilator used for treating bronchial asthma.

met·a·psy·chol·o·gy (mĕt′ə-sī-kŏl′ə-jē) *n.* **1.** Philosophical inquiry supplementing the empirical science of psychology. Metapsychology deals with aspects of the mind that cannot be evaluated on the basis of objective or empirical evidence. **2.** A comprehensive system of psychology involving several different approaches to mental processes as described in the Freudian theory of the mind.

met·a·ru·bri·cyte (mĕt′ə-rōō′brĭ-sīt′) *n.* A normo-

blast that stains whatever color it is exposed to histologically.

me·tas·ta·sis (mə-tăs′tə-sĭs) *n., pl.* **-ses** (-sēz′). **1.** Transmission of pathogenic microorganisms or cancerous cells from an original site to one or more sites elsewhere in the body, usually by way of the blood vessels or lymphatics. **2.** A secondary cancerous growth formed by transmission of cancerous cells from a primary growth elsewhere in the body. — **met′a·stat′ic** (mĕt′ə-stăt′ĭk) *adj.*

me·tas·ta·size (mə-tăs′tə-sīz′) *v.* **-sized, -siz·ing, -siz·es.** To be transmitted or transferred by or as if by metastasis.

metastatic abscess *n.* A secondary abscess formed at a distance from the primary abscess, due to the transport of pyogenic bacteria through the lymph or blood.

met·a·tar·sal (mĕt′ə-tär′səl) *adj.* Of or relating to the metatarsus. — *n.* Any of the five long bones that form the anterior portion of the foot and articulate posteriorly with the three cuneiform and the cuboid bones and anteriorly with the five proximal phalanges. — **met′a·tar′sal·ly** *adv.*

met·a·tar·sec·to·my (mĕt′ə-tär-sĕk′tə-mē) *n.* Surgical excision of the metatarsus.

met·a·tar·sus (mĕt′ə-tär′səs) *n., pl.* **-si** (-sī, -sē). The middle part of the human foot that forms the instep and includes the five bones between the toes and the ankle.

met·a·trop·ic dwarfism (mĕt′ə-trŏp′ĭk, -trō′pĭk) *n.* A congenital skeletal dysplasia in which the development of dwarfism changes with time; at birth the trunk lengthens relative to the limbs but later it begins to shorten.

met·a·zo·on·o·sis (mĕt′ə-zō-ŏn′ə-sĭs, -zō′ə-nō′-) *n.* A zoonosis that requires both a vertebrate and an invertebrate host for completion of the life cycle of the infective organism.

met·en·ceph·a·lon (mĕt′ĕn-sĕf′ə-lŏn′) *n.* The anterior part of the embryonic hindbrain, which gives rise to the cerebellum and pons. — **met′en·ce·phal′ic** (-sə-făl′ĭk) *adj.*

me·te·or·ism (mē′tē-ə-rĭz′əm) *n.* See **tympanites.**

me·ter (mē′tər) *n.* The standard unit of length in the International System, equivalent to 39.37 inches.

met·es·trus (mĕ-tĕs′trəs) *n.* The period of sexual inactivity that follows estrus.

meth·a·done hydrochloride (mĕth′ə-dōn′) *n.* A potent addictive synthetic narcotic drug used to alleviate pain and as a substitute narcotic in the treatment of heroin addiction.

meth·am·phet·a·mine hydrochloride (mĕth′-ăm-fĕt′ə-mēn′, -mĭn) *n.* A crystalline amine used as a central nervous system stimulant and in the treatment of obesity.

meth·a·qua·lone (mĕth′ə-kwä′lōn′) *n.* A potentially habit-forming drug used as a sedative and hypnotic.

met·hem·al·bu·min (mĕt′hē-măl-byōō′mĭn) *n.* An abnormal albumin-heme complex formed in the blood during diseases that are characterized by extensive hemolysis.

met·he·mo·glo·bin (mĕt-hē′mə-glō′bĭn) *n.* A brownish-red crystalline organic compound formed in the blood when hemoglobin is oxidated either by decomposition of the blood or by the action of various oxidizing drugs or toxic agents. It contains iron in the ferric state and cannot function as an oxygen carrier.

met·he·mo·glo·bi·ne·mi·a (mĕt′hē-mə-glō′bə-nē′mē-ə) *n.* The presence of methemoglobin in the blood.

met·he·mo·glo·bi·nu·ri·a (mĕt′hē-mə-glō′bə-nŏŏr′ē-ə, -nyŏŏr′-) *n.* The presence of methemoglobin in the urine.

me·the·na·mine (mə-thē′nə-mēn′, -mĭn) *n.* An organic compound used as a urinary tract antiseptic.

meth·i·cil·lin (mĕth′ĭ-sĭl′ĭn) *n.* A synthetic antibiotic related to penicillin and most commonly used in treatment of infections caused by penicillinase-producing staphylococci.

me·thi·o·nine (mə-thī′ə-nēn′) *n.* A sulfur-containing essential amino acid obtained from various proteins or prepared synthetically and used as a dietary supplement and in pharmaceuticals.

me·thox·y·flu·rane (mə-thŏk′sē-flŏŏr′ān′) *n.* A potent, nonflammable, nonexplosive inhalation anesthetic.

meth·yl·cel·lu·lose (mĕth′əl-sĕl′yə-lōs′, -lōz′) *n.* A powdery substance that swells in water to form a gel, is prepared synthetically by the methylation of natural cellulose, and is used as a food additive, a bulk-forming laxative, an emulsifier, and a thickener.

meth·yl·do·pa (mĕth′əl-dō′pə) *n.* A drug used in the treatment of high blood pressure.

meth·yl·phen·i·date (mĕth′əl-fĕn′ĭ-dāt′, -fē′nĭ-) *n.* A drug chemically related to amphetamine, that acts as a mild stimulant of the central nervous system and is used especially in the form of its hydrochloride for the treatment of narcolepsy in adults and hyperkinetic disorders in children.

meth·yl·pred·nis·o·lone (mĕth′əl-prĕd-nĭs′ə-lōn′) *n.* An anti-inflammatory steroid administered to children and adolescents to relieve pain induced by sickle-cell anemia.

meth·yl·tes·tos·ter·one (mĕth′əl-tĕs-tŏs′tə-rōn′) *n.* A synthetic methyl derivative of testosterone used in the treatment of male sex hormone deficiency.

met·my·o·glo·bin (mĕt-mī′ə-glō′bĭn) *n.* Myoglobin in which the ferrous ion of the heme prosthetic group is oxidized.

me·ton·y·my (mə-tŏn′ə-mē) *n.* In schizophrenia, a language disturbance in which an inappropriate but related word is used in place of the correct one.

met·o·pon (mĕt′ə-pŏn′) *n.* A narcotic drug derived from morphine and used in the form of its hydrochloride as an analgesic.

met·o·po·plas·ty (mĕt′ə-pō-plăs′tē, mə-tŏp′ə-plăs′tē) *n.* The surgical repair of the skin or bone of the forehead.

me·tra (mē′trə) *n., pl.* **-trae** (-trē). See **uterus.**

me·trat·ro·phy (mī-trăt′rə-fē) or **me·tra·tro·phi·a** (mē′trə-trō′fē-ə) *n.* Atrophy of the uterus.

me·tri·a (mē′trē-ə) *n.* An inflammatory condition following childbirth, such as pelvic cellulitis.

met·ric (mĕt′rĭk) *adj.* Of or relating to the meter or the metric system.

metric system *n.* A decimal system of units based on the meter as a unit length, the kilogram as a unit mass, and the second as a unit time.

me·tri·tis (mĭ-trī′tĭs) *n.* Inflammation of the walls of the uterus.

me·tro·cyte (mē′trə-sīt′) *n.* See **mother cell.**

me·tro·fi·bro·ma (mē′trə-fī-brō′mə) *n.* A fibroma of the uterus.

me·tro·ni·da·zole (mĕt′rə-nī′də-zōl′) *n.* A synthetic antimicrobial drug used in the treatment of vaginal trichomoniasis and intestinal amebiasis.

me·trop·a·thy (mī-trŏp′ə-thē) or **me·tro·path·i·a** (mē′trə-păth′ē-ə) *n.* A disease of the uterus. — **me′tro·path′ic** *adj.*

met·ro·plas·ty (mē′trə-plăs′tē) *n.* See **uteroplasty.**

me·tror·rha·gi·a (mē′trə-rā′jē-ə, -jə) *n.* Bleeding from the uterus that is not associated with menstruation.

me·tro·sal·pin·gog·ra·phy (mē′trō-săl′pĭng-gŏg′rə-fē, -pĭn-) *n.* See **hysterosalpingography.**

me·tro·scope (mē′trə-skōp′) *n.* See **hysteroscope.**

mg *abbr.* milligram

MI *abbr.* myocardial infarction

mi·cren·ceph·a·ly (mī′krĕn-sĕf′ə-lē) or **mi·cro·en·ceph·a·ly** (mī′krō-ĕn-) *n.* The condition of having an abnormally small brain.

mi·cro·ab·scess (mī′krō-ăb′sĕs′) *n.* A very small circumscribed collection of white blood cells in solid tissues.

mi·cro·ad·e·no·ma (mī′krō-ăd′n-ō′mə) *n.* A very small pituitary adenoma thought to cause hypersecretion syndromes.

mi·cro·a·nas·to·mo·sis (mī′krō-ə-năs′tə-mō′sĭs) *n.* Anastomosis of minute structures performed with the aid of a surgical microscope.

mi·cro·a·nat·o·my (mī′krō-ə-năt′ə-mē) *n.* See **histology.** — **mi′cro·a·nat′o·mist** *n.*

mi·cro·an·eu·rysm (mī′krō-ăn′yə-rĭz′əm) *n.* A focal dilation of the venous end of retinal capillaries occurring in diabetes mellitus, retinal vein obstruction, and absolute glaucoma.

mi·cro·an·gi·og·ra·phy (mī′krō-ăn′jē-ŏg′rə-fē) *n.* Radiography of the minute blood vessels of an organ obtained by injection of a contrast medium and enlargement of the resulting radiograph.

mi·cro·an·gi·op·a·thy (mī′krō-ăn′jē-ŏp′ə-thē) *n.* See **capillaropathy.** — **mi′cro·an′gi·o·path′ic** (-ə-păth′ĭk) *adj.*

mi·cro·As·trup method (mī′krō-ăs′trəp) *n.* A interpolation technique for acid-base measurement.

mi·crobe (mī′krōb) *n.* A microorganism, especially a bacterium that causes disease; a minute life form. Not in technical use. — **mi·cro′bi·al** (mī-krō′bē-əl) *adj.*

mi·cro·bi·ol·o·gy (mī′krō-bī-ŏl′ə-jē) *n.* The branch of biology that deals with microorganisms and their effects on other living organisms. — **mi′cro·bi′o·log′ic** (-ə-lŏg′ĭk) *adj.* — **mi′cro·bi·ol′o·gist** *n.*

mi·cro·blast (mī′krə-blăst′) *n.* A small nucleated red blood cell.

mi·cro·ble·phar·i·a (mī′krō-blĕ-fâr′ē-ə) or **mi·cro·bleph·a·rism** (-blĕf′ə-rĭz′əm) or **mi·cro·bleph·a·ron** (-blĕf′ə-rŏn′) *n.* A rare developmental anomaly characterized by eyelids that are abnormally short.

mi·cro·car·di·a (mī′krō-kär′dē-ə) *n.* Abnormal smallness of the heart.

mi·cro·ceph·a·ly (mī′krō-sĕf′ə-lē) *n.* Abnormal smallness of the head. — **mi′cro·ce·phal′ic** (-sə-făl′ĭk) *adj.*

mi·cro·cin·e·ma·tog·ra·phy (mī′krō-sĭn′ə-mə-tŏg′rə-fē) *n.* The use of motion pictures taken through magnifying lenses to study an organ or system in motion.

mi·cro·cir·cu·la·tion (mī′krō-sûr′kyə-lā′shən) *n.* The flow of blood or lymph through the smallest vessels of the body, such as the venules, capillaries, and arterioles.

mi·cro·co·lon (mī′krō-kō′lən) *n.* An abnormally small colon, often developing because of a decreased functional state.

mi·cro·cyst (mī′krə-sĭst′) *n.* A minute cyst, often only observable microscopically.

mi·cro·cyte (mī′krə-sīt′) *n.* An abnormally small red blood cell that is less than five micrometers in diameter and may occur in certain forms of anemia. — **mi′cro·cyt′ic** (-sĭt′ĭk) *adj.*

mi·cro·cy·the·mi·a (mī′krō-sī-thē′mē-ə) *n.* The presence of microcytes in the blood.

mi·cro·fil·a·re·mi·a (mī′krō-fĭl′ə-rē′mē-ə) *n.* Infection of the blood with microfilariae.

mi·cro·fi·lar·i·a (mī′krō-fə-lâr′ē-ə) *n., pl.* **-i·ae** (-ē-ē′). The minute larval form of a filarial worm. — **mi′cro·fi·lar′i·al** *adj.*

mi·cro·gas·tri·a (mī′krō-găs′trē-ə) *n.* Abnormal smallness of the stomach.

mi·cro·ge·ni·a (mī′krō-jē′nē-ə) *n.* Abnormal smallness of the chin.

mi·crog·li·a (mī-krŏg′lē-ə) *n.* Any of the small neuroglial cells of the central nervous system having long processes and ameboid and phagocytic activity at sites of neural damage or inflammation.

mi·crog·li·o·ma (mī-krŏg′lē-ō′mə, mī′krō-glī-ō′mə) *n.* A brain neoplasm derived from microglial cells that is structurally similar to reticulum cell sarcoma.

mi·cro·glos·si·a (mī′krō-glŏs′ē-ə) *n.* Abnormal smallness of the tongue.

mi·cro·gna·thi·a (mī′krō-nā′thē-ə, mī′krŏg-nā′-) *n.* Abnormal smallness of the jaws, especially of the mandible.

mi·cro·graph (mī′krə-grăf′) *n.* A drawing or photographic reproduction of an object as viewed through a microscope.

mi·cro·he·pat·i·a (mī′krō-hǐ-păt′ē-ə) *n.* Abnormal smallness of the liver.

mi·cro·in·ci·sion (mī′krō-ĭn-sĭzh′ən) *n.* The destruction of cellular organelles by laser beam.

mi·cro·in·jec·tion (mī′krō-ĭn-jĕk′shən) *n.* Injection of minute amounts of a substance into a microscopic structure, such as a single cell.

mi·cro·in·va·sion (mī′krō-ĭn-vā′zhən) *n.* Invasion of in-situ carcinoma into tissue that is immediately adjacent; the earliest stage of malignant neoplastic invasion.

mi·cro·lith (mī′krə-lĭth′) *n.* A minute calculus, usually multiple and resembling coarse sand.

mi·cro·li·thi·a·sis (mī′krō-lǐ-thī′ə-sĭs) *n.* The formation, presence, or discharge of minute calculi or gravel.

mi·cro·ma·nip·u·la·tion (mī′krō-mə-nĭp′yə-lā′-shən) *n.* The manipulation of minute instruments and needles under a microscope in order to perform delicate procedures, such as microsurgery.

mi·cro·me·li·a (mī′krō-mē′lē-ə) *n.* Abnormal shortness or smallness of limbs. — **mi′cro·mel′ic** (-mĕl′ĭk, -mē′lĭk) *adj.*

mi·cro·mere (mī′krō-mēr′) *n.* A very small blastomere.

mi·cro·me·tas·ta·sis (mī′krō-mə-tăs′tə-sĭs) *n.* The spread of cancer cells from the primary site with the secondary tumors being too small to be clinically detected. — **mi′cro·met′a·stat′ic** (-mĕt′-ə-stăt′ĭk) *adj.*

mi·cro·me·ter (mī′krō-mē′tər) *n.* A unit of length equal to one thousandth (10^{-3}) of a millimeter or one millionth (10^{-6}) of a meter.

mi·cro·my·e·li·a (mī′krō-mī-ē′lē-ə) *n.* Abnormal smallness or shortness of the spinal cord.

mi·cro·my·e·lo·blast (mī′krō-mī′ə-lə-blăst′) *n.* A small myeloblast, often the predominant cell in myeloblastic leukemia.

mi·cron (mī′krŏn′) *n., pl.* **-crons** or **-kra** (-krə). See **micrometer.**

mi·cro·nu·cle·us (mī′krō-nōō′klē-əs, -nyōō′-) *n.* **1.** A minute nucleus. **2.** The smaller of two nuclei in ciliate protozoans that contains genetic material and functions in reproduction.

mi·cro·nu·tri·ent (mī′krō-nōō′trē-ənt, -nyōō′-) *n.* A substance, such as a vitamin or mineral, that is essential in minute amounts for the proper growth and metabolism of a living organism.

mi·cro·nych·i·a (mī′krō-nĭk′ē-ə) *n.* Abnormal smallness of the fingernails or toenails.

mi·cro·or·gan·ism (mī′krō-ôr′gə-nĭz′əm) *n.* An organism of microscopic or submicroscopic size, especially a bacterium or protozoan.

mi·cro·pa·thol·o·gy (mī′krō-pă-thŏl′ə-jē) *n.* The microscopic study of disease changes.

mi·cro·phage (mī′krə-fāj′) *n.* A small phagocytic white blood cell.

mi·cro·pho·ni·a (mī′krō-fō′nē-ə) or **mi·croph·o·ny** (mī-krŏf′ə-nē) *n.* Weakness of voice.

mi·croph·thal·mi·a (mī′krŏf-thăl′mē-ə) *n.* A condition in which the eyeball is abnormally small.

mi·croph·thal·mos (mī′krŏf-thăl′mŏs′) *n.* See **microphthalmia.**

mi·cro·pi·pette (mī′krō-pī-pĕt′) *n*. **1.** A very small pipette used in microinjection. **2.** A pipette used to measure very small volumes of liquids.

mi·cro·pleth·ys·mog·ra·phy (mī′krō-plĕth′ĭz-mŏg′rə-fē) *n*. The technique of measuring and recording minute changes in the size of a limb or organ as a result of the volume of blood flowing into and out of it.

mi·cro·po·di·a (mī′krō-pō′dē-ə) *n*. Abnormal smallness of the feet.

mi·crop·si·a (mī-krŏp′sē-ə) *n*. A visual disorder in which objects appear much smaller than they actually are; it may be due to a retinal disorder but is often associated with hallucination or other psychological condition.

mi·cro·punc·ture (mī′krō-pŭngk′chər) *n*. See **microincision**.

mi·cro·res·pi·rom·e·ter (mī′krō-rĕs′pə-rŏm′-ĭ-tər) *n*. An apparatus for measuring the utilization of oxygen by isolated tissues or cells.

mi·cro·scope (mī′krə-skōp′) *n*. **1.** An optical instrument that uses a lens or a combination of lenses to produce magnified images of small objects, especially of objects too small to be seen by the unaided eye. **2.** An instrument, such as an electron microscope, that uses electronic or other processes to magnify objects.

mi·cro·scop·ic (mī′krə-skŏp′ĭk) or **mi·cro·scop·i·cal** (-ĭ-kəl) *adj*. **1.** Too small to be seen by the unaided eye but large enough to be studied under a microscope. **2.** Of, relating to, or concerned with a microscope. **3.** Being or characterized as exceedingly small; minute.

mi·cros·co·py (mī-krŏs′kə-pē) *n*. **1.** The use of microscopes. **2.** Investigation by means of a microscope.

mi·cro·some (mī′krə-sōm′) *n*. A small particle in the cytoplasm of a cell, typically consisting of fragmented endoplasmic reticulum to which ribosomes are attached.

mi·cro·so·mi·a (mī′krə-sō′mē-ə) *n*. Abnormal smallness of the whole body, as in dwarfism.

mi·cro·spec·tro·pho·tom·e·try (mī′krō-spĕk′-trō-fō-tŏm′ĭ-trē) *n*. **1.** The technique of measuring the light absorbed, reflected, or emitted by the microscopic specimen at different wavelengths. **2.** Such a technique used to characterize and quantify nucleoproteins in single cells or cell organelles on the basis of their natural ultraviolet absorption spectra or after binding in selective cytochemical staining reactions.

mi·cro·spec·tro·scope (mī′krō-spĕk′trə-skōp′) *n*. A spectroscope used with a microscope for observing the spectra of microscopic objects.

mi·cro·sphyg·my (mī′krō-sfĭg′mē) *n*. A weak pulse that is difficult to detect manually.

mi·cro·sple·ni·a (mī′krō-splē′nē-ə) *n*. Abnormal smallness of the spleen.

mi·cro·steth·o·scope (mī′krō-stĕth′ə-skōp′) *n*. A stethoscope that amplifies the sounds heard.

mi·cro·sur·ger·y (mī′krō-sûr′jə-rē) *n*. Surgery on minute body structures or cells performed with the aid of a microscope and other specialized instruments, such as a micromanipulator.

mi·cro·su·ture (mī′krō-sōō′chər) *n*. Suture material having a tiny caliber and used in microsurgery.

mi·cro·sy·ringe (mī′krō-sə-rĭnj′, -sĕr′ĭnj) *n*. A hypodermic syringe having a micrometer screw attached to the piston, allowing accurately measured minute quantities of fluid to be injected.

mi·cro·tome (mī′krə-tōm′) *n*. An instrument used to cut a specimen, as of organic tissue, into thin sections for microscopic examination.

mi·crot·o·my (mī-krŏt′ə-mē) *n*. The preparation of specimens with a microtome. — **mi′cro·tom′ic** (mī′krə-tŏm′ĭk) *adj*.

mi·cro·tu·bule (mī′krō-tōō′byōōl, -tyōō-) *n*. Any of the proteinaceous cylindrical hollow structures that are distributed throughout the cytoplasm of eukaryotic cells, providing structural support and assisting in cellular locomotion and transport.

mi·cro·vil·lus (mī′krō-vĭl′əs) *n*., *pl*. **-vil·li** (-vĭl′ī′). Any of the minute hairlike structures projecting from the surface of certain types of epithelial cells, especially those of the small intestine.

mic·tion (mĭk′shən) *n*. See **urination**.

mic·tu·rate (mĭk′chə-rāt′, mĭk′tə-) *v*. **-rat·ed, -rat·ing, -rates**. To urinate.

mic·tu·ri·tion (mĭk′chə-rĭsh′ən, -tə-) *n*. **1.** See **urination**. **2.** The desire to urinate. **3.** The frequency of urination.

mi·daz·o·lam (mĭ-dăz′ə-lăm′) *n*. A colorless crystalline derivative of diazepam with sedative and anxiolytic properties, usually used in its hydrochloride form as an intravenous anesthetic.

mid·bod·y (mĭd′bŏd′ē) *n*. **1.** One of several granules composed of microtubules that forms between daughter cells during the telophase of mitosis. **2.** The anatomical middle region of the trunk of the body.

mid·brain (mĭd′brān′) *n*. See **mesencephalon**.

mid·dle age (mĭd′l) *n*. The time of human life between youth and old age, usually reckoned as the years between 40 and 60.

middle ear *n*. The space between the eardrum and the inner ear that contains the three auditory ossicles, which convey vibrations through the oval window to the cochlea.

middle lobe syndrome *n*. Atelectasis with chronic pneumonitis in the middle lobe of the right lung due to compression of the middle-lobe bronchus, usually by enlarged lymph nodes.

midge (mĭj) *n*. Any of various gnatlike flies, some of which serve as vectors for parasitic diseases.

mid·gut (mĭd′gŭt′) *n*. The middle section of the digestive tract in a vertebrate embryo from which the ileum, jejunum, and portions of the duodenum and colon develop.

mid·life (mĭd′līf′) *n*. See **middle age**. — *adj*. Of, relating to, or characteristic of middle age.

mid·life crisis (mĭd′līf′) *n*. A period of psychological doubt and anxiety that some people experience in middle age.

mid·line (mĭd′lĭn′) *n.* A medial line, especially the medial line or plane of the body.

midline myelotomy *n.* Severing of the midline transverse fibers of the spinal cord.

mid·riff (mĭd′rĭf) *n.* See **diaphragm** (sense 1).

mid·sag·it·tal plane (mĭd-săj′ĭ-tl) *n.* See **median plane**.

mid·sec·tion (mĭd′sĕk′shən) *n.* A middle section, especially the midriff of the human body.

mid·wife (mĭd′wīf′) *n., pl.* **-wives** (-wīvz′). A person, usually a woman, who is trained to assist women in childbirth. — *v.* **-wifed** or **-wived, -wif·ing** or **-wiv·ing, -wifes** or **-wives**. To assist in the birth of a baby.

mid·wife·ry (mĭd-wīf′ə-rē, mĭd′wīf′rē, -wī′fə-rē) *n.* The techniques and practice of a midwife including childbirth assistance, the independent care of essentially normal healthy women and infants before, during, and after childbirth, and, in collaboration with medical personnel, the consultation, management, and referral of cases in which abnormalities develop.

mi·graine (mī′grān′) *n.* A severe, recurring headache, usually affecting only one side of the head, characterized by sharp pain, often accompanied by nausea, vomiting, and visual disturbances.

mi·gra·tion (mī-grā′shən) *n.* The moving from place to place, as of disease symptoms.

migration inhibition test *n.* An in vitro method that uses macrophage antigenic sensitivity to test for cellular immune response.

Mi·ku·licz disease (mĭk′ə-lĭch′, mē′kŏŏ-) *n.* Benign swelling of the lacrimal glands and usually also of the salivary glands as a result of infiltration and replacement of the normal gland structure by lymphoid tissue.

Mikulicz drain *n.* A drain made of several strings of gauze placed into a wound and held together by a single layer of gauze.

Mikulicz operation *n.* Excision of the bowel in two stages: the diseased area is first exteriorized, enclosed by the abdomen around it, and excised; then the spur is cut and the stoma closed.

Miles′ operation (mīlz) *n.* Resection of the abdomen and perineum in cases of carcinoma of the rectum.

mil·i·ar·i·a (mĭl′ē-âr′ē-ə) *n.* See **heat rash**.

mil·i·ar·y (mĭl′ē-ĕr′ē) *adj.* **1.** Having the appearance of grains derived from haylike millet grass. **2.** Characterized by the presence of small skin lesions that have the size and appearance of millet seeds.

miliary abscess *n.* Any of numerous minute collections of pus widely disseminated throughout an area or the whole body.

miliary fever *n.* An infectious disease characterized by fever, profuse sweating, and the production of small, fluid-filled vesicles in the epidermis.

mi·lieu (mĭl-yŏŏ′, mē-lyœ′) *n., pl.* **-lieus** or **-lieux** (-lyœ′). The social setting of a mental patient.

milieu therapy *n.* Psychotherapy in which the social environment is arranged for the benefit of the patient.

mil·i·um (mĭl′ē-əm) *n., pl.* **-i·a** (-ē-ə). A small, white or yellowish cystlike mass just below the surface of the skin, caused by retention of the secretion of a sebaceous gland.

milk (mĭlk) *n.* **1.** A whitish liquid containing proteins, fats, lactose, and various vitamins and minerals that is produced by the mammary glands of all mature female mammals after they have given birth and serves as nourishment for their young. **2.** The milk of cows, goats, or other animals, used as food by humans. **3.** A liquid, such as coconut milk or various medical emulsions, that is similar to milk in appearance. — *v.* **milked, milk·ing, milks. 1.** To draw milk from the teat or udder of a female mammal. **2.** To press out, drain off, or remove by or as if by milking.

milk-alkali syndrome *n.* A chronic disorder of the kidneys that resembles nephrosis and is induced by protracted therapy of peptic ulcer with alkalis and a high milk regimen; it is reversible in its early stages.

milk crust *n.* Seborrhea of the scalp of an infant.

milk duct *n.* See **lactiferous duct**.

milk fever *n.* A slight elevation of temperature following childbirth, possibly due to the establishment of the secretion of milk.

milk leg *n.* A painful swelling of the leg occurring in women after childbirth as a result of clotting and inflammation of the femoral veins.

milk of magnesia *n.* A milky white aqueous suspension of magnesium hydroxide used as an antacid and a laxative.

milk ring test *n.* See **abortus Bang ring test**.

milk sugar *n.* See **lactose** (senses 1, 2).

milk tooth *n.* See **deciduous tooth**.

mil·li·e·quiv·a·lent (mĭl′ē-ĭ-kwĭv′ə-lənt) *n.* One thousandth (10^{-3}) of a gram equivalent of a chemical element, ion, radical, or compound.

mil·li·gram (mĭl′ĭ-grăm′) *n.* A metric unit of mass equal to one thousandth (10^{-3}) of a gram.

mil·li·li·ter (mĭl′ə-lē′tər′) *n.* A unit of of volume equal to one thousandth (10^{-3}) of a liter, 1 cubic centimeter, or about 15 minims.

mil·li·me·ter (mĭl′ə-mē′tər) *n.* A unit of length equal to one thousandth (10^{-3}) of a meter (0.0394 inch).

mi·me·sis (mĭ-mē′sĭs, mī-) *n.* **1.** The appearance of symptoms of a disease not actually present, often caused by hysteria. **2.** Symptomatic imitation of one organic disease by another.

mi·met·ic (mĭ-mĕt′ĭk, mī-) *adj.* **1.** Of or exhibiting mimicry. **2.** Of or relating to mimesis. — **mi·met′i·cal·ly** *adv.*

mim·ic (mĭm′ĭk) *v.* **-icked, -ick·ing, -ics. 1.** To resemble closely; simulate. **2.** To take on the appearance of. — **mim′ic** *adj. & n.*

Min·a·ma·ta disease (mĭn′ə-mä′tə) *n.* A degenerative neurological disorder caused by poisoning with a mercury compound found in seafood obtained from waters contaminated with mercury-containing industrial waste, characterized by burning or tingling sensations, poor articulation of speech, and the loss of coordination and peripheral vision.

mind (mīnd) *n.* **1.** The human consciousness that originates in the brain and is manifested especially in thought, perception, emotion, will, memory, and imagination. **2.** The conscious and unconscious processes in a sentient organism that direct and influence mental and physical behavior.

mind·set or **mind-set** (mīnd′sĕt′) *n.* **1.** A fixed mental attitude or disposition that predetermines a person's responses to and interpretations of situations. **2.** An inclination or a habit.

min·er·al (mĭn′ər-əl) *n.* An inorganic element, such as calcium, iron, potassium, sodium, or zinc, that is essential to the nutrition of humans, animals, and plants.

min·er·al·o·cor·ti·coid (mĭn′ər-ə-lō-kôr′tĭ-koid′) *n.* Any of a group of steroid hormones, such as aldosterone, that are secreted by the adrenal cortex and regulate the balance of water and electrolytes in the body.

mineral oil *n.* **1.** Any of various light hydrocarbon oils, especially a distillate of petroleum. **2.** A refined distillate of petroleum, used as a laxative.

mineral water *n.* Naturally occurring or prepared water that contains dissolved mineral salts, elements, or gases, and is often used therapeutically.

min·er's lung (mī′nərz) *n.* See **anthracosis.**

min·i·lap·a·rot·o·my (mĭn′ē-lăp′ə-rŏt′ə-mē) *n.* A method of female sterilization by surgical ligation of the fallopian tubes, performed through a small incision above the pubic symphysis.

min·i·mal brain dysfunction (mĭn′ə-məl) *n.* A mild impairment of brain function that affects perception, behavior, and academic ability, and is characterized by dyslexia, difficulty in writing, hyperactivity, or mental retardation.

min·i·stroke (mĭn′ē-strōk′) *n.* See **transient ischemic attack.**

Min·ne·so·ta mul·ti·pha·sic personality inventory test (mĭn′ĭ-sō′tə mŭl′tə-fā′zĭk, mŭl′tē-, -tĭ-) *n.* A psychological test for persons 16 or more years of age, consisting of a questionnaire containing statements to be agreed or disagreed with and coded in 14 personality scales.

mi·nor (mī′nər) *adj.* **1.** Lesser or smaller in amount, extent, or size. **2.** Lesser in seriousness or danger.

mi·o·car·di·a (mī′ō-kär′dē-ə) *n.* See **systole.** — **mi′o·car′di·al** *adj.*

mi·o·sis or **my·o·sis** (mī-ō′sĭs) *n., pl.* **-ses** (-sēz). **1.** The period of decline of a disease in which the intensity of the symptoms begins to diminish. **2.** Constriction of the pupil of the eye, resulting from a normal response to an increase in light or caused by certain drugs or pathological conditions.

mir·a·cle drug (mĭr′ə-kəl) *n.* A usually new drug that proves extraordinarily effective.

mir·ror-im·age cell (mĭr′ər-ĭm′ĭj) *n.* **1.** A cell whose nuclei have identical features and are placed in the cytoplasm in similar fashion. **2.** A

binucleate form of Reed–Sternberg cell often found in Hodgkin's disease.

mis·car·riage (mĭs′kăr′ĭj, mĭs-kăr′-) *n.* Premature expulsion of a nonviable fetus, especially before the middle of the second trimester; spontaneous abortion.

mis·car·ry (mĭs′kăr′ē, mĭs-kăr′ē) *v.* **-ried, -ry·ing, -ries.** To have a miscarriage; abort.

mis·ci·ble (mĭs′ə-bəl) *adj.* Capable of being and remaining mixed in all proportions. Used of liquids. — **mis′ci·bil′i·ty** *n.*

mis·di·ag·no·sis (mĭs-dī′əg-nō′sĭs) *n., pl.* **-ses** (-sēz). A diagnosis that is incorrect. — **mis·di′ag·nose′** *v.*

missed abortion (mĭst) *n.* An abortion in which the fetus dies but is retained in the uterus for two months or longer.

missed labor *n.* A condition in which a pregnant woman experiences uterine contractions at the normal term, but the contractions soon stop, and the fetus is retained, usually lifeless, within the uterus for an indefinite period.

mis·sense (mĭs′sĕns′) *n.* A section within a strand of mRNA containing a codon altered by mutation so that it codes for a different amino acid.

missense mutation *n.* A mutation in which a base change or substitution results in a codon that causes insertion of a different amino acid into the growing polypeptide chain, giving rise to an altered protein.

mite (mīt) *n.* Any of numerous small or minute arachnids of the order Acarina, certain species of which are parasitic on animals and plants, infest stored food products, and in some cases transmit disease.

mit·i·gate (mĭt′ĭgāt′) *v.* **-gat·ed, -gat·ing, -gates.** To moderate in force or intensity; alleviate. — **mit′i·ga′tion** *n.* — **mit′i·ga·tive, mit′i·ga·to′ry** (-gə-tôr′ē) *adj.*

mi·to·chon·dri·on (mī′tə-kŏn′drē-ən) *n., pl.* **-dri·a** (-drē-ə). A spherical or elongated organelle in the cytoplasm of nearly all eukaryotic cells, containing genetic material and many enzymes important for cell metabolism, including those responsible for the conversion of food to usable energy. It consists of an outer membrane and an inner membrane arranged to form cristae. — **mi′to·chon′dri·al** (-drē-əl) *adj.*

mi·to·gen·e·sis (mī′tə-jĕn′ĭ-sĭs) *n.* Induction of mitosis in a cell.

mi·to·my·cin (mī′tə-mī′sĭn) *n.* Any of a group of antibiotics produced by the soil actinomycete *Streptomyces caespitosus* that inhibit DNA synthesis and are used against bacteria and cancerous tumor cells.

mi·to·sis (mī-tō′sĭs) *n., pl.* **-ses** (-sēz). **1.** The process in cell division by which the nucleus divides, typically consisting of four stages (prophase, metaphase, anaphase, and telophase) and normally resulting in two new nuclei, each of which has exactly the same chromosome and DNA content as the original cell. **2.** The entire process of cell division including division of the nucleus and the cytoplasm. — mi·tot'ic (-tŏt'ĭk) *adj.* — mi·tot'i·cal·ly *adv.*

mitotic division *n.* See mitosis (sense 1).

mitotic figure *n.* The microscopic appearance of a cell undergoing mitosis.

mitotic spindle *n.* The fusiform figure characteristic of a dividing cell, consisting of microtubules, some of which become attached to each chromosome at its centromere and provide the mechanism for chromosomal movement.

mi·to·xan·trone hydrochloride (mī'tō-zăn'-trōn') *n.* A synthetic antineoplastic drug used intravenously in the initial therapy for acute non-lymphocytic leukemia in adults.

mitral atresia (mī'trəl) *n.* The congenital absence of the normal mitral valve orifice.

mitral cell *n.* Any of the large triangular nerve cells in the olfactory bulb.

mitral insufficiency *n.* Valvular insufficiency involving the mitral valve.

mi·tral·i·za·tion (mī'trə-lĭ-zā'shən) *n.* A straightening of the left heart border in a chest x-ray due to increased prominence of the left atrial appendage and/or the pulmonary salient.

mitral murmur *n.* A murmur produced at the mitral valve. It can be either obstructive or regurgitant.

mitral stenosis *n.* A narrowing of the mitral valve, usually caused by rheumatic fever, resulting in an obstruction to the flow of blood from the left atrium to the left ventricle.

mitral valve *n.* A valve of the heart, composed of two triangular flaps, that is located between the left atrium and left ventricle and regulates blood flow between these chambers.

mitral valve prolapse *n.* A condition in which there is excessive retrograde movement of the mitral valve into the left atrium during left ventricular systole, often allowing mitral regurgitation.

mit·tel·schmerz (mĭt'l-shmûrts', -shmĕrts') *n.* Abdominal pain occurring at the time of ovulation, resulting from irritation of the peritoneum by bleeding from the ovulation site.

mixed aphasia *n.* Combined motor and sensory aphasia.

mixed astigmatism *n.* Astigmatism in which one meridian is hyperopic while the one at a right angle to it is myopic.

mixed connective-tissue disease *n.* A disease of the connective tissues, combining features of systemic lupus erythematosus and systemic sclerosis or polymyositis and characterized by the presence of serum antibodies to nuclear ribonucleoprotein.

mixed gland *n.* **1.** A gland containing both serous and mucous secretory units. **2.** A gland having both exocrine and endocrine portions.

mixed lymphocyte culture test *n.* A test for histocompatibility of HLA antigens in donor and recipient lymphocytes.

mixed nerve *n.* A nerve that contains both sensory and motor fibers.

mixed paralysis *n.* Combined motor and sensory paralysis.

mixed tumor *n.* A tumor composed of two or more types of tissue.

mix·ture (mĭks'chər) *n.* **1.** A composition of two or more substances that are not chemically combined with each other and are capable of being separated. **2.** A preparation consisting of a liquid holding an insoluble medicinal substance in suspension by means of some viscid material.

ml *abbr.* milliliter

M line *n.* A fine dark band in the center of the H band in the myofibrils of striated muscle fibers.

mm *abbr.* millimeter

mmol *abbr.* millimole

MMR *abbr.* measles, mumps, rubella vaccine

mo·bi·lize (mō'bə-līz') *v.* -lized, -liz·ing, -liz·es. **1.** To make mobile or capable of movement. **2.** To restore the power of motion to a joint. **3.** To release into the body, as glycogen from the liver. — mo'bi·li·za'tion (-lĭ-zā'shən) *n.*

Mö·bi·us disease (mō'bē-əs, mœ'bē-ōōs) *n.* A periodic migraine headache accompanied by paralysis of the muscles that move the eyes.

Mö·bi·us' sign (mō'bē-ə-sīz, mœ'bē-ōōs) *n.* An indication of Graves' disease in which ocular convergence is impaired.

mo·dal·i·ty (mō-dăl'ĭ-tē) *n.* **1.** A therapeutic method or agent, such as surgery, chemotherapy, or electrotherapy, that involves the physical treatment of a disorder. **2.** Any of the various types of sensation, such as vision or hearing.

mod·el·ing (mŏd'l-ĭng) *n.* **1.** The acquisition of a new skill by observing and imitating that behavior being performed by another individual. **2.** In behavior modification, a treatment procedure in which the therapist models the target behavior which the learner is to imitate. **3.** A continuous process by which a bone is altered in size and shape during its growth by resorption and formation of bone at different sites and rates.

mod·i·fi·ca·tion (mŏd'ə-fĭ-kā'shən) *n.* Any of the changes in an organism caused by environment or activity and not genetically transmissable to offspring.

mod·i·fied radical mastectomy (mŏd'ə-fīd') *n.* Surgical removal of the entire breast and the lymphatic-bearing tissue in the armpit.

mo·di·o·lus (mō-dī'ə-ləs) *n., pl.* -li (-lī'). The central conical bony core of the cochlea of the ear.

mod·u·la·tion (mŏj'ə-lā'shən) *n.* The functional and morphological fluctuation of cells in response to changing environmental conditions.

moi·e·ty (moi'ĭ-tē) *n.* One of two or more parts into which something may be divided, such as the various parts of a vitamin or molecule.

moist gangrene *n.* A form of gangrene in which the necrosed part is moist and soft.

mo·lar (mō'lər) *n.* A tooth having a crown with three, four, or five cusps on the grinding surface, a bifid root in the lower jaw, and three conical roots in the upper jaw. In permanent dentition, there are three on either side behind the premolars; in deciduous dentition, there are two on either side behind the canines. — *adj.* **1.** Of or relating to the molars. **2.** Capable of grinding.

mold[1] (mōld) *n.* **1.** A frame around which something is formed or shaped. **2.** The shape of an artificial tooth or teeth. — *v.* **mold·ed, mold·ing, molds.** To change in shape. Used especially of the adaptation of the fetal head to the pelvic canal. — **mold′a·ble** *adj.*

mold[2] *n.* Any of various filamentous fungi, generally a circular colony having a woolly or furry appearance, that grow on the surface of organic matter and contribute to its disintegration.

mole (mōl) *n.* A small congenital growth on the skin, usually slightly raised and dark and sometimes hairy, especially a pigmented nevus.

mo·lec·u·lar (mə-lĕk′yə-lər) *adj.* Of, relating to, or consisting of molecules.

molecular disease *n.* A disease in which there is an abnormality in or a deficiency of a particular molecule, such as hemoglobin in sickle-cell anemia.

molecular knife *n.* A synthetic enzmye capable of cutting out and destroying specific genes such as those in a virus that control its replication or the production of a protein.

molecular surgery *n.* A technique used to increase the drug susceptibility of tumor cells by introducing gene segments into such cells so as to alter their drug resistance.

molecular weight *n.* The sum of the atomic weights of all the atoms in a molecule.

mol·e·cule (mŏl′ĭ-kyōōl′) *n.* The smallest particle into which an element or a compound can be divided without changing its chemical and physical properties; a group of like or different atoms held together by chemical forces.

mol·li·ti·es (mə-lĭsh′ē-ēz) *n.* See **malacia.**

mol·lus·cum (mə-lŭs′kəm) *n., pl.* **-ca** (-kə). Any of various skin diseases marked by the occurrence of soft spherical tumors on the face or other parts of the body.

molluscum con·ta·gi·o·sum (kən-tā′jē-ō′səm) *n.* An infectious disease of the skin caused by a virus of the family Poxviridae and marked by the appearance of small, pearly, umbilicated papular epithelial lesions containing numerous inclusion bodies.

molt (mōlt) *v.* **molt·ed, molt·ing, molts.** To shed periodically part or all of a coat or an outer covering, such as feathers, cuticle, or skin, which is then replaced by a new growth. — *n.* **1.** The act or process of molting. **2.** The material cast off during molting.

mo·lyb·de·num (mə-lĭb′də-nəm) *n.* A hard metallic element with atomic number 42 that is an essential trace element in plant and animal nutrition and is used to toughen alloy steels.

mon·as·ter (mŏn-ăs′tər) *n.* The single-star formation of chromosomes that forms at the equatorial plate at the end of prophase in mitosis.

mon·au·ral (mŏn-ôr′əl) *adj.* Of or relating to

sound reception by one ear. — **mon·au′ral·ly** *adv.*

monaural diplacusis *n.* A form of diplacusis in which one sound is perceived as two in the same ear.

mongolian spot *n.* Any of a number of dark-bluish or mulberry-colored spots on the lower back, observed in newborn infants, that enlarge for a short time after birth and then gradually recede.

Mon·gol·oid or **mon·gol·oid** (mŏng′gə-loid′, mŏn′-) *adj.* Of or relating to Down syndrome. Not in technical use. — *n.* A person affected with Down syndrome. No longer in technical use.

mo·nil·e·thrix (mə-nĭl′ə-thrĭks′) *n.* A condition in which the hair is brittle and shows a series of constrictions, resembling strings of spindle-shaped beads.

mo·nil·i·id (mə-nĭl′ē-ĭd) *n.* A skin condition characterized by minute macular or papular lesions, occurring as an allergic reaction to infection with a fungus of the genus *Candida.*

mon·i·tor (mŏn′ĭ-tər) *n.* A usually electronic device used to record, regulate, or control a process or system. — *v.* **-tored, -tor·ing, -tors.**

mon·o (mŏn′ō) *n.* Infectious mononucleosis.

mon·o·am·ine oxidase (mŏn′ō-ăm′ēn, -ə-mēn′) *n.* An enzyme in the cells of most tissues that catalyzes the oxidative deamination of monoamines such as norepinephrine and serotonin.

mon·o·clo·nal (mŏn′ə-klō′nəl) *n.* Of or relating to a protein from a single clone of cells, all molecules of which are the same.

monoclonal antibody *n.* Any of a class of highly specific antibodies that are produced by the clones of a single hybrid cell formed in the laboratory by the fusion of a B cell with a tumor cell. Such a hybrid cell and its clones allow the production of large amounts of a single antibody molecule, as opposed to the wide range of antibodies produced by an immune response.

mo·noc·ro·tism (mə-nŏk′rə-tĭz′əm) *n.* The state in which the pulse has a simple beat and produces a tracing that is smooth and without a downward notch.

mon·o·cyte (mŏn′ə-sīt′) *n.* A large, circulating, phagocytic white blood cell, having a single well-defined nucleus and very fine granulation in the cytoplasm. Monocytes make up from 3 to 8 percent of the white blood cells in humans. — **mon′o·cyt′ic** (-sĭt′ĭk), **mon′o·cy′toid** (-sĭ′toid′) *adj.*

mon·o·cy·to·pe·ni·a (mŏn′ə-sī′tə-pē′nē-ə) *n.* An abnormally low number of monocytes in the circulating blood.

mon·o·cy·to·sis (mŏn′ə-sī-tō′sĭs) *n.* An abnormal increase of monocytes in the blood, occurring in infectious mononucleosis and certain bacterial infections such as tuberculosis.

mon·o·der·mo·ma (mŏn′ō-dər-mō′mə) *n.* A neoplasm composed of tissues from a single germ layer.

mon·o·gen·e·sis (mŏn′ə-jĕn′ĭ-sĭs) *n.* **1.** The production of similar organisms in each generation. **2.** Asexual reproduction, as by sporulation or parthenogenesis. **3.** The process of parasitizing a single host, in or on which the entire life cycle of the parasite is passed. — **mon′o·ge·net′ic** (-jə-nĕt′ĭk) *adj.*

mon·o·ma·ni·a (mŏn′ə-mā′nē-ə, -mān′yə) *n.* Pathological obsession with one idea or subject, as in paranoia. — **mon′o·ma′ni·ac′** (-mā′nē-ăk′) *n.* — **mon′o·ma·ni′a·cal** (-mə-nī′ə-kəl) *adj.*

mon·o·neu·ri·tis (mŏn′ō-nŏŏ-rī′tĭs, nyŏŏ-) *n.* Inflammation of a single nerve.

mon·o·neu·rop·a·thy (mŏn′ō-nŏŏ-rŏp′ə-thē, -nyŏŏ-) *n.* Disease involving a single nerve.

mon·o·nu·cle·ar phagocyte system (mŏn′ō-nŏŏ′klē-ər, -nyŏŏ′-) *n.* A widely distributed collection of both free and fixed macrophages derived from bone-marrow precursor cells by way of monocytes; their substantial phagocytic activity is mediated by immunoglobulin and by the serum complement system.

mon·o·nu·cle·o·sis (mŏn′ō-nŏŏ′klē-ō′sĭs, -nyŏŏ-) *n.* **1.** The presence of abnormally large numbers of mononuclear white blood cells in the circulating blood, especially forms that are not normal. **2.** Infectious mononucleosis.

mon·o·nu·cle·o·tide (mŏn′ō-nŏŏ′klē-ə-tīd′, -nyŏŏ′-) *n.* A nucleotide consisting of one molecule each of a phosphoric acid, a sugar, and either a purine or a pyrimidine base.

mo·nop·a·thy (mə-nŏp′ə-thē) *n.* **1.** A single uncomplicated disease. **2.** A local disease affecting only one organ or part. — **mon′o·path′ic** (mŏn′-ə-păth′ĭk) *adj.*

mon·o·pho·bi·a (mŏn′ō-fō′bē-ə) *n.* An abnormal fear of being alone.

mon·o·phy·let·ic (mŏn′ō-fī-lĕt′ĭk) *adj.* **1.** Of or being the theory that all blood cells are derived from one common stem cell. — **mon′o·phy′le·tism** (-fī′lĭ-tĭz′əm) *n.*

mon·o·ple·gi·a (mŏn′ə-plē′jē-ə, -plē′jə) *n.* Paralysis of a single limb, muscle, or muscle group. — **mon′o·ple′gic** (-plē′jĭk) *adj.*

mon·o·po·lar cautery (mŏn′ə-pō′lər) *n.* Cauterization using high frequency electrical current passed from a single electrode where cauterization occurs; the patient's body serves as a ground.

mon·or·chism (mŏn-ôr′kĭz′əm) or **mon·or·chid·ism** (mŏn-ôr′kĭ-dĭz′əm) *n.* A condition in which only one testis is apparent, the other being absent or undescended. — **mon′or·chid′ic, mon′or′chid** *adj.*

mon·o·sac·cha·ride (mŏn′ə-săk′ə-rīd′, -rĭd) *n.* A carbohydrate that cannot be decomposed to a simpler carbohydrate by hydrolysis, especially one of the hexoses.

mon·o·so·di·um glutamate (mŏn′ə-sō′dē-əm) *n.* A white, odorless, crystalline compound that is the monosodium salt of a form of glutamic acid; it is used as a flavor enhancer in foods, where it may cause Chinese restaurant syndrome in sensitive people, and used intravenously as an adjunct in treating encephalopathies associated with liver disease.

mon·o·some (mŏn′ə-sōm′) *n.* **1.** A chromosome

having no homologue, especially an unpaired X-chromosome. **2.** A single ribosome, especially one that is combined with a molecule of messenger RNA. — **mon′o·so′mic** (-sō′mĭk) *adj.* — **mon′o·so′my** *n.*

mon·o·ther·mi·a (mŏn′ō-thûr′mē-ə) *n.* Evenness of body temperature throughout the day.

mons (mŏnz) *n., pl.* **mon·tes** (mŏn′tēz). An anatomical prominence or slight elevation above the general level of the surface.

mons pu·bis (pyŏŏ′bĭs) *n., pl.* **montes pubis.** A rounded fleshy protuberance situated over the pubic bones that becomes covered with hair during puberty.

mons ve·ne·ris (vĕn′ər-ĭs) *n., pl.* **montes veneris.** The female mons pubis.

mood (mŏŏd) *n.* A state of mind or emotion.

mood swing *n.* Alternation of a person's emotional state between periods of euphoria and depression.

moon face *n.* The round usually red face seen in Cushing's disease or in hyperadrenocorticalism.

MOPP (mŏp) *n.* A cancer chemotherapy drug consisting of Mustargen, Oncovin, procarbozine hydrochloride (Metulane) and prednisone.

mor·bid (môr′bĭd) *adj.* **1.** Relating to or caused by disease; pathological or diseased. **2.** Psychologically unhealthy or unwholesome. — **mor′bid·ness** *n.*

mor·bid·i·ty (môr-bĭd′ĭ-tē) *n.* **1.** The quality of being morbid; morbidness. **2.** A diseased state. **3.** The incidence or prevalence of a disease. **4.** Morbidity rate.

morbidity rate *n.* The proportion of patients with a particular disease during a given year per given unit of population.

morbid obesity *n.* The condition of weighing at least twice the ideal weight.

mor·bil·li (môr-bĭl′ī) *pl.n.* Measles; rubeola.

mor·bus (môr′bəs) *n., pl.* **-bi** (-bī). A disease.

mor·cel·la·tion (môr′sə-lā′shən) *n.* Division into and removal of small pieces, as of a tumor.

morcellation operation *n.* Vaginal hysterectomy in which the uterus is removed by lateral halves after being split.

mor. dict. *abbr. Latin.* more dicto (as directed)

mor·ga·gni·an cyst (môr-gän′yē-ən) *n.* A fluid-filled cyst attached to the fimbriated end of the uterine tube or to the upper end of the testis; it is a remnant of the embryonic mesonephric duct.

Mor·ga·gni's prolapse (môr-gä′nyēz) *n.* Chronic inflammation of the recessed areas in the wall of the larynx between the vestibular and vocal folds.

Mor·gan's bacillus (môr′gənz) *n.* A gram-negative aerobic bacterium, *Proteus morganii*, that occurs in the intestinal tract of humans and is present in normal and diarrheal stools.

morgue (môrg) *n.* A place in which dead bodies are temporarily kept until identified and claimed or until arrangements for burial have been made.

mo·ri·a (môr′ē-ə) *n.* **1.** Dullness of mind; mental lethargy. **2.** A mental state characterized by frivolity, joviality, and the inability to take anything seriously.

mor·i·bund (môr′ə-bŭnd′) *n*. At the point of death; dying. — **mor′i·bun′di·ty** (-bŭn′dĭ-tē) *n*.

morn·ing-af·ter pill (môr′nĭng-ăf′tər) *n*. A pill containing a drug, especially an estrogen or estrogen substitute such as diethylstilbestrol, that prevents implantation of a fertilized ovum and is therefore effective as a contraceptive after sexual intercourse.

morning sickness *n*. Nausea and vomiting upon rising in the morning, especially during early pregnancy.

mo·ron (môr′ŏn′) *n*. A person of mild mental retardation having a mental age of 7 to 12 years. The term is no longer in use and is considered offensive. — **mo·ron′ic** (mə-rŏn′ĭk, mô-) *adj*. — **mo′ron′ism, mo·ron′i·ty** (mə-rŏn′ĭ-tē, mô-) *n*.

Mo·ro's reflex (môr′ōz) *n*. See **startle reflex** (sense 1).

mor·phe·a (môr-fē′ə) *n*. A localized form of scleroderma characterized by hardened, slightly depressed patches of dermal fibrous tissue.

mor·phine (môr′fēn′) *n*. A bitter crystalline alkaloid extracted from opium, the soluble salts of which are used in medicine as an analgesic, a light anesthetic, or a sedative.

mor·phin·ism (môr′fē-nĭz′əm, môr′fə-) *n*. **1.** Addiction to morphine. **2.** A diseased condition caused by habitual or addictive use of morphine.

mor·pho·gen·e·sis (môr′fō-jĕn′ĭ-sĭs) *n*. Differentiation of cells and tissues in the early embryo which results in establishing the form and structure of the various organs and parts of the body. — **mor′pho·ge·net′ic** (-jə-nĕt′ĭk), **mor′pho·gen′ic** *adj*.

morphogenetic movement *n*. The movement of cells in the early embryo that change the shape or form of differentiating cells and tissues.

mor·phol·o·gy (môr-fŏl′ə-jē) *n*. **1.** The branch of biology that deals with the form and structure of organisms without consideration of function. **2.** The form and structure of an organism or one of its parts. — **mor′pho·log′i·cal** (-fə-lŏj′ĭ-kəl), **mor′pho·log′ic** *adj*. — **mor′pho·log′o·gist** *n*.

mor·pho·sis (môr-fō′sĭs) *n., pl.* **-ses** (-sēz). The manner in which an organism or any of its parts changes form or undergoes development.

mors (môrz) *n*. Death.

mor. sol. *abbr. Latin.* more solito (as usual, as customary)

mor·tal (môr′tl) *n*. **1.** Liable or subject to death. **2.** Causing death; fatal.

mor·tal·i·ty (môr-tăl′ĭ-tē) *n*. **1.** The quality or condition of being mortal. **2.** Death rate.

mortality rate *n*. See **death rate**.

mor·ti·fi·ca·tion (môr′tə-fĭ-kā′shən) *n*. Death or decay of one part of a living body; gangrene or necrosis.

mor·ti·fy (môr′tə-fī′) *v*. **-fied, -fy·ing, -fies.** To undergo mortification; become gangrenous or necrosed.

mor·tu·ar·y (môr′chōō-ĕr′ē) *n*. A place, especially

a funeral home, where dead bodies are kept before burial or cremation.

mor·u·la (môr′yə-lə, môr′ə-) *n., pl.* **-lae** (-lē′). The spherical embryonic mass of blastomeres formed before the blastula and resulting from cleavage of the fertilized ovum. — **mor′u·lar** *adj*. — **mor′u·la′tion** *n*.

mo·sa·ic inheritance (mō-zā′ĭk) *n*. Inheritance in which the paternal influence is dominant in one group of cells and the maternal influence is dominant in another.

mo·sa·i·cism (mō-zā′ĭ-sĭz′əm) *n*. A condition in which tissues of genetically different types occur in the same organism.

mosaic wart *n*. A grouping of numerous, closely aggregated plantar warts on the sole of the foot.

mos·qui·to (mə-skē′tō) *n., pl.* **-toes** or **-tos.** Any of various two-winged insects of the family Culicidae, in which the female of most species is distinguished by a long proboscis for sucking blood. Some species are vectors of diseases such as malaria and yellow fever.

mosquito forceps or **mosquito clamp** *n*. A small, straight or curved hemostatic forceps used to hold delicate tissue or compress a bleeding vessel.

Mosz·ko·wicz's test (mŏs′kə-wĭts′, -wĭt′sĭz) *n*. A test for arteriosclerosis performed by monitoring the return of color to a limb that has had its blood flow inhibited for a short period.

Mo·tais operation (mō-tā′, mô-tĕ′) *n*. Transplantation of the middle third of the tendon of the superior rectus muscle of the eyeball into the upper lid to supplement the action of the levator muscle in cases of ptosis.

moth·er (mŭth′ər) *n*. **1.** A woman who conceives, gives birth to, or raises and nurtures a child. **2.** A female parent of an animal. **3.** A structure, such as a mother cell, from which other similar bodies are formed.

mother cell *n*. A cell that divides to produce two or more daughter cells.

mo·tile (mōt′l, mō′tīl′) *adj*. **1.** Moving or having the power to move spontaneously. **2.** Of or relating to mental imagery that arises primarily from sensations of bodily movement and position rather than from visual or auditory sensations. — **mo·til′i·ty** (mō-tĭl′ĭ-tē) *n*.

mo·tion (mō′shən) *n*. **1.** The act or process of changing position or place. **2.** The manner in which the body or a body part moves.

mo·tion sickness (mō′shən) *n*. Nausea and dizziness induced by motion, as in travel by aircraft, car, or ship.

mo·to·neu·ron (mō′tə-nŏŏr′ŏn′, -nyŏŏr′-) *n*. A motor neuron.

mo·tor (mō′tər) *adj*. **1.** Causing or producing motion. **2.** Of or being nerves that carry impulses from the nerve centers to the muscles. **3.** Involving or relating to movements of the muscles. **4.** Of or relating to an organism's overt reaction to a stimulus.

motor area *n*. See **motor cortex**.

motor ataxia *n*. Inability to perform coordinated

muscular movements necessary for moving the body, as for walking.

motor cortex *n.* The region of the cerebral cortex influencing movements of the face, neck and trunk, and arm and leg.

motor fiber *n.* Any of the fibers in a mixed nerve that transmit motor impulses.

motor image *n.* The cerebral image of possible body movements.

motor nerve *n.* An efferent nerve conveying an impulse that excites muscular contraction.

motor neuron *n.* A neuron that conveys impulses from the central nervous system to a muscle, gland, or other effector tissue.

motor neuron disease *n.* Any of various diseases of motor neurons, such as progressive muscular atrophy, amyotrophic lateral sclerosis, progressive bulbar paralysis, and primary lateral sclerosis.

motor paralysis *n.* Loss of the power of muscular contraction.

mount (mount) *v.* **mount·ed, mount·ing, mounts.** To prepare a specimen for microscopic examination, especially by positioning on a slide.

moun·tain sickness (moun′tən) *n.* Altitude sickness brought on by the diminished oxygen pressure at mountain elevations.

mouse-tooth forceps *n.* A forceps with one or two fine teeth at the tip of each blade that mesh with the tooth or teeth on the opposite blade.

mouth (mouth) *n.,* pl. **mouths** (mou*th*z). **1.** The oral cavity. **2.** The opening to any cavity or canal in an organ or a bodily part.

mouth-to-mouth respiration *n.* See **mouth-to-mouth resuscitation.**

mouth-to-mouth resuscitation *n.* A technique used to resuscitate a person who has stopped breathing, in which the rescuer presses his or her mouth against the mouth of the victim and, allowing for passive exhalation, forces air into the lungs at intervals of several seconds.

mouth·wash (mouth′wŏsh′) *n.* A medicated liquid used for cleaning the mouth and treating diseased states of its mucous membranes.

mov·a·ble joint (mōō′və-bəl) *n.* **1.** A joint in which the opposing bony surfaces are covered with a layer of hyaline cartilage or fibrocartilage and in which some degree of free movement is possible. **2.** A joint, either a synchondrosis or a symphysis, in which the apposed bony surfaces are united by cartilage.

movable testis *n.* A condition in which the testis tends to ascend to the upper part of the scrotum or into the inguinal canal.

move·ment (mōōv′mənt) *n.* **1.** The act or an instance of moving; a change in place or position. **2.** An evacuation of the bowels; defecation.

M protein *n.* A surface protein present on strep bacteria that prevents white blood cells from engulfing and destroying the bacteria.

MRI *abbr.* magnetic resonance imaging

mRNA (ĕm′är-ĕn-ā′) *n.* Messenger RNA; the form of RNA, synthesized from a DNA template during transcription, that mediates the transfer of genetic information from the cell nucleus to ribosomes in the cytoplasm, where it serves as a template for protein synthesis.

ms *abbr.* millisecond

MS *abbr.* multiple sclerosis

msec *abbr.* millisecond

MSG *abbr.* monosodium glutamate

mu·ci·lage (myōō′sə-lĭj) *n.* A viscid preparation consisting of a solution of a plant-based gum in water and used in pharmacy as a diluent or vehicle for a drug.

mu·cin (myōō′sĭn) *n.* Any of a group of glycoproteins found especially in the secretions of mucous membranes. — **mu′cin·ous** *adj.*

mu·ci·ne·mi·a (myōō′sə-nē′mē-ə) *n.* The presence of mucin in the blood.

mucinous carcinoma *n.* An adenocarcinoma in which the neoplastic cells secrete significant amounts of mucin.

muciparous gland *n.* See **mucous gland.**

mu·co·cele (myōō′kə-sēl′) *n.* **1.** A mucous polyp. **2.** A retention cyst of the lacrimal sac, paranasal sinuses, appendix, or gallbladder.

mu·co·lip·i·do·sis (myōō′kō-lĭp′ĭ-dō′sĭs) *n.* Any of a group of hereditary metabolic storage diseases resembling Hurler's syndrome but with normal urinary mucopolysaccharides.

mu·co·pol·y·sac·cha·ride (myōō′kō-pŏl′ē-săk′-ə-rīd′) *n.* Any of a group of polysaccharides with high molecular weight that contain amino sugars and often form complexes with proteins.

mu·co·pol·y·sac·cha·ri·do·sis (myōō′kō-pŏl′ē-săk′ə-rĭ-dō′sĭs) *n.* Any of several inherited diseases of mucopolysaccharide metabolism characterized by the accumulation of mucopolysaccharides in the tissues and their excretion in the urine and resulting in various defects of bone, cartilage, and connective tissue.

mu·co·pol·y·sac·cha·ri·du·ri·a (myōō′kō-pŏl′ē-săk′ə-rĭ-dōōr′ē-ə, -dyōōr′-) *n.* The excretion of mucopolysaccharides in the urine.

mu·co·pro·tein (myōō′kō-prō′tēn′, -prō′tē-ĭn) *n.* Any of a group of organic compounds, such as the mucins, that consist of a complex of proteins and glycosaminoglycons and are found in body tissues and fluids.

mu·co·sa (myōō-kō′sə) *n.,* pl. **-sas** or **-sae** (-sē). See **mucous membrane.** — **mu·co′sal** *adj.*

mu·co·sec·to·my (myōō′kə-sĕk′tə-mē) *n.* Excision of the mucosa, usually of the rectum prior to ileoanal anastomosis for treatment of ulcerative colitis.

mu·cous (myōō′kəs) *adj.* **1.** Containing, producing, or secreting mucus. **2.** Relating to, consisting of, or resembling mucus.

mucous cell *n.* A cell secreting mucus, such as a goblet cell.

mucous colitis *n.* A disease of the mucous membrane of the colon, characterized by colicky pain, constipation or diarrhea, and the passage of mucous or slimy pseudomembranous shreds and patches.

mucous connective tissue *n.* A gelatinous type of connective tissue, characteristically supporting the blood vessels of the umbilical cord.

mucous gland *n.* A gland that secretes mucus.

mucous membrane *n.* A membrane lining all body passages that communicate with the exterior, such as the respiratory, genitourinary, and alimentary tracts, and having cells and associated glands that secrete mucus.

mucous plug *n.* A mass of mucus and cells filling the cervical canal between menstrual periods or during pregnancy.

mu·cus (myōō′kəs) *n.* The viscous, slippery substance that consists chiefly of mucin, water, cells, and inorganic salts and is secreted as a protective lubricant coating by cells and glands of the mucous membranes.

mud fever *n.* Leptospirosis caused by spirochete, *Leptospira grippotyphosa.*

Muehr·cke's lines (mōōr′kəz, mür′-) *n.* Parallel white lines in the fingernails and toenails associated with hypoalbuminemia.

mül·le·ri·an duct (myōō-lêr′ē-ən, -lêr′-) *n.* Either of two embryonic tubes extending along the mesonephros that form the uterine tubes, uterus, and part of the vagina in the female and the prostatic utricle in the male.

mul·ti·ar·tic·u·lar (mŭl′tē-är-tĭk′yə-lər, mŭl′tī-) *adj.* Relating to or involving many joints.

mul·ti·cel·lu·lar (mŭl′tē-sĕl′yə-lər, -tī-) *adj.* Having or consisting of many cells. — **mul′ti·cel′lu·lar′i·ty** *n.*

mul·ti·fac·to·ri·al inheritance (mŭl′tĭ-făk-tôr′ē-əl) *n.* Inheritance involving many factors, of which at least one is genetic but none is of overwhelming importance, as in the causation of a disease by multiple genetic and environmental factors.

mul·ti·form (mŭl′tə-fôrm′) *adj.* Occurring in or having many forms or shapes; polymorphic. — **mul′ti·for′mi·ty** (-fôr′mĭ-tē) *n.*

mul·ti·grav·i·da (mŭl′tĭ-grăv′ĭ-də) *n.* A pregnant woman who has had one or more previous pregnancies.

mul·ti·in·fec·tion (mŭl′tē-ĭn-fĕk′shən, mŭl′tī-) *n.* A mixed infection with two or more varieties of microorganisms developing simultaneously.

mul·ti·la·mel·lar body (mŭl′tē-lə-mĕl′ər, -tī-) *n.* See **cytosome** (sense 2).

multinuclear leukocyte *n.* See **polymorphonuclear leukocyte.**

mul·tip·a·ra (mŭl-tĭp′ər-ə) *n.,* pl. **-ras** or **-rae** (-rē). A woman who has given birth two or more times.

mul·ti·par·i·ty (mŭl′tĭ-păr′ĭ-tē) *n.* The condition of being a multipara.

mul·ti·ple fission (mŭl′tə-pəl) *n.* Division of the nucleus, simultaneously or successively, into a number of daughter nuclei, followed by division of the cell body into an equal number of parts, each containing a nucleus.

multiple fracture *n.* The simultaneous fracture of several bones.

multiple myeloma *n.* A malignant proliferation of plasma cells in bone marrow causing numerous tumors and characterized by the presence of abnormal proteins in the blood.

multiple neurofibroma *n.* See **neurofibromatosis.**

multiple personality *n.* A dissociative disorder in which two or more distinct personalities exist in the same person, each of which prevails at a particular time.

multiple pregnancy *n.* The state of bearing two or more fetuses simultaneously.

multiple puncture tuberculin test *n.* A test in which the tuberculin or purified protein is inserted under the skin by repeated punctures with several needles or prongs.

multiple sclerosis *n.* A chronic degenerative disease of the central nervous system in which gradual destruction of myelin occurs in patches throughout the brain or spinal cord or both, interfering with nerve pathways and causing muscular weakness, loss of coordination, and speech and visual disturbances. It may be caused by an immune system defect of genetic or viral origin.

multiple vision *n.* See **polyopia.**

mul·ti·pli·ca·tion (mŭl′tə-plĭ-kā′shən) *n.* **1.** The act or process of multiplying or the condition of being multiplied. **2.** Propagation of plants and animals; procreation.

mul·ti·pli·ca·tive division (mŭl′tə-plĭk′ə-tĭv, mŭl′tə-plĭ-kā′tĭv) *n.* Reproduction by simultaneous division of a mother cell into a number of daughter cells.

mul·ti·ply (mŭl′tə-plī′) *v.* **-plied, -ply·ing, -plies. 1.** To increase the amount, number, or degree of. **2.** To breed or propagate.

mul·ti·vi·ta·min (mŭl′tə-vī′tə-mĭn) *adj.* Containing many vitamins. — *n.* A preparation containing many vitamins.

mum·mi·fi·ca·tion (mŭm′ə-fĭ-kā′shən) *n.* The shrivelling of a dead and retained fetus.

mumps (mŭmps) *pl.n.* An acute, inflammatory, contagious disease caused by a paramyxovirus and characterized by swelling of the salivary glands, especially the parotids, and sometimes of the pancreas, ovaries, or testes. It mainly affects children and can be prevented by vaccination.

mumps skin test antigen *n.* A sterile suspension of killed mumps virus used to determine mumps susceptibility or to confirm a tentative diagnosis.

mumps virus *n.* A virus of the genus *Paramyxovirus* that causes parotitis and is transmitted by infected salivary secretions.

mumps virus vaccine *n.* A vaccine containing live attenuated mumps virus prepared in chick embryo cell cultures, used to immunize against mumps.

Mun·chau·sen syndrome or **Munch·hau·sen syndrome** (mŭn′chou′zən, mŭnch′hou′-, mü̃nKH′hou′-) *n.* A psychological disorder characterized by the repeated fabrication of disease symptoms for the purpose of gaining medical attention.

Mun·ro's abscess (mən-rōz′) *n.* See **Munro's microabscess.**

Munro's microabscess *n.* A microscopic collection

of polymorphonuclear white blood cells found in the stratum corneum in psoriasis.

mu·ram·i·dase (myo͞o-răm′ĭ-dās′, -dāz′) *n.* See **lysozyme.**

mu·rine (myo͝or′īn′) *n.* Of, relating to, or transmitted by a member of the rodent family Muridae, including rats and mice.

murine typhus *n.* A comparatively mild, acute, endemic form of typhus caused by the microorganism *Rickettsia typhi,* transmitted from rats to humans by fleas and characterized by fever, headache, and muscular pain.

mur·mur (mûr′mər) *n.* An abnormal sound heard on auscultation of the heart, lungs, or blood vessels.

Mur·phy drip (mûr′fē) *n.* See **proctoclysis.**

mus·cae vol·i·tan·tes (mŭs′ē vŏl′ĭ-tăn′tēz, mŭs′-kē) *n.* An appearance of moving specks or threads before the eyes; floaters.

mus·cle (mŭs′əl) *n.* **1.** A tissue consisting predominantly of contractile cells and classified as skeletal, cardiac, or smooth, the last lacking transverse striations characteristic of the first two. **2.** Any of the contractile organs of the body by which movements of the various organs and parts are effected, and whose fibers are usually attached at each extremity to a bone or other structure by a tendon.

muscle fiber *n.* A cylindrical, multinucleate cell composed of numerous myofibrils that contracts when stimulated.

muscle hemoglobin *n.* See **myoglobin.**

mus·cu·lar (mŭs′kyə-lər) *adj.* **1.** Of, relating to, or consisting of muscle. **2.** Having well-developed muscles.

muscular anesthesia *n.* Loss of muscle sense, specifically loss of the ability to determine the position of a limb or to distinguish differences in weight.

muscular dystrophy *n.* **1.** Any of a group of progressive muscle disorders caused by a defect in one or more genes that control muscle function and characterized by gradual irreversible wasting of skeletal muscle. **2.** Pseudohypertrophic muscular dystrophy.

mus·cu·lar·i·ty (mŭs′kyə-lăr′ĭ-tē) *n.* The state or condition of having well-developed muscles.

muscular relaxant *n.* An agent that relaxes striated muscle.

muscular system *n.* All the muscles of the body collectively, especially the voluntary skeletal muscles.

mus·cu·la·ture (mŭs′kyə-lə-cho͝or′) *n.* The arrangement of the muscles in a part or in the body as a whole.

mus·cu·lo·skel·e·tal (mŭs′kyə-lō-skĕl′ĭ-tl) *adj.* Relating to or involving the muscles and the skeleton.

mus·cu·lo·spi·ral paralysis (mŭs′kyə-lō-spī′rəl) *n.* Paralysis of the muscles of the forearm due to injury of the radial nerve.

mu·si·co·ther·a·py (myo͞o′zĭ-cō-thĕr′ə-pē) *n.* The treatment of mental disorders by means of music.

Mus·set's sign (mo͞o-sāz′, mü-) *n.* An indication of aortic insufficiency in which the head rhythmically nods in synchrony with the heartbeat.

mus·si·ta·tion (mŭs′ĭ-tā′shən) *n.* Movements of the lips as if speaking, but without sound.

Mus·tard operation (mŭs′tərd) *n.* Correction of abnormal blood circulation due to the transposition of the great arteries through creation of an intra-arterial baffle that partitions the atrium.

mustard plaster *n.* A medicinal plaster made with a pastelike mixture of powdered black mustard, flour, and water, used especially as a counterirritant.

mu·ta·cism (myo͞o′tə-sĭz′əm) *n.* See **mytacism.**

mu·ta·gen (myo͞o′tə-jən, -jĕn′) *n.* An agent, such as ultraviolet light or a radioactive element, that can induce or increase the frequency of mutation in an organism. — **mu′ta·gen′ic** *adj.* — **mu′ta·gen′i·cal·ly** *adv.* — **mu′ta·ge·nic′i·ty** (-jə-nĭs′ĭ-tē) *n.*

mu·ta·gen·e·sis (myo͞o′tə-jĕn′ĭ-sĭs) *n., pl.* **-ses** (-sēz′). The formation or development of a mutation.

mu·ta·gen·ize (myo͞o′tə-jĕn′īz) *v.* **-ized, -iz·ing, -iz·es.** To cause or induce mutation in a cell or an organism.

mu·tant (myo͞ot′nt) *n.* An organism possessing one or more genes that have undergone mutation. — *adj.* Resulting from or undergoing mutation.

mutant gene *n.* A gene that has lost, gained, or exchanged some of the material it received from its parent, resulting in a permanent transmissible change in its function.

mu·ta·tion (myo͞o-tā′shən) *n.* **1.** The act or process of being altered or changed. **2.** A sudden structural change within a gene or chromosome of an organism resulting in the creation of a new character or trait not found in the parental type. **3.** The process by which such a sudden structural change occurs, either through an alteration in the nucleotide sequence of the DNA coding for a gene or through a change in the physical arrangement of a chromosome. **4.** A mutant. — **mu·ta′tion·al** *adj.* — **mu·ta′tion·al·ly** *adv.*

mute (myo͞ot) *adj.* Unable or unwilling to speak.

mu·tein (myo͞o′tēn′, -tē-ĭn) *n.* A protein arising as a result of a mutation.

mu·ti·la·tion (myo͞ot′l-ā′shən) *n.* Disfigurement or injury by removal or destruction of a conspicuous or essential body part. — **mu′ti·late′** *v.*

mut·ism (myo͞o′tĭz′əm) *n.* Absence of the faculty of speech.

mu·ton (myo͞o′tŏn′) *n.* The smallest unit of a chromosome in which alteration can be effective in causing a mutation.

mu·tu·al·ism (myo͞o′cho͞o-ə-lĭz′əm) *n.* A symbiotic relationship in which both species benefit. — **mu′tu·al·is′tic** *adj.*

my·al·gi·a (mī-ăl′jē-ə, -jə) *n.* Muscular pain or tenderness, especially when diffuse and nonspecific. — **my·al′gic** (-jĭk) *adj.*

my·as·the·ni·a (mī′əs-thē′nē-ə) *n.* **1.** Abnormal

muscular weakness or fatigue. **2.** Myasthenia gravis. — **my′as·then′ic** (-thĕn′ĭk) *adj.*

myasthenia grav·is (grăv′ĭs) *n.* A disease characterized by progressive fatigue and generalized weakness of the skeletal muscles, especially those of the face, neck, arms, and legs, caused by impaired transmission of nerve impulses following an autoimmune attack on acetylcholine receptors.

my·a·to·ni·a (mī′ə-tō′nē-ə) or **my·at·o·ny** (mī-ăt′ə-nē) *n.* Lack of muscle tone.

my·cete (mī′sēt) *n.* A fungus.

my·ce·to·ma (mī′sĭ-tō′mə) *n.* **1.** A chronic, slowly progressing bacterial or fungal infection usually of the foot or leg, characterized by nodules that discharge an oily pus. **2.** A tumor produced by filamentous fungi. — **my′ce·to′ma·tous** (-tō′mə-təs, -tŏm′ə-) *adj.*

my·co·bac·te·ri·o·sis (mī′kō-băk-tēr′ē-ō′sĭs) *n.* Infection with mycobacteria.

my·co·bac·te·ri·um (mī′kō-băk-tēr′ē-əm) *n.* Any of various slender, rod-shaped, aerobic bacteria of the genus *Mycobacterium*, which includes the bacteria that cause tuberculosis and leprosy.

Mycobacterium *n.* A genus of aerobic, nonmotile bacteria containing gram-positive rods and including both parasitic and saprophytic species.

my·co·der·ma·ti·tis (mī′kō-dûr′mə-tī′tĭs) *n.* A skin eruption of mycotic origin.

my·co·phage (mī′kə-fāj′) *n.* A virus that infects fungi.

my·co·plas·ma (mī′kō-plăz′mə) *n., pl.* **-mas** or **-ma·ta** (-mə-tə). A microorganism of the genus *Mycoplasma.* — **my′co·plas′mal** *adj.*

Mycoplasma *n.* A genus of nonmotile, parasitic, pathogenic microorganisms whose members lack a true cell wall, are gram-negative, and require sterols such as cholesterol for growth.

my·co·sis (mī-kō′sĭs) *n., pl.* **-ses** (-sēz). **1.** A disease caused by fungi. **2.** A fungal infection in or on a part of the body.

mycosis fun·goi·des (fŭng-goi′dēz) *n.* A chronic progressive lymphoma arising in the skin and initially simulating eczema or other inflammatory dermatoses.

my·cot·ic (mī-kŏt′ĭk) *adj.* **1.** Relating to mycosis. **2.** Relating to a fungus.

my·co·tox·in (mī′kō-tŏk′sĭn) *n.* A toxin produced by a fungus.

my·dri·a·sis (mĭ-drī′ə-sĭs) *n.* Prolonged abnormal dilation of the pupil of the eye induced by a drug or caused by disease.

my·ec·to·my (mī-ĕk′tə-mē) *n.* Surgical excision of a portion of muscle.

my·ec·to·py (mī-ĕk′tə-pē) or **my·ec·to·pi·a** (mī′-ĭk-tō′pē-ə) *n.* Dislocation of a muscle.

my·e·le·mi·a (mī′ə-lē′mē-ə) *n.* See **myelocytosis**.

my·e·lin (mī′ə-lĭn) or **my·e·line** (-lĭn, -lēn′) *n.* **1.** A white fatty material composed chiefly of alternating layers of lipids and lipoproteins that encloses the axons of myelinated nerve fibers. **2.** Droplets of lipid formed during autolysis and postmortem decomposition. — **my′e·lin′ic** *adj.*

my·e·li·nat·ed fiber (mī′ə-lə-nā′tĭd) *n.* An axon enveloped by a myelin sheath formed by oligodendroglia cells in the brain and spinal cord or by Schwann cells in the peripheral nerves.

my·e·li·na·tion (mī′ə-lə-nā′shən) or **my·e·li·ni·za·tion** (mī′ə-lə-nī-zā′shən) *n.* The acquisition, development, or formation of a myelin sheath around a nerve fiber.

myelin sheath *n.* The insulating envelope of myelin that surrounds the core of a nerve fiber or axon and facilitates the transmission of nerve impulses. In the peripheral nervous system, the sheath is formed from the cell membrane of the Schwann cell and, in the central nervous system, from oligodendrocytes.

my·e·li·tis (mī′ə-lī′tĭs) *n.* **1.** Inflammation of the spinal cord. **2.** Inflammation of the bone marrow. — **my′e·lit′ic** (-lĭt′ĭk) *adj.*

my·e·lo·blast (mī′ə-lə-blăst′) *n.* An immature cell of the bone marrow that is the precursor of a myelocyte.

my·e·lo·blas·te·mi·a (mī′ə-lō-blă-stē′mē-ə) *n.* The presence of myeloblasts in the blood.

my·e·lo·blas·to·ma (mī′ə-lō-blă-stō′mə) *n.* A malignant tumor consisting of myeloblasts.

my·e·lo·blas·to·sis (mī′ə-lō-blă-stō′sĭs) *n.* The presence of unusually large numbers of myeloblasts in the tissues or blood.

my·e·lo·cele (mī′ə-lə-sēl′) *n.* **1.** Protrusion of the spinal cord in cases of spina bifida. **2.** The central canal of the spinal cord.

my·e·lo·cyst (mī′ə-lə-sĭst′) *n.* A cyst that develops from a rudimentary medullary canal in the central nervous system.

my·e·lo·cyte (mī′ə-lə-sīt′) *n.* **1.** A large cell of the bone marrow that is a precursor of the mature granulocytes of the blood. **2.** A nerve cell of the gray matter of the brain or spinal cord. — **my′e·lo·cyt′ic** (-sĭt′ĭk) *adj.*

my·e·lo·cy·the·mi·a (mī′ə-lō-sī-thē′mē-ə) *n.* The presence of myelocytes in the blood, especially in persistently large numbers.

my·e·lo·cy·to·ma (mī′ə-lō-sī-tō′mə) *n., pl.* **-mas** or **-ma·ta** (-mə-tə). A nodular, circumscribed, relatively dense accumulation of myelocytes.

my·e·lo·cy·to·sis (mī′ə-lō-sī-tō′sĭs) *n.* The occurrence of abnormally large numbers of myelocytes in the tissues or blood.

my·e·lo·dys·pla·sia (mī′ə-lō-dĭs-plā′zhə, -zhē-ə) *n.* An abnormality in the development of the spinal cord.

my·e·lo·fi·bro·sis (mī′ə-lō-fī-brō′sĭs) *n.* Fibrosis of the bone marrow associated with myeloid metaplasia, leukoerythroblastosis, and thrombocytopenia.

my·e·lo·gen·e·sis (mī′ə-lō-jĕn′ĭ-sĭs) *n.* The development of bone marrow.

my·e·lo·gone (mī′ə-lə-gōn′) or **my·e·lo·go·ni·um** (mī′ə-lə-gō′nē-əm) *n.* An immature white blood cell of the bone marrow characterized by a relatively large, fairly deeply staining, finely reticulated nucleus that contains palely staining nucleoli, and a scant amount of rimlike, nongranular, moderately basophilic cytoplasm.

my·e·lo·gram (mī′ə-lə-grăm′) *n.* An x-ray of the spinal cord after injection of air or a radiopaque substance into the subarachnoid space. — **my′e·log′ra·phy** (-lŏg′rə-fē) *n.*

my·e·loid (mī′ə-loid′) *adj.* **1.** Of, relating to, or derived from the bone marrow. **2.** Of or relating to the spinal cord.

myeloid metaplasia *n.* A syndrome characterized by anemia, enlargement of the spleen, and the presence of nucleated red blood cells and immature granulocytes in the blood, with extramedullary hemopoiesis in the spleen and liver.

myeloid series *n.* The various stages of cell development as seen in the granulocytic and erythrocytic series.

myeloid tissue *n.* Bone marrow consisting of the developmental and adult stages of red blood cells, granulocytes, and megakaryocytes in a stroma of reticular cells and fibers, with sinusoidal vascular channels.

my·e·lo·ma (mī′ə-lō′mə) *n., pl.* **-mas** or **-ma·ta** (-mə-tə). A tumor composed of cells derived from hemopoietic tissues of the bone marrow.

my·e·lo·ma·to·sis (mī′ə-lō′mə-tō′sĭs) *n.* The occurrence of myelomas at various sites throughout the body.

my·e·lo·plast (mī′ə-lə-plăst′) *n.* Any of the leukocytic series of cells in the bone marrow, especially those in an early stage of development.

my·e·lo·poi·e·sis (mī′ə-lō-poi-ē′sĭs) *n.* The formation of bone marrow or of blood cells derived from bone marrow.

my·e·lo·pro·lif·er·a·tive syndrome (mī′ə-lō-prə-lĭf′ə-rā′tĭv) *n.* Any of a group of conditions resulting from a disorder in the rate of formation of cells of the bone marrow and including chronic granulocytic leukemia, erythremia, myelosclerosis, panmyelosis, and erythroleukemia.

my·e·lor·rha·phy (mī′ə-lôr′ə-fē) *n.* Suture of a wound of the spinal cord.

my·e·lo·sar·co·ma (mī′ə-lō-sär-kō′mə) *n.* A malignant tumor derived from bone marrow or from one of its cellular elements.

my·e·lo·scle·ro·sis (mī′ə-lō-sklə-rō′sĭs) *n.* See **myelofibrosis.**

my·e·lo·sis (mī′ə-lō′sĭs) *n.* **1.** Abnormal proliferation of bone marrow tissue. **2.** Abnormal proliferation of medullary tissue in the spinal cord.

my·e·lo·to·mog·ra·phy (mī′ə-lō-tō-mŏg′rə-fē) *n.* Tomographic depiction of the spinal subarachnoid space following injection of a contrast medium.

my·e·lot·o·my (mī′ə-lŏt′ə-mē) *n.* Incision of the spinal cord.

my·es·the·sia (mī′ĭs-thē′zhə) *n.* The sensation felt in a muscle when it is contracting.

my·ia·sis (mī′ə-sĭs, mī-ī′ə-sĭs) *n., pl.* **my·ia·ses** (mī′ə-sēz′). **1.** Infestation of tissue by fly larvae. **2.** A disease resulting from infestation of tissue by fly larvae.

my·o·blast (mī′ə-blăst′) *n.* A primitive muscle cell with the potential to develop into a muscle fiber.

my·o·blas·to·ma (mī′ō-blă-stō′mə) *n.* A tumor composed of immature muscle cells.

my·o·bra·di·a (mī′ə-brā′dē-ə) *n.* Sluggish reaction of muscle following stimulation.

myocardial infarction *n.* Necrosis of a region of the myocardium caused by an interruption in the supply of blood to the heart, usually as a result of occlusion of a coronary artery.

myocardial insufficiency *n.* See **heart failure** (sense 1).

my·o·car·di·o·graph (mī′ō-kär′dē-ə-grăf′) *n.* An instrument for making tracings of the movements of the heart muscle.

my·o·car·di·or·ra·phy (mī′ō-cär′dē-ôr′ə-fē) *n.* Suture of the myocardium.

my·o·car·di·tis (mī′ō-kär-dī′tĭs) *n.* See **carditis.**

my·o·car·di·um (mī′ō-kär′dē-əm) *n., pl.* **-di·a** (-dē-ə). The middle layer of the heart, consisting of cardiac muscle. — **my′o·car′di·al** *adj.*

my·oc·lo·nus (mī-ŏk′lə-nəs) *n.* A sudden shock-like twitching of muscles or parts of muscles, without any rhythm or pattern, occurring in various brain disorders. — **my′o·clon′ic** (mī′ə-klŏn′ĭk) *adj.*

my·o·cyte (mī′ə-sīt′) *n.* A muscle cell.

my·o·cy·to·ma (mī′ō-sī-tō′mə) *n., pl.* **-mas** or **-ma·ta** (-mə-tə). A benign tumor derived from muscle.

my·o·dyn·i·a (mī′ō-dĭn′ē-ə) *n.* See **myalgia.**

my·o·dys·to·ny (mī′ō-dĭs′tə-nē) *n.* A condition of slow relaxation interrupted by a succession of slight contractions following electrical stimulation of a muscle.

my·o·dys·tro·phy (mī′ō-dĭs′trə-fē) *n.* See **muscular dystrophy.**

my·o·e·de·ma (mī′ō-ĭ-dē′mə) *n.* Localized contraction of a degenerating muscle, occurring at the point of a sharp blow.

my·o·en·do·car·di·tis (mī′ō-ĕn′dō-kär-dī′tĭs) *n.* Inflammation of the muscular wall and lining membrane of the heart.

my·o·ep·i·the·li·um (mī′ō-ĕp′ə-thē′lē-əm) *n.* Contractile spindle-shaped cells arranged longitudinally or obliquely around sweat glands and around the secretory alveoli of the mammary gland. — **my′o·ep′i·the′li·al** *adj.*

my·o·fa·cial pain-dysfunction syndrome (mī′ō-fā′shəl) *n.* See **temporomandibular joint syndrome.**

my·o·fi·bril (mī′ə-fī′brəl, -fĭb′rəl) *n.* One of the threadlike longitudinal fibrils occurring in a skeletal or cardiac muscle fiber.

my·o·fi·bro·ma (mī′ō-fī-brō′mə) *n.* A benign tumor that consists chiefly of fibrous connective tissue, with variable numbers of muscle cells forming portions of the tumor.

my·o·fi·bro·sis (mī′ō-fī-brō′sĭs) *n.* Chronic myositis with diffuse hyperplasia of the interstitial connective tissue pressing upon and causing atrophy of the muscular tissue.

my·o·fil·a·ment (mī′ə-fĭl′ə-mənt) *n.* Any of the ultramicroscopic filaments, made up of actin and myosin, that are structural units of a myofibril.

my·o·gen·e·sis (mī′ə-jĕn′ĭ-sĭs) *n.* The formation of muscle cells or fibers.

my·o·gen·ic (mī′ə-jĕn′ĭk) or **my·o·ge·net·ic** (mī′-ō-jə-nĕt′ĭk) *adj.* **1.** Giving rise to or forming muscular tissue. **2.** Of muscular origin; arising from the muscles.

my·o·glo·bin (mī′ə-glō′bĭn) *n.* The oxygen-transporting protein of muscle, resembling blood hemoglobin in function, but containing only one heme as part of the molecule and with one fourth the molecular weight.

my·o·glo·bi·nu·ri·a (mī′ə-glō′bə-nŏŏr′ē-ə, -nyŏŏr′-) *n.* Excretion of myoglobin in the urine.

my·o·glob·u·lin (mī′ō-glŏb′yə-lĭn) *n.* Globulin present in muscle tissue.

my·o·glob·u·li·nu·ri·a (mī′ō-glŏb′yə-lə-nŏŏr′ē-ə, -nyŏŏr′-) *n.* Excretion of myoglobulin in the urine.

my·o·gram (mī′ə-grăm′) *n.* A tracing of muscular contractions. — **my′o·graph′** (-grăf′) *n.* — **my′o·graph′ic** *adj.* — **my·og′ra·phy** (mī-ŏg′rə-fē) *n.*

my·o·kin·e·sim·e·ter (mī′ō-kĭn′ĭ-sĭm′ĭ-tər, -kī′-nĭ′-) *n.* A device for registering the time and extent of the contraction of muscles in response to electric stimulation.

my·o·ky·mi·a (mī′ō-kī′mē-ə, -kĭm′ē-ə) *n.* A benign condition, often familial, characterized by irregular twitching of groups of muscle fibers giving a rippling appearance to the overlying skin.

my·o·li·po·ma (mī′ō-lĭ-pō′mə, -lī-) *n.* A benign tumor that consists chiefly of fat cells, with variable numbers of muscle cells forming portions of the tumor.

my·ol·o·gy (mī-ŏl′ə-jē) *n.* The scientific study of muscles. — **my′o·log′ic** (mī′ə-lŏj′ĭk) *adj.* — **my·ol′o·gist** *n.*

my·o·ma (mī-ō′mə) *n., pl.* **-mas** or **-ma·ta** (-mə-tə). A benign tumor of muscular tissue. — **my·o′ma·tous** (-ō′mə-təs, -ŏm′ə-) *adj.*

my·o·ma·la·ci·a (mī′ō-mə-lā′shē-ə, -shə) *n.* Pathological softening of muscular tissue.

my·o·mec·to·my (mī′ə-mĕk′tə-mē) *n.* Surgical removal of a myoma, especially of a uterine myoma.

my·o·mel·a·no·sis (mī′ō-mĕl′ə-nō′sĭs) *n.* Abnormal dark pigmentation of muscular tissue.

my·o·mere (mī′ə-mēr′) *n.* The segment within a metamere that develops into skeletal muscle.

my·om·e·ter (mī-ŏm′ĭ-tər) *n.* An instrument for measuring the extent of a muscular contraction.

my·o·me·tri·um (mī′ō-me′trē-əm) *n.* The muscular wall of the uterus.

my·o·ne·cro·sis (mī′ō-nə-krō′sĭs, -nĕ-) *n.* Necrosis of muscle.

my·o·neme (mī′ə-nēm′) *n.* A muscle fibril.

my·o·neu·ral blockade (mī′ə-nŏŏr′əl, -nyŏŏ′-) *n.* Inhibition of nerve impulse transmission at myoneural junctions by a drug such as curare.

my·o·neu·ral·gia (mī′ō-nŏŏ-răl′jə, -nyŏŏ-) *n.* Neuralgic pain in a muscle.

myoneural junction *n.* The synaptic connection of the axon of a motor neuron with a muscle fiber.

my·o·pal·mus (mī′ə-păl′məs) *n.* Twitching of a muscle.

my·o·pa·ral·y·sis (mī′ō-pə-răl′ĭ-sĭs) *n.* Muscular paralysis.

my·o·pa·re·sis (mī′ō-pə-rē′sĭs, -păr′ĭ-) *n.* Slight muscular paralysis.

my·op·a·thy (mī-ŏp′ə-thē) *n.* Any of various abnormal conditions or diseases of the muscular tissues, especially one involving skeletal muscle. — **my′o·path′ic** (mī′ə-păth′ĭk) *adj.*

my·o·per·i·car·di·tis (mī′ō-pĕr′ĭ-kär-dī′tĭs) *n.* Inflammation of the muscular wall of the heart and of the enveloping pericardium.

my·o·pi·a (mī-ō′pē-ə) *n.* A visual defect in which distant objects appear blurred because their images are focused in front of the retina rather than on it; nearsightedness; shortsightedness. — **my·op′ic** (-ŏp′ĭk, -ō′pĭk) *adj.*

myopic astigmatism *n.* Astigmatism in which one meridian is myopic while the one at a right angle to it is without refractive error.

my·o·plasm (mī′ə-plăz′əm) *n.* The contractile portion of the muscle cell.

my·o·plas·tic (mī′ə-plăs′tĭk) *adj.* **1.** Of or relating to plastic surgery of the muscles. **2.** Of or relating to the use of muscular tissue in correcting defects.

my·o·plas·ty (mī′ə-plăs′tē) *n.* Plastic surgery of muscular tissue.

my·or·rha·phy (mī-ôr′ə-fē) *n.* Suture of a muscle.

my·o·sar·co·ma (mī′ō-sär-kō′mə) *n.* A malignant tumor derived from muscular tissue.

my·o·sin (mī′ə-sĭn) *n.* The commonest protein in muscle cells, a globulin responsible for the elastic and contractile properties of muscle and combining with actin to form actomyosin.

my·o·si·tis (mī′ə-sī′tĭs) *n.* Inflammation of a muscle, especially a voluntary muscle, characterized by pain, tenderness, and sometimes spasm in the affected area.

myositis os·sif·i·cans (ŏ-sĭf′ĭ-kănz′) *n.* Ossification or the deposit of bone in muscle tissue, causing pain and swelling.

my·o·spasm (mī′ə-spăz′əm) *n.* Spasmodic contraction of a muscle.

my·ot·a·sis (mī-ŏt′ə-sĭs) *n.* Stretching of a muscle. — **my′o·tat′ic** (mī′ə-tăt′ĭk) *adj.*

myotatic contraction *n.* A contraction of a skeletal muscle that occurs as part of a myotatic reflex.

myotatic irritability *n.* The ability of a muscle to contract in response to the stimulus produced by a sudden stretching.

myotatic reflex *n.* Tonic contraction of the muscles in response to a stretching force, due to stimulation of muscle proprioceptors.

my·o·te·not·o·my (mī′ō-tĕ-nŏt′ə-mē) *n.* Cutting through the principal tendon of a muscle, with partial or complete division of the muscle itself.

my·ot·o·my (mī-ŏt′ə-mē) *n.* **1.** Dissection of the muscles. **2.** Surgical division of a muscle.

my·o·to·ni·a (mī′ə-tō′nē-ə) *n.* Delayed relaxation or temporary rigidity of a muscle after an initial contraction. — **my′o·ton′ic** (-tŏn′ĭk) *adj.*

my·ot·o·nus (mī-ŏt′n-əs) *n.* A tonic spasm or temporary rigidity of a muscle or group of muscles.

my·ot·o·ny (mī-ŏt′n-ē) *n.* Muscular tonus or tension.

My·o·tro·phin (mī′ə-trō′pĭn, -fĭn) A trademark for a genetically engineered protein used to slow nerve damage associated with amyotrophic lateral sclerosis.

my·ot·ro·phy (mī-ŏt′rə-fē) *n.* Nutrition of muscular tissue.

my·o·tube (mī′ə-tōōb′, -tyōōb′) *n.* A developing skeletal muscle fiber with a tubular appearance.

my·rin·ga (mə-rĭng′gə) *n.* See **eardrum**.

myr·in·gec·to·my (mĭr′ĭn-jĕk′tə-mē) *n.* Excision of the tympanic membrane of the ear.

myr·in·gi·tis (mĭr′ĭn-jī′tĭs) *n.* Inflammation of the tympanic membrane.

my·rin·go·dec·to·my (mə-rĭng′gō-dĕk′tə-mē) *n.* See **myringectomy**.

my·rin·go·plas·ty (mə-rĭng′gə-plăs′tē) *n.* Surgical repair of a damaged tympanic membrane.

my·rin·go·sta·pe·di·o·pex·y (mə-rĭng′gō-stā-pē′dē-ə-pĕk′sē) *n.* Tympanoplasty in which the tympanic membrane is brought into functional connection with the stapes.

myr·in·got·o·my (mĭr′ĭng-gŏt′ə-mē) *n.* Surgical puncture of the tympanic membrane, as for the removal of fluid or the drainage of pus.

my·rinx (mī′rĭngks′, mĭr′ĭngks′) *n.* See **eardrum**.

my·so·phil·i·a (mī′sə-fĭl′ē-ə) *n.* Sexual interest in excretions.

my·so·pho·bi·a (mī′sə-fō′bē-ə) *n.* An abnormal fear of dirt or contamination.

mytacism *n.* A form of stammering in which the letter *m* is frequently substituted for other consonants.

myx·as·the·ni·a (mĭk′săs-thē′nē-ə) *n.* Faulty secretion of mucus.

myx·e·de·ma (mĭk′sĭ-dē′mə) *n.* A disease caused by decreased activity of the thyroid gland in adults and characterized by dry skin, swellings around the lips and nose, mental deterioration, and a subnormal basal metabolic rate. — **myx′e·dem′a·tous** (-dĕm′ə-təs, -dē′mə-), **myx′e·dem′ic** (-dĕm′ĭk) *adj.*

myx·e·mi·a (mĭk-sē′mē-ə) *n.* See **mucinemia**.

myx·o·fi·bro·ma (mĭk′sō-fī-brō′mə) *n.* A benign tumor of fibrous connective tissue in which focal or diffuse degenerative changes result in portions that resemble primitive mesenchymal tissue.

myx·o·fi·bro·sar·co·ma (mĭk′sō-fī′brō-sär-kō′-mə) *n.* A fibrosarcoma in which degenerative change or growth of less differentiated anaplastic cells results in portions that resemble primitive mesenchymal tissue.

myx·o·ma (mĭk-sō′mə) *n., pl.* **-mas** or **-ma·ta** (-mə-tə). A benign tumor composed of connective tissue embedded in mucus. — **myx·o′ma·tous** (-sō′mə-təs, -sŏm′ə-) *adj.*

myx·o·ma·to·sis (mĭk-sō′mə-tō′sĭs) *n.* **1.** A condition characterized by the growth of many myxomas. **2.** A highly infectious, usually fatal disease of rabbits that is caused by a pox virus and is characterized by many skin tumors similar to myxomas.

myx·o·mem·bra·nous colitis (mĭk′sō-mĕm′-brə-nəs) *n.* See **mucous colitis**.

myx·o·poi·e·sis (mĭk′sō-poi-ē′sĭs) *n.* The production of mucus.

myx·o·sar·co·ma (mĭk′sō-sär-kō′mə) *n.* A sarcoma characterized by immature, relatively undifferentiated cells that grow rapidly and invade extensively, resulting in tissue that resembles primitive mesenchymal tissue.

myx·o·vi·rus (mĭk′sə-vī′rəs) *n.* Formerly, any of a group of RNA-containing viruses with an affinity for mucins, now included in the families of Orthomyxoviridae and Paramyxoviridae. These viruses include the influenza virus, parainfluenza virus, respiratory syncytial virus, and measles virus.

~~~~~ **N** ~~~~~

nab·i·lone (năb′ə-lōn′) *n.* A synthetic cannabinoid used in the treatment of nausea and vomiting associated with cancer chemotherapy.

NAD (ĕn′ā-dē′) *n.* Nicotinamide adenine dinucleotide; a coenzyme occurring in most living cells and used as an oxidizing or reducing agent in various metabolic processes.

NADP (ĕn-ā′dē-pē′) *n.* Nicotinamide adenine dinucleotide phosphate; a coenzyme occurring in most living cells and used similarly to NAD but interacting with different metabolites.

Nae·ge·li syndrome (nā′gə-lē) *n.* An inherited disorder characterized by reticular skin pigmentation, diminished sweating, the absence of one or more teeth, and hyperkeratosis of the palms and soles.

Naff·zi·ger operation (năf′zĭ-gər) *n.* Removal of the lateral and superior orbital walls for the relief of severe exophthalmos.

naf·ti·fine hydrochloride (năf′tə-fēn′) *n.* A broad-spectrum antifungal agent used in the topical treatment of tinea infections.

nail (nāl) *n.* **1.** A slender rod used in operations to fasten together the divided extremities of a broken bone. **2.** A fingernail or toenail.

nail bed *n.* The formative layer of cells at the base of the fingernail or toenail; the matrix.

na·li·dix·ic acid (nā′lĭ-dĭk′sĭk) *n.* A compound

used to treat infections of the genital and urinary tracts caused by gram-negative bacteria.

nal·or·phine (năl′ər-fēn′, năl-ôr′fēn) *n.* A drug derived from morphine that acts as an antagonist to the depressant and stimulatory effects of morphine and related narcotics and is used to counteract the respiratory depression produced by narcotic overdosage.

nal·ox·one hydrochloride (năl′ək-sōn′, nə-lŏk′-sōn) *n.* A drug used as an antagonist to narcotic drugs such as morphine.

NANB hepatitis *abbr.* non-A, non-B hepatitis

na·nism (nā′nĭz′əm, năn′ĭz′-) *n.* See **dwarfism.**

nan·oph·thal·mi·a (năn′ŏf-thăl′mē-ə) *n.* See **microphthalmia.**

na·nus (nā′nəs, năn′əs) *n.* A dwarf.

nape (nāp, năp) *n.* The back of the neck.

na·prox·en (nə-prŏk′sən) *n.* A drug used to reduce inflammation and pain, especially in the treatment of arthritis.

nar·cis·sism (när′sĭ-sĭz′əm) or **nar·cism** (när′sĭz′-əm) *n.* **1.** Excessive love or admiration of oneself. **2.** Erotic pleasure derived from contemplation or admiration of one's own body or self, especially as a fixation on or a regression to an infantile stage of development. — **nar′cis·sist** *n.* — **nar′cis·sis′tic** *adj.* — **nar′cis·sis′ti·cal·ly** *adv.*

nar·co·a·nal·y·sis (när′kō-ə-năl′ĭ-sĭs) *n., pl.* **-ses** (-sēz′). Psychotherapy conducted while the patient is in a sleeplike state induced by barbiturates or other drugs, especially as a means of releasing repressed feelings or thoughts. — **nar′co·an′a·lyt′ic** (-ăn′ə-lĭt′ĭk) *adj.*

nar·co·hyp·ni·a (när′kō-hĭp′nē-ə) *n.* General numbness sometimes experienced at the moment of waking.

nar·co·hyp·no·sis (när′kō-hĭp-nō′sĭs) *n.* Stupor or deep sleep induced by hypnosis.

nar·co·lep·sy (när′kə-lĕp′sē) *n.* A disorder characterized by sudden and uncontrollable, though often brief, attacks of deep sleep, sometimes accompanied by paralysis and hallucinations. — **nar′co·lep′tic** (-lĕp′tĭk) *adj. & n.*

nar·co·ma (när-kō′mə) *n.* Stupor induced by a narcotic.

nar·co·sis (när-kō′sĭs) *n., pl.* **-ses** (-sēz). General and nonspecific reversible depression of neuronal excitability, produced by a physical or chemical agent, usually resulting in stupor rather than in anesthesia.

nar·co·syn·the·sis (när′kō-sĭn′thĭ-sĭs) *n.* See **narcoanalysis.**

nar·co·ther·a·py (när′kō-thĕr′ə-pē) *n.* Psychotherapy conducted while a person is under the influence of a sedative or narcotic drug.

nar·cot·ic (när-kŏt′ĭk) *n.* A drug derived from opium or opiumlike compounds, with potent analgesic effects associated with significant alteration of mood and behavior, and with the potential for dependence and tolerance following repeated administration. — *adj.* Capable of inducing a state of stuporous analgesia.

nar·co·tism (när′kə-tĭz′əm) *n.* **1.** Addiction to narcotics such as opium, heroin, or morphine. **2.** Narcosis.

nar·co·tize (när′kə-tīz′) *v.* **-tized, -tiz·ing, -tiz·es.** To place under the influence of a narcotic. — **nar′co·ti·za′tion** (-tĭ-zā′shən) *n.*

nar·is (nâr′ĭs) *n., pl.* **-es** (-ēz). The anterior opening on either side of the nasal cavity; a nostril.

na·sal (nā′zəl) *adj.* Of, in, or relating to the nose.

nasal bone *n.* An elongated rectangular bone that forms the bridge of the nose.

nasal cavity *n.* The cavity on either side of the nasal septum, extending from the nares to the pharynx, and lying between the floor of the cranium and the roof of the mouth.

nasal concha *n.* See **ethmoidal crest.**

nasal meatus *n.* Any of the three passages, designated inferior, middle, and superior, in the nasal cavity formed by the projection of the ethmoidal crests.

nasal muscle *n.* A muscle that passes across the bridge of the nose and attaches to the ala of the nose, and whose action dilates the nostrils.

nasal pit *n.* One of a pair of depressions formed when the nasal placodes come to lie below the general external contour of the developing face as a result of the rapid growth of the adjacent nasal elevations.

nasal reflex *n.* Sneezing caused by irritation of the nasal mucous membrane.

nasal septum *n.* The wall dividing the nasal cavity into halves, composed of a central supporting skeleton covered by a mucous membrane.

na·so·lac·ri·mal duct (nā′zō-lăk′rə-məl) *n.* The passage leading downward from the lacrimal sac on each side of the nose, through which tears are conducted into the nasal cavity.

na·so·phar·yn·gi·tis (nā′zō-făr′ĭn-jī′tĭs) *n.* Inflammation of the nasal passages and of the upper part of the pharynx.

na·so·pha·ryn·go·la·ryn·go·scope (nā′zō-fə-rĭng′gō-lə-rĭng′gə-skōp′, -lə-rĭn′jə-) *n.* A fiberoptic endoscope used to visualize the upper airways and the pharynx.

na·so·phar·yn·gos·co·py (nā′zō-făr′ĭn-gŏs′kə-pē, -făr′ĭng-) *n.* Examination of the upper airways and the pharynx with an optical instrument.

na·so·phar·ynx (nā′zō-făr′ĭngks) *n.* The part of the pharynx above the soft palate that is continuous with the nasal passages. — **na′so·pha·ryn′ge·al** (-fə-rĭn′jē-əl, -jəl, -făr′ən-jē′əl) *adj.*

na·so·scope (nā′zə-skōp′) *n.* An instrument for examining the nasal passages; a rhinoscope.

na·so·si·nu·si·tis (nā′zō-sī′nə-sī′tĭs) *n.* Inflammation of the nasal cavities and accessory sinuses.

na·so·tra·che·al tube (nā′zō-trā′kē-əl) *n.* An endotracheal tube inserted through the nasal passages.

na·tal (nāt′l) *adj.* **1.** Of, relating to, or accompanying birth. **2.** Of or relating to the buttocks.

na·tal·i·ty (nā-tăl′ĭ-tē, nə-) *n.* The ratio of births to the general population; the birth rate.

na·ti·mor·tal·i·ty (nā′tə-môr-tăl′ĭ-tē) *n.* The proportion of fetal and neonatal deaths to the general natality; the perinatal death rate.

na·tive immunity (nā′tĭv) *n.* See **innate immunity**.

na·tre·mi·a (nā-trē′mē-ə) *n.* The presence of sodium in the blood.

na·tri·u·re·sis (nā′trə-yoō-rē′sĭs) *n.* Excretion of excessive amounts of sodium in the urine.

nat·u·ral antibody (năch′ər-əl, năch′rəl) *n.* See **normal antibody**.

natural childbirth *n.* A method of childbirth in which medical intervention is minimized and the mother often practices relaxation and breathing techniques to control pain and ease delivery.

natural immunity *n.* See **innate immunity**.

natural killer cell *n.* A killer cell that is activated by double-stranded RNA and fights off viral infections and tumors.

natural mutation *n.* See **spontaneous mutation**.

natural selection *n.* The process in nature by which, according to Darwin's theory of evolution, only the organisms best adapted to their environment tend to survive and transmit their genetic characters in increasing numbers to succeeding generations while those less adapted tend to be eliminated.

na·tur·op·a·thy (nā′chə-rŏp′ə-thē) *n.* A system of therapeutics in which neither surgical nor medicinal agents are used, dependence being placed only on natural remedies. — **na′tur·o·path′** (nā′-chər-ə-păth′, nə-choōr′-) *n.* — **na·tur′o·path′ic** (nə-choōr′ə-păth′ĭk) *adj.*

nau·se·a (nô′zē-ə, -zhə, -sē-ə, -shə) *n.* A feeling of sickness in the stomach characterized by an urge to vomit.

nausea grav·i·dar·um (grăv′ĭ-dâr′əm) *n.* See **morning sickness**.

nau·se·ate (nô′zē-āt′, -zhē-, -sē-, -shē-) *v.* **-at·ed, -at·ing, -ates.** To feel or cause to feel nausea.

nauseated *adj.* Affected with nausea.

nau·seous (nô′shəs, -zē-əs) *adj.* **1.** Causing nausea. **2.** Affected with nausea. — **nau′seous·ly** *adv.*

na·vel (nā′vəl) *n.* The mark on the surface of the abdomen where the umbilical cord was attached to the fetus during gestation.

na·vic·u·lar (nə-vĭk′yə-lər) *n.* **1.** A comma-shaped bone of the human wrist, located in the first row of carpals. **2.** A concave bone of the human foot, located between the talus and the metatarsals.

near point *n.* The nearest point of distinct vision.

near·sight·ed (nēr′sī′tĭd) *adj.* Unable to see distant objects clearly; myopic.

near·sight·ed·ness (nēr′sī′tĭd-nĭs) *n.* Myopia.

ne·ar·thro·sis (nē′är-thrō′sĭs) or **neoarthrosis** (x) *n.* **1.** A pseudarthrosis arising in an ununited fracture. **2.** A new joint resulting from a total joint replacement operation.

neb·u·la (nĕb′yə-lə) *n., pl.* **-las** or **-lae** (-lē′). **1.** A faint, foglike opacity of the cornea. **2.** A class of oily preparations for use in a nebulizer.

neb·u·liz·er (nĕb′yə-lī′zər) *n.* A device used to reduce liquid to an extremely fine cloud, especially for delivering medication to the deep part of the respiratory tract.

neck (nĕk) *n.* **1.** The part of the body joining the head to the shoulders or trunk. **2.** A narrow or constricted part of a structure, as of a bone or an organ, that joins its parts; a cervix.

ne·crec·to·my (nĭ-krĕk′tə-mē, nĕ-) *n.* Surgical removal of necrosed tissue.

nec·ro·bi·o·sis (nĕk′rō-bī-ō′sĭs) *n.* **1.** Physiological or normal death of cells or tissues as a result of changes associated with development, aging, or use. **2.** Necrosis of a small area of tissue. — **nec′ro·bi·ot′ic** (-ŏt′ĭk) *adj.*

necrobiosis li·poi·di·ca (lĭ-poi′dĭ-kə) *n.* A condition, sometimes associated with diabetes, in which one or more atrophic shiny lesions develop on the legs.

necrobiotic xanthogranuloma *n.* A cutaneous and subcutaneous xanthogranuloma with focal necroses that manifest as multiple large, sometimes ulcerated nodules, especially around the eyes; it is associated with paraproteinemia.

nec·ro·cy·to·sis (nĕk′rō-sī-tō′sĭs) *n.* The abnormal or pathological death of cells.

ne·crol·o·gy (nə-krŏl′ə-jē, nĕ-) *n.* The science of the collection, classification, and interpretation of mortality statistics. — **ne·crol′o·gist** *n.*

ne·crol·y·sis (nē-krŏl′ĭ-sĭs) *n.* Necrosis and loosening of tissue.

nec·ro·ma·ni·a (nĕk′rə-mā′nē-ə, -mān′yə) *n.* **1.** An abnormal tendency to dwell with longing on death. **2.** See **necrophilia** (sense 1).

nec·ro·phil·i·a (nĕk′rə-fĭl′ē-ə) *n.* **1.** An abnormal fondness for being in the presence of dead bodies. **2.** Sexual contact with or erotic desire for dead bodies. — **nec′ro·phil′i·ac′** (-ē-ăk′) *adj. & n.*

nec·ro·pho·bi·a (nĕk′rə-fō′bē-ə) *n.* An abnormal fear of death or corpses. — **nec′ro·pho′bic** *adj.*

nec·rop·sy (nĕk′rŏp′sē, -rəp-) *n.* See **autopsy**.

ne·crose (nĕ-krōs′, -krōz′, nĕk′rōs′, -rōz′) *v.* **-crosed, -cros·ing, -cros·es.** To undergo or cause to undergo necrosis.

ne·cro·sis (nə-krō′sĭs, nĕ-) *n., pl.* **-ses** (-sēz′). Death of cells or tissues through injury or disease, especially in a localized area of the body. — **ne·crot′ic** (-krŏt′ĭk) *adj.*

nec·ro·sper·mi·a (nĕk′rə-spûr′mē-ə) *n.* A condition in which there are dead or immobile spermatozoa in the semen.

necrotic inflammation *n.* Inflammation characterized by rapid necrosis throughout the affected tissue.

nec·ro·tize (nĕk′rə-tīz′) *v.* **-tized, -tiz·ing, -tiz·es.** To undergo necrosis or cause to necrose.

ne·crot·o·my (nə-krŏt′ə-mē, nĕ-) *n.* **1.** Surgical excision of dead tissue. **2.** Dissection of a dead body.

nee·dle (nēd′l) *n.* **1.** A slender, usually sharp-pointed instrument used for puncturing tissues, suturing, or passing a ligature around an artery. **2.** A hollow, slender, sharp-pointed instrument used for injection or aspiration. — *v.* To separate tissues by means of one or two needles in the dissection of small parts.

needle bath *n.* Water projected against the body in very fine sprays from many jets.

needle biopsy *n.* Removal of a specimen for biopsy by aspirating it through a needle or trocar that pierces the skin, or the external surface of an organ, and continues into the underlying tissue.

needle forceps *n.* See **needle-holder.**

needle-holder *n.* An instrument for grasping a needle used in suturing.

nee·dling (nēd′l-ĭng) *n.* Dissection of a soft or secondary cataract.

neg·a·tive (nĕg′ə-tĭv) *adj.* **1.** Marked by failure of response or absence of a reaction. **2.** Not indicating the presence of microorganisms, disease, or a specific condition. **3.** Moving or turning away from a stimulus, such as light.

negative accommodation *n.* Adjustment of the lens for distant vision by relaxation of the ciliary muscles of the eye.

negative convergence *n.* The outward divergence of the visual axes when the eyes are not required to be convergent, as when looking at the far point of normal vision or during sleep.

negative end-expiratory pressure *n.* A subatmospheric pressure at the airway at the end of expiration.

negative feedback *n.* Feedback that reduces the output of a system, as the action of heat on a thermostat to limit the output of a furnace.

negative scotoma *n.* A scotoma that is not ordinarily perceived and is detected only on examination of the visual field.

negative stain *n.* A stain forming an opaque or colored background against which the object to be demonstrated appears as a translucent or colorless area.

negative transfer *n.* The interference of previous learning in the process of learning something new.

neg·a·tiv·ism (nĕg′ə-tĭv-vĭz′əm) *n.* A tendency to do the opposite of what one is requested to do, or to resist stubbornly for no apparent reason. — **neg′a·tiv·ist** *n.* — **neg′a·tiv·is′tic** *adj.*

Neis·se·ri·a (nī-sēr′ē-ə) *n.* A genus of aerobic to facultatively anaerobic bacteria containing gram-negative cocci and including the causative agent of gonorrhea.

Né·la·ton catheter (nā-lə-tŏn′, -tôn′) *n.* A flexible catheter made of soft rubber.

Nel·son syndrome (nĕl′sən) *n.* A syndrome marked by skin hyperpigmentation of the skin and enlargment of the sphenoid bone of the skull, caused by the development of a pituitary tumor after adrenalectomy for Cushing's syndrome.

nem·a·line myopathy (nĕm′ə-līn′, -lĭn) *n.* Congenital, nonprogressive muscle weakness most evident in the proximal muscles, with characteristic threadlike rods seen in some muscle cells.

nem·a·to·cyst (nĕm′ə-tə-sĭst′, nĭ-măt′ə-) *n.* A capsule within specialized cells of certain coelenterates, such as jellyfish, containing a barbed, threadlike tube that delivers a paralyzing sting.

nem·a·tode (nĕm′ə-tōd′) *n.* A parasitic worm of the class Nematoda.

Nem·bu·tal (nĕm′byə-tôl′) A trademark used for pentobarbital sodium.

ne·o·an·ti·gen (nē′ō-ăn′tĭ-jən) *n.* See **tumor antigen.**

ne·o·cor·tex (nē′ō-kôr′tĕks′) *n.* See **isocortex.**

ne·o·cys·tos·to·my (nē′ō-sĭ-stŏs′tə-mē) *n.* A surgical procedure in which the ureter or a segment of the ileum is implanted into the bladder.

ne·o·dym·i·um (nē′ō-dĭm′ē-əm) *n.* A bright, silvery rare-earth metal with atomic number 60.

ne·o·gen·e·sis (nē′ō-jĕn′ĭ-sĭs) *n.* Regeneration of tissue. — **ne′o·ge·net′ic** (-jə-nĕt′ĭk) *adj.*

ne·ol·o·gism (nē-ŏl′ə-jĭz′əm) *n.* A meaningless word used by a psychotic. — **ne·ol′o·gis′tic, ne·ol′o·gis′ti·cal** *adj.*

ne·o·mem·brane (nē′ō-mĕm′brān′) *n.* See **false membrane.**

ne·o·my·cin (nē′ə-mī′sĭn) *n.* A broad-spectrum antibiotic produced from strains of the actinomycete *Streptomyces fradiae* and used especially in the form of its sulfate as an intestinal antiseptic in surgery.

ne·on (nē′ŏn′) *n.* A rare inert colorless gaseous element with atomic number 10 that glows reddish orange in an electric discharge and is used in display and television tubes.

ne·o·na·tal (nē′ō-nāt′l) *adj.* Of or relating to a newborn infant or to the first 28 days of an infant's life.

neonatal anemia *n.* See **erythroblastosis fetalis.**

neonatal medicine *n.* See **neonatology.**

neonatal mortality rate *n.* The ratio of the number of deaths in the first 28 days of life to the number of live births occurring in the same population during the same period of time.

ne·o·nate (nē′ə-nāt′) *n.* A neonatal infant.

ne·o·na·tol·o·gy (nē′ō-nā-tŏl′ə-jē) *n.* The branch of pediatrics that deals with the diseases and care of newborn infants. — **ne′o·na·tol′o·gist** *n.*

ne·o·pal·li·um (nē′ō-pāl′ē-əm) *n., pl* **-pal·li·ums** or **-pal·li·a** (-păl′ē-ə). See **isocortex.**

ne·o·pla·sia (nē′ō-plā′zhə, -zhē-ə) *n.* The pathological process that results in the formation and growth of a neoplasm.

ne·o·plasm (nē′ə-plăz′əm) *n.* An abnormal new growth of tissue that grows by cellular proliferation more rapidly than normal, continues to grow after the stimuli that initiated the new growth cease, exhibits a lack of structural organization and functional coordination with the normal tissue, and usually forms a distinct mass of tissue which may be benign or malignant; a tumor. — **ne′o·plas′tic** (-plăs′tĭk) *adj.*

ne·o·stig·mine (nē′ō-stĭg′mēn, -mĭn) *n.* Either of two related synthetic compounds that oppose the action of acetylcholinesterase and are used in the treatment of glaucoma, myasthenia gravis, and various postoperative conditions.

ne·o·vas·cu·lar·i·za·tion (nē′ō-văs′kyə-lər-ĭ-zā′-shən) *n.* **1.** Proliferation of blood vessels in tissue not normally containing them. **2.** Proliferation of blood vessels of a different kind than usual in tissue.

neph·e·lom·e·ter (něf'ə-lŏm'ĭ-tər) *n*. An apparatus used to measure the size and concentration of particles in a liquid by analysis of light scattered by the liquid. — **neph'e·lo·met'ric** (-lō-mět'rĭk) *adj*. — **neph'e·lom'e·try** *n*.

ne·phral·gi·a (nə-frăl'jē-ə, -jə) *n*. Pain in the kidney.

ne·phrec·ta·sis (nə-frěk'tə-sĭs) *n*. Dilation or distention of the pelvis of the kidney.

ne·phrec·to·my (nə-frěk'tə-mē) *n*. Surgical removal of a kidney.

neph·ric (něf'rĭk) *adj*. Relating to or connected with a kidney.

ne·phri·tis (nə-frī'tĭs) *n*., *pl*. **-phri·tis·es** or **-phrit·i·des** (-frĭt'ĭ-dēz'). Acute or chronic inflammation of the kidneys.

neph·ro·cap·sec·to·my (něf'rō-kăp-sěk'tə-mē) *n*. Surgical excision of the capsule of the kidney.

neph·ro·cele (něf'rə-sēl') *n*. Hernial displacement of a kidney.

neph·ro·gram (něf'rə-grăm') *n*. A radiograph of the kidney following the intravenous injection of a radiopaque substance. — **ne·phrog'ra·phy** (nə-frŏg'rə-fē, ně-) *n*.

neph·ro·li·thi·a·sis (něf'rō-lĭ-thī'ə-sĭs) *n*. The presence of calculi in the kidneys.

neph·ro·li·thot·o·my (něf'rō-lĭ-thŏt'ə-mē) *n*. Incision into the kidney to remove a renal calculus.

ne·phrol·o·gy (nə-frŏl'ə-jē) *n*. The medical science that deals with the kidneys, especially their functions or diseases. — **ne·phrol'o·gist** *n*.

ne·phrol·y·sis (nə-frŏl'ĭ-sĭs) *n*. **1.** The operation of freeing of the kidney from inflammatory adhesions, with preservation of the capsule. **2.** The destruction of renal cells. — **neph'ro·lyt'ic** (něf'rə-lĭt'ĭk) *adj*.

ne·phro·ma (nə-frō'mə) *n*., *pl*. **-mas** or **-ma·ta** (-mə-tə). A tumor arising from renal tissue.

neph·ron (něf'rŏn) *n*. The functional unit of the kidney, consisting of the renal corpuscle, the proximal convoluted tubule, the nephronic loop, and the distal convoluted tubule.

ne·phron·ic loop (ně-frŏn'ĭk) *n*. The U-shaped part of the nephron extending from the proximal to the distal convoluted tubules.

ne·phrop·a·thy (nə-frŏp'ə-thē) *n*. A disease of the kidney. — **neph'ro·path'ic** (něf'rə-păth'ĭk) *adj*.

neph·ro·pex·y (něf'rə-pěk'sē) *n*. Surgical fixation of a floating or mobile kidney.

neph·ro·py·e·lo·plas·ty (něf'rō-pī'ə-lə-plăs'tē) *n*. Plastic surgery of the kidney and renal pelvis.

neph·ro·py·o·sis (něf'rō-pī-ō'sĭs) *n*. Suppuration of the kidney.

neph·ror·rha·phy (něf-rôr'ə-fē) *n*. Suture of the kidney.

neph·ro·scle·ro·sis (něf'rō-sklə-rō'sĭs) *n*. Induration of the kidney from overgrowth and contraction of the interstitial connective tissue. — **neph'ro·scle·rot'ic** (-rŏt'ĭk) *adj*.

ne·phro·sis (nə-frō'sĭs) *n*., *pl*. **-ses** (-sēz). **1.** Disease of the kidneys marked by degeneration of renal tubular epithelium. **2.** See **nephrotic syndrome**. — **ne·phrot'ic** (-frŏt'ĭk) *adj*.

ne·phros·to·gram (nə-frŏs'tə-grăm') *n*. A radiograph of the kidney after a contrast agent has been administered. — **ne·phros'to·my** *n*.

ne·phrot·ic syndrome (nə-frŏt'ĭk) *n*. A clinical state characterized by edema, albuminuria, decreased plasma albumin, doubly refractile bodies in the urine, and usually increased blood cholesterol. It results from increased permeability of the glomerular capillary basement membranes.

neph·ro·to·mo·gram (něf'rō-tō'mə-grăm') *n*. A sectional radiograph of the kidneys following intravenous administration of contrast material to improve visualization of the renal parenchyma. — **neph'ro·to·mog'ra·phy** (-tō-mŏg'rə-fē) *n*.

ne·phrot·o·my (nə-frŏt'ə-mē) *n*. Incision into the kidney.

neph·ro·tox·ic·i·ty (něf'rō-tŏk-sĭs'ĭ-tē) *n*. The quality or state of being toxic to kidney cells.

neph·ro·tox·in (něf'rō-tŏk'sĭn) *n*. A cytotoxin specific for kidney cells. — **neph'ro·tox'ic** *adj*.

neph·ro·u·re·ter·ec·to·my (něf'rō-yŏŏ-rē'tə-rěk'tə-mē) *n*. Surgical removal of a kidney and its ureter.

neph·ro·u·re·ter·o·cys·tec·to·my (něf'rō-yŏŏ-rē'tə-rō-sĭ-stěk'tə-mē) *n*. Surgical removal of a kidney, ureter, and part or all of the bladder.

nep·tu·ni·um (něp-tōō'nē-əm, -tyōō'-) *n*. A metallic radioactive element with atomic number 93, found in trace quantities in uranium ores.

nerve (nûrv) *n*. **1.** Any of the cordlike bundles of nervous tissue made up of nerve fibers arranged in fascicles held together by a connective tissue sheath through which sensory stimuli and motor impulses pass between the brain or other parts of the central nervous system and the eyes, glands, muscles, and other parts of the body, forming a network of pathways for conducting information throughout the body. **2.** The sensitive tissue in the pulp of a tooth. **3. nerves**. Nervous agitation caused by fear, anxiety, or stress.

nerve avulsion *n*. The forcible disengagement of a portion of a nerve to produce paralysis.

nerve block anesthesia *n*. Conduction anesthesia in which the local anesthetic solution is injected about the peripheral nerves.

nerve cell *n*. **1.** See **neuron**. **2.** The body of a neuron without its axon and dendrites.

nerve conduction *n*. The transmission of an impulse along a nerve fiber.

nerve decompression *n*. The relief of pressure on a nerve trunk by the surgical excision of constricting bands or widening of the bony canal.

nerve fiber *n*. A threadlike process of a neuron, especially the prolonged axon that conducts nerve impulses.

nerve gas *n*. Any of various poisonous gases that interfere with the functioning of nerves by inhibiting cholinesterase.

nerve graft *n*. A graft in which a healthy nerve is used to replace a portion of a defective one.

nerve growth factor *n*. A protein that stimulates the growth of sympathetic and sensory nerve cells.

nerve impulse *n.* A wave of physical and chemical excitation along a nerve fiber in response to a stimulus, accompanied by a transient change in electric potential in the membrane of the fiber.

nerve plexus *n.* A plexus formed by nerves interlaced with numerous communicating branches.

nerve tissue *n.* A highly differentiated tissue composed of nerve cells, nerve fibers, dendrites, and neuroglia.

nerve trunk *n.* The main stem of a nerve, consisting of a bundle of nerve fibers bound together by a tough sheath of connective tissue.

ner·von·ic acid (nûr-vŏn′ĭk) *n.* A 24-carbon unsaturated fatty acid that occurs in cerebrosides and is formed through hydrolysis.

nerv·ous (nûr′vəs) *adj.* **1.** Of or relating to the nerves or nervous system. **2.** Stemming from or affecting the nerves or nervous system, as a disease. **3.** Easily agitated or distressed; high-strung or jumpy. — **nerv′ous·ness** *n.*

nervous bladder *n.* A urinary bladder condition in which there is a need to urinate frequently but failure to empty the bladder completely.

nervous breakdown *n.* A severe or incapacitating emotional disorder, especially when occurring suddenly and marked by depression.

nervous system *n.* The system of cells, tissues, and organs that regulates the body's responses to internal and external stimuli. In vertebrates it consists of the brain, spinal cord, nerves, ganglia, and parts of the receptor and effector organs.

net·il·mi·cin sulfate (nĕt′l-mī′sĭn) *n.* A parenteral aminoglycoside antibiotic used for short-term treatment of serious bacterial infections.

net·tle rash (nĕt′l) *n.* See **urticaria.**

neu·ral (nŏŏr′əl, nyŏŏr′-) *adj.* **1.** Of or relating to a nerve or the nervous system. **2.** Of, relating to, or located on the same side of the body as the spinal cord; dorsal.

neu·ral·gia (nŏŏ-răl′jə, nyŏŏ-) *n.* Sharp, severe paroxysmal pain extending along a nerve or group of nerves. — **neu·ral′gic** *adj.*

neu·ran·a·gen·e·sis (nŏŏr′ăn-ə-jĕn′ĭ-sĭs, nyŏŏr′-) *n.* Regeneration of a nerve.

neu·ra·prax·i·a (nŏŏr′ə-prăk′sē-ə, nyŏŏr′-) *n.* Injury to a nerve resulting in paralysis without degeneration and followed by rapid and complete recovery of function.

neu·ras·the·ni·a (nŏŏr′əs-thē′nē-ə, nyŏŏr′-) *n.* A complex of symptoms characterized by chronic fatigue and weakness, loss of memory, and generalized aches and pains. — **neu′ras·then′ic** (-thĕn′ĭk) *adj.*

neu·rax·is (nŏŏ-răk′sĭs, nyŏŏ-) *n.* The axial part of the central nervous system, including the spinal cord, rhombencephalon, mesencephalon, and diencephalon.

neu·rec·ta·sis (nŏŏ-rĕk′tə-sĭs, nyŏŏ-) or **neu·rec·ta·si·a** (nŏŏr′ĭk-tā′zē-ə, -zhə, nyŏŏr′-) *n.* Surgical stretching of a nerve or nerve trunk.

neu·rec·to·my (nŏŏ-rĕk′tə-mē, nyŏŏ-) *n.* Surgical removal of a nerve or part of a nerve.

neu·rex·er·e·sis (nŏŏr′ĕk-sĕr′ĭ-sĭs, nyŏŏr′-) *n.* Surgical extraction of a nerve.

neu·ri·lem·ma or **neu·ro·lem·ma** (nŏŏr′ə-lĕm′ə, nyŏŏr′-) *n.* The delicate membranous covering of a nerve fiber.

neurilemma cell or **neurolemma cell** *n.* See **Schwann cell.**

neu·ri·le·mo·ma or **neu·ri·lem·mo·ma** (nŏŏr′ə-lə-mō′mə, nyŏŏr′-) *n.* A benign, encapsulated neoplasm that may originate from a peripheral or sympathetic nerve or from cranial nerves.

neu·ri·no·ma (nŏŏr′ə-nō′mə, nyŏŏr′-) *n.* See **neurilemoma.**

neuritic plaque *n.* See **senile plaque.**

neu·ri·tis (nŏŏ-rī′tĭs, nyŏŏ-) *n.* Inflammation of a nerve or group of nerves, characterized by pain, loss of reflexes, and atrophy of the affected muscles. — **neu·rit′ic** (-rĭt′ĭk) *adj.*

neu·ro·a·nas·to·mo·sis (nŏŏr′ō-ə-năs′tə-mō′sĭs, nyŏŏr′-) *n.* Surgical formation of a junction between nerves.

neu·ro·ar·throp·a·thy (nŏŏr′ō-är-thrŏp′ə-thē, nyŏŏr′-) *n.* Disease of one or more joints caused by nerve injury or disease.

neu·ro·blast (nŏŏr′ə-blăst′, nyŏŏr′-) *n.* An embryonic cell from which a nerve develops.

neu·ro·blas·to·ma (nŏŏr′ō-blă-stō′mə, nyŏŏr′-) *n.* A malignant tumor composed of neuroblasts, originating in the autonomic nervous system or the adrenal medulla and occurring chiefly in infants and young children.

neu·roc·la·dism (nŏŏ-rŏk′lə-dĭz′əm, nyŏŏ-) *n.* The growth of axons from one segment of a cut nerve to bridge the gap to the other segment.

neu·ro·cra·ni·um (nŏŏr′ō-krā′nē-əm, nyŏŏr′-) *n.* The part of the skull enclosing the brain.

neu·ro·cyte (nŏŏr′ə-sīt′, nyŏŏr′-) *n.* See **neuron.**

neu·ro·cy·tol·y·sis (nŏŏr′ō-sī-tŏl′ĭ-sĭs, nyŏŏr′-) *n.* Destruction of nerve cells.

neu·ro·cy·to·ma (nŏŏr′ō-sī-tō′mə, nyŏŏr′-) *n.* See **ganglioneuroma.**

neu·ro·der·ma·ti·tis (nŏŏr′ō-dûr′mə-tī′tĭs, nyŏŏr′-) *n.* A chronic skin disorder characterized by localized or disseminated lichenified skin lesions that itch severely. It is thought to be a psychogenic disorder.

neu·ro·der·ma·to·sis (nŏŏr′ō-dûr′mə-tō′sĭs, nyŏŏr′-) *n.* See **neurodermatitis.**

neu·ro·dyn·i·a (nŏŏr′ō-dĭn′ē-ə, nyŏŏr′-) *n.* See **neuralgia.**

neu·ro·en·ceph·a·lo·my·e·lop·a·thy (nŏŏr′ō-ĕn-sĕf′ə-lō-mī′ə-lŏp′ə-thē, nyŏŏr′-) *n.* Disease of the brain, spinal cord, and nervous tissue.

neu·ro·fi·bril (nŏŏr′ə-fī′brəl, -fĭb′rəl, nyŏŏr′-) *n.* Any of the long, thin, microscopic fibrils that run through the body of a neuron and extend into the axon and dendrites, giving the neuron support and shape. — **neu′ro·fi′bril·lar** (-brə-lər) *adj.*

neu·ro·fi·bro·ma (nŏŏr′ō-fī-brō′mə, nyŏŏr′-) *n.* A moderately firm, benign, nonencapsulated tumor resulting from proliferation of Schwann cells in a disorderly pattern that includes portions of nerve fibers.

neu·ro·fi·bro·ma·to·sis (nŏŏr′ō-fī-brō′mə-tō′-sĭs, nyŏŏr′-) *n.* A genetic disease characterized by pigmented skin lesions and multiple skin neurofibromas, and sometimes accompanied by physical deformity and a predisposition to brain tumors and various forms of cancer.

neu·ro·fil·a·ment (nŏŏr′ə-fĭl′ə-mənt, nyŏŏr′-) *n.* Any of the long, fine threads that make up a neurofibril.

neu·ro·gan·gli·on (nŏŏr′ō-găng′glē-ən, nyŏŏr′-) *n.* See **ganglion** (sense 1).

neu·ro·gen·e·sis (nŏŏr′ə-jĕn′ĭ-sĭs, nyŏŏr′-) *n.* Formation of nervous tissue.

neu·ro·gen·ic (nŏŏr′ə-jĕn′ĭk, nyŏŏr′-) or **neu·ro·ge·net·ic** (-jə-nĕt′ĭk) *adj.* **1.** Originating in the nerves or nervous tissue. **2.** Caused or affected by the nerves or nervous system.

neurogenic bladder *n.* Defective functioning of the urinary bladder due to impaired nerve supply.

neu·rog·li·a (nŏŏ-rŏg′lē-ə, nyŏŏ-, nŏŏr′ə-glē′ə, -glī′-, nyŏŏr′-) *n.* The delicate network of branched cells and fibers supporting tissue of the central nervous system. — **neu·rog′li·al** *adj.*

neu·rog·li·o·ma·to·sis (nŏŏ-rŏg′lē-ō′mə-tō′sĭs, nyŏŏ-) *n.* See **gliomatosis**.

neu·ro·gram (nŏŏr′ə-grăm′, nyŏŏr′-) *n.* See **engram**.

neu·ro·hor·mone (nŏŏr′ō-hôr′mōn, nyŏŏr′-) *n.* A hormone secreted by or acting on a part of the nervous system.

neu·ro·hy·poph·y·sis (nŏŏr′ō-hī-pŏf′ĭ-sĭs, -hī-, nyŏŏr′-) *n., pl* **-ses** (-sēz′). The posterior portion of the pituitary gland, having a rich supply of nerve fibers and storing and releasing the hypothalamic hormones oxytocin and vasopressin. — **neu·ro·hy′po·phys′e·al, neu′ro·hy′po·phys′i·al** (-hī′pə-fīz′ē-əl, -hĭp′ə-, -hī-pŏf′ə-sē′əl) *adj.*

neu·roid (nŏŏr′oid′) *adj.* Relating to or resembling a nerve; nervelike.

neu·ro·lep·tan·al·ge·si·a (nŏŏr′ō-lĕp′tăn-əl-jē′zē-ə, -zhə, nyŏŏr′-) *n.* An intense analgesic and amnesic state produced by the combination of narcotic analgesics and neuroleptic drugs.

neu·ro·lep·tan·es·the·sia (nŏŏr′ō-lĕp′tăn-ĭs-thē′zhə, nyŏŏr′-) *n.* General anesthesia induced by intravenous administration of neuroleptic drugs combined with inhalation of a weak anesthetic.

neu·ro·lep·tic (nŏŏr′ə-lĕp′tĭk, nyŏŏr′-) *n.* A tranquilizing drug, especially one used in treating mental disorders. — *adj.* Having a tranquilizing effect.

neu·rol·o·gy (nŏŏ-rŏl′ə-jē, nyŏŏ-) *n.* The branch of medical science that deals with the nervous system and its disorders. — **neu·rol′o·gist** *n.*

neu·rol·y·sin (nŏŏ-rŏl′ĭ-sĭn, nyŏŏ-, nŏŏr′ə-lī′sĭn, nyŏŏr′-) *n.* A substance, such as a toxin, that destroys ganglion and cortical cells.

neu·rol·y·sis (nŏŏ-rŏl′ĭ-sĭs, nyŏŏ-) *n.* **1.** The breaking down or destruction of nerve tissue, especially as a result of disease. **2.** The surgical freeing of a nerve from inflammatory adhesions. — **neu′ro·lyt′ic** (nŏŏr′ə-lĭt′ĭk, nyŏŏr′-) *adj.*

neu·ro·ma (nŏŏ-rō′mə, nyŏŏ-) *n., pl.* **-mas** or **-ma·ta** (-mə-tə). A neoplasm from nerve tissue.

neuroma cu·tis (kyŏŏ′tĭs) *n.* Neurofibroma of the skin.

neu·ro·ma·la·ci·a (nŏŏr′ō-mə-lā′shē-ə, -shə, nyŏŏr′-) *n.* Softening of the nervous tissue as a result of disease.

neuroma tel·an·gi·ec·to·des (tĕl-ăn′jē-ĭk-tō′dēz) *n.* A neurofibroma having many blood vessels.

neu·ro·mus·cu·lar (nŏŏr′ō-mŭs′kyə-lər, nyŏŏr′-) *adj.* **1.** Of, relating to, or affecting both nerves and muscles. **2.** Having the characteristics of both nervous and muscular tissue.

neuromuscular blocking agent *n.* A compound, such as curare, that competes with acetylcholine and similar neurotransmitters for nerve cell receptor sites, thus preventing the contraction of skeletal muscles.

neuromuscular system *n.* The muscles of the body together with the nerves supplying them.

neu·ro·my·as·the·ni·a (nŏŏr′ō-mī′əs-thē′nē-ə, nyŏŏr′-) *n.* Muscular weakness, usually of emotional origin.

neu·ro·my·e·li·tis (nŏŏr′ō-mī′ə-lī′tĭs, nyŏŏr′-) *n.* Neuritis and inflammation of the spinal cord.

neu·ro·my·op·a·thy (nŏŏr′ō-mī-ŏp′ə-thē, nyŏŏr′-) *n.* A disorder or disease affecting nerves and associated muscle tissue.

neu·ron (nŏŏr′ŏn′, nyŏŏr′-) or **neu·rone** (-ōn′) *n.* Any of the impulse-conducting cells that constitute the brain, spinal column, and nerves, consisting of a nucleated cell body with one or more dendrites and a single axon.

neu·ro·ne·vus (nŏŏr′ō-nē′vəs, nyŏŏr′-) *n.* Any of various intradermal nevi containing nests of hyalinized nevus cells that resemble nerve bundles.

neu·ron·o·phage (nŏŏ-rŏn′ə-fāj′) *n.* A phagocyte that ingests neurons.

neu·ro·on·col·o·gy surgery (nŏŏr′ō-ŏn-kŏl′ə-jē, -ŏng-, nyŏŏr′-) *n.* Brain surgery that employs various techniques, such as sterotactic surgery, to locate, dislodge, and remove tumors.

neu·ro·o·tol·o·gy (nŏŏr′ō-ō-tŏl′ə-jē, nyŏŏr′-) *n.* The neurologic study of the ear.

neu·ro·pa·ral·y·sis (nŏŏr′ō-pə-răl′ĭ-sĭs, nyŏŏr′-) *n.* Paralysis resulting from a disease of the neurve supplying the affected part. — **neu′ro·par′a·lyt′ic** (-păr′ə-lĭt′ĭk) *adj.*

neu·ro·path·o·gen·e·sis (nŏŏr′ō-păth′ə-jĕn′ĭ-sĭs, nyŏŏr′-) *n.* The origin or development of a disease of the nervous system.

neu·ro·pa·thol·o·gy (nŏŏr′ō-pə-thŏl′ə-jē, nyŏŏr′-) *n.* The scientific study of diseases of the nervous system.

neu·rop·a·thy (nŏŏ-rŏp′ə-thē, nyŏŏ-) *n.* A disease or an abnormality of the nervous system, especially one affecting the cranial or spinal nerves. — **neu′ro·path′ic** (nŏŏr′ə-păth′ĭk, nyŏŏr′-) *adj.*

neu·ro·pep·tide (nŏŏr′ō-pĕp′tīd′, nyŏŏr′-) *n.* Any of a variety of peptides found in neural tissue, such as endorphins and enkephalins.

neu·ro·plas·ty (nŏŏr′ə-plăs′tē, nyŏŏr′-) *n.* Surgery to repair or restore nerve tissue.

neu·ro·po·di·a (nŏŏr′ə-pō′dē-ə, nyŏŏr′-) *pl.n.* See **axon terminals.**

neu·ro·psy·chi·a·try (nŏŏr′ō-sĭ-kī′ə-trē, -sī-, nyŏŏr′-) *n.* The medical science dealing with organic and psychic disorders of the nervous system.

neu·ro·psy·cho·log·ic disorder (nŏŏr′ō-sī′kə-lŏj′ĭk, nyŏŏr′-) *n.* A disturbance of mental function as a result of trauma that is associated with psychotic, neurotic, behavioral, or psychophysiologic disorders, and/or mental impairment.

neu·ro·psy·chop·a·thy (nŏŏr′ō-sī-kŏp′ə-thē, nyŏŏr′-) *n.* An emotional illness that is neurologic, functional, or both in origin.

neu·ro·ret·i·ni·tis (nŏŏr′ō-rĕt′n-ī′tĭs, nyŏŏr′-) *n.* Inflammation of the retina and optic nerve.

neu·ror·rha·phy (nŏŏ-rôr′ə-fē, nyŏŏ-) *n.* The surgical suturing of a divided nerve.

neu·ro·sar·co·clei·sis (nŏŏr′ō-sär′kō-klī′sĭs, nyŏŏr′-) *n.* Surgical procedure to relieve neuralgia in which a nerve traversing a wall of an osseous canal is transplanted into soft tissue.

neu·ro·sci·ence (nŏŏr′ō-sī′əns, nyŏŏr′-) *n.* Any of the sciences, such as neuroanatomy and neurobiology, that deal with the nervous system.

neu·ro·sis (nŏŏ-rō′sĭs, nyŏŏ-) *n., pl.* **-ses** (-sēz). **1.** Any of various mental or emotional disorders arising from no apparent organic lesion or change and involving symptoms such as insecurity, anxiety, depression, and irrational fears. **2.** Tension or irritability of the nervous system; any form of nervousness.

neu·ro·spasm (nŏŏr′ə-spăz′əm, nyŏŏr′-) *n.* A muscular spasm or twitching caused by or associated with a disordered nerve supply.

neu·ro·sthe·ni·a (nŏŏr′ō-sthē′nē-ə, nyŏŏr′-) *n.* A condition in which neurons respond with abnormal force or rapidity to slight stimuli.

neu·ro·sur·ger·y (nŏŏr′ō-sûr′jə-rē, nyŏŏr′-) *n.* Surgery on any part of the nervous system. — **neu′ro·sur′geon** (-jən) *n.* — **neu′ro·sur′gi·cal** (-jĭ-kəl) *adj.*

neu·ro·su·ture (nŏŏr′ō-sŏŏ′chər, nyŏŏr′-) *n.* See **neurorrhaphy.**

neu·ro·syph·i·lis (nŏŏr′ō-sĭf′ə-lĭs, nyŏŏr′-) *n.* Nervous system manifestations of syphilis including tabes dorsalis and general paresis.

neu·ro·the·ke·o·ma (nŏŏr′ō-thē′kē-ō′mə, nyŏŏr′-) *n.* A benign myxoma originating in the cutaneous nerve sheath.

neu·rot·ic (nŏŏ-rŏt′ĭk, nyŏŏ-) *adj.* Of, relating to, derived from, or affected with a neurosis. — *n.* A person suffering from a neurosis.

neu·rot·me·sis (nŏŏr′ŏt-mē′sĭs, nyŏŏr′-) *n.* The condition marked by complete division of a nerve.

neu·rot·o·my (nŏŏ-rŏt′ə-mē, nyŏŏ-) *n.* Surgical division of a nerve.

neu·rot·o·ny (nŏŏ-rŏt′n-ē, nyŏŏ-) *n.* See **neurectasis.** — **neu′ro·ton′ic** (nŏŏr′ə-tŏn′ĭk, nyŏŏr′-) *adj.*

neu·ro·tox·in (nŏŏr′ō-tŏk′sĭn, nyŏŏr′-) *n.* See **neurolysin.** — **neu′ro·tox′ic** *adj.*

neu·ro·trans·mit·ter (nŏŏr′ō-trăns′mĭt-ər,

-trănz′-, nyŏŏr′-) *n.* A chemical substance, such as acetylcholine or dopamine, that transmits nerve impulses across a synapse.

neu·ro·trip·sy (nŏŏr′ə-trĭp′sē, nyŏŏr′-) *n.* The surgical crushing of a nerve.

neu·rot·ro·phy (nŏŏ-rŏt′rə-fē, nyŏŏ-) *n.* The nutrition and metabolism of tissues under nervous influence. — **neu′ro·troph′ic** (nŏŏr′ə-trŏf′ĭk, -trō′fĭk, nyŏŏr′-) *adj.*

neu·rot·ro·py (nŏŏ-rŏt′rə-pē, nyŏŏ-) or **neu·rot·ro·pism** (-pĭz′əm) *n.* The tendency to affect, be attracted to, or attack nervous tissue. — **neu′ro·trop′ic** (nŏŏr′ə-trŏp′ĭk, nyŏŏr′-) *adj.*

neu·ro·vac·cine (nŏŏr′ō-văk-sēn′ -văk′sēn′, nyŏŏr′-) *n.* A vaccine virus, such as that in the smallpox vaccine, of known strength cultivated in vivo in the brains of rabbits.

neu·ro·vis·cer·al (nŏŏr′ō-vĭs′ər-əl, nyŏŏr′-) *adj.* Of or relating to innervation of the internal organs by the autonomic nervous system.

neu·ru·la·tion (nŏŏr′ə-lā′shən, -yə-lā′-, nyŏŏr′-) *n.* The formation of the embryonic neural plate and its transformation into the neural tube.

neu·ter (nŏŏ′tər, nyŏŏ′-) *adj.* **1.** Having undeveloped or imperfectly developed sexual organs. **2.** Sexually undeveloped. — *v.* **-tered, -ter·ing, -ters.** To castrate or spay.

neu·tral (nŏŏ′trəl, nyŏŏ′-) *adj.* **1.** Of or relating to a solution or compound that is neither acidic nor alkaline. **2.** Of or relating to a particle, an object, or a system that has neither positive nor negative electric charge. **3.** Of or relating to a particle, an object, or a system that has a net electric charge of zero.

neu·tral·i·za·tion (nŏŏ′trə-lĭ-zā′shən, nyŏŏ′-) *n.* **1.** A reaction between an acid and a base that yields a salt and water. **2.** The rendering ineffective of an action or substance, such as a drug.

neutralization plate *n.* A metal plate used for the internal fixation of a long-bone fracture to neutralize the forces producing displacement.

neu·tral·iz·ing antibody (nŏŏ′trə-lī′zĭng, nyŏŏ′-) *n.* An antibody that reacts with an infectious agent, usually a virus, and destroys or inhibits its infectiveness and virulence.

neutral mutation *n.* A mutation with a negligible impact on genetic fitness.

neu·tro·pe·ni·a (nŏŏ′trə-pē′nē-ə, nyŏŏ′-) *n.* The presence of a abnormally small numbers of neutrophils in the blood.

neu·tro·phil (nŏŏ′trə-fĭl′, nyŏŏ′-) or **neu·tro·phile** (-fĭl′) *n.* **1.** A neutrophil cell, especially an abundant type of granular white blood cell that destroys microorganisms. **2.** A cell or tissue that shows no special affinity for acid or basic dyes. — *adj.* Not stained strongly or definitely by either acid or basic dyes but stained readily by neutral dyes. Used especially of white blood cells. — **neu′tro·phile′** (-fĭl′), **neu′tro·phil′ic** (-fĭl′ĭk) *adj.*

neu·tro·phil·i·a (nŏŏ′trə-fĭl′ē-ə, nyŏŏ′-) *n.* An increase of neutrophilic white blood cells in blood or tissues.

neu·tro·phil·ic leukocyte (nōō'trə-fĭl'ĭk, nyōō'-) *n*. A highly phagocytic, polymorphonuclear white blood cells containing granules that do not stain deeply with acid or basic dyes.

neu·tro·tax·is (nōō'trə-tăk'sĭs, nyōō'-) *n*. A response shown by neutrophilic white blood cells when stimulated by a substance.

ne·vus (nē'vəs) *n., pl.* **-vi** (-vī'). **1.** A congenital circumscribed growth or mark on the skin, such as a mole or a birthmark, colored by hyperpigmentation or increased vascularity. **2.** A benign localized overgrowth of melanin-forming cells arising in the skin early in life.

nevus pig·men·to·sus (pĭg'mən-tō'səs, -mēn-) *n*. See **mole.**

nevus se·ba·ce·us (sə-bā'sē-əs) *n*. Congenital hyperplasia of the sebaceous glands with papillary acanthosis of the epidermis.

nevus spi·lus (spī'ləs) *n*. A flat mole.

nevus u·ni·us lat·er·is (yōō-nī'əs lăt'ər-ĭs, yōō'-nē-əs) *n*. A congenital linear nevus limited to one side of the body or to portions of the extremities on one side of the body.

nevus vas·cu·lar·is (văs'kyə-lâr'ĭs) or **nevus vas·cu·lo·sus** (-lō'səs) *n*. A congenital skin discoloration that is red-colored and irregular in shape, caused by overgrowth of cutaneous capillaries.

new·born (nōō'bôrn', nyōō'-) *adj*. Very recently born. — *n*. A neonate.

ng *abbr*. nanogram

ni·a·cin (nī'ə-sĭn) *n*. A white crystalline acid that is a component of the vitamin B complex found in meat, wheat germ, dairy products, and yeast and is used to treat and prevent pellagra.

niche (nĭch, nēsh) *n*. An eroded or ulcerated area detected by contrast radiography.

nick·el (nĭk'əl) *n*. A silvery hard ductile metallic element with atomic number 28.

nick·ing (nĭk'ĭng) *n*. A localized constriction in blood vessels of the retina of the eye.

nic·o·tin·a·mide adenine dinucleotide (nĭk'ə-tĭn'ə-mīd', -tē'nə-) *n*. NAD.

nicotinamide adenine dinucleotide phosphate *n*. NADP.

nic·o·tine (nĭk'ə-tēn') *n*. A colorless, poisonous alkaloid derived from the tobacco plant and used as an insecticide. It is the substance in tobacco to which smokers can become addicted.

nicotinic acid *n*. See **niacin.**

nic·o·tin·ism (nĭk'ə-tē-nĭz'əm) *n*. Nicotine poisoning, caused by excessive use of tobacco and marked by depression of the central and autonomic nervous systems.

nic·ti·ta·tion (nĭk'tĭ-tā'shən) *n*. The process of winking.

ni·da·tion (nī-dā'shən) *n*. The implantation of the early embryo in the uterine mucosa.

NIDD *abbr*. non-insulin-dependent diabetes

Nie·mann–Pick cell (nē'män'-) *n*. A rounded or polygonal mononuclear cell with indistinctly or palely staining, foamlike cytoplasm that contains numerous droplets of sphingomyelin; it is characteristic of Niemann–Pick disease.

Niemann–Pick disease *n*. An inherited disorder of lipid metabolism characterized by gastrointestinal disturbances and enlargement and abnormalities of blood-forming organs; it occurs primarily in infants of eastern European Jewish descent and leads to early death.

ni·fed·i·pine (nī-fĕd'ə-pēn') *n*. A coronary vasodilator and calcium-channel blocking agent that reduces calcium ions available to heart and smooth muscle, used in the treatment of angina pectoris.

night-blind *adj*. Affected with night blindness.

night blindness *n*. See **nyctalopia.**

night·mare (nīt'mâr') *n*. **1.** A dream arousing feelings of intense fear, horror, and distress. **2.** An event or experience that is intensely distressing.

night palsy *n*. Temporary numbness and paresis of an extremity due to its compression during sleep.

night terror *n*. A state of intense fear and agitation sometimes experienced, especially by children, on awakening from a stage of sleep not associated with dreaming but characterized by extremely vivid hallucinations.

night vision *n*. Vision occurring in dim light.

ni·gra (nī'grə) *n*. See **substantia nigra.**

ni·gri·ti·es (nī-grĭsh'ē-ēz') *n*. Black pigmentation, usually of the tongue.

ni·gro·sine (nī'grə-sēn', -sĭn) or **ni·gro·sin** (-sĭn) *n*. Any of a class of aniline dyes, varying from blue to black, used as histological stains for nervous tissue and as a negative stain for studying bacteria and spirochetes.

NIH *abbr*. National Institutes of Health

ni·hil·ism (nī'ə-lĭz'əm, nē'-) *n*. **1.** An extreme form of skepticism that denies all existence. **2.** A delusion, experienced in some mental disorders, that the world or one's mind, body, or self does not exist.

ninth cranial nerve *n*. See **glossopharyngeal nerve.**

ni·o·bi·um (nī-ō'bē-əm) *n*. A soft ductile metallic element with atomic number 41.

nip·ple (nĭp'əl) *n*. The projection at the apex of the mammary gland, on the surface of which the lactiferous ducts open, surrounded by the circular pigmented areola.

nipple shield *n*. A cap or dome placed over the nipple of the breast to protect it during nursing.

nit (nĭt) *n*. The egg or young of a parasitic insect, such as a louse.

ni·tri·tu·ri·a (nī'trī-tŏŏr'ē-ə, -tyŏŏr'-) *n*. The presence of nitrites, nitrates, or both in the urine.

ni·tro·fu·ran (nī'trō-fyŏŏr'ăn', -fyŏŏ-răn') *n*. Any of several drugs derived from furan that are used to inhibit bacterial growth.

ni·tro·fur·an·to·in (nī'trō-fyŏŏ-răn'tō-ĭn) *n*. A derivative of nitrofuran used in the treatment of bacterial infections of the urinary tract.

ni·tro·gen (nī'trə-jən) *n*. A nonmetallic element with atomic number 7 that constitutes nearly four fifths of the air by volume, occurs as a colorless, odorless, almost inert gas, and is in various minerals and all proteins and nucleic acids; it is soluble in blood and other body fluids.

nitrogen balance *n.* The difference between the amount of nitrogen taken into the body and the amount excreted or lost.

nitrogen equivalent *n.* The nitrogen content of protein, used in calculating the grams of protein metabolized by the body as a function of the grams of nitrogen excreted in the urine.

nitrogen lag *n.* The length of time between ingestion of a protein and urinary excretion of the amount of nitrogen equal to that in the protein.

nitrogen mustard *n.* Any of various toxic blistering compounds analogous to mustard gas but containing nitrogen rather than sulfur, sometimes used to control or check the growth of neoplastic cells.

nitrogen narcosis *n.* A condition of confusion or stupor resulting from increased levels of dissolved nitrogen in the blood, as that occurring in deepsea divers breathing air under high pressure.

ni·trog·e·nous (nī-trŏj′ə-nəs) *adj.* Relating to or containing nitrogen.

nitrogen partition *n.* The determination of the distribution of nitrogen in the urine among the various constituents.

ni·tro·glyc·er·in or **ni·tro·glyc·er·ine** (nī′trŏ-glĭs′ər-ĭn, -trə-) *n.* A thick, pale yellow liquid that is explosive on concussion or exposure to sudden heat. It is used as a vasodilator in medicine.

ni·tros·a·mine (nī-trŏ′sə-mēn′, nī′trŏs-ăm′ēn) *n.* Any of a class of organic compounds present in various foods and other products. Some have been found carcinogenic and mutagenic in laboratory animals.

ni·trous oxide (nī′trəs) *n.* A colorless, sweet-tasting gas used as a mild anesthetic in dentistry and surgery.

ni·zat·i·dine (nī-zăt′ĭ-dēn′) *n.* A histamine antagonist used to treat active duodenal ulcers.

NK cell *abbr.* natural killer cell

nm *abbr.* nanometer

NMR *abbr.* nuclear magnetic resonance

no·bel·i·um (nō-bĕl′ē-əm) *n.* A radioactive synthetic element with atomic number 102.

no·ble gas (nō′bəl) *n.* Any of the chemically inert gaseous elements in Group O of the periodic table, including helium, neon, argon, krypton, xenon, and radon.

No·car·di·a (nō-kär′dē-ə) *n.* A genus of aerobic, gram-positive, primarily saprophytic actinomycetes, transitional between bacteria and fungi, that form filaments that fragment to single nonmotile microorganisms, including some species that may be pathogenic to humans.

no·car·di·o·sis (nō-kär′dē-ō′sĭs) *n.* A generalized disease in humans caused by *Nocardia asteroides* or occasionally by *N. farcinica* and characterized by pulmonary lesions that may be subclinical or chronic and may spread to other organs of the body, especially the brain.

no·ci·cep·tive (nō′sĭ-sĕp′tĭv) *adj.* **1.** Causing pain. Used of a stimulus. **2.** Caused by or responding to a painful stimulus.

nociceptive reflex *n.* A reflex elicited by a painful stimulus.

no·ci·cep·tor (nō′sĭ-sĕp′tər) *n.* A sensory receptor that responds to pain.

no·ci·fen·sor (nō′sə-fĕn′sər) *n.* **1.** A process or mechanism that acts to protect the body from injury. **2.** A system of nerves in the skin and mucous membranes that react to adjacent injury by causing vasodilation.

no·ci·per·cep·tion (nō′sə-pər-sĕp′shən) *n.* The perception of injurious stimuli, such as by nerve centers.

noc·tam·bu·lism (nŏk-tăm′byə-lĭz′əm) *n.* See **sleepwalking.**

noct. maneq. *abbr. Latin.* nocte maneque (at night and in the morning)

noc·tu·ri·a (nŏk-tŏŏr′ē-ə, -tyŏŏr′-) *n.* Urination at night, especially if excessive.

noc·tur·nal (nŏk-tûr′nəl) *adj.* **1.** Of, relating to, or occurring in the night. **2.** Most active at night.

nocturnal enuresis *n.* See **bed-wetting.**

nocturnal myoclonus *n.* Involuntary muscular jerks occurring during sleep.

nod·al (nōd′l) *adj.* Of, relating to, resembling, being, or situated near or at a node.

nodal bradycardia *n.* See **atrioventricular nodal rhythm.**

nodal escape *n.* Cardiologic escape in which the atrioventricular node serves as pacemaker.

nodal extrasystole *n.* See **atrioventricular nodal extrasystole.**

nodal rhythm *n.* See **atrioventricular nodal rhythm.**

node (nōd) *n.* **1.** A knob, knot, protuberance, or swelling. **2.** A protuberant growth or swelling in a tissue. **3.** A knuckle or other swelling.

node of Ran·vier (rän′vyā, rän-vyā′, räɴ) *n.* A small gap in the myelin sheath along the axon of a neuron.

no·dose (nō′dōs′) *adj.* Having many nodes or knotlike swellings. —**no·dos′i·ty** (-dŏs′ĭ-tē) *n.*

nodose rheumatism *n.* Acute or subacute articular rheumatism accompanied by the formation of nodules on the tendons, ligaments, and periosteum in the area of the affected joints.

nod·u·lar (nŏj′ə-lər) *adj.* Characterized by the formation of nodules. —**nod′u·lar′i·ty** (lăr′ĭ-tē) *n.*

nodular fasciitis *n.* A tumorlike proliferation of fibroblasts with mild inflammatory exudation occurring in a fascia.

nod·u·la·tion (nŏj′ə-lā′shən) *n.* The formation or presence of nodules.

nod·ule (nŏj′ōōl) *n.* **1.** A small node. **2.** A small mass of tissue or aggregation of cells.

no·ma (nō′mə) *n.* A severe, often gangrenous inflammation of the lips and cheek or of the female genitals, occurring usually after an infectious disease and found most often in children in poor hygienic or malnourished condition.

no·men·cla·ture (nō′mən-klā′chər, nō-mĕn′klə-) *n.* A system of names used in a science, as of anatomical structures or biological organisms.

no·mi·fen·sine ma·le·ate (nō′mə-fĕn′sēn′ mā′lē-āt′, mə-lē′ət) *n.* An antidepressant and central nervous system stimulant.

non·ab·sorb·a·ble suture (nŏn′əb-sôr′bə-bəl, -zôr′-) *n.* A surgical suture made from a material unaffected by the biological activities of the body tissues, and therefore permanent unless removed.

non·al·co·hol·ic (nŏn′ăl-kə-hô′lĭk) *adj.* A beverage usually containing less than 0.5 percent alcohol by volume.

non-A, non-B hepatitis *n.* Hepatitis caused by a virus that is antigenically different from hepatitis viruses A and B.

non·com·pet·i·tive inhibition (nŏn′kəm-pĕt′ĭ-tĭv) *n.* A type of enzyme inhibition in which the inhibiting compound does not compete with the natural substrate for the active site on the enzyme, but inhibits reaction by combining with the enzyme-substrate complex after the complex is formed.

non com·pos men·tis (nŏn kŏm′pəs mĕn′tĭs) *adj.* Not of sound mind and hence not legally responsible; mentally incompetent.

non·e·lec·tro·lyte (nŏn′ĭ-lĕk′trə-līt′) *n.* A substance whose molecules in solution do not dissociate to ions and thus do not conduct an electric current.

non·es·sen·tial (nŏn′ĭ-sĕn′shəl) *adj.* Being a substance that is required for normal functioning but does not need to be included in the diet because of the body's ability to synthesize it from other nutrients.

non·es·sen·tial amino acid (nŏn′ĭ-sĕn′shəl) *n.* An alpha-amino acid that is both required for protein synthesis and produced by humans.

non·fat (nŏn′făt′) *adj.* Lacking fat solids or having the fat content removed.

non·fen·es·trat·ed forceps (nŏn-fĕn′ĭ-strā′tĭd) *n.* An obstetrical forceps without openings in the blades, thus facilitating rotation of the head.

non·gon·o·coc·cal urethritis (nŏn′gŏn-ə-kŏk′əl) *n.* Inflammation of the urethra similar to that of gonorrhea but usually caused by infection with the rickettsia *Chlamydia trachomatis* and occurring mostly in males.

non-Hodg·kin's lymphoma (nŏn-hŏj′kĭnz) *n.* Any of various malignant lymphomas characterized by the absence of Reed–Sternberg cells.

non·i·den·ti·cal (nŏn′ī-dĕn′tĭ-kəl) *adj.* **1.** Not being the same; different. **2.** Fraternal, as of twins.

non·im·mune serum (nŏn′ĭ-myōon′) *n.* Serum that does not contain antibodies to a given antigen.

non·im·mu·ni·ty (nŏn′ĭ-myōo′nĭ-tē) *n.* See **aphylaxis.**

non·in·su·lin-de·pend·ent diabetes (nŏn-ĭn′sə-lĭn-dĭ-pĕn′dənt) *n.* See **diabetes mellitus** (sense 2).

non·in·va·sive (nŏn′ĭn-vā′sĭv) *adj.* **1.** Not penetrating the body, as by incision or injection. Used especially of a diagnostic procedure. **2.** Not invading healthy tissue.

non·la·mel·lar bone (nŏn′lə-mĕl′ər) *n.* See **woven bone.**

non·med·ul·lat·ed fiber (nŏn-mĕd′l-ā′tĭd) *n.* See **unmyelinated fiber.**

non·os·te·o·gen·ic fibroma (nŏn′ŏs-tē-ə-jĕn′ĭk) *n.* See **fibrous cortical defect.**

non·ox·y·nol-9 (nŏn-ŏk′sə-nôl′-, -nôl′-) *n.* A spermicide widely used in contraceptive creams, foams, and lubricants.

non·pen·e·trance (nŏn-pĕn′ĭ-trəns) *n.* **1.** The state in which a genetic trait, although present in the appropriate genotype, fails to manifest itself in the phenotype. **2.** The obscuring of genetic traits by nongenetic mechanisms.

non·pen·e·trant trait (nŏn-pĕn′ĭ-trənt) *n.* A genetic trait that is not manifested phenotypically because of factors outside its own locus.

non·pen·e·trat·ing wound (nŏn-pĕn′ĭ-trā′tĭng) *n.* A wound, especially to the thorax or abdomen, produced without disruption of the body's surface.

non·pre·scrip·tion (nŏn′prĭ-skrĭp′shən) *adj.* Sold legally without a physician's prescription; over-the-counter.

non·pro·tein nitrogen (nŏn-prō′tēn′, -tē-ĭn) *n.* The nitrogen content of substances other than protein present in blood, tissues, and waste materials.

non·rap·id eye movement (nŏn-răp′ĭd) *n.* Slow oscillation of the eyes during the portion of the sleep cycle when dreaming does not take place.

non·re·breath·ing anesthesia (nŏn′rē-brē′thĭng) *n.* A technique for inhalation anesthesia in which valves exhaust all exhaled air from the circuit.

non·se·cre·tor (nŏn′sĭ-krē′tər) *n.* A person whose saliva does not contain antigens of the ABO blood group.

non·self (nŏn-sĕlf′) *n.* That which the immune system identifies as foreign to the body.

non·spe·cif·ic immunity (nŏn′spī-sĭf′ĭk) *n.* See **innate immunity.**

nonspecific protein *n.* A protein substance that elicits an immunological response not mediated by a specific antigen-antibody reaction.

nonspecific urethritis *n.* Urethritis not resulting from gonococcal or other identifiable infectious agents.

non·vi·a·ble (nŏn-vī′ə-bəl) *adj.* Not capable of living or developing independently. Used especially of an embryo or a fetus.

Noo·nan's syndrome (nōo′nənz) *n.* An inherited condition characterized by congenital heart disease, pulmonary stenosis, webbing of the neck, and pigeon breast.

nor·a·dren·a·lin (nôr′ə-drĕn′ə-lĭn) *n.* See **norepinephrine.**

nor·ep·i·neph·rine (nôr′ĕp-ə-nĕf′rĭn) *n.* A substance, both a hormone and neurotransmitter, secreted by the adrenal medulla and the nerve endings of the sympathetic nervous system to cause vasoconstriction and increases in heart rate, blood pressure, and the sugar level of the blood.

nor·eth·in·drone (nôr-ĕth′ĭn-drōn′) *n.* A progestational agent with some estrogenic and androgenic activity that is used as a substitute for progesterone and, in combination with an estrogen, as an oral contraceptive.

nor·flox·a·cin (nôr-flŏk′sə-sĭn) *n.* An oral broad-spectrum quinoline antibacterial agent used in the treatment of urinary tract infections.

nor·mal (nôr′məl) *adj.* **1.** Conforming with, adhering to, or constituting a norm, standard, pattern, level, or type; typical. **2.** Functioning or occurring in a natural way; lacking observable abnormalities or deficiencies. **3.** Occurring naturally and not because of disease, inoculation, or any experimental treatment. Used of immunity. **4.** Of, relating to, or being a solution having one gram equivalent weight of solute per liter of solution. **5.** Relating to or characterized by average intelligence or development. — *n.* The usual or expected state, form, amount, or degree.

normal human plasma *n.* Sterile plasma obtained by pooling the liquid portion of citrated whole blood from eight or more healthy adult humans and by exposing it to ultraviolet light to destroy bacterial and viral contaminants.

normal human serum albumin *n.* A sterile preparation of serum albumin obtained by fractionating blood plasma proteins from healthy persons and used as a transfusion material.

normal opsonin *n.* Opsonin normally present in the blood, without stimulation by a known specific antigen.

normal serum *n.* A nonimmune serum, especially serum obtained from a person prior to immunization.

normal values *pl.n.* A set of laboratory test values used to characterize apparently healthy individuals; they have now been replaced by reference values.

nor·mo·blast (nôr′mə-blăst′) *n.* A nucleated red blood cell, the immediate precursor of a normal red blood cell in humans.

nor·mo·cap·ni·a (nôr′mə-kăp′nē-ə) *n.* A state in which the arterial carbon dioxide pressure is normal.

nor·mo·chro·mi·a (nôr′mə-krō′mē-ə) *n.* Normal blood color because of normal amount of hemoglobin in the red blood cells.

nor·mo·cyte (nôr′mə-sīt′) *n.* A red blood cell having normal size, shape, or color.

nor·mo·cy·to·sis (nôr′mō-sī-tō′sĭs) *n.* A normal state of the blood with regard to its component formed elements.

nor·mo·gly·ce·mi·a (nôr′mō-glī-sē′mē-ə) *n.* See **euglycemia.** — *nor′mo·gly·ce′mic adj.*

nor·mo·ka·le·mi·a (nôr′mō-kā-lē′mē-ə) *n.* A normal level of potassium in the blood.

nor·mo·ka·le·mic periodic paralysis (nôr′mō-kā-lē′mĭk) *n.* An inherited form of periodic paralysis in which the serum potassium level is within normal limits during attacks.

nor·mo·ten·sive (nôr′mō-tĕn′sĭv) *adj.* Of or relating to a normal arterial blood pressure; normotonic. — *nor′mo·ten′sive n.*

nor·mo·ther·mi·a (nôr′mō-thûr′mē-ə) *n.* **1.** A condition of normal body temperature. **2.** An en-

vironmental temperature that does not cause increased or depressed activity of body cells. — *nor′mo·ther′mic adj.*

nor·mo·vo·le·mi·a (nôr′mō-vō-lē′mē-ə) *n.* A normal blood volume.

North·ern blot analysis (nôr′thərn) *n.* An electrophoretic procedure used to separate and identify RNA fragments.

nor·trip·ty·line (nôr-trĭp′tə-lēn′) *n.* A tricyclic compound used as a tranquilizer and an antidepressant.

nos·ca·pine (nŏs′kə-pēn′) *n.* An alkaloid occurring in opium that suppresses the cough reflex and is used as an antitussive.

nose (nōz) *n.* The part of the face that contains the nostrils and organs of smell and forms the beginning of the respiratory tract.

nose·bleed (nōz′blēd′) *n.* A nasal hemorrhage; bleeding from the nose.

nose job *n.* Plastic surgery on the nose, especially to improve its appearance; rhinoplasty.

nos·o·co·mi·al (nŏs′ə-kō′mē-əl) *adj.* **1.** Of or relating to a hospital. **2.** Of or being a secondary disorder associated with being treated in a hospital but unrelated to a primary condition.

nos·o·gen·e·sis (nŏs′ō-jĕn′ĭ-sĭs) or **no·sog·e·ny** (nō-sŏj′ə-nē) *n.* See **pathogenesis.**

no·sog·ra·phy (nō-sŏg′rə-fē, -zŏg′-) *n.* The systematic description of diseases.

nos·o·ma·ni·a (nŏs′ə-mā′nē-ə, -măn′yə) *n.* An unfounded, abnormal belief that one is suffering from some special disease.

nos·o·phil·i·a (nŏs′ə-fĭl′ē-ə) *n.* A desire to be ill; love of sickness.

nos·o·pho·bi·a (nŏs′ə-fō′bē-ə) *n.* An inordinate fear of disease.

nos·tril (nŏs′trəl) *n.* Either of the external openings of the nose; a naris.

notch (nŏch) *n.* **1.** An indentation at the edge of a structure; an incisure. **2.** An upstroke or peak on a pulse tracing.

no·ti·fi·a·ble disease (nō′tə-fī′ə-bəl) *n.* A disease that must be reported to public health authorities at the time it is diagnosed because of the danger it poses to human or animal health.

no·to·chord (nō′tə-kôrd′) *n.* A flexible rodlike structure in embryos, from which the spinal column develops. — *no′to·chord′al adj.*

nour·ish (nûr′ĭsh, nŭr′-) *v.* **-ished, -ish·ing, -ish·es.** To provide with food or other substances necessary for sustaining life and growth.

nour·ish·ment (nûr′ĭsh-mənt, nŭr′-) *n.* Something that nourishes; food.

No·vo·cain (nō′və-kān′) A trademark used for an anesthetic preparation of procaine.

nox·ious (nŏk′shəs) *adj.* Harmful to living things; injurious to health. — *nox′ious·ness n.*

NP *abbr.* neuropsychiatry

NREM *abbr.* non-rapid eye movement

nRNA (ĕn′är-ĕn-ā′) *n.* Nuclear RNA; RNA found in the nucleus either associated with chromosomes or in the nucleoplasm.

NSAID (ĕn′sād′) *n.* A nonsteroidal anti-inflammatory drug, such as aspirin or ibuprofen.

nu·cha (nōō′kə, nyōō′-) *n.* The back of the neck; the nape. — **nu′chal** *adj.*

nu·cle·ar (nōō′klē-ər, nyōō′-) *adj.* **1.** Of, relating to, or forming a nucleus. **2.** Of or relating to atomic nuclei.

nuclear envelope *n.* See **nuclear membrane.**

nuclear family *n.* A family unit consisting of a mother and father and their progeny.

nuclear hyaloplasm *n.* See **karyolymph.**

nuclear magnetic resonance *n.* The absorption of electromagnetic radiation of a specific frequency by an atomic nucleus that is placed in a strong magnetic field, used especially in spectroscopic studies of molecular structure and clinically as the technology that permits magnetic resonance imaging of soft tissue body structures.

nuclear medicine *n.* The branch of medicine that deals with the use of radionuclides in the diagnosis and treatment of disease.

nuclear membrane *n.* The double-layered membrane enclosing the nucleus of a cell.

nuclear pore *n.* An octagonal opening where the inner and outer membranes of the nuclear envelope are continuous.

nuclear RNA *n.* nRNA.

nuclear spindle *n.* See **mitotic spindle.**

nuclear stain *n.* A stain for cell nuclei, usually based on the binding of a basic dye to DNA or to histone-containing nucleoprotein.

nu·cle·ase (nōō′klē-ās′, -āz′, nyōō′-) *n.* Any of several enzymes, such as endonucleases and exonucleases, that hydrolize nucleic acids.

nu·cle·a·tion (nōō′klē-ā′shən, nyōō′-) *n.* The formation of cell nuclei.

nu·cle·ic acid (nōō-klē′ĭk, -klā′-, nyōō-) *n.* Any of a group of complex compounds found in all living cells and viruses, composed of purines, pyrimidines, carbohydrates, and phosphoric acid. Nucleic acids in the form of DNA and RNA control cellular function and heredity.

nu·cle·in (nōō′klē-ĭn, nyōō-) *n.* Any of the substances present in the nucleus of a cell, consisting chiefly of proteins, phosphoric acids, and nucleic acids.

nu·cle·o·lus (nōō-klē′ə-ləs, nyōō-) *n., pl.* **-li** (-lī′). A small, typically round granular body composed of protein and RNA in the nucleus of a cell, usually associated with a specific chromosomal site and involved in rRNA synthesis and the formation of ribosomes. — **nu·cle′o·lar** (-lər) *adj.*

nu·cle·on (nōō′klē-ŏn′, nyōō′-) *n.* A proton or a neutron, especially as part of an atomic nucleus. — **nu′cle·on′ic** *adj.*

nu·cle·o·plasm (nōō′klē-ə-plăz′əm, nyōō′-) *n.* The protoplasm of a cell nucleus.

nu·cle·o·pro·tein (nōō′klē-ō-prō′tēn′, -prō′tē-ĭn, nyōō′-) *n.* Any of a group of substances found in the nuclei of all living cells and in viruses, composed of a protein and a nucleic acid.

nu·cle·or·rhex·is (nōō′klē-ə-rěk′sĭs) *n.* Fragmentation of a cell nucleus.

nu·cle·o·si·dase (nōō′klē-ə-sī′dās′, -dāz′, -klē-ō′-

sĭ-, nyōō′-) *n.* Any of various enzymes that catalyze the hydrolysis of nucleosides, releasing their purine or pyrimidine base.

nu·cle·o·side (nōō′klē-ə-sīd′, nyōō′-) *n.* Any of various compounds consisting of a sugar, usually ribose or deoxyribose, and a purine or pyrimidine base, especially a compound obtained by hydrolysis of a nucleic acid, such as adenosine or guanine.

nu·cle·o·some (nōō′klē-ə-sōm′, nyōō′-) *n.* Any of the repeating subunits of chromatin, consisting of a DNA chain coiled around a core of histones. — **nu′cle·o·som′al** (-sō′məl) *adj.*

nu·cle·o·ti·dase (nōō′klē-ə-tī′dās, -dāz, nyōō′-) *n.* An enzyme that catalyzes the hydrolysis of a nucleotide to a nucleoside and phosphoric acid.

nu·cle·o·tide (nōō′klē-ə-tīd′, nyōō′-) *n.* Any of various compounds consisting of a nucleoside combined with a phosphate group and forming the basic constituent of DNA and RNA.

nu·cle·o·tox·in (nōō′klē-ə-tŏk′sĭn, nyōō′-) *n.* A toxin acting upon the cell nuclei.

nu·cle·us (nōō′klē-əs, nyōō′-) *n., pl.* **-cle·us·es** or **-cle·i** (-klē-ī′). **1.** A large, membrane-bound, usually spherical protoplasmic structure within a living cell, containing the cell's hereditary material and controlling its metabolism, growth, and reproduction. **2.** A membraneless structure in microorganisms that contains genetic material but does not itself replicate. **3.** A group of specialized nerve cells or a localized mass of gray matter in the brain or spinal cord. **4.** The substance around which a urinary or other calculus forms.

nu·clide (nōō′klīd′, nyōō′-) *n.* A type of atom specified by its atomic number, atomic mass, and energy state, such as carbon 14. — **nu·clid′ic** (nōō-klĭd′ĭk, nyōō-) *adj.*

null cell *n.* See **killer cell.**

nul·li·grav·i·da (nŭl′ĭ-grăv′ĭ-də) *n.* A woman who has never conceived a child.

nul·lip·a·ra (nə-lĭp′ər-ə) *n.* A woman who has never given birth. — **nul′li·par′i·ty** (nŭl′ə-păr′ĭ-tē) *n.* — **nul·lip′a·rous** (-rəs) *adj.*

numb (nŭm) *adj.* **1.** Unable or only partially able to feel sensation or pain; deadened or anesthetized. **2.** Emotionally unresponsive; indifferent. — *v.* **numbed, numb·ing, numbs.** To make or become numb. — **numb′ness** *n.*

num·mu·lar (nŭm′yə-lər) *adj.* **1.** Shaped like a coin; disk-shaped. Used of mucus or sputum in certain respiratory diseases. **2.** Arranged like stacks of coins. Used of red blood cells in rouleaux formation.

nurse (nûrs) *n.* **1.** A person trained to care for the sick or disabled, especially one who is educated in the scientific basis of human response to actual or potential health problems and who is trained to assist a physician. **2.** A wet nurse. **3.** A person who cares for an infant or young child; a nursemaid. — *v.* **nursed, nurs·ing, nurs·es. 1.** To serve as a nurse. **2.** To provide or take nourishment from the breast; suckle.

nurse anesthetist *n.* A person who, after completing basic educational requirements as a nurse, is further trained in the supervised administration of anesthetics.

nurse-midwife *n.* A person formally educated and certified to practice in the two disciplines of nursing and midwifery. — **nurse-midwifery** *n.*

nurse practitioner *n.* A registered nurse with advanced training for providing primary health care, including many tasks customarily performed by a physician.

nurse's aide (nûr′sĭz) *n.* A person who assists nurses at a hospital or other medical facility in tasks requiring little or no formal training or education.

nurs·ing (nûr′sĭng) *n.* **1.** The profession of a nurse. **2.** The tasks or care of a nurse. **3.** The act or practice of breast-feeding.

nursing home *n.* A private establishment that provides living quarters and care for the elderly or the chronically ill.

nu·ta·tion (nōō-tā′shən, nyōō-) *n.* The act of nodding the head, especially involuntarily.

nu·tri·ent (nōō′trē-ənt, nyōō′-) *n.* A source of nourishment, especially a nourishing ingredient found in food, such as carbohydrate, protein, or fat.

nutrient artery *n.* An artery of variable origin that supplies the medullary cavity of a long bone.

nutrient canal *n.* A canal in the shaft of a long bone or in other locations in irregular bones through which the nutrient artery enters.

nutrient foramen *n.* The external opening of the nutrient canal in a bone.

nutrient vessel *n.* An artery of variable origin that supplies the medullary cavity of a long bone.

nu·tri·ment (nōō′trə-mənt, nyōō′-) *n.* **1.** A source of nourishment; food. **2.** An agent that promotes growth or development.

nu·tri·tion (nōō-trĭsh′ən, nyōō-) *n.* **1.** The process by which a living organism assimilates food and uses it for growth, liberation of energy, and replacement of tissues; its successive stages include digestion, absorption, assimilation, and excretion. **2.** The science or study that deals with food and nourishment, especially in humans. — **nu·tri′tion·al** *adj.*

nu·tri·tion·ist (nōō-trĭsh′ə-nĭst, nyōō-) *n.* One who is trained or is an expert in the field of nutrition.

nu·tri·tion·ist's calorie *n.* See **calorie** (sense 1).

nu·tri·tious (nōō-trĭsh′əs, nyōō-) *adj.* Providing nourishment; nourishing.

nu·tri·tive equilibrium (nōō′trĭ-tĭv, nyōō-) *n.* A balance between intake and excretion of nutritive material, so that there is no gain or loss in weight.

nu·tri·ture (nōō′trə-chŏŏr′, -chər) *n.* **1.** The state or condition of the nutrition of the body. **2.** Nutritional status, especially with regard to a specific nutrient.

nyc·tal·gi·a (nĭk-tăl′jē-ə, -jə) *n.* Night pain, especially the bone pains of syphilis occurring at night.

nyc·ta·lo·pi·a (nĭk′tə-lō′pē-ə) *n.* A condition of the eyes in which vision is normal in daylight or other strong light but is abnormally weak or completely lost at night or in dim light, resulting from vitamin A deficiency, disease, or hereditary factors. — **nyc′ta·lo′pic** (-lō′pĭk, -lŏp′ĭk) *adj.*

nyc·to·phil·i·a (nĭk′tə-fĭl′ē-ə) *n.* A preference for the night or darkness.

nyc·to·pho·bi·a (nĭk′tə-fō′bē-ə) *n.* An abnormal fear of night or of the dark.

nym·pha (nĭm′fə) *n.*, *pl.* **-phae** (-fē). Either of the labia minora. — **nym′phal** *adj.*

nym·pho·ma·ni·a (nĭm′fə-mā′nē-ə, -mān′yə) *n.* Extreme or obsessive sexual desire in a woman. — **nym′pho·ma′ni·ac′** (-nē-ăk′) *adj. & n.* — **nym′pho·ma·ni′a·cal** (-mə-nī′ə-kəl) *adj.*

nym·phot·o·my (nĭm-fŏt′ə-mē) *n.* An incision into the labia minora or into the clitoris.

nys·tag·mus (nĭ-stăg′məs) *n.* A rapid, involuntary, oscillatory motion of the eyeball. — **nys·tag′mic** (-mĭk) *adj.*

nys·ta·tin (nĭs′tə-tĭn) *n.* An antibiotic produced by the actinomycete *Streptomyces noursei* and used especially in the treatment of candidiasis and other fungal infections.

Nys·ten's law (nē-stănz′) *n.* The principle that rigor mortis affects first the muscles of the head and spreads toward the hands and feet.

nyx·is (nĭk′sĭs) *n.* A pricking or puncture; paracentesis.

~ ~ ~ ~ ~ O ~ ~ ~ ~ ~ ~

O agglutinin (ō) *n.* An agglutinin that reacts with, and is formed as the result of stimulation by, the relatively thermostable antigens in the cells of microorganisms.

oat cell *n.* A short, bluntly spindle-shaped, anaplastic cell containing a relatively large, hyperchromatic nucleus and observed in some forms of undifferentiated bronchogenic carcinoma.

OB *abbr.* obstetrics

o·bese (ō-bēs′) *adj.* Extremely fat; very overweight.

o·be·si·ty (ō-bē′sĭ-tē) *n.* The condition of being obese; increased body weight caused by excessive accumulation of fat, usually from 20% to 30% over an individual's recommended weight.

ob-gyn or **OB/GYN** (ō′bē-jē′wī-ĕn′) *n.* **1.** The comhined practice or field of obstetrics and gynecology. **2.** An obstetrician-gynecologist.

ob·jec·tive (əb-jĕk′tĭv) *adj.* **1.** Based on observable phenomena; presented factually. **2.** Indicating a symptom or condition perceived as a sign of disease by someone other than the person affected. — **ob·jec′tive·ness** *n.*

objective sensation *n.* A sensation caused by some material object.

o·blique (ō-blēk′, ə-blēk′) *adj.* Situated in a slanting position; not transverse or longitudinal. — **o·blique′ness** *n.*

oblique fracture *n.* A fracture in which the line of break runs obliquely to the axis of the bone.

oblique muscle *n.* **1.** A flat muscle that forms the outer layer on each side of the abdominal wall; external oblique. **2.** A flat muscle that lies beneath the external oblique on each side of the abdominal wall; internal oblique.

o·bliq·ui·ty (ō-blĭk′wĭ-tē, ə-blĭk′-) *n.* See **asynclitism**.

o·blit·er·ate (ə-blĭt′ə-rāt′, ō-blĭt′-) *v.* **-at·ed, -at·ing, -ates. 1.** To remove a body organ or part completely, as by surgery, disease, or radiation. **2.** To blot out, especially through the filling of a natural space by fibrosis or inflammation. — **o·blit′er·a′tion** *n.*

o·blit·er·a·tive bronchitis (ə-blĭt′ə-rā′tĭv, -ər-ə-tĭv, ō-blĭt′-) *n.* Fibrinous bronchitis in which the exudate is not expectorated but becomes organized, obliterating the affected portion of the bronchial tubes.

ob·ses·sion (əb-sĕsh′ən, ŏb-) *n.* **1.** Compulsive preoccupation with an idea or an unwanted feeling or emotion, often accompanied by symptoms of anxiety. **2.** A compulsive, often unreasonable idea or emotion. — **ob·ses′sion·al** *adj.*

ob·ses·sive (əb-sĕs′ĭv, ŏb-) *adj.* Of, characteristic of, or causing an obsession. — **ob·ses′sive** *n.* — **ob·ses′sive·ness** *n.*

obsessive-compulsive *adj.* Having a tendency to dwell on unwanted thoughts or perform certain repetitious rituals, especially as a defense against anxiety from unconscious conflicts. — *n.* An obsessive-compulsive person.

obsessive-compulsive neurosis *n.* An anxiety disorder characterized by the persistent and repetitive intrusion of unwanted thoughts, urges, or actions that the person is unable to prevent.

ob·stet·ric (ŏb-stĕt′rĭk, əb-) or **ob·stet·ri·cal** (-rĭ-kəl) *adj.* Of or relating to obstetrics or the care of women during and after pregnancy.

obstetrical binder *n.* A garment covering the abdomen and providing support after childbirth.

obstetrical forceps *n.* Forceps used for gently grasping and pulling on or rotating the fetal head. The blades are introduced separately into the vaginal canal and joined after being placed in correct position.

ob·ste·tri·cian (ŏb′stĭ-trĭsh′ən) *n.* A physician who specializes in obstetrics.

obstetrician–gynecologist *n.* A physician who specializes in obstetrics and gynecology.

ob·stet·rics (ŏb-stĕt′rĭks, əb-) *n.* The branch of medicine that deals with the care of women during pregnancy, childbirth, and the recuperative period following delivery.

ob·sti·nate (ŏb′stə-nĭt) *adj.* Difficult to alleviate or cure. — **ob′sti·nate·ness** *n.*

ob·struct (əb-strŭkt′, ŏb-) *v.* **-struct·ed, -struct·ing, -structs.** To block or close a body passage so as to hinder or interrupt a flow. — **ob·struc′tive** *adj.*

ob·struc·tion (əb-strŭk′shən, ŏb-) *n.* **1.** The blocking of a body passage, as by clogging or stricture. **2.** The state of being obstructed. **3.** Something, such as a mass or stricture, that obstructs.

obstructive murmur *n.* A murmur caused by a narrowing of one of the valvular orifices.

ob·tu·ra·tor (ŏb′tə-rā′tər, -tyə-) *n.* **1.** A structure, such as the soft palate, that closes an opening in the body. **2.** A prosthetic device serving to close an opening or cleft, especially in the palate. **3.** The stylus or removable plug used during the insertion of many tubular instruments.

obturator foramen *n.* A large oval or irregularly triangular aperture in the hipbone, whose margins are formed by the pubis and ischium.

oc·cip·i·tal bone (ŏk-sĭp′ĭ-tl) *n.* A bone at the lower and posterior part of the skull, enclosing the great foramen.

occipital lobe *n.* The posterior lobe of each cerebral hemisphere, having the shape of a three-sided pyramid and containing the visual center of the brain.

oc·ci·put (ŏk′sə-pŭt′, -pət) *n., pl.* **-puts** or **oc·cip·i·ta** (ŏk-sĭp′ĭ-tə). The back part of the head or skull.

oc·clude (ə-klōōd′) *v.* **-clud·ed, -clud·ing, -cludes. 1.** To cause to become closed; obstruct. **2.** To prevent the passage of. **3.** To bring together the upper and lower teeth in proper alignment for chewing. **4.** To enclose a virus, as in an inclusion body. — **oc·clud′ent** *adj.*

oc·clu·sal (ə-klōō′zəl, -səl) *adj.* **1.** Of or relating to occlusion or closure. **2.** Relating to the contacting surfaces of opposing teeth, especially the biting or chewing surfaces.

oc·clu·sion (ə-klōō′zhən) *n.* **1.** The act of occluding or the state of being occluded. **2.** An obstruction or a closure of a body passage. **3.** Any contact between the cutting or chewing surfaces of opposing teeth. **4.** The alignment of the teeth of the upper and lower jaws when brought together. **5.** The inclusion of one substance within another.

oc·clu·sive (ə-klōō′sĭv, -zĭv) *adj.* **1.** Occluding or tending to occlude. **2.** Of or being a bandage or dressing that closes a wound and keeps it from the air.

occlusive dressing *n.* A dressing that seals a wound from air or bacteria.

oc·cult (ə-kŭlt′, ŏk′ŭlt′) *adj.* **1.** Detectable only by microscopic examination or chemical analysis, as a minute amount of blood in a stool sample. **2.** Not accompanied by readily detectable signs or symptoms.

occult blood *n.* Blood that is present in amounts too small to be seen and can be detected only by chemical analysis or microscopic eexamination.

occult fracture *n.* A fracture that does not appear in x-rays, although the bone shows new bone formation within three or four weeks.

oc·cu·pa·tion·al disease (ŏk′yə-pā′shə-nəl) *n.* A pathological condition resulting from a toxic agent, a hazard, or a repetitive operation encountered during the usual performance of one's occupation.

occupational medicine *n.* The branch of medicine that deals with the prevention and treatment of diseases and injuries occurring at work or in specific occupations.

occupational therapy *n.* The use of productive or creative activity in the treatment or rehabilitation of physically or emotionally disabled people. — **occupational therapist** *n.*

o·chro·no·sis (ō′krə-nō′sĭs) *n.* A pathological condition observed in certain patients with alkaptonuria, characterized by pigmentation of cartilage and sometimes of other tissues. — **o′chro·not′ic** (-nŏt′ĭk) *adj.*

oc·to·ge·nar·i·an (ŏk′tə-jə-nâr′ē-ən) *adj.* Being between 80 and 90 years of age. — *n.* A person between 80 and 90 years of age.

oc·u·lar (ŏk′yə-lər) *adj.* **1.** Of or relating to the eye or the sense of sight. **2.** Resembling the eye in form or function.

ocular humor *n.* Either of the two humors of the eye, the aqueous humor or the vitreous humor.

ocular hypertelorism *n.* Extreme width between the eyes due to an enlarged sphenoid bone, sometimes associated with other congenital deformities and mental retardation.

oc·u·lar·ist (ŏk′yə-lər-ĭst) *n.* One skilled in the design, fabrication, and fitting of artificial eyes and in the making of prostheses associated with the appearance or function of the eyes.

ocular tension *n.* Resistance of the tunics of the eye to deformation, estimated digitally or by an instrument that measures pressure or tension.

ocular vertigo *n.* Vertigo resulting from refractive errors or imbalance of the extrinsic eye muscles.

oc·u·list (ŏk′yə-lĭst) *n.* **1.** A physician who treats diseases of the eyes; an ophthalmologist. **2.** An optometrist.

oc·u·log·ra·phy (ŏk′yə-lŏg′rə-fē) *n.* A method of recording eye position and eye movements.

oc·u·lo·gy·ri·a (ŏk′yə-lō-jī′rē-ə) *n.* The limits of rotation of the eyeballs.

oc·u·lo·mo·tor nerve (ŏk′yə-lō-mō′tər) *n.* A nerve originating in the midbrain below the cerebral aqueduct, supplying most of the extrinsic muscles of the eye and supplying the elevator muscle of the upper eyelid, the ciliary muscle, and the sphincter muscle of the pupil.

oc·u·lus (ŏk′yə-ləs) *n., pl.* **-li** (-lī′). Eye.

OD *abbr.* O.D. Doctor of Optometry; *Latin.* oculus dexter (right eye); overdose

o·don·tec·to·my (ō′dŏn-tĕk′tə-mē) *n.* Removal of teeth by the bending back of a mucoperiosteal flap and excision of bone from around the root before the application of force to remove the tooth.

o·don·to·blast (ō-dŏn′tə-blăst′) *n.* One of the cells forming the outer surface of dental pulp that produces the dentin of a tooth. — **o·don′to·blas′tic** *adj.*

o·don·to·blas·to·ma (ō-dŏn′tə-blă-stō′mə) *n.* **1.** A tumor composed of neoplastic epithelial and mesenchymal cells that may differentiate into cells able to produce calcified tooth substances. **2.** An odontoma in its early formative stage.

o·don·to·clast (ō-dŏn′tə-klăst′) *n.* A cell believed to produce absorption of the roots of the deciduous teeth.

o·don·to·gen·e·sis (ō-dŏn′tə-jĕn′ĭ-sĭs) *n.* The formation and development of teeth.

odontogenesis im·per·fec·ta (ĭm′pər-fĕk′tə) *n.* An odontogenic developmental anomaly characterized by deficient formation of enamel and dentin causing the affected teeth to exhibit a marked reduction in radiopacity.

o·don·tog·e·ny (ō′dŏn-tŏj′ə-nē) *n.* See **odontogenesis.**

o·don·toid process (ō-dŏn′toid′) *n.* A small, toothlike, upward projection from the second vertebra of the neck around which the first vertebra rotates.

o·don·to·ma (ō′dŏn-tō′mə) *n., pl.* **-mas** or **-ma·ta** (-mə-tə). **1.** A tumor of odontogenic origin. **2.** A developmental anomaly of odontogenic origin, resembling a hard tumor and composed of enamel, dentin, cementum, and pulp tissue.

o·don·to·neu·ral·gia (ō-dŏn′tō-nōō-răl′jə, -nyōō-) *n.* Facial neuralgia caused by a decayed tooth.

o·don·top·a·thy (ō′dŏn-tŏp′ə-thē) *n.* A disease of the teeth or of their sockets.

o·don·to·sis (ō′dŏn-tō′sĭs) *n.* See **odontogenesis.**

o·dor (ō′dər) *n.* **1.** The property or quality of a thing that affects, stimulates, or is perceived by the sense of smell. **2.** A sensation, stimulation, or perception of the sense of smell.

o·dy·nom·e·ter (ō′də-nŏm′ĭ-tər) *n.* See **algesiometer.**

o·dyn·o·pha·gia (ō-dĭn′ə-fā′jə, -jē-ə) *n.* See **dysphagia.**

oe- For words beginning with *oe-* that are not found here, see under *e-*.

oedipal phase *n.* In psychoanalytic theory, the stage in psychosexual development, usually occurring between the ages of 3 and 7, characterized by manifestation of the Oedipal complex.

Oed·i·pus complex (ĕd′ə-pəs, ē′də-) *n.* In psychoanalytic theory, a subconscious sexual desire in a child, especially a male child, for the parent of the opposite sex.

off·spring (ôf′sprĭng′) *n.* **1.** The progeny or descendants of a person considered as a group. **2.** A child of particular parentage.

O·gu·chi's disease (ō-gōō′chēz) *n.* An inherited nonprogressive form of night blindness.

oh·ne Hauch (ō′nä houch′, houкн′) *n.* Somatic agglutination.

o·id·i·o·my·cin (ō-ĭd′ē-ō-mī′sĭn) *n.* **1.** An antigen used to demonstrate cutaneous hypersensitivity in patients infected with one of the *Candida* species of fungi. **2.** One of a series of antigens used to demonstrate an immunocompromised patient's capacity to react to any cutaneous antigen.

oil gland *n.* A gland, such as a sebaceous gland, that secretes an oily substance.

oint·ment (oint′mənt) *n.* A highly viscous or semisolid preparation usually containing medicinal substances and intended for external application.

OKT cell *abbr.* Ortho-Kung T cell

o·lec·ra·non (ō-lĕk′rə-nŏn′) *n.* The large process on the upper end of the ulna that projects behind the elbow joint and forms the point of the elbow. — **o·lec′ra·nal** (-nəl), **o′le·cra′ni·al** (ō′lĭ-krā′-nē-əl), **o′le·cra′ni·an** (-nē-ən) *adj.*

ol·fac·tion (ŏl-făk′shən, ōl-) *n.* The sense of smell.

ol·fac·to·ry (ŏl-făk′tə-rē, -trē, ōl-) *adj.* Of, relating to, or contributing to the sense of smell.

olfactory anesthesia *n.* See **anosmia**.

olfactory bulb *n.* The bulblike distal portion of a lobe of the brain where the olfactory nerves begin.

olfactory epithelium *n.* Pseudostratified epithelium containing olfactory, receptor, and nerve cells whose axons connect with the olfactory bulb.

olfactory gland *n.* Any of the branched, tubuloalveolar, mucus-secreting glands in the olfactory epithelium of the nasal cavity.

olfactory nerve *n.* Any of numerous olfactory filaments in the olfactory portion of the nasal mucosa that pass through the ethmoid bone and enter the olfactory bulb.

olfactory receptor cell *n.* Any of the specialized, nucleated cells of the mucous membrane of the nose that serve as the receptors for smell.

ol·i·ge·mi·a (ŏl′ĭ-gē′mē-ə) *n.* A deficiency in the amount of blood in the body. — **ol′i·ge′mic** (-gē′mĭk) *adj.*

ol·i·go·am·ni·os (ŏl′ĭ-gō-ăm′nē-ŏs′) *n.* A deficiency in the amount of amniotic fluid.

ol·i·go·hy·dru·ri·a (ŏl′ĭ-gō-hī-drŏŏr′ē-ə) *n.* Excretion of abnormally small quantities of urine, as in dehydration.

ol·i·go·nu·cle·o·tide (ŏl′ĭ-gō-nŏŏ′klē-ə-tīd, -nyŏŏ′-) *n.* A polymeric chain of two to ten nucleotides.

ol·i·go·ri·a (ŏl′ĭ-gôr′ē-ə) *n.* An abnormal lack of interest in one's surroundings or relationships, as in depression.

ol·i·go·sper·mi·a (ŏl′ĭ-gō-spûr′mē-ə) *n.* A subnormal concentration of spermatozoa in the ejaculated semen.

ol·i·go·zo·o·sper·mi·a (ŏl′ĭ-gō-zō′ə-spûr′mē-ə) *n.* See **oligospermia**.

ol·i·gu·ri·a (ŏl′ĭ-gyŏŏr′ē-ə) *n.* Abnormally slight or infrequent urination.

Ol·lier's disease (ŏl′ē-āz′, ô-lyäz′) *n.* See **enchondromatosis**.

Ollier–Thiersch graft (-tērsh′) *n.* A thin split-skin graft, usually in small pieces.

o·me·ga (ō-mĕg′ə, ō-mē′gə, ō-mā′-) *adj.* Of or characterizing a chemical group or position at the end of a molecular chain, such as omega-oxidation.

omega-3 fatty acid *n.* Any of various polyunsaturated fatty acids that are found primarily in fish, fish oils, vegetable oils, and leafy green vegetables, and that seem to reduce the risk of stroke and heart attack.

O·menn's syndrome (ō′mĕnz′) *n.* A rapidly fatal familial immunodeficiency disease characterized by widespread reddening of the skin, diarrhea, repeated infections, enlargement of the liver and spleen, and leukocytosis.

o·men·tal (ō-mĕn′tl) *adj.* Of or relating to the omentum.

omental bursa *n.* An isolated portion of the peritoneal cavity lying dorsal to the stomach and opening into the general peritoneal cavity at the epiploic foramen.

omental graft *n.* A segment of omentum, with its supplying blood vessels, transplanted as a free flap to a distant area.

o·men·tec·to·my (ō′mĕn-tĕk′tə-mē) *n.* Resection or surgical excision of the omentum.

o·men·ti·tis (ō′mĕn-tī′tĭs) *n.* Peritonitis involving the omentum.

o·men·to·fix·a·tion (ō-mĕn′tō-fĭk-sā′shən) *n.* Omentopexy.

o·men·to·pex·y (ō-mĕn′tə-pĕk′sē) *n.* **1.** Suture of the greater omentum to the abdominal wall. **2.** Suture of the omentum to another organ to increase arterial circulation.

o·men·to·plas·ty (ō-mĕn′tə-plăs′tē) *n.* A surgical procedure in which a portion of the greater omentum is used to cover or fill a defect, augment arterial or portal venous circulation, absorb effusions, or increase lymphatic drainage.

o·men·tor·rha·phy (ō′mĕn-tôr′ə-fē) *n.* Suture of an opening in the omentum.

o·men·tu·lum (ō-mĕn′tyə-ləm, -chə-) *n.* See **lesser omentum**.

o·men·tum (ō-mĕn′təm) *n., pl.* **-tums** or **-ta** (-tə). One of the peritoneal folds that connect the stomach with other abdominal organs, especially the greater omentum or the lesser omentum.

omn. hor. *abbr. Latin.* omni hora (every hour)

om·ni·fo·cal lens (ŏm′nə-fō′kəl) *n.* A lens that corrects for near and distant vision, the section for near vision is a continuously variable curve.

om·pha·lec·to·my (ŏm′fə-lĕk′tə-mē) *n.* Surgical excision of the navel or of a tumor connected with it.

om·phal·ic (ŏm-făl′ĭk) *adj.* Relating to the navel; umbilical.

om·pha·li·tis (ŏm′fə-lī′tĭs) *n.* Inflammation of the navel and surrounding parts.

om·phal·o·cele (ŏm-făl′ə-sĕl′, ŏm′fə-lō-) *n.* Congenital herniation of viscera into the base of the umbilical cord.

om·pha·lo·mes·en·ter·ic duct (ŏm′fə-lō-mĕz′ən-tĕr′ĭk, -mĕs′-) *n.* See **yolk stalk.**

om·pha·los (ŏm′fə-lŏs′, -ləs) *n., pl.* **-li** (-lī′). The navel.

om·pha·lot·o·my (ŏm′fə-lŏt′ə-mē) *n.* Cutting of the umbilical cord at birth.

o·nan·ism (ō′nə-nĭz′əm) *n.* **1.** See **coitus interruptus. 2.** Masturbation.

on·cho·cer·ci·a·sis (ŏng′kō-sər-kī′ə-sĭs) or **on·cho·cer·co·sis** (-sər-kō′sĭs) *n.* A disease occurring in tropical Africa and Central America, transmitted by black flies and caused by infestation with filarial worms of the genus *Onchocerca,* especially *O. volvulus,* and characterized by nodular swellings on the skin and lesions of the eyes.

on·co·cyte (ŏng′kə-sīt′) *n.* A large granular acidophilic tumor cell having numerous mitochondria.

on·co·cyt·ic hepatocellular tumor (ŏn′kə-sĭt′ĭk, ŏng′-) *n.* A tumor in which malignant hepatocytes are intersected by fibrous lamellated bands.

on·co·cy·to·ma (ŏng′kō-sī-tō′mə) *n., pl.* **-mas** or **-mata** (-mə-tə). A glandular tumor that is chiefly composed of oncocytes, occurring most often in the salivary glands.

on·co·fe·tal (ŏng′kō-fēt′l) *adj.* Relating to tumor-associated substances, such as oncofetal antigens, present in fetal tissue.

oncofetal antigen *n.* One of the tumor-associated antigens present in fetal tissue but not in normal adult tissue, such as alpha-fetoprotein and carcinoembryonic antigen.

oncofetal marker *n.* A tumor marker produced by tumor tissue and by fetal tissue of the same type as the tumor, but not by normal adult tissue from which the tumor arises.

on·co·gene (ŏn′kə-jēn, ŏng′-) *n.* A gene that causes the transformation of normal cells into cancerous tumor cells, especially a viral gene that transforms a host cell into a tumor cell.

on·co·gen·e·sis (ŏng′kō-jĕn′ĭ-sĭs) *n.* The formation and development of tumors.

on·co·gen·ic (ŏng′kō-jĕn′ĭk) or **on·cog·e·nous** (ŏng-kŏj′ə-nəs) *adj.* Causing or tending to cause the formation and development of tumors. **— on′co·ge·nic′i·ty** (-jə-nĭs′ĭ-tē) *n.*

oncogenic virus *n.* A virus capable of inducing the formation of tumors.

on·col·o·gy (ŏng-kŏl′ə-jē) *n.* The branch of medicine dealing with the physical, chemical, and biological properties of tumors, including study of their development, diagnosis, treatment, and prevention. **— on′co·log′i·cal** (-kə-lŏj′ĭ-kəl), **on′co·log′ic** (-lŏj′ĭk) *adj.* **— on·col′o·gist** *n.*

on·col·y·sis (ŏng-kŏl′ĭ-sĭs) *n.* **1.** The destruction of a tumor or tumor cells. **2.** The reduction of any swelling or mass. **— on′co·lyt′ic** (ŏng′kə-lĭt′ĭk) *adj.*

on·cor·na·vi·rus (ŏng-kôr′nə-vī′rəs) *n.* A virus of the subfamily Oncovirinae, an RNA tumor virus.

on·co·sis (ŏng-kō′sĭs) *n.* **1.** Formation of a tumor or tumors. **2.** A condition characterized by swelling.

on·cot·o·my (ŏng-kŏt′ə-mē) *n.* Surgical incision of an abscess, cyst, or tumor.

on·co·vi·rus (ŏng′kō-vī′rəs) *n.* See **oncornavirus.**

o·nei·ric (ō-nī′rĭk) *adj.* **1.** Of, relating to, or suggestive of dreams. **2.** Relating to the clinical state of oneirophrenia.

o·nei·rism (ō-nī′rĭz′əm) *n.* An abnormal state of consciousness in which dreamlike, often disturbing illusions are experienced while awake.

o·nei·ro·dyn·i·a (ō-nī′rō-dĭn′ē-ə) *n.* Intense mental disturbance or distress associated with dreaming.

o·nei·ro·phre·ni·a (ō-nī′rə-frē′nē-ə, -frĕn′ē-ə) *n.* A mental state characterized by hallucinations and other disturbances, associated with such conditions as prolonged deprivation of sleep, sensory isolation, or psychoactive drugs.

o·nei·ros·co·py (ō′nī-rŏs′kə-pē) *n.* See **dream analysis.**

on·lay (ŏn′lā′) *n.* A bone graft applied to the exterior surface of the bone.

on-off phenomenon *n.* A state in the treatment of Parkinson's disease with dopa in which there is a rapid fluctuation of akinetic and choreoathetotic movements.

on·set (ŏn′sĕt′) *n.* A beginning; a start, as of a cold.

on·to·gen·e·sis (ŏn′tō-jĕn′ĭ-sĭs) *n.* See **ontogeny.**

on·tog·e·ny (ŏn-tŏj′ə-nē) *n.* The origin and development of an organism from embryo to adult.

on·y·chec·to·my (ŏn′ĭ-kĕk′tə-mē) *n.* Surgical removal of a toenail or fingernail.

o·nych·i·a (ō-nĭk′ē-ə) *n.* Inflammation of the fingernail or toenail matrix.

on·y·choc·la·sis (ŏn′ĭ-kŏk′lə-sĭs) *n.* Breaking of the fingernails or toenails.

on·y·cho·dys·tro·phy (ŏn′ĭ-kō-dĭs′trə-fē) *n.* Dystrophic changes in fingernails or toenails, such as malformation or discoloration, occurring as a congenital defect or due to illness or injury.

on·y·cho·gry·po·sis (ŏn′ĭ-kō-grə-pō′sĭs) or **on·y·cho·gry·pho·sis** (-grə-fō′sĭs) *n.* Enlargement of the fingernails or toenails accompanied by increased thickening and curvature.

on·y·cho·ma·de·sis (ŏn′ĭ-kō′mə-dē′sĭs) *n.* Complete shedding of a fingernail or toenail, usually associated with a systemic illness.

on·y·cho·my·co·sis (ŏn′ĭ-kō-mī-kō′sĭs) *n.* A fungous infection of the fingernails or toenails, causing thickening, roughness, and splitting.

on·y·chop·a·thy (ŏn′ĭ-kŏp′ə-thē) *n.* A disease of the fingernails or toenails. **— on′y·cho·path′ic** (-kō-păth′ĭk) *adj.*

on·y·choph·a·gy (ŏn′ĭ-kŏf′ə-jē) or **on·y·cho·pha·gi·a** (-kō-fā′jē-ə, -jə) *n.* The habit of nail biting.

on·y·cho·plas·ty (ŏn′ĭ-kō-plăs′tē) *n.* A corrective or plastic operation on the matrix of a fingernail or toenail.

on·y·chot·il·lo·ma·ni·a (ŏn′ĭ-kŏt′l-ō-mā′nē-ə, -mān′yə, ŏn′ĭ-kō-tĭl′ə-) *n.* A tendency to pick at the fingernails or toenails.

on·y·chot·o·my (ŏn′ĭ-kŏt′ə-mē) *n.* Incision into a toenail or fingernail.

o·o·cyst (ō′ə-sĭst′) *n.* A thick-walled structure in

which sporozoan zygotes develop and that serves to transfer them to new hosts.

o·o·cyte (ō'ə-sīt') *n.* A cell from which an egg or ovum develops by meiosis; a female gametocyte.

o·o·gam·ete (ō'ə-găm'ēt', -gə-mēt') *n.* A female gamete, especially the larger of two gametes produced by an oogamous species.

o·o·gen·e·sis (ō'ə-jĕn'ĭ-sĭs) *n.* The formation and development of the ovum. — **o'o·ge·net'ic** (-jə-nĕt'ĭk) *adj.*

o·o·go·ni·um (ō'ə-gō'nē-əm) *n.,* pl. **-ni·ums** or **-ni·a** (-nē-ə). The primitive egg mother cell, from which the oocytes are developed. — **o'o·go'ni·al** (-nē-əl) *adj.*

o·o·ki·ne·sis (ō'ə-kə-nē'sĭs, -kī-) *n.* The chromosomal movements in the egg during maturation and fertilization.

o·o·lem·ma (ō'ə-lĕm'ə) *n.* See **zona pellucida.**

o·o·pho·rec·to·my (ō'ə-fə-rĕk'tə-mē) *n.* See **ovariectomy.**

o·o·pho·ri·tis (ō'ə-fə-rī'tĭs) *n.* Inflammation of an ovary.

o·oph·o·ro·cys·tec·to·my (ō-ŏf'ə-rō-sĭ-stĕk'tə-mē) *n.* Excision of an ovarian cyst.

o·oph·o·ro·hys·ter·ec·to·my (ō-ŏf'ə-rō-hĭs'tə-rĕk'tə-mē) *n.* See **ovariohysterectomy.**

o·oph·o·ron (ō-ŏf'ə-rŏn') *n.* See **ovary.**

o·oph·o·ro·pex·y (ō-ŏf'ə-rə-pĕk'sē) *n.* Surgical fixation or suspension of an ovary.

o·oph·o·ro·plas·ty (ō-ŏf'ə-rō-plăs'tē) *n.* Plastic surgery on an ovary.

o·oph·o·ros·to·my (ō-ŏf'ə-rŏs'tə-mē) *n.* See **ovariostomy.**

o·oph·o·rot·o·my (ō-ŏf'ə-rŏt'ə-mē) *n.* See **ovariotomy** (sense 2).

o·o·plasm (ō'ə-plăz'əm) *n.* The protoplasmic portion of the ovum.

o·o·sphere (ō'ə-sfîr') *n.* A large nonmotile female gamete or egg cell, formed in an oogonium and ready for fertilization.

o·pac·i·fi·ca·tion (ō-păs'ə-fĭ-kā'shən) *n.* **1.** The process of making opaque. **2.** The formation of opacities.

o·pac·i·ty (ō-păs'ĭ-tē) *n.* **1.** The quality or state of being opaque. **2.** An opaque or nontransparent area, as of the cornea.

o·pen biopsy *n.* Surgical incision or excision of the region from which a biopsy is taken.

open chest massage *n.* Cardiac massage in which the heart is compressed with the hand inside the thoracic cavity.

open circuit method *n.* A method for measuring oxygen consumption and carbon-dioxide production by collecting expired gas over a given period and determining its volume and composition.

open comedo *n.* See **blackhead.**

open drainage *n.* The admittance of air into a wound or cavity to facilitate drainage.

open-drop technique *n.* A technique for producing inhalation anesthesia in which drops of a liquid anesthetic, such as ether or chloroform, are placed on a gauze mask or cone applied over the mouth and nose.

open flap *n.* See **flat flap.**

open fracture *n.* A fracture in which broken bone fragments lacerate soft tissue and protrude through an open wound in the skin.

open-heart surgery *n.* Surgery in which the thoracic cavity is opened to expose the heart and the blood is recirculated and oxygenated by a heart-lung machine.

open hospital *n.* A hospital in which physicians who are not members of the attending and consulting staff may admit and treat patients.

o·pen·ing snap (ō'pə-nĭng) *n.* A sharp, high-pitched click in early diastole and related to the opening of the abnormal valve in cases of mitral stenosis.

open pneumothorax *n.* A free communication between the exterior and the pleural space either via the lung or through the chest wall, as through an open wound.

open reduction *n.* Reduction of a fractured bone by manipulation after incision into skin and muscle over the site of the fracture.

open wound *n.* A wound in which the injured tissues are exposed to the air.

op·er·a·ble (ŏp'ər-ə-bəl, ŏp'rə-) *adj.* Treatable by surgical operation with a reasonable degree of safety and an expectation for success. — **op'er·a·bil'i·ty** *n.*

op·er·ant (ŏp'ər-ənt) *adj.* **1.** Operating to produce effects; effective. **2.** Of, relating to, or being a response that occurs spontaneously and is identified by its reinforcing or inhibiting effects. —*n.* In operant conditioning, a behavior or specific response chosen by the experimenter or therapist.

op·er·ate (ŏp'ə-rāt') *v.* **-at·ed, -at·ing, -ates.** To perform surgery.

operating microscope *n.* See **surgical microscope.**

operating room *n.* A room equipped for performing surgical operations.

op·er·a·tion (ŏp'ə-rā'shən) *n.* A surgical procedure for remedying an injury, an ailment, a defect, or a dysfunction.

op·er·a·tive (ŏp'ər-ə-tĭv, -ə-rā'tĭv, ŏp'rə-) *adj.* **1.** Of, relating to, or resulting from a surgical operation. **2.** Functioning effectively; efficient.

op·er·a·tor gene (ŏp'ə-rā'tər) *n.* A gene that interacts with a specific repressor to control the functioning of adjacent structural genes.

o·per·cu·li·tis (ō-pûr'kyə-lī'tĭs) *n.* See **pericoronitis.**

o·per·cu·lum (ō-pûr'kyə-ləm) *n.,* pl. **-lums** or **-la** (-lə). **1.** Something resembling a lid or cover. **2.** The portions of the frontal, parietal, and temporal lobes covering the insula. **3.** A bit of mucus sealing the endocervical canal of the uterus after conception. **4.** The attached flap in cases of torn retinal detachment. — **o·per'cu·lar** (-lər) *adj.*

op·er·on (ŏp'ə-rŏn') *n.* A unit of gene activity consisting of a sequence of genetic material that functions in a coordinated manner to control production of messenger RNA and consists of an operator gene, a promoter, and two or more structural genes.

o·phri·tis (ŏ-frī′tĭs) or **oph·ry·i·tis** (ŏf′rē-ī′tĭs) *n.* Dermatitis in the region of the eyebrows.

oph·thal·mi·a (ŏf-thăl′mē-ə, ŏp-) *n.* **1.** Severe, often purulent, conjunctivitis. **2.** Inflammation of the deeper structures of the eye.

ophthalmia ne·o·na·to·rum (nē′ō-nā-tôr′əm) *n.* Any of various forms of conjunctivitis in newborn infants, usually contracted during birth from passage through the infected birth canal of the mother.

oph·thal·mic (ŏf-thăl′mĭk, ŏp-) *adj.* Of or relating to the eye; ocular.

ophthalmic nerve *n.* The ophthalmic branch of the trigeminal nerve that supplies sensation to the eye socket and its contents, the anterior part of the nasal cavity, and the skin of the nose and forehead.

ophthalmic solution *n.* A sterile solution, free from foreign particles, suitably compounded, and dispensed for eyedrops.

oph·thal·mi·tis (ŏf′thəl-mī′tĭs, ŏp′-) *n.* See **oph·thalmia** (sense 2).

oph·thal·mo·di·aph·a·no·scope (ŏf-thăl′mō-dī-ăf′ə-nə-skōp′, ŏp-) *n.* An instrument for viewing the interior of the eye by transmitted light.

oph·thal·mo·dy·na·mom·e·ter (ŏf-thăl′mō-dī′nə-mŏm′ĭ-tər, ŏp-) *n.* **1.** An instrument for determining the near point of convergence of the eyes. **2.** An instrument that measures the blood pressure in the retinal vessels. — **oph·thal′mo·dy′na·mom′e·try** *n.*

oph·thal·mog·ra·phy (ŏf′thəl-mŏg′rə-fē, -thăl-, ŏp′-) *n.* The recording of eye movements during reading by photographing a mark on the cornea or by making a tracing of light reflexes. — **oph·thal′mo·graph′** (ŏf-thăl′mə-grăf′, ŏp-) *n.*

oph·thal·mol·o·gist (ŏf′thəl-mŏl′ə-jĭst, -thăl-, ŏp′-) *n.* A physician who specializes in ophthalmology.

oph·thal·mol·o·gy (ŏf′thəl-mŏl′ə-jē, -thăl-, ŏp′-) *n.* The branch of medicine that deals with the anatomy, functions, pathology, and treatment of the eye. — **oph·thal′mo·log′ic** (-thăl′mə-lŏj′ĭk), **oph·thal′mo·log′i·cal** (-ĭ-kəl) *adj.*

oph·thal·mom·e·ter (ŏf′thəl-mŏm′ĭ-tər, -thăl-, ŏp′-) *n.* See **keratometer.**

oph·thal·mo·my·co·sis (ŏf-thăl′mō-mī-kō′sĭs, ŏp-) *n.* Any of various diseases of the eye or its appendages caused by a fungus.

oph·thal·mop·a·thy (ŏf′thəl-mŏp′ə-thē, -thăl-, ŏp′-) *n.* A disease of the eyes.

oph·thal·mo·ple·gi·a (ŏf-thăl′mō-plē′jē-ə, -jə, ŏp-) *n.* Paralysis of one or more of the muscles of the eye. — **oph·thal′mo·ple′gic** *adj.*

oph·thal·mo·scope (ŏf-thăl′mə-skōp′, ŏp-) *n.* An instrument for examining the interior structures of the eye, especially the retina, featuring a mirror that reflects light into the eye and a central hole through which the eye is examined.

oph·thal·mos·co·py (ŏf′thəl-mŏs′kə-pē, -thăl-, ŏp′-) *n.* Examination of the interior of the eye

through the pupil with an ophthalmoscope. — **oph·thal′mo·scope′** (ŏf-thăl′mə-skōp′, ŏp-) *n.* — **oph·thal′mo·scop′ic** (-skŏp′ĭk), **oph·thal′mo·scop′i·cal** (-ĭ-kəl) *adj.* — **oph′thal·mos′co·py** (ŏf′thăl-mŏs′kə-pē, ŏp′-) *n.*

o·pi·ate (ō′pē-ĭt, -āt′) *n.* **1.** Any of various sedative narcotics containing opium or one or more of its natural or synthetic derivatives. **2.** A drug, hormone, or other chemical substance having sedative or narcotic effects similar to those containing opium or its derivatives: — *adj.* **1.** Containing opium or any of its derivatives. **2.** Resembling opium or its derivatives in action. **3.** Inducing sleep or sedation; soporific. — *v.* **-at·ed, -at·ing, -ates.** (-āt′). To subject to the action of an opiate. — **o′pi·ate** (-ĭt, -āt′) *adj.*

opiate receptor *n.* Any of various cell membrane receptors that can bind with morphine and other opiates; concentrations of such receptors are especially high in regions of the brain having pain-related functions.

op·is·thor·chi·a·sis (ŏp′ĭs-thôr-kī′ə-sĭs, ō-pĭs′-thôr-) *n.* Infection of the biliary tract with trematodes of the genus *Opisthorchis;* cause by ingesting raw or inadequately cooked fish infected with the parasites.

o·pi·um (ō′pē-əm) *n.* A bitter, yellowish-brown, strongly addictive narcotic drug prepared from the opium poppy and containing alkaloids such as morphine, codeine, and papaverine.

opium poppy *n.* An annual plant *(Papaver somniferum)* native to Turkey and adjacent areas, cultivated as a source of opium.

Op·pen·heim's syndrome (ŏp′ən-hīmz′) *n.* See **amyotonia congenita.**

op·por·tun·is·tic (ŏp′ər-tōō-nĭs′tĭk, -tyōō-) *adj.* **1.** Of or relating to an organism capable of causing disease only in a host whose resistance is lowered. **2.** Of or relating to a disease caused by an opportunistic organism.

opportunistic infection *n.* An infection by a microorganism that normally does not cause disease but becomes pathogenic when the body's immune system is impaired and unable to fight off infection, as in AIDS and certain other diseases.

op·po·si·tion·al disorder (ŏp′ə-zĭsh′ə-nəl) *n.* A persistent pattern of disobedient, negativistic, and provocative opposition to authority figures that occurs between the ages of 3 and 18 and is characterized by temper tantrums, violation of minor rules, and argumentativeness.

op·sin (ŏp′sĭn) *n.* A protein of the retina, especially the protein constituent of rhodopsin, that makes up one of the visual pigments.

op·sin·o·gen (ŏp-sĭn′ə-jən, -jĕn′) *n.* A substance that stimulates the formation of opsonin.

op·si·u·ri·a (ŏp′sĭ-yōŏr′ē-ə) *n.* A more rapid excretion of urine during fasting than after a full meal.

op·so·gen (ŏp′sə-jən, -jĕn′) *n.* See **opsinogen.**

op·so·ma·ni·a (ŏp′sə-mā′nē-ə, -mān′yə) *n.* An intense longing for a particular food or flavor.

op·so·nin (ŏp′sə-nĭn) *n.* An antibody in blood serum that causes bacteria or other foreign cells to become more susceptible to phagocytes.

op·son·i·za·tion (ŏp′sə-nĭ-zā′shən) *n.* The process by which bacteria are altered so as to be more readily and more efficiently engulfed by phagocytes.

op·so·nize (ŏp′sə-nīz′) *v.* -nized, -niz·ing, -niz·es. To make bacteria or other cells more susceptible to the action of phagocytes.

op·tes·the·sia (ŏp′tĭs-thē′zhə) *n.* Visual sensibility to light stimuli.

op·tic (ŏp′tĭk) or **op·ti·cal** (ŏp′tĭ-kəl) *adj.* **1.** Of or relating to the eye or vision. **2.** Of or relating to the science of optics or optical equipment.

optical aberration *n.* The failure of light rays from a point source to form a perfect image after passing through an optical system.

optical allachesthesia *n.* See **visual allesthesia**.

optical image *n.* An image formed by the refraction or reflection of light.

optic center *n.* The point in the lens of the eye where light rays cross as they move from the cornea to the retina.

optic chiasm *n.* A flattened quadrangular body that is the point of crossing of the fibers of the optic nerves.

optic decussation *n.* See **optic chiasm**.

op·tic disk (ŏp′tĭk) *n.* The small optically insensitive region in the retina containing no rods or cones, where fibers of the optic nerve emerge from the eyeball.

op·ti·cian (ŏp-tĭsh′ən) *n.* One who practices opticianry.

op·ti·cian·ry (ŏp-tĭsh′ən-rē) *n.* The professional practice of filling prescriptions for ophthalmic lenses, dispensing eyeglasses, and fitting contact lenses.

optic keratoplasty *n.* Surgical transplantation of transparent corneal tissue to replace tissue that impaired vision, such as that from a scar.

optic lobe *n.* Either of two lobes of the dorsal mesencephalon, containing primary visual centers.

optic nerve *n.* A nerve that originates from the retina, passes out of the eye socket through the optic canal to the chiasm, and serves to conduct visual stimuli to the brain.

optic papilla *n.* See **optic disk**.

op·tics (ŏp′tĭks) *n.* The science concerned with the properties of light, its refraction and absorption, and the refracting media of the eye.

op·ti·mum dose (ŏp′tə-məm) *n.* The quantity of a radiological or pharmacological substance that will produce the desired effect without any unfavorable effects.

op·tom·e·ter (ŏp-tŏm′ĭ-tər) *n.* An instrument for determining the refraction of the eye.

op·tom·e·try (ŏp-tŏm′ĭ-trē) *n.* The health care profession concerned with the examination, diagnosis, treatment, and management of diseases and disorders of the eyes and related structures, and with the determination and correction of vision problems using lenses and other optical aids. — **op·tom′e·trist** *n.*

op·to·my·om·e·ter (ŏp′tō-mī-ŏm′ĭ-tər) *n.* An instrument for determining the relative power of the extrinsic muscles of the eye.

OPV *abbr.* oral poliovirus vaccine

o·ral (ôr′əl) *adj.* **1.** Of or relating to the mouth. **2.** Used in or taken through the mouth. **3.** Of or relating to the first stage of psychosexual development in psychoanalytic theory, during which the mouth is the chief focus of exploration and pleasure. — **o′ral·ly** *adv.*

oral biology *n.* The study of the biological phenomena associated with the mouth in health and in disease.

oral cavity *n.* The part of the mouth behind the teeth and gums that is bounded above by the hard and soft palates and below by the tongue and the mucous membrane connecting it with the inner part of the mandible.

oral contraceptive *n.* A pill, typically containing estrogen, progesterone, or both, that prevents conception or pregnancy.

oral hygiene *n.* See **dental hygiene**.

oral lactose tolerance test *n.* A test for lactase deficiency in which serum glucose is measured after a quantity of lactose has been taken orally.

oral phase *n.* In psychoanalytic theory, the first stage in psychosexual development, usually occurring in the first year, when the mouth is the focus of the infant's needs and pleasure.

oral poliovirus vaccine *n.* See **poliovirus vaccine** (sense 2).

oral rehydration therapy *n.* Treatment for diarrhea-related dehydration in which an electrolyte solution containing fluids and vital ions is administered.

oral surgery *n.* The branch of dentistry concerned with the surgical and adjunctive treatment of diseases, injuries, and deformities of the oral and maxillofacial region.

or·bic·u·lar muscle of the eye (ôr-bĭk′yə-lər) *n.* A muscle that consists of three parts: the orbital or external part; the palpebral or internal part; and the lacrimal part. The orbital part arises the frontal process of the maxilla and the nasal process of the frontal bone and encircles the aperture of the eye socket. The palpebral part arises from the medial palpebral ligament and passes through each eyelid. The lacrimal part arises from the posterior lacrimal crest and passes across the lacrimal sac to join the palpebral portion. The action of all three parts closes the eye and wrinkles the forehead vertically.

orbicular muscle of the mouth *n.* A muscle with origin from the septum of the nose, from the incisor fossa of the maxilla, and from the lower jaw on each side of the symphysis; the fibers surround the mouth between the skin and the mucous membrane of lips and cheeks; and whose action closes the lips.

orbicular zone *n.* The fibers of the articular capsule of the hip joint encircling the neck of the femur.

or·bit (ôr′bĭt) *n.* See **orbital cavity**.

or·bit·al cavity (ôr′bĭ-tl) *n.* The bony cavity containing the eyeball and its associated muscles, vessels, and nerves.

or·bi·tog·ra·phy (ôr′bĭ-tŏg′rə-fē) *n.* A diagnostic technique for radiographic evaluation in suspected blow-out fracture of the orbit.

or·bi·tot·o·my (ôr′bĭ-tŏt′ə-mē) *n.* Surgical incision into the orbit.

or·ce·in (ôr′sē-ĭn) *n.* A natural dye used in histologic staining methods as a purple dye complex.

or·chi·al·gi·a (ôr′kē-ăl′jē-ə, -jə) *n.* Testicular pain.

or·chi·ec·to·my (ôr′kē-ĕk′tə-mē) or **or·chi·dec·to·my** (-kĭ-dĕk′-) *n.* Surgical removal of one or both testes.

or·chi·o·cele (ôr′kē-ə-sēl′) *n.* **1.** A tumor of the testis. **2.** A testis retained in the inguinal canal.

or·chi·op·a·thy (ôr′kē-ŏp′ə-thē) *n.* Disease of a testis.

or·chi·o·pex·y (ôr′kē-ə-pĕk′sē) *n.* Surgical treatment of an undescended testicle by freeing it and implanting it into the scrotum.

or·chi·o·plas·ty (ôr′kē-ə-plăs′tē) *n.* Plastic surgery of the testis.

or·chi·ot·o·my (ôr′kē-ŏt′ə-mē) *n.* Incision into a testis.

or·chis (ôr′kĭs) *n.* See **testis.**

or·chi·tis (ôr-kī′tĭs) or **or·chi·di·tis** (ôr′kĭ-dī′tĭs) *n.* Inflammation of the testis. — **or·chit′ic** (ôr-kĭt′-ĭk) *adj.*

or·der (ôr′dər) *n.* A taxonomic category of organisms ranking above a family and below a class.

or·der·ly (ôr′dər-lē) *n.* An attendant in a hospital.

or·gan (ôr′gən) *n.* A differentiated part of the body that performs a specific function.

organ culture *n.* **1.** The maintenance or growth of tissues, organ primordia, or the parts or whole of an organ in vitro in such a way as to allow differentiation or preservation of the architecture or function. **2.** A culture of such tissue or organ.

or·gan·elle (ôr′gə-nĕl′) *n.* A differentiated structure within a cell, such as a mitochondrion or microsome, that performs a specific function.

or·gan·ic (ôr-găn′ĭk) *adj.* **1.** Of, relating to, or affecting organs or an organ of the body. **2.** Of or designating carbon compounds. **3.** Of, relating to, or derived from living organisms. — **or′gan·ic′i·ty** (ôr′gə-nĭs′ĭ-tē) *n.*

organic brain syndrome *n.* Any of a group of acute or chronic syndromes involving temporary or permanent impairment of brain function caused by trauma, infection, toxin, tumor, or tissue sclerosis, and causing mild-to-severe impairment of memory, orientation, judgment, intellectual functions, and emotional adjustment.

organic compound *n.* A compound containing hydrocarbon groups.

organic disease *n.* A disease in which there is a structural change to some tissue or organ.

or·gan·i·cism (ôr-găn′ĭ-sĭz′əm) *n.* **1.** The theory that all disease is associated with structural alterations of organs. **2.** The theory that the total organization of an organism, rather than the func-

tioning of specific organs, is the principal or exclusive determinant of every life process.

organic mental disorder *n.* Any of a group of mental disturbances resulting from temporary or permanent brain dysfunction caused by organic factors such as alcohol, infections, metabolic disorders, and aging.

organic murmur *n.* A murmur caused by an organic lesion.

organic vertigo *n.* Vertigo that is caused by a lesion of the brain.

or·gan·ism (ôr′gə-nĭz′əm) *n.* An individual form of life, such as a plant, an animal, a bacterium, a protist, or a fungus; a body made up of organs, organelles, or other parts that work together to carry on the various processes of life. — **or′gan·is′mal** (-nĭz′məl), **or′gan·is′mic** (-mĭk) *adj.*

or·ga·niz·er (ôr′gə-nī′zər) *n.* A group of cells that induces differentiation of cells in the embryo and controls the growth and development of adjacent parts through the action of an evocator.

organ of Corti *n.* See **spiral organ.**

or·gan·o·gen·e·sis (ôr′gə-nō-jĕn′ĭ-sĭs, ôr-găn′ə-) *n.* Formation and development of the organs of living things. — **or′gan·o·ge·net′ic** (-jə-nĕt′ĭk) *adj.*

or·gan·og·e·ny (ôr′gə-nŏj′ə-nē) *n.* See **organogenesis.** — **or′gan·o·gen′ic** (-nō-jĕn′ĭk) *adj.*

or·gan·oid tumor (ôr′gə-noid′) *n.* A tumor that is glandular in origin and contains epithelium, connective tissue, and other tissue structures that give it a complex structure similar to an organ.

organ-specific antigen *n.* A heterogenetic antigen that is specific to a particular organ, whether of a single species or of many species.

or·gasm (ôr′găz′əm) *n.* The highest point of sexual excitement, characterized by strong feelings of pleasure and marked normally by ejaculation of semen by the male and by vaginal contractions in the female. — **or·gas′mic** (ôr-găz′mĭk) *adj.*

o·ri·ent (ôr′ē-ənt, -ĕnt′) *v.* **-ent·ed, -ent·ing, -ents.** To align or position with respect to a point or system of reference.

o·ri·en·ta·tion (ôr′ē-ĕn-tā′shən, -ən-) *n.* **1.** The act of orienting or the state of being oriented. **2.** Sexual orientation. **3.** Introductory instruction concerning a new situation. **4.** Awareness of the objective world in relation to one's self.

orienting reflex *n.* An aspect of responding to environmental stimuli in which an organism's initial response to a change or novel stimulus makes the organism more sensitive to the stimulation, as when the pupil of the eye dilates in response to dim light.

orienting response *n.* See **orienting reflex.**

or·i·fice (ôr′ə-fĭs) *n.* An opening, especially to a cavity or passage of the body; a mouth or vent. — **or′i·fi′cial** (-fĭsh′əl) *adj.*

or·i·gin (ôr′ə-jĭn) *n.* **1.** The point at which something comes into existence or from which it derives or is derived. **2.** The point of attachment of a muscle that remains relatively fixed during contraction. **3.** The starting point of a cranial or spinal nerve.

o·rig·i·nate (ə-rĭj′ə-nāt′) v. **-nat·ed, -nat·ing, -nates. 1.** To bring into being; create. **2.** To come into being; start.

Orn abbr. ornithine

or·ni·thine (ôr′nə-thēn′) n. An amino acid formed by the hydrolysis of arginine; it is an important intermediate in the formation of urea.

or·ni·tho·sis (ôr′nə-thō′sĭs) n. A disease of birds caused by Chlamydia psittaci and contracted by humans through contact with infected birds.

o·r·o·pha·ryn·go·lar·yn·gi·tis (ôr′ō-fə-rĭng′gō-lăr′ĭn-jī′tĭs) n. Inflammation of the mucosa of the upper respiratory tract, as from inhalation or ingestion of chemical or physical agents.

o·ro·phar·ynx (ôr′ō-făr′ĭngks) n. The part of the pharynx between the soft palate and the epiglottis. — o′ro·pha·ryn′ge·al (-fə-rĭn′jē-əl, -jəl, -făr′-ĭn-jē′əl) adj.

o·ro·so·mu·coid (ôr′ə-sō-myōō′koid′) n. A glycoprotein in blood plasma.

o·ro·tra·che·al tube (ôr′ō-trā′kē-əl) n. An endotracheal tube inserted through the mouth.

O·ro·ya fever (ə-roi′ə, ô-rō′yä) n. An acute endemic disease of the central Andes caused by the bacterium Bartonella bacilliformis and marked by high fever, rheumatic pains, albuminuria, and progressive severe anemia.

or·phan drug (ôr′fən) n. Any of various drugs or biologicals that may be useful in treating disease but are not considered to be commercially viable.

or·ther·ga·si·a (ôr′thər-gā′zē-ə, -zhə) n. Normal intellectual and emotional adjustment.

or·the·sis (ôr-thē′sĭs) n. An orthopedic brace or appliance.

or·thet·ics (ôr-thĕt′ĭks) n. See **orthotics**. — **or·thet′ic** adj.

or·tho·don·tia (ôr′thə-dŏn′shə) n. See **orthodontics**.

or·tho·don·tics (ôr′thə-dŏn′tĭks) or **or·tho·don·ture** (ôr′thə-dŏn′chər) n. The dental specialty and practice of preventing and correcting irregularities of the teeth, as by the use of braces. — **or′tho·don′tic** adj.

or·tho·don·tist (ôr′thə-dŏn′tĭst) n. A specialist in orthodontics.

or·tho·dox sleep (ôr′thə-dŏks′) n. Sleep characterized by a slow alpha rhythm and the absence of REM.

or·tho·ker·a·tol·o·gy (ôr′thō-kĕr′ə-tŏl′ə-jē) n. A method of improving unaided vision by molding the cornea with contact lenses.

Or·tho–Kung T cell (ôr′-thō-kŭng′) n. Any of various classes of monoclonal antibodies to T-cell substrates.

or·tho·pe·dics or **or·tho·pae·dics** (ôr′thə-pē′dĭks) n. The branch of medicine that deals with the prevention and correction of injuries or disorders of the skeletal system and associated muscles, joints, and ligaments. — **or′tho·pe′dic** adj.

orthopedic surgery n. The branch of surgery that deals with the correction of injuries or disorders of the skeletal system and associated muscles, joints, and ligaments.

or·tho·pe·dist or **or·tho·pae·dist** (ôr′thə-pē′dĭst) n. A specialist in orthopedics.

or·tho·per·cus·sion (ôr′thō-pər-kŭsh′ən) n. Very light percussion of the chest, used to determine the size of the heart.

or·tho·pho·ri·a (ôr′thə-fôr′ē-ə) n. The normal condition of balance between the muscles of the eyes that permits the lines of sight to meet at an object being looked at.

or·tho·psy·chi·a·try (ôr′thō-sī-kī′ə-trē, -sī-) n. The psychiatric study, treatment, and prevention of emotional and behavioral problems, especially of those that arise during early development.

or·thop·tics (ôr-thŏp′tĭks) n. The study and treatment of defective binocular vision, of defects in the action of the ocular muscles, or of faulty visual habits. — **or·thop′tic** adj.

or·tho·scope (ôr′thə-skōp′) n. An instrument used to examine the eye that eliminates corneal refraction by means of a layer of water.

or·tho·scop·ic (ôr′thə-skŏp′ĭk) adj. **1.** Of or relating to an orthoscope. **2.** Having normal vision; free from visual distortion.

or·thos·co·py (ôr-thŏs′kə-pē) n. Examination of the eye with an orthoscope.

or·tho·sis (ôr-thō′sĭs) n., pl. **-ses** (-sēz). The straightening of a deformity, often by use of orthopedic appliances.

or·thot·ic (ôr-thŏt′ĭk) adj. Of or relating to orthotics. — n. An orthopedic appliance designed to straighten or support a body part.

or·thot·ics (ôr-thŏt′ĭks) n. The science that deals with the use of specialized mechanical devices to support or supplement weakened or abnormal joints or limbs.

or·thot·ist (ôr-thŏt′ĭst, ôr′thə-tĭst) n. A specialist in orthotics.

os¹ (ŏs) n., pl. **o·ra** (ôr′ə). **1.** An opening into a hollow organ or canal. **2.** The oral cavity; mouth.

os² (ŏs) n., pl. **os·sa** (ŏs′ə). Bone.

os·che·o·plas·ty (ŏs′kē-ə-plăs′tē) n. See **scrotoplasty**.

os·cil·late (ŏs′ə-lāt′) v. **-lat·ed, -lat·ing, -lates. 1.** To swing back and forth with a steady, uninterrupted rhythm. **2.** To vary between alternate extremes, usually within a definable period of time. — **os′cil·la′tor** n. — **os′cil·la·to′ry** (-lə-tôr′ē) adj.

os·cil·la·tion (ŏs′ə-lā′shən) n. **1.** The act of oscillating. **2.** A stage in inflammation in which the accumulation of white blood cells in the small vessels arrests the passage of blood, causing a to-and-fro movement of the blood at each cardiac contraction. — **os′cil·la′tion·al** adj.

oscillatory potential n. The variable voltage in the positive deflection of the electroretinogram of the dark-adapted eye arising from amacrine cells.

os·cil·lo·gram (ə-sĭl′ə-grăm′) n. **1.** The curve traced by an oscillograph. **2.** An instantaneous oscilloscope trace or photograph.

os·cil·lo·graph (ə-sĭl′ə-grăf′) n. A device that records oscillations, as of an electric current and voltage. — os·cil′lo·graph′ic adj. — os′cil·log′ra·phy (ŏs′ə-lŏg′rə-fē) n.

os·cil·lo·scope (ə-sĭl′ə-skōp′) n. An electronic instrument that produces an instantaneous trace on the screen of a cathode-ray tube corresponding to oscillations of voltage and current. — os·cil′lo·scop′ic (-skŏp′ĭk) adj.

os cox·ae (kŏk′sē) n. The hipbone.

os·cu·lum (ŏs′kyə-ləm) n., pl. -la (-lə). A pore or minute opening.

Os·good–Schlatter disease (ŏs′gŏŏd′-, ŏz′-) n. Osteochondrosis of the tibial tubercle.

OSHA (ō′shə) n. Occupational Safety and Health Administration, a branch of the U.S. department of Labor, responsible for establishing and enforcing safety and health standards in the workplace.

Os·ler′s sign (ŏs′lərz, ŏz′-) n. An indication of acute bacterial endocarditis in which small, circumscribed, painful, erythematous swellings appear on the skin and in the subcutaneous tissues of the hands and feet.

os·mics (ŏz′mĭks) n. The science that deals with smells and the olfactory sense.

os·mi·um (ŏz′mē-əm) n. A hard, brittle, grayish metallic element with atomic number 76.

os·mo·re·cep·tor¹ (ŏz′mō-rĭ-sĕp′tər, ŏs′-) n. A receptor in the central nervous system that responds to changes in the osmotic pressure of the blood.

osmoreceptor² n. A receptor that receives olfactory stimuli.

os·mo·reg·u·la·tion (ŏz′mə-rĕg′yə-lā′shən, ŏs′-) n. Maintenance of an optimal, constant osmotic pressure in the body of a living organism. — os′·mo·reg′u·la·to′ry (-lə-tôr′ē) adj.

os·mose (ŏz′mōs′, ŏs′-) v. -mosed, -mos·ing, -mos·es. To diffuse or cause to diffuse by osmosis.

os·mo·sis (ŏz-mō′sĭs, ŏs-) n., pl. -ses (-sēz). 1. Diffusion of fluid through a semipermeable membrane until there is an equal concentration of fluid on both sides of the membrane. 2. The tendency of fluids to diffuse in such a manner. — os·mot′ic (-mŏt′ĭk) adj.

osmotic pressure n. The pressure exerted by the flow of water through a semipermeable membrane separating two solutions with different concentrations of solute.

os·phre·sis (ŏs-frē′sĭs) n. The sense of smell.

os·se·in or os·se·ine (ŏs′ē-ĭn) n. The collagen component of bone.

os·se·ous (ŏs′ē-əs) adj. Composed of, containing, or resembling bone; bony.

osseous labyrinth n. A series of cavities in the petrous portion of the temporal bone, consisting of the cochlea, the vestibule and the semicircular canals, and lodging the membranous labyrinth.

osseous lacuna n. A cavity in bony tissue occupied by an osteocyte.

os·si·cle (ŏs′ĭ-kəl) n. A small bone, especially one of three bones of the middle ear that articulate to form a chain for transmitting sound from the tympanic membrane to the oval window. — os·sic′u·lar (ŏ-sĭk′yə-lər), os·sic′u·late (-lĭt) adj.

os·sic·u·lec·to·my (ŏ-sĭk′′yə-lĕk′tə-mē) n. Surgical removal of the ossicles of the middle ear.

os·si·cu·lot·o·my (ŏ-sĭk′yə-lŏt′ə-mē) n. Surgical division of a middle ear ossicle or of a fibrous band causing ankylosis between two ossicles.

os·si·fi·ca·tion (ŏs′ə-fĭ-kā′shən) n. 1. The natural process of bone formation. 2. The hardening or calcification of soft tissue into a bonelike material. 3. A mass or deposit of such material.

os·si·fy (ŏs′ə-fī′) v. -fied, -fy·ing, -fies. To change into bone.

os·te·al (ŏs′tē-əl) adj. 1. Bony; osseous. 2. Relating to bone or to the skeleton.

os·te·al·gi·a (ŏs′tē-ăl′jē-ə, -jə) n. Pain in a bone. — os·te·al′gic (-jĭk) adj.

os·tec·to·my (ŏs-tĕk′tə-mē) n. Surgical removal of a bone or part of a bone.

os·te·in or os·te·ine (ŏs′tē-ĭn) n. See ossein.

os·te·i·tis (ŏs′tē-ī′tĭs) or os·ti·tis (ŏ-stī′tĭs) n. Inflammation of bone or bony tissue.

osteitis de·for·mans (dē-fôr′mănz′) n. See Paget's disease (sense 1).

os·te·o·an·a·gen·e·sis (ŏs′tē-ō-ăn′ə-jĕn′ĭ-sĭs) n. The regeneration of bone tissue.

os·te·o·ar·thri·tis (ŏs′tē-ō-är-thrī′tĭs) n. A form of arthritis, occurring mainly in older persons, that is marked by chronic degeneration of the joint cartilage. — os′te·o·ar·thrit′ic (-thrĭt′ĭk) adj.

os·te·o·ar·throp·a·thy (ŏs′tē-ō-är-thrŏp′ə-thē) n. A disorder affecting bones and joints.

os·te·o·blast (ŏs′tē-ə-blăst′) n. A cell from which bone forms. — os′te·o·blas′tic adj.

os·te·o·blas·to·ma (ŏs′tē-ō-blă-stō′mə) n. A benign tumor of bone characterized by areas of osteoid and calcified tissue.

os·te·o·chon·dri·tis (ŏs′tē-ō-kŏn-drī′tĭs) n. Inflammation of a bone along with its cartilage.

os·te·o·chon·dro·ma (ŏs′tē-ō-kŏn-drō′mə) n. A benign cartilaginous neoplasm that consists of a pedicle of normal bone covered with a rim of proliferating cartilage cells.

os·te·o·chon·dro·sar·co·ma (ŏs′tē-ō-kŏn′drō-sär-kō′mə) n. A chondrosarcoma arising in bone.

os·te·o·chon·dro·sis (ŏs′tē-ō-kŏn-drō′sĭs) n. Any of a group of disorders of one or more ossification centers of the bones in children, characterized by degeneration or aseptic necrosis followed by reossification.

os·te·o·cla·sis (ŏs′tē-ŏk′lə-sĭs) n., pl. -ses (-sēz′). 1. The process of dissolution and resorption of bony tissue. 2. Surgical fracture of a bone, performed to correct a deformity.

os·te·o·clast (ŏs′tē-ə-klăst′) n. 1. A large multinucleate cell found in growing bone that resorbs bony tissue, as in the formation of canals and cavities. 2. An instrument used in surgical osteoclasis. — os′te·o·clas′tic adj.

osteoclast-activating factor n. A lymphokine that stimulates bone resorption and inhibits bone-collagen synthesis.

os·te·o·cyte (ŏs'tē-ə-sīt') *n.* A branched cell embedded in the matrix of bone tissue.

os·te·o·dyn·i·a (ŏs'tē-ō-dĭn'ē-ə) *n.* Pain in a bone.

os·te·o·dys·tro·phy (ŏs'tē-ō-dĭs'trə-fē) *n.* Defective formation of bone.

os·te·o·fi·bro·ma (ŏs'tē-ō-fī-brō'mə) *n.* A benign bone tumor, consisting chiefly of dense fibrous connective tissue and bone.

os·te·o·fi·bro·sis (ŏs'tē-ō-fī-brō'sĭs) *n.* Fibrosis of bone, mainly involving bone marrow.

os·te·o·gen (ŏs'tē-ə-jən, -jĕn') *n.* The substance forming the inner layer of the periosteum, from which new bone is formed.

os·te·o·gen·e·sis (ŏs'tē-ə-jĕn'ĭ-sĭs) *n.* The formation and development of bony tissue.

osteogenesis im·per·fec·ta (ĭm'pər-fĕk'tə) *n.* A hereditary disease marked by abnormal fragility and plasticity of bone, with recurring fractures resulting from minimal trauma; deformity of long bones; a bluish coloration of the sclerae; and, in many cases, otosclerotic development.

osteogenic sarcoma *n.* See **osteosarcoma**.

os·te·og·e·ny (ŏs'tē-ŏj'ə-nē) *n.* See **osteogenesis**.

os·te·oid osteoma (ŏs'tē-oid') *n.* A painful benign tumor usually originating in one of the bones of the lower extremities and characterized by a nidus composed of vascularized connective tissue and osteoid material and surrounded by a relatively large zone of thickened bone.

os·te·ol·y·sis (ŏs'tē-ŏl'ĭ-sĭs) *n.* Dissolution or degeneration of bone tissue resulting from disease. — **os'te·o·lyt'ic** (-ə-lĭt'ĭk) *adj.*

os·te·o·ma (ŏs'tē-ō'mə) *n., pl.* **-mas** or **-ma·ta** (-mə-tə). A benign tumor composed of bony tissue, often developing on the skull.

os·te·o·ma·la·cia (ŏs'tē-ō-mə-lā'shə, -shē-ə) *n.* A disease occurring primarily in adults that results from a deficiency in vitamin D or calcium and is characterized by a softening of the bones with accompanying pain and weakness.

os·te·o·ma·toid (ŏs'tē-ō'mə-toid') *n.* An abnormal nodule or small overgrowth of bone, usually occurring bilaterally and symmetrically in juxtaepiphysial regions, especially in long bones of the lower extremities.

os·te·o·my·e·li·tis (ŏs'tē-ō-mī'ə-lī'tĭs) *n.* Inflammation of bone and bone marrow.

os·te·o·my·e·lo·dys·pla·sia (ŏs'tē-ō-mī'ə-lō-dĭs-plā'zhə, -zhē-ə) *n.* A disease characterized by enlargement of the marrow cavities of the bones, thinning of the osseous tissue, large thin-walled vascular spaces, leukopenia, and irregular fever.

os·te·on (ŏs'tē-ŏn') or **os·te·one** (-ōn') *n.* A central canal and the concentric osseous lamellae encircling it, occurring in compact bone.

os·te·o·path (ŏs'tē-ə-păth') or **os·te·op·a·thist** (ŏs'tē-ŏp'ə-thĭst) *n.* A physician who practices osteopathy.

os·te·o·path·i·a stri·a·ta (ŏs'tē-ə-păth'ē-ə strī-ā'təs) *pl.n.* Linear striations, visible by radiographic examination, in the metaphyses of long or flat bones.

osteopathic medicine *n.* See **osteopathy** (sense 1).

osteopathic physician *n.* An osteopath.

os·te·op·a·thy (ŏs'tē-ŏp'ə-thē) *n.* **1.** A system of medicine based on the theory that disturbances in the musculoskeletal system affect other bodily parts, causing many disorders that can be corrected by various manipulative techniques in conjunction with conventional therapeutic procedures. **2.** A disease of a bone. — **os'te·o·path'ic** (-ə-păth'ĭk) *adj.*

os·te·o·pe·ni·a (ŏs'tē-ə-pē'nē-ə) *n.* A condition of bone in which decreased calcification, decreased density, or reduced mass occurs.

os·te·o·per·i·os·ti·tis (ŏs'tē-ō-pĕr'ē-ŏs-tī'tĭs) *n.* Inflammation of the periosteum and the underlying bone.

os·te·o·phage (ŏs'tē-ə-fāj') *n.* See **osteoclast** (sense 1).

os·te·o·phy·ma (ŏs'tē-ə-fī'mə) *n.* See **osteophyte**.

os·te·o·phyte (ŏs'tē-ə-fīt') *n.* A small, abnormal bony outgrowth.

os·te·o·plas·tic (ŏs'tē-ə-plăs'tĭk) *adj.* **1.** Of or relating to osteoplasty. **2.** Relating to or functioning in bone formation.

os·te·o·plas·ty (ŏs'tē-ə-plăs'tē) *n.* Surgical repair or alteration of bone.

os·te·o·po·ro·sis (ŏs'tē-ō-pə-rō'sĭs) *n., pl.* **-ses** (-sēz). A disease in which the bones become extremely porous, are subject to fracture, and heal slowly, occurring especially in women following menopause and often leading to curvature of the spine from vertebral collapse. — **os'te·o·po·rot'-ic** (-rŏt'ĭk) *adj.*

os·te·o·ra·di·o·ne·cro·sis (ŏs'tē-ō-rā'dē-ō-nə-krō'sĭs, -nĕ-) *n.* Necrosis of bone caused by exposure to ionizing radiation.

os·te·or·rha·phy (ŏs'tē-ôr'ə-fē) *n.* The surgical suturing or joining of fragments of broken bone, usually by wiring them together.

os·te·o·sar·co·ma (ŏs'tē-ō-sär-kō'mə) *n.* A malignant bone tumor.

os·te·o·scle·ro·sis (ŏs'tē-ō-sklə-rō'sĭs) *n.* Abnormal hardening of bone or bone marrow. — **os'te·o·scle·rot'ic** (-rŏt'ĭk) *adj.*

os·te·o·sis (ŏs'tē-ō'sĭs) or **os·to·sis** (-tō'sĭs) *n.* The formation of bony tissue, especially over connective or other tissue.

os·te·o·su·ture (ŏs'tē-ō-sōō'chər) *n.* See **osteorrhaphy**.

os·te·o·syn·the·sis (ŏs'tē-ō-sĭn'thĭ-sĭs) *n.* The process of mechanically bringing the ends of a fractured bone close together, as by wiring together or attaching to a metal plate.

os·te·o·throm·bo·sis (ŏs'tē-ō-thrŏm-bō'sĭs) *n.* Thrombosis in one or more of the veins of a bone.

os·te·o·tome (ŏs'tē-ə-tōm') *n.* A chisel-like instrument for cutting bone.

os·te·ot·o·my (ŏs'tē-ŏt'ə-mē) *n.* Surgical division or sectioning of bone.

os·te·o·tribe (ŏs'tē-ə-trīb') *n.* An instrument for filing or abrading away pieces of necrosed or decayed bone.

os·te·o·trite (ŏs'tē-ə-trīt') *n.* An instrument for grinding away decayed bone.

os·ti·um (ŏs′tē-əm) n., pl. -ti·a (-tē-ə). A small opening or orifice, as in a body organ or passage. — os′ti·al adj.

os·to·my (ŏs′tə-mē) n. Surgical construction of an artificial excretory opening, as a colostomy.

OT abbr. occupational therapy

o·tal·gi·a (ō-tăl′jē-ə, -jə) n. Pain in the ear; earache. — o·tal′gic adj.

OTC or O.T.C. abbr. over-the-counter

ot·he·ma·to·ma (ŏt′hē-mə-tō′mə) n. A purplish, rounded, hard swelling of the external ear.

o·tic (ō′tĭk, ŏt′ĭk) adj. Of, relating to, or located near the ear; auricular.

otic vesicle n. See auditory vesicle.

o·ti·tis (ō-tī′tĭs) n. Inflammation of the ear. — o·tit′ic (ō-tĭt′ĭk) adj.

otitis ex·ter·na (ĭk-stûr′nə) n. Inflammation of the external auditory canal.

otitis me·di·a (mē′dē-ə) n. Inflammation of the middle ear, occurring commonly in children as a result of infection and often causing pain and temporary hearing loss.

o·to·ceph·a·ly (ō′tō-sĕf′ə-lē) n. A congenital malformation of the head characterized by a markedly diminished or absent lower jaw and the joining or close approach of the ears on the front of the neck below the face.

o·to·clei·sis (ō′tō-klī′sĭs) n. The closing of the auditory tube of the ear either by a new growth or accumulation of cerumen.

o·to·cyst (ō′tə-sĭst′) n. The structure formed by invagination of the embryonic ectodermal tissue that develops into the inner ear. — o′to·cys′tic adj.

o·to·dyn·i·a (ō′tə-dĭn′ē-ə) n. Pain in the ear.

o·to·en·ceph·a·li·tis (ō′tō-ĕn-sĕf′ə-lī′tĭs) n. Inflammation of the brain caused by the extension of an infection from an inflamed middle ear.

o·to·lar·yn·gol·o·gy (ō′tō-lăr′ən-gŏl′ə-jē) n. The branch of medicine that deals with diagnosis and treatment of diseases of the ear, larynx, and upper respiratory tract. — o′to·lar′yn·gol′o·gist n.

o·to·lith (ō′tə-lĭth′) n. See otosteon (sense 2). — o′to·lith′ic adj.

o·tol·o·gy (ō-tŏl′ə-jē) n. The branch of medicine that deals with the structure, function, and pathology of the ear. — o·to·log′ic (ō′tə-lŏj′ĭk) adj. — o·tol′o·gist n.

o·to·my·co·sis (ō′tō-mī-kō′sĭs) n. A fungous infection of the external auditory canal.

o·top·a·thy (ō-tŏp′ə-thē) n. A disease of the ear.

o·to·plas·ty (ō′tə-plăs′tē) n. The surgical repair, restoration, or alteration of the auricle of the ear.

o·to·pol·y·pus (ō′tō-pŏl′ə-pəs) n. A polyp in the external auditory canal, usually arising from the middle ear.

o·to·py·or·rhe·a (ō′tō-pī′ə-rē′ə) n. Chronic otitis media resulting in perforation of the eardrum and a purulent discharge.

o·to·rhi·no·lar·yn·gol·o·gy (ō′tō-rī′nō-lăr′ĭng-gŏl′ə-jē) n. The medical specialty concerned with diseases of the ear, nose, and throat.

o·to·rhi·nol·o·gy (ō′tō-rī′nŏl′ə-jē) n. The branch

of medicine concerned with diseases of the ear and nose.

o·to·scle·ro·sis (ō′tō-sklə-rō′sĭs) n. A formation of spongy bone about the stapes and oval windows, causing progressive deafness.

o·to·scope (ō′tə-skōp′) n. An instrument for examining the interior of the ear, especially the eardrum, having a magnifying lens and a light.

o·tos·co·py (ō-tŏs′kə-pē) n. Examination of the ear by means of an otoscope.

ot·os·te·on (ō-tŏs′tē-ŏn′) n. 1. Any of the small bones of the middle ear. 2. A calcareous concretion in the inner ear.

o·tot·o·my (ō-tŏt′ə-mē) n. Surgical incision of the ear.

oua·ba·in (wä-bā′ĭn) n. A white poisonous glycoside extracted from the seeds of the African trees Strophanthus gratus and Acokanthera ouabaio and used as a heart stimulant.

ounce (ouns) n. 1. A unit of weight in the U.S. Customary System, an avoirdupois unit equal to 437.5 grains or 28.35 grams. 2. A unit of apothecary weight equal to 480 grains or 31.10 grams. 3. A fluid ounce.

out·er ear (ou′tər) n. See external ear.

out·pa·tient (out′pā′shənt) n. A patient who is admitted to a hospital or clinic for treatment that does not require an overnight stay.

out·put (out′pŏŏt′) n. The amount produced, ejected, or excreted by an organism or part in a specified period of time.

o·va·lo·cyte (ō′və-lō-sīt′, ō-văl′ə-) n. See ellipto-cyte.

o·val window (ō′vəl) n. An oval opening on the medial wall of the tympanic cavity, leading into the vestibule, to which the base of the stapes is connected and through which the ear ossicles transmit sound vibrations to the cochlea.

o·var·i·al·gi·a (ō-vâr′ē-ăl′jē-ə, -jə) n. Pain in the ovary.

ovarian cycle n. The normal sex cycle that includes development of an ovarian follicle, rupture of the follicle, discharge of the ovum, and formation and regression of a corpus luteum.

ovarian cyst n. A cystic tumor of the ovary, which is usually benign.

ovarian follicle n. A cavity in the ovary containing a maturing ovum and its encasing cells.

ovarian pregnancy n. An ectopic pregnancy developing in an ovarian follicle.

o·var·i·ec·to·my (ō-vâr′ē-ĕk′tə-mē) n. Surgical removal of one ovary or both ovaries.

o·var·i·o·cen·te·sis (ō-vâr′ē-ō-sĕn-tē′sĭs) n. Puncture of an ovary or an ovarian cyst.

o·var·i·o·cy·e·sis (ō-vâr′ē-ō-sī-ē′sĭs) n. See ovari-an pregnancy.

o·var·i·o·hys·ter·ec·to·my (ō-vâr′ē-ō-hĭs′tə-rĕk′tə-mē) n. Surgical removal of one ovary or both ovaries and the uterus.

o·var·i·or·rhex·is (ō-vâr′ē-ə-rĕk′sĭs) n. Rupture of an ovary.

o·var·i·o·sal·pin·gec·to·my (ō-vâr′ē-ō-săl′pĭn-jĕk′tə-mē) *n.* Surgical removal of an ovary and the corresponding oviduct.

o·var·i·o·sal·pin·gi·tis (ō-vâr′ē-ō-săl′pĭn-jī′tĭs) *n.* Inflammation of an ovary and the corresponding oviduct.

o·var·i·os·to·my (ō-vâr′ē-ŏs′tə-mē) *n.* Surgical formation of a temporary fistula to drain an ovarian cyst.

o·var·i·ot·o·my (ō-vâr′ē-ŏt′ə-mē) *n.* **1.** Ovariectomy. **2.** Surgical incision into an ovary, as to perform a biopsy or remove a tumor.

o·va·ri·tis (ō′və-rī′tĭs) *n.* See **oophoritis**.

o·va·ry (ō′və-rē) *n.* One of the paired female reproductive organs that produces ova and certain sex hormones, including estrogen and progesterone. — **o·var′i·an** (ō-vâr′ē-ən) *adj.*

o·ver·anx·ious disorder (ō′vər-ăngk′shəs, -ăng′-shəs) *n.* A generalized and persistent anxiety in children or adults that is not the result of separation or recent stress and is characterized by self-consciousness and obsessiveness over past behavior, future events, personal health, and competence in social or academic arenas.

o·ver·bite (ō′vər-bīt′) *n.* A malocclusion of the teeth in which the front upper incisor and canine teeth project over the lower.

o·ver·com·pen·sa·tion (ō′vər-kŏm′pən-sā′shən) *n.* **1.** Excessive compensation, especially the exertion of effort in excess of that needed to compensate for a physical or psychological characteristic or defect. **2.** A neurotic striving for power or prestige because of a feeling of inferiority.

o·ver·dose (ō′vər-dōs′) *n.* An excessive dose, especially of a narcotic.

o·ver·eat (ō′vər-ēt′) *v.* **-ate** (-āt′), **-eat·en** (-ēt′n), **-eat·ing, -eats.** To eat to excess, especially when habitual.

o·ver·ex·press (ō′vər-ĭk-sprĕs′) *v.* **-pressed, -pressing, -press·es.** Producing in excess, said of the genetic material of cancer cells.

o·ver·feed (ō′vər-fēd′) *v.* **-fed** (-fĕd′), **-feed·ing, -feeds.** To feed or eat too often or too much.

o·ver·lap (ō′vər-lăp′) *n.* **1.** A part or portion of a structure that extends or projects over another. **2.** The suturing of one layer of tissue above or under another layer to provide additional strength. — *v.* **-lapped, -lap·ping, -laps.** (ō′vər-lăp′). **1.** To lie over and partly cover something. **2.** To perform a surgical overlap on tissues.

o·ver·med·i·cate (ō′vər-mĕd′ĭ-kāt′) *v.* **-cat·ed, -cat·ing, -cates.** To medicate a patient excessively.

o·ver·pre·scribe (ō′vər-prĭ-skrīb′) *v.* **-scribed, -scrib·ing, -scribes.** To prescribe an excessive amount of a medication.

o·ver·re·act (ō′vər-rē-ăkt′) *v.* **-act·ed, -act·ing, -acts.** To react with unnecessary or inappropriate force, emotional display, or violence.

o·ver·rid·ing (ō′vər-rī′dĭng) *adj.* **1.** Of or relating to a fracture in which the broken ends of the bone slip past each other and are held in the overlap position by contracted muscles. **2.** Of or relating to a fetal head that is palpable above the pubic symphysis because of the disproportion between

the size of the fetal head and the size of the maternal pelvis.

o·ver·shoot (ō′vər-shōōt′) *n.* A change from steady state in response to a sudden change in some factor, as in electric potential or polarity when a cell or tissue is stimulated.

o·ver·stretch (ō′vər-strĕch′) *v.* **-stretched, -stretch·ing, -stretch·es. 1.** To stretch one's body or muscles to the point of strain or injury. **2.** To stretch or extend over.

o·ver-the-count·er (ō′vər-*th*ə-koun′tər) *adj.* That can be sold legally without a doctor's prescription.

o·vi·duct (ō′vĭ-dŭkt′) *n.* See **fallopian tube.** — **o′vi·duc′tal, o′vi·du′cal** (-dōō′kəl, -dyōō′-) *adj.*

o·vi·gen·e·sis (ō′və-jĕn′ĭ-sĭs) *n.* See **oogenesis.** — **o′vi·ge·net′ic** (-jə-nĕt′ĭk) *adj.*

o·vo·plasm (ō′və-plăz′əm) *n.* The cytoplasm of an unfertilized ovum.

ovular membrane *n.* See **vitelline membrane** (sense 1).

o·vu·late (ō′vyə-lāt′, ŏv′yə-) *v.* **-lat·ed, -lat·ing, -lates.** To produce ova; discharge eggs from the ovary.

o·vu·la·tion (ō′vyə-lā′shən, ŏv′yə-) *n.* The discharge of an ovum from the ovary.

o·vu·la·to·ry (ō′vyə-lə-tôr′ē, ŏv′yə-) *adj.* Of, relating to, or characterizing ovulation.

o·vule (ō′vyōōl, ŏv′yōōl) *n.* **1.** A small or immature ovum of a mammal. **2.** A small egglike structure. — **o′vu·lar** (ō′vyə-lər, ŏv′yə-), **o′vu·lar′y** (-lĕr′ē)

o·vu·lum (ō′vyə-ləm, ŏv′yə-) *n.* See **ovule** (sense 2).

o·vum (ō′vəm) *n., pl.* **o·va** (ō′və). The female reproductive cell or gamete; egg.

ox·a·cil·lin (ŏk′sə-sĭl′ĭn) *n.* A semisynthetic penicillin effective against penicillin-resistant bacteria, especially staphylococci.

ox·a·late calculus (ŏk′sə-lāt′) *n.* A hard urinary calculus composed of calcium oxalate; it can be smooth or covered with minute sharp spines.

ox·az·e·pam (ŏk-săz′ə-păm′) *n.* A tranquilizing drug related to benzodiazepine and used especially in the treatment of insomnia and alcohol withdrawal.

ox·i·da·tion (ŏk′sĭ-dā′shən) *n.* The combination of a substance with oxygen.

ox·i·da·tive (ŏk′sĭ-dā′tĭv) *adj.* Of, relating to, or characterized by oxidation.

oxidative phosphorylation *n.* The formation of ATP from the energy released by the oxidation of various substrates, especially the organic acids involved in the Krebs cycle.

ox·im·e·ter (ŏk-sĭm′ĭ-tər) *n.* A device for measuring the oxygen saturation of arterial blood. — **ox·im′e·try** *n.*

ox·o·lin·ic acid (ŏk′sə-lĭn′ĭk) *n.* An antibacterial agent used to urinary tract infections.

ox·y·ceph·a·ly (ŏk′sē-sĕf′ə-lē) *n.* A congenital abnormality of the skull in which the top of the head assumes a conical or pointed shape because of premature closing of the lambdoid and coronal sutures. — **ox′y·ce·phal′ic** (-sə-făl′ĭk), **ox′y·ceph′a·lous** (-sĕf′ə-ləs) *adj.*

ox·y·gen (ŏk′sĭ-jən) *n.* **1.** A colorless, odorless element with atomic number 8 that constitutes 21 percent of the atmosphere by volume, occurs as a gas, combines with most elements, is essential for plant and animal respiration, and is required for nearly all combustion. **2.** A medicinal gas containing oxygen.

oxygen affinity hypoxia *n.* Hypoxia due to the reduced ability of hemoglobin to release oxygen.

ox·y·gen·ase (ŏk′sĭ-jə-nās′, -nāz′) *n.* An enzyme that catalyzes the incorporation of molecular oxygen into its substrate.

ox·y·gen·ate (ŏk′sĭ-jə-nāt′) *or* **ox·y·gen·ize** (-jə-nīz′) *v.* **-at·ed** *or* **-ized, -at·ing** *or* **-iz·ing, -ates** *or* **-iz·es.** To treat, combine, or infuse with oxygen.

oxygenated hemoglobin *n.* See **oxyhemoglobin.**

ox·y·gen·a·tion (ŏk′sĭ-jə-nā′shən) *n.* The addition of oxygen to a chemical substance or physical system.

oxygen capacity *n.* The amount of oxygen a quantity of blood is able to absorb.

oxygen consumption *n.* An expression of the rate at which oxygen is used by tissues, usually given in microliters of oxygen consumed in 1 hour by 1 milligram dry weight of tissue.

oxygen debt *n.* The amount of extra oxygen required by muscle tissue to oxidize lactic acid and replenish depleted ATP and phosphocreatine following vigorous exercise.

oxygen mask *n.* A masklike device placed over the mouth and nose and through which oxygen is supplied from an attached storage tank.

oxygen tent *n.* A canopy placed over the head and shoulders or over the body of a patient to provide oxygen at a higher concentration than normal.

oxygen toxicity *n.* A condition resulting from breathing high partial pressures of oxygen, characterized by visual and hearing abnormalities, unusual fatigue, muscular twitching, anxiety, confusion, incoordination, and convulsions.

ox·y·he·mo·glo·bin (ŏk′sē-hē′mə-glō′bĭn) *n.* Hemoglobin in combination with oxygen, present in arterial blood.

ox·y·me·taz·o·line (ŏk′sē-mĭ-tăz′ə-lēn′, -mĕt′ə-zō-) *n.* A vasoconstricting drug that is used topically in the form of its hydrochloride salt to reduce nasal congestion.

ox·yn·tic (ŏk-sĭn′tĭk) *adj.* Forming or secreting acid, as the parietal cells of gastric glands.

oxyntic cell *n.* See **parietal cell.**

ox·y·phil·ic leukocyte (ŏk′sĭ-fĭl′ĭk) *n.* See **eosinophil** (sense 1).

ox·y·pho·ni·a (ŏk′sĭ-fō′nē-ə) *n.* Shrillness or high pitch of the voice.

ox·yt·a·lan (ŏk-sĭt′ə-lăn′) *n.* A type of connective tissue fiber, distinct from collagen or elastic fibers, and found in the periodontal membrane and gingivae of the mouth.

ox·y·tet·ra·cy·cline (ŏk′sē-tĕt′rə-sī′klĭn, -klēn′) *n.* A broad-spectrum antibiotic derived from the actinomycete *Streptomyces rimosus* and used to treat a variety of bacterial infections.

ox·y·to·ci·a (ŏk′sĭ-tō′shē-ə, -shə) *n.* An unusually rapid childbirth.

ox·y·to·cic (ŏk′sĭ-tō′sĭk) *adj.* Hastening or facilitating childbirth, especially by stimulating contractions of the uterus. Used of a drug. — *n.* An oxytocic drug.

ox·y·to·cin (ŏk′sĭ-tō′sĭn) *n.* A short polypeptide hormone released from the posterior lobe of the pituitary gland to stimulate the contraction of smooth muscle of the uterus during labor and facilitate release of milk during nursing.

oz *or* **oz.** *abbr.* ounce

o·ze·na (ō-zē′nə) *n.* A chronic disease of the nose characterized by intranasal crusting, atrophy, and a fetid odor.

o·zone (ō′zōn) *n.* A blue gaseous allotrope of oxygen formed naturally from diatomic oxygen by electric discharge or exposure to ultraviolet radiation.

o·zo·sto·mi·a *n.* Foul-smelling breath; halitosis.

~~~~~~ **P** ~~~~~~

p- *abbr.* para- (often italic)

PA *or* **P.A.** *abbr.* physician's assistant

PABA (pä′bə) *n.* Para-aminobenzoic acid; a crystalline para form of aminobenzoic acid that is part of the vitamin B complex, is required by many organisms for folic acid formation, and is widely used in sunscreens to absorb ultraviolet light.

pace·fol·low·er (pās′fŏl′ō-ər) *n.* A cell in excitable tissue that responds to stimuli from a pacemaker.

pace·mak·er (pās′mā′kər) *n.* **1.** A part of the body, such as the specialized mass of cardiac muscle fibers of the sinoatrial node, that sets the pace or

rhythm of physiological activity. **2.** Any of several usually miniaturized and surgically implanted electronic devices used to stimulate or regulate contractions of the heart muscle. — **pace′mak′-ing** *adj. & n.*

pach·y·bleph·a·ron (păk′ē-blĕf′ə-rŏn′) *n.* Thickening of the tarsal border of the eyelid.

pach·y·der·ma (păk′ĭ-dûr′mə) *n.* Abnormally thick skin.

pach·y·der·mo·per·i·os·to·sis (păk′ĭ-dûr′mō-pĕr′ē-ŏ-stō′sĭs) *n.* A hereditary syndrome characterized by clubbing of the digits, periostosis of the long bones, and coarsening of the facial features with thickening, furrowing, and oiliness of the skin of the face and forehead.

pach·y·men·in·gi·tis (păk′ē-mĕn′ĭn-jī′tĭs) *n.* Inflammation of the dura mater.

pach·y·me·nin·gop·a·thy (păk′ē-mĕn′ĭng-gŏp′ə-thē) *n.* Disease of the dura mater.

pa·chyn·sis (pă-kĭn′sĭs) *n.* A pathological thickening of a bodily organ, tissue, or structure. — **pa·chyn′tic** *adj.*

pach·y·o·nych·i·a con·gen·i·ta (păk′ē-ō-nĭk′ē-ə kən-jĕn′ĭ-tə) *n.* A hereditary syndrome characterized by abnormal thickness and elevation of the nail plates, palmar and plantar hyperkeratosis, and a whitish and glazed tongue due to papillary atrophy.

pach·y·so·mi·a (păk′ĭ-sō′mē-ə) *n.* Pathological thickening of the soft parts of the body, especially as occurring in acromegaly.

pach·y·tene (păk′ĭ-tēn′) *n.* The third stage of the prophase of meiosis during which the homologous chromosomes become short and thick and divide into four distinct chromatids.

pa·cif·a·rin (pə-sĭf′ər-ĭn) *n.* Any of various bacterial products that, introduced in small amounts, protect an organism from an infection or a disease without killing the infectious agent.

pac·ing catheter (pā′sĭng) *n.* A cardiac catheter having one or two electrodes at its tip that, when connected to a pulse generator and properly positioned in the right atrium or ventricle, will artificially pace the heart.

pack (păk) *v.* **packed, pack·ing, packs. 1.** To fill, stuff, plug, or tampon. **2.** To enwrap or envelop the body in a sheet, blanket, or other covering. **3.** To apply a dressing or covering to a surgical site. — *n.* **1.** The swathing of a patient or a body part in hot, cold, wet, or dry materials, such as cloth towels, sheets, or blankets. **2.** The materials so used. **3.** An ice pack; an ice bag.

packed-cell volume *n.* The volume of blood cells in a sample of blood after it has been centrifuged.

pack·er (păk′ər) *n.* An instrument for tamponing.

pack·ing (păk′ĭng) *n.* **1.** The insertion of gauze or other material into a body cavity or wound for therapeutic purposes. **2.** The material so used; a pack.

pac·li·tax·el (păk′lĭ-tăk′əl) *n.* A drug made from the toxin of various species of yew and used to kill dividing cells, especially tumor cells.

pad (păd) *n.* **1.** A soft material forming a cushion, used in applying or relieving pressure on a part, or in filling a depression so that dressings can fit snugly. **2.** A fatty mass of tissue acting as a cushion in the body, such as the fleshy underside of a finger or toe.

Pag·et's cell (păj′ĭts) *n.* Any of the large, epithelial cells with clear cytoplasm associated with Paget's disease of the breast or an apocrine gland cancer of the skin.

Paget's disease *n.* **1.** A disease, occurring chiefly in old age, in which the bones become enlarged and weakened, often resulting in fracture or deforma-

tion. **2.** A form of breast cancer affecting the areola and nipple. **3.** A form of skin cancer arising from apocrine sweat glands.

pain (pān) *n.* **1.** An unpleasant sensation occurring in varying degrees of severity as a consequence of injury, disease, or emotional disorder. **2.** One of the uterine contractions occurring in childbirth.

pain-pleasure principle *n.* See **pleasure principle.**

paint (pānt) *n.* A solution or suspension of one or more medicaments applied to the skin with a brush or large applicator. — *v.* **paint·ed, paint·ing, paints.** To apply medicine to; swab.

pal·a·tal reflex (păl′ə-təl) *n.* Swallowing reflex induced by stimulation of the palate.

pal·ate (păl′ĭt) *n.* The bony and muscular partition between the oral and nasal cavities; the roof of the mouth.

pal·a·tine (păl′ə-tīn′) *adj.* Of or relating to the palate.

palatine bone *n.* An irregularly shaped bone posterior to the maxilla, which forms part of the nasal cavity, the eye socket, and the hard palate.

palatine tonsil *n.* See **tonsil** (sense 2).

pal·a·ti·tis (păl′ə-tī′tĭs) *n.* Inflammation of the palate.

pal·a·to·phar·yn·gor·rha·phy (păl′ə-tō-făr′ĭng-gŏr′ə-fē) *n.* See **staphylopharyngorrhaphy.**

pal·a·to·plas·ty (păl′ə-tə-plăs′tē) *n.* Surgery of the palate to restore form and function.

pal·a·to·ple·gi·a (păl′ə-tō-plē′jē-ə) *n.* Paralysis of the muscle of the soft palate.

pal·a·tor·rha·phy (păl′ə-tôr′ə-fē) *n.* Suture of a cleft palate.

pal·i·ki·ne·sia (păl′ĭ-kə-nē′zhə, -kī-) *n.* Involuntary repetition of movements.

pal·i·la·li·a (păl′ə-lā′lē-ə) *n.* See **paliphrasia.**

pal·in·drome (păl′ĭn-drōm′) *n.* A segment of double-stranded DNA in which the nucleotide sequence of one strand reads in reverse order to that of the complementary strand. — **pal′in·dro′mic** (-drō′mĭk, -drŏm′ĭk) *adj.*

pal·in·dro·mi·a (păl′ĭn-drō′mē-ə) *n.* A relapse or recurrence of a disease.

pal·in·gen·e·sis (păl′ĭn-jĕn′ĭ-sĭs) *n.* The repetition by a single organism of various stages in the evolution of its species during embryonic development.

pal·i·nop·si·a (păl′ə-nŏp′sē-ə) *n.* Abnormally recurring visual imagery.

pal·i·phra·si·a (păl′ə-frā′zē-ə, -zhə) *n.* Involuntary repetition of words or sentences in talking.

pal·la·di·um (pə-lā′dē-əm) *n.* A soft ductile metallic element with atomic number 46, occurring naturally with platinum, especially in gold, nickel, and copper ores, and used as a basis for dental alloys and for metals used in surgical instruments.

pall·es·the·sia (păl′ĭs-thē′zhə) *n.* The perception of vibration; pressure sense most acute when a vibrating tuning fork is applied over a bony prominence. — **pall′es·thet′ic** (-thĕt′ĭk) *adj.*

pal·li·ate (păl′ē-āt′) *v.* **-at·ed, -at·ing, -ates.** To reduce the severity of; to relieve somewhat.

pal·li·a·tive (păl′ē-ā′tĭv, -ē-ə-tĭv) *adj.* Relieving or soothing the symptoms of a disease or disorder without effecting a cure. — **pal′li·a′tive·ly** *adv.*

palliative treatment *n.* Treatment to alleviate symptoms without curing the disease.

pal·li·um (păl′ē-əm) *n., pl.* **-li·ums** or **-li·a** (-lē-ə). The mantle of gray matter forming the cerebral cortex with the underlying white substance.

pal·lor (păl′ər) *n.* Paleness, as of the skin.

palm (päm) *n.* The inner surface of the hand that extends from the wrist to the base of the fingers.

pal·mar (păl′mər, päl′-, pä′mər) *adj.* Of, relating to, or corresponding to the palm of the hand.

palmar arch *n.* **1.** The deep arterial arch located below the long flexor tendons in the hand. **2.** The superficial arterial arch in the hand located above the long flexor tendons.

palmar digital artery *n.* **1.** Any of the three arteries arising from the superficial palmar arch and running to the interdigital clefts where each divides into the two proper palmar digital arteries. **2.** Any of the arteries that pass along the side of each finger.

palmar digital vein *n.* Any of the paired veins that accompany the digital arteries and empty into the venous arch located above the long flexor tendons of the hand.

pal·mus (păl′məs) *n., pl.* **-mi** (-mī). A rhythmical fibrillary contraction in a muscle.

pal·pa·ble (păl′pə-bəl) *adj.* **1.** Perceptible to touch; capable of being palpated. **2.** Evident; obvious.

pal·pate (păl′pāt′) *v.* **-pat·ed, -pat·ing, -pates.** To examine by feeling and pressing with the palms of the hands and the fingers. — **pal·pa′tion** *n.* — **pal′pa′tor** *n.* — **pal′pa·tor′y** (-pə-tôr′ē) *adj.*

palpatory percussion *n.* Finger percussion in which the resistance of the tissues under the finger as well as the sound elicited are used in aiding diagnosis.

pal·pe·bra (păl′pə-brə, păl-pē′-) *n., pl.* **-pe·bras** or **-pe·brae** (-pə-brē′, -pē′brē). See **eyelid.** — **pal′pe·bral** (păl′pə*brəl, păl-pē′brəl, -pēb′rəl) *adj.*

palpebral fissure *n.* The longitudinal opening between the upper and lower eyelids.

pal·pi·ta·tion (păl′pĭ-tā′shən) *n.* Perceptible forcible pulsation of the heart, usually with an increase in frequency or force, with or without irregularity in rhythm.

pal·sy (pôl′zē) *n.* Complete or partial muscle paralysis, often accompanied by loss of sensation and uncontrollable body movements or tremors.

pan·a·ce·a (păn′ə-sē′ə) *n.* A remedy claimed to be curative of all problems or disorders; a cure-all.

pan·ag·glu·ti·nin (păn′ə-glōōt′n-ĭn) *n.* An agglutinin that reacts with all human red blood cells.

pan·an·gi·i·tis (păn′ăn-jē-ī′tĭs) *n.* Inflammation involving all the coats of a blood vessel.

pan·ar·thri·tis (păn′är-thrī′tĭs) *n.* **1.** Inflammation involving all the tissues of a joint. **2.** Inflammation of all the joints of the body.

pan·at·ro·phy (păn-ăt′rə-fē) *n.* **1.** Atrophy of all the parts of a structure. **2.** General atrophy of the body.

pan·car·di·tis (păn′kär-dī′tĭs) *n.* Diffuse inflammation of the heart.

Pan·coast's operation (păn′kōsts′) *n.* Division of the trigeminal nerve at the oval foramen.

Pancoast syndrome *n.* A syndrome characterized by pain and tingling of the arm, constriction of the pupil, and paralysis of the muscle that raises the upper eyelid, caused by pressure on the brachial plexus by a malignant tumor near the superior pulmonary sulcus.

pan·co·lec·to·my (păn′kə-lĕk′tə-mē) *n.* Surgical removal of the entire colon.

pan·cre·as (păng′krē-əs, păn′-) *n., pl.* **pan·cre·a·ta** (păn-krē′ə-tə). A lobulated gland without a capsule, that extends from the concavity of the duodenum to the spleen, consists of a flattened head within the duodenal concavity, an elongated three-sided body extending transversely across the abdomen, and a tail touching the spleen, and secretes insulin and glucagon internally and pancreatic juice externally into the intestine. — **pan′cre·at′ic** (păng′krē-ăt′ĭk, păn′-) *adj.*

pan·cre·a·tal·gi·a (păng′krē-ə-tăl′jē-ə, -jə, păn′-) *n.* Pain that arises from, or is felt in or near, the pancreas.

pan·cre·a·tec·to·my (păng′krē-ə-tĕk′tə-mē, păn′-) *n.* Excision of the pancreas.

pancreatic digestion *n.* Digestion in the intestine by the enzymes of the pancreatic juice.

pancreatic duct *n.* The excretory duct of the pancreas, extending through the gland from tail to head, where it empties into the duodenum.

pancreatic juice *n.* A clear, alkaline secretion of the pancreas containing enzymes that aid in the digestion of proteins, carbohydrates, and fats.

pan·cre·a·tin (păng′krē-ə-tĭn, păn′-, păn-krē′ə-tĭn) *n.* A mixture of the enzymes of pancreatic juice, such as amylase, lipase, and trypsin, extracted from animals such as cattle or hogs and used as a digestive aid.

pan·cre·a·ti·tis (păng′krē-ə-tī′tĭs, păn′-) *n.* Inflammation of the pancreas.

pan·cre·a·to·du·o·de·nec·to·my (păng′krē-ə-tō-dōō′ō-də-nĕk′tə-mē, -dyōō′-, -dōō-ŏd′n-ĕk′-, -dyōō-, păn′-) *n.* Excision of all or part of the pancreas together with the duodenum.

pan·cre·a·to·du·o·de·nos·to·my (păng′krē-ə-tō-dōō′ə-də-nŏs′tə-mē, -dyōō′-, -dōō-ŏd′n-ŏs′-, -dyōō-, păn′-) *n.* Surgical anastomosis of a pancreatic duct, cyst, or fistula to the duodenum.

pan·cre·a·to·gas·tros·to·my (păng′krē-ə-tō-gă-strŏs′tə-mē, păn′-) *n.* Surgical anastomosis of a pancreatic cyst or fistula to the stomach.

pan·cre·a·tog·ra·phy (păng′krē-ə-tŏg′rə-fē, păn′-) *n.* Radiographic visualization of the pancreatic ducts after injection of radiopaque material into the collecting system.

pan·cre·a·to·je·ju·nos·to·my (păng′krē-ə-tō-jə-jōō′nŏs′tə-mē, -jē′jōō-, -jĕj′ōō-, păn′-) *n.* The surgical formation of an opening between the jejunum and a pancreatic duct, cyst, or fistula.

pan·cre·at·o·li·thec·to·my (păng′krē-ə-tō-lĭ-thĕk′tə-mē, păn′-, -ăt′ō-) *n.* See **pancreatolithot-omy**.

pan·cre·a·to·li·thi·a·sis (păng′krē-ə-tō-lĭ-thī′-ə-sĭs, păn′-, -ăt′ō-) *n.* The presence of concretions in the pancreatic duct system.

pan·cre·a·to·li·thot·o·my (păng′krē-ə-tō-thŏt′ə-mē, păn′-, -ăt′ō-) *n.* Surgical removal of a pancreatic concretion.

pan·cre·a·tol·y·sis (păng′krē-ə-tŏl′ĭ-sĭs, păn′-) *n.* Destruction of pancreatic tissue. — **pan′cre·at·o·lyt′ic** (-ăt′ə-lĭt′ĭk) *adj.*

pan·cre·a·top·a·thy (păng′krē-ə-tŏp′ə-thē, păn′-) *n.* Disease of the pancreas.

pan·cre·a·tot·o·my (păng′krē-ə-tŏt′ə-mē, păn′-) *n.* Incision of the pancreas.

pan·cy·to·pe·ni·a (păn′sī-tə-pē′nē-ə) *n.* A pronounced reduction in all of the formed elements of the blood.

pan·dem·ic (păn-dĕm′ĭk) *adj.* Epidemic over a wide geographic area. — *n.* A pandemic disease.

pan·en·ceph·a·li·tis (păn′ĕn-sĕf′ə-lī′tĭs) *n.* Encephalitis that affects both the gray and white matter of the brain, resulting in progressive loss of mental and motor functions.

pan·en·do·scope (păn-ĕn′də-skōp′) *n.* An illuminated instrument for inspecting the interior of the urethra as well as the bladder.

Pa·neth′s granular cell (pä′nāts, -nĕts) *n.* Any of the coarsely granular secretory cells located in the intestinal glands of the small intestine and appendix.

pan·hy·po·pi·tu·i·ta·rism (păn′hī-pō-pĭ-tōō′ĭ-tə-rĭz′əm, -tyōō′-) *n.* A state in which secretion of the anterior pituitary hormones is inadequate or absent, as a result of destruction of the anterior pituitary gland.

pan·ic (păn′ĭk) *n.* A sudden overpowering feeling of terror. — **pan′ic** *v.*

panic attack *n.* The sudden onset of intense apprehension, fear, terror, impending doom, depersonalization, and derealization, occurring in phobias, schizophrenia, and major depression.

panic disorder *n.* A neurosis characterized by the occurrence of intense attacks of anxiety in specific circumstances and situations and by such symptoms as shortness of breath, chest pain, sweating, dizziness, and fear of dying or of losing mental functioning.

pan·my·e·lo·sis (păn′mī-ə-lō′sĭs) *n.* Myeloid metaplasia with the presence of abnormal immature blood cells in the spleen and liver, associated with myelofibrosis.

pan·nic·u·lec·to·my (pə-nĭk′yə-lĕk′tə-mē) *n.* Surgical excision of superficial fat of the abdomen.

pan·nic·u·li·tis (pə-nĭk′yə-lī′tĭs) *n.* Inflammation of the subcutaneous fat, especially of the abdominal wall.

pan·nic·u·lus (pə-nĭk′yə-ləs) *n., pl.* **-li** (-lī′). A sheet or layer of tissue.

pan·nus (păn′əs) *n., pl.* **-ni** (păn′ī). **1.** A membrane of granulation tissue covering the surface of the articular cartilages in rheumatoid arthritis. **2.** A membrane of granulation tissue covering the surface of the cornea in trachoma.

pan·oph·thal·mi·a (păn′ŏf-thăl′mē-ə, -ŏp-) or **pan·oph·thal·mi·tis** (-thəl-mī′tĭs) *n.* Purulent inflammation of all parts of the eye.

pan·o·ram·ic x-ray film (păn′ə-răm′ĭk) *n.* A dental x-ray film that gives a view of the entire upper and lower dental arch and the temporomandibular joint.

pan·o·ti·tis (păn′ō-tī′tĭs) *n.* Inflammation of the entire ear.

pan·si·nus·i·tis (păn′sī-nə-sī′tĭs) *n.* Inflammation of all paranasal sinuses on one or both sides.

pan·sys·tol·ic murmur (păn′sĭ-stŏl′ĭk) *n.* A murmur extending through the entire systolic interval, from the first to the second sound.

pant (pănt) *v.* **pant·ed, pant·ing, pants.** To breathe rapidly and shallowly.

pan·tal·gi·a (păn-tăl′jē-ə, -jə) *n.* Pain involving the entire body.

pan·to·then·ic acid (păn′tə-thĕn′ĭk) *n.* A yellow, oily acid, widely distributed in plant and animal tissues, that is a component of coenzyme A and a part of the vitamin B_2 complex, and that functions as a growth factor.

pap (păp) *n.* Soft or semiliquid food, as for infants.

pa·pa·in (pə-pā′ĭn, -pī′ĭn) or **pa·pa·in·ase** (-ə-nās′, -nāz′) *n.* An enzyme, or a crude extract containing it, that digests protein, is obtained from the juice of the unripe papaya fruit, and is used as a digestive aid.

Pa·pa·ni·co·laou smear (pä′pə-nē′kə-lou′, păp′ə-nĭk′ə-lou′) *n.* See **Pap smear.**

Papanicolaou stain *n.* A method of staining used principally on exfoliated cytologic specimens from the respiratory, digestive, or genitourinary tract. It is important in cancer screening, especially of smears of the female genital tract.

Papanicolaou test *n.* The Pap smear.

pa·pav·er·ine (pə-păv′ə-rēn′, -ər-ĭn) *n.* A nonaddictive opium derivative used medicinally to relieve spasms of smooth muscle.

pa·per chromatography (pā′pər) *n.* A form of partition chromatography in which the moving phase is liquid and the stationary phase paper.

paper mill worker's disease *n.* An inflammation of alveoli of the lung caused by allergic reaction to air-borne spores of a fungi found in moldy wood pulp.

pa·pil·la (pə-pĭl′ə) *n., pl.* **-pil·lae** (-pĭl′ē). **1.** A small nipplelike projection, such as a protuberance on the skin, at the root of a hair, or at the base of a developing tooth. **2.** One of the small, round or cone-shaped protuberances on the top of the tongue that contain taste buds. **3.** A pimple or pustule. — **pap′il·lar′y** (păp′ə-lĕr′ē, pə-pĭl′ə-rē) *adj.* — **pap′il·late′** (păp′ə-lāt′, pə-pĭl′ĭt) *adj.* — **pap·il·lose** (păp′ə-lōs′, pə-pĭl′ōs′) *adj.*

papilla mam·mae (măm′ē) *n.* See **nipple.**

papilla of corium *n.* See **dermal papilla.**

papillary stasis *n.* See **papilledema.**

papillary tumor *n.* See **papilloma.**

pap·il·lec·to·my (păp'ə-lĕk'tə-mē) *n.* Surgical removal of any papilla.

pap·il·le·de·ma (păp'ə-lĭ-dē'mə, pə-pĭl'ĭ-) *n.* Edema of the optic disk.

pap·il·li·tis (păp'ə-lī'tĭs) *n.* **1.** Inflammation of the optic disk. **2.** Inflammation of a renal papilla.

pap·il·lo·car·ci·no·ma (păp'ə-lō-kär'sə-nō'mə) *n.* **1.** A papilloma that has become malignant. **2.** A carcinoma that is characterized by papillary, finger-like projections of neoplastic cells found in association with cores of fibrous stroma as a supporting structure.

pap·il·lo·ma (păp'ə-lō'mə) *n., pl.* **-mas** or **-ma·ta** (-mə-tə). A benign epithelial tumor consisting of villous or arborescent outgrowths of fibrovascular stroma covered by neoplastic cells. — **pap'il·lo'ma·tous** (-təs) *adj.*

pap·il·lo·ma·to·sis (păp'ə-lō'mə-tō'sĭs) *n.* **1.** The development of numerous papillomas. **2.** Papillary projections of the epidermis forming a microscopically undulating surface.

papilloma virus *n.* A DNA virus of the genus *Papillomavirus.*

pap·il·lo·ret·i·ni·tis (păp'ə-lō-rĕt'n-ī'tĭs) *n.* Papillitis with extension of the inflammation to neighboring parts of the retina.

pap·il·lot·o·my (păp'ə-lŏt'ə-mē) *n.* Incision into the major duodenal papilla.

Pap·pen·hei·mer body (păp'ən-hī'mər) *n.* A phagosome containing ferruginous granules, found in red blood cells in sideroblastic anemia, hemolytic anemia, and sickle cell anemia.

Pap smear (păp) *n.* **1.** A smear of vaginal or cervical cells obtained for a Pap test. **2.** A Pap test.

PAP technique (păp) *n.* An enzymatic technique used to detect antigen or antibody in tissue that has been embedded in paraffin.

Pap test *n.* A test for cancer, especially of the female genital tract, in which a smear of cells exfoliated or scraped from a mucosal surface is stained with Papanicolaou stain and examined under a microscope for pathological changes.

pap·u·la·tion (păp'yə-lā'shən) *n.* The formation of papules.

pap·ule (păp'yōōl) *n., pl.* **-ules** or **-u·lae** (-yə-lē'). A small, solid, usually inflammatory elevation of the skin that does not contain pus. — **pap'u·lar** (-yə-lər) *adj.*

pap·u·lo·sis (păp'yə-lō'sĭs) *n.* The occurrence of numerous widespread papules.

par·a (păr'ə) *n.* A woman who has given birth to an infant or infants.

par·a·a·mi·no·ben·zo·ic acid (păr'ə-ə-mē'nō-bĕn-zō'ĭk, -ăm'ə-) *n.* PABA.

par·a·a·mi·no·sal·i·cyl·ic acid (păr'ə-ə-mē'nō-săl'ĭ-sĭl'ĭk) *n.* A bacteriostatic agent used against tubercle bacilli.

par·a·bal·lism (păr'ə-băl'ĭz'əm) *n.* Severe jerking movements of both legs.

par·a·bi·o·sis (păr'ə-bī-ō'sĭs) *n.* **1.** The fusion of whole eggs or embryos, as occurs in conjoined twins. **2.** Surgical joining of the vascular systems of two organisms. — **par'a·bi·ot'ic** (-ŏt'ĭk) *adj.*

par·a·blast (păr'ə-blăst') *n.* The nutritive yolk of a meroblastic egg.

par·a·blep·si·a (păr'ə-blĕp'sē-ə) *n.* Abnormality of the vision, as in visual illusions or hallucination.

par·a·bu·li·a (păr'ə-bōō'lē-ə, -byōō'-) *n.* Abnormality of volition or will, as when one impulse is checked and replaced by another.

par·a·ce·nes·the·sia (păr'ə-sē'nĭs-thē'zhə) *n.* A deterioration in one's sense of bodily well-being.

par·a·cen·te·sis (păr'ə-sĕn-tē'sĭs) *n.* Surgical puncture or tapping of a fluid-filled body cavity, especially the abdomen, with a hollow needle or trochar to withdraw fluid. — **par'a·cen·tet'ic** (-tĕt'ĭk) *adj.*

par·a·chol·er·a (păr'ə-kŏl'ər-ə) *n.* A disease clinically resembling Asiatic cholera, but due to an organism different from *Vibrio cholerae.*

par·a·chro·ma (păr'ə-krō'mə) *n.* Abnormal coloration of the skin.

par·a·chro·ma·top·si·a (păr'ə-krō'mə-tŏp'sē-ə) *n.* See **dichromatism** (sense 2).

par·a·chro·ma·to·sis (păr'ə-krō'mə-tō'sĭs) *n.* See **parachroma**.

parachute reflex *n.* See **startle reflex** (sense 1).

par·a·coc·cid·i·oi·do·my·co·sis (păr'ə-kŏk-sĭd'ē-oi'dō-mī-kō'sĭs) *n.* A chronic mycosis caused by *Paracoccidioides brasiliensis,* characterized by primary lesions of the lungs with dissemination to many internal organs, by conspicuous ulcerative granulomas of the mucous membranes of the cheeks and nose with extensions to the skin, and by generalized lymphangitis.

par·a·co·li·tis (păr'ə-kə-lī'tĭs) *n.* Inflammation of the peritoneal coat of the colon.

par·a·cu·sis (păr'ə-kōō'sĭs, -kyōō'-) or **par·a·cu·si·a** (-zē-ə, -zhə) *n.* **1.** Impaired hearing. **2.** An auditory illusion or hallucination.

par·a·cys·ti·tis (păr'ə-sĭ-stī'tĭs) *n.* Inflammation of the connective tissue and other structures surrounding the urinary bladder.

par·a·dip·si·a (păr'ə-dĭp'sē-ə) *n.* An abnormal craving for fluids without relation to bodily need.

par·a·dox (păr'ə-dŏks') *n.* That which is apparently, though not actually, inconsistent with or opposed to the known facts in any case. — **par'a·dox'i·cal** *adj.* — **par'a·dox'i·cal·ly** *adv.*

paradoxical contraction *n.* A contraction of the shin muscles that occurs as a response to sudden backward flexing of the foot, as during a physical examination.

paradoxical diaphragm phenomenon *n.* A phenomenon occurring in pyopneumothorax, hydropneumothorax, and some cases of injury in which the diaphragm on the affected side rises during inspiration and falls during expiration.

paradoxical pulse *n.* An exaggeration of the normal variation in the pulse during respiration, in which the pulse becomes weaker as one inhales and stronger as one exhales; it is characteristic of constrictive pericarditis or pericardial effusion.

paradoxical reflex *n.* A reflex in which the usual response is reversed or does not conform to the pattern characteristic of the particular reflex.

paradoxical respiration *n.* The deflation of the lung during inspiration and its inflation during expiration, usually seen in the lung on the side of an open pneumothorax.

paradoxical sleep *n.* See **REM sleep.**

par·af·fi·no·ma (păr′ə-fə-nō′mə) *n.* A tumefaction, usually a granuloma, caused by the prosthetic or therapeutic injection of paraffin.

par·a·fol·lic·u·lar cell (păr′ə-fə-lĭk′yə-lər) *n.* Any of the cells rich in mitochondria occurring in the thyroid epithelium, especially around the follicle.

par·a·gan·gli·o·ma (păr′ə-găng′glē-ō′mə) *n.* A tumor usually derived from the chromoceptor or chromaffin tissue of a paraganglion or the medulla of the adrenal gland.

par·a·gan·gli·on (păr′ə-găng′glē-ən) *n., pl.* **-gli·a** (-glē-ə). A small round body containing chromaffin cells, found near the aorta and in the kidney, liver, heart, and gonads.

par·a·geu·si·a (păr′ə-gyōō′zē-ə, -zhə, -jōō′-) *n.* A disordered or abnormal sense of taste.

par·a·gon·i·mi·a·sis (păr′ə-gŏn′ə-mī′ə-sĭs) *n.* Infestation with a worm of the genus *Paragonimus,* especially *P. westermani.*

Par·a·gon·i·mus (păr′ə-gŏn′ə-məs) *n.* A genus of lung flukes parasitic in humans and other mammals that feed upon crustaceans.

par·a·gram·ma·tism (păr′ə-grăm′ə-tĭz′əm) *n.* See **paraphasia.**

par·a·graph·i·a (păr′ə-grăf′ē-ə) *n.* **1.** The loss of the ability to write from dictation, although the words are understood. **2.** Writing one word when another is intended.

par·a·he·mo·phil·i·a (păr′ə-hē′mə-fĭl′ē-ə, -fēl′yə) *n.* A congenital deficiency of factor V characterized by abnormally slow blood coagulation.

par·a·in·flu·en·za virus (păr′ə-ĭn′flōō-ĕn′zə) *n.* Any of five types of viruses of the genus *Paramyxovirus* that are similar to the viruses that cause influenza and are associated with various respiratory infections, especially in children.

par·a·ker·a·to·sis (păr′ə-kĕr′ə-tō′sĭs) *n.* Retention of nuclei in the cells of the stratum corneum of the epidermis. It is observed in scaly dermatoses such as psoriasis and exfoliative dermatitis.

par·a·ki·ne·sia (păr′ə-kə-nē′zhə, -kī-) or **par·a·ki·ne·sis** (-sĭs) *n.* An abnormality of motor function.

par·a·la·li·a (păr′ə-lā′lē-ə) *n.* A speech defect, especially one in which one sound is habitually substituted for another.

par·al·de·hyde (pə-răl′də-hīd′) *n.* A potent hypnotic and sedative suitable for oral, rectal, intravenous, and intramuscular administration.

par·a·lex·i·a (păr′ə-lĕk′sē-ə) *n.* Misapprehension in the reading of written or printed words and substitution of other meaningless words for them.

par·al·ge·si·a (păr′ăl-jē′zē-ə, -zhə) *n.* A disorder or abnormality of the sense of pain.

par·al·lax (păr′ə-lăks′) *n.* The apparent displacement of an object caused by a change in the position from which it is viewed. — **par·al·lac·tic** (-lăk′tĭk) *adj.*

parallax test *n.* Measurement of the deviation in strabismus by the alternate cover test, combined with neutralization of the deviation using prisms.

pa·ral·y·sis (pə-răl′ĭ-sĭs) *n., pl.* **-ses** (-sēz′). **1.** Loss of power of voluntary movement in a muscle through injury or disease of its nerve supply. **2.** Loss of sensation over a region of the body.

paralysis ag·i·tans (ăj′ĭ-tănz′) *n.* See **Parkinson's disease.**

par·a·lyt·ic (păr′ə-lĭt′ĭk) *adj.* **1.** Of or relating to paralysis. **2.** Affected with paralysis. — *n.* A person affected with paralysis.

par·a·lyze (păr′ə-līz′) *v.* **-lyzed, -lyz·ing, -lyz·es.** To affect with paralysis; cause to be paralytic.

par·a·med·ic (păr′ə-mĕd′ĭk) *n.* A person who is trained to give emergency medical treatment or assist medical professionals.

par·a·med·i·cal (păr′ə-mĕd′ĭ-kəl) *adj.* **1.** Of, relating to, or being a person trained to give emergency medical treatment or assist medical professionals. **2.** Relating to the medical profession in an adjunctive capacity, especially to the allied health fields.

par·a·me·ni·a (păr′ə-mē′nē-ə) *n.* A disorder or irregularity of menstruation.

pa·ram·e·ter (pə-răm′ĭ-tər) *n.* **1.** One of a set of measurable factors, such as temperature and pressure, that define a system and determine its behavior. **2.** A psychoanalytic tactic, other than interpretation, used by the analyst to further the patient's progress. — **par′a·met′ric** (păr′ə-mĕt′-rĭk), **par′a·met′ri·cal** *adj.*

par·a·me·tri·um (păr′ə-mē′trē-əm) *n., pl.* **-tri·a** (-trē-ə). The connective tissue surrounding the uterus.

par·a·mim·i·a (păr′ə-mĭm′ē-ə) *n.* The use of inappropriate or incorrect gestures in speaking.

par·am·ne·sia (păr′ăm-nē′zhə) *n.* A distortion of memory in which fantasy and objective experience are confused.

par·am·y·loid (pă-răm′ə-loid′) *n.* A variety of amyloid deposit seen in the lymph nodes in some chronic nonspecific inflammations and in primary localized amyloidosis.

par·am·y·loi·do·sis (pə-răm′ə-loi-dō′sĭs) *n.* A condition resulting from the abnormal accumulation of paramyloids.

par·a·my·o·to·ni·a (păr′ə-mī′ə-tō′nē-ə) *n.* An atypical form of myotonia.

par·a·myx·o·vi·rus (păr′ə-mĭk′sə-vī′rəs) *n.* A member of the genus *Paramyxovirus.*

par·a·na·sal sinus (păr′ə-nā′zəl) *n.* Any of the paired cavities, designated frontal, sphenoidal, maxillary, and ethmoidal, located in the bones of the face and lined by a mucous membrane continuous with that of the nasal cavity.

par·a·ne·o·pla·sia (păr′ə-nē′ō-plā′zhə, -zhē-ə) *n.* Hormonal, neurological, hematological, and other clinical and biochemical disturbances associated with malignant neoplasms but not directly related to invasion by the primary tumor or its metastases. — **par·a·ne·o·plas·tic** (-plăs′tĭk) adj.

par·a·neph·ros (păr′ə-nĕf′rŏs′) n., pl. **-neph·roi** (-nĕf′roi′). See **adrenal gland**. — **par·a·neph·ric** (-nĕf′rĭk) adj.

par·a·noi·a (păr′ə-noi′ə) n. **1.** A psychotic disorder characterized by the presence of systematized delusions, especially of persecution or grandeur, in the absense of other personality disorders. **2.** Extreme, irrational distrust of others.

par·a·noid (păr′ə-noid′) adj. Relating to, characteristic of, or affected with paranoia. —n. One affected with paranoia.

paranoid personality n. A personality disorder characterized by unwarranted mistrust and suspicion, hypersensitivity to the words or actions of others, and rigidity of emotions or behavior.

paranoid schizophrenia n. Schizophrenia characterized predominantly by megalomania and delusions of persecution.

par·a·no·mi·a (păr′ə-nō′mē-ə) n. Aphasia in which objects are called by the wrong names.

par·a·pa·re·sis (păr′ə-pə-rē′sĭs, -păr′ĭ-sĭs) n. Partial paralysis of the lower extremities. — **par′a·pa·ret′ic** (-rĕt′ĭk) adj.

par·a·pha·sia (păr′ə-fā′zhə) or **par·a·phra·si·a** (-frā′zē-ə, -zhə) n. Aphasia in which the patient has lost the power of speaking correctly, substitutes one word for another, and jumbles words and sentences in such a way as to make speech unintelligible. — **par′a·pha′sic** (-fā′zĭk) adj.

pa·ra·phi·a (pə-rā′fē-ə) n. A disorder of the sense of touch.

par·a·phi·mo·sis (păr′ă-fī- mō′sĭs) n. **1.** Constriction of the glans penis by a phimotic foreskin, which has been retracted behind the corona. **2.** Retraction of the lid behind a protruding eyeball.

par·a·ple·gi·a (păr′ə-plē′jē-ə, -jə) n. Complete paralysis of the lower half of the body including both legs, usually caused by damage to the spinal cord. — **par′a·ple′gic** (-plē′jĭk) adj. & n.

par·a·prax·i·a (păr′ə-prăk′sē-ə) or **par·a·prax·is** (-prăk′sĭs) n. Defective performance of purposive acts, such as the mislaying of an object, thought to reveal a subconscious motive.

par·a·pro·tein (păr′ə-prō′tēn′, -tē-ĭn) n. An abnormal plasma protein, such as a macroglobulin, cryoglobulin, or myeloma protein.

par·a·pro·tein·e·mi·a (păr′ə-prō′tē-nē′mē-ə, -tē-ə-nē′-) n. The presence of abnormal proteins in the blood.

pa·rap·si·a (pə-răp′sē-ə) n. See **paraphia**.

par·a·pso·ri·a·sis (păr′ə-sə-rī′ə-sĭs) n. A chronic dermatosis of unknown origin, with erythematous, papular, and scaling lesions appearing in persistent and often enlarging plaques.

par·a·psy·chol·o·gy (păr′ə-sī-kŏl′ə-jē) n. The study of extrasensory perception, such as telepathy, psychokinesis, and clairvoyance. — **par′a·psy′cho·log′i·cal** (-sī′kə-lŏj′ĭ-kəl) adj. — **par′a·psy·chol′o·gist** or n.

par·a·re·flex·i·a (păr′ə-rĭ-flĕk′sē-ə) n. A condition characterized by abnormal reflexes.

par·a·ro·san·i·lin (păr′ə-rō-zăn′ə-lĭn) n. A red bi-

ological stain used to detect cellular DNA, mucopolysaccharides, and proteins.

par·ar·rhyth·mi·a (păr′ə-rĭth′mē-ə) n. A cardiac dysrhythmia in which two independent rhythms coexist, but not as a result of AV block.

par·a·site (păr′ə-sīt′) n. **1.** An organism that grows, feeds, and is sheltered on or in a different organism while contributing nothing to the survival of its host. **2.** In a fetal inclusion or conjoined twins, the usually incomplete twin that derives its support from the more nearly normal fetus.

par·a·si·te·mi·a (păr′ə-sī-tē′mē-ə) n. The presence of parasites in the blood.

par·a·sit·ic (păr′ə-sĭt′ĭk) or **par·a·sit·i·cal** (-ĭ-kəl) adj. **1.** Of, relating to, or characteristic of a parasite. **2.** Caused by a parasite.

par·a·sit·ism (păr′ə-sĭ-tĭz′əm, -sī-) n. A mode of existence relationship in which one species, the parasite, benefits at the expense of the other, the host.

par·a·si·tize (păr′ə-sī-tīz′, -sī-) v. **-ized, -iz·ing, -iz·es.** To live on or in a host as a parasite.

par·a·si·tol·o·gy (păr′ə-sī-tŏl′ə-jē, -sī-) n. The scientific study of parasites and parasitism. — **par′a·si′to·log′ic** (-sī′to-lŏj′ĭk), **par′a·si′to·log′i·cal** (-ĭ-kəl) adj. — **par′a·si·tol′o·gist** n.

par·a·si·to·sis (păr′ə-sī-tō′sĭs, -sī-) n., pl. **-ses** (-sēz). Infestation with parasites.

par·a·som·ni·a (păr′ə-sŏm′nē-ə) n. Any of various sleep dysfunctions, such as somnambulism, night terrors, enuresis, or nocturnal seizures.

par·a·sta·sis (păr′ə-stā′sĭs, pə-răs′tə-sĭs) n. **1.** The relationship among causal mechanisms that can compensate for, or mask defects in, each other. **2.** In genetics, a relationship between non-alleles thought to be a form of epistasis.

par·a·sym·pa·thet·ic ganglion (păr′ə-sĭm′pə-thĕt′ĭk) n. Any of the ganglia of the autonomic nervous system composed of cholinergic neurons receiving afferent fibers originating from preganglionic visceral motor neurons in either the brainstem or the middle sacral segments of the spinal cord.

parasympathetic nerve n. One of the nerves of the parasympathetic nervous system.

parasympathetic nervous system n. The part of the autonomic nervous system originating in the brain stem and the lower part of the spinal cord that, in general, inhibits or opposes the physiological effects of the sympathetic nervous system, as in tending to stimulate digestive secretions, slow the heart, constrict the pupils, and dilate blood vessels.

par·a·sy·nap·sis (păr′ə-sĭ-năp′sĭs) n. Side-to-side union of homologous chromosomes in the process of reduction.

par·a·sy·no·vi·tis (păr′ə-sī′nə-vī′tĭs) n. Inflammation of the tissues immediately adjacent to a joint.

par·a·sys·to·le (păr′ə-sĭs′tə-lē) n. An arrhythmia characterized by a second automatic rhythm existing simultaneously with normal sinus rhythm.

par·a·tax·ic distortion (păr′ə-tăk′sĭk) n. An attitude toward another person based on a distorted evaluation, usually because of an identification of that person with emotionally significant individuals from the past.

par·a·ten·on (păr′ə-tĕn′ən, -ŏn′) *n.* The fatty or synovial material between a tendon and its sheath.

par·a·thi·on (păr′ə-thī′ŏn) *n.* A highly poisonous organic phosphate insecticide that is an irreversible inhibitor of cholinesterase.

par·a·thy·roid (păr′ə-thī′roid) *adj.* Of, relating to, or obtained from the parathyroid glands. — *n.* 1. Any of the parathyroid glands. 2. A parathyroid hormone.

par·a·thy·roid·ec·to·my (păr′ə-thī′roi-dĕk′tə-mē) *n.* Excision of the parathyroid glands.

parathyroid gland *n.* Any of usually four small kidney-shaped glands that lie in pairs near or within the posterior surface of the thyroid gland and secrete a hormone necessary for the metabolism of calcium and phosphorus.

parathyroid hormone *n.* A peptide hormone produced by the parathyroid glands that regulates the amount of calcium in the body.

parathyroid tetany *n.* Tetany following surgical injury to or excision of the parathyroid glands.

par·a·ty·phoid fever (păr′ə-tī′foid′) *n.* An acute intestinal disease, similar to typhoid fever but less severe, caused by food contaminated with bacteria of the genus *Salmonella.*

par·a·u·re·thral gland (păr′ə-yŏŏ-rē′thrəl) *n.* Any of several small mucus glands that deliver secretions into the female urethra near its opening and are homologous to the glandular tissue in the prostate gland of the male.

par·a·vag·i·ni·tis (păr′ə-văj′ə-nī′tĭs) *n.* Inflammation of the connective tissue alongside the vagina.

par·ax·on (pă-răk′sŏn′) *n.* A collateral branch of an axon.

par·e·gor·ic (păr′ə-gôr′ĭk, -gŏr′-) *n.* A camphorated tincture of opium, taken internally for the relief of diarrhea and intestinal pain.

pa·ren·chy·ma (pə-rĕng′kə-mə) *n.* The distinguishing or specific cells of a gland or organ, contained in and supported by the connective tissue framework or stroma. — **pa·ren′chy·mal, par′-en·chym′a·tous** (păr′ĕn-kĭm′ə-təs) *adj.* — **par′-en·chym′a·tous·ly** *adv.*

pa·ren·chy·ma·ti·tis (pə-rĕng′kə-mə-tī′tĭs) *n.* Inflammation of the parenchyma of a gland or organ.

par·ent (pâr′ənt, păr′-) *n.* 1. One who begets, gives birth to, or nurtures and raises a child; a father or a mother. 2. An ancestor; a progenitor. — *v.* **-ent·ed, -ent·ing, -ents. 1.** To act as a parent to; raise and nurture. **2.** To cause to come into existence; originate.

pa·ren·tal (pə-rĕn′tl) *adj.* Of, relating to, or characteristic of a parent.

parental generation *n.* The generation of individuals of different genotypes that are mated to produce hybrids.

par·en·ter·al (pă-rĕn′tər-əl) *adj.* 1. Located outside the alimentary canal. 2. Taken into the body or administered in a manner other than through the digestive tract, as by intravenous or intramuscular injection. — **par·en′ter·al·ly** *adv.*

par·en·ter·ic fever (păr′ən-tĕr′ĭk) *n.* Any of a group of fevers clinically resembling typhoid and paratyphoid fevers but caused by different bacteria.

pa·re·sis (pə-rē′sĭs, păr′ĭ-sĭs) *n.* **-ses** (-sēz). **1.** Slight or partial paralysis. **2.** General paresis. — **pa·ret′ic** (pə-rĕt′ĭk) *adj. & n.*

par·es·the·sia or **par·aes·the·sia** (păr′ĭs-thē′zhə) *n.* A skin sensation, such as burning, prickling, itching, or tingling, with no apparent physical cause. — **par′es·thet′ic** (-thĕt′ĭk) *adj.*

pa·reu·ni·a (pə-rōō′nē-ə, păr-yōō′-) *n.* Sexual intercourse.

pa·ri·es (pâr′ē-ēz′) *n., pl.* **pa·ri·e·tes** (pə-rī′ĭ-tēz′). A wall of a body part, organ, or cavity, as of the chest or abdomen. Often used in the plural.

pa·ri·e·tal (pə-rī′ĭ-təl) *adj.* **1.** Relating to or forming the wall of any cavity. **2.** Of or relating to either of the parietal bones.

parietal bone *n.* Either of two large, irregularly quadrilateral bones between the frontal and occipital bones that together form the sides and top of the skull.

parietal cell *n.* A cell of the gastric glands that secretes hydrochloric acid.

parietal lobe *n.* The middle portion of each cerebral hemisphere, located beneath each parietal bone.

pa·ri·e·tog·ra·phy (pə-rī′ĭ-tŏg′rə-fē) *n.* Radiographic imaging of the walls of an organ.

par·i·ty (păr′ĭ-tē) *n.* The state of having given birth to an infant or infants.

par·kin·so·ni·an (pär′kĭn-sō′nē-ən) *adj.* Relating to Parkinsonism.

Par·kin·son·ism or **par·kin·son·ism** (pär′kĭn-sə-nĭz′əm) *n.* **1.** Any of a group of nervous disorders similar to Parkinson's disease, marked by muscular rigidity, tremor, and impaired motor control and often having a specific cause, such as the use of certain drugs or frequent exposure to toxic chemicals. **2.** Parkinson's disease.

Par·kin·son's disease (pär′kĭn-sənz) *n.* A progressive nervous disease occurring most often after the age of 50, associated with the destruction of brain cells that produce dopamine and characterized by muscular tremor, slowing of movement, partial facial paralysis, peculiarity of gait and posture, and weakness.

par·om·phal·o·cele (păr′ŏm-făl′ə-sēl′, ŏm′fə-lō-) *n.* **1.** A tumor near the navel. **2.** A hernia through a defect in the abdominal wall near the navel.

par·o·nych·i·a (păr′ə-nĭk′ē-ə) *n.* Inflammation of the tissue surrounding a nail. — **par′o·nych′i·al** *adj.*

par·oph·thal·mi·a (păr′ŏf-thăl′mē-ə, -ŏp-) *n.* Inflammation of the tissues surrounding the eye.

par·o·rex·i·a (păr′ə-rĕk′sē-ə) *n.* Abnormal or inappropriate appetite, especially a craving for items unsuitable as food; pica.

pa·ros·mi·a (pə-rŏz′mē-ə) *n.* A distortion of the sense of smell, as in smelling odors that are not present.

par·os·te·o·sis (pă-rŏs′tē-ō′sĭs) or **par·os·to·sis** (păr′ŏs-tō′sĭs) *n.* **1.** Development of bone in an unusual location, as in the skin. **2.** Abnormal or defective ossification.

pa·rot·id (pə-rŏt′ĭd) *adj.* **1.** Situated near the ear. **2.** Of or relating to a parotid gland. — *n.* A parotid gland.

pa·rot·i·dec·to·my (pə-rŏt′ĭ-dĕk′tə-mē) *n.* Surgical removal of a parotid gland.

parotid gland *n.* Either of a pair of major salivary glands situated below and in front of each ear and opening into the parotid duct; the largest of the major salivary glands.

par·o·ti·tis (păr′ə-tī′tĭs) or **par·rot·i·di·tis** (pə-rŏt′-ĭ-dī′tĭs) *n.* Inflammation of the parotid glands, as in mumps. — **par′o·tit′ic** (-tĭt′ĭk) *adj.*

par·ous (păr′əs, pâr′-) *adj.* Having given birth one or more times.

par·ox·ysm (păr′ək-sĭz′əm) *n.* **1.** A sharp spasm or fit; a convulsion. **2.** A sudden onset of a symptom or disease, especially one with recurrent manifestations, such as the chills and fever of malaria. — **par′ox·ys′mal** (-ək-sĭz′məl) *adj.*

paroxysmal tachycardia *n.* A condition characterized by recurrent attacks of tachycardia, having abrupt onset and termination and originating from an ectopic focus.

paroxysmal trepidant abasia *n.* Abasia due to spastic stiffening of the legs.

par·rot fever (păr′ət) *n.* See **psittacosis**.

Par·rot's disease (pă-rŏz′, pă-) *n.* Pseudoparalysis of one or more of the extremities occurring in infants in whom congenital exposure to syphilis has caused inflammation of an epiphysis.

part (pärt) *n.* **1.** A portion, division, piece, or segment of a whole. **2.** An organ, a member, or another division of an organism. **3.** An anatomical part; pars. **4. parts.** The external genitalia.

part. *aeq. abbr. Latin.* partes aequales, partibus aequalibus (equal parts or amounts, in equal parts or amounts)

partial antigen *n.* See **hapten**.

partial denture *n.* A removable or fixed dental prosthesis that restores one or more, but less than all, of the natural teeth or associated parts and is supported by the teeth or the soft tissue.

partial-thickness flap *n.* See **split-thickness flap**.

partial-thickness graft *n.* See **split-thickness graft**.

par·ti·tion (pär-tĭsh′ən) *n.* **1.** The act or process of dividing something into parts. **2.** A wall, septum, or other separating membrane in an organism.

par·ti·tion chromatography (pär-tĭsh′ən) *n.* Separation of similar substances by repeated extraction by two immiscible liquids, so that the substances cross the partition between the liquids in opposite directions.

par·tu·ri·ent (pär-tŏŏr′ē-ənt, -tyŏŏr′-) *adj.* **1.** Of or relating to giving birth. **2.** About to bring forth young; being in labor.

parturient canal *n.* See **birth canal**.

par·tu·ri·fa·cient (pär-tŏŏr′ə-fā′shənt, -tyŏŏr′-) *n.* Inducing or accelerating childbirth; oxytocic. — *n.* A drug facilitating childbirth.

par·tu·ri·tion (pär′tyŏŏ-rĭsh′ən, -tŏŏ-, pär′chə-) *n.* The process of labor and delivery in the birth of a child; childbirth.

part. vic. *abbr. Latin.* partitis vicibus (in divided parts, amounts, or doses)

par·vo·vi·rus (pär′vō-vī′rəs) *n.* Any of a group of small viruses of the genus *Parvovirus* that cause disease in many vertebrates, especially mammals such as dogs and cattle.

pass (păs) *v.* **passed, pass·ing, pass·es. 1.** To go across; go through. **2.** To cause to move into a certain position. **3.** To cease to exist; die. **4.** To be voided from the body.

passage *n.* **1.** A movement from one place to another. **2.** The process of passing from one condition or stage to another; transition. **3.** A path, channel, or duct through, over, or along which something may pass. **4.** An act of emptying, as of the bowels. **5.** The process of passing or maintaining a group of microorganisms or cells through a series of hosts or cultures.

pas·sive (păs′ĭv) *n.* **1.** Accepting or submitting without resistance or objection. **2.** Of or being an inactive or submissive role in a relationship, especially a sexual relationship. — **pas′sive·ly** *adv.* — **pas′sive·ness** *n.*

passive-aggressive personality *n.* A personality disorder in which aggressive feelings are manifested in passive ways, especially through stubbornness, procrastination, and inefficiency so as to resist adequate social and occupational performance.

passive anaphylaxis *n.* An anaphylactic response in a nonsensitized person caused by inoculation with serum from a sensitized person.

passive clot *n.* A clot formed in an aneurysmal sac following the cessation of circulation through the aneurysm.

passive hemagglutination *n.* Passive agglutination in which red blood cells are used to adsorb soluble antigen onto their surface; the red blood cells then agglutinate in the presence of antiserum specific for the adsorbed antigen.

passive immunity *n.* Immunity acquired by the transfer of antibodies from another person, as through injection or placental transfer to a fetus.

passive movement *n.* Movement of a joint effected by another person, or by mechanical means, without participation or effort on the part of the subject.

passive transfer *n.* The transfer of skin-sensitizing antibodies from the blood of an allergic person to that of a nonallergic person in order to test the sensitized area for an allergic reaction to specific allergens.

passive tremor *n.* An involuntary tremor occurring when a person is at rest, and diminishing or ceasing during voluntary movement.

Pas·teu·rel·la (păs'chə-rĕl'ə, păs'tə-) *n.* A genus of aerobic to facultatively anaerobic, nonmotile bacteria of the family Vibrionaceae containing small gram-negative rods; they are parasites of humans and other animals.

Pasteurella pes·tis (pĕs'tĭs) *n.* See **Yersinia pestis**.

pas·teu·rel·lo·sis (păs'chər-ə-lō'sĭs, păs'tər-) *n.* Infection with bacteria of the genus *Pasteurella*.

pas·teur·i·za·tion (păs'chər-ĭ-zā'shən, păs'tər-) *n.* **1.** The process of heating a beverage, such as milk or beer, to a specific temperature for a specific period of time in order to kill microorganisms that could cause disease, spoilage, or undesired fermentation. **2.** The process of destroying most microorganisms in certain foods, such as fish or clam meat, by irradiating them with gamma rays or other radiation to prevent spoilage.

pas·teur·ize (păs'chə-rīz', păs'tə-) *v.* **-ized, -iz·ing, -iz·es.** To subject a beverage or other food to pasteurization.

Pas·teur treatment (păs-tûr', pă-stœr') *n.* A treatment for infection by the rabies virus in which a series of increasingly strong inoculations with attenuated virus is given to stimulate antibody production during the incubation period of the disease.

pas·tille (pă-stēl') or **pas·til** *n.* A small medicated or flavored tablet; a troche.

patch (păch) *n.* **1.** A small circumscribed area differing from the surrounding surface. **2.** A dressing or covering applied to protect a wound or sore. **3.** A transdermal patch.

patch test *n.* A test for allergic sensitivity in which a suspected allergen is placed on a small surgical pad applied to the skin for a period of time to determine if an allergic response is present.

pa·tel·la (pə-tĕl'ə) *n., pl.* **-tel·lae** (-tĕl'ē). **1.** A flat triangular bone located in the combined tendon of the extensors of the leg and covering the front surface of the knee joint. **2.** A pan-shaped anatomical formation. — **pa·tel'lar, pa·tel'late** (-tĕl'ĭt, -āt') *adj.*

patellar reflex *n.* A reflex contraction of the quadriceps muscle resulting in a sudden involuntary extension of the leg, produced by a sharp tap to the tendon below the patella.

pat·el·lec·to·my (păt'l-ĕk'tə-mē) *n.* Surgical excision of the patella.

pa·ten·cy (păt'n-sē) *n.* The state or quality of being open, expanded, or unblocked.

pat·ent (păt'nt) *adj.* **1.** Of, relating to, or being a nonprescription drug or other medical preparation that is often protected by a trademark. **2.** (păt'nt). Not blocked; open. **3.** (păt'nt). Spreading open; expanded.

patent ductus ar·te·ri·o·sus (är-tĕr'ē-ō'səs) *n.* A cardiovascular defect that is caused by failure of the arterial canal to close after birth and can be corrected by surgery.

pat·ent medicine (păt'nt) *n.* A nonprescription

drug or other medical preparation that is often protected by a trademark.

pa·ter·nal (pə-tûr'nəl) *adj.* **1.** Relating to or characteristic of a father or fatherhood; fatherly. **2.** Received or inherited from a father. **3.** Related through one's father.

pa·ter·ni·ty (pə-tûr'nĭ-tē) *n.* **1.** The state of being a father; fatherhood. **2.** Descent on a father's side; paternal descent.

paternity test *n.* A test using blood group identification of a mother, child, and putative father to establish the probability of paternity.

path·er·gy (păth'ər-jē) *n.* An abnormal reaction to an allergen; it may be either subnormal or abnormally severe.

path·find·er (păth'fīn'dər) *n.* A filiform bougie for introduction through a narrow stricture as a guide for the passage of a larger instrument.

path·o·clis·is (păth'ə-klĭs'ĭs) *n.* **1.** A specific tendency toward sensitivity to a particular toxin or toxins. **2.** A tendency for toxins to attack certain organs.

path·o·gen (păth'ə-jən) *n.* An agent that causes disease, especially a living microorganism such as a bacterium, virus, or fungus.

path·o·gen·e·sis (păth'ə-jĕn'ĭ-sĭs) or **pa·thog·e·ny** (pă-thŏj'ə-nē) *n.* The development of a disease or morbid condition.

path·o·gen·ic (păth'ə-jĕn'ĭk) or **path·o·ge·net·ic** (-jə-nĕt'ĭk) *adj.* **1.** Capable of causing disease. **2.** Originating or producing disease. **3.** Of or relating to pathogenesis. — **path'o·ge·nic'i·ty** (-jə-nĭs'ĭ-tē) *n.*

path·o·log·i·cal (păth'ə-lŏj'ĭ-kəl) or **path·o·log·ic** (-ĭk) *adj.* **1.** Of or relating to pathology. **2.** Relating to or caused by disease. — **path'o·log'i·cal·ly** *adv.*

pathologic calcification *n.* **1.** The presence of calculi in excretory or secretory passages. **2.** The calcification of tissues other than bone and teeth.

pathologic fracture *n.* A bone fracture occurring at a site weakened by disease, especially by a neoplasm or bone necrosis.

pathologic retraction ring *n.* A constriction located at the junction between the thinned lower uterine segment and the thick retracted upper uterine segment that is caused by obstructed labor; a sign of impending rupture of the uterus.

pa·thol·o·gist (pă-thŏl'ə-jĭst) *n.* A specialist in pathology who practices chiefly in the laboratory as a consultant to clinical colleagues.

pa·thol·o·gy (pă-thŏl'ə-jē) *n.* **1.** The medical science concerned with all aspects of disease with an emphasis on the essential nature, causes, and development of abnormal conditions, as well as with the structural and functional changes that result from disease processes. **2.** The anatomical or functional manifestations of a disease.

path·o·mi·me·sis (păth'ō-mĭ-mē'sĭs, -mī-) *n.* Mimicry of the symptoms or effects of a disease, whether intentional or unconscious.

path·o·phys·i·ol·o·gy (păth'ō-fĭz'ē-ŏl'ə-jē) *n.* **1.**

The functional changes associated with or resulting from disease or injury. **2.** The scientific study of such changes. — **path′o·phys′i·o·log′ic** (-ə-lŏj′ĭk), **path′o·phys′i·o·log′i·cal** (-ĭ-kəl) *adj.* — **path′o·phys′i·ol′o·gist** *n.*

pa·tho·sis (pă-thō′sĭs) *n., pl.* **-ses** (-sēz′). **1.** A state of disease. **2.** A diseased condition. **3.** A disease entity.

path·way (păth′wā′) *n.* **1.** A course usually followed by a body part or process. **2.** A chain of nerve fibers along which impulses normally travel. **3.** A sequence of enzymatic or other reactions by which one biological material is converted to another.

pa·tient (pā′shənt) *n.* One who receives medical attention, care, or treatment.

Pat·rick′s test (păt′rĭks) *n.* A test to determine the presence or absence of sacroiliac disease.

pat·tern·ing (păt′ər-nĭng) *n.* A method of physical therapy in which a rigid pattern of exercises is imposed to stimulate weak or paralyzed nerves and muscles to act on their own.

pat·u·lin (păch′ə-lĭn) *n.* A toxic antibiotic that is derived from the metabolites of certain fungi, such as *Aspergillus, Penicillium,* and *Gymnoascus,* and has carcinogenic activity.

paunch (pônch, pänch) *n.* The belly, especially a protruding one; a potbelly.

Pau·tri·er′s abscess (pō-trē-āz′) *n.* See **Pautrier′s microabscess.**

Pautrier′s microabscess *n.* A microscopic lesion in the epidermis, seen in mycosis fungoides.

pa·vor noc·tur·nus (pā′vər nŏk-tûr′nəs, pā′vôr′) *n.* Night terrors.

Payne operation (pān) *n.* A jejunoileal bypass for treating morbid obesity in which an anastomosis is created between the upper jejunum and the terminal ileum, with closure of the proximal end of the bypassed intestine.

Payr′s sign (pīrz) *n.* An indication of thrombophlebitis in which pain results when the sole of the foot receives pressure.

p.c. *abbr. Latin.* post cibum (after meals)

PCB (pē′sē-bē′) *n.* Polychlorinated biphenyl; any of a family of industrial compounds produced by chlorination of biphenyl, noted primarily as an environmental pollutant that accumulates in animal tissue with resultant pathogenic and teratogenic effects.

PCP *abbr.* phencyclidine; primary care physician

peak flow meter *n.* A portable instrument that detects minute decreases in air flow, used by people with asthma to monitor small changes in breathing capacity.

pearl·y tubercle (pûr′lē) *n.* See **milium.**

pec (pĕk) *n.* A pectoral muscle. Often used in the plural.

pec·te·ni·tis (pĕk′tə-nī′tĭs) *n.* Inflammation of the sphincter muscle of the anus.

pec·tin (pĕk′tĭn) *n.* Any of a group of water-soluble colloidal carbohydrates of high molecular weight found in ripe fruits, such as apples, plums, and grapefruit, and used to jell various foods, drugs, and cosmetics.

pec·tin·e·al muscle (pĕk-tĭn′ē-əl) *n.* A muscle with origin from the crest of the pubis, with insertion to the femur, and whose action adducts the thigh and assists in flexion.

pec·to·ral (pĕk′tər-əl) *adj.* **1.** Relating to or situated in the breast or chest. **2.** Useful in relieving disorders of the chest or respiratory tract.

pectoral girdle *n.* A bony or cartilaginous structure in humans, attached to and supporting the arms.

pec·tus (pĕk′təs) *n., pl.* **pec·to·ra** (pĕk′tə-rə). The chest, especially the anterior wall; breast; thorax.

pectus car·i·na·tum (kăr′ə-nā′təm) *n.* See **pigeon breast.**

pectus ex·ca·va·tum (ĕk′skə-vā′təm) *n.* See **funnel chest.**

pectus re·cur·va·tum (rē′kûr-vā′təm) *n.* See **funnel chest.**

pe·di·at·ric (pē′dē-ăt′rĭk) *adj.* Of or relating to pediatrics.

pe·di·a·tri·cian (pē′dē-ə-trĭsh′ən) or **pe·di·at·rist** (-ăt′rĭst) *n.* A physician who specializes in pediatrics.

pe·di·at·rics (pē′dē-ăt′rĭks) *n.* The branch of medicine that deals with the development and care of infants and children and the diagnosis and treatment of their diseases.

ped·i·cel (pĕd′ĭ-səl, -sĕl′) *n.* **1.** A small stalk, part, or organ, especially one serving as a support. **2.** The secondary process of a podocyte that helps form the visceral capsule of a renal corpuscle. — **ped′i·cel′lar** (-sĕl′ər) *adj.*

ped·i·cel·la·tion (pĕd′ĭ-sə-lā′shən) *n.* Formation of a pedicel, pedicle, or peduncle.

ped·i·cle (pĕd′ĭ-kəl) *n.* **1.** A slender footlike or stemlike stalk by which the base of a nonsessile tumor is attached to normal tissue. **2.** A stalk through which a skin flap receives its blood supply until the skin flap is transferred to its intended site of attachment.

pedicle flap *n.* A surgical flap sustained by a blood-carrying stem from the donor site during transfer.

pe·dic·u·la·tion (pə-dĭk′yə-lā′shən) *n.* Infestation with lice.

pe·dic·u·li·cide (pə-dĭk′yə-lĭ-sīd′) *n.* An agent used to destroy lice.

pe·dic·u·lo·sis (pə-dĭk′yə-lō′sĭs) *n.* The state of being infested with lice.

pe·dic·u·lus (pə-dĭk′yə-ləs) *n., pl.* **-li** (-lī′). A pedicle.

Pe·dic·u·lus (pə-dĭk′yə-ləs) *n.* A genus of parasitic lice of the family Pediculidae that live in the hair and feed periodically on the blood of animal hosts, including species that infest the human head and body.

ped·i·gree (pĕd′ĭ-grē′) *n.* An ancestral line of descent, especially as diagrammed on a chart, to show ancestral history and to analyze Mendelian inheritance of certain traits including familial diseases.

ped·o·phil·i·a (pĕd′ə-fĭl′ē-ə, pē′də-) *n.* The act or

fantasy on the part of an adult of engaging in sexual activity with a child or children. — **ped′o·phile′** (-fīl′) *n.* — **ped′o·phil′i·ac′** (-fīl′ē-ăk′) *adj. & n.* — **ped′o·phil′ic** *adj.*

pe·dun·cle (pĭ-dŭng′kəl, pē′dŭng′kəl) *n.* **1.** See **pedicle** (sense 1). **2.** See **pedunculus** (sense 2). — **pe·dun′cu·lar** (pĭ-dŭng′kyə-lər) *adj.*

pe·dun·cu·lot·o·my (pĭ-dŭng′kyə-lŏt′ə-mē) *n.* Total or partial surgical section of the cerebral peduncle.

pe·dun·cu·lus (pĭ-dŭng′kyə-ləs) *n., pl.* **-li** (-lī′). **1.** An anatomical stalk or stem, such as the stalklike base to which a tumor is attached to normal tissue. **2.** Any of several stalklike connecting structures in the brain, composed either of white matter or of white and gray matter.

peg-and-socket joint *n.* See **gomphosis.**

Pel–Ebstein disease (pĕl′-) *n.* Hodgkin's disease that includes periodic fevers.

Pel–Ebstein fever *n.* The remittent fever common in Hodgkin's disease.

pel·lag·ra (pə-lăg′rə, -lā′-, -lä′grə) *n.* A disease caused by a deficiency of niacin and protein in the diet and characterized by skin eruptions, digestive and nervous system disturbances, and eventual mental deterioration. — **pel·lag′rous** *adj.*

pel·lag·rin (pə-lăg′rĭn, -lā′-, -lä′grĭn) *n.* A person affected with pellagra.

pel·let (pĕl′ĭt) *n.* **1.** A small pill. **2.** A small rod-shaped or ovoid mass, as of compressed steroid hormones, intended for subcutaneous implantation in body tissues to provide timed release over an extended period of time.

pel·lu·cid (pə-lōō′sĭd) *adj.* Admitting the passage of light; transparent or translucent. — **pel·lu·cid′i·ty, pel·lu′cid·ness** *n.*

pel·vic (pĕl′vĭk) *adj.* Of, relating to, or near the pelvis.

pelvic arch *n.* See **pelvic girdle.**

pelvic cavity *n.* The space bounded by the bones of the pelvis and pelvic girdle.

pelvic girdle *n.* A bony or cartilaginous structure in humans, attached to and supporting the legs.

pelvic inflammatory disease *n.* Inflammation of the female genital tract, especially of the fallopian tubes, caused by any of several microorganisms, chiefly chlamydia and gonococci, and characterized by severe abdominal pain, high fever, vaginal discharge, and in some cases destruction of tissue that can result in sterility.

pelvic limb *n.* See **lower extremity.**

pelvic pole *n.* The breech end of the fetus.

pelvic version *n.* Version in which a transverse presentation or an oblique presentation is converted into a pelvic presentation by manipulating the buttocks of the fetus.

pel·vi·fix·a·tion (pĕl′və-fĭk-sā′shən) *n.* Surgical attachment of a floating pelvic organ to the wall of the cavity.

pel·vi·li·thot·o·my (pĕl′və-lĭ-thŏt′ə-mē) *n.* Surgical removal of a calculus from the kidney through an incision in the renal pelvis.

pel·vim·e·ter (pĕl-vĭm′ĭ-tər) *n.* An instrument shaped like calipers for measuring the dimensions of the pelvis.

pel·vim·e·try (pĕl-vĭm′ĭ-trē) *n.* Measurement of the dimensions and capacity of the pelvis, especially of the adult female pelvis.

pel·vi·o·plas·ty (pĕl′vē-ə-plăs′tē) *n.* Symphysiotomy or pubiotomy for enlargement of the pelvic outlet.

pel·vi·ot·o·my (pĕl′vē-ŏt′ə-mē) or **pel·vit·o·my** (pĕl-vĭt′ə-mē) *n.* **1.** See **symphysiotomy. 2.** See **pubiotomy. 3.** See **pyelotomy.**

pel·vis (pĕl′vĭs) *n., pl.* **-vis·es** or **-ves** (-vēz). **1.** A basin-shaped structure of the human skeleton, composed of the innominate bones on the sides, the pubis in front, and the sacrum and coccyx behind, that rests on the lower limbs and supports the spinal column. **2.** The cavity formed by this structure. **3.** A basinlike or cup-shaped anatomical cavity.

pem·phi·gus (pĕm′fĭ-gəs, pĕm-fī′gəs) *n.* Any of several acute or chronic skin diseases characterized by scaling patches or groups of itching blisters. — **pem′phi·gous** *adj.*

pen·e·trat·ing wound (pĕn′ĭ-trā′tĭng) *n.* A wound accompanied by disruption of the body surface that extends into the underlying tissue or into a body cavity.

pen·i·cil·lin (pĕn′ĭ-sĭl′ĭn) *n.* Any of a group of broad-spectrum antibiotic drugs obtained from penicillium molds or produced synthetically, most active against gram-positive bacteria and used in the treatment of various infections and diseases.

pen·i·cil·li·nase (pĕn′ĭ-sĭl′ĭ-nās′) *n.* Any of various enzymes, produced by certain bacteria, that hydrolyze and inactivate penicillin and are used in medicine to treat allergic reactions to penicillin.

pen·i·cil·li·um (pĕn′ĭ-sĭl′ē-əm) *n., pl.* **-cil·li·ums** or **-cil·li·a** (-sĭl′ē-ə). Any of various characteristically bluish-green fungi of the genus *Penicillium* that grow as molds on decaying fruits and ripening cheese and are used to produce penicillin.

pe·nile (pē′nīl′, -nəl) *adj.* Of or relating to the penis.

pe·nis (pē′nĭs) *n., pl.* **-nis·es** or **-nes** (-nēz). The male organ of copulation and of urinary excretion, formed by three columns of erectile tissue; the extremity is formed by an expansion of the urethral surface of the penis, covered by a free fold of skin.

pen·ta·me·tho·ni·um bromide (pĕn′tə-mĕ-thō′nē-əm) *n.* A ganglionic blocking agent used as an antihypertensive.

pen·ta·pi·per·i·um meth·yl·sul·fate (pĕn′tə-pī-pĕr′ē-əm mĕth′əl-sŭl′fāt′) *n.* An anticholinergic agent used in the treatment of peptic ulcer.

pen·ta·quine (pĕn′tə-kwēn′, -kwĭn) or **pen·ta·quin** (-kwĭn) *n.* A synthetic drug used with quinine in the prevention or treatment of malaria.

pen·taz·o·cine (pĕn-tăz′ə-sēn′) *n.* A synthetic narcotic drug used as a nonaddictive analgesic, often in place of morphine.

pen·tet·ic acid (pĕn-tĕt′ĭk) *n.* Diethylenetriamine

pentaacetic acid; a chelating agent, especially for iron but also showing an affinity for heavy metals that is used in the treatment of iron-storage disease and poisoning from heavy and radioactive metals.

pen·to·bar·bi·tal sodium (pĕn′tə-bär′bĭ-tôl′, -tăl′) *n.* A white crystalline or powdery barbiturate used as a hypnotic, a sedative, and an anticonvulsive drug.

pen·tose (pĕn′tōs′, -tōz′) *n.* Any of a class of monosaccharides having five carbon atoms per molecule and including ribose and several other sugars.

pen·to·su·ri·a (pĕn′tō-sŏor′ē-ə, -syŏor′-) *n.* The excretion of one or more pentoses in the urine.

pen·tox·if·yl·line (pĕn′tŏk-sĭf′ə-lēn′, -lĭn, pĕn-tŏk′sə-fĭl′ēn′, -ĭn) *n.* A bitter-tasting, colorless compound that decreases blood viscosity and improves blood flow, used in the treatment of intermittent claudication.

pe·o·til·lo·ma·ni·a (pē′ō-tĭl′ə-mā′nē-ə) *n.* A nervous tic consisting of a constant pulling of the penis.

pep·sin or **pep·sine** (pĕp′sĭn) *n.* **1.** Any of various digestive enzymes found in gastric juice that catalyze the hydrolysis of proteins to peptides. **2.** A substance containing pepsin, obtained from the stomachs of hogs and calves and used as a digestive aid.

pepsin A *n.* The principal digestive enzyme of gastric juice that is formed from pepsinogen and catalyzes the hydrolysis of peptide bonds to form proteases and peptones.

pep·sin·o·gen (pĕp-sĭn′ə-jən) *n.* The inactive precursor to pepsin, formed in the chief cells of the mucous membrane of the stomach and converted to pepsin by hydrochloric acid during digestion.

pep·tic (pĕp′tĭk) *adj.* **1.** Relating to or assisting digestion. **2.** Associated with the action of digestive secretions. **3.** Of or involving pepsin. **4.** Capable of digesting. — *n.* A digestive agent.

peptic cell *n.* See **zymogenic cell.**

peptic digestion *n.* See **gastric digestion.**

peptic esophagitis *n.* See **reflux esophagitis.**

peptic ulcer *n.* An ulcer of the upper digestive tract, usually in the stomach or duodenum, where the mucous membrane is exposed to acidic gastric secretions.

pep·ti·dase (pĕp′tĭ-dās′, -dāz′) *n.* An enzyme that catalyzes the hydrolysis of peptides into amino acids.

pep·tide (pĕp′tīd′) *n.* Any of various natural or synthetic compounds containing two or more amino acids linked by the carboxyl group of one amino acid and the amino group of another. — **pep·tid′ic** (-tĭd′ĭk) *adj.* — **pep·tid′i·cal·ly** *adv.*

peptide bond *n.* The chemical bond formed between the carboxyl groups and amino groups of neighboring amino acids, constituting the primary linkage of all protein structures.

pep·tol·y·sis (pĕp-tŏl′ĭ-sĭs) *n.* The hydrolysis of peptones.

pep·tone (pĕp′tōn′) *n.* Any of various soluble compounds that do not coagulate and are obtained by acid or enzyme hydrolysis of natural protein and are used as nutrients in culture media. — **pep·ton′ic** (-tŏn′ĭk) *adj.*

pep·to·nize (pĕp′tə-nīz′) *v.* **-nized, -niz·ing, -niz·es. 1.** To convert protein into a soluble peptone by enzymatic action. **2.** To dissolve food by means of a proteolytic enzyme. — **pep′to·ni·za′tion** (-nĭ-zā′shən) *n.*

per a·num (pər ā′nəm) *adv.* Through or by way of the anus, as in the administration of medication or nutrients.

per·ceive (pər-sēv′) *v.* **-ceived, -ceiv·ing, -ceives. 1.** To become aware of directly through any of the senses, especially sight or hearing. **2.** To achieve understanding of; apprehend. — **per·ceiv′a·ble** *adj.* — **per·ceiv′a·bly** *adv.* — **per·ceiv′er** *n.*

per·cept (pûr′sĕpt′) *n.* **1.** The object of perception. **2.** A mental impression of something perceived by the senses, viewed as the basic component in the formation of concepts; a sense datum.

per·cep·tion (pər-sĕp′shən) *n.* **1.** The process, act, or faculty of perceiving. **2.** Recognition and interpretation of sensory stimuli based chiefly on memory.

per·cep·tive (pər-sĕp′tĭv) *adj.* **1.** Of or relating to perception. **2.** Having the ability to perceive. — **per′cep·tiv′i·ty** (pûr′sĕp-tĭv′ĭ-tē), **per·cep′·tive·ness** *n.*

per·cep·tu·al (pər-sĕp′chŏo-əl) *adj.* Of, based on, or involving perception.

per con·tig·u·um (pər kən-tĭg′yŏo-əm) *adv.* By or through contiguity, as in the spread of infection or inflammation between adjacent structures.

per con·tin·u·um (pər kən-tĭn′yŏo-əm) *adv.* By or through continuity, as in the spread of infection or inflammation from one part to another through continuous tissue.

per·cuss (pər-kŭs′) *v.* **-cussed, -cuss·ing, -cuss·es.** To strike or tap firmly; perform percussion.

per·cus·sion (pər-kŭsh′ən) *n.* A method of medical diagnosis in which various areas of the body, especially the chest, back, and abdomen, are tapped with the finger or a plexor to determine by resonance the condition of internal organs.

per·cus·sor (pər-kŭs′ər) *n.* See **plexor.**

per·cu·ta·ne·ous (pûr′kyŏo-tā′nē-əs) *adj.* Passed, done, or effected through the unbroken skin. — **per′cu·ta′ne·ous·ly** *adv.*

percutaneous trans·lu·mi·nal angioplasty (trăns-lŏo′mə-nəl, trănz-) *n.* A procedure for enlarging a narrowed arterial lumen by peripheral introduction of a balloon-tip catheter followed by dilation of the lumen as the inflated catheter tip is withdrawn.

per·fec·tion·ism (pər-fĕk′shə-nĭz′əm) *n.* A tendency to set rigid high standards of performance for oneself. — **per·fec′tion·ist** *adj. & n.* — **per·fec′tion·is′tic** *adj.*

per·fo·rate (pûr′fə-rāt′) *v.* **-rat·ed, -rat·ing, -rates. 1.** To make a hole or holes in, as from injury, disease, or medical procedure. **2.** To pass into or through (a body structure or tissue). — *adj.* (pûr′fər-ĭt, -fə-rāt′). Having been perforated.

perforated ulcer *n.* An ulcer extending through the wall of an organ.

perforating abscess *n.* An abscess that penetrates tissue barriers and enters adjacent areas.

perforating fiber *n.* Any of the bundles of collagen fibers that pass into the outer circumferential lamellae of bone or into the cementum of teeth.

perforating wound *n.* A wound having an entrance and an exit.

per·fo·ra·tion (pûr′fə-rā′shən) *n.* **1.** The act of perforating or the state of being perforated. **2.** An abnormal opening in a hollow organ or viscus, as one made by rupture or injury.

per·fuse (pər-fyōōz′) *v.* **-fused, -fus·ing, -fus·es. 1.** To pour or diffuse a liquid over or through something. **2.** To force blood or other fluid to flow from the artery through the vascular bed of a tissue or to flow through the lumen of a hollow structure. — **per·fu′sive** (pər-fyōō′sĭv, -zĭv) *adj.*

per·fu·sion (pər-fyōō′zhən) *n.* **1.** The act of perfusing. **2.** The injection of fluid into a blood vessel in order to reach an organ or tissues, usually to supply nutrients and oxygen.

per·i·ad·e·ni·tis (pĕr′ē-ăd′n-ī′tĭs) *n.* Inflammation of the tissues surrounding a gland.

per·i·a·or·ti·tis (pĕr′ē-ā′ôr-tī′tĭs) *n.* Inflammation of the adventitia of the aorta and of the tissues surrounding it.

per·i·ap·i·cal curettage (pĕr′ē-ā′pĭ-kəl, -ăp′ĭ-) *n.* **1.** The removal of a cyst or granuloma from its pathological bony crypt with a curette. **2.** The removal of tooth fragments, pieces of dead bone, or debris from a tooth socket with a curette.

per·i·ar·te·ri·al sympathectomy (pĕr′ē-är-tĕr′ē-əl) *n.* Sympathectomy that is achieved by decortication of the arteries.

per·i·ar·te·ri·tis (pĕr′ē-är′tə-rī′tĭs) *n.* Inflammation of the outer coat of an artery.

per·i·ar·thri·tis (pĕr′ē-är-thrī′tĭs) *n.* Inflammation of the tissues surrounding a joint.

per·i·bron·chi·tis (pĕr′ə-brŏn-kī′tĭs, brŏng-) *n.* Inflammation of the tissues surrounding the bronchi or bronchial tubes.

pericardial cavity *n.* The fluid-filled space between the two layers of the pericardium.

pericardial decompression *n.* See **cardiac decompression.**

pericardial fremitus *n.* The vibration in the chest wall produced by the friction of opposing roughened surfaces of the pericardium.

pericardial friction sound *n.* An oscillating creaking sound heard on auscultation over the heart in some cases of pericarditis, caused by the rubbing together of inflamed pericardial surfaces as the heart contracts and relaxes.

pericardial murmur *n.* A friction sound, synchronous with the heart movements, heard in certain cases of pericarditis.

pericardial rub *n.* See **pericardial friction sound.**

per·i·car·di·ec·to·my (pĕr′ĭ-kär′dē-ĕk′tə-mē) *n.*
Surgical excision of a portion of the pericardium.

per·i·car·di·o·cen·te·sis (pĕr′ĭ-kär′dē-ō-sĕn-tē′sĭs) *n.* Paracentesis of the pericardium.

per·i·car·di·or·rha·phy (pĕr′ĭ-kär′dē-ôr′ə-fē) *n.* Suture of the pericardium.

per·i·car·di·os·to·my (pĕr′ĭ-kär′dē-ŏs′tə-mē) *n.* Surgical construction of an opening into the pericardium.

per·i·car·di·ot·o·my (pĕr′ĭ-kär′dē-ŏt′ə-mē) *n.* Surgical incision into the pericardium.

per·i·car·di·tis (pĕr′ĭ-kär-dī′tĭs) *n.* Inflammation of the pericardium.

pericarditis o·blit·er·ans (ə-blĭt′ə-rănz′) *n.* Inflammation of the pericardium leading to adhesion of the two layers, thus obliterating the sac.

per·i·car·di·um (pĕr′ĭ-kär′dē-əm) *n., pl.* **-di·a** (-dē-ə). The fibroserous sac enclosing the heart and the roots of the great vessels, consisting of two layers: the visceral layer or epicardium, immediately surrounding the heart; and the outer parietal layer, which forms the sac and is lined with a serous membrane. — **per′i·car′di·al** (-dē-əl), **per′i·car′di·ac′** (-dē-ăk′) *adj.*

perichondral bone *n.* A collar or cuff of osseous tissue that forms in the perichondrium of the cartilage in the development of a long bone.

per·i·chon·dri·um (pĕr′ĭ-kŏn′drē-əm) *n., pl* **-dri·a** (-drē-ə). The dense irregular fibrous membrane of connective tissue covering the surface of cartilage except at the endings of joints. — **per′i·chon′dri·al** (-drē-əl) *adj.*

per·i·co·li·tis (pĕr′ĭ-kə-lī′tĭs) or **per·i·co·lon·i·tis** (-kŏ′lə-nī′tĭs) *n.* Inflammation of the connective tissue or of the peritoneum around the colon.

per·i·cor·o·ni·tis (pĕr′ĭ-kôr′ə-nī′tĭs) *n.* Inflammation of the gingiva surrounding the crown of a tooth.

per·i·cra·ni·um (pĕr′ĭ-krā′nē-əm) *n., pl* **-ni·a** (-nē-ə). The external periosteum that covers the outer surface of the skull. — **per′i·cra′ni·al** *adj.*

per·i·cys·ti·tis (pĕr′ĭ-sĭ-stī′tĭs) *n.* Inflammation of the tissues surrounding the urinary bladder.

per·i·cyte (pĕr′ĭ-sīt′) *n.* A slender, relatively undifferentiated, connective tissue cell that occurs about capillaries or other small blood vessels.

per·i·des·mi·um (pĕr′ĭ-dĕz′mē-əm) *n.* The connective tissue membrane surrounding a ligament.

per·i·did·y·mis (pĕr′ĭ-dĭd′ə-mĭs) *n.* The thick white fibrous membrane forming the outer coat of the testis.

per·i·en·ceph·a·li·tis (pĕr′ē-ĕn-sĕf′ə-lī′tĭs) *n.* Inflammation of the cerebral membranes, especially of the pia mater.

per·i·en·ter·i·tis (pĕr′ē-ĕn′tə-rī′tĭs) *n.* Inflammation of the peritoneal coat of the intestine.

per·i·gas·tri·tis (pĕr′ĭ-gă-strī′tĭs) *n.* Inflammation of the peritoneal coat of the stomach.

per·i·hep·a·ti·tis (pĕr′ə-hĕp′ə-tī′tĭs) *n.* Inflammation of the serous or peritoneal covering of the liver.

per·i·in·farc·tion block (pĕr′ē-ĭn-färk′shən) *n.* An electrocardiographic abnormality associated with an old myocardial infarct and caused by delayed activation of the myocardium in the region of the infarct.

per·i·lar·yn·gi·tis (pĕr′ə-lăr′ən-jī′tĭs) *n.* Inflammation of the tissues around the larynx.

per·i·lymph (pĕr′ə-lĭmf′) *n.* The fluid in the space between the membranous and bony labyrinths of the inner ear.

per·i·men·in·gi·tis (pĕr′ə-mĕn′ĭn-jī′tĭs) *n.* See **pachymeningitis**.

pe·rim·e·ter (pə-rĭm′ĭ-tər) *n.* **1.** The outer limits of an area. **2.** An instrument used to measure field of vision.

per·i·me·tri·um (pĕr′ə-mē′trē-əm) *n., pl.* **-tri·a** (-trē-ə). The serous peritoneal coat of the uterus.

pe·rim·e·try (pə-rĭm′ĭ-trē) *n.* The determination of the limits of the visual field.

per·i·my·si·um (pĕr′ə-mĭzh′ē-əm, -mĭz′ē-əm) *n., pl.* **-my·si·a** (-mĭzh′ē-ə, -mĭz′ē-ə). The fibrous sheath enveloping each of the primary bundles of skeletal muscle fibers. — **per′i·my′si·al** *adj.*

per·i·na·tal (pĕr′ə-nāt′l) *adj.* Of, relating to, or being the period around childbirth, especially the five months before and one month after birth. — **per′i·na′tal·ly** *adv.*

perinatal medicine *n.* The branch of medicine concerned with the care of the mother and fetus during pregnancy, labor, and delivery.

per·i·na·tol·o·gy (pĕr′ə-nā-tŏl′ə-jē) *n.* The subspecialty of obstetrics concerned with the care of the mother, fetus, and infant during the perinatal period. — **per′i·na·tol′o·gist** *n.*

perineal section *n.* A surgical incision through the perineum, especially external urethrotomy.

per·i·ne·o·plas·ty (pĕr′ə-nē′ə-plăs′tē) *n.* Reparative or plastic surgery of the perineum.

per·i·ne·or·rha·phy (pĕr′ə-nē-ôr′ə-fē) *n.* Suture of the perineum.

per·i·ne·os·to·my (pĕr′ə-nē-ŏs′tə-mē) *n.* Urethrostomy through an incision in the perineum.

per·i·ne·ot·o·my (pĕr′ə-nē-ŏt′ə-mē) *n.* Surgical incision into the perineum, as in external urethrotomy or lithotomy or to facilitate childbirth.

per·i·ne·phri·tis (pĕr′ə-nə-frī′tĭs) *n.* Inflammation of the tissues surrounding a kidney.

per·i·ne·um (pĕr′ə-nē′əm) *n., pl.* **-ne·a** (-nē′ə). **1.** The portion of the body in the pelvis occupied by urogenital passages and the rectum, bounded in front by the pubic arch, in the back by the coccyx, and laterally by part of the hipbone. **2.** The region between the scrotum and the anus in males, and between the posterior vulva junction and the anus in females. — **per′i·ne′al** (-nē′əl) *adj.*

per·i·neu·ral anesthesia (pĕr′ə-nŏŏr′əl, nyŏŏr′-) *n.* Injection of an anesthetic agent about a nerve.

per·i·neu·ri·tis (pĕr′ə-nŏŏ-rī′tĭs, -nyŏŏ-) *n.* Inflammation of the perineurium.

per·i·neu·ri·um (pĕr′ə-nŏŏr′ē-əm, -nyŏŏr′-) *n., pl.* **-neu·ri·a** (-nŏŏr′ē-ə, -nyŏŏr′-). The sheath of connective tissue enclosing a bundle of nerve fibers. — **per′i·neu′ri·al** *adj.*

pe·ri·od (pîr′ē-əd) *n.* **1.** An interval of time characterized by the occurrence of a certain con-

dition, event, or phenomenon. **2.** One of the stages of a disease. **3.** A menstrual period; menses.

pe·ri·od·ic (pîr′ē-ŏd′ĭk) *adj.* **1.** Having or marked by repeated cycles. **2.** Recurring at regular intervals.

periodic disease *n.* A disease for which symptoms tend to recur at regular intervals.

pe·ri·o·dic·i·ty (pîr′ē-ə-dĭs′ĭ-tē) *n.* The quality or state of being periodic; recurrence at regular intervals.

periodic table *n.* A tabular arrangement of the elements according to their atomic numbers so that elements with similar chemical properties are in the same column.

per·i·o·don·tal (pĕr′ē-ə-dŏn′tl) *adj.* **1.** Surrounding or encasing a tooth. **2.** Relating to or affecting tissues and structures surrounding and supporting the teeth.

per·i·o·don·tist (pĕr′ē-ə-dŏn′tĭst) *n.* A dentist who specializes in periodontics.

per·i·o·don·ti·tis (pĕr′ē-ō′dŏn-tī′tĭs) *n.* Disease of the periodontium characterized by inflammation of the gingivae, resorption of the alveolar bone, and degeneration of the periodontal membrane.

per·i·o·don·to·sis (pĕr′ē-ō′dŏn-tō′sĭs) *n.* A degenerative disease of the periodontal ligament and tooth sockets, characterized by looseness and migration of teeth.

per·i·o·nych·i·um (pĕr′ē-ə-nĭk′ē-əm) *n., pl.* **-i·a** (-ē-ə). The border of epidermal tissue surrounding a fingernail or toenail.

per·i·or·chi·tis (pĕr′ē-ôr-kī′tĭs) *n.* Inflammation of the sheath surrounding the testes and epididymides.

periosteal graft *n.* A graft of periosteum, usually placed on bare bone.

per·i·os·te·o·ma (pĕr′ē-ŏs′tē-ō′mə) *n.* A neoplasm derived from the periosteum of a bone.

per·i·os·te·o·my·e·li·tis (pĕr′ē-ŏs′tē-ō-mī′ə-lī′tĭs) *n.* Inflammation of the entire bone, including the periosteum and the marrow.

per·i·os·te·o·sis (pĕr′ē-ŏs′tē-ō′sĭs) or **per·i·os·to·sis** (-ō-stō′sĭs) *n.* Formation of a periosteoma.

per·i·os·te·ot·o·my (pĕr′ē-ŏs′tē-ŏt′ə-mē) *n.* Surgical incision of the periosteum.

per·i·os·te·um (pĕr′ē-ŏs′tē-əm) *n., pl.* **-te·a** (-tē-ə). The thick fibrous membrane covering the entire surface of a bone except its articular cartilage and serving as an attachment for muscles and tendons. — **per′i·os′te·al** (-tē-əl), **per′i·os′te·ous** (-tē-əs) *adj.*

pe·riph·er·al (pə-rĭf′ər-əl) *adj.* **1.** Related to, located in, or constituting an outer boundary or periphery. **2.** Perceived or perceiving near the outer edges of the retina. **3.** Of or relating to the surface or outer part of a body or organ; external. **4.** Of, relating to, or being part of the peripheral nervous system.

peripheral motor neuron *n.* See **postganglionic motor neuron**.

peripheral nervous system *n.* The part of the nervous system constituting the nerves outside the central nervous system and including the cranial nerves, the spinal nerves, and the sympathetic and parasympathetic nervous systems.

peripheral ossifying fibroma *n.* A gingival fibroma derived from cells of the periodontal ligament and usually developing in response to local irritants such as plaque and calculus.

peripheral scotoma *n.* A scotoma outside of the central 30° of the visual field.

peripheral vision *n.* Vision produced by light rays falling on areas of the retina beyond the macula.

per·i·phle·bi·tis (pĕr′ə-flĭ-bī′tĭs) *n.* Inflammation of the outer coat of a vein or of the tissues surrounding it.

per·i·proc·ti·tis (pĕr′ə-prŏk-tī′tĭs) *n.* Inflammation of the areolar tissue about the rectum.

per·i·sal·pin·gi·tis (pĕr′ĭ-săl′pĭn-jī′tĭs) *n.* Inflammation of the peritoneal covering of the fallopian tube.

per·i·sal·pinx (pĕr′ĭ-săl′pĭngks) *n.* The peritoneal covering of a fallopian tube.

per·i·spon·dy·li·tis (pĕr′ĭ-spŏn′dl-ī′tĭs) *n.* Inflammation of the tissues about a vertebra.

per·i·stal·sis (pĕr′ĭ-stôl′sĭs, -stăl′-) *n., pl.* **-ses** (-sēz). The wavelike muscular contractions of the intestine or other tubular structure that propel the contents onward by alternate contraction and relaxation. — **per′i·stal′tic** (-stôl′tĭk, -stăl′-) *adj.*

pe·ris·to·le (pə-rĭs′tə-lē) *n.* The tonic contractions of the walls of the stomach about its contents. — **per′i·stol′ic** (pĕr′ĭ-stŏl′ĭk) *adj.*

per·i·tec·to·my (pĕr′ĭ-tĕk′tə-mē) *n.* The removal of a pericorneal strip of the conjunctiva to correct pannus.

per·i·the·li·um (pĕr′ə-thē′lē-əm) *n., pl.* **-li·a** (-lē-ə). The connective tissue surrounding small blood vessels and capillaries.

per·i·thy·roid·i·tis (pĕr′ə-thī′roi-dī′tĭs) *n.* Inflammation of the capsule or tissues surrounding the thyroid gland.

pe·rit·o·my (pə-rĭt′ə-mē) *n.* **1.** See **peritectomy. 2.** See **circumcision.**

peritoneal cavity *n.* The potential space between the parietal and visceral layers of the peritoneum.

peritoneal dialysis *n.* The removal of soluble substances and water from the body by transfer across the peritoneum, utilizing a solution which is intermittently introduced into and removed from the peritoneal cavity.

per·i·to·ne·o·cen·te·sis (pĕr′ĭ-tn-ē′ō-sĕn-tē′sĭs) *n.* **1.** Paracentesis of the peritoneal cavity. **2.** Paracentesis of the abdominal cavity; abdominocentesis.

per·i·to·ne·oc·ly·sis (pĕr′ĭ-tn-ē-ŏk′lĭ-sĭs, -ē′ə-klī′sĭs) *n.* Irrigation of the abdominal cavity.

per·i·to·ne·op·a·thy (pĕr′ĭ-tn-ē-ŏp′ə-thē) *n.* Disease of the peritoneum.

per·i·to·ne·o·plas·ty (pĕr′ĭ-tn-ē′ə-plăs′tē) *n.* The surgical loosening of adhesions in the abdominal viscera and the covering of the resultant raw surfaces with peritoneum to prevent recurrence.

per·i·to·ne·o·scope (pĕr′ĭ-tn-ē′ə-skōp′) *n.* See **laparoscope.**

per·i·to·ne·os·co·py (pĕr′ĭ-tn-ē-ŏs′kə-pē) *n.* Internal examination of the peritoneum with a peritoneoscope passed through an incision in the abdominal wall.

per·i·to·ne·ot·o·my (pĕr′ĭ-tn-ē-ŏt′ə-mē) *n.* Incision of the peritoneum.

per·i·to·ne·o·ve·nous shunt (pĕr′ĭ-tn-ē′ō-vē′nəs) *n.* A shunt between the peritoneal cavity and the venous system, usually by means of a catheter.

per·i·to·ne·um or **per·i·to·nae·um** (pĕr′ĭ-tn-ē′əm) *n., pl.* **-to·ne·a** or **-to·nae·a** (-tn-ē′ə). The serous sac consisting of mesothelium and a thin layer of irregular connective tissue that lines the abdominal cavity and covers most of its viscera, and itself forms two sacs, the peritoneal sac and the omental bursa, which are connected by the epiploic foramen. — **per′i·to·ne′al** *adj.*

per·i·to·ni·tis (pĕr′ĭ-tn-ī′tĭs) *n.* Inflammation of the peritoneum.

per·i·ton·sil·lar abscess (pĕr′ĭ-tŏn′sə-lər) *n.* An abscess formed usually above and behind the tonsil, due to extension of infection beyond the tonsillar capsule.

per·lèche (pər-lĕsh′, pĕr-) *n.* See **angular cheilitis.**

per·ma·nent cartilage (pûr′mə-nənt) *n.* Cartilage that does not become converted into bone.

permanent dentition *n.* See **secondary dentition.**

permanent tooth *n.* Any of the teeth of the secondary dentition.

per·me·a·ble (pûr′mē-ə-bəl) *adj.* That can be permeated or penetrated, especially by liquids or gases.

per·me·ate (pûr′mē-āt′) *v.* **-at·ed, -at·ing, -ates. 1.** To spread or flow throughout; pervade. **2.** To pass through the openings or interstices of, as a liquid through a membrane. — *n.* (-ĭt, -āt′). One that can permeate. — **per′me·ant** (-ənt), **per′me·a′tive** (-ā′tĭv) *adj.*

per·me·a·tion (pûr′mē-ā′shən) *n.* The process of spreading through or penetrating, as in the extension of a malignant neoplasm by continuous proliferation of the cells along the blood or lymph vessels.

per·ni·cious (pər-nĭsh′əs) *adj.* Tending to cause death or serious injury; deadly.

pernicious anemia *n.* A severe form of anemia most often affecting older adults, caused by failure of the stomach to absorb vitamin B_{12} and characterized by abnormally large red blood cells, gastrointestinal disturbances, and lesions of the spinal cord.

pe·ro·dac·ty·ly (pĕr′ə-dăk′tə-lē) *n.* A congenital condition marked by deformed fingers or toes.

pe·ro·me·li·a (pĕr′ə-mē′lē-ə) *n.* Severe congenital malformations of the limbs, including the absence of a hand or foot.

per·o·ne·al (pĕr′ə-nē′əl) *adj.* Of or relating to the fibula or to the outer portion of the leg.

per·o·ral (pər-ôr′əl) *adj.* Performed or administered through or by way of the mouth.

per os (pər ŏs) *adv.* By way of the mouth, as in the administration of medication.

per·ox·ide (pə-rŏk′sīd′) *n.* **1.** A compound, such

as sodium peroxide, that contains a peroxy group and yields hydrogen when treated with an acid. **2.** Hydrogen peroxide.

per·ox·y (pə-rŏk′sē) *adj.* Containing the group O_2.

per·phen·a·zine (pər-fĕn′ə-zēn′) *n.* A crystalline compound used as a tranquilizer especially in the treatment of psychosis and to prevent or alleviate nausea and vomiting.

per rec·tum (pər rĕk′təm) *adv.* By way of the rectum, as in the administration of medication.

per·sev·er·a·tion (pər-sĕv′ə-rā′shən) *n.* **1.** Uncontrollable repetition of a particular response, such as a word, phrase, or gesture, despite the absence or cessation of a stimulus, usually caused by brain injury or other organic disorder. **2.** The tendency to continue or repeat an act or activity after the cessation of the original stimulus.

per·sis·tence (pər-sĭs′təns, -zĭs′-) *n.* **1.** Continuance of an effect after the cause is removed. **2.** Continuance of a part or an organ, rather than having it disappear in an early stage of development.

per·son (pûr′sən) *n.* **1.** A living human. **2.** The composite of characteristics that make up an individual personality. **3.** The living body of a human. **4.** Physique and general appearance.

per·so·na (pər-sō′nə) *n., pl.* **-nas** or **-nae** (-nē). The role that one assumes or displays in public or society; one's public image or personality, as distinguished from the inner self.

per·son·al care (pûr′sə-nəl) *n.* The occupation of attending to the physical needs of people who are disabled or otherwise unable to take care of themselves, including tasks such as bathing, management of bodily functions, and cooking.

per·son·al equation (pûr′sə-nəl) *n.* A constant but slight error in judgment, perceptual response, or action that is specific to an individual and is so constant that it is usually possible to allow for it when assessing that person's statements or conclusions, thus arriving at approximate exactness.

per·son·al·i·ty (pûr′sə-năl′ĭ-tē) *n.* **1.** The quality or condition of being a person. **2.** The totality of qualities and traits, as of character or behavior, that are peculiar to a specific person. **3.** The pattern of collective character, behavioral, temperamental, emotional, and mental traits of a person.

personality disorder *n.* Any of a group of disorders in which patterns of perceiving, relating to, and thinking about one's self and one's environment interfere with one's long-term functioning, often manifested in deviant behavior.

personality inventory *n.* A questionnaire that is scored to yield a profile of the particular traits or characteristics that make up the respondent's personality.

personality profile *n.* **1.** A method of presenting the results of psychological testing in graphic form. **2.** A brief description of the personality of an individual.

personality test *n.* A test, usually involving a standardized series of questions or tasks, used to describe or evaluate a subject's personality characteristics.

per·spi·ra·tion (pûr′spə-rā′shən) *n.* **1.** The fluid, consisting of water with small amounts of urea and salts, that is excreted through the pores of the skin by the sweat glands; sweat. **2.** The act or process of excreting this fluid through the pores of the skin. — **per·spir′a·to′ry** (pər-spīr′ə-tôr′ē, pûr′spər-ə-) *adj.*

per·spire (pər-spīr′) *v.* **-spired, -spir·ing, -spires.** To excrete perspiration through the pores of the skin.

per tu·bam (pər tōō′bəm, tyōō′-) *adv.* Through a tube, as in the administration of food, liquids, or medication.

per·tus·sis (pər-tŭs′ĭs) *n.* See **whooping cough.**

pertussis immune globulin *n.* A sterile solution of globulins derived from the plasma of adult human donors who have been immunized against and have formed antibodies to pertussis, used in the prevention and treatment of pertussis.

pertussis vaccine *n.* A vaccine containing inactivated *Bordetella pertussis* bacteria, often used in the diphtheria, tetanus toxoids, and pertussis vaccine to immunize against whooping cough.

per·va·sive developmental disorder (pər-vā′sĭv, -zĭv) *n.* Any of a group of disorders of infancy, childhood, or adolescence that are characterized by distortions in the development of the basic psychological functions such as language, social skills, attention, perception, reality testing, and movement.

per·ver·sion (pər-vûr′zhən, -shən) *n.* A practice or act, especially one that is sexual in nature, considered abnormal or deviant.

per vi·as na·tu·ra·les (pər vī′əs năch′ə-rā′lēz) *adv.* Through the natural passages, as in a vaginal delivery of a child.

pes (pās) *n., pl.* **pe·des** (pĕd′ās′). **1.** The foot. **2.** A footlike or basal structure or part. **3.** Clubfoot.

pes an·se·ri·nus (ăn′sə-rī′nəs) *n.* The tendinous expansions of the sartorius, gracilis, and semitendinous muscles at the medial border of the tuberosity of the tibia.

pes·sa·ry (pĕs′ə-rē) *n.* **1.** Any of various devices worn in the vagina to support or correct the position of the uterus or rectum. **2.** A contraceptive diaphragm. **3.** A medicated vaginal suppository.

pest (pĕst) *n.* **1.** An injurious plant or animal, especially one harmful to humans. **2.** A deadly epidemic disease; a pestilence.

pes·ti·lence (pĕs′tə-ləns) *n.* **1.** A usually fatal epidemic disease, especially bubonic plague. **2.** An epidemic of such a disease.

PET *abbr.* positron emission tomography

pe·te·chi·a (pə-tē′kē-ə) *n., pl.* **-chi·ae** (-kē-ī′). A small purplish spot on a body surface, such as the skin or a mucous membrane, caused by a minute hemorrhage and often seen in typhus. — **pe·te′·chi·al** *adj.*

Pe·ters' ovum (pē′tərz, pā′tərs) *n.* A fertilized ovum that is 13 to 14 days into its development as an embryo.

pet·it mal (pĕt′ē mäl′, măl′) *n.* A form of epilepsy, occurring most often in adolescents and children, characterized by frequent but transient lapses of consciousness and only rare spasms or falling.

pe·tri dish (pē′trē) *n.* A shallow circular dish with a loose-fitting cover, used to culture bacteria or other microorganisms.

pé·tris·sage (pā-trē-säzh′) *n.* A manipulation in massage in which the muscles are kneaded.

pe·tro·le·um jelly (pə-trō′lē-əm) *n.* A colorless-to-amber semisolid mixture of hydrocarbons obtained from petroleum and used in lubricants and medicinal ointments.

pe·tro·sa (pə-trō′sə) *n., pl.* **-sae** (-sē). The petrous portion of the temporal bone; petrosal bone; petrous bone.

pet·ro·si·tis (pĕt′rə-sī′tĭs) *n.* Inflammation of the petrous portion of the temporal bone and its air cells.

PET scan (pĕt) *n.* A cross-sectional image produced by a PET scanner.

PET scanner *n.* A device that produces cross-sectional x-rays of metabolic processes by means of positron emission tomography.

Peutz–Jeghers syndrome (pŏŏts′-, pœts′-) *n.* Inherited polyposis of the intestinal tract, characterized by multiple harmartomas, especially of the jejunum, and associated with melanin spots on the lips, buccal mucosa, and fingers.

pex·is (pĕk′sĭs) *n.* **1.** Surgical fixation. **2.** The fixation of substances in the tissues, as for histologic examination.

PFB (pē′ĕf-bē′) *n.* A skin disorder in which tightly curled beard hairs that have been sharpened by shaving reenter the skin, causing inflammation, bumps, and infection.

pg *abbr.* picogram

pH (pē′āch′) *n.* A measure of the acidity or alkalinity of a solution, numerically equal to 7 for neutral solutions, increasing with increasing alkalinity and decreasing with increasing acidity. The pH scale commonly in use ranges from 0 to 14.

PH or **P.H.** *abbr.* public health

phac·o·an·a·phy·lax·is (făk′ō-ăn′ə-fə-lăk′sĭs) *n.* Hypersensitivity to protein of the lens of the eye.

phac·o·cele (făk′ə-sēl′) *n.* Hernia of the lens of the eye.

phac·o·cys·tec·to·my (făk′ō-sĭ-stĕk′tə-mē) *n.* Surgical removal of a portion of the capsule of the lens of the eye.

phac·o·e·mul·si·fi·ca·tion (făk′ō-ĭ-mŭl′sə-fĭ-kā′shən) *n.* Removal of a cataract by emulsifying the lens ultrasonically.

phac·o·er·y·sis (făk′ō-ĕr′ĭ-sĭs) *n.* Extraction of a cataract of the lens of the eye using suction.

pha·col·y·sis (fă-kŏl′ĭ-sĭs) *n.* The surgical breakdown and removal of the lens of the eye. — **phac′o·lyt′ic** (făk′ə-lĭt′ĭk) *adj.*

pha·co·ma or **pha·ko·ma** (fă-kō′mə) *n.* **-mas** or **-ma·ta** (-mə-tə). A hamartoma occurring in phacomatosis.

phac·o·ma·la·ci·a (făk′ō-mə-lā′shē-ə, -shə) *n.* Softening of the lens of the eye.

phac·o·ma·to·sis or **phak·o·ma·to·sis** (făk′ō-mə-tō′sĭs) *n.* Any of a group of congenital and hereditary diseases characterized by the development of hamartomas in various tissues and including neurofibromatosis, Lindau's disease, Sturge-Weber syndrome, and tuberous sclerosis.

phac·o·scope (făk′ə-skōp′) *n.* An instrument used to observe changes in the crystalline lens during accommodation.

phae·o·hy·pho·my·co·sis (fē′ō-hī′fō-mī-kō′sĭs) *n.* Any of a group of superficial and deep infections caused by fungi that form filaments and yeastlike cells in tissue.

phage (fāj) *n.* See **bacteriophage**.

phag·e·de·na (făj′ĭ-dē′nə) *n.* An ulcer that rapidly spreads peripherally, destroying tissues as it increases in size. — **phag′e·den′ic** (-dĕn′ĭk) *adj.*

phagedenic ulcer *n.* A rapidly spreading cutaneous ulcer marked by extensive sloughing of necrotic tissue.

phag·o·cyte (făg′ə-sīt′) *n.* A cell, such as a white blood cell, that engulfs and absorbs waste material, harmful microorganisms, or other foreign bodies in the bloodstream and tissues.

phag·o·cy·tize (făg′ə-sī-tīz′, -sĭ′-) *v.* **-tized, -tiz·ing, -tiz·es**. To ingest by phagocytosis.

phag·o·cy·tol·y·sis (făg′ə-sī-tŏl′ĭ-sĭs) *n.* The destruction of phagocytes or white blood cells that occurs during the process of blood coagulation or as the result of the introduction of certain antagonistic foreign substances into the body. — **phag′o·cy′to·lyt′ic** (făg′ə-sī′tə-lĭt′ĭk) *adj.*

phag·o·cy·to·sis (făg′ə-sī-tō′sĭs) *n.* The engulfing and ingestion of bacteria or other foreign bodies by phagocytes. — **phag′o·cy·tot′ic** (-tŏt′ĭk) *adj.*

pha·kic eye (fā′kĭk) *n.* An eye containing the natural lens.

pha·lan·ge·al (fə-lăn′jē-əl, fā-) or **pha·lan·gal** (fə-lăng′gəl, fā-) or **pha·lan·ge·an** (fə-lăn′jē-ən, fā-) *adj.* Of or relating to a phalanx or phalanges.

phalangeal joint *n.* See **digital joint**.

phal·an·gec·to·my (făl′ən-jĕk′tə-mē) *n.* Surgical excision of one or more phalanges of the hand or foot.

pha·lanx (fā′lăngks′, făl′ăngks′) *n., pl.* **pha·lanx·es** or **pha·lan·ges** (fə-lăn′jēz, fā-). Any of the long bones of the fingers or toes, numbering 14 for each hand or foot: two for the thumb or big toe, and three each for the other four digits.

phal·lec·to·my (fă-lĕk′tə-mē) *n.* Surgical removal of the penis.

phal·lic (făl′ĭk) *adj.* **1.** Of, relating to, or resembling a phallus. **2.** Of or relating to the third stage of psychosexual development in psychoanalytic theory during which the genital organs first become the focus of sexual feeling.

phallic phase *n.* In psychoanalytic theory, the stage in psychosexual development, usually occurring between the ages of 3 and 7, when a child's interest and curiosity are centered around the genital organs.

phal·lo·dyn·i·a (făl′ō-dĭn′ē-ə) *n.* Pain in the penis.

phal·loi·din (fă-loid′n) *n.* A heat-stable, toxic, cyclic peptide produced by the poisonous mushroom *Amanita phalloides* that acts by binding actin and causes vomiting, convulsions, diarrhea, asthenia, and death.

phal·lo·plas·ty (făl'ə-plăs'tē) *n*. Reparative or plastic surgery of the penis.

phal·lot·o·my (fă-lŏt'ə-mē) *n*. Surgical incision into the penis.

phal·lus (făl'əs) *n., pl.* **phal·lus·es** or **-li** (făl'ī'). **1.** The penis. **2.** The sexually undifferentiated tissue in an embryo that becomes the penis or clitoris. **3.** The immature penis considered in psychoanalysis as the libidinal object of infantile sexuality in the male.

phan·tasm (făn'tăz'əm) *n*. **1.** Something apparently seen but having no physical reality; an apparition. **2.** An illusory mental image.

phan·tas·ma·go·ri·a (făn-tăz'mə-gôr'ē-ə) or **phan·tas·ma·go·ry** (făn-tăz'mə-gôr'ē) *n*. **-ri·as** or **-ries**. **1.** A fantastic sequence of haphazardly associative imagery, as seen in dreams or fever. **2.** A constantly changing scene composed of numerous elements.

phan·tom or **fan·tom** (făn'təm) *n*. **1.** Something apparently seen, heard, or sensed, but having no physical reality. **2.** An image that appears only in the mind; an illusion. **3.** A model, especially a transparent one, of the human body or any of its parts. *—adj.* Resembling, characteristic of, or being a phantom; illusive.

phantom limb *n*. The sensation that an amputated limb is still attached, often associated with painful paresthesia.

phantom limb pain *n*. Pain or discomfort felt by an amputee in the area of the missing limb.

phantom tumor *n*. An accumulation of fluid in the interlobar spaces of the lung occurring as a result of congestive heart failure and appearing radiologically as a neoplasm.

phar·ma·ceu·ti·cal (făr'mə-sōō'tĭ-kəl) or **phar·ma·ceu·tic** (-tĭk) *adj*. Of or relating to pharmacy or pharmacists. *—n*. A pharmaceutical product or preparation.

phar·ma·cist (făr'mə-sĭst) *n*. One who prepares and dispenses drugs; a druggist.

phar·ma·col·o·gy (făr'mə-kŏl'ə-jē) *n*. **1.** The science of drugs, including their composition, uses, and effects. **2.** The characteristics or properties of a drug, especially those that make it medically effective. *— **phar'ma·co·log'ic** (-kə-lŏj'ĭk) adj. — **phar'ma·col'o·gist** n.*

phar·ma·co·poe·ia or **phar·ma·co·pe·ia** (făr'mə-kə-pē'ə) *n*. **1.** A book containing an official list of medicinal drugs together with articles on their preparation and use. **2.** A collection or stock of drugs.

phar·ma·co·psy·cho·sis (făr'mə-kō-sī-kō'sĭs) *n*. A psychosis caused by taking a drug.

phar·ma·co·ther·a·py (făr'mə-kō-thĕr'ə-pē) *n*. Treatment of disease through the use of drugs.

phar·ma·cy (făr'mə-sē) *n*. **1.** The art of preparing and dispensing drugs. **2.** A place where drugs are sold; a drugstore.

phar·yn·gal·gi·a (făr'ĭn-găl'jē-ə, -jə, făr'ĭng-) *n*. Pain in the pharynx.

pha·ryn·ge·al (fə-rĭn'jē-əl, -jəl, făr'ĭn-jē'əl) or **pha·ryn·gal** (fə-rĭng'gəl) *adj*. Of, relating to, located in, or coming from the pharynx.

pharyngeal reflex *n*. **1.** See **swallowing reflex. 2.** See **vomiting reflex.**

pharyngeal tonsil *n*. A collection of aggregated lymphoid nodules on the posterior wall of the nasopharynx, hypertrophy of which constitutes adenoids.

phar·yn·gec·to·my (făr'ĭn-jĕk'tə-mē) *n*. Surgical removal of all or part of the pharynx.

phar·yn·gis·mus (făr'ĭn-jĭz'məs) *n*. A spasm of the muscles of the pharynx.

phar·yn·gi·tis (făr'ĭn-jī'tĭs) *n*. Inflammation of the pharynx. *— **phar'yn·git'ic** (-jĭt'ĭk) adj.*

pha·ryn·go·cele (fə-rĭng'gə-sēl') *n*. Protrusion of mucous membrane through the wall of the pharynx; hernia of the pharynx.

pha·ryn·go·con·junc·ti·val fever (fə-rĭng'gō-kŏn'jŭngk-tī'vəl) *n*. An epidemic disease caused by an adenovirus and characterized by fever, pharyngitis, and conjunctivitis.

pha·ryn·go·dyn·i·a (fə-rĭng'gō-dĭn'ē-ə) *n*. See **pharyngalgia.**

pha·ryn·go·ker·a·to·sis (fə-rĭng'gō-kĕr'ə-tō'sĭs) *n*. A thickening of the lining of the lymphoid follicles of the pharynx and the formation of a pseudomembranous exudate.

pha·ryn·go·lar·yn·gi·tis (fə-rĭng'gō-lăr'ĭn-jī'tĭs) *n*. Inflammation of the pharynx and the larynx.

pha·ryn·go·lith (fə-rĭng'gə-lĭth') *n*. A concretion occurring in the pharynx.

phar·yn·gol·o·gy (făr'ĭn-gŏl'ə-jē, făr'ĭng-) *n*. The medical study of the pharynx and its diseases.

phar·yn·gop·a·thy (făr'ĭn-gŏp'ə-thē, făr'ĭng-) *n*. Disease of the pharynx.

pha·ryn·go·pe·ris·to·le (fə-rĭng'gō-pə-rĭs'tə-lē) *n*. A narrowing of the lumen of the pharynx.

pha·ryn·go·plas·ty (fə-rĭng'gə-plăs'tē) *n*. Plastic surgery of the pharynx.

pha·ryn·go·ple·gi·a (fə-rĭng'gō-plē'jē-ə, -jə) *n*. Paralysis of the muscles of the pharynx.

pha·ryn·go·rhi·ni·tis (fə-rĭng'gō-rī-nī'tĭs) *n*. Inflammation of the mucous membrane of the pharynx and the nasal cavity.

pha·ryn·go·scope (fə-rĭng'gə-skōp') *n*. An instrument used in examining the pharynx. *— **phar'yn·gos'co·py** (făr'ĭn-gŏs'kə-pē, făr'ĭng-) n.*

pha·ryn·go·spasm (fə-rĭng'gō-spăz'əm) *n*. See **pharyngismus.**

pha·ryn·go·ste·no·sis (fə-rĭng'gō-stə-nō'sĭs) *n*. Stricture of the pharynx.

phar·yn·got·o·my (făr'ĭn-gŏt'ə-mē, făr'ĭng-) *n*. Surgical incision of the pharynx.

phar·ynx (făr'ĭngks) *n., pl.* **phar·ynx·es** or **phar·yng·es** (fə-rĭn'jēz). The upper section of the alimentary canal that extends from the mouth and nasal cavities to the larynx, where it becomes continuous with the esophagus.

phase (fāz) *n*. **1.** A characteristic form, appearance, or stage of development that occurs in a cycle. **2.**

A discrete homogeneous part of a material system that is mechanically separable from the rest, as is ice from water. **3.** Any of the forms or states, solid, liquid, gas, or plasma, in which matter can exist, depending on temperature and pressure. **4.** A distinct part in a course or development, as of a disease. — *v.* To introduce, one stage at a time.

Ph.D. *abbr. Latin.* Philosophiae Doctor (Doctor of Philosophy)

Phe *abbr.* phenylalanine

Phem·is·ter graft (fĕm′ĭ-stər) *n.* An autogenous bone graft applied on the outside of an injured bone, used in treating delayed union of a fracture.

phe·na·caine (fē′nə-kān′, fĕn′ə-) *n.* A white crystalline compound used in the form of its hydrochloride as a local anesthetic in ophthalmology.

phe·neth·i·cil·lin potassium (fə-nĕth′ĭ-sĭl′ĭn) *n.* A semisynthetic oral penicillin preparation that is stable in gastric acid and is rapidly but only partially absorbed from the gastrointestinal tract.

phe·no·bar·bi·tal (fē′nō-bär′bĭ-tôl′, -tăl′) *n.* A crystalline barbiturate used as a sedative, a hypnotic, and an anticonvulsant.

phe·no·cop·y (fē′nə-kŏp′ē) *n.* **1.** An environmentally induced, nonhereditary variation in an organism, closely resembling a genetically determined trait. **2.** An individual exhibiting such a variation.

phe·no·de·vi·ant (fē′nō-dē′vē-ənt) *n.* An individual with a phenotype significantly different from that of the population to which it belongs.

phe·nol (fē′nôl′, -nōl′, -nŏl′) *n.* **1.** A caustic, poisonous, white crystalline compound derived from benzene and used in pharmaceuticals and in dilute form as a disinfectant and antiseptic. **2.** Any of a class of aromatic organic compounds having at least one hydroxyl group attached directly to the benzene ring.

phe·nol·phthal·ein (fē′nōl-thăl′ēn′, -thăl′ē-ĭn, -thā′lēn′, -thā′lē-ĭn) *n.* A white or pale yellow crystalline powder used as an acid-base indicator, in making dyes, and in medicine as a laxative.

phe·nom·e·non (fĭ-nŏm′ə-nŏn′, -nən) *n., pl.* **-na** (-nə) An occurrence, a circumstance, or a fact that is perceptible by the senses, especially one in relation to a disease.

phe·no·thi·a·zine (fē′nō-thī′ə-zēn′, -nə-) *n.* **1.** A yellow organic compound used in insecticides, veterinary anthelmintics, and dyes. **2.** Any of a group of drugs derived from this compound and used as tranquilizers in the treatment of psychiatric disorders, such as schizophrenia.

phe·no·type (fē′nə-tīp′) *n.* **1.** The observable physical or biochemical characteristics of an organism, as determined by both genetic makeup and environmental influences. **2.** The expression of a specific trait, such as stature or blood type, based on genetic and environmental influences. **3.** An individual or group of organisms exhibiting a particular phenotype. — **phe′no·typ′ic** (-tĭp′ĭk) *adj.*

phe·nox·y·ben·za·mine (fē-nŏk′sē-bĕn′zə-mēn′) *n.* A long-acting alpha blocker used in the form of

its hydrochloride as a vasodilator in the treatment of peripheral vascular diseases.

phen·pro·ba·mate (fĕn-prō′bə-māt′) *n.* A skeletal muscle relaxant that also has antianxiety action.

phen·yl·a·ce·tic acid (fĕn′əl-ə-sē′tĭk, fē′nəl-) *n.* An abnormal product of phenylalanine catabolism that appears in the urine in phenylketonuria.

phen·yl·al·a·nine (fĕn′əl-ăl′ə-nēn′, fē′nəl-) *n.* An essential amino acid that occurs as a constituent of many proteins and is normally converted to tyrosine in the human body. It is necessary for growth in infants and for nitrogen equilibrium in adults.

phen·yl·bu·ta·zone (fĕn′əl-byōō′tə-zōn′) *n.* A white or light yellow compound used as an antiinflammatory and analgesic drug in the treatment of arthritis, bursitis, and gout.

phen·yl·eph·rine (fĕn′əl-ĕf′rēn, fē′nəl-) *n.* An adrenergic drug that is a powerful vasoconstrictor and is used to relieve nasal congestion, dilate the pupils, and maintain blood pressure during anesthesia.

phen·yl·ke·to·nu·ri·a (fĕn′əl-kēt′n-ŏŏr′ē-ə, -yŏŏr′-, fē′nəl-) *n.* A genetic disorder in which the body lacks the enzyme necessary to metabolize phenylalanine to tyrosine. If untreated, the disorder can cause brain damage and mental retardation as a result of accumulation of phenylalanine and its breakdown products.

phen·yl·lac·tic acid (fĕn′əl-lăk′tĭk, fē′nəl-) *n.* A product of phenylalanine catabolism that occurs in the urine in phenylketonuria.

phen·yl·pro·pa·nol·a·mine (fĕn′əl-prō′pə-nŏl′ə-mēn′, fē′nəl-) *n.* An adrenergic drug that acts as a vasoconstrictor and is used as a nasal decongestant, a bronchodilator, an appetite suppressant, and a mild stimulant.

phen·y·to·in (fĕn′ĭ-tō′ĭn, fə-nĭt′ō-) *n.* An anticonvulsant drug chemically related to the barbiturates and used most commonly in the treatment of epilepsy.

phe·o·chro·mo·cyte (fē′ō-krō′mə-sīt′) *n.* A chromaffin cell of a sympathetic paraganglion, of a pheochromocytoma, or of the adrenal medulla.

phe·o·chro·mo·cy·to·ma (fē′ō-krō′mō-sī-tō′mə) *n., pl.* **-mas** or **-ma·ta** (-mə-tə). A usually benign tumor of the adrenal medulla or the sympathetic nervous system in which the affected cells secrete increased amounts of epinephrine or norepinephrine.

phe·re·sis (fə-rē′sĭs, fĕr′ĭ-) *n.* Apheresis.

Phil·a·del·phi·a chromosome (fĭl′ə-dĕl′fē-ə) *n.* An abnormal minute chromosome formed by a rearrangement of chromosomes 9 and 22; it is found in the white blood cells in many cases of chronic myelocytic leukemia.

Phil·lips catheter (fĭl′ĭps) *n.* A urethral catheter with a woven filiform guide.

phi·mo·sis (fī-mō′sĭs, fĭ-) *n., pl.* **-ses** (-sēz). A constriction of the foreskin that prevents it from being drawn back to uncover the glans penis.

phleb·ar·ter·i·ec·ta·si·a (flĕb′är-tĕr′ē-ĕk-tā′zē-ə, -zhə) *n.* See **vasodilation.**

phleb·ec·ta·si·a (flĕb′ĕk-tā′zē-ə, -zhə) *n.* Dilation of the veins.

phle·bec·to·my (flĭ-bĕk′tə-mē) *n.* Surgical excision of a segment of a vein.

phleb·em·phrax·is (flĕb′ĕm-frăk′sĭs) *n.* Venous thrombosis.

phle·bis·mus (flĭ-bĭz′məs) *n.* Venous congestion and dilation.

phle·bi·tis (flĭ-bī′tĭs) *n.* Inflammation of a vein. — **phle·bit′ic** (-bĭt′ĭk) *adj.*

phle·boc·ly·sis (flĭ-bŏk′lĭ-sĭs, flĕb′ə-klī′sĭs) *n.* Intravenous injection of an isotonic solution of dextrose or other substances.

phleb·o·gram (flĕb′ə-grăm′) *n.* A graphic tracing of the jugular venous pulse.

phleb·o·graph (flĕb′ə-grăf′) *n.* An instrument for making a graphic recording of the venous pulse.

phle·bog·ra·phy (flĭ-bŏg′rə-fē) *n.* The process of recording the venous pulse.

phleb·o·ma·nom·e·ter (flĕb′ō-mă-nŏm′ĭ-tər) *n.* A manometer for measuring venous pressure.

phleb·o·phle·bos·to·my (flĕb′ō-flĭ-bŏs′tə-mē) *n.* See **venovenostomy.**

phleb·o·plas·ty (flĕb′ə-plăs′tē) *n.* Surgical repair of a vein.

phleb·or·rha·gi·a (flĕb′ə-rā′jē-ə, -jə) *n.* Venous hemorrhage.

phle·bor·rha·phy (flĭ-bôr′ə-fē) *n.* The surgical suturing of a vein.

phleb·or·rhex·is (flĕb′ə-rĕk′sĭs) *n.* Rupture of a vein.

phleb·o·scle·ro·sis (flĕb′ō-sklə-rō′sĭs) *n.* The thickening or hardening of the walls of a vein.

phle·bos·ta·sis (flĭ-bŏs′tə-sĭs) *n.* **1.** The abnormally slow motion of blood in veins, usually with venous distention. **2.** The compression of the proximal veins of an extremity using tourniquets.

phleb·o·ste·no·sis (flĕb′ō-stə-nō′sĭs) *n.* Narrowing of the lumen of a vein.

phleb·o·throm·bo·sis (flĕb′ō-thrŏm-bō′sĭs) *n.* Thrombosis in a vein without primary inflammation.

phle·bot·o·mist (flĭ-bŏt′ə-mĭst) *n.* One who draws blood for analysis or transfusion.

phle·bot·o·mus fever (flə-bŏt′ə-məs) *n.* An infectious but not contagious denguelike disease occurring in parts of southern Europe, caused by an arbovirus introduced by the bite of the sand fly *Phlebotomus papatasi.*

phle·bot·o·my (flĭ-bŏt′ə-mē) *n.* The act or practice of opening a vein by incision or puncture to remove blood.

phlegm (flĕm) *n.* Thick, sticky, stringy mucus secreted by the mucous membrane of the respiratory tract, as during a cold or other respiratory infection. — **phlegm′y** *adj.*

phleg·ma·sia (flĕg-mā′zhə, -zē-ə) *n.* Inflammation, especially when acute and severe.

phleg·mat·ic (flĕg-măt′ĭk) or **phleg·mat·i·cal** (-ĭ-kəl) *adj.* **1.** Of or relating to phlegm. **2.** Having or suggesting a calm, sluggish temperament; unemotional.

phleg·mon (flĕg′mŏn′) *n.* Acute suppurative inflammation of the subcutaneous connective tissue. — **phleg′mon·ous** (-mə-nəs) *adj.*

phlyc·te·na or **phlyc·tae·na** (flĭk-tē′nə) *n., pl.* **-nae** (-nē). A small blister or vesicle, especially one of multiple blisters caused by a mild burn. — **phlyc′ten′ar** (flĭk′tĕn′ər) *adj.*

phlyc·ten·u·la (flĭk-tĕn′yə-lə) *n., pl.* **-lae** (-lē). A small red nodule of lymphoid cells, with an ulcerated apex, occurring in the conjunctiva of the eye. — **phlyc·ten′u·lar** (-lər) *adj.*

phlyc·ten·ule (flĭk′tĕn′-yōōl, -tə-nyōōl′) *n.* See **phlyctenula.**

phlyc·ten·u·lo·sis (flĭk-tĕn′yə-lō′sĭs) *n.* A nodular hypersensitive disease of the corneal and conjunctival epithelium of the eye caused by an endogenous toxin.

pho·bi·a (fō′bē-ə) *n.* **1.** A persistent, abnormal, or irrational fear of a specific thing or situation that compels one to avoid the feared stimulus. **2.** A strong fear, dislike, or aversion.

pho·bic (fō′bĭk) *adj.* Of, relating to, arising from, or having a phobia. — *n.* One who has a phobia.

pho·co·me·li·a (fō′kō-mē′lē-ə, -mēl′yə) *n.* A birth defect in which the upper portion of a limb is absent or poorly developed, so that the hand or foot attaches to the body by a short, flipperlike stump. — **pho′co·me′lic** (-mē′lĭk) *adj.*

phocomelic dwarf *n.* A dwarf in whom the shafts of the long bones are extremely short or in whom the intermediate parts of the limbs are absent.

pho·nas·the·ni·a (fō′năs-thē′nē-ə) *n.* Difficult or abnormal voice production characterized by enunciation that is too high, too loud, or too hard.

pho·nate (fō′nāt′) *v.* **-nat·ed, -nat·ing, -nates.** To utter speech sounds; vocalize.

pho·na·tion (fō-nā′shən) *n.* The utterance of sounds through the use of the vocal cords; vocalization. — **pho′na·to′ry** (fō′nə-tôr′ē) *adj.*

pho·nen·do·scope (fō-nĕn′də-skōp′) *n.* A stethoscope that intensifies auscultatory sounds.

pho·ni·at·rics (fō′nē-ăt′rĭks) *n.* The scientific study of speech and speech habits.

pho·no·an·gi·og·ra·phy (fō′nō-ăn′jē-ŏg′rə-fē) *n.* The recording and analysis of the audible frequency-intensity components of the bruit of turbulent arterial blood flow through an atherosclerotic stenotic lesion.

pho·no·car·di·o·gram (fō′nə-kär′dē-ə-grăm′) *n.* A graphic record of heart sounds and murmurs that is produced by a phonocardiograph.

pho·no·car·di·o·graph (fō′nə-kär′dē-ə-grăf′) *n.* An instrument consisting of microphones and recording equipment used to monitor and record heart sounds and murmurs. — **pho′no·car′di·og′ra·phy** (-ŏg′rə-fē) *n.*

pho·no·cath·e·ter (fō′nō-kăth′ĭ-tər) *n.* A cardiac catheter with a miniature microphone in its tip used in recording sounds and murmurs from within the heart and great blood vessels.

pho·no·gram (fō′nə-grăm′) *n.* A graphic tracing of the duration and intensity of a sound.

pho·nom·e·ter (fə-nŏm′ĭ-tər, fō-) *n.* An instrument used to measure the pitch and intensity of sounds.

pho·no·my·oc·lo·nus (fō'nō-mī-ŏk'lə-nəs) *n*. A condition characterized by fibrillary contractions of a muscle that can be heard on auscultation even though they are not visible.

pho·nop·a·thy (fə-nŏp'ə-thē, fō-) *n*. Any of various diseases of the vocal organs that affect speech.

pho·no·pho·tog·ra·phy (fō'nō-fə-tŏg'rə-fē) *n*. The process of graphically recording the movements sound waves impart to a diaphragm.

pho·nop·si·a (fə-nŏp'sē-ə, fō-) *n*. A condition in which hearing certain sounds elicits a subjective sensation of color.

pho·no·re·cep·tion (fō'nō-rĭ-sĕp'shən) *n*. Perception of or response to sound waves.

pho·no·re·cep·tor (fō'nō-rĭ-sĕp'tər) *n*. A receptor for sound stimuli.

pho·no·re·no·gram (fō'nō-rē'nə-grăm') *n*. A sound recording of the renal arterial pulse produced by means of a phonocatheter placed in the renal pelvis.

pho·ri·a (fôr'ē-ə) *n*. The relative directions assumed by the eyes during binocular fixation on a given object in the absence of an adequate fusion stimulus.

pho·ro·op·tom·e·ter (fôr'ō-ŏp-tŏm'ĭ-tər) *n*. An instrument for determining phorias, ductions, and refractive states of the eyes.

pho·rop·ter (fə-rŏp'tər) *n*. A device containing different lenses used for refraction of the eye during sight testing.

phos·phate (fŏs'fāt') *n*. A salt of phosphoric acid.

phos·pha·te·mi·a (fŏs'fə-tē'mē-ə) *n*. An abnormally high concentration of inorganic phosphates in the blood.

phos·pha·tide (fŏs'fə-tīd') *n*. See **phospholipid.**

phos·pha·ti·dyl·cho·line (fŏs'fə-tīd'l-kō'lēn') *n*. A phospholipid that is a major component of cellular membranes and functions in the transport of lipoproteins in tissues.

phos·pha·ti·dyl·glyc·er·ol (fŏs'fə-tīd'l-glĭs'ə-rôl', -rōl') *n*. A phosphatidic acid that is a constituent in human amniotic fluid and is used as an indicator of fetal lung maturity when present in the last trimester of gestation.

phos·pha·tu·ri·a (fŏs'fə-tōōr'ē-ə, -tyŏŏr'-) *n*. An excess of phosphates in the urine.

phos·phene (fŏs'fēn') *n*. A sensation of light caused by excitation of the retina by mechanical or electrical means rather than by light, as when the eyeballs are pressed through closed lids.

phos·pho·cre·a·tine (fŏs'fō-krē'ə-tēn') or **phos·pho·cre·a·tin** (-tĭn) *n*. An organic compound found in muscle tissue and capable of storing and providing energy for muscular contraction.

phos·pho·lip·id (fŏs'fō-lĭp'ĭd) *n*. Any of various phosphorus-containing lipids that are composed mainly of fatty acids, a phosphate group, and a simple organic molecule; found in cell membranes.

phos·phor·ic acid (fŏs-fôr'ĭk) *n*. A clear colorless

liquid used in fertilizers, detergents, food flavoring, and pharmaceuticals.

phos·pho·rism (fŏs'fə-rĭz'əm) *n*. Chronic phosphorus poisoning.

phos·pho·rus (fŏs'fər-əs) *n*. **1.** A highly reactive nonmetallic element with atomic number 15, occurring naturally in phosphates. An essential constituent of protoplasm, cell membranes, bone, and teeth. **2.** A phosphorescent substance.

phos·pho·ryl·a·tion (fŏs'fər-ə-lā'shən) *n*. The addition of phosphate to an organic compound through the action of a phosphorylase or kinase.

pho·tal·gi·a (fō-tăl'jē-ə, -jə) *n*. Pain caused by light.

pho·tism (fō'tĭz'əm) *n*. The production of a sensation of light or color by a stimulus to another sense organ, such as that of hearing or touch.

pho·to·chro·mic lens (fō'tə-krō'mĭk) *n*. A light-sensitive eyeglass lens that automatically darkens in sunlight and clears in reduced light.

pho·to·co·ag·u·la·tion (fō'tō-kō-ăg'yə-lā'shən) *n*. Surgical coagulation of tissue by means of intense light energy, such as a laser beam, performed to destroy abnormal tissues or to form adhesive scars, especially in ophthalmology. **— pho′to·co·ag′u·late′** *v*.

pho·to·co·ag·u·la·tor (fō'tō-kō-ăg'yə-lā'tər) *n*. An apparatus, such as a laser, used in photocoagulation.

pho·to·der·ma·ti·tis (fō'tō-dûr'mə-tī'tĭs) *n*. Dermatitis caused by exposure to ultraviolet light.

pho·to·dis·tri·bu·tion (fō'tō-dĭs'trə-byōō'shən) *n*. The areas on the skin that receive the greatest exposure to sunlight and are involved in eruptions due to photosensitivity.

pho·to·fluor·o·gram (fō'tə-flŏŏr'ə-grăm', -flôr'-) *n*. A photograph made by photofluorography.

pho·to·fluo·rog·ra·phy (fō'tō-flŏŏ-rŏg'rə-fē, -flô-) *n*. The photographic record of x-ray images produced by a fluoroscope. **— pho′to·fluor′o·graph′ic** (-flŏŏr'ə-grăf'ĭk, -flôr'-, -flôr'-) *adj*.

pho·to·gas·tro·scope (fō'tō-găs'trə-skōp') *n*. An instrument for taking photographs of the interior of the stomach.

pho·to·gene (fō'tə-jēn') *n*. See **afterimage.**

pho·to·in·ac·ti·va·tion (fō'tō-ĭn-ăk'tə-vā'shən) *n*. Inactivation, as of a substance, by light.

pho·to·lu·mi·nes·cent (fō'tō-lōō'mə-nĕs'ənt) *adj*. Having the ability to become luminescent upon exposure to visible light. **— pho′to·lu′mi·nes′cence** *n*.

pho·tol·y·sis (fō-tŏl'ĭ-sĭs) *n*. Chemical decomposition induced by light or other radiant energy. **— pho′to·lyt′ic** (fō'tə-lĭt'ĭk) *adj*.

pho·ton (fō'tŏn') *n*. The quantum of electromagnetic energy, generally regarded as a discrete particle having zero mass, no electric charge, and an indefinitely long lifetime. **— pho·ton′ic** *adj*.

pho·to·patch test (fō'tō-păch') *n*. A test for contact photosensitization in which a patch containing the suspected sensitizer is applied to the skin for 48 hours and, depending on the skin's reaction, exposed to a reddening dose of ultraviolet light.

pho·to·pe·ri·od (fō'tō-pîr'ē-əd) *n.* The duration of a person's daily exposure to light, considered especially with regard to the effect of the exposure on growth and development. — **pho'to·pe'·ri·od'ic** (-ŏd'ĭk), **pho'to·pe'ri·od'i·cal** (-ĭ-kəl) *adj.*

pho·to·pe·ri·od·ism (fō'tō-pîr'ē-ə-dĭz'əm) or **pho·to·pe·ri·o·dic·i·ty** (-pîr'ē-ə-dĭs'ĭ-tē) *n.* The response of a person to changes in its photoperiod, especially as indicated by vital processes.

pho·to·pho·bi·a (fō'tə-fō'bē-ə) *n.* **1.** An abnormal sensitivity to or intolerance of light, especially by the eyes, as may be caused by eye inflammation, lack of pigmentation in the iris, or various diseases. **2.** An abnormal or irrational fear of light.

pho·toph·thal·mi·a (fō'tŏf-thăl'mē-ə, -ŏp-) *n.* An inflammatory reaction of the external parts of the eye caused by intense light, as in snow blindness.

pho·to·pi·a (fō-tō'pē-ə) *n.* Vision in bright light, mediated by cone cells of the retina; daylight vision. — **pho·to'pic** (-tō'pĭk, -tŏp'ĭk) *adj.*

photopic adaptation *n.* See **light adaptation.**

photopic eye *n.* See **light-adapted eye.**

photopic vision *n.* See **photopia.**

pho·top·sin (fō-tŏp'sĭn) *n.* The protein component of the pigment iodopsin in the cones of the retina of the eye.

pho·to·ptar·mo·sis (fō'tō-tär-mō'sĭs) *n.* Reflex sneezing in response to bright light striking the retina.

pho·to·ra·di·a·tion (fō'tō-rā'dē-ā'shən) *n.* A treatment for cancer in which a laser is injected with a photosensitizing agent and the cancerous tissue is exposed to visible light, often by means of a fiberoptic probe.

pho·to·re·cep·tion (fō'tō-rĭ-sĕp'shən) *n.* The detection, absorption, and use of light, as for vision. — **pho'to·re·cep'tive** (-tĭv) *adj.*

pho·to·re·cep·tor (fō'tō-rĭ-sĕp'tər) *n.* A nerve ending, cell, or group of cells specialized to sense or receive light.

photoreceptor cell *n.* **1.** Any of the rod cells in the retina of the eye. **2.** Any of the cone cells in the retina.

pho·to·ret·i·ni·tis (fō'tō-rĕt'n-ī'tĭs) *n.* See **photoretinopathy.**

pho·to·ret·i·nop·a·thy (fō'tō-rĕt'n-ŏp'ə-thē) *n.* A macular burn from excessive exposure to sunlight or other intense light, causing reduced visual acuity.

pho·to·scan (fō'tə-skăn') *n.* See **scintigram.**

pho·to·sen·si·tive (fō'tō-sĕn'sĭ-tĭv) *adj.* **1.** Sensitive or responsive to light or other radiant energy. **2.** Abnormally sensitive or reactive to light.

pho·to·sen·si·tiv·i·ty (fō'tō-sĕn'sĭ-tĭv'ĭ-tē) *n.* **1.** Sensitivity or responsiveness to light. **2.** An abnormally heightened response, especially of the skin, to sunlight or ultraviolet radiation, caused by certain disorders or chemicals and characterized by a toxic or allergic reaction.

pho·to·sen·si·tize (fō'tō-sĕn'sĭ-tīz') *v.* **-tized, -tiz·**

ing, -tiz·es. To make an organism, a cell, or a substance photosensitive.

pho·to·steth·o·scope (fō'tō-stĕth'ə-skōp') *n.* A device that converts sound into flashes of light, used for continuous observation of the fetal heart.

pho·to·syn·the·sis (fō'tō-sĭn'thĭ-sĭs) *n.* The process in green plants and certain other organisms by which carbohydrates are synthesized from carbon dioxide and water using light as an energy source. Most forms of photosynthesis release oxygen as a byproduct. — **pho'to·syn·thet'ic** (-sĭn-thĕt'ĭk) *adj.*

pho·to·tax·is (fō'tō-tăk'sĭs) *n.* The movement of an organism or a cell toward or away from a source of light. — **pho'to·tac'tic** (-tăk'tĭk) *adj.*

pho·to·ther·a·py (fō'tō-thĕr'ə-pē) *n.* The treatment of a disorder, especially of the skin, by exposure to light, including ultraviolet and infrared radiation.

pho·to·tox·ic (fō'tō-tŏk'sĭk) *adj.* Rendering the skin susceptible to damage by light. Used of certain medications and cosmetics. — **pho'to·tox·ic'i·ty** (-tŏk-sĭs'ĭ-tē) *n.*

phre·nal·gi·a (frə-nǎl'jē-ə, -jə) *n.* **1.** See **psychalgia** (sense 1). **2.** Pain in the diaphragm.

phren·em·phrax·is (frĕn'ĕm-frăk'sĭs) *n.* See **phreniclasia.**

phren·ic (frĕn'ĭk, frē'nĭk) *adj.* **1.** Of or relating to the mind. **2.** Of or relating to the diaphragm.

phren·i·cec·to·my (frĕn'ĭ-sĕk'tə-mē) *n.* Surgical excision of a portion of the phrenic nerve.

phren·i·cla·sia (frĕn'ĭ-klā'zhə, -zē-ə) *n.* Surgical crushing of a section of the phrenic nerve as a substitute for phrenicotomy.

phrenic nerve *n.* A nerve that arises mainly from the fourth cervical nerve and is primarily the motor nerve of the diaphragm but also sends sensory fibers to the pericardium.

phren·i·co·ex·er·e·sis (frĕn'ĭ-kō-ĕk-sĕr'ĭ-sĭs) *n.* See **phrenicectomy.**

phren·i·cot·o·my (frĕn'ĭ-kŏt'ə-mē) *n.* Surgical division of the phrenic nerve to cause paralysis of the diaphragm on one side.

phren·i·co·trip·sy (frĕn'ĭ-kō-trĭp'sē) *n.* See **phreniclasia.**

phre·ni·tis (frĭ-nī'tĭs) *n.* Inflammation of the diaphragm. — **phre·nit'ic** (-nĭt'ĭk) *adj.*

phren·o·car·di·a (frĕn'ə-kär'dē-ə) *n.* Precordial pain and dyspnea of psychogenic origin.

phren·o·col·o·pex·y (frĕn'ō-kŏl'ə-pĕk'sē, -kō'-lə-) *n.* Suture of a displaced or prolapsed transverse colon to the diaphragm.

phryn·o·der·ma (frĭn'ə-dûr'mə) *n.* A follicular hyperkeratotic eruption thought to be due to deficiency of vitamin A.

PHS *abbr.* Public Health Service

phthi·ri·a·sis (thĭ-rī'ə-sĭs, thī-) *n.* Infestation with lice, especially crab lice; pediculosis.

phthiriasis pu·bis (pyōō'bĭs) *n.* Infestation of the pubic hair and sometimes the eyelashes with crab lice.

phthi·sis (thĭ'sĭs, tī'-) or **phthis·ic** (tĭz'ĭk, thĭz'-) *n.*

A disease characterized by the wasting away or atrophy of the body or a part of the body.

phy·co·my·cete (fī'kō-mī'sēt, -mī-sēt') *n.* Any of various fungi that resemble algae, including certain molds and mildews. — **phy'co·my·ce'tous** *adj.*

phy·lax·is (fĭ-lăk'sĭs) *n.* Protection against infection.

phy·lo·gen·e·sis (fī'lō-jĕn'ĭ-sĭs) *n.* See **phylogeny** (sense 1).

phy·log·e·ny (fī-lŏj'ə-nē) *n.* **1.** The evolutionary development and history of a species or higher taxonomic grouping of organisms. **2.** The evolutionary development of an organ or other part of an organism. — **phy'lo·gen'ic** (-jĕn'ĭk) *adj.*

phy·lum (fī'ləm) *n., pl.* **-la** (-lə). A taxonomic category that is a primary division of a kingdom and ranks next above a class in size.

phys·a·lis (fĭs'ə-lĭs) *n.* A vacuole in a giant cell found in certain malignant neoplasms, such as chondroma.

phys·i·at·rics (fĭz'ē-ăt'rĭks) *n.* **1.** See **physical medicine**. **2.** See **physical therapy**.

phys·i·at·rist (fĭz'ē-ăt'rĭst, fĭ-zī'ə-trĭst) *n.* **1.** A physician who specializes in physical medicine. **2.** A health care professional who administers physical therapy; a physical therapist.

phys·i·at·ry (fĭz'ē-ăt'rē, fĭ-zī'ə-trē) *n.* See **physical medicine**.

phys·ic (fĭz'ĭk) *n.* **1.** A medicine or drug, especially a cathartic. **2.** *Archaic.* The art or profession of medicine.

phys·i·cal (fĭz'ĭ-kəl) *adj.* **1.** Of or relating to the body. **2.** Involving or characterized by vigorous bodily activity. **3.** Of or relating to matter and energy or the sciences dealing with them, especially physics. — *n.* A physical examination. — **phys'i·cal'i·ty** (-kăl'ĭ-tē) *adj.*

physical diagnosis *n.* Diagnosis based on a physical examination of a patient.

physical education *n.* Education in the care and development of the body, stressing athletics and including hygiene.

physical examination *n.* A medical examination to determine the condition of a person's health or physical fitness, especially for a specified activity or service.

physical medicine *n.* The branch of medicine that deals with the treatment, prevention, and diagnosis of disease by essentially physical means, including manipulation, massage, and exercise, often with mechanical devices, and the application of heat, cold, electricity, radiation, and water.

physical sign *n.* Any of various signs that are elicited by auscultation, percussion, or palpation.

physical therapy *n.* The treatment of physical dysfunction or injury by the use of therapeutic exercise and the application of modalities intended to restore or facilitate normal function or development. — **physical therapist** *n.*

phy·si·cian (fĭ-zĭsh'ən) *n.* **1.** A person licensed to practice medicine; a medical doctor. **2.** A person

who practices general medicine as distinct from surgery.

phy·si·cian's assistant (fĭ-zĭsh'ənz) *n., pl.* **physicians' assistants.** A person trained and licensed to provide basic medical services, usually under the supervision of a physician.

phys·ics (fĭz'ĭks) *n.* **1.** The science of matter and energy and of interactions between the two, grouped in traditional fields such as acoustics, optics, and mechanics, as well as in modern extensions including atomic and nuclear physics. **2.** Physical properties, interactions, processes, or laws.

phys·i·og·no·my (fĭz'ē-ŏg'nə-mē, -ŏn'ə-mē) *n.* **1.** Facial features, especially when considered as an indicator of character or as a factor in diagnosis. **2.** Estimation of one's character and mental qualities by a study of the face and general bodily carriage.

phys·i·o·log·i·cal (fĭz'ē-ə-lŏj'ĭ-kəl) or **phys·i·o·log·ic** (-ĭk) *adj.* **1.** Of or relating to physiology. **2.** Being in accord with or characteristic of the normal functioning of a living organism. **3.** Relating to the action of a drug when given to a healthy person, as distinguished from its therapeutic action.

physiological saline *n.* A sterile solution of sodium chloride that is isotonic to body fluids, used to maintain living tissue temporarily and as a solvent for parenterally administered drugs.

physiologic dwarf *n.* An undersized but not deformed person whose development has been symmetrical and at a normal rate, but less extensive than normal.

physiologic equilibrium *n.* See **nutritive equilibrium**.

physiologic hypertrophy *n.* A temporary increase in size of an organ or part to provide for a natural increase of function such as occurs in the walls of the uterus and in the mammary glands during pregnancy.

physiologic leukocytosis *n.* Leukocytosis not directly related to a pathological condition but instead occurring in apparently normal conditions.

physiologic rest position *n.* The habitual postural position of the mandible when at rest in the upright position and the condyles are in a neutral unstrained position in the mandibular fossae.

physiologic retraction ring *n.* A ridge on the inner uterine surface at the boundary between the upper and lower uterine segments that occurs in the course of normal uterine labor.

physiologic scotoma *n.* See **blind spot** (sense 2).

physiologic unit *n.* The smallest division of an organ that will perform its specific function.

phys·i·ol·o·gy (fĭz'ē-ŏl'ə-jē) *n.* **1.** The biological study of the functions of living organisms and their parts. **2.** All the functions of a living organism or any of its parts. — **phys'i·ol'o·gist** *n.*

phys·i·o·pa·thol·o·gy (fĭz'ē-ō-pə-thŏl'ə-jē) *n.* See **pathophysiology**.

phys·i·o·ther·a·py (fĭz'ē-ō-thĕr'ə-pē) *n.* See **phys-**

ical therapy. — **phys′i·o·ther′a·peu′tic** (-thĕr′ə-pyōō′tĭk) *adj.* — **phys′i·o·ther′a·pist** *n.*

phy·sique (fĭ-zēk′) *n.* The body considered with reference to its proportions, muscular development, and appearance.

phy·so·cele (fī′sə-sēl′) *n.* **1.** A swelling filled with gas. **2.** A hernial sac distended with gas.

phy·so·stig·mine (fī′sō-stĭg′mēn′) or **phy·so·stig·min** (-mĭn) *n.* A crystalline alkaloid extracted from the Calabar bean, used in medicine as a miotic and cholinergic agent and to enhance memory in patients with Alzheimer's disease.

phy·to·ag·glu·ti·nin (fī′tō-ə-glōōt′n-ĭn) *n.* A lectin that causes agglutination of red blood cells or white blood cells.

phy·to·der·ma·ti·tis (fī′tō-dûr′mə-tī′tĭs) *n.* Dermatitis caused by various mechanisms including mechanical and chemical injury, allergy, or photosensitization at skin sites previously exposed to plants.

phy·to·he·mag·glu·ti·nin (fī′tō-hē′mə-glōōt′-n-ĭn) *n.* A hemagglutinin extracted from a plant.

phy·to·lec·tin (fī′tō-lĕk′tĭn) *n.* See **phytohemag-glutinin.**

phy·to·mi·to·gen (fī′tō-mī′tə-jən, -jĕn′) *n.* A mitogenetic lectin causing lymphocyte transformation accompanied by mitotic proliferation of the resulting blast cells identical to that produced by antigenic stimulation.

phy·to·tox·in (fī′tō-tŏk′sĭn) *n.* A toxin produced by a plant.

pi·a (pī′ə, pē′ə) *n.* The pia mater. — **pi′al** *adj.*

pi·a·a·rach·noid (pī′ə-ə-răk′noid′, pē′ə-) or **pi·a·rach·noid** (pī′ə-răk′noid′, pē′-) *n.* See **leptom-eninges.**

pia ma·ter (pī′ə mā′tər, pē′ə mä′tər) *n.* The fine vascular membrane that closely envelops the brain and spinal cord under the arachnoid and the dura mater.

pi·an (pē-än′, pyän) *n.* See **yaws.**

pi·ca (pī′kə) *n.* An abnormal craving or appetite for nonfood substances, such as dirt, paint, or clay.

Pick cell (pĭk) *n.* See **Niemann–Pick cell.**

Pick's atrophy (pĭks) *n.* Circumscribed atrophy of the cerebral cortex.

Pick's disease *n.* See **Pick's atrophy.**

pick·wick·i·an syndrome (pĭk-wĭk′ē-ən) *n.* A syndrome characterized by extreme obesity, hypoventilation, and general debility.

pi·co·me·ter (pē′kə-mē′tər, pī′-) *n.* One-trillionth (10^{-12}) of a meter.

pi·cor·na·vi·rus (pē-kôr′nə-vī′rəs, pĭ-) *n.* Any of several single-stranded RNA viruses of the family Picornaviridae, including the polioviruses, coxsackieviruses, and echoviruses.

pic·ro·tox·in (pĭk′rə-tŏk′sĭn) *n.* A bitter crystalline compound derived from the seed of an East Indian woody vine (*Animirta cocculus*) and used as a stimulant, especially in treating barbiturate poisoning.

PID *abbr.* pelvic inflammatory disease

pie·bald·ness (pī′bôld′nĭs) *n.* A skin disorder characterized by pigmentless patches of scalp hair, giving the hair a streaked appearance.

Pierre Ro·bin syndrome (pyĕr′ rô-băn′) *n.* Abnormal smallness of the jaw and tongue, often accompanied by cleft palate and bilateral eye defects such as myopia and congenital glaucoma.

pi·e·ses·the·sia (pī-ē′sĭs-thē′zhə, -zĭs-, pī′ĭs-ĭs-, pī′ĭz-ĭs-) *n.* See **pressure sense.**

pi·geon breast (pĭj′ən) *n.* A chest deformity marked by a projecting sternum, often occurring as a result of infantile rickets.

pig·ment (pĭg′mənt) *n.* **1.** A substance used as coloring. **2.** A substance, such as chlorophyll or melanin, that produces a characteristic color in plant or animal tissue. **3.** A medicinal preparation applied to the skin like paint. — *v.* **-ment·ed, -ment·ing, -ments.** To color with pigment.

pig·men·tar·y retinopathy (pĭg′mən-tĕr′ē) *n.* See **retinitis pigmentosa.**

pig·men·ta·tion (pĭg′mən-tā′shən) *n.* **1.** Coloration of tissues by pigment. **2.** Deposition of pigment by cells.

pigment cell *n.* See **chromatophore.**

pig·ment·ed (pĭg′mən-tĭd, -mĕn′-) *adj.* Colored as the result of a deposit of pigment.

pigmented vil·lo·nod·u·lar synovitis (vĭl′ō-nŏj′-ə-lər) *n.* Diffuse outgrowths of the synovial membrane of a joint, usually the knee.

pig·men·to·ly·sin (pĭg′mən-tŏl′ĭ-sĭn, -mĕn-) *n.* An antibody that destroys pigment.

pig·men·tum ni·grum (pĭg-mĕn′təm nī′grəm) *n.* Melanin of the choroid coat of the eye.

pi·lar tumor of the scalp (pī′lər) *n.* A benign solitary tumor occurring on the scalp in elderly women.

pile (pīl) *n.* A hemorrhoid.

pi·le·ous gland (pī′lē-əs) *n.* A sebaceous gland emptying into a hair follicle.

pill (pĭl) *n.* **1.** A small pellet or tablet of medicine, often coated, taken by swallowing whole or by chewing. **2.** *Informal.* An oral contraceptive.

pil·lar (pĭl′ər) *n.* A structure or part that provides support and resembles a column or pillar.

pil·low splint (pĭl′ō) *n.* A splint that is inflatable or that is made from unusually bulky fabric.

pi·lo·car·pine (pī′lō-kär′pēn′) *n.* A colorless or yellow poisonous compound obtained from the leaves of South American shrubs of the genus *Pilocarpus* and used to induce sweating, promote salivation, and treat glaucoma.

pi·lo·e·rec·tion (pī′lō-ĭ-rĕk′shən) *n.* Erection of hair.

pi·lo·jec·tion (pī′lə-jĕk′shən) *n.* The process of shooting a stiff mammalian hair into a saccular aneurysm in the brain to produce thrombosis, used in treating the aneurysm.

pi·lo·ma·trix·o·ma (pī′lō-mā′trĭk-sō′mə) *n.* A benign tumor of the skin and the tissue just below the skin that usually calcifies, often occurs as a single lesion on the face or upper extremities.

pi·lo·mo·tor reflex (pī′lō-mō′tər) *n.* Contraction of the smooth muscle of the skin caused by mild application of a tactile stimulus or by local cooling and resulting in goose bumps.

pi·lus (pī′ləs) *n., pl.* **li** (lī′). **1.** A hair. **2.** A fine filamentous appendage, somewhat analogous to the flagellum, that occurs on some bacteria.

pi·min·o·dine (pī-mĭn′ə-dēn′, pī-) *n.* A potent narcotic pain killer having a duration of action shorter than that of morphine.

pim·o·zide (pĭm′ō-zīd′) *n.* An antipshycotic drug used in the treatment of chronic schizophrenia and in the management of Tourette's syndrome.

pim·ple (pĭm′pəl) *n.* A small red swelling of the skin, usually caused by acne; a papule or pustule. — **pim′pled, pim′ply** *adj.*

pin (pĭn) *n.* A thin rod for securing the ends of fractured bones. — *v.* **pinned, pin·ning, pins.** To fasten or secure with a pin or pins.

Pi·nard's maneuver (pē-närz′) *n.* A method for delivering a fetus in breech position in which one leg is bent and its foot is brought down and out by being passed along the thigh of the other leg.

pince·ment (păns-män′, păNS-) *n.* A pinching manipulation in massage.

pinch graft *n.* A graft made with small bits of partial-thickness or full-thickness skin.

pin·do·lol (pĭn′də-lôl′, -lōl′) *n.* A beta-blocker used in the treatment of hypertension.

pin·e·al body (pĭn′ē-əl, pī′nē-) *n.* A small, unpaired, flattened glandular structure lying in the depression between the two superior colliculi of the brain and secreting the hormone melatonin.

pin·e·al·ec·to·my (pĭn′ē-ə-lĕk′tə-mē, pī′nē-) *n.* Surgical removal of the pineal body.

pineal gland *n.* See **pineal body.**

pin·e·a·lo·ma (pĭn′ē-ə-lō′mə, pī′nē-) *n.* -mas or -ma·ta (-mə-tə). A neoplasm derived from the pineal body and characterized by large, round, or polygonal cells with large nuclei and small cells that resemble lymphocytes.

pink·eye (pĭngk′ī′) *n.* See **acute contagious conjunctivitis.**

pink·ie or **pink·y** (pĭng′kē) *n.* The little finger.

pin·na (pĭn′ə) *n., pl.* **pin·nae** (pĭn′ē). See **auricle** (sense 2). — **pin′nal** *adj.*

pin·o·cyte (pĭn′ə-sīt′, pī′nə-) *n.* A cell that exhibits pinocytosis.

pin·o·cy·to·sis (pĭn′ə-sī-tō′sĭs, -sī-, pī′nə-) *n.* Introduction of fluids into a cell by invagination of its membrane, followed by formation of vesicles within the cells. — **pin′o·cy·tot′ic** (-tōt′ĭk) *adj.*

pin·o·some (pĭn′ə-sōm′, pī′nə-) *n.* A fluid-filled vacuole formed by pinocytosis.

pint (pīnt) *n.* **1.** A unit of volume or capacity in the U.S. Customary System, used in liquid measure, equal to 16 fluid ounces, 28.875 cubic inches, or 473.166 cubic centimeters. **2.** A unit of volume or capacity in the U.S. Customary System, used in dry measure, equal to ½ quart or 0.5506 liter. **3.** A unit of volume or capacity in the British Imperial System, used in dry and liquid measure, equal to 20 fluid ounces, 34.659 cubic inches, or 567.94 cubic centimeters.

pin·ta (pĭn′tə, pēn′tä) *n.* A contagious skin disease prevalent in tropical America, caused by the spirochete *Treponema carateum* and characterized

by extreme thickening and spotty discoloration of the skin.

pin·worm (pĭn′wûrm′) *n.* Any of various small nematode worms of the family Oxyuridae that are human parasites, especially *Enterobius vermicularis*, which infests the intestines and rectum.

pi·per·a·cil·lin sodium (pī-pĕr′ə-sĭl′ĭn) *n.* A semisynthetic broad-spectrum antibiotic related to penicillin and active against a variety of grampositive and gram-negative bacteria.

pi·per·a·zine (pī-pĕr′ə-zēn′, pī-) *n.* A colorless crystalline compound used as an antihistamine and an anthelmintic.

pi·per·o·caine hydrochloride (pī′pə-rō-kān′, pĭp′ə-, pī-pĕr′ə-kān′) *n.* A rapidly acting local anesthetic for infiltration and spinal anesthesia.

pi·pette or **pi·pet** (pī-pĕt′) *n.* A narrow, usually calibrated glass tube into which small amounts of liquid are suctioned for transfer or measurement.

pir·bu·ter·ol (pīr-byōō′tə-rôl′, -rōl′) *n.* An analogue of albuterol that acts as a bronchodilator and is used in the treatment of asthma.

pir·o·plas·mo·sis (pīr′ə-plăz-mō′sĭs) *n.* See **babesiosis.**

pi·rox·i·cam o·la·mine (pī-rŏk′sĭ-kăm′ ō′lə-mēn′) *n.* A nonsteroidal anti-inflammatory agent with analgesic and antipyretic actions.

pi·si·form (pī′sə-fôrm′) *n.* A small bone in the proximal row of the wrist, lying on the anterior surface of the triquetrum, with which it alone articulates.

pit (pĭt) *n.* **1.** A natural hollow or depression in the body or an organ. **2.** A small indented scar left in the skin by smallpox or other eruptive disease; a pockmark. **3.** A sharp-pointed depression in the enamel surface of a tooth, caused by faulty or incomplete calcification or formed by the confluent point of two or more lobes of enamel. — *v.* **pit·ted, pit·ting, pits.** **1.** To mark with cavities, depressions, or scars. **2.** To retain an impression after being indented. Used of the skin.

pitch wart *n.* A precancerous keratotic epidermal tumor that is common among persons who work with pitch and coal tar derivatives.

pith (pĭth) *n.* The soft inner substance of a hair.

pit·ting (pĭt′ĭng) *n.* The formation of well-defined, relatively deep depressions in a surface.

pitting edema *n.* Edema that retains for a time the indentation produced by pressure.

Pitts·burgh pneumonia (pĭts′bûrg′) *n.* A form of Legionnaires' disease caused by *Legionella micdadei.*

pi·tu·i·cyte (pī-tōō′ĭ-sīt′, -tyōō′-) *n.* A small branching cell of the posterior lobe of the pituitary gland.

pi·tu·i·ta·rism (pī-tōō′ĭ-tə-rĭz′əm, -tyōō′-) *n.* Pituitary dysfunction.

pi·tu·i·tar·y (pī-tōō′ĭ-tĕr′ē, -tyōō′-) *n.* **1.** The pituitary gland. **2.** An extract from the anterior or posterior lobes of the pituitary gland, prepared for therapeutic use. — *adj.* **1.** Of or relating to the pituitary gland. **2.** Of or secreting phlegm or mucus; mucous.

pituitary basophilism *n.* See **Cushing's syndrome.**

pituitary dwarfism *n.* A rare form of dwarfism caused by the absence of a functional anterior pituitary gland.

pituitary gland *n.* A small, oval endocrine gland attached to the base of the brain and having an anterior and a posterior lobe, the secretions of which control the other endocrine glands and influence growth, metabolism, and maturation.

pituitary gonadotropic hormone *n.* See **anterior pituitary gonadotropin.**

pituitary growth hormone *n.* See **somatotropin.**

pit·y·ri·a·sis (pĭt′ĭ-rī′ə-sĭs) *n., pl.* **-ses** (-sēz′). Any of various skin diseases characterized by epidermal shedding of flaky scales. — **pit′y·ri′a·sic** (-sĭk) *adj.*

piv·ot joint (pĭv′ət) *n.* See **trochoid joint.**

PKU *abbr.* phenylketonuria

pla·ce·bo (plə-sē′bō) *n., pl.* **-bos** or **-boes. 1.** A substance containing no medication and prescribed or given to reinforce a patient's expectation to get well. **2.** An inactive substance or preparation used as a control in an experiment or test to determine the effectiveness of a medicinal drug.

placebo effect *n.* A beneficial effect in a patient following a particular treatment that arises from the patient's expectations concerning the treatment rather than from the treatment itself.

pla·cen·ta (plə-sĕn′tə) *n., pl.* **-tas** or **-tae** (-tē). The membranous vascular organ in female mammals that permits metabolic interchange between fetus and mother. It develops from the chorion of the embryo and the decidua basalis of the maternal uterus and permits the absorption of oxygen and nutritive materials into the fetal blood and the release of carbon dioxide and nitrogenous waste from it, without the direct mixing of maternal and fetal blood. — **pla·cen′tal** *adj.*

placental barrier *n.* The semipermeable layer of tissue in the placenta that serves as a selective membrane to substances passing from maternal to fetal blood.

placental circulation *n.* Circulation of blood through the placenta during intrauterine life, serving the needs of the fetus for aeration, absorption, and excretion.

placental dystocia *n.* The retention or difficult passage of the placenta following delivery.

placental growth hormone *n.* See **human placental lactogen.**

placental lobe *n.* The part of the placenta, incompletely separated by septa, that contains the fetal cotyledon or cotyledons and the surrounding blood-filled intervillous space.

placental membrane *n.* The semipermeable layer of tissue separating maternal blood from fetal blood in the placenta.

placental souffle *n.* See **uterine souffle.**

placenta pre·vi·a (prē′vē-ə) *n.* A condition in which the placenta is implanted low in the uterus so that it is adjacent to or obstructs the internal opening of the cervix. It may cause maternal hemorrhage prior to or during labor.

placenta spu·ri·a (spyoͅor′ē-ə) *n.* A mass of placental tissue that has no vascular connection with the main placenta.

plac·en·ta·tion (plăs′ən-tā′shən) *n.* **1.** Formation of a placenta in the uterus. **2.** The type or structure of a placenta.

plac·en·ti·tis (plăs′ən-tī′tĭs) *n.* Inflammation of the placenta.

plac·en·tog·ra·phy (plăs′ən-tŏg′rə-fē) *n.* Radiography of the placenta following injection of a radiopaque substance.

plac·en·to·ma (plăs′ən-tō′mə) *n.* See **deciduoma.**

Pla·ci·do's disk (plä-sē′dōz, plä′sē-dōͅoz) *n.* See **keratoscope.**

plac·ode (plăk′ōd′) *n.* An area of thickening in the embryonic epithelial layer from which some organ or structure later develops.

plague (plāg) *n.* A highly infectious, usually fatal, epidemic disease, especially bubonic plague.

plague vaccine *n.* A vaccine prepared from live, killed, or attenuated *Yersinia pestis,* used to immunize against bubonic plague.

plane (plān) *n.* **1.** A flat or level surface. **2.** An imaginary surface formed by extension through any axis of the body or through two definite points on the body.

plane joint *n.* A synovial joint in which the opposing surfaces are nearly planes and in which there is only a slight, gliding motion.

pla·nig·ra·phy (plə-nĭg′rə-fē) *n.* See **tomography.**

plan·ing (plā′nĭng) *n.* See **dermabrasion.**

Planned Parenthood A service mark for an organization that offers family planning services.

pla·nog·ra·phy (plə-nŏg′rə-fē, plā-) *n.* See **tomography.**

plan·ta (plăn′tə) *n., pl.* **-tae** (-tē). The sole of the foot.

plan·tal·gi·a (plăn-tăl′jē-ə, -jə) *n.* Pain on the sole of the foot over the plantar fascia.

plan·tar (plăn′tər, -tär′) *adj.* Of, relating to, or occurring on the sole of the foot.

plantar fibromatosis *n.* Nodular fibroblastic proliferation in the sole of one or both feet, rarely associated with contracture.

plantar reflex *n.* Contraction of the toes in response to tactile stimulation of the ball of the foot.

plantar wart *n.* A wart occurring on the sole of the foot.

plaque (plăk) *n.* **1.** A small disk-shaped formation or growth; a patch. **2.** A deposit of fatty material on the inner lining of an arterial wall, characteristic of atherosclerosis. **3.** Dental plaque. **4.** A scaly patch formed on the skin by psoriasis. **5.** A sharply defined zone of demyelination characteristic of multiple sclerosis.

plasm (plăz′əm) *n.* Germ plasm.

plas·ma (plăz′mə) or **plasm** (plăz′əm) *n.* **1.** The clear, yellowish fluid portion of blood, lymph, or intramuscular fluid in which cells are suspended. **2.** Cell-free, sterilized blood plasma, used in transfusions. **3.** Protoplasm or cytoplasm. — **plas·mat′ic** (plăz-măt′ĭk), **plas′mic** (-mĭk) *adj.*

plas·ma·blast (plăz′mə-blăst′) *n*. The precursor or stem cell of a plasma cell.

plasma cell *n*. An antibody-producing lymphocyte derived from a B cell upon reaction with a specific antigen.

plas·ma·crit (plăz′mə-krĭt′) *n*. The percentage of the volume of blood occupied by plasma.

plasmacrit test *n*. A serologic screening method used as an aid in the diagnosis of syphilis.

plas·ma·cyte or **plas·mo·cyte** (plăz′mə-sīt′) *n*. See **plasma cell**.

plas·ma·cy·to·ma (plăz′mə-sī-tō′mə) *n*. -**mas** or -**ma·ta** (-mə-tə). A discrete, usually solitary mass of neoplastic plasma cells in bone or in one of various extramedullary sites.

plas·ma·cy·to·sis (plăz′mə-sī-tō′sĭs) *n*. **1.** The presence of plasma cells in the blood. **2.** The presence of unusually large proportions of plasma cells in the tissues or exudates.

plasma fibronectin *n*. An adhesive glycoprotein that circulates in the plasma and functions as an opsonin.

plas·ma·gene (plăz′mə-jēn′) *n*. A self-replicating hereditary structure thought to exist in cytoplasm and function in a manner analogous to, but independent of, chromosomal genes.

plas·ma·lem·ma (plăz′mə-lĕm′ə) *n*. See **cell membrane**.

plasma membrane *n*. See **cell membrane**.

plas·ma·phe·re·sis (plăz′mə-fə-rē′sĭs, -fĕr′ə-) *n*. A process in which plasma is taken from donated blood and the remaining components, mostly red blood cells, are returned to the donor.

plasma protein *n*. Any of the various dissolved proteins of blood plasma, including antibodies and blood-clotting proteins, that act by holding fluid in blood vessels by osmosis.

plasma renin activity *n*. The estimation of renin in plasma by measuring the rate of formation of angiotensin.

plas·mid (plăz′mĭd) *n*. A circular, double-stranded unit of DNA that replicates within a cell independently of the chromosomal DNA and is most often found in bacteria; it is used in recombinant DNA research to transfer genes between cells.

plas·min (plăz′mĭn) *n*. An enzyme that hydrolyzes peptides and esters of arginine and histidine and converts fibrin to soluble products. It occurs in plasma as plasminogen and is activated to plasmin by organic solvents.

plas·min·o·gen (plăz-mĭn′-ə-jən) *n*. The inactive precursor to plasmin that is found in body fluids and blood plasma.

plasminogen activator *n*. See **urokinase**.

plas·mo·di·um (plăz-mō′dē-əm) *n., pl*. -**di·a** (-dē-ə). A protozoan of the genus *Plasmodium*, which includes the parasites that cause malaria.

plas·mol·y·sis (plăz-mŏl′ĭ-sĭs) *n., pl*. -**ses** (-sēz′). Shrinkage or contraction of the protoplasm away from the wall of a living plant or bacterial cell, caused by loss of water through osmosis. — **plas′mo·lyt′ic** (plăz′mə-lĭt′ĭk) *adj*.

plas·mo·lyze (plăz′mə-līz′) *v*. -**lyzed, -lyz·ing, -lyz·es**. To subject to or undergo plasmolysis.

plas·mon (plăz′mŏn′) *n*. The aggregate of cytoplasmic or extranuclear genetic material in an organism.

plas·mor·rhex·is (plăz′mə-rĕk′sĭs) *n*. The splitting open of a cell from pressure of the protoplasm.

plas·mos·chi·sis (plăz-mŏs′kĭ-sĭs) *n*. The splitting of protoplasm into fragments.

plas·mot·ro·pism (plăz-mŏt′rə-pĭz′əm) *n*. A condition in which the bone marrow, spleen, and liver contain strongly hemolytic bodies that cause the destruction of the red blood cells, which are not affected while in the circulating blood.

plas·ter (plăs′tər) *n*. **1.** Plaster of Paris. **2.** A pastelike mixture applied to a part of the body for healing or cosmetic purposes.

plaster bandage *n*. A roller bandage impregnated with plaster of Paris and applied moist to make a rigid dressing for a fracture or a diseased joint.

plaster cast *n*. See **cast** (sense 1).

plaster of Par·is (păr′ĭs) *n*. Any of a group of gypsum cements, essentially hemihydrated calcium sulfate, a white powder that forms a paste when mixed with water and hardens into a solid, used in making casts and molds.

plas·tic surgery (plăs′tĭk) *n*. Surgery to remodel, repair, or restore body parts, especially by the transfer of tissue.

plas·tid (plăs′tĭd) *n*. Any of various granules of foreign or differentiated matter, food particles, or waste material in cells.

plate (plāt) *n*. **1.** A thin flat layer, part, or structure. **2.** A thin metallic or plastic support fitted to the gums to anchor artificial teeth. **3.** A metal bar applied to a fractured bone in order to maintain the ends in apposition. **4.** The agar layer within a Petri dish or similar vessel. — *v*. **plat·ed, plat·ing, plates.** To form a very thin layer of a bacterial culture by streaking it on the surface of agar to isolate individual organisms from which a colonial clone will develop.

pla·teau pulse (plă-tō′) *n*. The slow, sustained pulse of aortic stenosis, producing a prolonged flat-topped curve in the sphygmogram.

plate·let (plāt′lĭt) *n*. A minute, disklike cytoplasmic body found in the blood plasma of mammals that promotes blood clotting; it has no definite nucleus, no DNA, and no hemoglobin.

platelet-activating factor *n*. See **platelet-aggregating factor**.

platelet-aggregating factor *n*. A substance released from rabbit basophilic white blood cells that causes aggregation of platelets and is involved in the deposition of immune complexes.

platelet aggregation test *n*. A test of the ability of platelets to adhere to one another and form a hemostatic plug to prevent bleeding by quantifying the decrease in turbidity that occurs in platelet-rich plasma following the addition of one or several platelet-aggregating agents in vitro.

platelet-derived growth factor *n*. A substance in

platelets that is mitogenic for cells at the site of a wound, causing endothelial proliferation.

platelet factor 3 *n.* A phospholipid lipoprotein blood coagulation factor derived from platelets that acts with certain plasma thromboplastin factors to convert prothrombin to thrombin.

plate·let·phe·re·sis (plăt′lĭt-fə-rē′sĭs, -fĕr′ə-) *n.* A process in which platelets are removed from donated blood and the remaining components are returned to the donor.

platelet tissue factor *n.* See **thromboplastin.**

plat·i·num (plăt′n-əm) *n.* A ductile malleable metallic element with atomic number 78, usually occurring with other metals such as iridium or nickel and used as a catalyst and in alloys.

plat·y·hel·minth (plăt′ĭ-hĕl′mĭnth) *n.* See **flatworm.**

pla·typ·ne·a (plă-tĭp′nē-ə) *n.* Difficulty in breathing when erect, relieved by lying down.

pla·tys·ma (plə-tĭz′mə) *n., pl.* **-mas** or **-ma·ta** (-mə-tə). A platelike muscle in the neck extending to the lower face with origin from the subcutaneous layer and fascia covering the greater pectoral and deltoid muscles, with insertion to the lower border of the mandible and the platysma of the opposite side, and whose action depresses the lower lip and wrinkles the skin of the neck and the upper chest.

play therapy *n.* A form of psychotherapy used with children to help them express or act out their experiences, feelings, and problems by playing with dolls, toys, and other play material, under the guidance or observation of a therapist.

pleas·ure principle (plĕzh′ər) *n.* In psychoanalysis, the tendency or drive immediately to achieve pleasure and avoid pain as the chief motivating force in behavior.

pled·get (plĕj′ĭt) *n.* A small, flat absorbent pad used to medicate, drain, or protect a wound or sore.

pleiotropic gene *n.* A gene that causes a number of distinct but seemingly unrelated phenotypic effects.

plei·ot·ro·pism (plī-ŏt′rə-pĭz′əm) or **plei·ot·ro·py** (-pē) *n.* The control by a single gene of several distinct and seemingly unrelated phenotypic effects. — **plei′o·trop′ic** (plī′ə-trŏp′ĭk, -trō′pĭk) *adj.*

ple·o·cy·to·sis (plē′ō-sī-tō′sĭs) *n.* The presence of a greater number of cells than normal, as in the cerebrospinal fluid.

ple·o·mor·phic lipoma (plē′ə-môr′fĭk) *n.* See **atypical lipoma.**

ple·o·nasm (plē′ə-năz′əm) *n.* An excess in the number or size of parts.

ple·ro·cer·coid (plĕr′ō-sûr′koid′) *n.* The infective larva of some tapeworms, characterized by its solid elongated body.

pleth·o·ra (plĕth′ər-ə) *n.* **1.** An excess of blood in the circulatory system or in one organ or area. **2.** An excess of any of the body fluids. — **ple·thor′ic** (plĕ-thôr′ĭk) *adj.*

ple·thys·mo·gram (plē-thĭz′mə-grăm′, plə-) *n.* A record or tracing produced by a plethysmograph.

ple·thys·mo·graph (plē-thĭz′mə-grăf′, plə-) *n.* An instrument that measures variations in the size of an organ or body part on the basis of the amount of blood passing through or present in the part. — **ple·thys′mo·graph′ic** *adj.*

pleth·ys·mog·ra·phy (plĕth′ĭz-mŏg′rə-fē) *n.* The use of a plethysmograph.

pleth·ys·mom·e·try (plĕth′ĭz-mŏm′ĭ-trē) *n.* Measurement of the fullness of a hollow organ.

pleu·ra (ploŏr′ə) *n., pl.* **pleu·rae** (ploŏr′ē). The thin serous membrane that envelops each lung and folds back to make a lining for the chest cavity. — **pleu′ral** *adj.*

pleural cavity *n.* The potential space between the parietal and visceral layers of the pleura.

pleural fluid *n.* The thin film of fluid between the visceral and parietal pleurae.

pleural fremitus *n.* The vibration in the chest wall produced by the rubbing together of the roughened opposing surfaces of the pleura.

pleu·ral·gi·a (ploŏ-răl′jē-ə, -jə) *n.* See **pleurodynia** (sense 2).

pleural space *n.* See **pleural cavity.**

pleu·rec·to·my (ploŏ-rĕk′tə-mē) *n.* Surgical excision of the pleura.

pleu·ri·sy (ploŏr′ĭ-sē) *n.* Inflammation of the pleura, usually occurring as a complication of a disease such as pneumonia, accompanied by accumulation of fluid in the pleural cavity, chills, fever, and painful breathing and coughing.

pleu·rit·ic rub (ploŏ-rĭt′ĭk) *n.* A friction sound heard on auscultation that is produced by the rubbing together of the roughened surfaces of the costal and visceral pleurae.

pleu·ri·tis (ploŏ-rī′tĭs) *n.* See **pleurisy.**

pleu·ro·cele (ploŏr′ə-sēl′) *n.* See **pneumonocele.**

pleu·ro·cen·te·sis (ploŏr′ō-sĕn-tē′sĭs) *n.* See **thoracentesis.**

pleu·roc·ly·sis (ploŏ-rŏk′lĭ-sĭs) *n.* Washing out of the pleural cavity.

pleu·rod·e·sis (ploŏ-rŏd′ĭ-sĭs) *n.* The surgical creation of a fibrous adhesion between the visceral and parietal layers of the pleura, thus obliterating the pleural cavity. It is performed as a treatment in cases of recurrent spontaneous pneumothorax, malignant pleural effusion, and chylothorax.

pleu·ro·dyn·i·a (ploŏr′ə-dĭn′ē-ə) *n.* **1.** Pleuritic pain in the chest. **2.** Paroxysmal pain and soreness of muscles between the ribs, usually due to muscular rheumatism. **3.** Epidemic pleurodynia.

pleu·rog·ra·phy (ploŏ-rŏg′rə-fē) *n.* Radiography of the pleural cavity.

pleu·ro·hep·a·ti·tis (ploŏr′ō-hĕp′ə-tī′tĭs) *n.* Hepatitis with extension of the inflammation to the neighboring portion of the pleura.

pleu·ro·lith (ploŏr′ə-lĭth′) *n.* A concretion in the pleural cavity.

pleu·rol·y·sis (ploŏ-rŏl′ĭ-sĭs) *n.* Surgical division of pleural adhesions.

pleu·ro·per·i·car·di·tis (ploŏr′ō-pĕr′ĭ-kär-dī′tĭs) *n.* Inflammation of the pericardium and pleura.

pleu·ro·pneu·mo·ni·a (ploŏr′ō-noŏ-mōn′yə, -nyoŏ-)

n. Inflammation of the pleura and lungs; pneumonia aggravated by pleurisy.

pleuropneumonia-like organism *n.* See **mycoplasma.**

pleu·rot·o·my (plŏō-rŏt′ə-mē) *n.* See **thoracotomy.**

plex·ec·to·my (plĕk-sĕk′tə-mē) *n.* Surgical excision of a plexus.

plex·im·e·ter (plĕk-sĭm′ĭ-tər) or **ples·sim·e·ter** (plĕ-sĭm′-) or **plex·om·e·ter** (plĕk-sŏm′-) *n.* A small thin plate held against the body and struck with a plexor in diagnosis by percussion.

plex·o·gen·ic (plĕk′sə-jĕn′ĭk) *adj.* Giving rise to weblike structures.

plex·or (plĕk′sər) or **ples·sor** (plĕs′ər) *n.* A small, usually rubber-headed hammer used alone or with a pleximeter in examination or diagnosis by percussion.

plex·us (plĕk′səs) *n., pl.* **plexus** or **-us·es.** **1.** A structure in the form of a network, especially of nerves, blood vessels, or lymphatics. **2.** A combination of interlaced parts; a network.

pli·ca (plī′kə) *n., pl.* **pli·cae** (plī′sē, -kē). **1.** A fold or ridge, as of skin or membrane. **2.** See **false membrane.** — **pli′cal** *adj.*

pli·ca·tion (plī-kā′shən) *n.* **1.** An operation for reducing the size of a hollow structure by taking folds or tucks in its walls. **2.** The state of being folded.

pli·cot·o·my (plī-kŏt′ə-mē) *n.* Surgical division of the posterior fold of the tympanic membrane.

ploi·dy (ploi′dē) *n.* A multiple of the basic number of chromosomes in a cell.

plom·bage (pləm-bäzh′, plôm-) *n.* The use of an inert material to fill an abnormal cavity in the body.

PLSS *abbr.* portable life-support system

plug (plŭg) *n.* A dense mass of material filling a hole or closing an orifice. — *v.* **plugged, plugging, plugs.** To fill tightly with a plug.

Plum·mer–Vin·son syndrome (plŭm′ər-vĭn′sən) *n.* Difficulty in swallowing caused by degeneration of the muscle of the esophagus, atrophy of the tongue papillae, and hypochromic anemia.

plus cyclophoria *n.* See **excyclophoria.**

plu·to·ni·um (plŏō-tō′nē-əm) *n.* A radioactive metallic element with atomic number 94, occurring in uranium ores or produced artificially by neutron bombardment of uranium, used as a reactor fuel and in nuclear weapons.

P-mi·tra·le (-mī-trā′lē) *n.* An electrocardiographic syndrome consisting of broad, notched P waves in many leads with a prominent late negative component in the P wave. It is presumed to be characteristic of mitral valvular disease.

PMS *abbr.* premenstrual syndrome

pneu·mar·thro·gram (nŏō-mär′thrə-grăm′, nyŏō-) *n.* A radiograph produced by pneumarthrography.

pneu·mar·throg·ra·phy (nŏō′mär-thrŏg′rə-fē, nyŏō′-) or **pneu·mo·ar·throg·ra·phy** (nŏō′mō-är-) *n.* Radiographic examination of a joint fol-

lowing the introduction of air, with or without another contrast medium.

pneu·mar·thro·sis (nŏō′mär-thrō′sĭs, nyŏō′-) *n.* The presence of air in a joint.

pneu·mat·ic (nŏō-măt′ĭk, nyŏō-) *adj.* **1.** Of or relating to air or other gases. **2.** Relating to respiration. **3.** Relating to a structure filled with air.

pneu·ma·ti·za·tion (nŏō′mə-tĭ-zā′shən, nyŏō′-) *n.* The development of air cells or cavities, such as those of the mastoid and ethmoidal bones.

pneu·ma·to·car·di·a (nŏō′mə-tō-kär′dē-ə, nyŏō′-) *n.* The presence of air bubbles or gas in the blood of the heart.

pneu·ma·to·cele (nŏō′mə-tō-sēl′, nyŏō′-, nŏō-măt′ə-, nyŏō-) *n.* **1.** An emphysematous or gaseous swelling. **2.** See **pneumonocele. 3.** A thin-walled cavity formed within the lung, characteristic of staphylococcus pneumonia.

pneu·ma·tom·e·ter (nŏō′mə-tŏm′ĭ-tər, nyŏō′-) *n.* An instrument for measuring the force or volume of inspiration or expiration in the lungs.

pneu·ma·tor·rha·chis (nŏō′mə-tôr′ə-kĭs, nyŏō′-) *n.* See **pneumorrhachis.**

pneu·ma·to·sis (nŏō′mə-tō′sĭs, nyŏō′-) *n.* Abnormal accumulation of gas in any tissue or other part of the body.

pneu·ma·tu·ri·a (nŏō′mə-tŏŏr′ē-ə, nyŏō′mə-tyŏŏr′-) *n.* Passage of gas or air from the urethra during or after urination.

pneu·mo·an·gi·og·ra·phy (nŏō′mō-ăn′jē-ŏg′rə-fē, nyŏō′-) *n.* The radiographic study of the pulmonary and bronchial blood vessels.

pneu·mo·ba·cil·lus (nŏō′mō-bə-sĭl′əs, nyŏō′-) *n., pl.* **-cil·li** (-sĭl′ī′). A nonmotile, gram-negative bacterium *(Klebsiella pneumoniae)* that causes a severe form of pneumonia and is associated with other respiratory infections.

pneu·mo·cele (nŏō′mə-sēl′, nyŏō′-) *n.* See **pneumonocele.**

pneu·mo·ceph·a·lus (nŏō′mō-sĕf′ə-ləs, nyŏō′-) *n.* The presence of air or gas in the cranial cavity.

pneu·mo·coc·cal vaccine (nŏō′mə-kŏk′əl, nyŏō′-) *n.* A vaccine containing purified capsular polysaccharide antigen from the most common infectious types of *Streptococcus pneumoniae,* used to immunize against pneumonococcal disease.

pneu·mo·coc·ce·mi·a (nŏō′mō-kŏk-sē′mē-ə, nyŏō′-) *n.* The presence of pneumococci in the blood.

pneu·mo·coc·co·sis (nŏō′mə-kŏ-kō′sĭs, nyŏō′-) *n.* Infection with pneumococci.

pneu·mo·coc·co·su·ri·a (nŏō′mə-kŏk′ə-sŏŏr′ē-ə, nyŏō′-) *n.* The presence of pneumococci or of their specific capsular substance in the urine.

pneu·mo·coc·cus (nŏō′mə-kŏk′əs, nyŏō′-) *n., pl.* **-coc·ci** (-kŏk′sī′, -kŏk′ī′). A nonmotile, gram-positive bacterium *(Streptococcus pneumoniae)* that is the most common cause of bacterial pneumonia and is associated with meningitis and other infectious diseases. — **pneu′mo·coc′cal** (-kŏk′əl) *adj.*

pneu·mo·co·ni·o·sis (nŏō′mō-kō′nē-ō′sĭs, nyŏō′-)

n., pl. **-ses** (-sēz). A disease of the lungs, such as asbestosis or silicosis, caused by long-term inhalation of dusts, especially mineral or metallic dusts.

pneu·mo·cra·ni·um (nōō'mō-krā'nē-əm, nyōō'-) *n.* The presence of air between the cranium and the dura mater.

Pneu·mo·cys·tis ca·ri·nii pneumonia (nōō'mə-sĭs'tĭs, nyōō' kə-rī'-nē-ē) *n.* Pneumonia resulting from infection with *Pneumocystis carinii.* It is particularly frequent among immunologically compromised individuals and is characterized by alveoli filled with a network of acidophilic material within which the organisms are enmeshed.

pneu·mo·cys·tog·ra·phy (nōō'mō-sĭ-stŏg'rə-fē, nyōō'-) *n.* Radiography of the bladder following the injection of air.

pneu·mo·cys·to·sis (nōō'mō-sĭ-stō'sĭs, nyōō'-) *n.* See **Pneumocystis carinii pneumonia.**

pneu·mo·der·ma (nōō'mə-dûr'mə, nyōō'-) *n.* See **subcutaneous emphysema.**

pneu·mo·dy·nam·ics (nōō'mō-dī-năm'ĭks, nyōō'-) *n.* The mechanics of respiration.

pneu·mo·en·ceph·a·log·ra·phy (nōō'mō-ĕn-sĕf'ə-lŏg'rə-fē, nyōō'-) *n.* Radiographic visualization of the cerebral ventricles and subarachnoid spaces after the injection of air or gas. — **pneu'·mo·en·ceph'a·lo·gram'** (-ə-lə-grăm', -ə-lō-) *n.*

pneu·mo·gram (nōō'mə-grăm', nyōō'-) *n.* A radiograph of an organ inflated with air.

pneu·mog·ra·phy (nōō-mŏg'rə-fē, nyōō-) *n.* Radiography of the lungs. — **pneu'mo·graph'** (nōō'mə-grăf', nyōō'-), **pneu·mat'o·graph'** (nōō-măt'ə-grăf', nyōō-) *n.*

pneu·mo·hy·dro·me·tra (nōō'mō-hī'drō-mē'trə, nyōō'-) *n.* The presence of gas and serum in the uterine cavity.

pneu·mo·hy·dro·per·i·car·di·um (nōō'mō-hī'drō-pĕr'ĭ-kär'dē-əm, nyōō'-) *n.* See **hydropneumopericardium.**

pneu·mo·lith (nōō'mə-lĭth', nyōō'-) *n.* A calculus in the lung.

pneu·mo·li·thi·a·sis (nōō'mō-lĭ-thī'ə-sĭs, nyōō'-) *n.* The formation of calculi in the lungs.

pneu·mo·me·di·as·ti·num (nōō'mō-mē'dē-ə-stī'nəm, nyōō'-) *n.* The escape of air into the mediastinal tissues, usually from interstitial emphysema or from a ruptured pulmonary bleb.

pneu·mo·my·e·log·ra·phy (nōō'mō-mī'ə-lŏg'rə-fē, nyōō'-) *n.* Radiographic examination of the spinal canal after the injection of air or gas.

pneu·mo·nec·to·my (nōō'mə-nĕk'tə-mē, nyōō'-) or **pneu·mec·to·my** (nōō-mĕk'tə-mē, nyōō-) *n.* Surgical removal of all or part of a lung.

pneu·mo·nia (nōō-mōn'yə, nyōō-) *n.* An acute or chronic disease marked by inflammation of the lungs and caused by viruses, bacteria, or other microorganisms and sometimes by physical and chemical irritants.

pneu·mon·ic (nōō-mŏn'ĭk, nyōō-) *adj.* **1.** Relating to, affected by, or similar to pneumonia. **2.** Of, affecting, or relating to the lungs; pulmonary.

pneumonic plague *n.* A frequently fatal form of bubonic plague in which the lungs are infected and the disease is transmissible by coughing.

pneu·mo·ni·tis (nōō'mə-nī'tĭs, nyōō'-) *n.* Inflammation of lung tissue.

pneu·mo·no·cele (nōō'mə-nō-sēl', nyōō'-, nōō-mŏn'ə-, nyōō-) *n.* Protrusion of a portion of the lung through a defect in the chest wall.

pneu·mo·no·cen·te·sis (nōō'mə-nō-sĕn-tē'sĭs, nyōō'-) or **pneu·mo·cen·te·sis** (nōō'mō-, nyōō'-) *n.* Paracentesis of the lung.

pneu·mo·no·coc·cal (nōō'mə-nō-kŏk'əl, nyōō'-) *adj.* Relating to or associated with *Streptococcus pneumoniae.*

pneu·mo·no·cyte (nōō'mə-nō-sīt', nyōō'-, nōō-mŏn'ə-, nyōō-) *n.* Any of the cells lining the alveoli in the respiratory part of the lung.

pneu·mo·no·pex·y (nōō'mə-nō-pĕk'sē, nyōō'-, nōō-mŏn'ə-, nyōō-) *n.* Surgical fixation of the lung by suturing the costal and pulmonary pleurae or otherwise causing adhesion of the layers.

pneu·mo·nor·rha·phy (nōō'mə-nôr'ə-fē, nyōō'-) *n.* Suture of the lung.

pneu·mo·not·o·my (nōō'mə-nŏt'ə-mē, nyōō'-) *n.* Incision of the lung.

pneu·mo·or·bi·tog·ra·phy (nōō'mō-ôr'bĭ-tŏg'rə-fē, nyōō'-) *n.* Radiographic visualization of the eye socket after the injection of a gas.

pneu·mo·per·i·car·di·um (nōō'mō-pĕr'ĭ-kär'dē-əm, nyōō'-) *n.* The presence of gas in the pericardial sac.

pneu·mo·per·i·to·ne·um (nōō'mō-pĕr'ĭ-tn-ē'əm, nyōō'-) *n.* The presence of air or gas in the peritoneal cavity as a result of disease, or produced artificially for treatment of certain conditions.

pneu·mo·per·i·to·ni·tis (nōō'mō-pĕr'ĭ-tn-ī'tĭs, nyōō'-) *n.* Inflammation of the peritoneum, with an accumulation of gas in the peritoneal cavity.

pneu·mo·pleu·ri·tis (nōō'mō-plŏō-rī'tĭs, nyōō'-) *n.* Pleurisy with the presence of air or gas in the pleural cavity.

pneu·mo·py·e·log·ra·phy (nōō'mō-pī'ə-lŏg'rə-fē, nyōō'-) *n.* Radiographic examination of the kidney after a gas has been injected into the kidney pelvis.

pneu·mo·py·o·tho·rax (nōō'mō-pī'ə-thôr'ăks', nyōō'-) *n.* See **pyopneumothorax.**

pneu·mo·ra·di·og·ra·phy (nōō'mō-rā'dē-ŏg'rə-fē, nyōō'-) *n.* Radiographic study of an organ or part after air has been injected into it.

pneu·mo·ret·ro·per·i·to·ne·um (nōō'mō-rĕt'rō-pĕr'ĭ-tn-ē'əm, nyōō'-) *n.* Escape of air into the retroperitoneal tissues.

pneu·mor·rha·chis (nōō'mə-rā'kĭs, nyōō'-, nōō-môr'ə-kĭs, nyōō-) *n.* The presence of gas in the spinal canal.

pneu·mo·tach·o·gram (nōō'mə-tăk'ə-grăm', nyōō'-) *n.* A record produced by a pneumotachograph.

pneu·mo·tach·o·graph (nōō'mə-tăk'ə-grăf', nyōō'-) *n.* An apparatus for recording the rate of airflow to and from the lungs.

pneu·mo·ta·chom·e·ter (nōō'mō-tə-kŏm'ĭ-tər, nyōō'-) *n.* See **pneumotachograph.**

pneu·mo·tho·rax (nōō'mō-thôr'ăks', nyōō'-) *n.* Accumulation of air or gas in the pleural cavity, occurring as a result of disease or injury, or sometimes induced to collapse the lung in the treatment of tuberculosis and other lung diseases.

pneu·mot·o·my (nōō-mŏt'ə-mē, nyōō-) *n.* See **pneumonotomy.**

pock (pŏk) *n.* **1.** The characteristic pustular cutaneous lesion of smallpox. **2.** A mark or scar left in the skin by such a pustule; a pockmark.

pock·et (pŏk'ĭt) *n.* **1.** In anatomy, a cul-de-sac or pouchlike cavity. **2.** A diseased space between the inflamed gum and the surface of a tooth. **3.** A collection of pus in a nearly closed sac. — *v.* **-et·ed, -et·ing, -ets. 1.** To enclose within a confined space. **2.** To approach the surface at a localized spot, as with the thinned out wall of an abscess which is about to rupture.

pocketed calculus *n.* See **encysted calculus.**

pock·mark (pŏk'märk') *n.* A pitlike scar left on the skin by smallpox or another eruptive disease. — **pock'marked'** *adj.*

po·dag·ra (pə-dăg'rə) *n.* Gout, especially of the big toe. — **po·dag'ral, po·dag'ric** *adj.*

po·dal·gi·a (pō-dăl'jē-ə, -jə) *n.* Pain in the foot.

po·dal·ic version (pō-dăl'ĭk) *n.* Version resulting in delivery of the fetus by the feet.

pod·e·de·ma (pŏd'ĭ-dē'mə) *n.* Edema of the feet and ankles.

podiatric medicine *n.* See **podiatry.**

po·di·a·try (pə-dī'ə-trē) *n.* The branch of medicine concerned with the diagnosis and medical, surgical, mechanical, physical, and adjunctive treatment of the diseases, injuries, and defects of the human foot. — **po'di·at'ric** (pō'dē-ăt'rĭk) *adj.* — **po·di'a·trist** *n.*

pod·o·cyte (pŏd'ə-sīt') *n.* An epithelial cell of the renal glomerulus, attached to the outer surface of the glomerular capillary basement membrane by cytoplasmic foot processes.

pod·o·dy·na·mom·e·ter (pŏd'ō-dī'nə-mŏm'ĭ-tər) *n.* An instrument for measuring the strength of the muscles of the foot or leg.

pod·o·dyn·i·a (pŏd'ə-dĭn'ē-ə) *n.* See **podalgia.**

pod·o·gram (pŏd'ə-grăm') *n.* An imprint or an outline tracing of the sole of the foot.

pod·o·mech·a·no·ther·a·py (pŏd'ō-měk'ə-nō-thĕr'ə-pē) *n.* The treatment of foot conditions with mechanical devices such as arch supports.

pod·o·phyl·lin (pŏd'ə-fĭl'ĭn) *n.* A bitter-tasting resin obtained from the dried root of the May apple and used as a cathartic and caustic.

pod·o·phyl·lo·tox·in (pŏd'ə-fĭl'ə-tŏk'sĭn) *n.* A toxic polycyclic substance having cathartic properties and antineoplastic activity.

po·go·ni·a·sis (pō'gə-nī'ə-sĭs) *n.* **1.** Growth of a beard on a woman. **2.** Excessive hairiness of the face in men.

poi·ki·lo·blast (poi'kə-lə-blăst', poi-kĭl'ə-) *n.* A nucleated red blood cell of irregular shape.

poi·ki·lo·cyte (poi'kə-lə-sīt', poi-kĭl'ə-) *n.* A red blood cell of irregular shape.

poi·ki·lo·cy·the·mi·a (poi'kə-lō-sī-thē'mē-ə) *n.* See **poikilocytosis.**

poi·ki·lo·cy·to·sis (poi'kə-lō-sī-tō'sĭs) *n.* The presence of poikilocytes in the peripheral blood.

poi·ki·lo·der·ma (poi'kə-lō-dûr'mə) *n.* A variegated hyperpigmentation and telangiectasia of the skin, followed by atrophy.

poi·ki·lo·ther·mic (poi'kə-lō-thûr'mĭk) or **poi·ki·lo·ther·mal** (-mal) or **poi·ki·lo·ther·mous** (-məs) *adj.* **1.** Of or relating to an organism having a body temperature that varies with the temperature of its surroundings; cold-blooded. **2.** Capable of existence and growth in mediums of varying temperatures. — **poi'ki·lo·ther'mi·a, poi'ki·lo·ther'mism** *n.*

point (point) *n.* A stage or condition reached. — *v.* **point·ed, point·ing, points.** To become ready to open, as an abscess or boil.

point angle *n.* The junction of three surfaces, as of the crown of a tooth or the walls of a cavity.

point epidemic *n.* An epidemic in which several cases of a disease occur within a few days or hours due to exposure to a common source of infection such as food or water.

poin·til·lage (pwăn-tē-yäzh') *n.* A massage manipulation with the tips of the fingers.

point mutation *n.* A mutation that involves a single nucleotide and may consist of loss of a nucleotide, substitution of one nucleotide for another, or the insertion of an additional nucleotide.

point of fixation *n.* The point on the retina at which the light rays coming directly from an object are focused.

point-system test types *pl.n.* A near vision test chart containing test types that are multiples of a point (¹⁄₂ inch), lower-case letters being one-half the designated point size; reading 4-point type at a distance of 16 inches is normal.

Poi·seuille's space (pwä-zœ'yēz) *n.* See **still layer.**

poi·son (poi'zən) *n.* **1.** A substance taken internally or applied externally that is injurious to health or dangerous to life. **2.** A chemical substance that inhibits another substance or a reaction. — *v.* **-soned, -son·ing, -sons.** To kill or harm with poison.

poison ivy *n.* A North American shrub or vine (*Rhus radicans*) that has compound leaves with three leaflets, small green flowers, and whitish berries and that causes a rash on contact.

poison oak *n.* **1.** Either of two shrubs, *Rhus toxicodendron* of the southeast United States or *R. diversiloba* of western North America, related to poison ivy and causing a rash on contact. **2.** See **poison ivy.**

poison sumac *n.* A swamp shrub (*Rhus vernix*) of the southeast United States, having compound leaves and greenish-white berries and causing an itching rash on contact with the skin.

po·lar (pō'lər) *adj.* Having poles. Used of certain nerve cells having one or more processes.

polar body *n.* Either of two small cells formed by the ovum during its maturation, the first usually released just before ovulation and the second released after the ovum has been discharged from the ovary and penetrated by a sperm cell.

po·lar·i·ty (pō-lăr′ĭ-tē, pə-) *n.* The property of having two opposite poles or of having opposite properties or characteristics.

po·lar·i·za·tion (pō′lər-ĭ-zā′shən) *n.* **1.** The production or condition of polarity. **2.** The development of differences in potential between two points in living tissues, as between the inside and outside of the cell wall.

pol·i·clin·ic (pŏl′ē-klĭn′ĭk) *n.* The department of a hospital or health care facility that treats outpatients.

po·li·o (pō′lē-ō′) *n.* poliomyelitis.

po·li·o·dys·tro·phy (pō′lē-ō-dĭs′trə-fē) *n.* Wasting of the gray matter of the nervous system.

po·li·o·en·ceph·a·li·tis (pō′lē-ō-ĕn-sĕf′ə-lī′tĭs) *n.* An acute infectious inflammation of the gray matter of the brain, either of the cortex or of the central nuclei.

po·li·o·en·ceph·a·lo·me·nin·go·my·e·li·tis (pō′lē-ō-ĕn-sĕf′ə-lō-mə-nĭng′gō-mī′ə-lī′tĭs) *n.* Inflammation of the gray matter of the brain and spinal cord and of their meningeal covering.

po·li·o·my·e·li·tis (pō′lē-ō-mī′ə-lī′tĭs) *n.* A highly infectious viral disease that chiefly affects children and, in its acute forms, causes inflammation of motor neurons of the spinal cord and brainstem, leading to paralysis, muscular atrophy, and often deformity. Through vaccination, the disease is preventable.

poliomyelitis immune globulin *n.* A sterile solution of globulins containing antibodies normally present in adult human blood that is used as a passive immunological agent to confer temporary protection against paralytic polio and to attenuate or prevent poliomyelitis, measles, and infectious hepatitis.

poliomyelitis virus *n.* The picornavirus that causes poliomyelitis in humans. Serologic types 1, 2, and 3 are recognized, type 1 being responsible for most cases of paralytic poliomyelitis and most epidemics.

po·li·o·my·e·lo·en·ceph·a·li·tis (pō′lē-ō-mī′ə-lō-ĕn-sĕf′ə-lī′tĭs) *n.* Acute anterior poliomyelitis with encephalitis.

po·li·o·vi·rus (pō′lē-ō-vī′rəs) *n.* See poliomyelitis virus.

poliovirus vaccine or **poliomyelitis vaccine** *n.* **1.** An aqueous suspension of inactivated strains of poliomyelitis virus given by injection, now largely replaced by the oral vaccine. **2.** An aqueous suspension of live attenuated strains of poliomyelitis virus, given orally for active immunization against poliomyelitis.

Po·lit·zer bag (pō′lĭt-sər) *n.* A pear-shaped rubber bag used to force air through the eustachian tube.

po·lit·zer·i·za·tion (pō′lĭt-sər-ĭ-zā′shən, pŏl′ĭt-) *n.* Inflation of the auditory tube and middle ear with a Politzer bag.

pol·len (pŏl′ən) *n.* Microspores of seed plants carried by wind or insects prior to fertilization; many airborne types are allergens.

pollen count *n.* The average number of pollen grains, usually of ragweed, in a cubic yard or other standard volume of air over a 24-hour period at a specified time and place.

pol·lex (pŏl′ĕks′) *n., pl.* **pol·li·ces** (pŏl′ĭ-sēz′). The thumb.

pol·li·ci·za·tion (pŏl′ĭ-sĭ-zā′shən) *n.* Surgical construction of a substitute thumb.

pol·li·no·sis or **pol·le·no·sis** (pŏl′ə-nō′sĭs) *n.* Hay fever caused by an allergic reaction to pollen of various plants.

po·lo·ni·um (pə-lō′nē-əm) *n.* A radioactive metallic element with atomic number 84, occurring in minute quantities in uranium ores and produced by bombarding bismuth with neutrons.

pol·y·ad·e·ni·tis (pŏl′ē-ăd′n-ī′tĭs) *n.* Inflammation of many lymph nodes.

pol·y·ad·e·nop·a·thy (pŏl′ē-ăd′n-ŏp′ə-thē) or **pol·y·ad·e·no·sis** (-ō′sĭs) *n.* A disorder affecting many lymph nodes.

pol·y·a·mine (pŏl′ē-ə-mēn′, -ăm′ēn) *n.* Any of a group of organic compounds that contain two or more amino groups.

pol·y·an·gi·i·tis (pŏl′ē-ăn′jē-ī′tĭs) *n.* Inflammation of more than one type of blood vessel.

pol·y·ar·te·ri·tis (pŏl′ē-är′tə-rī′tĭs) *n.* Simultaneous inflammation of a number of arteries.

pol·y·ar·thri·tis (pŏl′ē-är-thrī′tĭs) *n.* Simultaneous inflammation of several joints.

polyarthritis chron·i·ca vil·lo·sa (krŏn′ĭ-kə vĭ-lō′sə) *n.* Chronic inflammation confined to the synovial membrane and involving a number of joints.

pol·y·blast (pŏl′ē-blăst′) *n.* One of a group of ameboid, mononucleated, phagocytic cells found in inflammatory exudates.

pol·y·chlo·rin·at·ed biphenyl (pŏl′ē-klôr′ə-nā′tĭd) *n.* PCB.

pol·y·chon·dri·tis (pŏl′ē-kŏn-drī′tĭs) *n.* Simultaneous inflammation of many cartilages.

pol·y·chro·ma·si·a (pŏl′ē-krō-mā′zē-ə, -zhə) *n.* See polychromatophilia.

pol·y·chro·mat·ic cell (pŏl′ē-krō-măt′ĭk) *n.* See polychromatophil.

pol·y·chro·mat·o·cyte (pŏl′ē-krō-măt′ə-sīt′, -krō′mə-tə-) *n.* See polychromatophil.

pol·y·chro·mat·o·phil (pŏl′ē-krō-măt′ə-fĭl′, -krō′mə-tə-) *n.* A young or degenerated red blood cell staining with both acid and basic dyes. *— adj.* Staining readily with acidic, neutral, or basic dyes.

pol·y·chro·mat·o·phil·i·a (pŏl′ē-krō-măt′ə-fĭl′ē-ə, -krō′mə-tə-) or **pol·y·chro·mo·phil·i·a** (pŏl′ē-krō′mə-fĭl′ē-ə) *n.* Affinity for more than one type of stain, especially for both basic and acidic stains. **— pol′y·chro·mat′o·phil′ic** (-fĭl′ĭk), **pol′y·chro·mat′o·phile′** (-fīl′) *adj.*

pol·y·chro·me·mi·a (pŏl′ē-krō-mē′mē-ə) *n.* An increase in the total amount of hemoglobin in the blood.

pol·y·clin·ic (pŏl′ē-klĭn′ĭk) *n.* A clinic, hospital, or health care facility that treats various types of diseases and injuries.

pol·y·clone (pŏl′ē-klōn′) *n.* A clone descended from one or more small groups of cells, especially ones of genetically different origins. — **pol′y·clo′nal** *adj.* — **pol′y·clo′nal·ly** *adv.*

po·lyc·ro·tism (pə-lĭk′rə-tĭz′əm) *n.* A condition in which the sphygmographic tracing shows several upward breaks in the descending wave.

pol·y·cy·e·sis (pŏl′ē-sī-ē′sĭs) *n.* The state of bearing two or more fetuses simultaneously.

pol·y·cys·tic kidney (pŏl′ē-sĭs′tĭk) *n.* An inherited progressive disease characterized by formation of multiple cysts of varying size scattered diffusely throughout both kidneys and resulting in destruction of the kidney parenchyma, hypertension, bloody urine, and uremia.

pol·y·cy·the·mi·a (pŏl′ē-sī-thē′mē-ə) *n.* A condition characterized by an abnormally high number of red blood cells in the blood.

pol·y·dac·ty·ly (pŏl′ē-dăk′tə-lē) or **pol·y·dac·tyl·ism** (-tə-lĭz′əm) *n.* The condition of having more than five digits on a hand or foot.

pol·y·dip·si·a (pŏl′ē-dĭp′sē-ə) *n.* Excessive or abnormal thirst. — **pol′y·dip′sic** *adj.*

pol·y·dys·pla·sia (pŏl′ē-dĭs-plā′zhə, -zhē-ə) *n.* Abnormal development in several types of tissue.

pol·y·e·lec·tro·lyte (pŏl′ē-ĭ-lĕk′trə-līt′) *n.* An electrolyte, such as a protein or polysaccharide, having a high molecular weight.

pol·y·em·bry·o·ny (pŏl′ē-ĕm′brē-ə-nē, -ĕm-brī′-) *n.* Development of more than one embryo from a single egg or ovule.

pol·y·ga·lac·ti·a (pŏl′ē-gə-lăk′tē-ə, -shē-ə) *n.* Excessive secretion of breast milk, especially at the weaning period.

pol·y·gene (pŏl′ē-jēn′) *n.* One of a group of nonallelic genes acting together to produce quantitative variations of a particular character.

pol·y·graph (pŏl′ē-grăf′) *n.* An instrument that simultaneously records changes in physiological processes such as heartbeat, blood pressure, and respiration.

pol·y·gy·ri·a (pŏl′ĭ-jī′rē-ə) *n.* The presence of an excessive number of convolutions in the brain.

pol·y·hy·dram·ni·os (pŏl′ē-hī-drăm′nē-ŏs′) *n.* An excess in the amount of amniotic fluid.

pol·y I:C (pŏl′ē ī′sē′) *n.* A synthetic chemical that resembles the RNA of infectious viruses and is used to stimulate the production of interferon by the immune system.

pol·y·men·or·rhe·a (pŏl′ē-mĕn′ə-rē′ə) *n.* The occurrence of menstrual cycles of greater than usual frequency.

pol·y·mer (pŏl′ə-mər) *n.* Any of numerous natural and synthetic compounds of usually high molecular weight consisting of up to millions of repeated linked units, each a relatively light and simple molecule.

pol·y·mer·ase (pŏl′ə-mə-rās′, -rāz′) *n.* Any of various enzymes that catalyze polymerization, especially those that catalyze the synthesis of polynucleotides of DNA or RNA using an existing strand of DNA or RNA as a template.

pol·y·me·ri·a (pŏl′ĭ-mêr′ē-ə) *n.* An excessive number of parts, limbs, or organs of the body.

pol·y·mer·ic (pŏl′ə-mĕr′ĭk) *adj.* **1.** Having the properties of a polymer. **2.** Of or relating to polymeria.

pol·y·mor·phism (pŏl′ē-môr′fĭz′əm) *n.* The occurrence of different forms, stages, or types in individual organisms or in organisms of the same species, independent of sexual variations. — **pol′y·mor′phic, pol′y·mor′phous** *adj.*

polymorphonuclear leukocyte *n.* A white blood cell, usually neutrophilic, having a nucleus that is divided into lobes connected by strands of chromatin.

pol·y·my·al·gi·a (pŏl′ē-mī-ăl′jē-ə, -jə) *n.* Pain in several muscle groups.

pol·y·my·o·si·tis (pŏl′ē-mī′ə-sī′tĭs) *n.* Inflammation of several voluntary muscles simultaneously.

pol·y·myx·in (pŏl′ē-mĭk′sĭn) *n.* Any of various mainly toxic antibiotics derived from strains of the soil bacterium *Bacillus polymyxa* and used to treat infections with gram-negative bacteria.

pol·y·neu·ral·gia (pŏl′ē-nōō-răl′jə, -nyōō-) *n.* Simultaneous neuralgia of several nerves.

pol·y·neu·ri·tis (pŏl′ē-nōō-rī′tĭs, -nyōō-) *n.* Inflammation of several nerves at one time, marked by paralysis, pain, and muscle wasting. — **pol′y·neu·rit′ic** (-rĭt′ĭk) *adj.*

pol·y·neu·rop·a·thy (pŏl′ē-nōō-rŏp′ə-thē, -nyōō-) *n.* A disease process involving several peripheral nerves.

pol·y·nu·cle·o·tide (pŏl′ē-nōō′klē-ə-tīd′, -nyōō′-) *n.* A polymer containing a chain of nucleotides.

pol·y·on·co·sis (pŏl′ē-ŏng-kō′sĭs) *n.* The formation of multiple tumors.

pol·y·o·nych·i·a (pŏl′ē-ō-nĭk′ē-ə) *n.* The presence of supernumerary nails on the fingers or toes.

pol·y·o·pi·a (pŏl′ē-ō′pē-ə) *n.* The perception of several visual images of one object.

pol·y·or·chism (pŏl′ē-ôr′kĭz′əm) or **pol·y·or·chi·dism** (-ôr′kĭ-dĭz′əm) *n.* The presence of one or more supernumerary testes.

pol·y·o·ti·a (pŏl′ē-ō′shē-ə) *n.* The presence of a supernumerary auricle on one or both sides of the head.

pol·y·o·vu·la·to·ry (pŏl′ē-ō′vyə-lə-tôr′ē, -ŏv′yə-) *n.* Discharging several ova in one ovulatory cycle.

pol·yp (pŏl′ĭp) *n.* A usually nonmalignant growth of tissue protruding from the mucous lining of an organ such as the nose, bladder, or intestine, often causing obstruction. — **pol′yp·oid′** *adj.*

pol·yp·ec·to·my (pŏl′ə-pĕk′tə-mē) *n.* Excision of a polyp.

pol·y·pep·tide (pŏl′ē-pĕp′tīd′) *n.* A peptide containing many molecules of amino acids, typically between 10 and 100.

pol·y·pha·gi·a (pŏl′ē-fā′jē-ə, -jə) *n.* Excessive eating; gluttony.

pol·y·pho·bi·a (pŏl′ĭ-fō′bē-ə) *n.* An abnormal fear of many things; a condition marked by the presence of many phobias.

pol·y·phra·si·a (pŏl′ĭ-frā′zē-ə, -zhə) *n.* Extreme talkativeness.

pol·y·phy·let·ic (pŏl′ē-fī-lĕt′ĭk) *adj.* **1.** Descended or derived from more than one ancestral stock or source. **2.** Of or being the theory that blood cells are derived from several different stem cells, depending on the particular blood cell type. — **pol′-y·phy′le·tism** (-fī′lĭ-tĭz′əm) *n.*

pol·y·ple·gi·a (pŏl′ē-plē′jē-ə, -jə) *n.* Paralysis of several muscles.

pol·yp·ne·a (pŏl′ĭp-nē′ə) *n.* See **tachypnea**.

pol·y·po·si·a (pŏl′ē-pō′zē-ə) *n.* Sustained excessive consumption of fluids.

pol·yp·o·sis (pŏl′ə-pō′sĭs) *n.* The presence of several polyps.

pol·y·pous (pŏl′ə-pəs) *adj.* Relating to, resembling, or characterized by the presence of a polyp or polyps.

polypous gastritis *n.* Chronic gastritis marked by irregular atrophy of the mucous membrane forming knobby or polypoid projections.

pol·y·ptych·i·al (pŏl′ē-tĭk′ē-əl, -tī′kē-əl) *adj.* Folded or arranged to form more than one layer.

pol·y·pus (pŏl′ə-pəs) *n., pl.* **-pi** (-pī′). See **polyp**.

pol·y·ra·dic·u·lo·neu·rop·a·thy (pŏl′ē-rə-dĭk′-yə-lō-nŏŏ-rŏp′ə-thē, -nyŏŏ-) *n.* See **acute idiopathic polyneuritis**.

pol·y·ri·bo·some (pŏl′ē-rī′bə-sōm′) *n.* A cluster of ribosomes connected by a strand of mRNA and functioning as a unit in protein synthesis.

pol·y·sac·cha·ride (pŏl′ē-săk′ə-rīd′) or **pol·y·sac·cha·rid** (-rĭd) or **pol·y·sac·cha·rose** (-rōs′, -rōz′) *n.* Any of a class of carbohydrates, such as starch and cellulose, consisting of a number of monosaccharides joined by glycosidic bonds.

pol·y·se·ro·si·tis (pŏl′ē-sĕr′ō-sī′tĭs) *n.* Chronic inflammation of several serous membranes with effusions in serous cavities resulting in fibrous thickening of the serosa and constrictive pericarditis.

pol·y·si·nus·i·tis (pŏl′ē-sī′nə-sī′tĭs) *n.* Simultaneous inflammation of two or more sinuses.

pol·y·some (pŏl′ē-sōm′) *n.* See **polyribosome**.

pol·y·so·mi·a (pŏl′ē-sō′mē-ə) *n.* A fetal malformation involving two or more imperfect and partially fused bodies.

pol·y·som·no·gram (pŏl′ē-sŏm′nə-grăm′) *n.* The recorded physiological functions obtained in polysomnography.

pol·y·som·nog·ra·phy (pŏl′ē-sŏm-nŏg′rə-fē) *n.* Simultaneous and continuous monitoring of relevant normal and abnormal physiological activity during sleep.

pol·y·so·my (pŏl′ē-sō′mē) *n.* The state of a cell nucleus in which a specific chromosome is represented more than twice.

pol·y·sor·bate (pŏl′ē-sôr′bāt′) *n.* Any of a class of emulsifiers used in food preparation and in some pharmaceuticals.

pol·y·sper·mi·a (pŏl′ē-spûr′mē-ə) *n.* **1.** An abnormally profuse spermatic secretion. **2.** See **polyspermy**.

pol·y·sper·my (pŏl′ē-spûr′mē) *n.* The entrance of more than one spermatozoon into the ovum.

pol·y·syn·dac·ty·ly (pŏl′ē-sĭn-dăk′tə-lē) *n.* A con-

genital condition in which multiple fingers or toes are webbed.

pol·y·ten·di·ni·tis (pŏl′ē-tĕn′də-nī′tĭs) *n.* Inflammation of several tendons at the same time.

pol·y·to·mog·ra·phy (pŏl′ē-tō-mŏg′rə-fē) *n.* Tomography of several sectional planes of the body using a machine specifically designed to effect complex motion.

pol·y·trich·i·a (pŏl′ē-trĭk′ē-ə) *n.* Excessive hairiness.

pol·y·un·sat·u·rat·ed (pŏl′ē-ŭn-săch′ə-rā′tĭd) *adj.* Of or relating to long-chain carbon compounds, especially fats, having many unsaturated bonds.

pol·y·u·ri·a (pŏl′ē-yŏŏr′ē-ə) *n.* Excessive passage of urine, as in diabetes.

pol·y·va·lent (pŏl′ē-vā′lənt) *adj.* Acting against or interacting with more than one kind of antigen, antibody, toxin, or microorganism. — **pol′y·va′-lence, pol′y·va′len·cy** *n.*

polyvalent serum *n.* An antiserum obtained from an animal that has been inoculated with several species or strains of a bacterium.

Pom·er·oy's operation (pŏm′ə-roiz′) *n.* Excision of a ligated portion of the fallopian tubes.

POMP (pē′ō-ĕm-pē′) *n.* A cancer chemotherapy drug consisting of purinethol (6-mercaptopurine), Oncovin (vincristine sulfate), methotrexate, and prednisone.

pons (pŏnz) *n., pl.* **pon·tes** (pŏn′tēz). **1.** The part of the brainstem that is intermediate between the medulla oblongata and the mesencephalon and is composed of a ventral part and the tegmentum. **2.** A bridgelike formation connecting two disjoined parts of a structure or organ.

pons Va·ro·li·i (və-rō′lē-ī′) *n.* A band of nerve fibers on the ventral surface of the brain stem that links the medulla oblongata and the cerebellum with upper portions of the brain.

pon·tine angle tumor (pŏn′tīn′, -tēn) *n.* A tumor growing in the proximal portion of the acoustic nerve, in the angle formed by the cerebellum and the lateral pons.

pontine nuclei *pl.n.* The very large mass of gray matter filling the pons and serving as a major way station in impulse conduction from the cerebral cortex of one hemisphere to the posterior lobe of the opposite cerebellar hemisphere.

pool (pōŏl) *n.* A collection of blood in any region of the body due to dilation and retardation of the circulation in capillaries and veins.

poor·ly differentiated lymphocytic lymphoma (pŏŏr′lē) *n.* A B-cell lymphoma with nodular or diffuse lymph node or bone marrow involvement by large lymphoid cells.

pop·les (pŏp′lēz) *n., pl.* **pop·li·tes** (pŏp′lĭ-tēz). The back part of the knee.

pop·lit·e·al artery (pŏp-lĭt′ē-əl, pŏp′lĭ-tē′əl) *n.* An artery that is the continuation of the femoral artery in the space behind the knee bifurcating at the lower border of the popliteus into the anterior and posterior tibial arteries, with branches to the knee and calf arteries.

popliteal ligament *n.* **1.** A broad fibrous band attached above to the lateral condyle of the femur and passing medially and downward in the posterior part of the capsule of the knee joint, arching over the tendon of the popliteus. **2.** A fibrous band that extends across the back of the knee from the insertion of the semimembranosus to the medial condyle of the tibia to the lateral condyle of the femur.

popliteal vein *n.* A vein that arises at the lower border of the popliteus by union of the anterior and posterior tibial veins, ascends through the space behind the knee and enters the great adductor muscle to become the femoral vein.

popliteus (păp′lĭ-tē′əs, pă-plə′tē-əs) *n.* A muscle with origin from the lateral condyle of the femur, with insertion into the posterior surface of the tibia and whose action flexes the leg and rotates it medially.

pop·py (pŏp′ē) *n.* **1.** Any of numerous plants of the genus *Papaver*, having showy red, orange, or white flowers, a milky juice, and capsules that dehisce through terminal pores. **2.** Any of several similar or related plants, such as the California poppy. **3.** An extract from the sap of unripe poppy seedpods, used in medicine and narcotics.

pop·u·la·tion (pŏp′yə-lā′shən) *n.* **1.** The total number of people inhabiting a specific area. **2.** The set of individuals, items, or data from which a statistical sample is taken.

pore (pôr) *n.* **1.** A minute opening in a tissue. **2.** One of the minute openings of the sweat glands of the skin.

por·en·ceph·a·li·tis (pôr′ĕn-sĕf′ə-lī′tĭs) *n.* Chronic inflammation of the brain with the formation of cavities in the brain substance.

por·en·ceph·a·ly (pôr′ĕn-sĕf′ə-lē) *n.* Occurrence of cavities in the brain substance, usually communicating with the lateral ventricles. — **por′en·ce·phal′ic** (-ĕn′sə-făl′ĭk), **por′en·ceph′a·lous** (-sĕf′ə-ləs) *adj.*

po·ro·ker·a·to·sis (pôr′ō-kĕr′ə-tō′sĭs) *n.* A rare dermatosis characterized by thickening of the stratum corneum together with progressive centrifugal atrophy.

po·ro·ma (pə-rō′mə, pô-) *n.* **1.** See **callosity**. **2.** See **exostosis**. **3.** Induration following inflammation of subcutaneous connective tissue. **4.** A tumor of cells lining the skin openings of sweat glands.

po·ro·sis (pə-rō′sĭs, pô-) *n., pl.* **-ses** (-sēz). A porous condition, as of the bones.

po·ros·i·ty (pə-rŏs′ĭ-tē, pô-) *n.* **1.** The state or property of being porous. **2.** A structure or part that is porous. **3.** A cavity or perforation.

po·rot·o·my (pə-rŏt′ə-mē, pô-) *n.* See **meatotomy**.

po·rous (pôr′əs) *adj.* **1.** Full of or having pores. **2.** Admitting the passage of gas or liquid through pores. — **po′rous·ness** *n.*

por·phyr·i·a (pôr-fĕr′ē-ə) *n.* Any of several disorders of porphyrin metabolism, usually hereditary, characterized by the presence of large amounts of porphyrins in the blood and urine.

por·phy·rin (pôr′fə-rĭn) *n.* Any of various heterocyclic compounds, derived from pyrrole, that occur universally in protoplasm, contain a central metal atom, and provide the foundation structure for hemoglobin, chlorophyll, and certain enzymes.

por·phy·rin·o·gen (pôr′fə-rĭn′ə-jən, -jĕn′) *n.* Any of the various intermediates in the biosynthesis of heme.

por·phy·ri·nu·ri·a (pôr′fə-rə-nŏŏr′ē-ə, -nyŏŏr′-) *n.* Excretion of abnormal levels of porphyrins and related compounds in the urine.

por·ta (pôr′tə) *n., pl.* **-tae** (-tē). See **hilum**.

por·ta·ca·val shunt (pôr′tə-kā′vəl) *n.* Any of various communications or anastomoses between the portal vein and the general circulation, especially a surgical anastomosis between the portal vein and the vena cava.

por·tal (pôr′tl) *adj.* **1.** Of or relating to a porta or hilum. **2.** Of or relating to the portal vein or the portal system. **3.** Of or relating to a point of entrance to an organ, especially the transverse fissure of the liver, through which the blood vessels enter. — *n.* **1.** The portal vein. **2.** The point of entry into the body of a pathogenic microorganism.

portal canal *n.* Any of the various spaces in the liver that contain connective tissue and the branchings of the bile ducts, portal vein, hepatic artery, nerves, and lymphatics.

portal circulation *n.* Circulation of blood to the liver from the small intestine via the portal vein.

portal fissure *n.* A transverse fissure on the visceral surface of the liver, lodging the portal vein, hepatic artery, hepatic nerve plexus, hepatic ducts, and lymphatic vessels.

portal hypertension *n.* Hypertension in the portal system as seen in cirrhosis of the liver and other conditions causing obstruction to the portal vein.

portal system *n.* A system of vessels in which blood, after passing through one capillary bed, is conveyed through a second capillary network.

portal vein *n.* A wide short vein that is formed by the superior mesenteric and splenic veins behind the pancreas, ascends in front of the inferior vena cava, and divides at the right end of the transverse fissure of the liver into right and left branches that ramify within the liver.

Por·ter's sign (pôr′tərz) *n.* An indication of aneurysm of the aortic arch marked by pulsation of the trachea when the cricoid cartilage of the larynx is drawn upward with the thumb and forefinger while the person sits with the head thrown back and mouth closed.

por·to·en·ter·os·to·my (pôr′tō-ĕn′tə-rŏs′tə-mē) *n.* A surgical procedure for the treatment of biliary atresia in which a Roux-en-Y loop of the jejunum is anastomosed to the hepatic end of the divided extravascular portal structures, including the rudimentary bile ducts.

por·to·gram (pôr′tə-grăm′) *n.* A radiographic image obtained by portography.

por·tog·ra·phy (pôr-tŏg′rə-fē) *n.* X-ray visualization of the portal circulation using radiopaque material introduced into the spleen or into the portal vein.

port-wine stain *n.* A purplish area of the skin, usually on the head and neck, appearing at birth and caused by an overgrowth of the cutaneous capillaries.

po·si·tion (pə-zĭsh′ən) *n.* **1.** A bodily attitude or posture, especially a posture assumed by a patient to facilitate the performance of diagnostic, surgical, or therapeutic procedures. **2.** The relation of an arbitrarily chosen portion of the fetus to the right or left side of the mother. — **position** *v.* — **po·si′tion·al** *adj.*

position effect *n.* Variation in the expression of a gene resulting from changes in its position along a chromosome.

position sense *n.* See **posture sense.**

pos·i·tive (pŏz′ĭ-tĭv) *adj.* **1.** Indicating the presence of a particular disease, condition, or organism. **2.** Indicating or characterized by response or motion toward the source of a stimulus, such as light. — **pos′i·tive·ness, pos′i·tiv′i·ty** *n.*

positive accommodation *n.* Accomodation for near vision by contraction of the ciliary muscles of the eye.

positive convergence *n.* The inward deviation of the visual axes.

positive declination *n.* See **extorsion** (sense 2).

positive end-expiratory pressure *n.* A technique used in respiratory therapy in which pressure is maintained in the airway so that the lungs empty less completely in expiration.

positive-negative pressure breathing *n.* Inflation of the lungs with positive pressure and deflation with negative pressure by an automatic ventilator.

positive scotoma *n.* A scotoma that is perceived as a black spot within the field of vision.

positron emission tomography *n.* Tomography in which a computer-generated image of local metabolic and physiological functions in tissues is produced through the detection of gamma rays that are emitted when introduced radionuclides decay and release positrons.

post·ca·va (pōst-kā′və) *n.* See **inferior vena cava.** — **post·ca′val** *adj.*

post·co·i·tus (pōst-kō′ĭ-təs, -kō-ē′-) *n.* The period immediately after coitus.

pos·te·ri·or (pŏ-stēr′ē-ər, -pō-) *adj.* **1.** Located behind a part or toward the rear of a structure. **2.** Relating to the dorsal side of the body. **3.** Near the tail or caudal end of certain embryos. — **pos·te′ri·or·ly** *adv.*

posterior chamber of the eye *n.* The ringlike space filled with aqueous humor between the iris, the crystalline lens, and the ciliary body.

posterior column of the spinal cord *n.* The dorsolateral ridge of gray matter in each lateral half of the spinal cord.

posterior horn *n.* **1.** The occipital division of the lateral ventricle of the brain, extending backward

into the occipital lobe. **2.** The posterior gray column of the spinal cord in cross section.

posterior lobe of the hypophysis *n.* See **neurohypophysis.**

posterior rhinoscopy *n.* Examination of the nasopharynx and posterior portion of the nasal cavity using a rhinoscope or a nasopharyngoscope.

posterior root *n.* See **dorsal root.**

posterior scleritis *n.* Scleritis with a tendency to extend posteriorly to the sheath of eyeball and to cause chemosis.

posterior staphyloma *n.* A bulging of a weakened sclera at the posterior of the eyeball resulting from loss of the choroid lining.

post·gan·gli·on·ic motor neuron (pōst′găng-glē-ŏn′ĭk) *n.* A motor neuron that forms a synapse with one or more preganglionic motor neurons; it is located outside the central nervous system with its cell body and dendrites in the autonomic ganglion and its unmyelinated axon ending in smooth muscle, cardiac muscle, or a gland.

pos·thi·o·plas·ty (pŏs′thē-ə-plăs′tē) *n.* Reparative or plastic surgery of the prepuce.

pos·thi·tis (pŏs-thī′tĭs) *n.* Inflammation of the prepuce.

posthypnotic suggestion *n.* A suggestion made to a hypnotized person that specifies an action to be performed after awakening, often in response to a cue.

post·men·o·paus·al (pōst′mĕn-ə-pô′zəl) *adj.* Of or occurring in the time following menopause.

post·men·stru·al (pōst-mĕn′strōō-əl) *adj.* Of or occurring in the time following menstruation.

post·mor·tem (pōst-môr′təm) *adj.* Relating to or occurring during the period after death. — *n.* See **autopsy.**

postmortem delivery *n.* The extraction of a fetus after its mother has died.

postmortem examination *n.* See **autopsy.**

postmortem rigidity *n.* See **rigor mortis.**

post·na·sal (pōst-nā′zəl) *adj.* **1.** Located or occurring posterior to the nose or the nasal cavity. **2.** Relating to the posterior portion of the nasal cavity.

postnasal drip *n.* The chronic secretion of mucus from the posterior nasal cavities, often caused by a cold or an allergy.

post·na·tal (pōst-nāt′l) *adj.* Of or occurring after birth, especially during the period immediately after birth.

post·op·er·a·tive (pōst-ŏp′ər-ə-tĭv, -ŏp′rə-, -ŏp′ə-rā′-) *adj.* Happening or done after a surgical operation.

post·par·tum (pōst-pär′təm) *adj.* Of or occurring in the period shortly after childbirth.

postpartum hemorrhage *n.* Hemorrhage from the birth canal in excess of 500 ml during the first 24 hours after birth.

post·per·fu·sion lung (pōst′pər-fyōō′zhən) *n.* A condition in which abnormal pulmonary function develops following cardiac surgery in which extracorporeal circulation was used.

post·po·li·o syndrome (pōst-pō′lē-ō′) *n.* A condition affecting poliomyelitis patients several decades after the initial attack, characterized by fatigue, muscular deterioration, pain in the joints, and respiratory problems.

post·pran·di·al (pōst-prăn′dē-əl) *adj.* Following a meal, especially dinner. — **post·pran′di·al·ly** *adv.*

postprandial lipemia *n.* See **alimentary lipemia.**

post·syn·ap·tic membrane (pōst′sĭ-năp′tĭk) *n.* The part of the cell membrane of a neuron or muscle fiber with which an axon terminal forms a synapse.

post-term infant (pōst′tûrm′) *n.* An infant born after the 42nd week of gestation.

post·trau·mat·ic neck syndrome (pōst′trou-măt′ĭk, -trô-) *n.* A syndrome characterized by pain, tenderness, tight neck musculature, vasomotor instability, dizziness, and blurred vision, resulting from injury to the neck.

posttraumatic stress disorder *n.* An anxiety disorder resulting from profound emotional trauma, such as torture, rape, or military combat, characterized by recurrent flashbacks of the traumatic event, nightmares, eating disorders, anxiety, fatigue, forgetfulness, and social withdrawal.

posttraumatic syndrome *n.* A syndrome characterized by headache, dizziness, neurasthenia, hypersensitivity to stimuli, and diminished concentration, caused by injury to the head.

pos·tur·al (pŏs′chər-əl) *adj.* Relating to or involving posture.

postural contraction *n.* The maintenance of muscular tension sufficient to maintain posture.

postural drainage *n.* A therapeutic technique for drainage, used in bronchiectasis and lung abscess, in which the patient is placed head downward so that the trachea is down and below the affected area.

postural position *n.* See **physiologic rest position.**

postural syncope *n.* A syncope that occurs upon assuming an upright position and is caused by inadequate blood flow to the brain resulting from failure of normal vasoconstrictive mechanisms.

postural vertigo *n.* Vertigo that occurs with a change of position, usually from a lying or sitting to a standing position.

pos·ture (pŏs′chər) *n.* **1.** A position of the body or of body parts. **2.** A characteristic or prescribed way of bearing one's body; carriage.

posture sense *n.* The ability to recognize the position in which a limb is passively placed without visual perception.

post·val·var (pōst-văl′vər) or **post·val·vu·lar** (-văl′vyə-lər) *adj.* Relating to a position distal to the pulmonary or aortic valves.

po·ta·ble (pō′tə-bəl) *adj.* Fit to drink; drinkable.

po·tas·si·um (pə-tăs′ē-əm) *n.* A metallic element with atomic number 19, occurring in nature, especially combined in minerals; it is the principal positive ion in intracellular fluid and is involved in nerve impulse conduction and muscle contraction.

potassium bicarbonate *n.* A compound in the form of a white powder or colorless crystals, used

in baking powder and as an antacid medicine.

potassium bitartrate *n.* A white, acid, crystalline solid or powder used in baking powder, the tinning of metals, and laxatives.

potassium bromide *n.* A white crystalline solid or powder used as a sedative.

potassium hydroxide *n.* A caustic white solid used as a bleach and in the manufacture of soaps, dyes, and many pharmaceuticals.

potassium sodium tartrate *n.* A colorless efflorescent crystalline compound used as a laxative.

pot·bel·ly (pŏt′bĕl′ē) *n.* A protruding abdomen.

po·ten·cy (pōt′n-sē) *n.* **1.** The quality or condition of being potent. **2.** The pharmacological activity of a compound.

po·tent (pōt′nt) *adj.* **1.** Exerting strong physiological or chemical effects. **2.** Able to perform sexual intercourse. Used of a male.

po·ten·tial (pə-tĕn′shəl) *n.* The potential energy of a unit charge at any point in an electric circuit measured with respect to a reference point in the circuit; voltage.

potential cautery *n.* An agent, such as potassium hydroxide, that causes the formation of an eschar by chemical means.

po·tion (pō′shən) *n.* A liquid medicinal dose or drink.

Pot·ter's facies (pŏt′ərz) *n.* The facial appearance characteristic of bilateral renal agenesis and other severe renal malformations, consisting of ocular hypertelorism, low-set ears, receding chin, and flattening of the nose.

Potter's syndrome *n.* A combination of birth defects characterized by the absence of one or both kidneys, underdeveloped lungs, and Potter's facies, and resulting in neonatal respiratory distress, circulatory abnormalities, acidosis, cyanosis, edema, and death.

Pott's fracture (pŏts) *n.* A fracture of the lower part of the fibula and of the bony prominence near the ankle joint, causing the foot to turn out.

Potts' operation *n.* Direct side-to-side anastomosis between the aorta and the pulmonary artery as a palliative procedure in congenital malformation of the heart.

pouch (pouch) *n.* A pocketlike space in the body.

pou·drage (poō-dräzh′) *n.* The surgical application of powder, such as the dusting of opposing pleural surfaces with a slightly irritating powder in order to secure adhesion.

poul·tice (pōl′tĭs) *n.* A soft, moist adhesive mass, as of clay, that is usually heated, spread on cloth, and applied to warm, moisten, or stimulate an aching or inflamed part of the body. — **poul′tice** *v.*

pound (pound) *n.* **1.** A unit of weight that is the basis of the avoirdupois system, equal to 16 ounces or 453.592 grams. **2.** A unit of apothecary weight equal to 12 ounces or 373.242 grams.

Pow·as·san encephalitis (pə-wä′sən) *n.* An acute disease of children varying clinically from undifferentiated febrile illness to encephalitis, caused by a tick-borne virus.

pow·der (pou′dər) *n.* **1.** A dry mass of pulverized

or finely dispersed solid particles. **2.** Any of various medicinal or cosmetic preparations in the form of powder. **3.** A single dose of a powdered drug.

pow·er (pou′ər) *n.* **1.** The capacity to perform or act effectively. **2.** Strength or force exerted or capable of being exerted. **3.** The rate at which work is done, expressed as the amount of work per unit time and commonly measured in units such as the watt and horsepower. **4.** A measure of the magnification of an optical instrument, such as a microscope or telescope.

Pow·er·Walk·ing (pou′ər-wô′kĭng) *n.* See **race walking**.

pox (pŏks) *n.* **1.** A disease such as chickenpox or smallpox, characterized by purulent skin eruptions that may leave pockmarks. **2.** Syphilis.

pox·vi·rus (pŏks′vī′rəs) *n.* A DNA virus of the family Poxviridae, including the vaccinia and variola viruses.

ppb *abbr.* parts per billion

ppm *abbr.* parts per million

PPO *abbr.* preferred provider organization

PPPPPP *abbr.* pain, pallor, paresthesia, pulselessness, paralysis, and prostration (symptom complex of acute arterial occlusion)

ppt *abbr.* parts per thousand; parts per trillion

prac·ti·cal nurse (prăk′tĭ-kəl) *n.* **1.** A licensed practical nurse. **2.** A person who has had practical experience in nursing care but who is not a graduate of a degree program in nursing.

prac·tice (prăk′tĭs) *v.* **-ticed, -tic·ing, -tic·es.** To engage in the profession of medicine or one of the allied health professions. — *n.* **1.** The exercise of the profession of medicine. **2.** The business of a practicing physician or group of physicians, including facilities and customary patients.

prac·ti·tion·er (prăk-tĭsh′ə-nər) *n.* One who practices medicine or an allied health profession.

Pra·der–Wil·li syndrome (prä′dər-wĭl′ē, prä′dər-vĭl′ē) *n.* A congenital syndrome of unknown cause characterized by short stature, mental retardation, excessive eating and obesity, and sexual infantilism.

prag·mat·ag·no·si·a (prăg′mə-tăg-nō′zē-ə, -zhə) *n.* Loss of the power of recognizing objects.

prag·mat·am·ne·sia (prăg′mə-tăm-nē′zhə) *n.* Loss of the memory of the appearance of objects.

Prague maneuver (präg) *n.* A method for delivering a fetus in breech position in which the infant's shoulders are grasped from below by one hand while the other hand supports the legs.

pran·di·al (prăn′dē-əl) *adj.* Of or relating to a meal.

pra·se·o·dym·i·um (prā′zē-ō-dĭm′ē-əm, prā′sē-) *n.* A soft malleable metallic element used in metallic alloys, having atomic number 59.

Praus·nitz–Küst·ner reaction (prous′nĭts-küst′-nər) *n.* A reaction based on passive transfer of allergic sensitivity in which serum from an allergic person is injected into cutaneous sites on a normal person and the injected sites are then exposed to antigens to which the donor is allergic.

prav·a·stat·in (prăv′ə-stăt′ĭn) *n.* A statin that acts to block the body's synthesis of cholesterol and is administered especially to persons who are at risk for heart disease.

pra·zi·quan·tel (prā′zĭ-kwän′tĕl′) *n.* A synthetic heterocyclic broad-spectrum anthelmintic agent effective against all schistosome species parasitic in humans as well as most other trematodes and adult cestodes.

pra·zo·sin (prā′zō-sĭn) *n.* A crystalline vasodilator used in the form of its hydrochloride to treat hypertension.

pre·ad·o·les·cence (prē′ăd-l-ĕs′əns) *n.* The period between childhood and the onset of puberty, often designated as between the ages of 10 and 12 in girls and 11 and 13 in boys.

pre·a·dult (prē′ə-dŭlt′) *adj.* Of or relating to the period preceding adulthood or the adult stage of the life cycle.

pre·ax·i·al (prē-ăk′sē-əl) *adj.* **1.** Situated in front of or superior to the median axis of the body or a body part. **2.** Of or being the portion of a limb bud lying cranial to the axis of the limb. — **pre·ax′i·al·ly** *adv.*

pre·can·cer (prē′kăn′sər) *n.* A lesion from which a malignant tumor is presumed to develop in a significant number of instances and that may or may not be recognizable clinically or by microscopic changes in the affected tissue.

pre·can·cer·ous (prē-kăn′sər-əs) *adj.* Of, relating to, or being a condition or lesion that typically precedes or develops into a cancer.

pre·ca·va (prē-kā′və, -kä′-) *n., pl* **-vae** (-vē). See **superior vena cava.** — **pre·ca′val** *adj.*

pre·cep·tor (prĭ-sĕp′tər, prē′sĕp′tər) *n.* An expert or a specialist, such as a physician, who gives practical experience and training to a student, especially of medicine or nursing.

pre·cep·tor·ship (prĭ-sĕp′tər-shĭp′) *n.* A period of practical experience and training for a student, especially of medicine or nursing, that is supervised by a specialist in a particular field.

pre·cip·i·tate (prĭ-sĭp′ĭ-tāt′, -tĭt) *n.* A punctate opacity on the posterior surface of the cornea developing from inflammatory cells in the vitreous body. — *v.* **-tat·ed, -tat·ing, -tates.** (-tāt′). **1.** To cause a solid substance to be separated from a solution. **2.** To be separated from a solution as a solid.

precipitate labor *n.* Labor that results in rapid expulsion of the fetus.

pre·cip·i·tin (prĭ-sĭp′ĭ-tĭn) *n.* An antibody that under suitable conditions combines with and causes a specific soluble antigen to precipitate; a precipitating antibody.

precipitin reaction *n.* See **precipitin test**.

precipitin test *n.* A serologic test in which antibody reacts with a specific soluble antigen and forms a solid that precipitates from solution.

pre·clin·i·cal (prē-klĭn′ĭ-kəl) *adj.* **1.** Of or relating to the period of a disease before the appearance of symptoms. **2.** Of or being a period in medical education before the student is involved with patients and clinical work.

pre·co·cious (prĭ-kō′shəs) *adj.* Showing unusually early development or maturity. — **pre·coc′i·ty** (-kŏs′ĭ-tē), **pre·co′cious·ness** *n.*

pre·cog·ni·tion (prē′kŏg-nĭsh′ən) *n.* Knowledge of something before its occurrence, especially by extrasensory perception. — **pre·cog′ni·tive** *adj.*

pre·con·cep·tu·al stage (prē′kən-sĕp′chōō-əl) *n.* The stage of development in an infant's life in which sensorimotor activity predominates.

pre·cor·di·a (prē-kôr′dē-ə) *pl.n.* The precordium.

precordial lead (lēd) *n.* **1.** A lead of an electrocardiograph that has one electrode placed in any of six standard positions on the chest and another electrode placed on a limb. **2.** A record obtained from such a lead.

pre·cor·di·um (prē-kôr′dē-əm) *n.* The part of the body comprising the epigastrium and anterior surface of the lower part of the thorax. — **pre·cor′di·al** *adj.*

pre·cur·so·ry cartilage (prĭ-kûr′sə-rē) *n.* See **temporary cartilage.**

pre·den·tin (prē-dĕn′tən) *n.* The organic fibrillar matrix of the dentin before its calcification.

pre·di·a·be·tes (prē′dī-ə-bē′tĭs, -tēz) *n.* The condition of having a hereditary tendency or high probability for developing diabetes mellitus, although neither symptoms nor test results confirm the presence of the disease.

pre·di·as·to·le (prē-dī-ăs′tə-lē) *n.* The interval in the cardiac rhythm immediately preceding diastole. — **pre′di·as·tol′ic** (-dī-ə-stŏl′ĭk) *adj.*

pre·di·gest (prē′dī-jĕst′, -dī-) *v.* **-gest·ed, -gest·ing, -gests.** To subject food to partial digestion, usually through an enzymatic or chemical process, before being eaten. — **pre′di·ges′tion** *n.*

pre·dis·pose (prē′dĭ-spōz′) *v.* **-posed, -pos·ing, -pos·es.** To make susceptible, as to a disease.

pre·dis·po·si·tion (prē′dĭs-pə-zĭsh′ən) *n.* A condition of special susceptibility, as to a disease.

pred·nis·o·lone (prĕd-nĭs′ə-lōn′) *n.* A synthetic steroid similar to hydrocortisone and used in various compounds as an anti-inflammatory, immunosuppressive, antiallergy, and anticancer drug.

pred·ni·sone (prĕd′nĭ-sōn′,-zōn′) *n.* A synthetic steroid similar to cortisone that is used as an antiallergy, immunosuppressive, and anticancer drug and as an anti-inflammatory agent in the treatment of rheumatoid arthritis.

pre·e·clamp·si·a (prē′ĭ-klămp′sē-ə) *n.* A condition of hypertension occurring in pregnancy or immediately following pregnancy, typically accompanied by edema and proteinuria but without the coma and convulsions of eclampsia. — **pre′e·clamp′tic** (-tĭk) *adj.*

pre·e·jec·tion period (prē′ĭ-jĕk′shən) *n.* The interval in the electrocardiogram between the onset of the QRS complex and cardiac ejection.

pre·em·bry·o (prē-ĕm′brē-ō′) *n.* A fertilized ovum up to 14 days old, before it becomes implanted in the uterus.

pree·mie or **pre·mie** (prē′mē) *n.* A prematurely born infant.

pre·ferred provider organization (prĭ-fûrd′) *n.* A medical insurance plan in which members receive more coverage if they choose health care providers approved by or affiliated with the plan.

pre·fron·tal (prē-frŭn′tl) *adj.* **1.** Of, relating to, or situated in the anterior part of the frontal lobe. **2.** Situated anterior to the frontal bone.

prefrontal lobotomy *n.* A lobotomy in which the white fibers that connect the thalamus to the prefrontal and frontal lobes of the brain are severed, performed as a treatment for intense anxiety or violent behavior.

pre·gan·gli·on·ic motor neuron (prē-găng′glē-ŏn′ĭk) *n.* A motor neuron having a cell body located in the brain or spinal cord and a myelinated axon that travels out of the central nervous system as part of a cranial or spinal nerve before terminating in an autonomic ganglion.

preg·nan·cy (prĕg′nən-sē) *n.* **1.** The condition of a woman from conception until birth; the condition of being pregnant. **2.** The period during which a woman is pregnant.

pregnancy gingivitis *n.* Inflammatory changes in the gum tissue appearing in the mother during pregnancy.

preg·nane (prĕg′nān′) *n.* A crystalline steroid hydrocarbon that is the parent compound of corticosteroids and progesterones.

preg·nant (prĕg′nənt) *adj.* Carrying developing offspring within the body.

pre·hen·sile (prē-hĕn′səl, -sīl′) *adj.* Adapted for seizing, grasping, or holding, especially by wrapping around an object. — **pre′hen·sil′i·ty** (-sĭl′-ĭ-tē) *n.*

pre·hen·sion (prē-hĕn′shən) *n.* The act of grasping or seizing.

pre·hor·mone (prē-hôr′mōn′) *n.* A glandular secretory product that is a precursor of a hormone but has little or no inherent biological potency itself.

pre·im·plan·ta·tion diagnosis (prē-ĭm′plăn-tā′-shən) *n.* A procedure in which embryos generated using in vitro fertilization techniques are screened for the presence of the gene for a particular characteristic or defect, such as the cystic fibrosis gene, prior to uterine implantation.

pre·load (prē′lōd′) *n.* The load to which a muscle is subjected before shortening.

pre·log·i·cal thinking (prē-lŏj′ĭ-kəl) *n.* A form of concrete thinking characteristic of children, to which schizophrenic persons are sometimes said to regress.

pre·ma·lig·nant (prē′mə-lĭg′nənt) *adj.* Precancerous.

pre·ma·ture (prē′mə-tyŏŏr′, -tŏŏr′, -chŏŏr′) *adj.* **1.** Occurring or developing before the usual or expected time. **2.** Born after a gestation period of less than the normal time, especially, in human infants, after a period of less than 37 weeks. — **pre′ma·tu′ri·ty, pre′ma·ture′ness** *n.*

premature birth *n.* The birth of an infant after the period of viability but before full term.

premature delivery *n.* The birth of a premature baby.

premature ejaculation *n.* During sexual intercourse, more rapid achievement of climax and ejaculation in the male than he or his partner wishes.

premature labor *n.* The onset of labor before the 37th completed week of pregnancy.

pre·med (prē'mĕd') *adj.* Premedical.

pre·med·i·cal (prē-mĕd'ĭ-kəl) *adj.* Preparing for or relating to the studies that prepare one for the study of medicine.

pre·med·i·ca·tion (prē'mĕd-ĭ-kā'shən) *n.* **1.** Administration of drugs prior to anesthesia to allay apprehension, produce sedation, and facilitate the administration of anesthesia to the patient. **2.** A drug or drugs used for such purposes.

pre·me·no·paus·al (prē'mĕn-ə-pô'zəl) *adj.* Of or relating to the years or the stage of life immediately before the onset of menopause.

pre·men·stru·al (prē-mĕn'strōō-əl) *adj.* Of or occurring in the period just before menstruation.

premenstrual syndrome *n.* A group of symptoms, including abdominal bloating, breast tenderness, headache, fatigue, irritability, and depression, that occur in many women from 2 to 14 days before the onset of menstruation.

premenstrual tension *n.* See **premenstrual syndrome.**

pre·men·stru·um (prē-mĕn'strōō-əm) *n.* The period just preceding menstruation.

pre·mo·lar (prē-mō'lər) *n.* Any of eight bicuspid teeth located in pairs on each side of the upper and lower jaws behind the canines and in front of the molars.

pre·mon·o·cyte (prē-mŏn'ə-sīt') *n.* An immature monocyte not normally present in the blood.

pre·mu·ni·tion (prē'myōō-nĭsh'ən) *n.* See **infection immunity.** — **pre·mune'** (prē-myōōn') *adj.* — **pre·mu'ni·tive** *adj.*

pre·my·e·lo·blast (prē-mī'ə-lə-blăst') *n.* The earliest recognizable precursor of the myeloblast.

pre·my·e·lo·cyte (prē-mī'ə-lə-sīt') *n.* See **myeloblast.**

pre·na·tal (prē-nāt'l) *adj.* Preceding birth.

pre·op·er·a·tive (prē-ŏp'ər-ə-tĭv, -ŏp'rə-, -ŏp'ə-rā'-) *adj.* Preceding a surgical operation.

pre·ox·y·gen·a·tion (prē'ŏk-sĭ-jə-nā'shən) *n.* Administration of pure oxygen prior to induction of general anesthesia in order to eliminate nitrogen from the lungs and body tissues.

prep (prĕp) *v.* **prepped, prep·ping, preps.** To prepare someone for a medical examination or surgical procedure.

prep·a·ra·tion (prĕp'ə-rā'shən) *n.* A substance, such as a medicine, prepared for a particular purpose.

pre·po·ten·tial (prē'pə-tĕn'shəl) *n.* The slow depolarization of a cell membrane that occurs between action potentials.

pre·pu·ber·ty (prē-pyōō'bər-tē) *n.* The period of life immediately before puberty, often marked by accelerated physical growth.

pre·pu·bes·cence (prē'pyōō-bĕs'əns) *n.* Prepuberty.

pre·pu·bes·cent (prē'pyōō-bĕs'ənt) *adj.* Of or characteristic of prepuberty. — *n.* A prepubescent child.

pre·puce (prē'pyōōs') *n.* **1.** See **foreskin. 2.** A loose fold of skin covering the glans clitoridis.

pre·pu·tial gland (prē-pyōō'shəl) *n.* Any of the small sebaceous glands of the corona of the penis and the inner surface of the prepuce that secrete smegma.

pre·pu·ti·ot·o·my (prē-pyōō'shē-ŏt'ə-mē) *n.* Surgical incision of the prepuce.

pre·pu·ti·um (prē-pyōō'shē-əm) *n.,* pl. **-ti·a** (-shē-ə). The prepuce.

pre·sa·cral neurectomy (prē-sā'krəl) *n.* Surgical removal of the presacral plexus to relieve severe dysmenorrhea.

presacral sympathectomy *n.* See **presacral neurectomy.**

pres·by·at·rics (prĕz'bē-ăt'rĭks, prĕs'-) *n.* See **geriatrics.**

pres·by·o·pi·a (prĕz'bē-ō'pē-ə, prĕs'-) *n.* Inability of the eye to focus sharply on nearby objects, resulting from loss of elasticity of the crystalline lens with advancing age. — **pres'by·op'ic** (-ŏp'-ĭk, -ō'pĭk) *adj.*

pre·scribe (prĭ-skrīb') *v.* **-scribed, -scrib·ing, -scribes.** To give directions, either orally or in writing, for the preparation and administration of a remedy to be used in the treatment of a disease.

pre·scrip·tion (prĭ-skrĭp'shən) *n.* **1.** A written order, especially by a physician, for the preparation and administration of a medicine or other treatment. **2.** A prescribed medicine or other treatment. **3.** An ophthalmologist's or optometrist's written instruction, as for the grinding of corrective lenses.

pre·se·nile dementia (prē-sē'nīl', -sĕn'īl') *n.* Any of various forms of dementia developing before old age.

pre·se·nil·i·ty (prē'sĭ-nĭl'ĭ-tē) *n.* The condition of one affected with the physical and mental characteristics of old age at an abnormally young age; premature old age.

pre·sent (prĭ-zĕnt') *v.* **-sent·ed, -sent·ing, -sents. 1.** To appear or be felt first during birth. Used of the part of the fetus that proceeds first through the birth canal. **2.** To come before a doctor or nurse, as with a medical problem or condition. **3.** To manifest a symptom.

pres·en·ta·tion (prĕz'ən-tā'shən, prē'zən-) *n.* **1.** The position of the fetus in the uterus at the beginning of labor, described in terms of the part that emerges or is felt first. **2.** The part of the fetal body in advance during birth.

pre·sent·a·tive (prĭ-zĕn'tə-tĭv) *n.* **1.** Having the capacity or function of bringing an idea or image to mind. **2.** Perceived or capable of being perceived directly rather than through association. **3.** Having the ability to so perceive.

pre·ser·va·tive (prĭ-zûr′və-tĭv) *n.* A substance added to foods or to organic solutions to prevent decomposition due to chemical change or bacterial action.

pres·sor (prĕs′ôr′, -ər) *adj.* **1.** Producing increased blood pressure. **2.** Causing constriction of the blood vessels.

pres·so·re·cep·tive (prĕs′ō-rĭ-sĕp′tĭv) *adj.* Capable of receiving as stimuli changes in pressure, especially changes of blood pressure.

pres·so·re·cep·tor (prĕs′ō-rĭ-sĕp′tər) *n.* See **baro-receptor.**

pressor nerve *n.* An afferent nerve that when stimulated causes the constriction of a blood vessel, thereby raising the blood pressure.

pres·sure (prĕsh′ər) *n.* **1.** The act of pressing or condition of being pressed. **2.** Force applied uniformly over a surface.

pressure dressing *n.* A dressing that exerts pressure on the area covered to prevent the collection of fluids in the underlying tissues, usually used after skin grafting and in the treatment of burns.

pressure paralysis *n.* Paralysis due to compression of a nerve or nerve trunk or the spinal cord.

pressure point *n.* **1.** Any of the various locations on the body where pressure may be applied to control bleeding. **2.** A point of extreme sensitivity to pressure.

pressure reversal *n.* Cessation of anesthesia by hyperbaric pressure.

pressure sense *n.* The ability to discriminate various degrees of pressure on the surface of one's body.

pressure sore *n.* See **bedsore.**

pre·ster·num (prē-stûr′nəm) *n.* See **episternum.**

pre·syn·ap·tic membrane (prē′sĭ-năp′tĭk) *n.* The part of the cell membrane of an axon terminal that faces the cell membrane of the neuron or muscle fiber with which the axon terminal establishes a synapse.

pre·sys·to·le (prē-sĭs′tə-lē) *n.* The interval in the cardiac rhythm immediately preceding systole. — **pre′sys·tol′ic** (-sĭ-stŏl′ĭk) *adj.*

presystolic gallop *n.* A heart gallop rhythm in which an abnormal fourth heart sound occurs in late diastole.

presystolic murmur *n.* A murmur heard at the end of ventricular diastole, during atrial systole, usually due to obstruction at one of the atrioventricular orifices.

pre·teen (prē′tēn′) *adj.* **1.** Relating to or designed for children especially between the ages of 9 and 12. **2.** Being a child especially between the ages of 9 and 12; preadolescent. — *n.* A preadolescent boy or girl.

pre·term (prē′tûrm′, prē-tûrm′) *adj.* Occurring or appearing before the expected time at the end of a full-term pregnancy. — *n.* An infant born prematurely.

pre·term infant (prē′tûrm′) *n.* An infant born before the 37th week of gestation.

pre·tib·i·al fever (prē-tĭb′ē-əl) *n.* A mild disease caused by *Leptospira autumalis* and characterized by fever, splenomegaly, and a rash on the front of the legs.

prev·a·lence (prĕv′ə-ləns) *n.* The total number of cases of a disease in a given population at a specific time.

pre·ven·tive (prĭ-vĕn′tĭv) or **pre·ven·ta·tive** (-tə-tĭv) *adj.* Preventing or slowing the course of an illness or a disease; prophylactic. — *n.* A preventive agent or treatment.

preventive medicine *n.* The branch of medical science concerned with the prevention of disease and the promotion of physical and mental health through the study of the etiology and epidemiology of disease processes.

preventive treatment *n.* See **prophylactic treatment.**

pri·a·pic (prī-ā′pĭk, -ăp′ĭk) or **pri·a·pe·an** (prī′ə-pē′ən) *adj.* **1.** Of, relating to, or resembling a phallus; phallic. **2.** Relating to or overly concerned with masculinity.

pri·a·pism (prī′ə-pĭz′əm) *n.* Persistent, usually painful erection of the penis, especially as a consequence of disease and not related to sexual arousal.

Price-Jones curve (prīs′jōnz′) *n.* A curve indicating the distribution of red blood cells according to the length of their diameters.

prick·le cell (prĭk′əl) *n.* One of the cells of the spinous layer of the skin having numerous intercellular bridges that give the separated cells a prickly appearance.

prick·ly heat (prĭk′lē) *n.* See **heat rash.**

pri·mal (prī′məl) *adj.* **1.** Being first in time; original. **2.** Of first or central importance; primary. — **pri·mal′i·ty** (-măl′ĭ-tē) *n.*

primal therapy *n.* A method of psychotherapy that treats neurosis by teaching patients to relive early traumatic experiences and to express feelings through angry screaming and other verbal or physical acts of aggression.

pri·ma·quine phosphate (prī′mə-kwĭn, -kwēn′) *n.* An antimalarial agent especially effective against *Plasmodium vivax,* the most common malarial parasite of humans.

pri·mar·y (prī′mĕr′ē, -mə-rē) *adj.* **1.** Occurring first in time or sequence. **2.** Preliminary to a later stage of development; primordial; embryonic. **3.** Immediate; direct. **4.** Of, relating to, or being a sequence of amino acids in a protein.

primary adhesion *n.* See **healing by first intention.**

primary care *n.* The medical care a patient receives upon first contact with the health care system, before referral elsewhere within the system.

primary care physician *n.* A physician, such as a general practioner or internist, chosen by a person to serve as his or her health-care professional and capable of handling a range of health-related problems, of keeping a medical history and medical records on the person, and of referring the person to specialists as needed.

primary dentition *n.* **1.** The first set of teeth, 20 in all, that usually erupt between the 6th and 28th month. **2.** The eruption of the first set of teeth.

primary digestion *n.* Digestion in the alimentary canal.

primary disease *n.* A disease arising spontaneously and not associated with or caused by a previous disease or injury.

primary gain *n.* Alleviation of anxiety from conversion of emotional conflict into demonstrably organic illnesses.

primary herpetic stomatitis *n.* First infection of oral tissues with herpes simplex virus, marked by gingival inflammation, vesicles, and ulcers.

primary lysosome *n.* A cytoplasmic body produced at the Golgi apparatus where hydrolytic enzymes are incorporated.

primary oocyte *n.* An oocyte during its growth phase and prior to completion of the first maturation division.

primary process *n.* In psychoanalysis, the mental process directly related to the functions of the id and characteristic of unconscious mental activity, marked by unorganized, illogical thinking.

primary reaction *n.* See **vaccinia** (sense 2).

primary sex character *n.* Any of various anatomical structures, such as the testes or ovaries, concerned directly with reproduction.

primary spermatocyte *n.* The spermatocyte arising by a growth phase from a spermatogonium.

primary tooth *n.* See **deciduous tooth.**

primary union *n.* See **healing by first intention.**

pri·mate (prī′māt′) *n.* A mammal of the order Primates, which includes humans, apes, and monkeys, characterized by refined development of the hands and feet, a shortened snout, and a large brain. — **pri·ma′tial** (-mā′shəl) *adj.*

pri·mi·grav·i·da (prī′mĭ-grăv′ĭ-də) *n.* A woman in her first pregnancy.

pri·mip·a·ra (prī-mĭp′ər-ə) *n., pl.* **-a·ras** or **-a·rae** (-ə-rē′). **1.** A woman who is pregnant for the first time. **2.** A woman who has given birth for the first time to an infant or infants, alive or stillborn. — **pri′mi·par′i·ty** (-mĭ-pār′ĭ-tē) *n.* — **pri·mip′a·rous** *adj.*

prim·i·tive (prĭm′ĭ-tĭv) *adj.* **1.** Primary; basic. **2.** Of or being an earliest or original stage.

primitive costal arch *n.* Any of the arches formed from the costal processes or elements that give rise to the ribs in the thoracic region of the embryonic vertebral column.

primitive knot *n.* See **primitive node.**

primitive node *n.* A knotlike thickening at the anterior end of the primitive streak of the blastoderm at the point of origin of the embryonic head.

primitive streak *n.* An ectodermal ridge in the midline at the caudal end of the embryonic disk from which the intraembryonic mesoderm arises.

pri·mor·di·al (prī-môr′dē-əl) *adj.* **1.** Being or happening first in sequence of time; primary; original. **2.** Belonging to or characteristic of the earliest stage of development of an organism or a part. **3.** Relating to a primordium.

pri·mor·di·um (prī-môr′dē-əm) *n., pl.* **-di·a** (-dē-ə). An aggregation of cells in the embryo indicating the first trace of an organ or structure.

P–R interval *n.* The time elapsing between the beginning of the P wave and the beginning of the QRS complex in an electrocardiogram; it corresponds to the atriocarotid interval of the venous pulse.

pri·on (prē′ŏn) *n.* A microscopic protein particle similar to a virus but lacking nucleic acid, possibly the infectious agent for certain degenerative diseases of the nervous system.

prism bar (prĭz′əm) *n.* A graduated series of prisms mounted on a frame and used in ocular diagnosis.

pri·vate duty nurse (prī′vĭt) *n.* A nurse who is not a member of a hospital staff but is called upon to take special care of one patient.

private parts *pl.n.* The external organs of sex and excretion.

priv·i·leged site (prĭv′ə-lĭjd, prĭv′lĭjd) *n.* An area in the body lacking lymphatic drainage, such as the cornea of the eye, in which rejection of foreign tissue grafts does not occur.

PRL *abbr.* prolactin

p.r.n. or **PRN** *abbr. Latin.* pro re nata (as the situation demands)

Pro *abbr.* proline

pro·ac·ro·so·mal granule (prō′ăk-rə-sō′məl) *n.* One of the small carbohydrate-rich granules appearing in vesicles of the Golgi apparatus of spermatids and coalescing to form an acrosomal granule.

pro·ac·ti·va·tor (prō-ăk′tə-vā′tər) *n.* A substance that, when enzymatically split, yields a fragment capable of rendering another substance or process active.

pro·band (prō′bănd′) *n.* An individual or member of a family being studied in a genetic investigation.

pro·bang (prō′băng′) *n.* A long, slender, flexible rod having a tuft or sponge at the end, used chiefly to remove foreign bodies from or apply medication to the larynx or esophagus.

probe (prōb) *n.* A slender flexible surgical instrument with a blunt bulbous tip, used to explore a wound or body cavity.

pro·ben·e·cid (prō-běn′ĭ-sĭd) *n.* A uricosuric drug derived from benzoic acid and used chiefly in the treatment of gout.

pro·caine (prō′kān′) *n.* A white crystalline powder used chiefly in its hydrochloride form as a local anesthetic.

pro·cap·sid (prō-kăp′sĭd) *n.* A protein shell lacking a virus genome.

pro·car·ba·zine (prō-kär′bə-zēn) *n.* A potent antineoplastic drug used to treat advanced Hodgkin's disease.

pro·car·box·y·pep·ti·dase (prō′kär-bŏk′sē-pĕp′tĭ-dās′, -dāz′) *n.* The inactive precursor of a carboxypeptidase.

pro·ce·dure (prə-sē′jər) *n.* **1.** A series of steps taken to accomplish an end. **2.** A surgical operation or technique.

pro·cen·tri·ole (prō-sĕn′trē-ōl′) *n.* The early phase in development of centrioles or basal bodies from the cytoplasmic mass surrounding the centriole.

proc·ess (prŏs′ĕs′, prō′sĕs′) *n., pl.* **proc·ess·es** (prŏs′ĕs′ĭz, prō′sĕs′-, prŏs′ĭ-sēz′, prō′sĭ-). **1.** Advance or progress, as of a disease. **2.** An outgrowth of tissue; a projecting part, as of a bone. — **proc′ess** *adj.* — **proc′ess** *v.*

pro·chy·mo·sin (prō-kī′mə-sĭn) *n.* The precursor of chymosin.

pro·co·ag·u·lant (prō′kō-ăg′yə-lənt) *n.* **1.** The precursor of any of various blood factors necessary for coagulation. **2.** An agent that promotes the coagulation of blood.

pro·cre·ate (prō′krē-āt′) *v.* **-at·ed, -at·ing, -ates.** To beget and conceive offspring; to reproduce. — **pro′cre·a′tion** *n.*

pro·cre·a·tive (prō′krē-ā′tĭv) *adj.* **1.** Capable of reproducing; generative. **2.** Of or directed to procreation.

proc·tal·gi·a (prŏk-tăl′jē-ə, -jə) *n.* Pain at the anus or in the rectum.

proc·ta·tre·sia (prŏk′tə-trē′zhə, -zhē-ə) *n.* See **anal atresia**.

proc·tec·ta·si·a (prŏk′tĭk-tā′zē-ə, -zhə) *n.* Dilation of the anus or rectum.

proc·tec·to·my (prŏk-tĕk′tə-mē) *n.* Surgical resection of the rectum.

proc·teu·ryn·ter (prŏk′tyŏŏ-rĭn′tər) *n.* An inflatable bag used to dilate the rectum.

proc·ti·tis (prŏk-tī′tĭs) *n.* Inflammation of the rectum or anus.

proc·to·cele (prŏk′tə-sēl′) *n.* **1.** Prolapse of the rectum. **2.** Herniation of the rectum.

proc·to·cly·sis (prŏk-tŏk′lĭ-sĭs) *n.* The slow, continuous, drop-by-drop administration of saline solution into the rectum and sigmoid colon.

proc·to·coc·cy·pex·y (prŏk′tō-kŏk′sə-pĕk′sē) *n.* Surgical fixation of a prolapsed rectum to the tissues anterior to the coccyx.

proc·to·co·lec·to·my (prŏk′tō-kə-lĕk′tə-mē) *n.* Surgical removal of the rectum and all or part of the colon.

proc·to·co·lon·os·co·py (prŏk′tō-kō′lə-nŏs′-kə-pē) *n.* Inspection of the interior of the rectum and the lower colon.

proc·to·col·po·plas·ty (prŏk′tō-kŏl′pə-plăs′tē) *n.* Surgical closure of a rectovaginal fistula.

proc·to·cys·to·plas·ty (prŏk′tō-sĭs′tə-plăs′tē) *n.* Surgical closure of a rectovesical fistula.

proc·to·cys·tot·o·my (prŏk′tō-sĭ-stŏt′ə-mē) *n.* Surgical incision into the bladder from the rectum.

proc·tol·o·gy (prŏk-tŏl′ə-jē) *n.* The branch of medicine that deals with the diagnosis and treatment of disorders affecting the colon, rectum, and anus. — **proc′to·log′ic** (-tə-lŏj′ĭk) *adj.* — **proc·tol′o·gist** *n.*

proc·to·pa·ral·y·sis (prŏk′tō-pə-răl′ĭ-sĭs) *n.* Paralysis of the anus.

proc·to·pex·y (prŏk′tə-pĕk′sē) *n.* Surgical fixation of a prolapsed rectum.

proc·to·plas·ty (prŏk′tə-plăs′tē) *n.* Reparative or plastic surgery of the anus or of the rectum.

proc·to·ple·gi·a (prŏk′tə-plē′jē-ə, -jə) *n.* Paralysis of the anus and the rectum resulting from paraplegia.

proc·top·to·si·a (prŏk′tŏp-tō′sē-ə) or **proc·top·to·sis** (-tō′sĭs) *n.* Prolapse of the rectum and the anus.

proc·tor·rha·phy (prŏk-tôr′ə-fē) *n.* Surgical suturing of a lacerated rectum or anus.

proc·tor·rhe·a (prŏk′tə-rē′ə) *n.* A mucoserous discharge from the rectum.

proc·to·scope (prŏk′tə-skōp′) *n.* An instrument for examining the rectum consisting of a tube or speculum equipped with a light. — **proc·tos′co·py** (-tŏs′kə-pē) *n.*

proc·to·sig·moid·ec·to·my (prŏk′tō-sĭg′moi-dĕk′tə-mē) *n.* Surgical excision of the rectum and the sigmoid colon.

proc·to·sig·moid·i·tis (prŏk′tō-sĭg′moi-dī′tĭs) *n.* Inflammation of the sigmoid colon and rectum.

proc·to·sig·moid·os·co·py (prŏk′tō-sĭg′moi-dŏs′kə-pē) *n.* Direct inspection of the rectum and the sigmoid colon using a sigmoidoscope.

proc·to·spasm (prŏk′tə-spăz′əm) *n.* **1.** Spasmodic stricture of the anus. **2.** Spasmodic contraction of the rectum.

proc·to·ste·no·sis (prŏk′tō-stə-nō′sĭs) *n.* Stricture of the rectum or the anus.

proc·tos·to·my (prŏk-tŏs′tə-mē) *n.* Surgical formation of an artificial opening into the rectum.

proc·tot·o·my (prŏk-tŏt′ə-mē) *n.* Surgical incision into the rectum.

proc·to·tre·sia (prŏk′tə-trē′zhə, -zhē-ə) *n.* Surgical correction of an imperforate anus.

proc·to·val·vot·o·my (prŏk′tə-văl-vŏt′ə-mē) *n.* Surgical incision of the rectal valves.

pro·drome (prō′drōm′) *n., pl.* **-dromes** or **-dro·ma·ta** (-drō′mə-tə). An early symptom indicating the onset of an attack or a disease. — **pro·dro′mal** (-drō′məl), **pro·drom′ic** (-drŏm′ĭk) *adj.*

prod·uct (prŏd′əkt) *n.* **1.** Something produced by human or mechanical effort or by a natural process. **2.** A substance resulting from a chemical reaction.

pro·duc·tive (prə-dŭk′tĭv, prō-) *adj.* **1.** Producing or capable of producing mucus or sputum. **2.** Forming new tissue, as of an inflammation.

productive cough *n.* A cough that expels mucus or sputum from the respiratory tract.

pro·en·zyme (prō-ĕn′zīm′) *n.* The inactive or nearly inactive precursor of an enzyme, converted into an active enzyme by proteolysis.

pro·e·ryth·ro·blast (prō′ĭ-rĭth′rə-blăst′) *n.* See **pronormoblast**.

pro·e·ryth·ro·cyte (prō′ĭ-rĭth′rə-sīt′) *n.* An immature nucleated red blood cell.

pro·es·trus (prō-ĕs′trəs) *n.* The period immediately before estrus, characterized by development of the endometrium and ovarian follicles.

pro·fi·bri·nol·y·sin (prō′fī-brə-nŏl′ĭ-sĭn) *n.* See **plasminogen**.

pro·file (prō′fīl′) *n.* **1.** A side view of an object or a structure, especially of the human head. **2.** A formal summary or analysis of data, as of blood, representing distinctive features or characteristics, often in the form of a graph or table.

pro·gen·i·tor (prō-jĕn'ĭ-tər) *n.* **1.** A direct ancestor. **2.** An originator of a line a descent.

prog·e·ny (prŏj'ə-nē) *n., pl.* **progeny** or **-nies. 1.** One born of, begotten by, or derived from another; an offspring or a descendant. **2.** Offspring or descendants considered as a group.

pro·ge·ri·a (prō-jēr'ē-ə) *n.* A rare congenital disorder of childhood characterized by gross retardation of growth after the first year and by rapid onset of the physical changes typical of old age, usually resulting in death before the age of 20.

pro·ges·ter·one (prō-jĕs'tə-rōn') *n.* **1.** A steroid hormone secreted by the corpus luteum of the ovary and by the placenta, that acts to prepare the uterus for implantation of the fertilized ovum, to maintain pregnancy, and to promote development of the mammary glands. **2.** A drug prepared from natural or synthetic progesterone, used to prevent miscarriage and to treat menstrual disorders.

pro·ges·tin (prō-jĕs'tĭn) *n.* A natural or synthetic progestational substance that mimics some or all of the actions of progesterone.

pro·ges·to·gen (prō-jĕs'tə-jən) *n.* Any of various substances having progestational effects; a progestin.

pro·glot·tid (prō-glŏt'ĭd) or **pro·glot·tis** (-glŏt'ĭs) *n., pl.* **-glot·tids** or **-glot·ti·des** (-glŏt'ĭ-dēz'). One of the segments of a tapeworm, containing both male and female reproductive organs.

pro·glot·tis (prō-glŏt'ĭs) *n.* See **proglottid.**

prog·na·thous (prŏg'nə-thəs, prŏg-nā'-) or **prog·nath·ic** (prŏg-năth'ĭk, -nā'thĭk) *adj.* Having jaws that project forward to a marked degree. — **prog'na·thism** (-nə-thĭz'əm) *n.*

prog·no·sis (prŏg-nō'sĭs) *n., pl.* **-ses** (-sēz). **1.** A prediction of the probable course and outcome of a disease. **2.** The likelihood of recovery from a disease. — **prog'nos·ti'cian** (-nŏs-tĭsh'ən) *n.*

prog·nos·tic (prŏg-nŏs'tĭk) *adj.* **1.** Of, relating to, or useful in prognosis. **2.** Of or relating to prediction; predictive. — *n.* **1.** A sign or symptom indicating the future course of a disease. **2.** A sign of a future happening; a portent.

prog·nos·ti·cian (prog- nos-tish'ŭn) *n.* One skilled in prognosis.

pro·gran·u·lo·cyte (prō-grăn'yə-lō-sīt') *n.* See **promyelocyte.**

pro·gres·sive (prə-grĕs'ĭv) *adj.* **1.** Moving forward; advancing. **2.** Proceeding in steps; continuing steadily by increments, as of a course of treatment. **3.** Tending to become more severe or wider in scope, as of a disease or paralysis.

progressive bulbar paralysis *n.* The progressive atrophy and paralysis of the muscles of the tongue, lips, palate, pharynx, and larynx due to atrophic degeneration of the neurons innervating these muscles, usually occurring later in life.

pro·hor·mone (prō-hôr'mōn') *n.* An intraglandular precursor of a hormone.

project *v.* **-ject·ed, -ject·ing, -jects** or prə-jĕkt'. **1.** To extend forward or out; jut out: **2.** In psychology, to externalize and attribute something, such as an emotion, to someone or something else.

pro·jec·tile vomiting (prə-jĕk'təl, -tīl') *n.* Expulsion of the contents of the stomach with great force.

pro·jec·tion (prə-jĕk'shən) *n.* **1.** A thing or part that extends outward beyond a prevailing line or surface. **2.** The attribution of one's own attitudes, feelings, or suppositions to others. **3.** The attribution of one's own attitudes, feelings, or desires to someone or something as a naive or unconscious defense against anxiety or guilt. **4.** Any of the systems of nerve fibers by which a group of nerve cells discharges its nerve impulses to one or more other cell groups.

projection fiber *n.* Any of the nerve fibers connecting the cerebral cortex with other centers in the brain or spinal cord.

pro·jec·tive test (prə-jĕk'tĭv) *n.* A psychological test in which a subject's responses to ambiguous or unstructured standard stimuli, such as a series of cartoons, abstract patterns, or incomplete sentences, are analyzed in order to determine underlying personality traits, feelings, or attitudes.

pro·kar·y·ote or **pro·car·y·ote** (prō-kăr'ē-ōt') *n.* An organism of the kingdom Prokaryotae, constituting the bacteria and cyanobacteria, characterized by the absence of a nuclear membrane and by DNA that is not organized into chromosomes. — **pro·kar'y·ot'ic** (-ŏt'ĭk) *adj.*

pro·lac·tin (prō-lăk'tĭn) *n.* A pituitary hormone that stimulates and maintains the secretion of milk.

pro·lapse (prō-lăps') *v.* **-lapsed, -laps·ing, -laps·es.** To fall or slip out of place, as of an organ or part. — *n.* or **pro·lap·sus** (prō'lăp'səs) (prō'lăps', prō-lăps'). The falling down or slipping out of place of an organ or part, such as the uterus.

prolapse of the umbilical cord *n.* A condition in which part of the umbilical cord appears before the fetus during delivery; it may cause fetal death due to compression of the cord between the presenting part of the fetus and the maternal pelvis.

prolapse of the uterus *n.* Displacement of the uterus downward due to laxity and atony of the muscles and fascia of the pelvic floor.

pro·lep·sis (prō-lĕp'sĭs) *n.* **-ses** (-sēz). The return of paroxysms of a recurrent disease at intervals that progressively become shorter. — **pro·lep'tic** (-lĕp'tĭk) *adj.*

pro·leu·ko·cyte (prō-lōō'kə-sīt') *n.* See **leukoblast.**

pro·lif·er·ate (prə-lĭf'ə-rāt') *v.* **-at·ed, -at·ing, -ates.** To grow or multiply by rapidly producing new tissue, parts, cells, or offspring.

proliferating systematized angioendotheliomatosis *n.* A rare generalized cutaneous and visceral intracapillary proliferation of endothelial cells, accompanied by vascular thrombosis and obstruction.

pro·lif·er·a·tion (prə-lĭf'ə-rā'shən) *n.* The growth and reproduction of similar cells.

pro·lif·er·a·tive (prə-lĭf'ə-rā'tĭv, -lĭf'ər-ə-) or **pro·lif·er·ous** (-ər-əs) *adj.* Tending to proliferate.

proliferative inflammation *n.* Inflammation characterized by an increase in the number of tissue cells.

pro·line (prō'lēn') *n.* An amino acid that is found in most proteins and is a major constituent of collagen.

pro·meg·a·lo·blast (prō-mĕg'ə-lō-blăst') *n.* The first of four maturation stages of the megaloblast.

pro·met·a·phase (prō-mĕt'ə-fāz') *n.* The stage of mitosis or meiosis in which the nuclear membrane disintegrates, the centrioles reach the poles of the cell, and the chromosomes continue to contract.

pro·me·thi·um (prə-mē'thē-əm) *n.* A radioactive rare-earth element with atomic number 61, obtained as a product of the fission of uranium.

prom·i·nence (prŏm'ə-nəns) *n.* A small projection or protuberance.

prom·i·nent (prŏm'ə-nənt) *adj.* **1.** Projecting outward or upward; protuberant. **2.** Immediately noticeable; conspicuous.

prominent heel *n.* A condition marked by a tender swelling on the heel caused by a thickening of the periosteum or fibrous tissue covering the back of the calcaneus.

pro·mon·o·cyte (prō-mŏn'ə-sīt') *n.* See **premonocyte.**

prom·on·to·ry (prŏm'ən-tôr'ē) *n.* A projecting part.

pro·mot·er (prə-mō'tər) *n.* **1.** A substance that increases the activity of a catalyst. **2.** A DNA molecule to which RNA polymerase binds, initiating the transcription of mRNA. **3.** A chemical thought to promote carcinogenicity or mutagenicity.

pro·mo·tion (prə-mō'shən) *n.* The stimulation of the progress or growth of a tumor following initiation by a promoter, which may itself be noncarcinogenic.

pro·my·e·lo·cyte (prō-mī'ə-lə-sīt') *n.* A cell containing a few granules formed in the transition from myeloblast to myelocyte during the development of a granular white blood cell; it is the predominant cell type seen in granulocytic leukemia.

pro·nate (prō'nāt') *v.* **-nat·ed, -nat·ing, -nates. 1.** To turn or rotate the hand or forearm so that the palm faces down or back. **2.** To turn or rotate the sole of the foot by abduction and eversion so that the inner edge of the sole bears the body's weight. **3.** To turn or rotate a limb so that the inner surface faces down or back. **4.** To place in a prone position.

pro·na·tion (prō-nā'shən) *n.* **1.** The act of pronating. **2.** The condition of being pronated, especially the condition of having flat feet.

pro·na·tor (prō'nā'tər) *n.* A muscle that effects or assists in pronation.

prone (prōn) *adj.* **1.** Lying with the front or face downward. **2.** Having a tendency; inclined. — *adv.* In a prone manner.

pro·neph·ros (prō-nĕf'rəs, -rŏs') *n., pl.* **-roi** (-roi) or **-ra** (-rə). A kidneylike organ, being either part of the most anterior pair of three pairs of organs in an embryo but disappearing early in embryonic development.

pro·nor·mo·blast (prō-nôr'mə-blăst') *n.* The first of four stages in development of the normoblast.

pro·nu·cle·us (prō-nōō'klē-əs, -nyōō'-) *n.* **1.** One of two nuclei undergoing fusion in karyogamy. **2.** The haploid nucleus of a sperm or egg before fusion of the nuclei in fertilization.

prop·a·gate (prŏp'ə-gāt') *v.* **-gat·ed, -gat·ing, -gates. 1.** To cause an organism to multiply or breed. **2.** To breed offspring. **3.** To transmit characteristics from one generation to another.

prop·a·ga·tion (prŏp'ə-gā'shən) *n.* **1.** Multiplication or increase, as by natural reproduction. **2.** The act or process of propagating, especially the process by which an impulse is transmitted along a nerve fiber.

prop·a·ga·tive (prŏp'ə-gā'tĭv) *adj.* **1.** Of, relating to, or involved in propagation. **2.** Relating to the germ cells as distinguished from the somatic cells.

pro·pa·no·ic acid (prō'pə-nō'ĭk) *n.* See **propionic acid.**

pro·pep·sin (prō-pĕp'sĭn) *n.* See **pepsinogen.**

pro·per·din (prō-pûr'dĭn) *n.* A natural protein in blood serum that participates in the body's immune response by working in conjunction with the complement system.

properdin system *n.* An alternative system by which, in the absence of antibodies bound to immunoglobulins and components of complement, the immunological cascade occurs, with the activation of critical components of complement aided by the stabilizing properties of properdin.

pro·phase (prō'fāz') *n.* **1.** The first stage of mitosis, during which the chromosomes condense and become visible, the nuclear membrane breaks down, and the spindle apparatus forms at opposite poles of the cell. **2.** The first stage of meiosis, during which the DNA replicates, homologous chromosomes undergo synapsis, chiasmata form, and the chromosomes contract. — **pro·pha'sic** (-fā'zĭk) *adj.*

pro·phy·lac·tic (prō'fə-lăk'tĭk, prŏf'ə-) *n.* **1.** A prophylactic agent, device, or measure, such as a vaccine or drug. **2.** A contraceptive device, especially a condom. — *adj.* Acting to defend against or prevent something, especially disease; protective.

prophylactic treatment *n.* The institution of measures to protect a person from a disease to which he or she has been, or may be, exposed.

pro·phy·lax·is (prō'fə-lăk'sĭs, prŏf'ə-) *n., pl.* **-lax·es** (-lăk'sēz'). Prevention of or protective treatment for disease.

pro·pi·o·ma·zine (prō'pē-ō'mə-zēn') *n.* A drug

used intramuscularly or intravenously as a sedative prior to the administration of anesthesia.

pro·pi·on·ic acid (prō'pē-ŏn'ĭk) *n.* A fatty acid found naturally in sweat and as a product of bacterial fermentation, used chiefly in the form of its propionates as a mold inhibitor in bread.

pro·pi·on·ic·ac·i·de·mi·a (prō'pē-ŏn'ĭ-kăs'ĭ-dē'-mē-ə) *n.* An abnormally high concentration of propionic acid in the blood, caused by the deficiency of an enzyme and characterized by vomiting, lethargy, ketoacidosis, and leukopenia.

pro·pos·i·tus (prō-pŏz'ĭ-təs) *n., pl.* **-ti** (-tī'). See **proband.**

pro·pox·y·phene (prō-pŏk'sə-fēn') *n.* A nonnarcotic analgesic drug used for the relief of mild to moderate pain.

pro·pran·o·lol (prō-prăn'ə-lôl', -lōl') *n.* A drug that blocks beta-adrenergic activity, used to treat hypertension, angina pectoris, and cardiac arrhythmia.

pro·pri·e·tar·y (prə-prī'ĭ-tĕr'ē) *adj.* **1.** Exclusively owned; private, as of a hospital. **2.** Owned by a private individual or corporation under a trademark or patent, as of a drug. —*n.* A proprietary medicine.

proprietary hospital *n.* A hospital operated as a profit-making business and owned by a corporation, investment group, or by physicians who use it primarily for their own patients.

pro·pri·o·cep·tion (prō'prē-ō-sĕp'shən) *n.* The unconscious perception of movement and spatial orientation arising from stimuli within the body itself.

proprioceptive mechanism *n.* The mechanism controlling position and movement, by which one is able to adjust muscular movements accurately and to maintain one's balance.

proprioceptive reflex *n.* A reflex induced by stimulation of proprioceptors.

pro·pri·o·cep·tor (prō'prē-ō-sĕp'tər) *n.* A sensory receptor, found chiefly in muscles, tendons, joints, and the inner ear, that detects the motion or position of the body or a limb by responding to stimuli arising within the organism. —**pro'pri·o·cep'tive** *adj.*

prop·to·sis (prŏp-tō'sĭs) *n., pl.* **-ses** (-sēz). Forward displacement of an organ, especially an eyeball. —**prop·tot·ic** (-tŏt'ĭk) *adj.*

pro·pul·sion (prə-pŭl'shən) *n.* **1.** A driving or propelling force. **2.** The leaning or falling forward characteristic of the festination of Parkinsonism.

pro·pyl alcohol (prō'pĭl) *n.* A clear colorless liquid used as a solvent and as an antiseptic.

pro·pyl·i·o·done (prō'pəl-ī'ə-dōn') *n.* A radiopaque material used for bronchography.

pro·pyl·thi·o·u·ra·cil (prō'pəl-thī'ō-yŏŏr'ə-sĭl') *n.* An agent that inhibits the synthesis of thyroid hormones and is used in the treatment of hyperthyroidism.

pro rat. aet. *abbr. Latin.* pro ratione aetatis (according to (the patient's) age)

pro·ren·nin (prō-rĕn'ĭn) *n.* See **prochymosin.**

pro·ru·bri·cyte (prō-rōō'brĭ-sīt') *n.* A basophilic normoblast.

pro·se·cre·tin (prō'sĭ-krēt'n) *n.* The inactive precursor of secretin.

pros·en·ceph·a·lon (prŏs'ĕn-sĕf'ə-lŏn') *n.* **1.** The most anterior of the three primary regions of the embryonic brain, from which the telencephalon and diencephalon develop. **2.** The segment of the adult brain that develops from the embryonic forebrain and includes the cerebrum, thalamus, and hypothalamus. —**pros'en·ce·phal'ic** (-sə-făl'ĭk) *adj.*

pros·o·pag·no·sia (prŏs'ə-păg-nō'zhə, -zē-ə) *n.* An inability or difficulty in recognizing familiar faces; it may be congenital or result from injury or disease of the brain.

pros·o·pla·sia (prŏs'ə-plā'zhə, -zē-ə) *n.* Progressive transformation to a higher level of function or complexity, such as in the cells of the salivary ducts as they become secreting cells.

pros·o·po·di·ple·gia (prŏs'ə-pō-dī-plē'jə, -jē-ə) *n.* Paralysis affecting both sides of the face.

pros·o·po·neu·ral·gia (prŏs'ə-pō-nŏŏ-răl'jə, -nyŏŏ-) *n.* See **trigeminal neuralgia.**

pros·o·po·spasm (prŏs'ə-pō-spăz'əm) *n.* See **facial tic.**

pro·sper·mi·a (prō-spûr'mē-ə) *n.* See **premature ejaculation.**

pros·ta·glan·din (prŏs'tə-glăn'dĭn) *n.* Any of a group of potent hormonelike substances produced in various tissues that are derived from fatty acids and mediate a wide range of physiological functions, such as control of blood pressure and smooth muscle contraction and modulation of inflammation.

pros·ta·tal·gi·a (prŏs'tə-tăl'jē-ə, -jə) *n.* Pain in the prostate gland.

pros·tate (prŏs'tāt') *n.* The prostate gland. —*adj.* Of or relating to the prostate gland. —**pro·stat'ic** (prō-stăt'ĭk) *adj.*

pros·ta·tec·to·my (prŏs'tə-tĕk'tə-mē) *n.* Surgical removal of all or part of the prostate gland.

prostate gland *n.* A chestnut-shaped body that surrounds the beginning of the male urethra at the base of the bladder, consists of two lateral lobes and a middle lobe lying above and between the ejaculatory ducts, controls the release of urine from the bladder, and whose milky fluid secretion is discharged by excretory ducts into the prostatic urethra during emission of semen.

prostatic ductule *n.* Any of the minute canals that receive the prostatic secretion from the glandular tubules and discharge it through openings on either side of the urethral crest in the posterior wall of the urethra.

prostatic fluid *n.* A whitish secretion that is one of the constituents of semen.

prostatic massage *n.* **1.** The expression of prostatic secretions by applying pressure on the prostate with a finger in the rectum. **2.** The emptying of prostatic grooves and ducts by repeated downward compression maneuvers, used in the treatment of inflammatory conditions of the prostate.

prostatic utricle *n.* A minute pouch in the prostate opening; it is the male analogue of the uterus and vagina and consists of the remains of the fused caudal ends of the embryonic excretory ducts.

pros·ta·tism (prŏs′tə-tĭz′əm) *n.* A disorder characterized by decreased force of urination and dysuria, usually resulting from enlargement of the prostate gland. — **pros′ta·tit′ic** *adj.*

pros·ta·ti·tis (prŏs′tə-tī′tĭs) *n.* Inflammation of the prostate gland. — **pros′ta·tit′ic** (-tĭt′ĭk) *adj.*

pros·ta·to·cys·ti·tis (prŏs′tə-tō-sĭ-stī′tĭs) *n.* Inflammation of the prostate and the bladder.

pros·ta·to·cys·tot·o·my (prŏs′tə-tō-sĭ-stŏt′ə-mē) *n.* Surgical incision through the prostate and bladder wall with drainage through the perineum.

pros·ta·to·meg·a·ly (prŏs′tə-tō-mĕg′ə-lē) *n.* Enlargement of the prostate gland.

pros·ta·tot·o·my (prŏs′tə-tŏt′ə-mē) *n.* Surgical incision into the prostate.

pros·ta·to·ve·sic·u·lec·to·my (prŏs′tə-tō-və-sĭk′yə-lĕk′tə-mē, -və-) *n.* Surgical removal of the prostate gland and the seminal vesicles.

pros·ta·to·ve·sic·u·li·tis (prŏs′tə-tō-və-sĭk′yə-lī′tĭs, -və-) *n.* Inflammation of the prostate gland and the seminal vesicles.

pros·the·sis (prŏs-thē′sĭs) *n., pl.* **-ses** (-sēz). **1.** An artificial device used to replace a missing body part, such as a limb, a tooth, an eye, or a heart valve. **2.** Replacement of a missing body part with such a device.

pros·thet·ic (prŏs-thĕt′ĭk) *adj.* **1.** Serving as or relating to a prosthesis. **2.** Of or relating to prosthetics.

prosthetic group *n.* The nonprotein component of a conjugated protein, as the heme group in hemoglobin.

pros·thet·ics (prŏs-thĕt′ĭks) *n.* The branch of medicine or surgery that deals with the production and application of artificial body parts. — **pros′the·tist** (prŏs′thĭ-tĭst) *n.*

pros·tho·don·tics (prŏs′thə-dŏn′tĭks) *n.* The branch of dentistry dealing with the replacement of missing teeth and related mouth or jaw structures by artificial devices.

pros·tra·tion (prŏ-strā′shən) *n.* Total exhaustion or weakness; collapse.

pro·tac·tin·i·um (prō′tăk-tĭn′ē-əm) *n.* A rare, extremely toxic radioactive element having atomic number 91.

pro·ta·mine (prō′tə-mēn′, -mĭn) or **pro·ta·min** (-mĭn) *n.* Any of a group of simple proteins found in fish sperm that are soluble in water and not coagulated by heat. In purified form, they are used in a long-acting formulation of insulin and to neutralize the anticoagulant effects of heparin.

pro·ta·no·pi·a (prō′tə-nō′pē-ə) *n.* A form of colorblindness characterized by defective perception of red and confusion of red with green or bluish green.

pro·te·ase (prō′tē-ās′, -āz′) *n.* Any of various enzymes, including the proteinases and peptidases, that catalyze the hydrolysis of proteins.

protease inhibitor *n.* An anti-HIV drug that blocks the action of the enzyme protease, which is needed for viral replication.

pro·tec·tive laryngeal reflex (prə-tĕk′tĭv) *n.* Closure of the glottis to prevent entry of foreign substances into the respiratory tract.

pro·tein (prō′tēn′, -tē-ĭn) *n.* Any of a group of complex organic macromolecules that contain carbon, hydrogen, oxygen, nitrogen, and usually sulfur and are composed of one or more chains of alpha-amino acids. Proteins are fundamental components of all living cells and include many substances, such as enzymes, hormones, and antibodies, that are necessary for the proper functioning of an organism. They are essential in the diet of animals for the growth and repair of tissue and can be obtained from foods such as meat, fish, eggs, milk, and legumes. — **pro′tein·a′ceous** (prōt′n-ā′shəs, prō′tē-nā′-) *adj.*

pro·tein·ase (prōt′n-ās′, -āz′, prō′tē-nās-, -nāz′) *n.* A protease that begins the hydrolytic breakdown of proteins usually by splitting them into polypeptide chains.

protein-bound iodine *n.* Thyroid hormone in its circulating form, consisting of one or more of the iodothyronines bound to one or more of the serum proteins.

protein-bound iodine test *n.* A test of thyroid function in which serum protein-bound iodine is measured to provide an estimate of hormone bound to protein in the peripheral blood.

protein C *n.* A vitamin-K dependent plasma protein that enzymatically cleaves activated forms of coagulation factors, thus inhibiting blood coagulation and interfering with the regulation of intravascular clot formation.

protein metabolism *n.* Decomposition and synthesis of proteins in tissue.

pro·tein·o·sis (prō′tē-nō′sĭs, -tē-ə- nō′-) *n.* A condition characterized by disordered protein formation and distribution, especially as manifested by the deposition of abnormal proteins in tissues.

pro·tein·u·ri·a (prōt′n-ōōr′ē-ə, -yōōr′-, prō′tē-nōōr′-, -nyōōr′-) *n.* **1.** The presence of excessive amounts of protein in the urine. **2.** See **albuminuria.**

pro·te·o·gly·can (prō′tē-ō-glī′kăn′, -kən) *n.* Any of various mucopolysaccharides bound to protein chains in covalent complexes and occurring in the extracellular matrix of connective tissue.

pro·te·o·lip·id (prō′tē-ō-lĭp′ĭd, -lī′pĭd) *n.* Any of a class of lipid-soluble proteins.

pro·te·ol·y·sis (prō′tē-ŏl′ĭ-sĭs) *n.* The hydrolytic breakdown of proteins into simpler, soluble substances, as occurs in digestion.

pro·te·o·me·tab·o·lism (prō′tē-ō-mĭ-tăb′ə-lĭz′-əm) *n.* See **protein metabolism.** — **pro′te·o·met′a·bol′ic** (-mĕt′ə-bŏl′ĭk) *adj.*

pro·te·ose (prō′tē-ōs′, -ōz′) *n.* Any of various water-soluble compounds that are produced during digestion by the hydrolytic breakdown of proteins.

Pro·te·us (prō′tē-əs) *n.* A genus of gram-negative,

rod-shaped aerobic bacteria of the family Enterobacteriaceae that includes species associated with human enteritis and urinary tract infections.

pro·throm·bin (prō-thrŏm'bĭn) *n.* A glycoprotein formed by and stored in the liver and present in the blood plasma that is converted to thrombin in the presence of thromboplastin and calcium ion during blood clotting.

prothrombin test *n.* A method for determining prothrombin concentrations in blood based on the clotting time of oxalated blood plasma in the presence of thromboplastin and calcium chloride.

pro·tist (prō'tĭst) *n.* A unicellular, colonial, or multicellular eukaroytic organism belonging to the taxonomic kingdom Protista, which includes protozoans, slime molds, and certain algae.

pro·to·col (prō'tə-kôl', -kŏl', -kōl') *n.* The plan for a course of medical treatment or for a scientific experiment.

pro·to·di·a·stol·ic gallop (prō'tō-dī'ə-stŏl'ĭk) *n.* A heart gallop rhythm in which an abnormal third heart sound occurs in early diastole.

pro·to·on·co·gene (prō'tō-ŏn'kə-jēn', -ŏng'kə-) *n.* A normal gene that has the potential to become an oncogene.

pro·to·path·ic sensibility (prō'tə-păth'ĭk) *n.* Sensibility to low level and poorly localized stimulations of pain and temperature.

pro·to·plasm (prō'tə-plăz'əm) *n.* The complex, semifluid, translucent substance that constitutes the living matter of cells and manifests essential cellular life functions. Composed of proteins, fats, and other molecules suspended in water, it includes the nucleus and cytoplasm. — **pro'to·plas'mic** (-plăz'mĭk) *adj.*

pro·to·por·phyr·i·a (prō'tō-pôr-fēr'ē-ə) *n.* Enhanced fecal excretion of protoporphyrin.

pro·to·por·phy·rin (prō'tō-pôr'fə-rĭn) *n.* A metalfree porphyrin that combines with iron to form the heme of hemoglobin, myoglobin, cytochrome, and other iron-containing proteins.

pro·to·spasm (prō'tə-spăz'əm) *n.* A spasm beginning in one limb or one muscle that gradually becomes more generalized.

pro·to·zo·an (prō'tə-zō'ən) or **pro·to·zo·on** (-ŏn') *n., pl.* **-zo·ans** or **-zo·a** or **-zo·ons.** Any of a large group of single-celled, usually microscopic, eukaryotic organisms, such as amoebas, ciliates, flagellates, and sporozoans. — **pro'to·zo'an, pro'to·zo'al, pro'to·zo'ic** *adj.*

pro·tract (prō-trăkt', prə-) *v.* **-tract·ed, -tract·ing, -tracts.** To extend or protrude a body part.

pro·trac·tion (prō-trăk'shən, prə-) *n.* Extension of teeth or other maxillary or mandibular structures into a position anterior to the normal position.

pro·trac·tor (prō-trăk'tər, prə-) *n.* A muscle that extends a limb or other part.

pro·trude (prō-trōōd') *v.* **-trud·ed, -trud·ing, -trudes. 1.** To push or thrust outward. **2.** To jut out; project.

pro·tru·sion (prō-trōō'zhən) *n.* **1.** The act of protruding. **2.** The state of being protruded. **3.** A position of the mandible forward from centric relation.

pro·tru·sive occlusion (prō-trōō'sĭv, prə-) *n.* Occlusion that results when the lower jaw is protruded forward from its centric position.

pro·tu·ber·ance (prō-tōō'bər-əns, -tyōō'-, prə-) *n.* **1.** Something, such as a bulge, knob, or swelling, that protrudes. **2.** The condition of being protuberant.

pro·tu·ber·ant (prō-tōō'bər-ənt, -tyōō'-, prə-) *adj.* Swelling outward; bulging. — **pro·tu'ber·ant·ly** *adv.*

protuberant abdomen *n.* Unusual or prominent convexity of the abdomen, due to excessive subcutaneous fat, poor muscle tone, or an increase in the contents of the abdomen.

Pro·ven·til (prō-věn'tl, prō'věn'tl) A trademark for albuterol.

prox·i·mal (prŏk'sə-məl) *adj.* Nearer to a point of reference such as an origin, a point of attachment, or the midline of the body.

prox·i·mo·a·tax·i·a (prŏk'sə-mō-ə-tăk'sē-ə) *n.* Lack of muscular coordination in the proximal portions of the extremities.

Pro·zac (prō'zăk') A trademark for fluoxetine hydrochloride.

pro·zone (prō'zōn') *n.* The phenomenon in which mixtures of specific antigen and antibody do not agglutinate or precipitate visibly because of an excess of either antibody or antigen.

pru·ri·go (prōō-rī'gō) *n.* A chronic skin disease having various causes, marked by the eruption of pale, dome-shaped papules that itch severely. — **pru·rig'i·nous** (-rĭj'ə-nəs) *adj.*

pru·ri·tus (prōō-rī'təs) *n.* Severe itching, often of undamaged skin. — **pru·rit'ic** (-rĭt'ĭk) *adj.*

pruritus a·ni (ā'nī) *n.* Itching of varying intensity localized at the anus.

pruritus vul·vae (vŭl'vē) *n.* Itching of the external female genitalia.

psam·mo·ma (să-mō'mə) *n., pl.* **-mas** or **-ma·ta** (-mə-tə). A firm fibrous neoplasm of the meninges of the brain and spinal cord characterized by calcareous bodies.

psammoma body *n.* **1.** A mineralized body occurring in the meninges, choroid plexus, and in certain meningiomas. **2.** See **brain sand. 3.** See **calcospherite.**

psam·mo·ma·tous meningioma (sə-mō'mə-təs) *n.* See **psammoma.**

pseud·a·graph·i·a (sōō'də-grăf'ē-ə) or **pseu·do·a·graph·i·a** (sōō'dō-ā-grăf'e-ə, -ə-grăf'-) *n.* Partial agraphia in which one cannot produce original writing but can copy correctly.

pseud·es·the·sia (sōō'dĭs-thē'zhə) or **pseu·do·es·the·sia** (sōō'dō-ĭs-) *n.* A subjective sensation not arising from an external stimulus. **2.** See **phantom limb.**

pseu·do·ac·an·tho·sis ni·gri·cans (sōō'dō-ăk'-ăn-thō'sĭs nī'grĭ-kănz', nĭg'rĭ-) *n.* Acanthosis nigricans occurring secondary to maceration of the skin from excessive sweating, or in obese and dark-complexioned adults, or in association with endocrine disorders.

pseu·do·al·lele (soō'dō-ə-lēl') *n.* A gene exhibiting pseudoallelism. **— pseu'do·al·le'lic** (-lē'lĭk, -lĕl'ĭk) *adj.*

pseu·do·al·le·lism (soō'dō-ə-lē'lĭz'əm, -lĕl'ĭz'-) *n.* The state in which two or more genes appear to occupy the same locus under certain conditions but can be shown to occupy closely linked loci under other conditions.

pseu·do·an·eu·rysm (soō'dō-ăn'yə-rĭz'əm) *n.* A dilation of an artery with actual disruption of one or more layers of its walls, rather than with expansion of all the layers of the wall.

pseu·do·bul·bar paralysis (soō'dō-bŭl'bər, -bär') *n.* Paralysis of the lips and tongue, with uncontrolled laughing or crying and difficulty in speaking and swallowing. It simulates progressive bulbar paralysis, and is due to cerebral lesions with bilateral involvement of the upper motor neurons.

pseu·do·car·ti·lage (soō'dō-kär'tl-ĭj) *n.* See **chondroid tissue** (sense 1). **— pseu'do·car'ti·lag'i·nous** (-kär'tl-ăj'ə-nəs) *adj.*

pseu·do·cast (soō'də-kăst') *n.* An elongated ribbonlike mucous thread occurring in the urine, having poorly defined edges and pointed or split ends and resembling a urinary cast.

pseu·do·chan·cre (soō'dō-shăng'kər) *n.* A nonspecific indurated sore resembling a chancre, usually located on the penis.

pseu·do·chro·mes·the·sia (soō'dō-krō'mĕs-thē'zhə) *n.* **1.** A form of synesthesia in which printed vowels or vowel sounds produce imaginary sensations of color. **2.** See **color hearing.**

pseu·do·cyl·in·droid (soō'dō-sĭl'ən-droid') *n.* A shred of mucus or other substance in the urine resembling a renal cast.

pseu·do·cy·e·sis (soō'dō-sī-ē'sĭs) *n.* A usually psychosomatic condition, occurring in both males and females, in which the physical symptoms of pregnancy are manifested but conception has not taken place.

pseu·do·cyst (soō'dō-sĭst') *n.* **1.** An abnormal sac that resembles a cyst but has no membranous lining. **2.** A cyst whose wall is formed by a host cell and not by a parasite. **3.** A cyst consisting of a host cell enclosing a mass of *Toxoplasma* parasites, usually found in the brain.

pseu·do·de·men·tia (soō'dō-dĭ-mĕn'shə) *n.* A condition of exaggerated indifference to one's surroundings without actual mental impairment.

pseu·do·frac·ture (soō'dō-frăk'chər) *n.* A condition in which an x-ray shows formation of new bone with thickening of periosteum at the site of an injury to bone.

pseu·do·gan·gli·on (soō'dō-găng'glē-ən) *n.* A localized thickening of a nerve trunk having the appearance of a ganglion.

pseu·do·gene (soō'də-jēn') *n.* A segment of DNA resembling a gene but lacking a genetic function.

pseu·do·geu·si·a (soō'dō-gyoō'zē-ə, -zhə, -joō'-)

n. A taste sensation not produced by an external stimulus.

pseu·do·her·maph·ro·dit·ism (soō'dō-hər-măf'rə-dī-tĭz'əm) *n.* A state in which a person possesses the internal reproductive organs of one sex while exhibiting some of the external physical characteristics of the opposite sex.

pseu·do·her·ni·a (soō'dō-hûr'nē-ə) *n.* Inflammation of the scrotal tissues or of an inguinal gland, simulating a strangulated hernia.

pseu·do·hy·per·par·a·thy·roid·ism (soō'dō-hī'-pər-păr'ə-thī'roi-dĭz'əm) *n.* Hypercalcemia occurring in association with a malignant neoplasm but without skeletal metastases or primary hyperparathyroidism; it is believed to be caused by the formation of parathyroid hormone by nonparathyroid tumor tissue.

pseu·do·hy·per·tro·phy (soō'dō-hī-pûr'trə-fē) *n.* Increase at the site of an organ or a part that is the result of an increase in the size or number of some other tissue, not of the specific functional elements. **— pseu'do·hy'per·tro'phic** (-trō'fĭk, -trŏf'ĭk) *adj.*

pseu·do·hy·po·na·tre·mi·a (soō'dō-hī'pō-nə-trē'mē-ə) *n.* A low serum sodium concentration resulting from volume displacement by massive hyperlipidemia or hyperproteinemia, or by hyperglycemia.

pseu·do·hy·po·par·a·thy·roid·ism (soō'dō-hī'-pō-păr'ə-thī'roi-dĭz'əm) *n.* A sex-linked disorder resembling hypoparathyroidism, but which is unresponsive to treatment with parathyroid hormone; it is characterized by short stature, round face, achondroplasia, mental deficiency, and parathyroid tissue that is hyperplastic.

pseu·do·ic·ter·us (soō'dō-ĭk'tər-əs) *n.* Discoloration of the skin not caused by bile pigments, as in Addison's disease.

pseu·do·lo·gi·a (soō'də-lō'jē-ə) *n.* Pathological lying in speech or writing.

pseudologia fan·tas·ti·ca (făn-tăs'tĭ-kə) *n.* An elaborate and often fantastic account of exploits that is completely false but that the teller believes to be true.

pseu·do·ma·lig·nan·cy (soō'dō-mə-lĭg'nən-sē) *n.* A benign tumor that appears, clinically or histologically, to be a malignant neoplasm.

pseu·do·ma·ni·a (soō'dō-mā'nē-ə, -măn'yə) *n.* **1.** Feigned insanity. **2.** A mental disorder in which a person alleges to have committed a crime, but has not. **3.** The pathological impulse to falsify.

pseu·do·mem·brane (soō'dō-mĕm'brān') *n.* See **false membrane.**

pseu·do·mem·bra·nous (soō'dō-mĕm'brə-nəs) *adj.* Relating to or marked by the presence of a false membrane.

pseudomembranous bronchitis *n.* See **fibrinous bronchitis.**

pseudomembranous colitis *n.* See **pseudomembranous enterocolitis.**

pseudomembranous enterocolitis *n.* Enterocolitis with the formation and passage of pseudomembranous material in the stools; a common sequel to prolonged antibiotic therapy.

pseudomembranous gastritis *n.* Gastritis characterized by the formation of a false membrane.

pseudomembranous inflammation *n.* A form of exudative inflammation characterized by the formation of a false membrane on a mucosal surface.

pseu·do·mo·nad (sōō′də-mō′năd′) *n.* A member of the large genus *Pseudomonas*.

Pseu·do·mo·nas (sōō′də-mō′nəs, sōō-dŏm′ə-nəs) *n.* A phylum of gram-negative, rod-shaped, mostly aerobic flagellated bacteria, commonly found in soil, water, and decaying matter and including some species that are human pathogens.

pseu·do·myx·o·ma (sōō′dō-mĭk-sō′mə) *n.* A gelatinous mass resembling a myxoma but composed of epithelial mucus.

pseudomyxoma per·i·to·ne·i (pĕr′ĭ-tn-ē′ī) *n.* The accumulation of large quantities of mucoid or mucinous material in the peritoneal cavity, either as a result of rupture of a mucocele of the appendix or of rupture of a benign or malignant cystic neoplasm of the ovary.

pseu·do·ne·o·plasm (sōō′dō-nē′ə-plăz′əm) *n.* See **pseudotumor** (sense 2).

pseu·do·neu·ri·tis (sōō′dō-nŏŏ-rī′tĭs, -nyŏŏ-) *n.* Congenital reddish appearance of the optic disk simulating optic neuritis.

pseu·do·pa·ral·y·sis (sōō′dō-pə-răl′ĭ-sĭs) *n.* A voluntary restriction or inhibition of motion because of pain, incoordination, or other cause, not due to actual muscular paralysis.

pseu·do·par·a·ple·gi·a (sōō′dō-păr′ə-plē′jē-ə, -jə) *n.* Apparent paralysis in the lower extremities, in which the tendon and skin reflexes and the electrical reactions are normal.

pseu·do·plate·let (sōō′dō-plāt′lĭt) *n.* Any of the various fragments of neutrophils that may be mistaken for platelets, especially in peripheral blood smears of leukemic patients.

pseu·do·pod (sōō′də-pŏd′) *n.* A temporary projection of the cytoplasm of certain cells, such as phagocytes, or of certain unicellular organisms, especially amoebas, that serves in locomotion and phagocytosis.

pseu·do·pol·yp (sōō′dō-pŏl′ĭp) *n.* A projecting mass of granulation tissue, such as the masses that may develop in ulcerative colitis.

pseu·do·preg·nan·cy (sōō′dō-prĕg′nən-sē) *n.* See **pseudocyesis**.

pseu·dop·si·a (sōō-dŏp′sē-ə) *n.* Visual hallucinations, illusions, or false perceptions.

pseu·do·pte·ryg·i·um (sōō′dō-tə-rĭj′ē-əm) *n.* A pterygium of irregular shape that may appear at any part of the corneal margin of the eye and that occurs following diphtheria, a burn, or other injury of the conjunctiva.

pseu·do·re·ac·tion (sōō′dō-rē-ăk′shən) *n.* A reaction not caused by the substances used in a given test but rather by impurities or other materials in the test medium; a false reaction.

pseu·do·ro·sette (sōō′dō-rō-zĕt′) *n.* The radial arrangement of neoplastic cells around a small blood vessel.

pseu·do·scar·la·ti·na (sōō′dō-skär′lə-tē′nə) *n.* Erythema with fever resulting from causes other than infection with *Streptococcus pyogenes*.

pseu·dos·mi·a (sōō-dŏz′mē-ə) *n.* Subjective sensation of an odor that is not present.

pseu·do·stra·bis·mus (sōō′dō-strə-bĭz′məs) *n.* The appearance of strabismus caused by epicanthus, abnormality in interorbital distance, or corneal light reflex not corresponding to the center of the pupil.

pseu·do·strat·i·fied epithelium (sōō′dō-străt′ə-fīd′) *n.* Epithelium made up of cells that reach the basement membrane and appear to be stratified because their nuclei are at different levels.

pseu·do·trun·cus ar·te·ri·o·sus (sōō′dō-trŭng′-kəs är-tēr′ē-ō′səs) *n.* A congenital cardiovascular deformity characterized by atresia of the pulmonic valve and the lack of a main pulmonary artery with the lungs being supplied with blood either through an arterial duct or via bronchial arteries arising from the aorta.

pseu·do·tu·ber·cu·lo·sis (sōō′dō-tŏŏ-bûr′kyə-lō′sĭs, -tyŏŏ-) *n.* Any of several diseases characterized by granulomas that resemble tubercular nodules but that are not caused by the tubercle bacillus.

pseu·do·tu·mor (sōō′dō-tŏŏ′mər, -tyŏŏ′-) *n.* **1.** An enlargement of nonneoplastic character that clinically resembles a true neoplasm. **2.** A circumscribed fibrous exudate of inflammatory origin. **3.** A condition characterized by cerebral edema with narrowed small ventricles but with increased intracranial pressure and frequently with papilledema, commonly associated with obesity in females between the ages of 13 and 40.

pseu·do·xan·tho·ma e·las·ti·cum (sōō′dō-zăn-thō′mə ĭ-lăs′tĭ-kəm) *n.* See **elastoma**.

P-sin·is·tro·car·di·a·le (sĭn′ĭ-strō-kär′dē-ä′lē) *n.* An electrocardiographic syndrome characteristic of overloading of the left atrium of the heart.

psit·ta·co·sis (sĭt′ə-kō′sĭs) *n.* An infectious disease of parrots and related birds caused by the bacterium *Chlamydia psittaci*, that is communicable to humans, in whom it produces high fever, severe headache, and symptoms similar to pneumonia.

pso·ra·len (sôr′ə-lən) *n.* Any of a group of chemical compounds found naturally in certain plants that are used in treating psoriasis and vitiligo.

pso·rel·co·sis (sôr′əl-kō′sĭs) *n.* Ulceration of the skin resulting from scabies.

pso·ri·a·sis (sə-rī′ə-sĭs) *n.* A noncontagious inflammatory skin disease characterized by recurring reddish patches covered with silvery scales.

psy·chal·gi·a (sī-kăl′jē-ə, -jə) *n.* **1.** Psychological or emotional pain or distress that accompanies a mental effort, especially in depression. **2.** Physical pain believed to be of psychological origin.

psy·che (sī′kē) *n.* The mind functioning as the center of thought, emotion, and behavior and consciously or unconsciously mediating the body's responses to the social and physical environment.

psy·chi·at·ric hospital (sī′kē ăt′rĭk) *n.* A hospital for the care and treatment of patients affected with acute or chronic mental illness.

psy·chi·a·trist (sī-kī′ə-trĭst, sī-) *n.* A physician who specializes in psychiatry.

psy·chi·a·try (sī-kī′ə-trē, sī-) *n.* The branch of medicine that deals with the diagnosis, treatment, and prevention of mental and emotional disorders.

psy·chic (sī′kĭk) *adj.* **1.** Of, relating to, affecting, or influenced by the human mind or psyche; mental. **2.** Capable of extraordinary mental processes, such as extrasensory perception and mental telepathy. **3.** Of or relating to such mental processes. —*n.* A person apparently responsive to psychic forces.

psychic trauma *n.* An upsetting experience precipitating or aggravating an emotional or mental disorder.

psy·cho·ac·tive (sī′kō-ăk′tĭv) *adj.* Affecting the mind or mental processes. Used of a drug.

psy·cho·a·nal·y·sis (sī′kō-ə-năl′ĭ-sĭs) *n., pl.* **-ses** (-sēz′). **1.** The method of psychiatric therapy originated by Sigmund Freud in which free association, dream interpretation, and analysis of resistance and transference are used to explore repressed or unconscious impulses, anxieties, and internal conflicts. **2.** The theory of personality developed by Freud that focuses on repression and unconscious forces and includes the division of the psyche into the id, ego, and superego. **3.** Psychiatric treatment incorporating this method and theory. —**psy′cho·an′a·lyt′ic** (-ăn′ə-lĭt′ĭk), **psy′·cho·an′a·lyt′i·cal** (-ĭ-kəl) *adj.*

psy·cho·an·a·lyst (sī′kō-ăn′ə-lĭst) *n.* A psychotherapist, usually a psychiatrist or a clinical psychologist, who is trained in psychoanalysis and employs its methods in treating emotional disorders.

psychoanalytic therapy *n.* See **psychoanalysis.**

psy·cho·an·a·lyze (sī′kō-ăn′ə-līz′) *v.* **-lyzed, -lyz·ing, -lyz·es.** To analyze and treat by psychoanalysis.

psy·cho·bab·ble (sī′kō-băb′əl) *n.* Psychological jargon, especially that of psychotherapy.

psy·cho·dra·ma (sī′kə-drä′mə, -drăm′ə) *n.* **1.** A psychotherapeutic and analytic technique in which people are assigned roles to be played spontaneously within a dramatic context devised by a therapist. **2.** A dramatization in which this technique is employed.

psy·cho·gen·e·sis (sī′kō-jĕn′ĭ-sĭs) *n.* **1.** The origin and development of psychological processes, personality, or behavior. **2.** Development of a physical disorder or illness resulting from psychic, rather than physiological, factors. —**psy′cho·ge·net′ic** (-jə-nĕt′ĭk) *adj.*

psychogenic vomiting *n.* Vomiting associated with emotional distress and anxiety, occurring usually during meals but without weight loss.

psy·cho·ki·ne·sis (sī′kō-kĭ-nē′sĭs, -kī-) *n., pl.* **-ses** (-sēz). An uncontrolled, maniacal outburst, re-

sulting from defective inhibition. —**psy′cho·ki·net′ic** (-kĭ-nĕt′ĭk, -kī-) *adj.*

psy·cho·lep·sy (sī′kə-lĕp′sē) *n.* A condition characterized by sudden mood changes accompanied by feelings of hopelessness and lethargy.

psy·cho·lin·guis·tics (sī′kō-lĭng-gwĭs′tĭks) *n.* The study of the influence of psychological factors on the development, use, and interpretation of language. —**psy′cho·lin′guist** *n.* —**psy′cho·lin·guis′tic** *adj.*

psy·cho·log·i·cal moment (sī′kə-lŏj′ĭ-kəl) *n.* The time at which the mental state of a person is most likely to produce a desired response.

psy·chol·o·gist (sī-kŏl′ə-jĭst) *n.* A person trained and educated to perform psychological research, testing, and therapy.

psy·chol·o·gize (sī-kŏl′ə-jīz′) *v.* **-gized, -giz·ing, -giz·es.** **1.** To explain behavior in psychological terms. **2.** To investigate, reason, or speculate in psychological terms.

psy·chol·o·gy (sī-kŏl′ə-jē) *n.* **1.** The science that deals with mental processes and behavior. **2.** The emotional and behavioral characteristics of an individual, a group, or an activity.

psy·cho·met·rics (sī′kə-mĕt′rĭks) *n.* The branch of psychology that deals with the design, administration, and interpretation of quantitative tests for the measurement of psychological variables such as intelligence.

psy·chom·e·try (sī-kŏm′ĭ-trē) *n.* See **psychometrics.**

psy·cho·mo·tor (sī′kō-mō′tər) *adj.* **1.** Of or relating to movement or muscular activity associated with mental processes. **2.** Relating to the combination of psychic and motor events, including disturbances.

psy·cho·neu·ro·sis (sī′kō-nŏŏ-rō′sĭs, -nyŏŏ-) *n., pl.* **-ses** (-sēz). Neurosis. —**psy′cho·neu·rot′ic** (-rŏt′ĭk) *adj.*

psy·cho·path (sī′kə-păth′) *n.* A person with an antisocial personality disorder, especially one manifested in aggressive, perverted, criminal, or amoral behavior.

psy·cho·path·ic (sī′kə-păth′ĭk) *adj.* **1.** Of, relating to, or characterized by psychopathy. **2.** Relating to or affected with an antisocial personality disorder that is usually characterized by aggressive, perverted, criminal, or amoral behavior.

psy·cho·phys·i·o·log·ic disorder (sī′kō-fĭz′ē-ə-lŏj′ĭk) *n.* See **psychosomatic disorder.**

psy·cho·sex·u·al development (sī′kō-sĕk′-shŏŏ-əl) *n.* In Freudian psychoanalytic theory, the influence that sexual growth has on personality development from birth to adult life.

psychosexual dysfunction *n.* A disturbance of sexual functioning, such as impotence, premature ejaculation, or anorgasmy, that is believed to be caused by mental and emotional difficulties concerning sexuality rather than physical disorders.

psy·cho·sis (sī-kō′sĭs) *n., pl.* **-ses** (-sēz). A severe mental disorder, with or without organic damage, characterized by derangement of personality and loss of contact with reality and causing deterioration of normal social functioning.

psy·cho·so·mat·ic (sī'kō-sō-măt'ĭk) *adj*. **1.** Of or relating to a disorder having physical symptoms but originating from mental or emotional causes. **2.** Relating to or concerned with the influence of the mind on the body, especially with respect to disease.

psychosomatic disorder *n*. A disorder characterized by physical symptoms resulting from psychological factors, usually involving one system of the body such as the gastrointestinal, respiratory, or genitourinary system.

psychosomatic medicine *n*. The branch of medicine that studies and treats diseases and disorders by investigating and exploiting the psychological processes that influence the body.

psy·cho·sur·ger·y (sī'kō-sûr'jə-rē) *n*. Brain surgery used to treat severe, intractable mental or behavioral disorders. — **psy'cho·sur'geon** (-sûr'jən) *n*.

psy·cho·ther·a·peu·tics (sī'kō-thĕr'ə-pyōō'tĭks) *n*. See **psychotherapy**.

psy·cho·ther·a·pist (sī'kō-thĕr'ə-pĭst) *n*. A person, usually a psychiatrist or clinical psychologist, professionally trained to practice psychotherapy.

psy·cho·ther·a·py (sī'kō-thĕr'ə-pē) *n*. The treatment of mental and emotional disorders through the use of psychological techniques designed to encourage communication of conflicts and insight into problems, with the goal being personality growth and behavior modification. — **psy'cho·ther'a·peu'tic** (-pyōō'tĭk) *adj*.

psy·chot·ic (sī-kŏt'ĭk) *adj*. Of, relating to, or affected by psychosis. — *n*. A person affected by psychosis.

psy·cho·tro·pic (sī'kə-trō'pĭk, -trŏp'ĭk) *adj*. Having an altering effect on perception or behavior. Used especially of a drug. — *n*. A psychotropic drug or other agent.

psy·chro·al·gi·a (sī'krō-ăl'jē-ə, -jə) *n*. A painful sensation of cold.

psy·chro·phore (sī'krə-fôr') *n*. A catheter having two tubes through which cold water is circulated to apply cold to a canal or cavity.

psyl·li·um (sĭl'ē-əm) *n*. **1.** An annual Eurasian plant (*Plantago psyllium*) having opposite leaves and small flowers borne in dense spikes. **2.** The seeds of this plant, widely used as a mild bulk laxative and sometimes added to foods as a dietary source of soluble fiber.

PT *abbr*. physical therapy

pter·op·ter·in (tĕr-ŏp'tər-ĭn) *n*. A crystalline conjugate of folic acid containing three molecules of glutamic acid instead of one and having the general properties of a polypeptide; formerly used as an antineoplastic agent.

pter·o·yl·glu·tam·ic acid (tĕr'ō-ĭl-glōō-tăm'ĭk) *n*. Folic acid.

pte·ryg·i·um (tə-rĭj'ē-əm) *n., pl.* **-i·ums** or **-i·a** (-ē-ə). An abnormal mass of tissue arising from the conjunctiva of the inner corner of the eye that obstructs vision by growing over the cornea. — **pte·ryg'i·al** (-əl) *adj*.

Pthir·us (thîr'əs, thī'rəs) *n*. A genus of parasitic lice of the family Pediculidae that includes the crab louse, *Pediculus pubis*.

pti·lo·sis (tĭ-lō'sĭs) *n*. Loss of the eyelashes.

pto·maine (tō'mān', tō-mān') *n*. A basic nitrogenous organic compound produced by bacterial putrefaction of protein.

ptomaine poisoning *n*. Food poisoning, erroneously believed to be the result of ptomaine ingestion. Not in technical use.

pto·sis (tō'sĭs) *n., pl.* **-ses** (-sēz). Abnormal lowering or drooping of an organ or a part, especially a drooping of the upper eyelid caused by muscle weakness or paralysis.

pty·a·lin (tī'ə-lĭn) *n*. A form of amylase present in saliva and acting to catalyze the hydrolysis of starch into maltose and dextrin.

pty·a·lism (tī'ə-lĭz'əm) *n*. Excessive flow of saliva.

pu·bar·che (pyōō-bär'kē) *n*. The onset of puberty, particularly as manifested by the appearance of pubic hair.

pu·ber·ty (pyōō'bər-tē) *n*. The stage of adolescence in which a person becomes physiologically capable of sexual reproduction.

pu·bes (pyōō'bēz) *n., pl.* **pubes**. **1.** The lower part of the abdomen, especially the region surrounding the external genitalia. **2.** The hair that appears on this region at puberty.

pu·bes·cence (pyōō-bĕs'əns) *n*. **1.** The state of being pubescent. **2.** The attainment or onset of puberty. **3.** The presence of downy or fine short hair.

pu·bes·cent (pyōō-bĕs'ənt) *adj*. **1.** Reaching or having reached puberty. **2.** Covered with short hairs or soft down.

pu·bic (pyōō'bĭk) *adj*. **1.** Of, relating to, or located in the region of the pubis or the pubes. **2.** Relating to the pubic region of the abdomen.

pubic arch *n*. The arch formed by the inferior rami of the pubic bones.

pubic bone *n*. The forward portion of either of the hipbones, at the juncture forming the front arch of the pelvis.

pubic region *n*. The lowest of the three median regions of the abdomen, lying below the umbilical region and between the inguinal regions.

pubic symphysis *n*. The firm fibrocartilaginous joint between the two pubic bones.

pu·bi·ot·o·my (pyōō'bē-ŏt'ə-mē) *n*. Surgical severance of the pubic bone a few centimeters lateral to the symphysis, especially to increase the capacity of a contracted pelvis sufficiently to permit the passage of a fetus during childbirth.

pu·bis (pyōō'bĭs) *n., pl.* **-bes** (-bēz). **1.** See **pubic bone**. **2.** The hair of the pubic region just above the external genitals. **3.** A pubic hair. **4.** See **mons pubis**.

pub·lic health (pŭb'lĭk) *n*. The science and practice of protecting and improving the health of a community, as by preventive medicine, health education, control of communicable diseases, application of sanitary measures, and monitoring of environmental hazards.

pu·bo·coc·cyg·e·al muscle (pyōō'bō-kŏk-sĭj'-ē-əl) *n.* A muscle formed of the fibers of the elevator muscle of the anus, arising from the pelvic surface of the body of the pubis, and attaching to the coccyx.

pu·bo·pros·tat·ic (pyōō'bō-prŏ-stăt'ĭk) *adj.* Relating to the pubic bone and the prostate gland.

pu·den·dum (pyōō-děn'dəm) *n., pl.* **-da** (-də). The human external genitalia, especially of a woman.

pu·er·il·ism (pyōō'ər-ə-lĭz'əm, pyōōr'ə-) *n.* Childish behavior in an adult, especially as a symptom of mental illness.

pu·er·per·a (pyōō-ûr'pər-ə) *n., pl.* **-per·ae** (-pər-ē'). A woman who has just given birth.

pu·er·per·al (pyōō-ûr'pər-əl) *adj.* Relating to, connected with, or occurring during childbirth or the period immediately following childbirth.

puerperal fever *n.* An illness resulting from infection of the endometrium following childbirth or abortion, marked by fever and septicemia and usually caused by unsterile technique.

pu·er·pe·ri·um (pyōō'ər-pēr'ē-əm) *n., pl.* **-pe·ri·a** (-pēr'ē-ə). **1.** The state of a woman during childbirth or immediately thereafter. **2.** The approximate six-week period lasting from childbirth to the return of normal uterine size.

pul·mo·nar·y (pōōl'mə-něr'ē, pŭl'-) *adj.* Of, relating to, or affecting the lungs.

pulmonary artery *n.* **1.** An artery that is one of the two branches of the pulmonary trunk and enters the hilus of the right lung, with branches distributed with the bronchi; right pulmonary artery. **2.** An artery that enters the hilus of the left lung, with branches accompanying the bronchi; left pulmonary artery.

pulmonary atresia *n.* The congenital absence of the normal valvular orifice into the pulmonary artery.

pulmonary capillary wedge pressure *n.* An indirect indication of left atrial pressure obtained by wedging a catheter into a small pulmonary artery tightly enough to block flow from behind and thus to sample the pressure beyond.

pulmonary circulation *n.* The passage of blood from the right ventricle through the pulmonary artery to the lungs and back through the pulmonary veins to the left atrium.

pulmonary edema *n.* Edema of the lungs usually resulting from mitral stenosis or left ventricular failure.

pulmonary embolism *n.* The obstruction of pulmonary arteries, usually by detached fragments of a clot from a leg or pelvic vein.

pulmonary emphysema *n.* See **emphysema** (sense 1).

pulmonary hypertension *n.* Hypertension in the pulmonary circulation; it may be primary or secondary to pulmonary or cardiac disease.

pulmonary insufficiency *n.* Valvular insufficiency involving the pulmonary valve.

pulmonary murmur or **pulmonic murmur** *n.* An obstructive or regurgitant murmur produced at the pulmonary orifice of the heart.

pulmonary opening *n.* The opening of the pulmonary trunk, opening from the right ventricle and guarded by the pulmonary valve.

pulmonary stenosis *n.* Narrowing of the right ventricular opening into the pulmonary artery.

pulmonary trunk *n.* An arterial trunk with origin from the right ventricle of the heart, and dividing into the right and left pulmonary arteries, which enter the corresponding lungs and branch with the bronchi.

pulmonary tuberculosis *n.* Tuberculosis of the lungs.

pulmonary valve *n.* A valve with semilunar cusps at the entrance to the pulmonary trunk from the right ventricle of the heart.

pulmonary vein *n.* A vein that carries oxygenated blood from the lungs to the left atrium of the heart.

pulmonary ventilation *n.* The total volume of gas per minute inspired or expired.

pul·mo·tor (pōōl'mō'tər, pŭl'-) *n.* A device used to inflate and deflate the lungs during resuscitation.

pulp (pŭlp) *n.* **1.** A soft, moist, shapeless mass of matter. **2.** Dental pulp.

pulp amputation *n.* See **pulpotomy**.

pulp calcification *n.* The presence of calcified nodules or amorphous deposits in the pulp of a tooth.

pul·pec·to·my (pŭl-pĕk'tə-mē) *n.* Removal of the entire pulp structure of a tooth, including that in the roots.

pul·pi·fac·tion (pŭl'pə-făk'shən) *n.* Reduction of tissue to a pulpy condition.

pul·pot·o·my (pŭl-pŏt'ə-mē) *n.* Surgical removal of a portion of the tooth pulp, usually of the coronal portion.

pulp stone *n.* A calcified mass of dentin within the pulp of a tooth.

pul·sate (pŭl'sāt') *v.* **-sat·ed, -sat·ing, -sates.** To expand and contract rhythmically; beat.

pul·sa·tion (pŭl-sā'shən) *n.* **1.** The act of pulsating. **2.** A single beat, throb, or vibration.

pulse (pŭls) *n.* The rhythmical dilation of arteries produced when blood is pumped outward by regular contractions of the heart, especially as palpated at the wrist or in the neck.

pulse deficit *n.* The difference between the heart rate and the palpable pulse, as is often seen in atrial fibrillation.

pulse generator *n.* A device that produces an electrical discharge at regular intervals, which can be modified as needed as in an electronic pacemaker.

pulse·less disease (pŭls'lĭs) *n.* A progressive inflammatory disease that causes the arteries arising from the aortic arch to collapse, making it impossible to detect a pulse in the arms and neck, and resulting in a variety of symptoms associated with ischemia, such as temporary loss of consciousness and blindness.

pulse pressure *n.* The variation in blood pressure

occurring in an artery during the cardiac cycle; the difference between the systolic or maximum and diastolic or minimum pressures.

pulse rate *n.* The rate of the pulse as observed in an artery, expressed as beats per minute.

pulse therapy *n.* A short, intensive course of pharmacotherapy, usually given at intervals such as weekly or monthly, often used in treating cancer.

pulse wave *n.* The progressive increase of pressure radiating through the arteries that occurs with each contraction of the left ventricle of the heart.

pul·sion (pŭl'shən) *n.* A swelling or pushing outward.

pul·sus (pŭl'səs) *n.* A pulse.

pulsus alternans *n.* See **alternating pulse.**

pulsus cel·er (sĕl'ər) *n.* A pulse beat swift to rise and fall.

pulsus dif·fer·ens (dĭf'ə-rĕnz') *n.* A condition in which the pulses in the two radial arteries differ in strength.

pulsus rar·us (râr'əs) *n.* A pulse beat slow to rise and fall.

pulsus tar·dus (tär'dəs) *n.* See **pulsus rarus.**

pump (pŭmp) *n.* **1.** A machine or device for raising, compressing, or transferring fluids. **2.** A molecular mechanism for the active transport of ions or molecules across a cell membrane. — *v.* **pumped, pump·ing, pumps. 1.** To raise or cause to flow by means of a pump. **2.** To transport ions or molecules against a concentration gradient by the expenditure of chemically stored energy.

pump lung *n.* See **shock lung.**

pump-ox·y·gen·a·tor (pŭmp-ŏk'sĭ-jə-nā'tər) *n.* A mechanical device that can substitute for both the heart and lungs during open-heart surgery.

punch biopsy *n.* Removal of a small cylindrical specimen for biopsy by means of a special instrument that either directly pierces the tissue or enters through the skin or a small incision in it.

punch-drunk syndrome *n.* A condition seen in boxers and alcoholics, caused by repeated cerebral concussions and characterized by weakness in the lower limbs, unsteadiness of gait, slowness of muscular movements, hand tremors, hesitancy of speech, and mental dullness.

punch graft *n.* A small graft of the full thickness of the scalp, removed with a circular punch and transplanted in large numbers to a bald area to grow hair.

punc·tate (pŭngk'tāt') *adj.* Having tiny spots, points, or depressions.

punc·tum (pŭngk'təm) *n., pl.* **-ta** (-tə). **1.** The tip of a sharp anatomical process. **2.** A minute round spot differing in color or appearance from the surrounding tissues; a point.

punc·ture (pŭngk'chər) *v.* **-tured, -tur·ing, -tures.** To pierce with a pointed object, as with a needle. — *n.* A hole or depression made by a sharp object.

puncture wound *n.* A wound that is deeper than it is wide, produced by a narrow pointed object.

pu·pil (pyo͞o'pəl) *n.* The apparently black circular opening in the center of the iris of the eye,

through which light passes to the retina. — **pu'·pi·lar** *adj.*

pu·pil·lar·y (pyo͞o'pə-lĕr'ē) *adj.* Of or affecting the pupil of the eye.

pupillary distance *n.* The distance between the center of each pupil, used in fitting eyeglass frames and lenses.

pupillary reflex *n.* A reflex resulting in change in the diameter of the pupil of the eye.

pupillary-skin reflex *n.* Dilation of the pupil following scratching of the skin of the neck.

pu·pil·los·co·py (pyo͞o'pə-lŏs'kə-pē) *n.* See **retinoscopy.**

pu·pil·lo·ton·ic pseudostrabismus (pyo͞o'pə-lō-tŏn'ĭk) *n.* See **Holmes–Adie syndrome.**

PUPPP (pē'yo͞o-pē'pē-pē') *n.* Pruritic urticarial papules and plaques of pregnancy; an intensely itching and occasionally vesicular eruption of the trunk and arms appearing in the third trimester of pregnancy. Spontaneous healing occurs within ten days of term.

pur·ga·tive (pûr'gə-tĭv) *n.* An agent used for purging the bowels. — *adj.* Tending to cause evacuation of the bowels. — **pur'ga·tive** *adj.*

purge (pûrj) *v.* **purged, purg·ing, purg·es.** To cause evacuation of the bowels. — *n.* **1.** The act or process of purging. **2.** Something that purges, especially a medicinal purgative.

pu·rine (pyo͞or'ēn) *n.* **1.** A colorless crystalline organic base that is the parent compound of various biologically important derivatives. **2.** Any of a group of organic compounds derived from or structurally related to purine, including uric acid, caffeine, and the nucleic acid constituents adenine and guanine.

Pur·kin·je cell (pər-kĭn'jē, po͞or'kĭn-yē) *n.* Any of numerous neurons of the cerebral cortex having large flask-shaped cell bodies with massive dendrites and one slender axon.

Purkinje fiber *n.* Any of the specialized cardiac muscle fibers, part of the impulse-conducting network of the heart, that rapidly transmit impulses from the atrioventricular node to the ventricles.

pur·pu·ra (pûr'pə-rə, -pyə-) *n.* A condition characterized by hemorrhages in the skin and mucous membranes that result in the appearance of purplish spots or patches.

pursed lips breathing (pûrsd) *n.* A technique, used by patients with chronic obstructive pulmonary disease, in which air is inhaled slowly through the nose and mouth and exhaled slowly through pursed lips.

purse-string instrument (pûrs'strĭng') *n.* An intestinal clamp with jaws at an angle to the handle, used in performing a purse-string suture of the bowel.

purse-string suture *n.* A continuous circular suture that is pulled together to invert or close an opening.

pu·ru·lence (pyo͞or'ə-ləns, pyo͞or'yə-) *n.* **1.** The condition of containing or discharging pus. **2.** Pus.

pu·ru·lent (pyo͞or'ə-lənt, pyo͞or'yə-) *adj.* Containing, discharging, or causing the production of pus.

purulent inflammation *n.* An acute form of exudative inflammation in which the enzymes produced by white blood cells cause liquefaction of the affected tissues, resulting in pus formation.

pus (pŭs) *n.* A generally viscous, yellowish-white fluid formed in infected tissue, consisting of white blood cells, cellular debris, and necrotic tissue.

pus·tu·lar (pŭs′chə-lər, pŭs′tyə-) *adj.* Of, relating to, or consisting of pustules.

pus·tu·late (pŭs′chə-lāt′, pŭs′tyə-) *v.* **-lat·ed, -lat·ing, -lates.** To form or cause to form pustules.

pus·tu·la·tion (pŭs′chə-lā′shən, pŭs′tyə-) *n.* The formation or appearance of pustules.

pus·tule (pŭs′chōol, pŭs′tyōol) *n.* **1.** A small inflamed elevation of the skin that is filled with pus; a pimple. **2.** A small swelling similar to a blister or pimple.

pus·tu·lo·sis (pŭs′chə-lō′sĭs, pŭs′tyə-) *n.* An eruption of pustules.

pu·tre·fac·tion (pyōo′trə-făk′shən) *n.* **1.** Decomposition of organic matter, especially protein, by microorganisms, resulting in production of foul-smelling matter. **2.** Putrefied matter. **3.** The condition of being putrefied.

pu·tre·fy (pyōo′trə-fī′) *v.* **-fied, -fy·ing, -fies. 1.** To become decayed or cause to decay and have a foul odor. **2.** To make or become gangrenous.

pu·tres·cence (pyōo-trĕs′əns) *n.* **1.** A putrescent character or condition. **2.** Putrid matter.

pu·tres·cine (pyōo-trĕs′ēn) *n.* A crystalline, mildly poisonous, colorless, foul-smelling ptomaine produced by the decarboxylation of ornithine, especially in decaying animal tissue.

pu·trid (pyōo′trĭd) *adj.* **1.** Decomposed and foul-smelling; rotten. **2.** Proceeding from, relating to, or exhibiting putrefaction.

Put·ti–Platt operation (pōo′tē-plăt′) *n.* A surgical procedure to correct recurrent dislocation of a shoulder joint.

PUVA (pōo′və, pyōo′-) *n.* Psoralen and ultraviolet light; a treatment for psoriasis combining the oral administration of psoralen with subsequent exposure to long wavelength ultraviolet light.

PVC *abbr.* polyvinyl chloride

P wave *n.* A deflection in an electrocardiogram indicating depolarization in the atria.

py·e·li·tis (pī′ə-lī′tĭs) *n.* Acute inflammation of the pelvis of the kidney, caused by bacterial infection. — **py′e·lit′ic** (-lĭt′ĭk) *adj.*

py·e·lo·cal·i·ec·ta·sis (pī′ə-lō-kăl′ē-ĕk′tə-sĭs, -kā′lē-) *n.* See **calicectasis.**

py·e·lo·cys·ti·tis (pī′ə-lō-sĭ-stī′tĭs) *n.* Inflammation of the renal pelvis and the urinary bladder.

py·e·lo·fluo·ros·co·py (pī′ə-lō-flōo-rŏs′kə-pē, -flô-) *n.* Fluoroscopic examination of the renal pelves.

py·e·lo·gram (pī′ə-lə-grăm′) *n.* An x-ray obtained by pyelography.

py·e·log·ra·phy (pī′ə-lŏg′rə-fē) *n.* X-ray photography of the pelvis of the kidney and associated structures after injection with a radiopaque dye.

py·e·lo·li·thot·o·my (pī′ə-lō-lĭ-thŏt′ə-mē) *n.* See **pelvilithotomy.**

py·e·lo·ne·phri·tis (pī′ə-lō-nə-frī′tĭs) *n.* Inflammation of the kidney and its pelvis, caused by bacterial infection. — **py′e·lo·ne·phrit′ic** (-frĭt′-ĭk) *adj.*

py·e·lo·ne·phro·sis (pī′ə-lō-nə-frō′sĭs) *n.* Disease of the pelvis of the kidney.

py·e·lo·plas·ty (pī′ə-lə-plăs′tē) *n.* Plastic or reconstructive surgery of the pelvis of the kidney to correct an obstruction.

py·e·lo·pli·ca·tion (pī′ə-lō-plĭ-kā′shən) *n.* A surgical procedure of taking tucks in the wall of the renal pelvis, formerly performed to treat hydronephrosis.

py·e·los·co·py (pī′ə-lŏs′kə-pē) *n.* Fluoroscopic observation of the pelvis and the calices of the kidney after injection of a contrast medium through the ureter.

py·e·los·to·my (pī′ə-lŏs′tə-mē) *n.* Surgical formation of an opening into the pelvis of the kidney to allow drainage of urine.

py·e·lot·o·my (pī′ə-lŏt′ə-mē) *n.* Surgical incision into the pelvis of the kidney.

py·e·lo·u·re·ter·og·ra·phy (pī′ə-lō-yōo-rē′tə-rŏg′rə-fē, -yōor′ĭ-) *n.* See **pyelography.**

py·em·e·sis (pī-ĕm′ĭ-sĭs) *n.* The vomiting of pus.

py·e·mi·a (pī-ē′mē-ə) *n.* Septicemia caused by pyogenic microorganisms in the blood, often resulting in the formation of multiple abscesses. — **py·e′mic** *adj.*

pyemic abscess *n.* A hematogenous abscess resulting from pyemia, septicemia, or bacteremia.

py·le·phle·bi·tis (pī′lə-flĭ-bī′tĭs) *n.* Inflammation of the portal vein or any of its branches.

py·lo·rec·to·my (pī′lə-rĕk′tə-mē) *n.* Surgical removal of the pylorus.

py·lor·ic (pī-lôr′ĭk, -pī-) *adj.* Of or relating to the pylorus.

pyloric gland *n.* Any of several coiled, tubular, mucus-secreting glands situated in the mucus membrane near the pyloric end of the stomach.

pyloric sphincter *n.* A thickening of the circular layer of the gastric musculature encircling the gastroduodenal junction.

pyloric stenosis *n.* Narrowing of the gastric pylorus, especially by congenital muscular hypertrophy or by scarring resulting from a peptic ulcer.

pyloric valve *n.* A fold of mucous membrane at the gastroduodenal junction, enclosing the pylorus.

py·lo·ri·ste·no·sis (pī-lôr′ĭ-stə-nō′sĭs, pī-) or **py·lo·ro·ste·no·sis** (pī-lôr′ō-) *n.* Stricture or narrowing of the orifice of the pylorus.

py·lo·ro·di·o·sis (pī-lôr′ō-dī-ō′sĭs) *n.* Surgical dilation of the pylorus.

py·lo·ro·my·ot·o·my (pī-lôr′ō-mī-ŏt′ə-mē) *n.* Longitudinal incision through the anterior wall of the pyloric canal to the level of the submucosa, performed as a treatment for hypertrophic pyloric stenosis.

py·lo·ro·plas·ty (pī-lôr′ō-plăs′tē) *n.* The surgical widening of the pyloric canal to facilitate emptying of gastric contents into the duodenum.

py·lo·ro·spasm (pī-lôr′ə-spăz′əm) *n.* Spasmodic contraction of the pylorus.

py·lo·ros·to·my (pī′lə-rŏs′tə-mē) *n.* Surgical formation of a fistula from the abdominal surface into the stomach near the pylorus.

py·lo·rot·o·my (pī′lə-rŏt′ə-mē) *n.* Surgical incision of the pylorus.

py·lo·rus (pī-lôr′əs) *n., pl.* **-lo·ri** (-lôr′ī′). **1.** The passage at the lower end of the stomach that opens into the duodenum. **2.** A muscular or myovascular structure that opens or closes an orifice or lumen of an organ.

py·o·cele (pī′ə-sēl′) *n.* An accumulation of pus in a body cavity, such as the scrotum.

py·o·ceph·a·lus (pī′ō-sĕf′ə-ləs) *n.* The presence of purulent fluid in the brain.

py·o·cyst (pī′ə-sĭst′) *n.* A cyst that contains pus.

py·o·der·ma (pī′ə-dûr′mə) *n.* A pyogenic skin disease. — **py′o·der′mic** *adj.*

py·o·he·mo·tho·rax (pī′ō-hē′mə-thôr′ăks′) *n.* The presence of pus and blood in the pleural cavity.

py·o·me·tri·tis (pī′ō-mĭ-trī′tĭs) *n.* Suppurative inflammation of the uterus.

py·o·my·o·si·tis (pī′ō-mī′ə-sī′tĭs) *n.* Suppurative inflammation of muscle tissue characterized by abscesses, carbuncles, or infected sinuses.

py·o·ne·phri·tis (pī′ō-nə-frī′tĭs) *n.* Suppurative inflammation of the kidney.

py·o·ne·phro·sis (pī′ō-nə-frō′sĭs) *n.* Distention of the pelvis and calices of the kidney, accompanied by suppuration and usually obstruction.

py·o·per·i·car·di·tis (pī′ō-pĕr′ĭ-kär-dī′tĭs) *n.* Suppurative inflammation of the pericardium.

py·o·per·i·to·ni·tis (pī′ō-pĕr′ĭ-tn-ī′tĭs) *n.* Suppurative inflammation of the peritoneum.

py·o·pneu·mo·tho·rax (pī′ō-nōō′mō-thôr′ăks′, -nyōō′-) *n.* The presence of gas and pus in the pleural cavity.

py·o·tho·rax (pī′ə-thôr′ăks′) *n.* Empyema in a pleural cavity.

pyr·a·mid (pĭr′ə-mĭd) *n.* A structure or part suggestive of a pyramid in shape. — **py·ram′i·dal** (pĭ-răm′ĭ-dl) *adj.*

pyramidal bone *n.* See **triquetrum.**

pyramidal fracture *n.* A fracture of the midfacial bones, especially the upper jawbone, in which the principal fracture lines meet at a point above the nasal bones, forming a triangular section that is detached from the skull.

pyramidal tract *n.* A bundle of fibers that origi-

nates from the precentral motor cortex and the postcentral motor cortex and crosses the medulla oblongata, descending the length of the spinal cord to innervate the muscles of the distal extremities.

pyramid of light *n.* A triangular area of reflected light at the lower part of the eardrum seen on examination of the ear.

pyramid sign *n.* Any of the various signs indicating a pathological condition of the pyramidal tracts.

py·re·to·gen·e·sis (pī′rĭ-tō-jĕn′ĭ-sĭs, pĭr′ĭ-) *n.* The origin and mode of production of fever. — **py′re·to·ge·net′ic** (-jə-nĕt′ĭk) *adj.*

py·rex·i·a (pī-rĕk′sē-ə) *n.* See **fever** (sense 1). — **py·rex′i·al, py·rex′ic** *adj.*

pyr·i·dox·ine (pĭr′ĭ-dŏk′sēn, -sĭn) or **pyr·i·dox·in** (-dŏk′sĭn) *n.* A water-soluble vitamin of the B complex group, occurring especially in cereals, yeast, liver, and fish, and serving as a coenzyme in amino acid metabolism.

py·rim·i·dine (pī-rĭm′ĭ-dēn′, pĭ-) *n.* **1.** A crystalline organic base that is the parent substance of various biologically important derivatives. **2.** Any of several basic compounds derived from or structurally related to pyrimidine, especially the nucleic acid constituents uracil, cytosine, and thymine.

py·ro·cat·e·chol (pī′rō-kăt′ĭ-kôl′, -kōl′) *n.* A biologically important organic phenol, having two hydroxyl groups attached to the benzene ring; used as a topical antiseptic.

py·ro·gen·ic (pī′rō-jĕn′ĭk) or **py·rog·e·nous** (pī-rŏj′ə-nəs) *adj.* **1.** Producing or produced by fever. **2.** Caused by or generating heat.

py·ro·glob·u·lin (pī′rō-glŏb′yə-lĭn) *n.* Any of various immunoglobulins that coagulate when heated, usually associated with multiple myeloma or macroglobulinemia.

py·rol·y·sis (pī-rŏl′ĭ-sĭs) *n.* Decomposition of a chemical compound caused by heat.

py·ro·ma·ni·a (pī′rō-mā′nē-ə, -mān′yə) *n.* An uncontrollable impulse to start fires. — **py′ro·ma′ni·ac′** (-mā′nē-ăk′) *adj. & n.*

py·ro·sis (pī-rō′sĭs) *n.* See **heartburn.**

pyr·role (pĕr′ōl′) *n.* A five-membered heterocyclic ring compound that has an odor similar to chloroform and is the parent compound of hemoglobin, chlorophyll, and many other complex biologically active substances.

py·ru·vic acid (pī-rōō′vĭk, pī-) *n.* A colorless organic liquid formed as a fundamental intermediate in protein and carbohydrate metabolism.

py·u·ri·a (pī-yŏŏr′ē-ə) *n.* The presence of pus in the urine, usually a sign of urinary tract infection.

Q

q.d. *abbr. Latin.* quaque die (every day)

Q fever *n.* An infectious disease caused by the rickettsia *Coxiella burnetii*, characterized by fever, malaise, and muscular pains.

q.h. *abbr. Latin.* quaque hora (every hour)

q.i.d. *abbr. Latin.* quater in die (four times a day)

q.l. *abbr. Latin.* quantum libet (as much as desired)

QRS complex (kyōō′är-ĕs′) *n.* The principal deflection in the electrocardiogram, representing ventricular depolarization.

q.s. *abbr. Latin.* quantum satis (as much as is enough); *Latin.* quantum sufficiat (as much as shall suffice)

Q–T interval *n.* The time elapsing from the beginning of the QRS complex to the end of the T wave in an electrocardiogram; it represents the total duration of electrical activity of the ventricles.

Quaa·lude (kwä′lōōd′) A trademark formerly used for methaqualone.

quack (kwăk) *n.* **1.** An untrained person who poses as a physician and dispenses medical advice and treatment. **2.** A charlatan. — **quack′er·y** *n.*

quad·rant (kwŏd′rənt) *n.* **1.** A circular arc of 90 degrees; one fourth of the circumference of a circle. **2.** A quarter of any roughly circular anatomical area such as the abdomen. The quartering of the region occurs along imaginary axes that are at right angles to each other.

quad·rate (kwŏd′rāt′, -rĭt) *adj.* Having four sides and four angles; square or rectangular.

quadrate muscle of the thigh *n.* A muscle with origin from the tuberosity of the ischium, with insertion into the crest of the trochanter, and whose action rotates the thigh laterally.

quadrate pronator muscle *n.* A muscle with origin from the anterior surface of the ulna, with insertion into the anterior surface of the radius, and whose action pronates the forearm.

quad·ri·ceps (kwŏd′rĭ-sĕps′) *n.* The large four-part extensor muscle at the front of the thigh. — *adj.* Having four heads, said of certain muscles.

quadriceps muscle of the thigh *n.* A muscle with origin by four heads: the rectus muscle of the thigh, and the lateral, intermediate, and medial vastus muscles; with insertion into the patella; and whose action extends the leg and flexes the thigh.

quadriceps reflex *n.* See **patellar reflex**.

quad·ri·gem·i·nal (kwŏd′rə-jĕm′ə-nəl) *adj.* Consisting of four parts; fourfold.

quadrigeminal rhythm *n.* A cardiac dysrhythmia in which heartbeats occur in groups of four, usually composed of one sinus beat followed by three extrasystolic beats.

quad·ri·ped·al extensor reflex (kwŏd′rə-pĕd′l, -pēd′l) *n.* Extension of the arm on the affected side in hemiplegia when the patient is positioned to be on all fours.

quad·ri·ple·gi·a (kwŏd′rə-plē′jē-ə, -jə) *n.* Paralysis of all four limbs. — **quad′ri·ple′gic** *adj. & n.*

quad·ru·plet (kwŏ-drŭp′lĭt, -drōō′plĭt, kwŏd′rə-plĭt) *n.* **1.** One of four offspring born in a single birth. **2.** A group or combination of four associated by common properties or behavior.

qual·i·ta·tive analysis (kwŏl′ĭ-tā′tĭv) *n.* The testing of a substance or mixture to determine the characteristics of its chemical constituents.

quan·ti·ta·tive analysis (kwŏn′tĭ-tā′tĭv) *n.* The testing of a substance or mixture to determine the amounts and proportions of its chemical constituents.

quar·an·tine (kwôr′ən-tēn′) *n.* **1.** A period of time during which a vehicle, person, or material suspected of carrying a contagious disease is detained at a port of entry under enforced isolation to prevent disease from entering a country. **2.** A place for such detention. **3.** Enforced isolation or restriction of free movement imposed to prevent the spread of contagious disease. **4.** A condition of enforced isolation. **5.** A period of 40 days. — *v.* **-tined, -tin·ing, -tines.** To isolate in or as if in quarantine.

quart (kwôrt) *n.* **1.** A unit of volume or capacity in the U.S. Customary System, used in liquid measure, equal to ¼ gallon or 32 ounces (0.946 liter). **2.** A unit of volume or capacity in the U.S. Customary System, used in dry measure, equal to ⅛ peck or 2 pints (1.101 liters). **3.** A unit of volume or capacity in the British Imperial System, used in liquid and dry measure, equal to 1.201 U.S. liquid quarts or 1.032 U.S. dry quarts (1.136 liters).

quar·tan (kwôrt′n) *adj.* Recurring every fourth day, counting inclusively, or every 72 hours. Used of a fever. — *n.* A malarial fever recurring every 72 hours.

quartz (kwôrts) *n.* A hard crystalline form of silicon dioxide used in optical instruments.

qua·si·dom·i·nance (kwä′zī-dŏm′ə-nəns, -sī-, kwä′zē-, -sē-) *n.* The appearance of a recessive trait in generation after generation of a population as a result of repeated consanguineous matings; false dominance. — **qua′si·dom′i·nant** *adj.*

qua·ze·pam (kwä′zə-păm′) *n.* A benzodiazepine derivative used as a sedative and hypnotic.

quea·sy or **quea·zy** (kwē′zē) *adj.* **1. -si·er** or **-zi·er, -si·est** or **-zi·est.** Experiencing nausea; nauseated. **2.** Easily nauseated. **3.** Causing nausea.

Queck·en·stedt–Stookey test (kwĕk′ən-stĕd′-, kvĕk′ən-shtĕt′-) *n.* A test to detect the blockage of subarachnoid channels in which the jugular vein is compressed; in a healthy person compression causes a rapid increase in the pressure of the spinal fluid and an equally rapid fall to normal on release of the pressure; when there is blockage of subarachnoid channels, compression causes little or no increase in the pressure of the spinal fluid.

quer·ce·tin (kwûr'sǐ-tǐn) *n.* A yellow, powdered crystalline compound produced synthetically or occurring as a glycoside in the rind and bark of numerous plants, and used medicinally to treat abnormal capillary fragility.

quick (kwǐk) *n.* Sensitive or raw exposed flesh, as under the fingernails. — *adj.* **quick·er, quick·est.** **1.** Pregnant. **2.** Alive.

quick·en (kwǐk'ən) *v.* **-ened, -en·ing, -ens. 1.** To become more rapid. **2.** To reach the stage of pregnancy when the fetus can be felt to move.

quick·en·ing (kwǐk'ə-nǐng) *n.* The initial signs of fetal life felt by the mother as a result of the movements by the fetus.

Quick's method (kwǐks) *n.* See prothrombin test.

Quick's test *n.* See prothrombin test.

qui·es·cent (kwē-ěs'ənt, kwī-) *adj.* Being quiet, still, or at rest; inactive.

qui·et lung (kwī'ǐt) *n.* The deliberate collapsing of a lung during thoracic operations to facilitate surgical procedure by absence of movement.

quin·a·crine hydrochloride (kwǐn'ə-krēn', -krǐn) *n.* The dihydrochloride form of an acridine derivative used as an antimalarial, an anthelmintic, and especially as a stain for Y chromatin in fluorescent microscopy.

Quinck·e's disease (kwǐn'kēz, kwǐng'-, kvǐn'kəz) *n.* See angioneurotic edema.

Quincke's pulse *n.* Capillary pulsation, as shown by alternate reddening and blanching of the nailbed with each heartbeat; it is a sign of arteriolar dilation and aortic insufficiency.

Quincke's sign *n.* See Quincke's pulse.

quin·i·dine (kwǐn'ǐ-dēn') *n.* A colorless crystalline alkaloid that is a stereoisomer of quinine and is used as a treatment for malaria and cardiac arrhythmias.

qui·nine (kwī'nīn') *n.* **1.** A bitter, colorless, amorphous powder or crystalline alkaloid derived from cinchona bark and used to treat malaria. **2.** Any of various compounds or salts of quinine.

qui·noi·dine (kwī-noi'dēn', -dǐn) *n.* A brownish-black mixture of alkaloids remaining after extraction of crystalline alkaloids from cinchona bark, used as a quinine substitute.

quin·o·line (kwǐn'ə-lēn', -lǐn) *n.* An aromatic organic base synthesized or obtained from coal tar and used in making antiseptics.

qui·none (kwǐ-nōn', kwǐn'ōn') *n.* Any of various biologically important compounds that act as coenzymes and vitamins.

quin·sy (kwǐn'zē) *n.* See peritonsillar abscess.

quin·tan (kwǐn'tən) *adj.* Recurring every fifth day. Used of a fever.

quin·tu·plet (kwǐn-tŭp'lǐt, -tōō'plǐt, -tyōō'-, kwǐn'tə-plǐt) *n.* **1.** One of five offspring born in a single birth. **2.** A group or combination of five associated by common properties or behavior.

quo·tid·i·an (kwō-tǐd'ē-ən) *adj.* Recurring daily. Used especially of attacks of malaria.

quotidian malaria *n.* Malaria in which the paroxysms occur daily, because of infection by two distinct groups of *Plasmodium* that sporulate alternately every 48 hours.

quo·tient (kwō'shənt) *n.* The number obtained by dividing one quantity by another.

Q wave *n.* The initial downward deflection of the QRS complex in the electrocardiogram.

~ ~ ~ ~ ~ ~ **R** ~ ~ ~ ~ ~ ~

℞ or **R** *abbr. Latin.* recipe (take)

rab·bet·ing (răb'ǐ-tǐng) *n.* The making of congruous stepwise cuts on apposing bone surfaces for impaction of a fractured bone.

rab·id (răb'ǐd) *adj.* Of or affected by rabies.

ra·bies (rā'bēz) *n.* An infectious, highly fatal viral disease of warm blooded animals that attacks the cental nervous system; symptoms include excitement, aggressiveness, and dementia, followed by paralysis and death. — **ra'bi·et'ic** (-ět'ǐk) *adj.*

rabies immune globulin *n.* Specific globulin fraction of pooled plasma from human donors immunized against rabies and having a high titer of antibodies to the rabies virus.

rabies vaccine *n.* **1.** A vaccine introduced by Pasteur as a method of treatment for the bite of a rabid animal, consisting of 23 daily injections of virus that are increased serially from noninfective to fully infective fixed virus. **2.** A similar vaccine prepared from rabies virus grown in duck embryos and then inactivated, requiring fewer injections to administer; it has largely replaced the vaccine introduced by Pasteur.

rabies virus *n.* A rather large, bullet-shaped virus of the genus *Lyssavirus* that causes rabies.

race (rās) *n.* **1.** A local geographic or global human population distinguished as a more or less distinct group by genetically transmitted physical characteristics. **2.** A population of organisms differing from others of the same species in the frequency of hereditary traits; a subspecies. — **ra'·cial** (rā'shəl) *adj.*

rac·e·mose gland (răs'ə-mōs') *n.* A gland having a clustered structure similar to that of a bunch of grapes.

race walking *n.* The sport of walking for speed, the

ra·chi·cen·te·sis (rā′kĭ-sĕn-tē′sĭs) *n*. See **lumbar puncture**.

ra·chil·y·sis (rā-kĭl′ĭ-sĭs, rə-) *n*. Forcible correction of lateral curvature of the spine by lateral pressure against the convexity of the curve.

ra·chi·o·cen·te·sis (rā′kē-ō-sĕn-tē′sĭs) *n*. See **lumbar puncture**.

ra·chi·ot·o·my (rā′kē-ŏt′ə-mē) *n*. See **laminectomy**.

ra·chis (rā′kĭs) *n., pl*. **ra·chis·es** or **rach·i·des** (răk′ĭ-dēz′, rā′kĭ-). See **spinal column**.

ra·chi·tis (rə-kī′tĭs) *n*. See **rickets**. — **ra·chit′ic** (-kĭt′ĭk) *adj*.

rad (răd) *n*. A unit of energy absorbed from ionizing radiation.

ra·dar·ky·mog·ra·phy (rā′där-kī-mŏg′rə-fē) *n*. Video tracking of heart motion by means of image intensification and closed circuit television during fluoroscopy, enabling cardiac motion to be graphically traced and measured.

ra·dec·to·my (rā-dĕk′tə-mē) or **ra·di·ec·to·my** (rā′dē-ĕk′tə-mē) or **ra·di·sec·to·my** (rā′dĭ-sĕk′-tə-mē) *n*. See **root amputation**.

ra·di·a·bil·i·ty (rā′dē-ə-bĭl′ĭ-tē) *n*. The property of being radiable.

ra·di·a·ble (rā′dē-ə-bəl) *adj*. Capable of being penetrated or examined by rays, especially x-rays.

ra·di·al (rā′dē-əl) *adj*. **1.** Of, relating to, or near the radius or forearm. **2.** Moving or directed along a radius. **3.** Radiating from or converging to a common center. — **ra′di·al·ly** *adv*.

radial artery *n*. **1.** An artery with its origin in the brachial artery, with branches to the radial side of the forearm, the wrist, the dorsal side of the fingers, the thumb, and the palm. **2.** An artery with its origin in the radial artery and branches to the radial side of the index finger.

radial keratotomy *n*. Surgical modification of corneal curvature to correct myopia by making multiple symmetrical incisions into but not through the cornea.

radial nerve *n*. A nerve that arises from the posterior cord of the brachial plexus and divides into two terminal branches, designated superficial and deep, that supply muscular and cutaneous branches to the dorsal aspect of the arm and forearm.

radial vein *n*. Any of several veins of the forearm that accompany the radial artery and open into the brachial veins.

ra·di·ate (rā′dē-āt′) *v*. **-at·ed, -at·ing, -ates. 1.** To spread out in all directions from a center. **2.** To emit or be emitted as radiation. — **ra′di·a′tive** *adj*.

ra·di·a·tion (rā′dē-ā′shən) *n*. **1.** The act or condition of diverging in all directions from a center. **2.** Energy radiated or transmitted in the form of rays, waves, or particles. **3.** A stream of particles or electromagnetic waves emitted by the atoms and molecules of a radioactive substance as a result of nuclear decay. **4.** Radiotherapy. **5.** Radial arrangement of anatomical or histological parts.

radiation sickness *n*. Illness induced by ionizing radiation, ranging in severity from nausea, vomiting, headache, and diarrhea to loss of hair and teeth, reduction in red and white blood cell counts, hemorrhaging, sterility, and death.

radiation therapy *n*. Radiotherapy.

rad·i·cal (răd′ĭ-kəl) *n*. Free radical. — *adj*. **1.** Of or being medical treatment by extreme, drastic, or innovative measures. **2.** Designed to act on or eliminate the root or cause of a pathological process.

radical hysterectomy *n*. Complete surgical removal of the uterus, upper vagina, and parametrium.

radical mastectomy *n*. Surgical removal of the entire breast, the pectoral muscles, the lymphatic-bearing tissue in the armpit, and other neighboring tissues.

rad·i·cle (răd′ĭ-kəl) *n*. A small structure, such as a fibril of a nerve, that resembles a root.

rad·i·cot·o·my (răd′ĭ-kŏt′ə-mē) *n*. See **rhizotomy**.

ra·dic·u·la (rə-dĭk′yə-lə) *n., pl* **-lae** (-lē′). A spinal nerve root.

ra·dic·u·lal·gi·a (rə-dĭk′yə-lăl′jē-ə, -jə) *n*. Neuralgia due to irritation of the sensory root of a spinal nerve.

ra·dic·u·lec·to·my (rə-dĭk′yə-lĕk′tə-mē) *n*. See **rhizotomy**.

ra·dic·u·li·tis (rə-dĭk′yə-lī′tĭs) *n*. **1.** Inflammation of the intradural portion of a spinal nerve root prior to its entrance into the intervertebral foramen. **2.** Inflammation of the portion of a spinal nerve root between the intervertebral foramen and the nerve plexus.

ra·dic·u·lo·gan·gli·o·ni·tis (rə-dĭk′yə-lō-găng′-glē-ə-nī′tĭs) *n*. See **acute idiopathic polyneuritis**.

ra·dic·u·lo·neu·rop·a·thy (rə-dĭk′yə-lō-no͝o-rŏp′ə-thē, -nyo͝o-) *n*. Disease of the spinal nerves and nerve roots.

ra·dic·u·lop·a·thy (rə-dĭk′yə-lŏp′ə-thē) *n*. Disease of the spinal nerve roots.

ra·di·o·ac·tive (rā′dē-ō-ăk′tĭv) *adj*. Of or exhibiting radioactivity.

radioactive iodine *n*. Any of the radioisotopes of iodine, especially ^{131}I, ^{125}I, or ^{123}I, used as tracers.

radioactive isotope *n*. An isotope having an unstable nucleus that emits radiation as it spontaneously decomposes to a stable nuclear composition.

ra·di·o·ac·tiv·i·ty (rā′dē-ō-ăk-tĭv′ĭ-tē) *n*. **1.** Spontaneous emission of radiation, either directly from unstable atomic nuclei or as a consequence of a nuclear reaction. **2.** The radiation emitted by a radioactive substance.

ra·di·o·al·ler·go·sor·bent test (rā′dē-ō-ăl′ər-gō-sôr′bənt, -zôr′-) *n*. A radioimmunoassay test to detect IgE-bound allergens responsible for tissue hypersensitivity.

ra·di·o·au·to·graph (rā′dē-ō-ô′tə-grăf′) *n.* See **autoradiograph.**

ra·di·o·bi·ol·o·gy (rā′dē-ō-bī-ŏl′ə-jē) *n.* The study of the effects of radiation on living organisms.

ra·di·o·cin·e·ma·tog·ra·phy (rā′dē-ō-sĭn′ə-mə-tŏg′rə-fē) *n.* The cinematic recording of the movements of organs during radiographic examination.

ra·di·o·den·si·ty (rā′dē-ō-děn′sĭ-tē) *n.* See **radiopacity.**

ra·di·o·der·ma·ti·tis (rā′dē-ō-dûr′mə-tī′tĭs) *n.* Dermatitis due to exposure to ionizing radiation.

ra·di·o·di·ag·no·sis (rā′dē-ō-dī′əg-nō′sĭs) *n.* Diagnosis by means of x-rays.

ra·di·o·gram (rā′dē-ō-grăm′) *n.* A radiograph.

ra·di·o·graph (rā′dē-ō-grăf′) *n.* An image produced on a radiosensitive surface, such as a photographic film, by radiation other than visible light, especially by x-rays passed through an object or by photographing a fluoroscopic image.

ra·di·og·ra·phy (rā′dē-ŏg′rə-fē) *n.* The process by which radiographs are made.

ra·di·o·im·mu·ni·ty (rā′dē-ō-ĭ-myōō′nĭ-tē) *n.* Reduced sensitivity to radiation.

ra·di·o·im·mu·no·as·say (rā′dē-ō-ĭm′yə-nō-ăs′ā, -ĭm-yōō′-) *n.* The immunoassay of a radiolabeled substance, such as a hormone or an enzyme.

ra·di·o·im·mu·no·dif·fu·sion (rā′dē-ō-ĭm′yə-nō-dĭ-fyōō′zhən, -ĭm-yōō′-) *n.* A method for the study of antigen-antibody reactions by gel diffusion using radioisotope-labeled antigen or antibody.

ra·di·o·im·mu·no·e·lec·tro·pho·re·sis (rā′dē-ō-ĭm′yə-nō-ĭ-lĕk′trə-fə-rē′sĭs, -ĭ-myōō′-) *n.* Immunoelectrophoresis in which the antigen or antibody is labeled with a radioisotope.

ra·di·o·im·mu·no·pre·cip·i·ta·tion (rā′dē-ō-ĭm′yə-nō-prī-sĭp′ĭ-tā′shən, -ĭ-myōō′-) *n.* Immunoprecipitation using a radioisotope-labeled antibody or antigen.

ra·di·o·i·so·tope (rā′dē-ō-ī′sə-tōp′) *n.* A naturally or artificially produced radioactive isotope of an element.

ra·di·o·li·gand (rā′dē-ō-lī′gənd, -lĭg′ənd) *n.* A molecule with a radionuclide tracer attached, usually used for radioimmunoassay procedures.

ra·di·ol·o·gy (rā′dē-ŏl′ə-jē) *n.* **1.** The branch of medicine that deals with the use of radioactive substances in diagnosis and treatment of disease. **2.** The use of ionizing radiation for medical diagnosis, especially the use of x-rays in medical radiography or fluoroscopy. — **ra′di·o·log′i·cal** (-ə-lŏj′ĭ-kəl), **ra′di·o·log′ic** (-lŏj′ĭk) *adj.* — **ra′di·ol′o·gist** *n.*

ra·di·o·lu·cent (rā′dē-ō-lōō′sənt) *adj.* Allowing the passage of x-rays or other radiation; not radiopaque. — **ra′di·o·lu′cen·cy** *n.*

ra·di·ol·y·sis (rā′dē-ŏl′ĭ-sĭs) *n., pl* **-ses** (-sēz′). Molecular decomposition of a substance as a result of radiation. — **ra′di·o·lyt′ic** (-ə-lĭt′ĭk) *adj.*

ra·di·o·ne·cro·sis (rā′dē-ō-nə-krō′sĭs, -nĕ-) *n.* Necrosis due to excessive exposure to radiation.

ra·di·o·neu·ri·tis (rā′dē-ō-nōō-rī′tĭs, -nyōō-) *n.* Neuritis due to excessive exposure to radiation.

ra·di·o·nu·clide (rā′dē-ō-nōō′klīd′, -nyōō′-) *n.* A nuclide of artificial or natural origin that exhibits radioactivity.

ra·di·o·pac·i·ty (rā′dē-ō-păs′ĭ-tē) *n.* The quality or state of being radiopaque.

ra·di·o·paque (rā′dē-ō-pāk′) *adj.* Relatively impenetrable by x-rays or other forms of radiation.

ra·di·o·phy·lax·is (rā′dē-ō-fə-lăk′sĭs) *n.* The lessened effect of a dose of radiation when administered after a previous smaller dose.

ra·di·o·pro·tec·tion (rā′dē-ō-prə-tĕk′shən) *n.* Protection against the harmful effects of radiation. — **ra′di·o·pro·tec′tive** *adj.*

ra·di·o·re·cep·tor (rā′dē-ō-rĭ-sĕp′tər) *n.* A receptor that normally responds to radiant energy such as light or heat.

ra·di·os·co·py (rā′dē-ŏs′kə-pē) *n.* See **fluoroscopy.**

ra·di·o·ther·a·peu·tics (rā′dē-ō-thĕr′ə-pyōō′tĭks) *n.* The study and use of ionizing radiation for therapeutic purposes.

ra·di·o·ther·a·py (rā′dē-ō-thĕr′ə-pē) *n.* Treatment of disease with radiation, especially by selective irradiation with x-rays or other ionizing radiation and by ingestion of radioisotopes. — **ra′di·o·ther′a·pist** *n.*

ra·di·o·ther·my (rā′dē-ō-thûr′mē) *n.* Diathermy using heat from radiant sources.

ra·di·o·tox·e·mi·a (rā′dē-ō-tŏk-sē′mē-ə) *n.* Radiation sickness caused by the products of disintegration produced by the action of x-rays or other forms of radiation and by the depletion of certain cells and enzyme systems.

ra·di·o·tox·ic (rā′dē-ō-tŏk′sĭk) *adj.* Of or being a radioactive substance that is toxic to living cells or tissues. — **ra′di·o·tox·ic′i·ty** (-tŏk-sĭs′ĭ-tē) *n.*

ra·di·o·trop·ic (rā′dē-ō-trŏp′ĭk, -trō′pĭk) *adj.* Moving or reacting in response to radiation. — **ra′di·ot′ro·pism** (-ŏt′rə-pĭz′əm) *n.*

ra·di·um (rā′dē-əm) *n.* A luminescent, highly radioactive metallic element with atomic number 88, found in minute amounts in uranium ores, and used in the treatment of cancer.

radium therapy *n.* The use of radium in radiotherapy, especially in treating cancer.

ra·di·us (rā′dē-əs) *n., pl.* **-di·us·es** or **-di·i** (-dē-ī′). A long, prismatic, slightly curved bone, the shorter and thicker of the two forearm bones, located on the lateral side of the ulna.

ra·dix (rā′dĭks) *n., pl* **ra·dix·es** or **ra·dic·es** (răd′ĭ-sēz′, rā′dĭ-). The primary or beginning portion of a part or organ, as of a nerve at its origin from the brainstem or spinal cord.

ra·don (rā′dŏn) *n.* A radioactive, largely inert gaseous element with atomic number 86, formed by the radioactive decay of radium and used as a radiation source in radiotherapy and research.

rag·weed (răg′wēd′) *n.* Any of various weeds of the genus *Ambrosia* producing abundant pollen that is one of the chief causes of hay fever.

rale or **râle** (räl) *n.* An abnormal or pathological respiratory sound heard on auscultation.

ram·i·fi·ca·tion (răm′ə-fĭ-kā′shən) *n.* A branching shape or arrangement.

ram·i·fy (răm′ə-fī′) *v.* **-fied, -fy·ing, -fies.** To branch.

ram·i·sec·tion (răm′ĭ-sĕk′shən) *n.* Surgical section of the communicating branches of the sympathetic nervous system.

ra·mi·tis (ră-mī′tĭs) *n.* Inflammation of a ramus.

Ram·stedt operation (răm′stĕt, räm′shtĕt) *n.* See **pyloromyotomy.**

ram·u·lus (răm′yə-ləs) *n., pl.* **-li** (-lī′). Any of the terminal divisions of a ramus.

ra·mus (rā′məs) *n., pl.* **-mi** (-mī′). **1.** Any of the primary divisions of a nerve or blood vessel. **2.** A part of an irregularly shaped bone that is thicker than a process and forms an angle with the main body, especially the ascending part of the lower jaw that makes a joint at the temple. **3.** Any of the primary divisions of a cerebral sulcus.

ran·cid (răn′sĭd) *adj.* Having the disagreeable odor or taste of decomposing oils or fats. — **ran·cid′i·ty, ran′cid·ness** *n.*

ran·dom mating (răn′dəm) *n.* Mating in which the pairing of a male and female with certain traits occurs with the frequency that would be predicted by chance or the same frequency with which the traits occur in the overall population.

range (rānj) *n.* In statistics, the difference or interval between the smallest and largest values in a frequency distribution.

range of accommodation *n.* The distance between one object viewed with minimal refractivity of the eye and another one viewed with maximal accommodation.

ran·u·la (răn′yə-lə) *n.* A cyst on the underside of the tongue or the floor of the mouth caused by obstruction of a duct of a salivary gland. — **ran′u·lar** (-lər) *adj.*

rape (rāp) *n.* The crime of forcing another person to submit to sex acts, especially sexual intercourse. — *v.* **raped, rap·ing, rapes.** To commit rape on. — **rap′ist** *n.*

ra·phe or **rha·phe** (rā′fē) *n., pl* **-phae** (-fē′). A seamless line or ridge between two similar parts of a body organ, as in the scrotum.

rap·id canities (răp′ĭd) *n.* The whitening of hair overnight or in the period of a few days.

rapid eye movement *n.* The rapid, periodic, jerky movement of the eyes during certain stages of the sleep cycle when dreaming takes place.

rapid plasma reagin test *n.* Any of a group of serologic tests for syphilis in which unheated serum or plasma is reacted with a standard test antigen containing charcoal particles; a positive test yields a flocculation.

Rap·o·port test (răp′ə-pôrt′) *n.* A test used in the evaluation of a suspected decrease in renal blood flow.

rap·port (ră-pôr′, rə-) *n.* Relationship, especially one of mutual trust.

rap·ture of the deep (răp′chər) *n.* See **nitrogen narcosis** (sense 2).

rare earth *n.* See **lanthanide.**

rare-earth element *n.* See **lanthanide.**

rash (răsh) *n.* A skin eruption.

ras·pa·to·ry (răs′pə-tôr′ē) *n.* An instrument used for scraping bone.

RAST *abbr.* radioallergosorbent test

rat (răt) *n.* Any of various long-tailed rodents of the genus *Rattus* and related genera, including certain species that are vectors for various diseases, including bubonic plague.

rat-bite fever *n.* Headache, fever, lymphangitis, and lymphadenitis following the bite of a rat or other rodent, due either to a spirillum or to the bacterium *Streptobacillus moniliformis.*

rate (rāt) *n.* **1.** A quantity measured with respect to another measured quantity. **2.** A measure of a part with respect to a whole; a proportion.

ra·tio (rā′shō, rā′shē-ō′) *n., pl.* **-tios. 1.** Relation in degree or number between two similar things. **2.** The relation between two quantities expressed as the quotient of one divided by the other.

ra·tion·al (răsh′ə-nəl) *adj.* **1.** Having or exercising the ability to reason. **2.** Influenced by reasoning rather than by emotion. **3.** Of sound mind; sane. **4.** Based on scientific knowledge or theory rather than practical observation.

ra·tion·al·ize (răsh′ə-nə-līz′) *v.* **-ized, -iz·ing, -iz·es. 1.** To make rational. **2.** To devise self-satisfying but false or inconsistent reasons for one's behavior, especially as an unconscious defense mechanism through which irrational acts or feelings are made to appear rational to oneself. — **ra′tion·al·i·za′tion** (răsh′ə-nə-lĭ-zā′shən) *n.*

rational therapy *n.* Psychotherapy based on the premise that a lack of information or illogical thought patterns are the basic causes of the patient's difficulties.

ray (rā) *n.* **1.** A narrow beam of light or other radiant energy. **2.** A stream of electromagnetic radiation or particles, as an x-ray. **3.** A structure or part having the form of a straight line extending from a point.

Ray·naud's phenomenon (rā-nōz′, rĕ-) *n.* Sensitivity of the hands and fingers to cold due to spasms of the digital arteries, resulting in blanching and numbness of the fingers.

Raynaud's syndrome *n.* A circulatory disorder that affects the hands and fingers, caused by insufficient blood supply to these parts and resulting in cyanosis, numbness, pain, and, in extreme cases, gangrene.

RBC or **rbc** *abbr.* red blood cell; red blood count

RBF *abbr.* renal blood flow

RD *abbr.* Registered Dietician

RDA *abbr.* recommended daily allowance

RDH *abbr.* Registered Dental Hygienist

RDS *abbr.* respiratory distress syndrome

RE *abbr.* right eye

re·act (rē-ăkt′) *v.* **-act·ed, -act·ing, -acts. 1.** To act in response to a stimulus. **2.** To undergo a chemical reaction.

re·ac·tant (rē-ăk′tənt) *n.* A substance participating in a chemical reaction, especially a directly reacting substance present at the start of the reaction.

re·ac·tion (rē-ăk′shən) *n.* **1.** A response of an organism or living tissue to a stimulus. **2.** The state resulting from such a response. **3.** A chemical change or transformation in which a substance decomposes, combines with other substances, or interchanges constituents with other substances. **4.** The response of cells or tissues to an antigen, as in a test for immunization. **5.** A pattern of behavior constituting a mental disorder or personality type.

reaction formation *n.* A defense mechanism by which an objectionable impulse is expressed in an opposite or contrasting factor.

reaction time *n.* The interval between the presentation of a stimulus and the response to it.

re·ac·ti·vate (rē-ăk′tə-vāt′) *v.* **-vat·ed, -vat·ing, -vates. 1.** To make active again, as inactivated immune serum to which normal serum complement has been added. **2.** To restore the ability to function or the effectiveness of. — **re·ac′ti·va′tion** *n.*

re·ac·tive (rē-ăk′tĭv) *adj.* **1.** Tending to be responsive or to react to a stimulus. **2.** Characterized by reaction. **3.** Tending to participate readily in chemical reactions.

re·ac·tive depression (rē-ăk′tĭv) *n.* Depression precipitated by an intensely sad or distressing event or situation.

re·ac·tiv·i·ty (rē′ăk-tĭv′ĭ-tē) *n.* **1.** The property of reacting. **2.** The process of reacting.

read·through (rēd′thrōō′) *n.* Transcription of a nucleic acid sequence beyond its normal termination sequence.

re·a·gent (rē-ā′jənt) *n.* A substance used in a chemical reaction to detect, measure, examine, or produce other substances.

re·a·gin (rē-ā′jĭn) *n.* **1.** An antibody found in the blood of persons having a genetic predisposition to allergies such as asthma and hay fever. **2.** A substance present in the blood of persons having a positive serological test for syphilis. — **re′a·gin′ic** (rē′ə-jĭn′ĭk) *adj.*

re·a·gin·ic antibody (rē′ə-jĭn′ĭk) *n.* See **homocytotropic antibody.**

re·al·i·ty (rē-ăl′ĭ-tē) *n.* **1.** The quality or state of being actual or true. **2.** The totality of all things possessing actuality, existence, or essence. **3.** That which exists objectively and in fact.

reality testing *n.* In psychoanalytic theory, the ego function by which the objective or real world and one's relationship to it are evaluated and appreciated by the self.

real-time ultrasound *n.* The use of a rapid succession of individual images to produce a moving video display.

ream·er (rē′mər) *n.* A rotating tool used to shape or enlarge holes.

re·bound phenomenon (rē′bound′, rĭ-bound′) *n.* See **Stewart–Holmes sign.**

rebound tenderness *n.* Pain or tenderness felt when pressure, especially abdominal pressure, is released suddenly.

re·breath·ing (rē-brē′thĭng) *n.* The partial or complete inhalation of previously exhaled gases.

rebreathing anesthesia *n.* A technique for inhalation anesthesia in which a portion or all of the gases that are exhaled are subsequently inhaled after carbon dioxide has been removed by the anesthetic apparatus.

rebreathing technique *n.* Use of a breathing or anesthesia circuit in which exhaled air is afterwards inhaled either with or without removal of carbon dioxide from the exhaled air.

re·cal·ci·fi·ca·tion (rē-kăl′sə-fĭ-kā′shən) *n.* The restoration of lost calcium salts to body tissues.

re·call (rĭ-kôl′) *n.* (also rē′kôl′). The ability to remember information or experiences.

re·can·a·li·za·tion (rē-kăn′ə-lĭ-zā′shən) *n.* **1.** The restoration of the lumen of a blood vessel following thrombotic occlusion by organization of the thrombus through the formation of new channels. **2.** Spontaneous restoration of the lumen of an occluded duct or tube.

re·cep·tive aphasia (rĭ-sĕp′tĭv) *n.* See **sensory aphasia.**

re·cep·tor (rĭ-sĕp′tər) *n.* **1.** A specialized cell or group of nerve endings that responds to sensory stimuli. **2.** A molecular structure or site on the surface or interior of a cell that binds with substances such as hormones, antigens, drugs, or neurotransmitters.

receptor protein *n.* An intracellular protein or protein fraction having a high specific affinity for binding agents known to stimulate cellular activity, such as a steroid hormone or cyclic AMP.

re·cess (rē′sĕs′, rĭ-sĕs′) *n.* A small hollow or indentation.

re·ces·sion (rĭ-sĕsh′ən) *n.* The withdrawal or retreating of tissue from its normal position.

re·ces·sive (rĭ-sĕs′ĭv) *adj.* **1.** Tending to go backward or recede. **2.** Of, relating to, or designating an allele that does not produce a characteristic effect when present with a dominant allele. **3.** Of or relating to a trait that is expressed only when the determining allele is present in the homozygous condition. — *n.* **1.** A recessive allele or trait. **2.** An organism having a recessive trait.

recessive character *n.* An inherited character determined by a recessive gene.

recessive gene *n.* A gene that is phenotypically expressed in the homozygous state, but has its expression masked by a dominant gene.

recessive inheritance *n.* Inheritance in which a trait is expressed only when the determining allele is present in the homozygous condition.

re·cid·i·va·tion (rĭ-sĭd′ə-vā′shən) *n.* See **recidivism.**

re·cid·i·vism (rĭ-sĭd′ə-vĭz′əm) *n.* **1.** A tendency to lapse into a previous pattern of behavior. **2.** The relapse of a disease or symptom.

re·cip·i·ent (rĭ-sĭp′ē-ənt) *adj.* Functioning as a receiver; receptive. — *n.* One who receives blood, tissue, or an organ from a donor.

re·cip·ro·cal (rĭ-sĭp′rə-kəl) *adj.* Of or relating to a neuromuscular phenomenon in which the excitation of one group of muscles is accompanied by the inhibition of another.

re·cip·ro·cal transfusion (rĭ-sĭp′rə-kəl) *n.* An attempt to confer immunity by transfusing blood taken from a donor just recovered from an infectious disease into a recipient suffering from the same disease, the balance being maintained by transfusing an equal amount from the sick to the well person.

reciprocal translocation *n.* Translocation without demonstrable loss of genetic material.

rec·li·na·tion (rĕk′lə-nā′shən) *n.* Surgical turning of a cataractous lens into the vitreous chamber to remove it from the line of vision.

rec·og·ni·tion (rĕk′əg-nĭsh′ən) *n.* **1.** An awareness that something perceived has been perceived before. **2.** The ability of one molecule to attach itself to another molecule having a complementary shape, as in enzyme-substrate and antibody-antigen interactions.

rec·og·ni·tion factor (rĕk′əg-nĭsh′ən) *n.* Any of the factors that allow polymorphonuclear neutrophil white blood cells to recognize target antigens.

re·com·bi·nant (rē-kŏm′bə-nənt) *n.* **1.** An organism or a cell in which genetic recombination has taken place. **2.** Genetic material produced by gene-splicing. — *adj.* **1.** Formed by or showing recombination, as a chromosome. **2.** Of or relating to recombinant DNA.

recombinant DNA *n.* Genetically engineered DNA prepared by transplanting or splicing one or more segments of DNA into the chromosomes of an organism from a different species. Such DNA becomes part of the host's genetic makeup and is replicated.

re·com·bine (rē′kəm-bīn′) *v.* **-bined, -bin·ing, -bines.** To undergo or cause genetic recombination; form new combinations.

rec·om·mend·ed daily allowance (rĕk′ə-mĕn′dĭd) *n.* The amounts of nutrients and calories a person is recommended to consume daily, especially of vitamins and minerals recommended by the Food and Nutrition Board of the National Research Council.

re·con (rē′kŏn′) *n.* The smallest genetic unit capable of recombination.

re·con·struc·tive mammaplasty (rē′kən-strŭk′tĭv) *n.* The making of a simulated breast by plastic surgery for replacement of one that has been removed.

reconstructive surgery *n.* Plastic surgery.

re·cord (rĭ-kôrd′) *v.* **-cord·ed, -cord·ing, -cords. 1.** To set down for preservation in writing or other permanent form. **2.** To register or indicate. — *n.*

rec·ord (rĕk′ərd). **1.** An account, as of information or facts, set down especially in writing as a means of preserving knowledge. **2.** A medical record. **3.** In dentistry, a registration of desired jaw relations in a plastic material or on a device so that such relations may be transferred to an articulator.

re·cov·er·y room (rĭ-kŭv′ə-rē) *n.* A hospital room equipped for the care and observation of patients immediately following surgery.

rec·re·a·tion·al drug (rĕk′rē-ā′shə-nəl) *n.* A drug used nonmedically for personal enjoyment.

re·cru·des·cence (rē′krōō-dĕs′əns) *n.* A recurrence of a pathological process or its symptoms after a period of improvement or quiesence. — re′cru·desce′ *v.* — re′cru·des′cent *adj.*

re·cruit·ment (rĭ-krōōt′mənt) *n.* **1.** An abnormal disproportionate sensation of loudness to sounds of increasing intensity. **2.** The activation of additional motor neurons in response to sustained stimulation of a given receptor or afferent nerve.

rec·tal (rĕk′təl) *adj.* Of, relating to, or situated near the rectum.

rectal anesthesia *n.* General anesthesia following instillation of liquid anesthetics into the rectum.

rec·tec·to·my (rĕk-tĕk′tə-mē) *n.* See **proctectomy**.

rec·ti·tis (rĕk-tī′tĭs) *n.* See **proctitis**.

rec·to·cele (rĕk′tə-sēl′) *n.* See **proctocele**.

rec·to·coc·cy·pex·y (rĕk′tō-kŏk′sə-pĕk′sē) *n.* See **proctococcypexy**.

rec·to·pex·y (rĕk′tə-pĕk′sē) *n.* See **proctopexy**.

rec·to·plas·ty (rĕk′tə-plăs′tē) *n.* See **proctoplasty**.

rec·to·scope (rĕk′tə-skōp′) *n.* See **proctoscope**.

rec·to·sig·moid (rĕk′tō-sĭg′moid′) *n.* **1.** The rectum and the sigmoid colon considered as a unit. **2.** The junction of the rectum and sigmoid colon.

rec·tos·to·my (rĕk-tŏs′tə-mē) *n.* See **proctostomy**.

rec·tot·o·my (rĕk-tŏt′ə-mē) *n.* See **proctotomy**.

rec·tum (rĕk′təm) *n., pl.* **-tums** or **-ta** (-tə). The terminal portion of the large intestine, extending from the sigmoid flexure to the anal canal.

rec·tus muscle of the abdomen (rĕk′təs) *n.* A muscle with origin from the pubis, with insertion into the xiphoid process and the fifth to seventh costal cartilages, and whose action flexes the vertebral column and draws the chest downward.

rectus muscle of the thigh *n.* A muscle with origin from the anterior inferior spine of the ilium and the upper margin of the acetabulum, with insertion into the quadriceps muscle of the thigh.

re·cum·bent (rĭ-kŭm′bənt) *adj.* Lying down, especially in a position of comfort; reclining. — re·cum′bence, re·cum′ben·cy *n.*

re·cu·per·ate (rĭ-kōō′pə-rāt′, -kyōō′-) *v.* **-at·ed, -at·ing, -ates.** To return to health or strength; recover.

re·cur (rĭ-kûr′) *v.* **-curred, -cur·ring, -curs.** To happen, come up, or show up again or repeatedly.

re·cur·rence (rĭ-kûr′əns, -kûr′-) *n.* **1.** A return of symptoms as part of the natural progress of a disease, as in relapsing fever. **2.** See **relapse**.

recurrence risk *n.* Risk that a disease will occur elsewhere in a pedigree, given that at least one member of the pedigree exhibits the disease.

re·cur·rent (rĭ-kûr′ənt, -kûr′-) *adj.* **1.** Occurring or appearing again or repeatedly. **2.** Turning in a reverse direction. Used of blood vessels and nerves.

recurrent herpetic stomatitis *n.* Reactivation of

herpes simplex virus in the oral tissues, characterized by vesicles and ulceration.

recurring digital fibroma of childhood *n.* Any of several fibrous flesh-colored nodules on the the tips of the fingers and toes of infants and young children, composed of spindle cells containing cytoplasmic inclusions.

re·cur·va·tion (rē′kər-vā′shən) *n.* A backward bending or flexure. — **re·cur′vate′** (rĭ-kûr′vāt′, -vĭt) *adj.*

red blood cell *n.* A disk-shaped, biconcave cell in the blood that contains hemoglobin, lacks a nucleus, and transports oxygen and carbon dioxide to and from the tissues.

red bone marrow *n.* Bone marrow in which the meshes of the reticular network contain the developmental stages of red blood cells, white blood cells, and megakaryocytes.

red bug or **redbug** *n.* See chigger (sense 1).

red cell *n.* See red blood cell.

red corpuscle *n.* See red blood cell.

Red Crescent *n.* **1.** A branch of the Red Cross organization operating in a Moslem country. **2.** The crescent-shaped emblem of such a branch.

Red Cross *n.* **1.** An international organization that cares for the wounded, sick, and homeless in wartime and during and following natural disasters. **2.** A national branch of this organization. **3.** The emblem of this organization.

red hepatization *n.* The first stage of hepatization of lung tissue in pneumonia, in which the exudate is blood-stained.

red·in·te·gra·tion (rĕd-ĭn′tĭ-grā′shən, rĭ-dĭn′-) *n.* **1.** The restoration of a lost or injured part. **2.** Evocation of a particular state of mind resulting from the recurrence of one of the elements that made up the original experience.

red muscle *n.* A muscle in which small dark fibers predominate and in which myoglobin and mitochondria are abundant.

red reflex *n.* See light reflex (sense 2).

re·duce (rĭ-dōōs′, -dyōōs′) *v.* **-duced, -duc·ing, -duc·es.** **1.** To bring down, as in extent, amount, or degree; diminish. **2.** To restore a fractured or displaced body part to a normal condition or position. **3.** To remove oxygen from a compound. **4.** To add hydrogen to a compound. **5.** To lose weight, as by dieting. **6.** To undergo meiosis. — **re·duc′er** *n.* — **re·duc′i·bil′i·ty** *n.* — **re·duc′i·ble** *adj.*

reduced hematin *n.* See heme.

reduced hemoglobin *n.* Hemoglobin in red blood cells after the oxygen of oxyhemoglobin is released in the tissues.

re·duc·tase (rĭ-dŭk′tās′, -tāz′) *n.* An enzyme that promotes reduction of an organic compound.

re·duc·tion (rĭ-dŭk′shən) *n.* **1.** The act, process, or result of reducing. **2.** The amount by which something is lessened or diminished. **3.** Restoration of an injured or dislocated part to its normal anatomical relation by surgery or manipulation. **4.** The first meiotic division, in which the chromosome number is reduced. — **re·duc′tion·al** *adj.*

reduction mammaplasty *n.* Plastic surgery on the breast to reduce its size and often to change its shape and position.

re·du·pli·ca·tion (rĭ-dōō′plĭ-kā′shən, -dyōō′-) *n.* **1.** A duplication or doubling, as of the sounds of the heart in certain diseased states. **2.** The abnormal presence of two parts instead of a single part. **3.** A fold or duplicature. — **re·du′pli·cate′** *v.*

Reed–Sternberg cell (rēd′-) *n.* A giant binucleated or multinucleated acidophilic cell found in tissues in Hodgkin's disease.

reef·ing (rē′fĭng) *n.* Surgical reduction of the extent of a tissue by folding it and securing with sutures, as in plication.

ref·er·ence values (rĕf′ər-əns, rĕf′rəns) *pl.n.* A set of laboratory test values obtained from an individual or from a group in a defined state of health.

re·ferred pain (rĭ-fûrd′) *n.* Pain that is felt in a part of the body at a distance from its area of origin, as pain in the right shoulder derived from the presence of a gallstone in the bladder.

referred sensation *n.* A sensation felt in a place other than the site at which a stimulus was applied.

re·flect (rĭ-flĕkt′) *v.* **-flect·ed, -flect·ing, -flects.** To throw or bend back light, heat, or sound from a surface.

re·flec·tion (rĭ-flĕk′shən) *n.* **1.** Something, such as light, radiant heat, sound, or an image, that is reflected. **2.** The folding of a membrane from the wall of a cavity over an organ and back to the wall. **3.** The folds so made. — **re·flec′tion·al** *adj.*

reflection coefficient *n.* A measure of the relative permeability of a particular membrane to a particular solute.

re·flec·tor (rĭ-flĕk′tər) *n.* A surface that reflects light, heat, or sound.

re·flex (rē′flĕks) *n.* **1.** An involuntary physiological response to a stimulus. **2.** An unlearned or instinctive response to a stimulus. **3.** Something, such as light or heat, that is reflected. — *adj.* **1.** Being an involuntary action or response, such as a sneeze, blink, or hiccup. **2.** Bent, turned, or thrown back; reflected. — *v.* **-flexed, -flex·ing, -flex·es.** (rĭ-flĕks′). **1.** To cause to undergo a reflex process. **2.** To bend, turn back, or reflect.

reflex arc *n.* The route followed by nerve impulses to produce a reflex act, from the periphery through the afferent nerve to the nervous system, and thence through the efferent nerve to the effector organ.

reflex inhibition *n.* A decrease in reflex activity caused by sensory stimuli.

re·flex·o·graph (rĭ-flĕk′sə-grăf′) *n.* An instrument for graphically recording a reflex.

re·flex·ol·o·gy (rē′flĕk-sŏl′ə-jē) *n.* **1.** The study of reflex responses, especially as they affect behavior. **2.** A method of massage that relieves nervous tension through the application of finger pressure, especially to the feet.

re·flex·om·e·ter (rē′flĕk-sŏm′ĭ-tər) *n.* An instrument for measuring the force necessary to excite a reflex.

reflex sensation *n.* See **referred sensation.**

re·flux (rē'flŭks') *n.* **1.** A flowing back. **2.** Regurgitation, as of gastric contents.

reflux esophagitis *n.* Inflammation of the lower esophagus from regurgitation of acid gastric contents, characterized by substernal pain and usually due to malfunction of the lower esophageal sphincter.

re·fract (rĭ-frăkt') *v.* **-fract·ed, -fract·ing, -fracts.** To determine the refraction of an eye or a lens.

re·frac·tion (rĭ-frăk'shən) *n.* **1.** The turning or bending of any wave, such as a light or sound wave, when it passes from one medium into another of different density. **2.** The ability of the eye to bend light so that an image is focused on the retina. **3.** Determination of the refractive characteristics of the eye and often the correction of refractive defects with lenses. — **re·frac'tion·al, re·frac'tive** *adj.* — **re·frac'tive·ness, re·frac·tiv'i·ty** (rē'frăk-tĭv'ĭ-tē) *n.*

re·frac·tion·ist (rĭ-frăk'shə-nĭst) *n.* A person trained to measure the refraction of the eye and to determine the proper corrective lenses.

refractive keratotomy *n.* Surgical modification of corneal curvature by incising the cornea to minimize hyperopia, myopia, or astigmatism.

re·frac·tom·e·ter (rē'frăk-tŏm'ĭ-tər) *n.* Any of several instruments used to measure the index of refraction of a substance.

re·frac·tom·e·try (rē'frăk-tŏm'ĭ-trē) *n.* **1.** Measurement of the refractive index of a substance with a refractometer. **2.** Use of a refractometer in determining the refractive error of the eye.

re·frac·to·ry (rĭ-frăk'tə-rē) *adj.* **1.** Resistant to treatment, as a disease. **2.** Unresponsive to stimuli, as a muscle or nerve fiber. — **re·frac'to·ri·ness** *n.*

refractory period *n.* The period following effective stimulation, during which excitable tissue fails to respond to a stimulus of threshold intensity.

refractory state *n.* Subnormal excitability of a muscle or nerve immediately following a response to previous excitation.

re·frac·ture (rē-frăk'chər) *n.* The breaking of a bone that has united after a previous fracture.

re·fresh (rĭ-frĕsh') *v.* **-freshed, -fresh·ing, -freshes. 1.** To cause to recuperate; revive. **2.** To renew by stimulation. **3.** To pare or scrape the edges of a wound to promote healing.

re·frig·er·a·tion anesthesia (rĭ-frĭj'ə-rā'shən) *n.* See **cryoanesthesia.**

re·frin·gence (rĭ-frĭn'jəns) *n.* See **refraction** (sense 3).

re·fu·sion (rĭ-fyoō'zhən) *n.* The return of blood to circulation following its temporary stoppage by the ligature of a limb.

re·gen·er·a·tion (rĭ-jĕn'ə-rā'shən) *n.* Regrowth of lost or destroyed parts or organs.

re·gen·er·a·tive polyp (rĭ-jĕn'ə-rā'tĭv, -ər-ə-tĭv) *n.* A hyperplastic polyp of the gastric mucosa.

re·gime (rā-zhēm', rĭ-) *n.* A regulated system, as of diet and exercise; a regimen.

reg·i·men (crĕj'ə-mən, -mĕn') *n.* **1.** A regulated system, as of diet, therapy, or exercise, intended to promote health or achieve another beneficial effect. **2.** A course of intense physical training.

re·gion (rē'jən) *n.* **1.** An area of the body having natural or arbitrarily assigned boundaries. **2.** A portion of the body having a special nervous or vascular supply. **3.** A part of an organ having a special function.

re·gion·al anesthesia (rē'jə-nəl) *n.* The use of a local anesthetic solution or solutions to produce circumscribed areas of loss of sensation.

regional enteritis *n.* Enteritis of unknown cause that is usually limited to the terminal ileum but can progress to other intestinal segments, characterized by nodule formation and fibrous tissue buildup, abdominal pain, and patchy deep ulceration.

regional hypothermia *n.* Perfusion with cold blood or local refrigeration to cool an organ being subjected to ischemia in order to reduce its metabolic requirements.

reg·is·tered nurse (rĕj'ĭ-stərd) *n.* A nurse who has graduated from an accredited school of nursing and has been registered and licensed to practice by a state authority.

reg·is·trar (rĕj'ĭ-strär', rĕj'ĭ-strär') *n.* An admitting officer in a hospital.

re·gres·sion (rĭ-grĕsh'ən) *n.* **1.** A subsidence of the symptoms of a disease. **2.** A relapse of symptoms. **3.** Reversion to an earlier or less mature pattern of feeling or behavior. **4.** Relapse to a less perfect or developed state.

re·gres·sive (rĭ-grĕs'ĭv) *adj.* **1.** Tending to return or revert. **2.** Characterized by regression. — **re·gres'sive·ness** *n.*

reg·u·lar astigmatism (rĕg'yə-lər) *n.* Astigmatism in which the curvature in each meridian is equal throughout its course, and the meridians of greatest and least curvature are at right angles to each other.

reg·u·late (rĕg'yə-lāt') *v.* **-lat·ed, -lat·ing, -lates. 1.** To adjust to a particular specification or requirement. **2.** To adjust a mechanism for accurate and proper functioning. — **reg'u·la'tive, reg'u·la·to'ry** (-lə-tôr'ē) *adj.* — **reg'u·la'tor** *n.*

reg·u·la·tion (rĕg'yə-lā'shən) *n.* **1.** The act of regulating or the state of being regulated. **2.** The capacity of an embryo to continue normal development following injury to or alteration of a structure.

re·gur·gi·tant murmur (rē-gûr'jĭ-tənt) *n.* A murmur due to leakage or backward flow at one of the valvular orifices of the heart.

re·gur·gi·tate (rē-gûr'jĭ-tāt') *v.* **-tat·ed, -tat·ing, -tates. 1.** To rush or surge back. **2.** To cause to pour back, especially to cast up partially digested food. — **re·gur'gi·tant** (-tənt) *adj.* — **re·gur'gi·ta'tion** *n.* — **re·gur'gi·ta'tive** *adj.*

re·hab (rē'hăb') *n. Informal.* Rehabilitation.

re·ha·bil·i·tant (rē'hə-bĭl'ĭ-tənt) *n.* One who is undergoing rehabilitation, as for a disability.

re·ha·bil·i·tate (rē'hə-bĭl'ĭ-tāt') *v.* **-tat·ed, -tat·ing, -tates. 1.** To restore to good health or useful life, as through therapy and education. **2.** To restore to good condition, operation, or capacity. **— re'ha·bil'i·ta'tion** *n.* **— re'ha·bil'i·ta'tive** *adj.*

re·hears·al (rĭ-hûr'səl) *n.* The process of repeating information, such as a name or a list of words, in order to remember it. **— re·hearse'** *v.*

re·hy·drate (rē-hī'drāt') *v.* **-drat·ed, -drat·ing, -drates. 1.** To cause something dehydrated to take up fluid. **2.** To replenish body fluids.

re·hy·dra·tion (rē'hī-drā'shən) *n.* **1.** The restoration of fluid to a dehydrated substance. **2.** The replenishment of bodily fluids.

Rei·fen·stein's syndrome (rī'fən-stīnz') *n.* A familial form of male pseudohermaphroditism characterized by ambiguous genitalia or hypospadias, postpubertal development of abnormally large breasts, and infertility associated with sclerosis of the seminal tubules.

re·im·plan·ta·tion (rē'ĭm-plăn-tā'shən) *n.* See **replantation.**

re·in·fec·tion (rē'ĭn-fĕk'shən) *n.* A second infection that follows recovery from a previous infection by the same causative agent.

re·in·force (rē'ĭn-fôrs') *v.* **-forced, -forc·ing, -forces. 1.** To give more force or effectiveness to something; strengthen. **2.** To reward an individual, especially an experimental subject, with a reinforcer subsequent to a desired response or performance. **3.** To stimulate a response by means of a reinforcer.

re·in·force·ment (rē'ĭn-fôrs'mənt) *n.* **1.** The act or process of reinforcing. **2.** Something that reinforces. **3.** The occurrence or experimental introduction of an unconditioned stimulus along with a conditioned stimulus. **4.** The strengthening of a conditioned response by such means. **5.** An event, a circumstance, or a condition that increases the likelihood that a given response will recur in a situation like that in which the reinforcing condition originally occurred.

re·in·forc·er (rē'ĭn-fôr'sər) *n.* A stimulus, such as a reward, that in operant conditioning maintains or strengthens a desired response.

re·in·ner·va·tion (rē'ĭn-ər-vā'shən) *n.* Restoration of nerve control of a paralyzed muscle or organ by means of the regrowth of nerve fibers, either spontaneously or after anastomosis.

reins (rānz) *pl.n.* The kidneys, loins, or lower back.

re·in·te·gra·tion (rē'ĭn-tĭ-grā'shən) *n.* **1.** Restoration to a condition of integration or unity. **2.** The return to well-adjusted functioning following mental illness. **— re·in'te·grate'** *v.* **— re·in'te·gra'tive** *adj.*

Rei·ter's syndrome (rī'tərz) *n.* A triad of disorders that can appear consecutively or concurrently and include inflammation of the urethra, the iris and ciliary body, and the joints.

re·ject (rĭ-jĕkt') *v.* **-ject·ed, -ject·ing, -jects. 1.** To refuse to accept, submit to, believe, or make use of something. **2.** To spit out or vomit. **3.** To resist immunologically the introduction of a transplanted organ or tissue; fail to accept as part of one's own body.

re·jec·tion (rĭ-jĕk'shən) *n.* **1.** The act of rejecting or the state of being rejected. **2.** The failure of a recipient's body to accept a transplanted tissue or organ as the result of immunological incompatability.

re·lapse (rĭ-lăps') *v.* **-lapsed, -laps·ing, -laps·es. 1.** To regress after partial recovery from illness. **2.** To fall or slide back into a former state. **— n.** (rē'-lăps, rĭ-lăps'). A falling back into a former state, especially the return of symptoms after apparent recovery.

re·laps·ing fever (rĭ-lăp'sĭng) *n.* An acute infectious disease caused by a strain of *Borrelia*, transmitted by lice or ticks, and marked by recurring febrile attacks lasting about six days and separated from one other by apyretic intervals of about the same length.

re·la·tion (rĭ-lā'shən) *n.* **1.** A logical or natural association between two or more things. **2.** The connection of people by blood or marriage; kinship. **3.** A person connected to another by blood or marriage; a relative. **4.** The positional relationship of the teeth or other structures in the mouth.

re·la·tion·ship (rĭ-lā'shən-shĭp') *n.* **1.** The condition or fact of being related; connection or association. **2.** Connection by blood or marriage; kinship.

rel·a·tive accommodation (rĕl'ə-tĭv) *n.* The quantity of accomodation required for binocular vision for any distance or for any degree of convergence.

relative leukocytosis *n.* An increased proportion of one or more types of white cells in the blood without an actual increase in the total number of such cells.

relative scotoma *n.* A scotoma in which the visual impairment is not complete.

relative specificity *n.* The specificity of a medical screening test as determined by comparison with an established test of the same type.

relax *v.* **-laxed, -lax·ing, -lax·es. 1.** To make or become lax or loose. **2.** To relieve or become relieved from tension or strain.

re·lax·ant (rĭ-lăk'sənt) *adj.* Something, such as a drug or therapeutic treatment, that relaxes or relieves muscular or nervous tension. **— adj.** Tending to relax or to relieve tension.

re·lax·a·tion (rē'lăk-sā'shən) *n.* **1.** The act of relaxing or the state of being relaxed. **2.** A loosening or slackening. **3.** The lengthening of inactive muscle or muscle fibers.

relaxation suture *n.* A suture arranged so that it may be loosened if the tension of the wound becomes excessive.

re·lax·in (rĭ-lăk'sĭn) *n.* A female hormone secreted by the corpus luteum that helps soften the cervix and relax the pelvic ligaments in childbirth.

re·learn·ing (rē-lûr'nĭng) *n.* The process of regaining a skill or ability that has been partially or entirely lost. — **re·learn'** v.

rel·ict (rĕl'ĭkt, rĭ-lĭkt') n. Something that has survived; a remnant.

re·lieve (rĭ-lēv') v. **-lieved, -liev·ing, -lieves. 1.** To lessen or alleviate something, such as pain or a symptom. **2.** To free from pain, anxiety, or distress. — **re·liev'a·ble** adj. — **re·liev'er** n.

rem (rĕm) n. **1.** The amount of ionizing radiation required to produce the same biological effect as one rad of high-penetration x-rays. **2.** A unit for measuring absorbed doses of radiation, equivalent to one roentgen of x-rays or gamma rays; roentgen-equivalent-man.

REM abbr. rapid eye movement

Re·mak's sign (rā'mäks, -mäks) n. An indication of tabes dorsalis and polyneuritis in which there is a dissociation of the sensations of touch and of pain.

rem·e·dy (rĕm'ĭ-dē) n. Something, such as medicine or therapy, that relieves pain, cures disease, or corrects a disorder. — v. **-died, -dy·ing, -dies.** To relieve or cure a disease or disorder.

re·mem·ber (rĭ-mĕm'bər) v. **-bered, -ber·ing, -bers. 1.** To recall to the mind; think of again. **2.** To retain in memory. **3.** To return to original shape or form after being deformed or altered.

re·min·er·al·i·za·tion (rē-mĭn'ər-ə-lĭ-zā'shən) n. The restoration of lost mineral constituents to the body, especially to bone.

re·mis·sion (rĭ-mĭsh'ən) n. **1.** Abatement or subsiding of the symptoms of a disease. **2.** The period during which the symptoms of a disease abate or subside.

re·mit (rĭ-mĭt') v. **-mit·ted, -mit·ting, -mits.** To diminish; abate.

re·mit·tent (rĭ-mĭt'nt) adj. Characterized by temporary abatement in severity. Used especially of diseases. — **re·mit'tence, re·mit'ten·cy** n.

re·mod·el·ing (rē-mŏd'l-ĭng) n. A cyclical process by which bone maintains a dynamic steady state through resorption and formation of a small amount of bone at the same site.

REM sleep (rĕm) n. A stage in the normal sleep cycle during which dreams occur and the body undergoes various physiological changes, including rapid eye movement, loss of reflexes, and increased pulse rate and brain activity.

ren (rĕn) n., pl. **re·nes** (rē'nēz). A kidney.

re·nal (rē'nəl) adj. Of, relating to, or in the region of the kidneys.

renal artery n. An artery with its origin in the aorta, with branches to the ureter, adrenal gland, and associated structures, and with distribution to the kidney.

renal cast n. Any of various casts that are formed in the renal tubule and found in the urine and consist of materials such as albumin, cells, and blood.

renal clearance n. The volume of plasma completely cleared of a specific compound per unit time and measured as a test of kidney function.

renal glycosuria n. Recurring or persistent glyco-

suria in association with blood levels that are in the normal range, resulting from the failure of renal tubules to reabsorb glucose at a normal rate from the glomerular filtrate.

renal hypertension n. Hypertension that is secondary to kidney disease.

renal pelvis n. A hollow flattened funnel-shaped expansion of the upper end of the ureter into which urine is discharged before entering the ureter, located at the upper end of the ureter and whose apex is continuous with it.

renal rickets n. A form of rickets occurring in children in association with, and apparently caused by, renal disease with hyperphosphatemia.

renal tubular acidosis n. A syndrome characterized by the inability to excrete acidic urine and by low plasma bicarbonate and high plasma chloride concentrations, often with hypokalemia.

renal tubule n. A tubule of the kidney, such as a collecting or convoluted tubule.

renal vein n. Any of the veins that accompany the renal arteries and open at right angles into the vena cava at the level of the second lumbar vertebra.

re·nin (rē'nĭn, rĕn'ĭn) n. A protein-digesting enzyme that is released by the kidneys and hydrolyzes angiotensinogen.

ren·nin (rĕn'ĭn) n. A milk-coagulating enzyme found especially in the gastric juice of young animals, used in making cheeses.

re·no·gram (rē'nə-grăm') n. **1.** A graphic record of the renal excretion of a radioactive tracer that has been injected into the renal system. **2.** A radiograph of a kidney.

re·nog·ra·phy (rē-nŏg'rə-fē) n. Radiography of the kidney.

re·no·meg·a·ly (rē'nō-mĕg'ə-lē) n. Enlargement of the kidney.

re·nop·a·thy (rē-nŏp'ə-thē) n. See **nephropathy.**

Re·o·vi·rus (rē'ō-vī'rəs) n. A genus of viruses having double-stranded RNA, associated with infections of the respiratory and gastrointestinal tracts.

rep (rĕp) n. Roentgen-equivalent-physical; a unit of absorbed radiation dose.

re·pair (rĭ-pâr') v. **-paired, -pair·ing, -pairs.** To restore to a healthy or functioning condition after damage or injury. — n. Restoration of diseased or damaged tissues naturally or by surgical means.

re·place·ment therapy (rĭ-plās'mənt) n. Therapy designed to compensate for a lack or deficiency arising from inadequate nutrition, from certain dysfunctions, or from losses, as by the administration of natural or synthetic substances.

re·plant (rē-plănt') v. **-plant·ed, -plant·ing, -plants.** To reattach an organ, limb, or other body part surgically to the original site. — n. (rē'plănt'). An organ, limb, or body part that has been replanted.

re·plan·ta·tion (rē'plăn-tā'shən) n. Replacement of an organ or part into its original site and the reestablishment of circulation.

re·ple·tion (rĭ-plē'shən) n. **1.** The condition of being fully supplied or completely filled. **2.** A state of excessive fullness.

rep·li·cate (rĕp′lĭ-kāt′) v. **-cat·ed, -cat·ing, -cates. 1.** To duplicate, copy, reproduce, or repeat. **2.** To reproduce or make an exact copy or copies of genetic material, a cell, or an organism. — n. A repetition of an experiment or a procedure.

rep·li·ca·tion (rĕp′lĭ-kā′shən) n. **1.** The act or process of duplicating or reproducing something. **2.** Autoreproduction.

rep·li·con (rĕp′lĭ-kŏn′) n. A genetic element that undergoes replication as an autonomous unit.

rep·li·some (rĕp′lĭ-sōm′) n. Any of the sites on the matrix of a cell nucleus that contains a series of enzyme complexes where DNA replication is thought to occur.

re·po·lar·i·za·tion (rē-pō′lər-ĭ-zā′shən) n. The restoration of a polarized state across a membrane, as in a muscle fiber following contraction.

re·port·a·ble disease (rĭ-pôr′tə-bəl) n. See notifiable disease.

re·po·si·tion·ing (rē′pə-zĭsh′ə-nĭng) n. See reduction (sense 3).

re·pos·i·tor (rĭ-pŏz′ĭ-tər) n. An instrument used to reposition a displaced organ, especially a prolapsed uterus.

re·press (rĭ-prĕs′) v. **-pressed, -press·ing, -press·es. 1.** To hold back by an act of volition. **2.** To exclude something, such as a painful or unpleasant memory, from the conscious mind.

re·pres·sion (rĭ-prĕsh′ən) n. **1.** The act of repressing or the state of being repressed. **2.** The unconscious exclusion of painful impulses, desires, or fears from the conscious mind.

re·pro·duce (rē′prə-dōōs′, -dyōōs′) v. **-duced, -duc·ing, -duc·es. 1.** To generate offspring by sexual or asexual means. **2.** To bring something, such as a memory, to mind again. **3.** To produce a counterpart, an image, or a copy of something.

re·pro·duc·tion (rē′prə-dŭk′shən) n. **1.** The act of reproducing or the condition or process of being reproduced. **2.** Recall of a memory. **3.** The sexual or asexual process by which organisms generate others of the same kind.

re·pro·duc·tive (rē′prə-dŭk′tĭv) adj. **1.** Of or relating to reproduction. **2.** Tending to reproduce.

reproductive cycle n. The cycle of physiological changes that begins with conception and extends through gestation and parturition.

reproductive system n. The complex of male or female gonads, associated ducts, and external genitalia concerned with sexual reproduction.

re·pul·sion (rĭ-pŭl′shən) n. **1.** A feeling of extreme dislike or repugnance. **2.** The tendency of particles or bodies of the same electric charge or magnetic polarity to separate.

re·sect (rĭ-sĕkt′) v. **-sect·ed, -sect·ing, -sects.** To perform a resection on a part of the body.

re·sec·tion (rĭ-sĕk′shən) n. **1.** Surgical removal of part of an organ or a structure. **2.** Removal of the articular ends of one or both bones forming a joint.

re·sec·to·scope (rĭ-sĕk′tə-skōp′) n. A surgical instrument for performing a resection without an opening or incision other than that made by the instrument.

re·ser·pine (rĭ-sûr′pēn, -pĭn, rĕs′ər-pĭn, -pēn′, rĕz′-) n. A white to yellowish powder used as a sedative and an antihypertensive.

re·serve (rĭ-zûrv′) v. **-served, -serv·ing, -serves.** To set or cause to be set apart for a particular person or use. — n. Something kept back or saved for future use or a special purpose. — adj. Held back, set aside, or saved.

reserve force n. The energy residing in an organ or in any of its parts above that required for its normal functioning.

res·er·voir (rĕz′ər-vwär′, -vwôr′, -vôr′) n. **1.** A fluid-containing sac or cavity. **2.** An organism or a population that directly or indirectly transmits a pathogen while being virtually immune to its effects.

reservoir bag n. See breathing bag.

reservoir host n. A host that serves as a source of infection and potential reinfection of humans and as a means of sustaining a parasite when it is not infecting humans.

reservoir of spermatozoa n. The distal portion of the tail of the epididymis and the beginning of the vas deferens, where spermatozoa are stored.

res·i·dence (rĕz′ĭ-dəns, -dĕns′) n. A medical residency.

res·i·den·cy (rĕz′ĭ-dən-sē, -dĕn′-) n. The period during which a physician receives specialized clinical training.

res·i·dent (rĕz′ĭ-dənt, -dĕnt′) n. A physician receiving specialized clinical training for a specified period of time.

re·sid·u·al abscess (rĭ-zĭj′ōō-əl) n. An abscess recurring at the site of a former abscess as a result of the persistence of microbes and pus.

residual air n. See residual volume.

residual capacity n. See residual volume.

residual urine n. Urine remaining in the bladder at the end of micturition, as in cases of prostatic obstruction or bladder atony.

residual volume n. The volume of air remaining in the lungs after a maximal expiratory effort.

res·i·due (rĕz′ĭ-dōō′, -dyōō′) n. The remainder of something after removal of parts or a part.

re·sid·u·um (rĭ-zĭj′ōō-əm) n., pl. **-u·a** (-ōō-ə). Something remaining after removal of a part; a residue.

re·sis·tance (rĭ-zĭs′təns) n. **1.** The capacity of an organism to defend itself against a disease. **2.** The capacity of an organism, a tissue, or a cell to withstand the effects of a harmful physical or environmental agent. **3.** In psychoanalysis, a process in which the ego opposes the conscious recall of repressed unpleasant experiences.

resistance factor n. See resistance plasmid.

resistance plasmid n. Any of various plasmids carrying genes that allow bacteria to resist the effects of antibiotics and other bacteriostatic agents.

res·o·lu·tion (rĕz′ə-lōō′shən) n. **1.** The subsiding

or termination of an abnormal condition, such as a fever or an inflammation. **2.** The act or process of separating or reducing something into its constituent parts.

re·solve (rĭ-zŏlv′) *v.* **-solved, -solv·ing, -solves. 1.** To cause resolution of an abnormal condition. **2.** To render parts of an image visible and distinct.

res·o·nance (rĕz′ə-nəns) *n.* **1.** The sound produced by diagnostic percussion of the normal chest. **2.** Intensification of vocal tones during articulation, as by the air cavities of the mouth and nasal passages. **3.** Intensification and prolongation of sound produced by sympathetic vibration after percussion.

re·sorb (rē-sôrb′, -zôrb′) *v.* **-sorbed, -sorb·ing, -sorbs. 1.** To absorb again. **2.** To dissolve and assimilate, as of bone tissue.

res·or·cin·ol (rĭ-zôr′sə-nôl′, -nōl′) or **res·or·cin** (-sĭn) *n.* A white crystalline compound used primarily as an antiseptic in skin diseases such as psoriasis and ringworm, but also used to treat nausea, asthma, whooping cough, and diarrhea.

re·sorp·tion (rē-sôrp′shən, -zôrp′-) *n.* The act or process of resorbing.

resorption lacuna *n.* See **Howship's lacuna.**

res·pi·ra·ble (rĕs′pər-ə-bəl, rĭ-spīr′-) *adj.* Fit for breathing, as of air.

res·pi·ra·tion (rĕs′pə-rā′shən) *n.* **1.** The act or process of inhaling and exhaling; breathing. **2.** The oxidative process occurring within living cells by which the chemical energy of organic molecules is released in a series of metabolic steps involving the consumption of oxygen and the liberation of carbon dioxide and water.

respiration rate *n.* Frequency of breathing, expressed as the number of breaths per minute.

res·pi·ra·tor (rĕs′pə-rā′tər) *n.* **1.** A device that supplies oxygen or a mixture of oxygen and carbon dioxide for breathing, used especially in artificial respiration. **2.** A screenlike device worn over the mouth or nose or both to protect the respiratory tract.

res·pi·ra·to·ry (rĕs′pər-ə-tôr′ē, rĭ-spīr′ə-) *adj.* Of, relating to, used in, or affecting respiration.

respiratory acidosis *n.* Acidosis caused by retention of carbon dioxide, due to inadequate pulmonary ventilation or hypoventilation, with a decrease in blood pH unless compensated for by renal retention of bicarbonate.

respiratory alkalosis *n.* Alkalosis resulting from abnormal loss of carbon dioxide due to hyperventilation.

respiratory bronchiole *n.* The smallest subdivision of a bronchiole, connecting a terminal bronchiole to an alveolar duct.

respiratory capacity *n.* See **vital capacity.**

respiratory center *n.* The region of neurons in the brain that receives afferent information that is then translated to signals controlling the sequence of breathing.

respiratory distress syndrome *n.* A respiratory disease of newborn infants, especially premature infants, characterized by reduced amounts of lung surfactant, cyanosis, the formation of a glassy membrane over the alveoli of the lungs, and pulmonary collapse.

respiratory enzyme *n.* An enzyme, such as oxidase, that transfers electrons from its substrate to molecular oxygen during cellular respiration.

respiratory pause *n.* Cessation of air flow during respiration for less than ten seconds.

respiratory pigment *n.* Any of the oxygen-carrying substances in the blood and tissues, such as hemoglobin and myoglobin.

respiratory quotient *n.* The ratio of carbon dioxide produced by tissue metabolism to oxygen consumed in the same metabolism.

respiratory syncytial virus *n.* An RNA-containing virus that causes minor respiratory infections in adults and bronchitis and bronchopneumonia in children.

respiratory system *n.* The integrated system of organs involved in the intake and exchange of oxygen and carbon dioxide between the body and the environment and including the nasal passages, larynx, trachea, bronchial tubes, and lungs.

respiratory tract *n.* The air passages from the nose to the pulmonary alveoli, including the pharynx, larynx, trachea, and bronchi.

re·spire (rĭ-spīr′) *v.* **-spired, -spir·ing, -spires. 1.** To breathe in and out; inhale and exhale. **2.** To undergo the metabolic process of respiration. **3.** To breathe easily again, as after a period of exertion or trouble.

res·pi·rom·e·ter (rĕs′pə-rŏm′ĭ-tər) *n.* An instrument for measuring the degree and nature of respiration.

re·sponse (rĭ-spŏns′) *n.* A reaction, as that of an organism or any of its parts, to a specific stimulus.

rest (rĕst) *n.* **1.** Cessation of work, exertion, or activity. **2.** Peace, ease, or refreshment resulting from sleep or the cessation of an activity. **3.** Sleep or quiet relaxation. **4.** Mental or emotional tranquility. **5.** A device used as a support, as for the back. **6.** A group of embryonic cells or a portion of fetal tissue that has become displaced during development. **7.** An extension from a prosthesis that gives vertical support to a dental restoration. — *v.* **rest·ed, rest·ing, rests. 1.** To cease motion, work, or activity. **2.** To lie down, especially to sleep. **3.** To be supported or based; lie, lean, or sit against.

re·ste·no·sis (rē′stə-nō′sĭs) *n.* Recurrence of stenosis after corrective surgery on a heart valve.

rest home *n.* An establishment where the elderly or frail are housed and cared for.

resting cell *n.* A cell that is not actively in the process of dividing.

resting tidal volume *n.* The tidal volume under normal resting conditions.

res·ti·tu·tion (rĕs′tĭ-tōō′shən, -tyōō′-) *n.* A return to or restoration of a previous state or position, especially the return of the rotated head of a fetus to its natural alignment with the fetal body following delivery.

rest·less legs syndrome (rĕst′lĭs) *n.* Discomfort or twitching in the legs that occurs after going to bed and often leads to insomnia.

res·to·ra·tion (rĕs′tə-rā′shən) *n.* **1.** Any of various dental fittings, such as an inlay, crown, bridge, partial denture, or complete denture, that restore or replace lost tooth structure, teeth, or oral tissues. **2.** A substance used to restore the missing portion of a tooth.

re·stor·a·tive (rĭ-stôr′ə-tĭv) *adj.* Of or relating to restoration. — *n.* A medicine or other agent that helps to restore health, strength, or consciousness.

re·straint (rĭ-strānt′) *n.* **1.** An instrument or a means of restraint to prevent the infliction of harm to self or others, such as a straightjacket. **2.** Control or repression of feelings; constraint.

re·stric·tion enzyme (rĭ-strĭk′shən) *n.* Any of a group of enzymes that cleave DNA at specific sites to produce discrete fragments, used especially in gene-splicing.

restriction fragment length polymorphism *n.* Intraspecies variations in the length of DNA fragments generated by the action of restriction enzymes caused by mutations that alter the sites at which these enzymes can act, thus changing the length, number, or even production of such fragments.

restriction-site polymorphism *n.* A form of DNA polymorphism in which one of the two nucleotide sequence contains a recognition site for a particular endonuclease but the second nucleotide sequence lacks such a site.

re·sus·ci·tate (rĭ-sŭs′ĭ-tāt′) *v.* **-tat·ed, -tat·ing, -tates.** To restore consciousness, vigor, or life to.

re·sus·ci·ta·tion (rĭ-sŭs′ĭ-tā′shən) *n.* The act of resuscitating or the state of being resuscitated.

re·sus·ci·ta·tor (rĭ-sŭs′ĭ-tā′tər) *n.* One that resuscitates, as an apparatus that forces oxygen or a mixture of oxygen and carbon dioxide into the lungs of a person who has undergone partial asphyxiation.

re·tain·er (rĭ-tā′nər) *n.* **1.** One that retains, as a device, frame, or groove that restrains or guides, especially for a prosthesis. **2.** An appliance used to hold teeth in position after orthodontic treatment.

re·tar·da·tion (rē′tär-dā′shən) *n.* **1.** The condition of being relatively slow in mental, emotional, or physical development. **2.** The extent to which something is held back or delayed. **3.** Mental retardation.

retch (rĕch) *v.* **retched, retch·ing, retch·es.** To try to vomit.

re·te (rē′tē) *n., pl.* **re·ti·a** (rē′tē-ə, rē′shə). An anatomical mesh, network, or structure, as of veins, arteries, or nerves. — **re′ti·al** (-tē-əl, -shəl)

rete tes·tis (tĕs′tĭs) *n.* The network of canals at the termination of the seminiferous tubules.

re·ten·tion (rĭ-tĕn′shən) *n.* **1.** Involuntary withholding by the body of wastes or secretions that are normally eliminated. **2.** The holding by the body of what normally belongs in it, such as food

in the stomach. **3.** An ability to recall or recognize what has been learned or experienced; memory.

retention cyst *n.* A cyst caused by an obstruction to the excretory duct of a gland.

retention suture *n.* A heavy, reinforcing suture placed deep within the muscles and fasciae of the abdominal wall to relieve tension on the primary suture line and avoid postsurgical wound disruption.

re·tic·u·lar (rĭ-tĭk′yə-lər) or **re·tic·u·lat·ed** (-lā′tĭd) *adj.* Resembling a net in form; netlike. — **re·tic′- u·la′tion** *n.*

reticular activating system *n.* The part of the reticular formation in the brainstem that plays a central role in bodily and behavioral alertness; its ascending connections affect the function of the cerebral cortex and its descending connections transmit its activating influence upon bodily posture and reflex mechanisms.

reticular cell *n.* Any of the cells forming the stroma of bone marrow and lymphatic tissues whose processes contact similar cells to form a network.

reticular fiber *n.* Any of the small, branching, intercellular fiber elements that may be continuous with collagen fibers.

reticular formation *n.* A massive but vaguely delimited neural apparatus composed of closely intermingled gray and white matter, extending throughout the length of the spinal cord and upward into the diencephalon, and dominating the control of autonomic and endocrine functions, bodily posture, skeletomuscular reflex activity, and general behavioral states.

reticular membrane *n.* The membrane formed by cuticular plates of the cells of the spiral organ.

reticular substance *n.* **1.** A filamentous plasmatic material beaded with granules that is visible upon vital staining in the immature red blood cells. **2.** See **reticular formation.**

reticular tissue *n.* A form of connective tissue in which reticular fibers form a branching network; it usually has a network of reticular cells associated with the fibers.

re·tic·u·lat·ed bone (rĭ-tĭk′yə-lā′tĭd) *n.* See **woven bone.**

re·tic·u·lin (rĭ-tĭk′yə-lĭn) *n.* A scleroprotein present in the connective-tissue framework of the lymphatic tissues.

re·tic·u·lo·cyte (rĭ-tĭk′yə-lō-sīt′) *n.* An immature red blood cell that contains a network of basophilic filaments.

re·tic·u·lo·cy·to·pe·ni·a (rĭ-tĭk′yə-lō-sī′tə-pē′- nē-ə) *n.* An abnormal decrease in the number of reticulocytes in the blood.

re·tic·u·lo·cy·to·sis (re-tik′yū-lō- sī-tō′sis) *n.* An increase in the number of reticulocytes in the blood.

re·tic·u·lo·en·do·the·li·al system (rĭ-tĭk′yə-lō- ĕn′dō-thē′lē-əl) *n.* The diffuse system constituting all phagocytic cells of the body except granulocytic leukocytes. It includes the cells lining the sinusoids of the spleen, lymph nodes, and bone marrow along with the fibroblastic reticular cells of hematopoietic tissues.

re·tic·u·lo·en·do·the·li·o·ma (rĭ-tĭk′yə-lō-ĕn′dō-thē′lē-ō′mə) *n.* A neoplasm derived from reticuloendothelium.

re·tic·u·lo·en·do·the·li·um (rĭ-tĭk′yə-lō-ĕn′dō-thē′lē-əm) *n.* The cells and tissues making up the reticuloendothelial system.

re·tic·u·lo·sis (rĭ-tĭk′yə-lō′sĭs) *n.* An increase in histiocytes, monocytes, or other reticuloendothelial elements.

re·tic·u·lo·spi·nal tract (rĭ-tĭk′yə-lō-spī′nəl) *n.* Any of several fiber tracts descending to the spinal cord from the reticular formation of the pons and medulla oblongata. Some fibers conduct impulses from the neural mechanisms regulating cardiovascular and respiratory functions and others form links in extrapyramidal motor mechanisms affecting muscle tonus and somatic movement.

re·tic·u·lum (rĭ-tĭk′yə-ləm) *n., pl.* **-la** (-lə). **1.** A fine network formed by cells, or by certain structures within cells, or by connective-tissue fibers between cells. **2.** See **neuroglia.**

re·ti·form tissue (rē′tə-fôrm′, rĕt′ə-) *n.* See **reticular tissue.**

ret·i·na (rĕt′n-ə) *n., pl.* **ret·i·nas** or **ret·i·nae** (rĕt′-n-ē′). The delicate, multilayered, light-sensitive membrane lining the inner posterior chamber of the eyeball containing the rods and cones and connected by the optic nerve to the brain. — **ret′-i·nal** *adj.*

ret·i·nac·u·lum (rĕt′n-ăk′yə-ləm) *n., pl.* **-la** (-lə). A band or bandlike structure that holds an organ or a part in place. — **ret′i·nac′u·lar** (-lər) *adj.*

ret·i·nal (rĕt′n-ăl′, -ôl′) *n.* See **retinaldehyde.**

retinal adaptation *n.* Adjustment of the eye to the degree of illumination.

retinal cone *n.* See **cone cell.**

ret·i·nal·de·hyde (rĕt′n-ăl′də-hīd′) *n.* A yellow to orange aldehyde derivative of vitamin A that acts on the retina to form the visual pigments of the rods and cones.

ret·i·ni·tis (rĕt′n-ī′tĭs) *n.* Inflammation of the retina.

retinitis pig·men·to·sa (pĭg′mən-tō′sə, -mĕn-) *n.* A hereditary degenerative disease of the retina producing conditions such as night blindness, pigmentation changes in the retina, narrowing of the visual field, and the eventual loss of vision.

ret·i·no·blas·to·ma (rĕt′n-ō-blă-stō′mə) *n., pl.* **-mas** or **-ma·ta** (-mə-tə). A hereditary malignant tumor of the retina, transmitted as a dominant trait and occurring chiefly among infants.

ret·i·no·cer·e·bral angiomatosis (rĕt′n-ō-sĕr′ə-brəl, -sə-rē′-) *n.* See **Lindau's disease.**

ret·i·no·cho·roid·i·tis (rĕt′n-ō-kôr′oi-dī′tĭs) *n.* See **chorioretinitis.**

ret·i·no·di·al·y·sis (rĕt′n-ō-dī-ăl′ĭ-sĭs) *n.* Detachment of the retina.

ret·i·no·ic acid (rĕt′n-ō′ĭk) *n.* An acid formed in the oxidation of retinaldehyde and used as a topical treatment for acne.

ret·i·nol (rĕt′n-ôl′, -ōl′) *n.* See **vitamin A.**

ret·i·no·pap·il·li·tis (rĕt′n-ō-păp′ə-lī′tĭs) *n.* See **papilloretinitis.**

ret·i·nop·a·thy (rĕt′n-ŏp′ə-thē) *n.* A noninflammatory degenerative disease of the retina.

ret·i·no·pex·y (rĕt′n-ō-pĕk′sē) *n.* Surgical correction of a detachment of the retina by forming chorioretinal adhesions around the torn part of the retina.

ret·i·no·scope (rĕt′n-ə-skōp′) *n.* An optical instrument for examining refraction of light in the eye.

ret·i·nos·co·py (rĕt′n-ŏs′kə-pē) *n.* A method of detecting errors of refraction of the eye by illuminating the retina and noting the direction of movement of the light on the retinal surface. — **ret′i·no·scop′ic** (-ə-skŏp′ĭk) *adj.*

re·trac·tion (rĭ-trăk′shən) *n.* **1.** The act of drawing back or in; shrinking. **2.** The act of pulling apart, usually as part of a surgical procedure.

re·trac·tor (rĭ-trăk′tər) *n.* **1.** A surgical instrument used to hold back organs or the edges of an incision. **2.** A muscle, such as a flexor, that retracts an organ or a part.

re·trench·ment (rĭ-trĕnch′mənt) *n.* The cutting away of superfluous tissue.

re·triev·al (rĭ-trē′vəl) *n.* The third stage in the memory process, after encoding and storage, involving mental processes associated with bringing stored information back into consciousness.

ret·ro·bul·bar anesthesia (rĕt′rō-bŭl′bər, -bär′) *n.* Injection of a local anesthetic behind the eye to produce sensory denervation of the eye.

ret·ro·ces·sion (rĕt′rō-sĕsh′ən) *n.* **1.** A relapse, as of a disease. **2.** Cessation of the external symptoms of a disease, followed by signs of involvement of an internal organ or part. **3.** Backward displacement of the uterus or other organ.

ret·ro·clu·sion (rĕt′rō-klōō′zhən) *n.* A form of acupressure used to halt bleeding, especially of a cut artery.

ret·ro·col·lic spasm (rĕt′rō-kŏl′ĭk) *n.* Torticollis in which the spasm affects the posterior neck muscles.

ret·ro·col·lis (rĕt′rō-kŏl′ĭs) *n.* See **retrocollic spasm.**

ret·ro·con·duc·tion (rĕt′rō-kən-dŭk′shən) *n.* Conduction backward from the ventricles or from the atrioventricular node into and through the atria.

ret·ro·cus·pid papilla (rĕt′rō-kŭs′pĭd) *n.* A small tag of tissue on the mandibular gingiva, lingual to the cuspid teeth. It usually occurs bilaterally, is more commonly seen in children, and is considered a normal anatomic structure.

ret·ro·de·vi·a·tion (rĕt′rō-dē′vē-ā′shən) *n.* A backward bending or inclining.

ret·ro·dis·place·ment (rĕt′rō-dĭs-plās′mənt) *n.* A backward displacement, such as retroversion or retroflexion of the uterus.

ret·ro·flex·ion (rĕt′rō-flĕk′shən) *n.* A backward bending, especially of the body of the uterus toward the cervix.

ret·ro·gnath·ism (re′t′rō-năth′ĭz′əm) *n.* A condition of facial disharmony in which one or both jaws are posterior to their normal positions. — ret′ro·gnath′ic adj.

ret·ro·grade (rĕt′rə-grād′) adj. **1.** Moving or tending backward. **2.** Opposite to the usual order; inverted or reversed. **3.** Reverting to an earlier or inferior condition. — v. **-grad·ed, -grad·ing, -grades. 1.** To move or seem to move backward; recede. **2.** To decline to an inferior state; degenerate.

retrograde amnesia n. A condition in which events that occurred before the onset of amnesia cannot be recalled.

retrograde beat n. A beat occurring as a contraction of a portion of a heart chamber cephalad to the chamber of origin, such as an atrial beat initiated by an impulse originating in the ventricle.

retrograde embolism n. The obstruction of a vein by a mass carried in a direction opposite that of the normal blood current.

retrograde hernia n. A hernia of two loops of intestine, with the portion of intestine between the loops lying in the abdominal cavity.

retrograde urography n. X-ray examination of the urinary tract following the injection of a contrast agent directly into the bladder, ureter, or renal pelvis.

ret·ro·gres·sion (rĕt′rə-grĕsh′ən) n. **1.** The act or process of deteriorating or declining. **2.** A return to a less complex or more primitive biological state or stage.

ret·ro·jec·tion (rĕt′rə-jĕk′shən) n. The washing out of a cavity using the backward flow of an injected fluid.

ret·ro·per·i·to·ni·tis (rĕt′rō-pĕr′ĭ-tn-ī′tĭs) n. Inflammation of the cellular tissue behind the peritoneum.

ret·ro·pla·sia (rĕt′rō-plā′zhə, -zhē-ə) n. A decreased state of activity of a cell or tissue that is usually associated with retrogressive changes.

ret·ro·po·si·tion (rĕt′rō-pə-zĭsh′ən) n. Simple backward displacement of a structure or organ, such as the uterus, without retroversion or retroflexion.

ret·ro·pul·sion (rĕt′rō-pŭl′shən) n. **1.** An involuntary backward walking or running, as seen in parkinsonism. **2.** A pushing back of a part or organ.

ret·ro·spon·dy·lo·lis·the·sis (rĕt′rō-spŏn′də-lō-lĭs-thē′sĭs) n. Backward slippage of the body of a vertebra that moves it out of alignment with adjacent vertebrae.

ret·ro·trans·po·son (rĕt′rō-trăns-pō′zŏn) n. A DNA fragment capable of replication, mutation, and movement along a chromosome.

ret·ro·ver·si·o·flex·ion (rĕt′rō-vûr′sē-ō-flĕk′-shən, -vûr′zhō-) n. Retroversion and retroflexion of the uterus.

ret·ro·ver·sion (rĕt′rō-vûr′zhən, -shən) n. **1.** A turning or tilting backward, as of the uterus. **2.** The state of being turned or tilted back. — ret′ro·vert′ed adj.

ret·ro·vi·rus (rĕt′rō-vī′rəs, rĕt′rə-vī′-) n., pl. **-rus·**

es. Any of a group of viruses, many of which produce tumors, that contain RNA and reverse transcriptase. The virus that causes AIDS is a retrovirus

re·tru·sion (rĭ-trōō′zhən) n. Retraction from any given point, especially the backward movement of the mandible.

Rett's syndrome (rĕts) n. A progressive brain disorder occurring principally in girls, characterized by autism, dementia, ataxia, and purposeless hand movements, and associated with abnormally high levels of ammonia in the blood.

re·turn extrasystole (rĭ-tûrn′) n. A form of reciprocal rhythm in which the impulse, having arisen in the ventricle, ascends toward the atria, but before reaching the atria is reflected back to the ventricles to produce a second ventricular contraction.

re·vas·cu·lar·i·za·tion (rē-văs′kyə-lər-ĭ-zā′shən) n. Reestablishment of blood supply to a part or organ.

re·ver·sal (rĭ-vûr′səl) n. **1.** The act or instance of turning in the opposite direction, as of a disease, symptom, or a state. **2.** A condition in which a person has difficulty distinguishing the lowercase printed or written characters of particular letters: p from q; g or b from d; or s from z.

re·verse Colles′ fracture (rĭ-vûrs′) n. See **Smith′s fracture.**

re·versed Prausnitz–Küstner reaction (rĭ-vûrst′) n. The reaction at the site of injection when serum containing reaginic antibody is injected into the skin of a person in whom the antigen is already present.

reverse Eck fistula n. Side-to-side anastomosis of the portal vein with the inferior vena cava, and ligation of the vena cava above the anastomosis but below the hepatic veins. The blood from the lower part of the body is thus directed through the hepatic circulation.

reverse passive hemagglutination n. A diagnostic technique for virus infection using agglutination by viruses of red blood cells that previously have been coated with antibody specific to the virus.

reverse transcriptase n. A polymerase that catalyzes the formation of DNA on an RNA template, found in oncogenic viruses containing RNA, especially the retroviruses.

re·ver·sion (rĭ-vûr′zhən) n. **1.** The return of a trait or characteristic peculiar to a remote ancestor, especially one that has been suppressed for one or more generations. **2.** A return to the normal phenotype, usually by a second mutation.

re·vert (rĭ-vûrt′) v. **-vert·ed, -vert·ing, -verts. 1.** To return to a former condition, practice, subject, or belief. **2.** To undergo genetic reversion.

re·vive (rĭ-vīv′) v. **-vived, -viv·ing, -vives.** To bring back to life or consciousness; resuscitate.

re·viv·i·fi·ca·tion (rē-vĭv′ə-fĭ-kā′shən) n. Refreshening the edges of a wound by paring or scraping to promote healing.

re·ward (rĭ-wôrd′) n. The return for performance

of a desired behavior; positive reinforcement. — re·ward′ v.

Reye's syndrome (rīz, rāz) n. An acute encephalopathy characterized by fever, vomiting, fatty infiltration of the liver, disorientation, and coma, occurring mainly in children and usually following a viral infection, such as chicken pox.

R factor n. See resistance plasmid.

Rh (är′āch′) adj. Of or relating to the Rh factor.

Rho(D) immune globulin n. A specific globulin fraction derived from serum of human blood donors immunized to produce antibodies against the Rh_0 antigen (D antigen), the most common antigen of the Rh blood group, used to prevent Rh-sensitization of an Rh-negative woman after delivery of an Rh-positive fetus.

rhab·do·my·o·blast (răb′dō-mī′ə-blăst′) n. Large spindle-shaped or strap-shaped cells found in some rhabdomyosarcomas.

rhab·do·my·ol·y·sis (răb′dō-mī-ŏl′ĭ-sĭs) n. An acute, fulminating, potentially fatal disease that destroys skeletal muscle and is often accompanied by the excretion of myoglobin in the urine.

rhab·do·my·o·ma (răb′dō-mī-ō′mə) n. A benign tumor derived from striated muscle.

rhab·do·my·o·sar·co·ma (răb′dō-mī′ō-sär-kō′mə) n. A malignant tumor derived from skeletal muscle. It is characterized in adults by poorly differentiated cells with large hyperchromatic nuclei.

rhab·do·sar·co·ma (răb′dō-sär-kō′mə) n. See rhabdomyosarcoma.

rhab·do·vi·rus (răb′dō-vī′rəs) n., pl. -rus·es. A virus of the family Rhabdoviridae of rod- or bullet-shaped RNA viruses, including the rabies virus.

rhag·a·des (răg′ə-dēz′) n. Chips, cracks, or fissures occurring especially around the mouth and at other mucocutaneous junctions. They are seen in vitamin deficiency diseases and in congenital syphilis.

rheg·ma (rĕg′mə) n. A rent or fissure.

rhe·ni·um (rē′nē-əm) n. A rare dense metallic element with atomic number 75.

rhes·to·cy·the·mi·a (rĕs′tō-sī-thē′mē-ə) n. The presence of broken down red blood cells in the peripheral circulation.

Rhesus factor (rē′səs) n. Rh factor.

rheum (rōōm) n. A watery or thin mucous discharge from the eyes or nose.

rheu·ma·tal·gi·a (rōō′mə-tăl′jē-ə, -jə) n. Rheumatic pain.

rheu·mat·ic (rōō-măt′ĭk) adj. Relating to or characterized by rheumatism. —n. One who is affected by rheumatism.

rheumatic fever n. An acute inflammatory disease occurring during recovery from infection with group A streptococci, having an onset marked by fever and joint pain. It is associated with polyarthritis, Sydenham's chorea, and endocarditis, and is frequently followed by scarring of the heart valves.

rheumatic heart disease n. Permanent damage to

the valves of the heart usually caused by repeated attacks of rheumatic fever.

rheu·ma·tid (rōō′mə-tĭd′) n. A rheumatic nodule or other eruption accompanying rheumatism.

rheu·ma·tism (rōō′mə-tĭz′əm) n. **1.** Any of several pathological conditions of the muscles, tendons, joints, bones, or nerves, characterized by discomfort and disability. **2.** Rheumatoid arthritis.

rheumatoid arthritis n. A chronic and progressive systemic disease, especially common in women, characterized by stiffness and inflammation of the joints and sometimes leading to deformity and disability.

rheumatoid factor n. Any of the globulins that are thought to be antibodies of the IgG and IgM classes, are found in the serum of individuals with rheumatoid arthritis, and enhance agglutination of suspended particles coated with pooled human gamma globulin.

rheu·ma·tol·o·gy (rōō′mə-tŏl′ə-jē) n. The medical science that deals with the study and treatment of rheumatic diseases. — **rheu′ma·tol′o·gist** n.

rhex·is (rĕk′sĭs) n., pl. **rhex·es** (rĕk′sēz). Bursting or rupture of an organ or vessel.

Rh factor n. Any of several substances on the surface of red blood cells that induce a strong antigenic response in individuals lacking the substance.

rhi·nal·gi·a (rī-năl′jē-ə, -jə) n. Pain in the nose.

rhi·ne·de·ma (rī′nĭ-dē′mə) n. Swelling of the nasal mucous membrane.

rhi·nen·ceph·a·lon (rī′nĕn-sĕf′ə-lŏn′, -lən) n., pl. **-la** (-lə). The olfactory region of the brain, located in the cerebrum. — **rhi′nen·ce·phal′ic** (-sə-făl′ĭk) adj.

rhi·ni·tis (rī-nī′tĭs) n. Inflammation of the nasal mucous membranes.

rhi·no·can·thec·to·my (rī′nō-kăn-thĕk′tə-mē) n. Excision of the inner canthus of the eye.

rhi·no·chei·lo·plas·ty or **rhi·no·chi·lo·plas·ty** (rī′nō-kī′lə-plăs′tē) n. Plastic or reparative surgery of the nose and upper lip.

rhi·no·dac·ry·o·lith (rī′nō-dăk′rē-ə-lĭth′) n. A calculus in the nasolacrimal duct.

rhi·no·dyn·i·a (rī′nə-dĭn′ē-ə) n. See rhinalgia.

rhi·no·ky·phec·to·my (rī′nō-kī-fĕk′tə-mē) n. Plastic surgery to correct rhinokyphosis.

rhi·no·ky·pho·sis (rī′nō-kī-fō′sĭs) A humpback deformity of the nose.

rhi·no·lar·yn·gi·tis (rī′nō-lăr′ĭn-jī′tĭs) n. Inflammation of the nasal and laryngeal mucous membranes.

rhi·no·lar·yn·gol·o·gy (rī′nō-lăr′ən-gŏl′ə-jē) n. The anatomy, physiology, and pathology of the nose and larynx.

rhi·nol·o·gy (rī-nŏl′ə-jē) n. The anatomy, physiology, and pathology of the nose.

rhi·no·ma·nom·e·ter (rī′nō-mă-nŏm′ĭ-tər) n. A manometer used to determine the presence and amount of nasal obstruction.

rhi·no·ma·nom·e·try (rī′nō-mă-nŏm′ĭ-trē) n. **1.** The study and measurement of nasal airflow and pressures. **2.** The use of a rhinomanometer.

rhi·no·my·co·sis (rī'nō-mī-kō'sĭs) *n.* Fungal infection of the nasal mucous membranes.

rhi·nop·a·thy (rī-nŏp'ə-thē) *n.* Disease of the nose.

rhi·no·phy·ma (rī'nō-fī'mə) *n.* Hypertrophy of the nose with follicular dilation resulting from hyperplasia of sebaceous glands accompanied by fibrosis and increased vascularity.

rhi·no·plas·ty (rī'nō-plăs'tē, -nə-) *n.* Plastic surgery of the nose.

rhi·nor·rha·gi·a (rī'nə-rā'jē-ə, -jə) *n.* Nosebleed, especially one in which bleeding is profuse.

rhi·nor·rhe·a (rī'nə-rē'ə) *n.* A discharge from the nasal mucous membrane, especially if excessive.

rhi·no·scle·ro·ma (rī'nō-sklə-rō'mə) *n.* A chronic granulomatous process involving the nose, upper lip, mouth, and upper air passages that is believed to be caused by a bacterium, such as a strain of *Klebsiella.*

rhi·nos·co·py (rī-nŏs'kə-pē) *n.* Examination of the nasal passages. — **rhi'no·scope'** (rī'nə-skōp') *n.* — **rhi'no·scop'ic** (-skŏp'ĭk) *adj.*

rhi·no·spo·rid·i·o·sis (rī'nō-spə-rĭd'ē-ō'sĭs, -spō-) *n.* A chronic granulomatous disease of the mucous membranes of the nasal cavity characterized by polyps or other forms of hyperplasia and caused by a yeastlike microorganism *Rhinosporidium seeberi.*

rhi·no·ste·no·sis (rī'nō-stə-nō'sĭs) *n.* Obstruction of the nasal passages.

rhi·not·o·my (rī-nŏt'ə-mē) *n.* Incision into the nose, especially incision along one side to allow viewing of the nasal passages for radical sinus operations.

rhi·no·vi·rus (rī'nō-vī'rəs) *n.* Any of a group of picornaviruses that are causative agents of disorders of the respiratory tract, such as the common cold.

rhi·zo·me·li·a (rī'zə-mē'lē-ə, -mēl'yə) *n.* A disproportion in the length of the upper arms and thighs. — **rhi'zo·me'lic** (-mē'lĭk, -mēl'ĭk) *adj.*

rhi·zo·me·nin·go·my·e·li·tis (rī'zō-mə-nĭng'gō-mī'ə-lī'tĭs) *n.* Inflammation of the nerve roots, the meninges, and the spinal cord.

rhi·zot·o·my (rī-zŏt'ə-mē) *n.* Surgical severance of spinal nerve roots, as for the relief of pain.

Rh-negative *adj.* Lacking an Rh factor.

Rho·de·sian trypanosomiasis (rō-dē'zhən) *n.* An acute type of African trypanosomiasis that progresses rapidly, caused by *Trypanosoma brucei rhodesiense,* and are transmitted by tsetse flies.

rho·di·um (rō'dē-əm) *n.* A hard durable metallic element with atomic number 45.

rho·do·gen·e·sis (rō'də-jĕn'ĭ-sĭs) *n.* The regeneration of rhodopsin; the process occurs in darkness.

rho·do·phy·lax·is (rō'dō-fə-lăk'sĭs) *n.* The action of the pigment cells of the choroid of the eye in preserving or facilitating the regeneration of rhodopsin. — **rho'do·phy·lac'tic** (-lăk'tĭk) *adj.*

rho·dop·sin (rō-dŏp'sĭn) *n.* A thermolabile protein that is sensitive to red light and is found in the external segments of the rods of the retina.

rhom·ben·ceph·a·lon (rŏm'bĕn-sĕf'ə-lŏn', -lən) *n.* The portion of the embryonic brain from which the metencephalon and myelencephalon develop, including the pons, cerebellum, and the medulla oblongata.

rhon·chus (rŏng'kəs) *n., pl.* **-chi** (-kī). A coarse rattling sound somewhat like snoring, usually caused by secretion in a bronchial tube. — **rhon'chal** (-kəl) *adj.*

Rh-positive *adj.* Containing an Rh factor.

rhythm (rĭth'əm) *n.* Movement or variation characterized by the regular recurrence or alternation of different quantities or conditions, as in the heartbeat.

rhythm method *n.* A birth-control method dependent on abstinence during the period of ovulation.

rhyt·i·dec·tomy (rĭt'ĭ-dĕk'tə-mē) *n.* See **face-lift.**

rhyt·i·do·plas·ty (rĭt'ĭ-dō-plăs'tē) *n.* See **face-lift.**

rib (rĭb) *n.* One of a series of long curved bones occurring in 12 pairs in humans and extending from the spine to or toward the sternum.

rib cage *n.* The enclosing structure formed by the ribs and the bones to which they are attached.

ri·bo·fla·vin (rī'bō-flā'vĭn, -bə-) *n.* An orange-yellow crystalline compound that is the principal growth-promoting factor in the vitamin B complex, naturally occurring in milk, leafy vegetables, fresh meat, and egg yolks.

ri·bo·nu·cle·ase (rī'bō-nōō'klē-ās', -āz', -nyōō'-) *n.* Any of various enzymes that catalyze the hydrolysis of RNA.

ri·bo·nu·cle·ic acid (rī'bō-nōō-klē'ĭk, -klā'-, -nyōō-) *n.* See **RNA.**

ri·bo·nu·cle·o·pro·tein (rī'bō-nōō'klē-ō-prō'tēn, -tē-ĭn, -nyōō'-) *n.* A nucleoprotein that contains RNA.

ri·bo·nu·cle·o·side (rī'bō-nōō'klē-ə-sīd', -nyōō'-) *n.* A nucleoside that contains ribose as its sugar component.

ri·bo·nu·cle·o·tide (rī'bō-nōōklē-ə-tīd', -nyōō'-) *n.* A nucleotide that contains ribose as its sugar and usually occurs as a component of RNA.

ri·bose (rī'bōs') *n.* A pentose sugar occurring as a component of riboflavin, nucleotides, and nucleic acids.

ribosomal RNA *n.* rRNA.

ri·bo·some (rī'bə-sōm') *n.* A minute round particle composed of RNA and protein and found in the cytoplasm of living cells; it is the site of protein synthesis as directed by mRNA. — **ri'bo·so'mal** (-sō'məl) *adj.*

ri·bo·su·ri·a (rī'bō-sŏŏr'ē-ə) *n.* Excretion of an excessive amount of ribose in the urine, usually a manifestation of muscular dystrophy.

ri·bo·zyme (rī'bə-zīm') *n.* A strand of RNA that attaches to specific sites on other RNA strands and lyses the strands.

rick·ets (rĭk'ĭts) *n.* A deficiency disease resulting from a lack of vitamin D or calcium and from insufficient exposure to sunlight, characterized by defective bone growth and occurring chiefly in children.

Rick·ett·si·a (rĭ-kĕt'sē-ə) *n.* A genus of gram-negative bacteria carried as parasites by many ticks, fleas, and lice, that cause diseases such as typhus, scrub typhus, and Rocky Mountain spotted fever.

rick·ett·si·al (rĭ-kĕt'sē-əl) *adj.* Relating to or caused by Rickettsiae.

rick·ett·si·al·pox (rĭ-kĕt'sē-əl-pŏks') *n.* An acute nonfatal disease caused by *Rickettsia akari* and transmitted by mites; it is characterized by a papule in the skin and symptoms that develop about a week after the appearance of the papule, consisting of fever, chills, headache, backache, sweating, and local adenitis.

Rickettsia pro·wa·zek·i·i (prō'və-zĕk'ē-ī') *n.* A species of *Rickettsia* that causes epidemic typhus fever.

Rickettsia rick·ett·si·i (rĭ-kĕt'sē-ī') *n.* A species of *Rickettsia* that causes a variety of spotted fevers including Rocky Mountain spotted fever.

rid·er's bone (rī'dərz) *n.* Ossification of the tendon of the long adductor muscle of the leg from strain in horseback riding.

ridge (rĭj) *n.* A long, narrow, or crested part of the body, as on the nose.

Rie·der cell (rē'dər) *n.* An anaplastic cell, thought to be a type of white blood cell or a granulocyte, that occurs in acute leukemia.

Rie·gel's pulse (rē'gəlz) *n.* A pulse that diminishes in volume during exhalation.

rif·am·pin (rĭ-făm'pĭn) or **ri·fam·pi·cin** (-pĭ-sĭn) *n.* A semisynthetic antibiotic derived from a form of rifamycin that interferes with the synthesis of RNA and is used to treat bacterial and viral diseases.

rif·a·my·cin (rĭf'ə-mī'sĭn) *n.* Any of a group of antibiotics originally isolated from a strain of the soil microorganism *Streptomyces mediterranei,* used in the treatment of leprosy, tuberculosis, and other bacterial diseases.

Riggs' disease (rĭgz) *n.* Inflammation of the tissues surrounding and supporting the teeth.

right atrioventricular valve *n.* See **tricuspid valve**.

right brachiocephalic vein *n.* A vein that receives the right vertebral and internal thoracic veins, and the right lymphatic duct.

right brain *n.* The cerebral hemisphere to the right of the corpus callosum, controlling the left side of the body.

right heart *n.* The right atrium and right ventricle.

right hepatic duct *n.* The duct that conveys bile to the common hepatic duct from the right half of the liver.

right·ing reflex (rī'tĭng) *n.* Any of various reflexes that tend to bring the body into normal position in space and resist forces acting to displace it out of normal position.

right-to-die *adj.* Advocating or expressing, as in a living will, a person's right to refuse extraordinary life-sustaining measures intended to prolong life artificially when the person is deemed by his or her physicians to be terminally or incurably ill.

right-to-left shunt *n.* **1.** The passage of blood

from the right side of the heart into the left, as through a septal defect. **2.** The passage of blood from the pulmonary artery into the aorta, as through a patent ductus arteriosus.

right ventricle *n.* The chamber on the right side of the heart that receives venous blood from the right atrium and forces it into the pulmonary artery.

right ventricular failure *n.* Congestive heart failure manifested by distention of the neck veins, enlargement of the liver, and dependent edema.

right ventricular opening *n.* An opening that leads from the right atrium into the right ventricle of the heart.

ri·gid·i·ty (rĭ-jĭd'ĭ-tē) *n.* **1.** The quality or state of stiffness or inflexibility. **2.** An aspect of the personality characterized by resistance to change.

rig·or (rĭg'ər) *n.* **1.** See **rigidity** (sense 1). **2.** Shivering or trembling, as caused by a chill. **3.** A state of rigidity in living tissues or organs that prevents response to stimuli.

rigor mor·tis (môr'tĭs) *n.* Muscular stiffening following death.

rim (rĭm) *n.* The border, edge, or margin of an organ or a part.

ri·ma (rī'mə) *n., pl.* **-mae** (-mē). A slit or elongated opening between two symmetrical parts.

rim·u·la (rĭm'yə-lə) *n., pl.* **-lae** (-lē'). A minute slit or fissure.

ring abscess (rĭng) *n.* An acute purulent inflammation of the cornea which often progresses to panophthalmia.

Ring·er's solution (rĭng'ərz) *n.* **1.** A solution resembling blood serum in its salt constituents, containing sodium chloride, potassium chloride, and calcium chloride in water, used topically for burns and wounds. **2.** A salt solution usually used in combination with naturally occurring body substances or with more complex chemically defined nutritive solutions for culturing cells.

ring finger *n.* The third finger of the left hand.

ring-knife *n.* A circular or oval ring with an internal cutting edge used to shave off tumors in the nasal and other cavities.

ring scotoma *n.* An annular area of blindness in the visual field surrounding the fixation point, associated with glaucoma and pigmentary degeneration of the retina.

ring·worm (rĭng'wûrm') *n.* Any of a number of contagious fungal skin diseases characterized by ring-shaped, scaly, itching patches on the skin.

Rin·ne's test (rĭn'ĕz, -əz) *n.* A hearing test in which a vibrating tuning fork is held against the mastoid process until the sound is lost and then brought close to the auditory orifice.

Ri·o·lan's anastomosis (rē'ō-länz') *n.* A surgical connection of the superior and inferior mesenteric arteries.

risk (rĭsk) *n.* **1.** The possibility of suffering a harmful event. **2.** A factor or course involving uncertain danger, as with smoking or exposure to radiation.

ri·sus ca·ni·nus (rī'səs kā-nī'nəs) *n.* The semblance of a grin caused by facial spasm, especially in tetanus.

Rit·a·lin (rĭt′l-ĭn) A trademark used for methylphenidate.

rite of passage *n.* A ritual or ceremony signifying an event in a person's life indicative of a transition from one stage to another, as from adolescence to adulthood.

rit·u·al (rĭch′ōō-əl) *n.* A detailed act or series of acts carried out by an individual to relieve anxiety or to forestall the development of anxiety.

ri·val·ry (rī′vəl-rē) *n.* The state or condition of competition or antagonism.

riv·er blindness (rĭv′ər) *n.* See **onchocerciasis**.

RNA (är′ĕn-ā′) *n.* A polymeric constituent of all living cells and many viruses, consisting of a long, usually single-stranded chain of alternating phosphate and ribose units with the bases adenine, guanine, cytosine, and uracil bonded to the ribose. The structure and base sequence of RNA are determinants of protein synthesis and the transmission of genetic information.

RNA splicing *n.* See **splicing** (sense 2).

RNA tumor virus *n.* An oncornavirus containing RNA.

RNA virus *n.* A virus whose nucleic acid core is composed of RNA, such as any of the reoviruses, retroviruses, and paramyxoviruses.

Rock·y Moun·tain spotted fever (rŏk′ē moun′tən) *n.* An acute infectious disease that is caused by a microorganism *(Rickettsia rickettsii)* transmitted by ticks, is characterized by muscular pains, high fever, and skin eruptions, and is endemic throughout North America.

rod (rŏd) *n.* **1.** A rod cell. **2.** An elongated bacterium; a bacillus.

rod cell *n.* Any of various cylindrically-shaped cells in the retina that respond to dim light.

ro·dent ulcer (rŏd′nt) *n.* A slowly enlarging ulcerated basal cell carcinoma, usually on the face.

rod granule *n.* The nucleus of a retinal cell connecting with one of the rods.

roent·gen or **rönt·gen** (rĕnt′gən, -jən, rŭnt′-) *n.* A unit of radiation exposure equal to the quantity of ionizing radiation that will produce one electrostatic unit of electricity in one cubic centimeter of dry air at 0°C and standard atmospheric pressure.

roent·ge·nism (rĕnt′gə-nĭz′əm, -jə-, rŭnt′-) *n.* **1.** The use of x-rays in the diagnosis and treatment of disease. **2.** A damaging effect of x-rays on tissues.

roent·gen·o·gram (rĕnt′gə-nə-grăm′, -jə-, rŭnt′-) *n.* A photograph made with x-rays.

roent·gen·o·graph (rĕnt′gə-nə-grăf′, -jə-, rŭnt′-) *n.* See **roentgenogram**.

roent·gen·og·ra·phy (rĕnt′gə-nŏg′rə-fē, -jə-, rŭnt′-) *n.* Photography with the use of x-rays. — **roent′gen·o·graph′ic** (-gə-nə-grăf′ĭk, -jə-) *adj.*

roent·gen·ol·o·gy (rĕnt′gə-nŏl′ə-jē, -jə-, rŭnt′-) *n.* Radiology employing x-rays. — **roent′gen·ol′o·gist** *n.*

Ro·ger's disease (rō-zhäz′) *n.* A congenital defect in the septum that separates the ventricles of the heart.

Roger's murmur *n.* A loud pansystolic murmur heard at the left sternal border, caused by a small ventricular septal defect.

Ro·lan·do's area (rō-län′dōz) *n.* See **motor cortex**.

role or **rôle** (rōl) *n.* The characteristic and expected social behavior of a person.

role model *n.* A person who serves as a model in a particular behavioral or social role for another person to emulate.

role-play (rōl′plā′) *v.* **-played, -play·ing, -plays.** To assume deliberately the part or role of; act out. — *n.* Role-playing.

role-playing *n.* A psychotherapeutic technique in which participants act out particular behavioral roles in order to expand their awareness of differing points of view.

Rolf·ing (rōl′fĭng) A service mark used for a technique of deep muscular manipulation and massage for the relief of bodily and emotional tension.

roll·er bandage (rō′lər) *n.* A strip of material, of variable width, rolled into a compact cylinder to facilitate application.

rom·berg·ism (rŏm′bər-gĭz′əm) *n.* See **Romberg's sign**.

Rom·berg's sign (rŏm′bərgz) *n.* A sign indicating loss of proprioceptive control in which increased unsteadiness occurs when standing with the eyes closed compared with standing with the eyes open.

ron·geur (rôn-zhœr′, rôn-) *n.* A heavy-duty forceps for removing small pieces of bone.

roof plate or **roof·plate** (rōōf′plāt, rōōf′-) *n.* The thin layer of the embryonic neural tube connecting the lateral plates dorsally.

root (rōōt, rŏŏt) *n.* **1.** The embedded part of an organ or structure such as a hair, tooth, or nerve, that serves as a base or support. **2.** A primary source; an origin; radix.

root amputation *n.* Surgical removal of one or more roots of a multirooted tooth.

root canal *n.* **1.** The chamber of the dental pulp lying within the root portion of a tooth. **2.** A treatment in which diseased tissue from this part of the tooth is removed and the resulting cavity is filled with an inert material.

root·ing reflex (rōō′tĭng, rŏŏt′ĭng) *n.* A reflex in infants in which rubbing or scratching about the mouth causes the infant to turn its head toward the stimulus.

root of the lung *n.* All the structures entering or leaving the lung at the hilum, forming a pedicle invested with the pleura.

root of the nail *n.* The proximal end of the nail, concealed under a fold of skin.

root of the penis *n.* The proximal attached part of the penis, including the two crura and the bulb.

root of the tooth *n.* The part of a tooth below the neck of the tooth, covered by cementum rather than enamel, and attached by the periodontal ligament to the alveolar bone.

root resection *n.* See **apicoectomy.**

ro·sa·ce·a (rō-zā′shē-ə) *n.* A chronic dermatitis of the face, especially of the nose and cheeks, characterized by a red or rosy coloration with deep-seated papules and pustules, caused by dilation of capillaries.

rose ben·gal (rōz′ běn-gôl′, běng-, běn′gəl, běng′-) *n.* A bluish red dye used as a stain for bacteria, as a stain in the diagnosis of keratitis sicca, and in tests of liver function.

rose cold *n.* See **rose fever.**

rose fever *n.* A spring or early summer hay fever.

ro·se·o·la (rō-zē′ə-lə, rō′zē-ō′lə) *n.* A rose-colored skin rash, sometimes occurring with diseases such as measles, syphilis, or scarlet fever.

rose spots *pl.n.* The characteristic rose-colored spots of typhoid fever.

ro·sette (rō-zět′) *n.* **1.** The segmented or mature phase of *Plasmodium malariae.* **2.** A grouping of cells, characteristic of neoplasms of neuroblastic or neuroectodermal origin, in which a number of nuclei form a ring from which neurofibrils extend to interlace in the center.

Ros·so·li·mo's reflex (rŏs′ə-lē′mōz) *n.* **1.** Flexion of the toes in response to flicking the tips of the underside of the toes, indicative of lesions of the pyramidal tracts. **2.** Flexion of the fingers by tapping the tips of the fingers on their volar surfaces.

Rossolimo's sign *n.* See **Rossolimo's reflex.**

Ross River virus (rôs) *n.* A mosquito-borne alphavirus that causes epidemic polyarthritis.

ros·trum (rŏs′trəm) *n., pl.* **-trums** or **-tra** (-trə) A beaklike or snoutlike projection. — **ros′tral** (-trəl) *adj.*

ro·ta·ry joint (rō′tə-rē) or **ro·ta·to·ry joint** (rō′tə-tôr′ē) *n.* See **trochoid joint.**

ro·ta·tion (rō-tā′shən) *n.* **1.** The act or process of turning around a center or an axis. **2.** Regular and uniform variation in a sequence or series, as in the recurrence of symptoms of a disease.

rotation flap *n.* A pedicle flap rotated from the donor site to an adjacent recipient area, usually as a direct flap.

ro·ta·tor (rō′tā′tər) *n.* A muscle that serves to rotate a part of the body.

rotator cuff *n.* A set of muscles and tendons that secures the arm to the shoulder joint and permits rotation of the arm.

rotator muscle *n.* Any of a number of short transversospinal muscles chiefly developed in cervical, lumbar, and thoracic regions, arising from the transverse process of one vertebra and inserted into the root of the spinous process of the next two or three vertebrae above, and whose actions rotate the vertebral column.

ro·ta·vi·rus (rō′tə-vī′rəs) *n., pl.* **-rus·es.** Any of a group of wheel-shaped RNA viruses, of the family Reoviridae, including the human gastroenteritis viruses that cause infant diarrhea.

rote learning *n.* Learning or memorization by repetition, often without an understanding of the reasoning or relationships involved in the material that is learned.

Roth·mund's syndrome (rôth′məndz, rōt′-mŏonts) *n.* An inherited syndrome characterized by atrophy, pigmentation, and telangiectasia of the skin, and usually accompanied by juvenile cataract, saddle nose, congenital bone defects, disturbance of hair growth, and hypogonadism.

ro·to·tome (rō′tə-tōm′) *n.* A rotating cutting instrument used in arthroscopic surgery.

Rou·get cell (rōō-zhā′) *n.* Any of numerous branching, contractile cells on the external wall of a capillary.

rough·age (rŭf′ĭj) *n.* See **fiber** (sense 5).

rou·leaux formation (rōō-lō′) *n.* A stacklike arrangement of red cells in blood or in diluted suspensions of blood in which their biconcave surfaces are next to each other.

round ligament of the uterus *n.* A fibromuscular band attached to the uterus on either side in front of and below the opening of the fallopian tube and passing through the inguinal canal to the labia majora.

round window *n.* An opening on the medial wall of the middle ear that leads into the cochlea and is covered by the secondary tympanic membrane.

round·worm (round′wûrm′) *n.* See **nematode.**

Roux-en-Y anastomosis (rōō′ĕn-wī′) *n.* A Y-shaped surgical connection that divides the small intestine and connects one end to the stomach, bile duct, or other structure and connects the opposite end to the small intestine at a point below the first connection.

RPh *abbr.* Registered Pharmacist

RPR test *n.* See **rapid plasma reagin test.**

R.Q. *abbr.* respiratory quotient

rRNA (är′är′ĕn-ā′) *n.* Ribosomal RNA; the RNA that is a permanent structural part of a ribosome.

Rs virus *abbr.* respiratory syncytial virus

RU 486 (är′yōō fôr′ā-tē-sĭks′) *n.* Drug that chemically terminates a pregnancy.

rub (rŭb) *n.* **1.** The application of friction and pressure. **2.** Such a procedure applied to the body, as in massage.

ru·be·do (rōō-bē′dō) *n.* A temporary redness of the skin.

ru·be·fa·cient (rōō′bə-fā′shənt) *adj.* Producing redness, as of the skin. — *n.* A substance that irritates the skin, causing redness. — **ru′be·fac′tion** (-fāk′shən) *n.*

ru·bel·la (rōō-bĕl′ə) *n.* A mild contagious eruptive disease caused by the rubella virus and capable of producing congenital defects in infants born to mothers infected during the first three months of pregnancy.

rubella HI test *n.* A hemagglutination inhibition test for rubella in which the presence of hemagglutination inhibition titer in the absence of disease indicates previous infection and therefore immunity to reinfection.

rubella virus *n.* An RNA virus of the genus *Rubivirus* that causes German measles.

rubella virus vaccine *n.* A vaccine containing live

attenuated rubella virus prepared in duck embryo or human diploid cell culture and administered as a single subcutaneous injection to immunize against rubella.

ru·be·o·la (rōō-bē′ə-lə, rōō′bē-ō′lə) *n.* See **measles** (sense 1). — **ru·be′o·lar** *adj.*

rubeola virus *n.* See **measles virus.**

ru·be·o·sis (rōō′bē-ō′sĭs) *n.* A condition characterized by reddish discoloration, as of the skin.

ru·bid·i·um (rōō-bĭd′ē-əm) *n.* A soft metallic element of the alkali group with atomic number 37.

Ru·bin test (rōō′bĭn) *n.* A test of patency of the fallopian tubes in which carbon dioxide gas is passed through a cannula into the cervix.

ru·bor (rōō′bôr′) *n.* Redness, especially as a sign of inflammation.

ru·di·ment (rōō′də-mənt) *n.* **1.** An imperfectly or incompletely developed organ or part. **2.** *Often* **rudiments.** Something in an incipient or undeveloped form.

ru·ga (rōō′gə) *n., pl.* **-gae** (-gē′, -gī′). A fold, crease, or wrinkle, as in the lining of the stomach. Often used in the plural. — **ru′gate′** (-gāt′) *adj.*

ru·gine (rōō-zhēn′) *n.* See **raspatory.**

ru·gose (rōō′gōs′) or **ru·gous** (-gəs) *adj.* Having many wrinkles or creases; ridged.

ru·gos·i·ty (rōō-gŏs′ĭ-tē) *n.* The state or condition of being rugose.

ru·pi·a (rōō′pē-ə) *n.* **1.** Ulcers of late secondary syphilis, covered with yellowish or brown crusts. **2.** See **yaws.** — **ru′pi·al** *adj.*

rup·ture (rŭp′chər) *n.* **1.** The process of breaking open or bursting. **2.** A hernia, especially of the groin or intestines. **3.** A tear in an organ or a tissue. — *v.* **-tured, -tur·ing, -tures.** To break open; burst.

ruptured disk *n.* See **herniated disk.**

Rus·sell's sign (rŭs′əlz) *n.* An indication of bulemia in which abrasions and scars occur on the back of the hands as a result of manual attempts to induce vomiting.

Russell's syndrome *n.* Failure of infants and young children to thrive due to brain lesions in the region above the pituitary gland, characterized by emaciation and loss of body fat.

Russell's viper venom *n.* A venom used as a coagulant in the arrest of hemorrhage from accessible sites in hemophilia.

rust (rŭst) *n.* Any of a group of parasitic fungi of the order Uredinales that are plant pathogens, especially of cereal grains, and that can produce allergy in humans when inhaled in large numbers.

rust·y sputum (rŭs′tē) *n.* A reddish-brown, blood-stained expectoration characteristic of lobar pneumonia.

ru·the·ni·um (rōō-thē′nē-əm) *n.* A hard acid-resistant metallic element with atomic number 44.

ruth·er·for·di·um (rŭth′ər-fôr′dē-əm, -fôr′-) *n.* An artificially produced radioactive element with atomic number 104.

R wave *n.* The initial positive (upward) deflection of the QRS complex in the electrocardiogram.

~ ~ ~ ~ ~ ~ **S** ~ ~ ~ ~ ~ ~

S–A *abbr.* sinoatrial

sa·ber shin (sā′bər) *n.* A sharp-edged anteriorly convex tibia characteristic of congenital syphilis.

Sa·bin vaccine (sā′bĭn) *n.* An oral vaccine containing live attenuated polioviruses, used to immunize against poliomyelitis.

sac (săk) *n.* **1.** A pouch or bursa. **2.** An encysted abscess at the root of a tooth. **3.** The capsule of a tumor or the envelope of a cyst.

sac·cade (să-käd′, sə-) *n.* A rapid intermittent eye movement, as that which occurs when the eyes fix on one point after another in the visual field. — **sac·cad′ic** (-kä′dĭk) *adj.*

sac·cha·rase (săk′ə-rās′, -rāz′) *n.* See **invertase.**

sac·cha·ride (săk′ə-rīd′) *n.* Any of a series of compounds of carbon, hydrogen, and oxygen in which the atoms of the latter two elements are in the ratio of 2:1.

sac·cha·rin (săk′ər-ĭn) *n.* A white crystalline powder having a taste about 500 times sweeter than cane sugar, used as a calorie-free sweetener.

sac·char·ic acid (sə-kăr′ĭk) *n.* A white crystalline acid formed by the oxidation of glucose, sucrose, or starch.

sac·cha·ro·me·tab·o·lism (săk′ə-rō-mĭ-tăb′ə-lĭz′əm) *n.* The cellular process by which sugar is metabolized. — **sac′cha·ro·met′a·bol′ic** (-mĕt′ə-bŏl′ĭk) *adj.*

sac·cha·ro·my·ces (să′kə-rō-mī′sēz′) *n.* Any of various unicellular yeasts of the genus *Saccharomyces* that lack a true mycelium and many of which ferment sugar.

sac·cu·la·tion (săk′yə-lā′shən) *n.* **1.** A structure formed by a group of sacs. **2.** The formation of a sac or pouch.

sac·cule (săk′yōōl) or **sac·cu·lus** (-yə-ləs) *n., pl* **saccules** or **sac·cu·li** (săk′yə-lī′). **1.** A small sac. **2.** The smaller of two membranous sacs in the vestibule of the inner ear.

sa·cral (sā′krəl) *adj.* Of or relating to the sacrum.

sacral canal *n.* The continuation of the vertebral canal in the sacrum.

sacral crest *n.* Any of five rough irregular ridges on the posterior surface of the sacrum.

sa·cral·gi·a (sā-krăl′jē-ə, -jə) *n*. Pain in the sacral region.

sa·cral·i·za·tion (sā′krə-lĭ-zā′shən) *n*. A developmental abnormality in which the first sacral vertebra fuses with the fifth lumbar verterba.

sacral foramen *n*. Any of the openings between the fused vertebrae of the sacrum transmitting the sacral nerves.

sacral nerve *n*. Any of five nerves emerging from the sacral foramina: the first three enter into the formation of the sacral plexus, and the second two into the coccygeal plexus.

sa·crec·to·my (sā-krĕk′tə-mē) *n*. Resection of a portion of the sacrum.

sac·ro·il·i·ac (săk′rō-ĭl′ē-ăk′, sā′krō-) *adj*. Of, relating to, or affecting the sacrum and ilium and their articulation or associated ligaments. —*n*. The sacroiliac region or cartilage.

sa·crum (sā′krəm, săk′rəm) *n., pl*. **sa·cra** (sā′krə, săk′rə). The triangular segment of the spinal column that forms part of the pelvis, is formed by the fusion of five originally separate sacral vertebrae, and articulates with the last lumbar vertebra, the coccyx, and the hipbone on either side.

SAD *abbr*. seasonal affective disorder

sad·dle back (săd′l) *n*. See **lordosis**.

saddle block anesthesia *n*. A form of spinal anesthesia limited in effect to the buttocks, perineum, and inner surfaces of the thighs.

saddle nose *n*. A nose with a markedly depressed bridge.

sa·dism (sā′dĭz′əm, săd′ĭz′-) *n*. **1.** The act or an instance of deriving sexual gratification from infliction of pain on others. **2.** A psychological disorder in which sexual gratification is derived from infliction of pain on others. **3.** Delight in cruelty. —**sa′dist** *n*. —**sa·dis′tic** (sə-dĭs′tĭk) *adj*.

sa·do·mas·och·ism (sā′dō-măs′ə-kĭz′əm, săd′ō-) *n*. The perversion of deriving pleasure, especially sexual pleasure, from simultaneous sadism and masochism. —**sa′do·mas′o·chist** *n*. —**sa′do·mas′o·chis′tic** *adj*.

Sae·misch's operation (sā′mĭsh′ĭz) *n*. Incision of the cornea to evacuate pus.

safe period *n*. The period in the menstrual cycle when conception is least likely to occur, typically from ten days before to ten days after the onset of menstruation.

safe sex *n*. Sexual activity with safeguards, such as the use of a condom, to avoid acquiring or spreading a sexually transmitted disease.

safe·ty lens (sāf′tē) *n*. A lens that meets government specifications for impact resistance.

saf·ra·nine (săf′rə-nēn′, -nĭn) or **saf·ra·nin** (-nĭn) *n*. Any of a family of dyes based on phenazine, used as biological stains.

sag·it·tal (săj′ĭ-tl) *adj*. **1.** Of or relating to the suture uniting the two parietal bones of the skull. **2.** Of or relating to the sagittal plane.

sagittal plane *n*. A longitudinal plane that divides the body into right and left sections.

Saint An·tho·ny's fire (sānt ăn′thə-nēz) *n*. See **erysipelas**.

Saint Lou·is encephalitis (lōō′ĭs) *n*. A viral encephalitis occurring in parts of North America and transmitted by a culex mosquito.

Saint Louis encephalitis virus *n*. An arbovirus that causes St. Louis encephalitis and is transmitted by a mosquito.

Saint Vi·tus' dance or **Saint Vi·tus's dance** (vītəs, -tə-sĭz) *n*. See **Sydenham's chorea**.

sal·bu·ta·mol (săl-byōō′tə-môl′, -mōl′) *n*. A sympathomimetic agent used as a bronchodilator, especially in the treatment of asthma.

sal·i·cyl·a·mide (săl′ĭ-sĭl′ə-mīd′) *n*. The crystalline amide of salicylic acid used as an analgesic, antipyretic, and antiarthritic.

sal·i·cyl·ic acid (săl′ĭ-sĭl′ĭk) *n*. A white crystalline acid used as a topical antiseptic and disinfectant, and, in pharmaceuticals such as aspirin, as an antipyretic and analgesic.

sa·line (sā′lēn′, -līn′) *adj*. **1.** Of, relating to, or containing salt; salty. **2.** Of or relating to chemical salts. —*n*. **1.** A salt of magnesium or of the alkalis, used in medicine as a cathartic. **2.** A saline solution, especially one that is isotonic to blood.

saline agglutinin *n*. An antibody that causes agglutination of Rh-positive red blood cells when they are suspended in a saline or protein medium.

sa·li·va (sə-lī′və) *n*. The watery mixture of secretions from the salivary and oral mucous glands that lubricates chewed food, moistens the oral walls, and contains ptyalin.

sal·i·var·y (săl′ə-vĕr′ē) *adj*. **1.** Of, relating to, or producing saliva. **2.** Of or relating to a salivary gland.

salivary digestion *n*. Conversion of starch into sugar by the action of salivary amylase.

salivary duct *n*. A type of intralobular duct found in salivary glands and involved in the production and transport of their secretions.

salivary fistula *n*. An opening between a salivary duct or gland and the cutaneous surface or the oral cavity.

salivary gland *n*. A exocrine gland that secretes saliva, especially any of major salivary glands or minor salivary glands.

sal·i·vate (săl′ə-vāt′) *v*. **-vat·ed, -vat·ing, -vates. 1.** To secrete or produce saliva. **2.** To produce excessive salivation in.

sal·i·va·tion (săl′ə-vā′shən) *n*. **1.** The act or process of secreting saliva. **2.** See **ptyalism**.

Salk vaccine (sôlk) *n*. A vaccine containing inactivated polioviruses, used to immunize against poliomyelitis.

sal·me·ter·ol xi·naf·o·ate (săl-mē′tə-rôl′ zĭ-năf′-ō-āt′) *n*. An inhalant drug used in the treatment of asthma and having physiological activity similar to albuterol but longer lasting and more effective in preventing subsequent attacks.

sal·mo·nel·la (săl′mə-nĕl′ə) *n., pl*. **-nel·lae** (-nĕl′ē) or **-nel·las** or **salmonella**. Any of various bacteria of the genus *Salmonella*, many of which cause food poisoning, typhoid, and paratyphoid fever.

Sal·mo·nel·la (săl′mə-nĕl′ə) *n*. A genus of aerobic

to facultatively anaerobic gram-negative, rod-shaped bacteria.

Salmonella poisoning *n.* Gastroenteritis caused by food contaminated with various strains of *Salmonella* which multiply freely in the gastrointestinal tract but do not produce septicemia. Symptoms include fever, headache, nausea, vomiting, diarrhea, and abdominal pain.

sal·mo·nel·lo·sis (săl′mə-nĕ-lō′sĭs) *n.* Infection with bacteria of the genus *Salmonella*, characterized by gastroeneritis and fever, and caused especially by eating improperly stored or undercooked foods.

sal·ol (săl′ôl′, -ōl′) *n.* A white crystalline powder derived from salicylic acid and used as an analgesic and antipyretic.

sal·pin·gec·to·my (săl′pĭn-jĕk′tə-mē) *n.* Surgical removal of a fallopian tube.

sal·pin·gem·phrax·is (săl′pĭn-jĕm-frăk′sĭs) *n.* Obstruction of a eustachian or fallopian tube.

sal·pin·gi·tis (săl′pĭn-jī′tĭs) *n.* Inflammation of a fallopian tube or eustachian tube.

sal·pin·go·cele (săl-pĭng′gə-sēl′) *n.* Hernia of a fallopian tube.

sal·pin·gog·ra·phy (săl′pĭng-gŏg′rə-fē) *n.* Radiographic visualization of the fallopian tubes after injection of a radiopaque substance.

sal·pin·gol·y·sis (săl′pĭng-gŏl′ĭ-sĭs) *n.* A surgical procedure for freeing a fallopian tube from adhesions.

sal·pin·go-o·o·pho·rec·to·my (săl-pĭng′gō-ō′ə-fə-rĕk′tə-mē) *n.* Surgical removal of an ovary and its fallopian tube.

sal·pin·go-o·o·pho·ri·tis (săl-pĭng′gō-ō′ə-fə-rī′tĭs) *n.* Inflammation of a fallopian tube and its ovary.

sal·pin·go·per·i·to·ni·tis (săl-pĭng′gō-pĕr′ĭ-tn-ī′tĭs) *n.* Inflammation of a fallopian tube, the perisalpinx, and the peritoneum.

sal·pin·go·pex·y (săl-pĭng′gə-pĕk′sē) *n.* Surgical fixation of an oviduct.

sal·pin·go·plas·ty (săl-pĭng′gə-plăs′tē) *n.* Plastic surgery on a fallopian tube.

sal·pin·gor·rha·phy (săl′pĭng-gôr′ə-fē) *n.* Suture of a fallopian tube.

sal·pin·gos·to·my (săl′pĭng-gŏs′tə-mē) *n.* Surgical formation of an opening in a fallopian tube that has been closed by inflammation.

sal·pin·got·o·my (săl′pĭng-gŏt′ə-mē) *n.* Incision of a fallopian tube.

sal·pinx (săl′pĭngks) *n., pl.* **sal·pin·ges** (săl-pĭn′-jēz). **1.** See **fallopian tube. 2.** See **eustachian tube.**

salt (sôlt) *n.* **1.** A colorless or white crystalline solid, chiefly sodium chloride, used as a food seasoning and preservative. **2.** A chemical compound replacing all or part of the hydrogen ions of an acid with metal ions or electropositive radicals. **3. salts.** Any of various mineral salts, such as magnesium sulfate, sodium sulfate, or potassium sodium tartrate, used as laxatives or cathartics. **4. salts.** Smelling salts. **5. salts.** Epsom salts.

sal·ta·tion (săl-tā′shən, sôl-) *n.* **1.** Discontinuous movement, transition, or development; advance-

ment by leaps. **2.** A single mutation that drastically alters the phenotype.

saltatory conduction *n.* A form of nerve impulse conduction in which the impulse jumps from one node of Ranvier to the next, rather than traveling the entire length of the nerve fiber.

Sal·ter–Harris classification (sôl′tər-) *n.* The classification of epiphysial fractures into five groups (I to V), according to different prognoses regarding the effects of the injury on subsequent growth and subsequent deformity of the epiphysis.

salt substitute *n.* A low-sodium food additive that tastes like salt, such as potassium chloride, and is used as a dietary alternative to salt.

sal·u·re·sis (săl′yə-rē′sĭs) *n.* The presence of sodium in the urine.

salve (săv, säv) *n.* An analgesic or medicinal ointment. — **salve** *v.*

sa·mar·i·um (sə-mâr′ē-əm, -măr′-) *n.* A metallic rare-earth element with atomic number 62.

san·a·to·ri·um (săn′ə-tôr′ē-əm) or **san·a·tar·i·um** (-târ′ē-əm) *n., pl.* **-to·ri·ums** or **-to·ri·a** (-tôr′ē-ə) or **-tar·i·ums** or **-tar·i·a** (-târ′ē-ə). **1.** An institution for the treatment of chronic diseases or for medically supervised recuperation. **2.** An institution for improvement or maintenance of health, especially for convalescents.

sand flea (sănd) *n.* See **chigoe** (sense 1).

sand fly *n.* Any of various small biting flies of the genus *Phlebotomus* of tropical areas, some of which transmit diseases.

Sand·hoff's disease (sănd′hôfs′) *n.* A form of gangliosidosis that resembles Tay–Sachs disease but does not affect persons of Jewish descent, characterized by a defect in the production of two forms of hexosaminidase.

sand tumor *n.* See **psammoma.**

sane (sān) *adj.* Of sound mind; mentally healthy. — **sane′ness** *n.*

San·fi·lip·po's syndrome (săn′fə-lĭp′ōz) *n.* An inherited disorder of mucopolysaccharide metabolism, characterized by the presence of heparitin sulfate in the urine, enlargement of the liver, and severe mental retardation.

san·gui·fi·ca·tion (săng′gwə-fĭ-kā′shən) *n.* See **hematopoiesis.**

san·guine (săng′gwĭn) *adj.* Of a healthy, reddish color; ruddy.

sa·ni·es (sā′nē-ēz′) *n., pl.* **sanies.** A thin, fetid, blood-tinged fluid consisting of serum and pus discharged from a wound, an ulcer, or a fistula.

san·i·tar·i·an (săn′ĭ-târ′ē-ən) *n.* A public health or sanitation expert.

san·i·tar·i·um (săn′ĭ-târ′ē-əm) *n.* See **sanatorium.**

san·i·tar·y (săn′ĭ-tĕr′ē) *adj.* **1.** Of or relating to health. **2.** Free from elements, such as filth or pathogens, that endanger health; hygienic.

sanitary napkin *n.* A disposable pad of absorbent material worn to absorb menstrual flow.

san·i·ta·tion (săn′ĭ-tā′shən) *n.* **1.** Formulation and application of measures designed to protect public health. **2.** Disposal of sewage.

san·i·ti·za·tion (săn′ĭ-tĭ-zā′shən) *n.* The process of

making something sanitary, as by cleaning or disinfecting. — **san′i·tize′** (-tīz′) v.

san·i·ty (săn′ĭ-tē) n. **1.** The quality or condition of being sane. **2.** Soundness of judgment or reason.

S–A node n. The sinoatrial node.

san·pa·ku (săn-pä′kōō) n. A condition in which the white of the eye is visible below the iris as well as on either side.

san·to·nin (săn′tə-nĭn) n. A colorless crystalline compound used as an anthelmintic.

sa·phe·na (sə-fē′nə) n., pl. **-nae** (-nē′). Either of two main superficial veins of the leg, one larger than the other, that begin at the foot.

sa·phe·nous (să-fē′nŭs) adj. Relating to or associated with the saphena (denoting a number of structures in the leg).

saphenous nerve n. A branch of the femoral nerve that supplies cutaneous branches to the skin of the leg and foot.

sa·pre·mi·a or **sa·prae·mi·a** (sə-prē′mē-ə) n. Blood poisoning resulting from the absorption of the products of putrefaction.

sap·ro·gen·ic (săp′rə-jĕn′ĭk) or **sa·prog·e·nous** (sə-prŏj′ə-nəs) adj. Of, producing, or resulting from putrefaction.

sap·ro·phyte (săp′rə-fīt′) n. An organism, especially a fungus or bacterium, that grows on and derives its nourishment from dead or decaying organic matter.

sap·ro·zo·on·o·sis (săp′rə-zō-ŏn′ə-sĭs, -zō′ə-nō′-) n. A zoonosis whose causative agent requires both a vertebrate host and a nonanimal reservoir for completion of its life cycle.

sar·co·blast (sär′kə-blăst′) n. See **myoblast.**

sar·co·car·ci·no·ma (sär′kō-kär′sə-nō′mə) n. See **carcinosarcoma.**

sar·co·cele (sär′kə-sēl′) n. A fleshy tumor or sarcoma of the testis.

sar·coid (sär′koid′) adj. Of or resembling flesh. — n. **1.** A tumor resembling a sarcoma. **2.** See **sarcoidosis.**

sar·coid·o·sis (sär′koi-dō′sĭs) n., pl. **-ses** (-sēz). A disease of unknown origin marked by the formation of granulomatous lesions that appear especially in the liver, lungs, skin, and lymph nodes.

sar·co·lac·tic acid (sär′kə-lăk′tĭk) n. An isomeric form of lactic acid produced by muscle tissue during the anaerobic metabolism of glucose.

sar·co·lem·ma (sär′kə-lĕm′ə) n. A thin membrane enclosing a striated muscle fiber. — **sar′co·lem′mal** adj.

sar·co·ma (sär-kō′mə) n., pl. **-mas** or **-ma·ta** (-mə-tə). A malignant tumor arising from connective tissues. — **sar·co′ma·toid′** (-mə-toid′), **sar·co′ma·tous** (-təs) adj.

sar·co·ma·to·sis (sär-kō′mə-tō′sĭs) n. Formation of numerous sarcomas in various body parts.

sar·co·mere (sär′kə-mĕr′) n. One of the segments into which a fibril of striated muscle is divided.

sar·co·plasm (sär′kə-plăz′əm) n. The cytoplasm of a striated muscle fiber. — **sar′co·plas·mat′ic** (-plăz-măt′ĭk), **sar′co·plas′mic** (-mĭk) adj.

sarcoplasmic reticulum n. The form of endoplasmic reticulum found in striated muscle fibers.

Sar·cop·tes (sar-kŏp′tēz) n. A genus of acarids that includes the itch mite.

sar·cop·tid (sär-kŏp′tĭd) n. A mite of the family Sarcoptidae that includes species that are parasitic on the skin of humans.

sar·co·sine (sär′kə-sēn′, -sĭn) n. An amino acid made synthetically or formed naturally during the decomposition of creatine.

sar·co·si·ne·mi·a (sär′kə-sə-nē′mē-ə) n. A hereditary disorder of amino acid metabolism, marked by elevated levels of sarcosine in blood plasma and excretion of sarcosine in the urine, failure to thrive, irritability, muscle tremors, and retarded motor and mental development.

sar·co·sis (sär-kō′sĭs) n. **1.** An abnormal increase of body tissue. **2.** A growth of fleshy tumors. **3.** A diffuse sarcoma involving an entire organ.

sar·co·some (sär′kə-sōm′) n. A large specialized mitochondrion found in striated muscle.

sar·cos·to·sis (sär′kŏ-stō′sĭs) n. Ossification of muscular tissue.

sar·co·style (sär′kə-stīl′) n. See **myofibril.**

sar·co·tu·bules (sär′kō-tōō′byōōl, -tyōō′-) pl.n. Membranous tubules that constitute a continuous system in striated muscle, corresponding to the smooth endoplasmic reticulum of other cells.

sar·to·ri·us muscle (sär-tôr′ē-əs) n. A muscle with origin from the anterior superior spine of the ilium, with insertion into the tuberosity of the tibia, and whose action flexes the thigh and leg and rotates the leg medially and the thigh laterally.

sat·el·lite cell (săt′l-īt′) n. Any of the cells that encapsulate the bodies of nerve cells in many ganglia.

satellite DNA n. A portion of DNA in animal cells whose density differs from that of the other DNA, consisting of short, repeating sequences of nucleotide pairs near the region of the centromere.

sa·ti·a·tion (sā′shē-ā′shən) n. The state produced by having had a specific need, such as hunger or thirst, fulfilled. — **sa′ti·ate′** v.

sat·is·fac·tion (săt′ĭs-făk′shən) n. **1.** The fulfillment or gratification of a desire, a need, or an appetite. **2.** Pleasure or contentment derived from such gratification.

sat·is·fac·to·ry (săt′ĭs-făk′tə-rē) adj. Providing satisfaction sufficient to meet a demand or requirement.

sat·u·rate (săch′ə-rāt′) v. **-rat·ed, -rat·ing, -rates.** **1.** To imbue or impregnate thoroughly. **2.** To soak or fill to capacity. **3.** To cause a substance to unite with the greatest possible amount of another substance. **4.** To satisfy all the chemical affinities of a substance. **5.** To dissolve a substance up to that concentration beyond which the addition of more results in a second phase.

saturated compound n. An organic compound in which all the carbon atoms are connected by single bonds.

saturated fat n. A fat, most often of animal origin, having chains of saturated fatty acids. An excess of these fats in the diet is thought to raise the cholesterol level in the bloodstream.

saturated fatty acid *n.* A fatty acid, such as stearic acid, whose carbon chain contains no ethylenic or other unsaturated linkages between carbon atoms and hence cannot incorporate any more hydrogen atoms.

sat·u·ra·tion (săch'ə-rā'shən) *n.* **1.** The act or process of saturating. **2.** The condition of being saturated. **3.** The condition of being full to or beyond satisfaction; satiety. **4.** Filling of all the available sites on an enzyme molecule by its substrate, or on a hemoglobin molecule by molecular oxygen or carbon monoxide.

sat·urn·ism (săt'ər-nĭz'əm) *n.* See **lead poisoning.**

sau·cer·i·za·tion (sô'sər-ĭ-zā'shən) *n.* Surgical excavation of tissue to form a shallow depression to facilitate drainage from infected areas of a wound.

Saund·by's test (sônd'bēz) *n.* A test for blood in the stool.

s.c. *abbr. Latin.* sub cutem, sub cute (under the skin, subcutaneously.)

scab (skăb) *n.* **1.** A crust formed from and covering a healing wound. **2.** Scabies or mange in domestic animals or livestock, especially sheep. —*v.* **scabbed, scab·bing, scabs.** To become covered with scabs or a scab.

scab·by (skăb'ē) *adj.* **-bi·er, -bi·est. 1.** Having, consisting of, or covered with scabs. **2.** Affected with scab or scabies.

sca·bies (skā'bēz) *n.* **1.** A contagious skin disease caused by a parasitic mite *(Sarcoptes scabiei)* and characterized by intense itching. **2.** A similar disease in animals, especially sheep.

sca·la (skā'lə) *n., pl.* **-lae** (-lē). Any of the spiral cavities of the cochlea winding around the modiolus of the ear.

scald (skôld) *v.* **scald·ed, scald·ing, scalds.** To burn with a hot liquid or steam. —*n.* A body injury caused by scalding.

scale¹ (skāl) *n.* A dry, thin flake of epidermis shed from the skin. —*v.* **scaled, scal·ing, scales. 1.** To come off in scales or layers; flake. **2.** To become encrusted. **3.** To remove tartar from tooth surfaces with a pointed instrument.

scale² *n.* **1.** A system of ordered marks at fixed intervals used as a reference standard in measurement. **2.** An instrument or device bearing such marks. **3.** A standard of measurement or judgment; a criterion.

scale³ *n.* **1.** An instrument or a machine for weighing. **2.** Either of the pans, trays, or dishes of a balance.

sca·le·nec·to·my (skā'lə-nĕk'tə-mē) *n.* Resection of a scalene muscle.

sca·lene muscle (skā'lēn', skā-lēn') *n.* Any of three muscles on each side of the neck that serve to bend and rotate it and that assist breathing by raising or fixing the first two ribs.

sca·le·not·o·my (skā'lə-nŏt'ə-mē) *n.* Surgical division or section of the anterior scalene muscle.

scall (skôl, skäl) or **scald** (skôld, skäld) *n.* A scaly eruption of the skin or scalp.

scalp (skălp) *n.* The skin covering the top of the human head.

scal·pel (skăl'pəl) *n.* A small straight knife with a thin sharp blade used in surgery and dissection.

scal·prum (skăl'prəm) *n.* **1.** A large strong scalpel. **2.** See **raspatory.**

scal·y (skā'lē) *adj.* **1.** Covered or partially covered with scales. **2.** Shedding scales or flakes; flaking.

scan (skăn) *v.* **scanned, scan·ning, scans. 1.** To move a finely focused beam of light or electrons in a systematic pattern over a surface in order to reproduce or sense and subsequently transmit an image. **2.** To examine a body or a body part with a CAT scanner or similar scanning apparatus. —*n.* **1.** The act or an instance of scanning. **2.** Examination of a body or body part by a CAT scanner or similar scanning apparatus. **3.** A picture or an image produced by this means. — **scan'na·ble** *adj.* — **scan'ner** *n.*

scan·di·um (skăn'dē-əm) *n.* A highly reactive metallic element with atomic number 21.

scanning electron microscope *n.* An electron microscope that forms a three-dimensional image on a cathode-ray tube by moving a beam of focused electrons across an object and reading both the electrons scattered by the object and the secondary electrons produced by it.

Scan·zo·ni's maneuver (skän-zō'nēz, skän-tsō'-nēz) *n.* A method of applying an obstetrical forceps to rotate a fetus.

scap·u·la (skăp'yə-lə) *n., pl.* **-las** or **-lae** (-lē'). Either of two large, flat, triangular bones forming the back part of the shoulder.

scap·u·lec·to·my (skăp'yə-lĕk'tə-mē) *n.* Surgical removal of the scapula.

scap·u·lo·cos·tal syndrome (skăp'yə-lō-kŏs'təl) *n.* Pain in the upper or posterior part of the shoulder radiating into the neck, head, arm or chest, caused by an abnormal relationship between the scapula and the posterior wall of the thorax.

scap·u·lo·pex·y (skăp'yə-lō-pĕk'sē) *n.* Surgical fixation of the scapula to the chest wall or to the spinous process of the vertebrae.

scar (skär) *n.* A mark left on the skin after a surface injury or wound has healed. —*v.* **scarred, scar·ring, scars. 1.** To mark with a scar or become marked with a scar. **2.** To form scar.

scar·i·fi·ca·tor (skăr'ə-fĭ-kā'tər) *n.* A surgical instrument with several spring-operated lancets, used to scarify the skin.

scar·i·fy (skăr'ə-fī') *v.* **-fied, -fy·ing, -fies.** To make shallow cuts in the skin, as when vaccinating. — **scar'i·fi·ca'tion** (-fĭ-kā'shən) *n.*

scar·la·ti·na (skär'lə-tē'nə) *n.* See **scarlet fever.** — **scar'la·ti'nal** *adj.*

scar·la·ti·nel·la (skär'lə-tə-nĕl'ə) *n.* See **fourth disease.**

scar·let fever (skär'lĭt) *n.* An acute contagious disease caused by a hemolytic streptococcus, occurring predominantly among children and marked by a scarlet skin eruption and high fever.

scar tissue *n.* Dense, fibrous connective tissue that forms over a healed wound or cut.

sca·te·mi·a (skă-tē′mē-ə) *n.* Toxemia resulting from the absorption of toxins in the intestines.

sca·tol·o·gy (skă-tŏl′ə-jē, skə-) *n.* **1.** The study and analysis of feces for physiological and diagnostic purposes. **2.** An obsession with excrement or excretory functions. **3.** The psychiatric study of such an obsession. — **scat′o·log′i·cal** (skăt′l-ŏj′ĭ-kəl), **scat′o·log′ic** (-ĭk) *adj.*

sca·toph·a·gy (skă-tŏf′ə-jē) *n.* The eating of excrement.

sca·tos·co·py (skă-tŏs′kə-pē) *n.* Examination of the feces for diagnostic purposes.

scat·ter (skăt′ər) *v.* **-tered, -ter·ing, -ters. 1.** To cause to separate and go in different directions. **2.** To separate and go in different directions; disperse. **3.** To deflect radiation or particles.

Scheie's syndrome (shīz) *n.* An inherited syndrome that is a form of Hurler's syndrome and is characterized by corneal clouding and deformity of the hands; stature and intelligence usually remain normal.

sche·ma (skē′mə) *n., pl.* **sche·mas** or **sche·ma·ta** (skē-mä′tə, skĭ-măt′ə). A pattern imposed on complex reality or experience to assist in explaining it, mediate perception, or guide response.

Schick test (shĭk) *n.* An intracutaneous test for detecting immunity or susceptibility to diphtheria.

Schick test toxin *n.* The inoculated dose of the toxin produced by *Corynebacterium diptheriae* and used in the Schick test.

Schil·der's disease (shĭl′dərz) *n.* A degenerative fatal brain disease occurring chiefly in children, marked by destruction of myelin, progressive dementia, convulsions, hearing loss, spastic paralysis, and blindness.

Schil·ler's test (shĭl′ərz) *n.* A test for cancer of the cervix, in which the cervix is stained with a solution of iodine and potassium iodide.

Schil·ling's blood count (shĭl′ĭngz) *n.* A method of counting blood cells in which the polymorphonuclear neutrophils are separated into four groups according to the number and arrangement of the nuclear masses in each cell.

Schilling's index *n.* See **Schilling's blood count**.

Schil·ling test (shĭl′ĭng) *n.* A test for determining the amount of vitamin B_{12} excreted in the urine, in which vitamin B_{12} tagged with a radioisotope is taken orally and quantified in urine samples.

schis·to·cyte (shĭs′tə-sīt′, skĭs′-) *n.* A red blood cell having an abnormal shape due to fragmentation that occurs as the cell passes through damaged small vessels.

schis·to·cy·to·sis (shĭs′tə-sī-tō′sĭs, skĭs′-) *n.* **1.** The presence or accumulation of schistocytes in the blood. **2.** Fragmentation of a red blood cell.

Schis·to·so·ma (shĭs′tə-sō′mə, skĭs′-) *n.* A genus of digenetic trematodes, including the blood flukes that cause schistosomiasis.

schis·to·some (shĭs′tə-sōm′, skĭs′-) *n.* Any of several chiefly tropical trematodes of the genus *Schis-*

tosoma, many of which are human blood parasites.

schistosome dermatitis *n.* An inflammation of the skin caused by parasitic larvae of certain schistosomes that penetrate the skin of persons who bathe in infested water.

schis·to·so·mi·a·sis (shĭs′tə-sə-mī′ə-sĭs, skĭs′-) *n., pl.* **-ses** (-sēz′). Any of various generally tropical diseases caused by schistosomes ingested through use of contaminated water, and marked by infection and gradual destruction of the tissues of the kidneys, liver, and other organs.

schiz·oid (skĭt′soid′) *adj.* **1.** Schizophrenic. **2.** Of, relating to, or having a personality marked by extreme shyness, seclusiveness, and an inability to form close relationships. — *n.* A schizoid or schizophrenic person.

schizoid personality *n.* A personality disorder characterized by long-term emotional coldness, indifference to praise, criticism, or the feelings of others, and an inability to form close friendships with more than one or two people.

schiz·o·nych·i·a (skĭz′ə-nĭk′ē-ə) *n.* A condition marked by irregular splitting of the nails.

schiz·o·pha·sia (skĭt′sə-fā′zhə, -zē-ə) *n.* The characteristic disordered speech of a schizophrenic person.

schiz·o·phre·ni·a (skĭt′sə-frē′nē-ə, -frĕn′ē-ə) *n.* Any of a group of psychotic disorders usually characterized by withdrawal from reality, illogical thought patterns, delusions, and hallucinations, and accompanied by other emotional, behavioral, or intellectual disturbances. It is often associated with dopamine imbalances in the brain and defects of the frontal lobe.

schiz·o·phren·ic (skĭt′sə-frĕn′ĭk) *adj.* Of, relating to, or affected by schizophrenia. — *n.* One who is affected with schizophrenia.

schiz·o·trich·i·a (skĭz′ə-trĭk′ē-ə) *n.* A splitting of the hairs at the ends.

schiz·o·typ·i·cal personality (skĭt′sə-tĭp′ĭ-kəl) *n.* A personality disorder characterized by eccentricities of thought, appearance, behavior, and speech, although the eccentricities are not severe enough to be considered psychotic.

school phobia *n.* The aversion to or fear of attending school that occurs in young children, usually considered a manifestation of separation anxiety.

Schultz–Charl·ton reaction (shōŏlts′chärl′tən) *n.* The specific blanching of a scarlatinal rash at the site of an intracutaneous injection of scarlatina antiserum.

Schütz rule (shüts) *n.* A rule for determining the activity of an enzyme, especially of pepsin, by calculating the rate of the enzyme's reaction as proportional to the square root of the enzyme's concentration.

Schwach·man syndrome (shwăch′mən, shwäch′-) *n.* An inherited disorder characterized by sinusitis and bronchiectasis accompanied by pancreatic insufficiency and resulting in malnutrition.

Schwann cell (shwän, shvän) *n.* Any of the cells

that cover the nerve fibers in the peripheral nervous system and form the myelin sheath.

schwan·no·ma (shwä-nō′mə) *n.* **1.** See **neurofibroma. 2.** See **neurilemoma.**

schwan·no·sis (shwä-nō′sĭs) *n.* A non-neoplastic proliferation of Schwann cells in the spaces around the blood vessels of the spinal cord.

sci·age (sē-äzh′) *n.* In massage, a to-and-fro sawlike movement of the hand.

sci·at·ic (sī-ăt′ĭk) *adj.* **1.** Of or relating to the ischium or to the region of the hipbone in which it is located. **2.** Of or relating to sciatica.

sci·at·i·ca (sī-ăt′ĭ-kə) *n.* Pain along the sciatic nerve that radiates from the lower back to the buttocks and back of the thigh and is usually caused by a herniated disk of the lumbar region of the spine.

sciatic foramen Either of two foramina, designated greater and lessor, formed by ligaments that cross the sciatic notch of the hipbone.

sciatic hernia *n.* Protrusion of intestine through the greater sciatic foramen.

sciatic nerve *n.* A nerve that arises from the sacral plexus and passes through the greater sciatic foramen to about the middle of thigh where it divides into the common peroneal and tibial nerves.

SCID *abbr.* severe combined immunodeficiency

sci·ence (sī′əns) *n.* **1.** The observation, identification, description, experimental investigation, and theoretical explanation of phenomena. **2.** Such activities restricted to a class of natural phenomena. **3.** Such activities applied to an object of inquiry or study. **4.** Knowledge, especially that gained through experience.

sci·en·tif·ic method (sī′ən-tĭf′ĭk) *n.* The principles and empirical processes of discovery and demonstration considered characteristic of or necessary for scientific investigation, generally involving the observation of phenomena, the formulation of a hypothesis concerning the phenomena, experimentation to demonstrate the truth or falseness of the hypothesis, and a conclusion that validates or modifies the hypothesis.

scim·i·tar sign (sĭm′ĭ-tər, -tär′) *n.* A radiologic indication of anomalous pulmonary venous drainage in which a curvilinear structure is seen in the base of the lung.

scin·ti·cis·ter·nog·ra·phy (sĭn′tĭ-sĭs′tər-nŏg′rə-fē) *n.* Cisternography performed with a radiopharmaceutical and recorded with a stationary imaging device.

scin·ti·gram (sĭn′tĭ-grăm′) *n.* A two-dimensional record of the distribution of a radioactive tracer in a tissue or organ, obtained by means of a scanning scintillation counter.

scin·ti·graph (sĭn′tĭ-grăf′) *n.* **1.** A device for producing a scintigram; a scintiscanner. **2.** See **scintigram. —scin′ti·graph′ic** *adj.*

scin·tig·ra·phy (sĭn-tĭg′rə-fē) *n.* See **scintiphotography.**

scin·til·lat·ing scotoma (sĭn′tl-ā′tĭng) *n.* A localized area of blindness that may follow the appearance of brilliantly colored shimmering lights and is associated with the aura of migraine.

scin·til·la·tion (sĭn′tl-ā′shən) *n.* A flash of light produced in a phosphorescent substance by absorption of an ionizing particle or photon.

scin·til·la·tor (sĭn′tl-ā′tər) *n.* A substance that glows when hit by high-energy particles or photons.

scin·ti·pho·tog·ra·phy (sĭn′tə-fə-tŏg′rə-fē) *n.* The process of obtaining a scintigram.

scin·ti·scan (sĭn′tĭ-skăn′) *n.* See **scintigram.**

scin·ti·scan·ner (sĭn′tĭ-skăn′ər) *n.* The apparatus used to make a scintigram.

scir·rhus (skĭr′əs, sĭr′-) *n., pl.* **scir·rhus·es** or **scir·rhi** (skĭr′ī, sĭr′ī) *n.* A hard, dense cancerous growth usually arising from connective tissue.

scis·sure (sĭzh′ər, sĭsh′-) *n.* A split or opening in an organ or part.

scle·ra (sklēr′ə) *n., pl.* **scle·ras** or **scle·rae** (sklēr′ē). The tough fibrous tunic forming the outer envelope of the eye and covering all the eye except the cornea; white of the eye. **—scle′ral** *adj.*

scler·ad·e·ni·tis (sklēr′ăd-n-ī′tĭs) *n.* Inflammatory induration of a gland.

scleral staphyloma *n.* See **equatorial staphyloma.**

scleral vein *n.* Any of the tributaries to the anterior ciliary veins, draining the sclera.

scler·ec·ta·sia (sklēr′ĕk-tā′zē-ə, -zhə) *n.* Localized bulging of the sclera lined with uveal tissue.

scle·rec·to·ir·i·dec·to·my (sklə-rĕk′tō-ĭr′ĭ-dĕk′tə-mē, ĭ′rĭ-) *n.* Excision of a portion of the sclera and the iris in the treatment of glaucoma.

scle·rec·to·ir·i·do·di·al·y·sis (sklə-rĕk′tō-ĭr′ĭ-dō-dī-ăl′ĭ-sĭs, -ĭ′rĭ-) *n.* A surgical procedure used in treating glaucoma that combines sclerectomy and iridodialysis.

scle·rec·to·my (sklə-rĕk′tə-mē) *n.* **1.** Surgical excision of a portion of the sclera. **2.** Surgical removal of the fibrous adhesions formed in chronic otitis media.

scler·e·de·ma (sklēr′ĭ-dē′mə) *n.* Hard nonpitting edema of the skin, having a waxy appearance with no sharp demarcation and occurring mainly in females with diabetes mellitus.

scle·re·ma (sklə-rē′mə) *n.* **1.** Induration of the subcutaneous fat. **2.** Sclerema neonatorum.

sclerema ne·o·na·to·rum (nē′ō-nā-tôr′əm) *n.* Necrosis of subcutaneous fat appearing at birth or in early infancy as sharply demarcated indurated plaques, usually on the cheeks, buttocks, shoulders, and calves.

scler·i·rit·o·my (sklēr′ī-rĭt′ə-mē) *n.* Incision of the iris and sclera.

scle·ri·tis (sklə-rī′tĭs) *n.* Inflammation of the sclera.

scle·ro·blas·te·ma *n.* The embryonic tissue that forms bones.

scle·ro·cho·roid·i·tis (sklēr′ō-kôr′oi-dī′tĭs) *n.* Inflammation of the scleral and choroid coats of the eye.

scle·ro·con·junc·ti·val (sklēr′ō-kŏn′jŭngk-tī′vəl) *adj.* Of or relating to the sclera and the conjunctiva.

scle·ro·cor·ne·a (sklēr′ō-kôr′nē-ə) *n.* **1.** The cornea and sclera regarded as forming together the hard outer coat of the eye. **2.** A congenital anomaly in which all or part of the cornea is opaque and resembles the sclera.

scle·ro·cor·ne·al junction (sklēr'ō-kôr'nē-əl) *n.* See **corneal margin.**

scle·ro·der·ma (sklēr'ə-dûr'mə) *n.* A pathological thickening and hardening of the skin caused by swelling and thickening of fibrous tissue. — **scle·ro·der'ma·tous** (-mə-təs), **scle·ra·der'mous** (-məs)

scle·ro·ker·a·ti·tis (sklēr'ō-kĕr'ə-tī'tĭs) *n.* Inflammatory infiltration of the sclera and cornea.

scle·ro·ma (sklə-rō'mə) *n., pl.* **-mas** or **-ma·ta** (-mə-tə). An indurated patch of body tissue especially in the upper respiratory tract.

scle·ro·myx·e·de·ma (sklēr'ō-mĭk'sĭ-dē'mə) *n.* Lichen myxedematosus with diffuse thickening of the skin underlying the papules.

scle·ro·nych·i·a (sklēr'ō-nĭk'ē-ə) *n.* Induration and thickening of the nails.

scle·ro·o·o·pho·ri·tis (sklēr'ō-ō'ə-fə-rī'tĭs) *n.* Inflammatory induration of the ovary.

scle·ro·pro·tein (sklēr'ō-prō'tēn', -tē-ĭn) *n.* Any of a class of generally insoluble proteins, such as collagen, found in skeletal and connective tissue.

scle·ro·sant (sklə-rō'sənt, -zənt) *n.* An injectable irritant used in the treatment of varicose veins that causes inflammation and subsequent fibrosis, thus obliterating the lumen of the vein.

scle·rose (sklə-rōz', -rōs') *v.* **-rosed, -ros·ing, -ros·es.** To harden; undergo sclerosis.

sclerosing adenosis *n.* A benign nodular breast lesion occurring most frequently in young women and consisting of hyperplastic distorted lobules of acinar tissue with increased collagenous stroma.

scle·ro·sis (sklə-rō'sĭs) *n., pl.* **-ses** (-sēz). **1.** The hardening of a tissue or part due to chronic inflammation. **2.** A thickening or hardening of a body part or system, especially from excessive formation of fibrous interstitial or glial tissue. **3.** Any of various diseases characterized by thickening or hardening, such as arteriosclerosis.

scle·ro·ste·no·sis (sklēr'ō-stə-nō'sĭs) *n.* Induration and contraction of the tissues, as around an orifice.

scle·ros·to·my (sklə-rŏs'tə-mē) *n.* Surgical perforation of the sclera, as in glaucoma treatment.

scle·ro·ther·a·py (sklēr'ō-thĕr'ə-pē) *n.* Treatment, as for varicose veins, involving injection of a sclerosing solution into vessels or tissues.

scle·rot·ic (sklə-rŏt'ĭk) *adj.* **1.** Affected or marked by sclerosis. **2.** Of or relating to the sclera of the eye. — *n.* also **scle·rot·i·ca** (-rŏt'ĭ-kə) See **sclera.**

scle·rot·o·my (sklə-rŏt'ə-mē) *n.* Incision through the sclera of the eye.

sco·lex (skō'lĕks') *n., pl.* **-lex·es** or **-li·ces** or **-le·ces** (-lĭ-sēz'). The knoblike anterior end of a tapeworm, having suckers or hooklike parts that in the adult stage serve as organs of attachment to the host.

sco·li·o·ky·pho·sis (skō'lē-ō-kī-fō'sĭs) *n.* A combination of lateral and posterior curvature of the spine.

sco·li·o·sis (skō'lē-ō'sĭs, skŏl'ē-) *n.* A condition of lateral curvature of the spine, which may have just one curve or primary and secondary compensatory curves and may be fixed or mobile.

scom·broid poisoning (skŏm'broid') *n.* Poisoning from ingestion of heat-stable toxins produced by bacterial action on inadequately preserved fish of the order Scombroidea, including tuna, bonito, and mackerel. It is characterized by epigastric pain, nausea and vomiting, headache, thirst, difficulty in swallowing, and urticaria.

sco·pol·a·mine (skə-pŏl'ə-mēn', -mĭn) *n.* A thick, syrupy, colorless alkaloid used as a mydriatic, sedative, and truth serum.

sco·po·phil·i·a (skō'pə-fĭl'ē-ə) *n.* See **voyeurism.**

sco·po·pho·bi·a (skō'pə-fō'bē-ə) *n.* An abnormal fear of being looked at or seen.

score (skôr) *n.* A result of a test or examination, usually expressed numerically.

sco·to·ma (skə-tō'mə) *n., pl.* **-mas** or **-ma·ta** (-mə-tə). An area of diminished vision within the visual field.

sco·tom·e·ter (skə-tŏm'ĭ-tər) *n.* An instrument used in scotometry.

sco·tom·e·try (skə-tŏm'ĭ-trē) *n.* The plotting and measuring of a scotoma.

sco·to·phil·i·a (skō'tə-fĭl'ē-ə) *n.* See **nyctophilia.**

sco·to·pho·bi·a (skō'tə-fō'bē-ə) *n.* See **nyctophobia.**

sco·to·pi·a (skə-tō'pē-ə) *n.* See **scotopic vision.**

sco·to·pic adaptation (skə-tō'pĭk, -tŏp'ĭk) *n.* See **dark adaptation.**

scotopic eye *n.* See **dark-adapted eye.**

scotopic vision *n.* Vision that occurs when the eye is dark-adapted.

sco·top·sin (skə-tŏp'sĭn) *n.* The protein component of the pigment in the rods of the retina.

Scott operation (skŏt) *n.* A jejunoileal bypass for treating morbid obesity in which the upper jejunum is joined to the terminal ileum, with the bypassed intestine closed proximally and anastomosed distally to the colon.

scratch test (skrăch) *n.* A test for allergy performed by scratching the skin and applying an allergen to the wound.

screen (skrēn) *n.* **1.** One that serves to protect, conceal, or divide. **2.** A screen memory. — *tr.v.* **screened, screen·ing, screens. 1.** To process a group of people in order to select or separate certain individuals from it. **2.** To test or examine for the presence of disease or infection.

screen·ing (skrē'nĭng) *n.* **1.** The examination of a group of usually asymptomatic individuals to detect those with a high probability of having or developing a given disease, typically by means of an inexpensive diagnostic test. **2.** The initial evaluation of a person, intended to determine suitability for a particular treatment modality.

screening test *n.* A test designed to identify and eliminate those who are not affected by a disease.

screen memory *n.* In psychoanalysis, the memory of an unacceptable but tolerable experience that unconsciously serves to conceal the memory of an associated experience that is more significant but emotionally more difficult to recall.

screw·worm (skrōō'wûrm') *n.* The larva of the screwworm fly *(Cochliomyia hominivorax),* which breeds in the sores, wounds, or nostrils of humans.

scrof·u·la (skrŏf'yə-lə) *n.* A form of tuberculosis affecting the lymph nodes, especially of the neck, that is most common in children and is usually spread by drinking unpasteurized milk from infected cows.

scrotal septum *n.* An incomplete wall of connective tissue and nonstriated muscle dividing the scrotum into two sacs, each containing a testis.

scro·tec·to·my (skrō-tĕk'tə-mē) *n.* Surgical removal of part of the scrotum.

scro·ti·tis (skrō-tī'tĭs) *n.* Inflammation of the scrotum.

scro·to·plas·ty (skrō'tə-plăs'tē) *n.* Reparative or plastic surgery of the scrotum.

scro·tum (skrō'təm) *n., pl.* **-tums** or **-ta** (-tə). The musculocutaneous sac that encloses the testes and is formed of skin, a network of nonstriated muscular fibers, cremasteric fascia, the cremaster muscle, and the serous coverings of the testes and epididymides. — **scro′tal** (skrōt′l) *adj.*

scrub nurse *n.* A nurse who assists the surgeon in the operating room.

scrub typhus *n.* An acute infectious disease common in Asia caused by *Rickettsia tsutsugamushi* and transmitted by mites; it is characterized by sudden fever, painful swelling of the lymph glands, skin lesions, and skin rash.

Scul·te·tus bandage (skəl-tē'təs) *n.* See **many-tailed bandage.**

scurf (skûrf) *n.* Scaly or shredded dry skin, such as dandruff.

scur·vy (skûr'vē) *n.* A disease caused by deficiency of vitamin C, characterized by spongy and bleeding gums, bleeding under the skin, and extreme weakness.

scu·tu·lum (skyōō'chə-ləm) *n., pl.* **-la** (-lə). The characteristic lesion of favus, appearing as a yellow saucer-shaped crust.

scyb·a·lum (sĭb'ə-ləm) *n., pl.* **-la** (-lə). A hard round mass of inspissated feces.

sea·bor·gi·um (sē-bôr'gē-əm) *n.* An artifically produced radioactive element with atomic number 106.

search·er (sûr'chər) *n.* A sounding instrument used to determine the presence of a calculus in the bladder.

sea·sick·ness (sē'sĭk'nĭs) *n.* Motion sickness resulting from the pitching and rolling of a ship or boat in water, especially at sea.

sea·son·al affective disorder (sē'zə-nəl) *n.* A mild form of depression occurring at certain seasons of the year, especially one recurring in winter that is characterized by loss of energy and sexual drive, restlessness, and often a craving for carbohydrates.

se·ba·ceous (sĭ-bā'shəs) *adj.* **1.** Of, relating to, or resembling fat or sebum; fatty. **2.** Secreting fat or sebum.

sebaceous cyst *n.* A harmless cyst, especially on the scalp or face, containing the fatty secretion of a sebaceous gland.

sebaceous gland *n.* Any of the numerous holocrine glands in the dermis that empty into a hair follicle and produce and secrete sebum.

seb·o·lith (sĕb'ə-lĭth') *n.* A concretion in a sebaceous follicle.

seb·or·rhe·a or **seb·or·rhoe·a** (sĕb'ə-rē'ə) *n.* Overactivity of the sebaceous glands characterized by excessive secretion of sebum or an alteration in its quality, resulting in an oily coating, crusts, or scales on the skin.

seb·or·rhe·ic dermatitis (sĕb'ə-rē'ĭk) *n.* A chronic form of dermatitis characterized by oily scales, crusty yellow patches, and itching, and occurring primarily on the scalp and face.

seborrheic keratosis *n.* A superficial, benign, verrucose lesion consisting of proliferating epidermal cells enclosing horn cysts, usually appearing on the face, trunk, or extremities in adulthood.

se·bum (sē'bəm) *n.* The semifluid secretion of the sebaceous glands, consisting chiefly of fat, keratin, and cellular material.

Seck·el syndrome (sĕk'əl) *n.* An inherited disorder characterized by low birth weight, dwarfism, microcephaly, large eyes, beaked nose, receding chin, and mental retardation.

sec·o·bar·bi·tal (sĕk'ō-bär'bĭ-tôl', -tăl') *n.* A white, odorless barbiturate used in the form of its sodium salt as a sedative and hypnotic.

sec·ond·ar·y (sĕk'ən-dĕr'ē) *adj.* **1.** Of the second rank; not primary. **2.** Minor; lesser. **3.** Of, relating to, or being a degree of health care intermediate between that offered in a physician's office and that available at a research hospital, as the care typically offered at a clinic or community hospital. — **sec′ond·ar′i·ly** (-där'ə-lē) *adv.* — **sec′ond·ar′i·ness** *n.*

secondary abdominal pregnancy *n.* A condition in which the embryo or fetus continues to grow in the abdominal cavity after its expulsion from the tube or other site of its primary development.

secondary cartilage *n.* Cartilage, as in certain joints, that changes directly into bone.

secondary dentition *n.* **1.** The set of 32 permanent teeth whose eruptions begin from the fifth to the seventh year, lasting until the 17th to the 23rd year, when the last of the wisdom teeth appear. **2.** The eruption of the permanent teeth.

secondary digestion *n.* Digestion of nutrients by the cells of the body, especially through metabolic activity, as opposed to the breakdown of nutrients by primary digestion.

secondary disease *n.* **1.** A disease that follows and results from an earlier disease, injury, or event. **2.** A wasting disorder that follows the successful transplantation of bone marrow into a patient whose immune system has been destroyed by radiation, usually accompanied by fever, diarrhea, and dermatitis.

secondary follicle *n.* See **Graafian follicle**.

secondary gain *n.* Interpersonal or social advantages gained indirectly from organic illness, such as an increase in attention from others.

secondary lysosome *n.* A lysosome formed by the combination of a primary lysosome and a membrane-bound vesicle, such as a pinosome, and in which lysis takes place through the activity of hydrolytic enzymes.

secondary oocyte *n.* An oocyte in which the first meiotic division is completed. The second meiotic division usually stops short of completion unless fertilization occurs.

secondary process *n.* In psychoanalysis, the mental process directly related to the functions of the ego, marked by logical thinking and by the tendency to delay gratification by regulation of actions based on instinctual demands.

secondary saturation *n.* A technique of nitrous oxide anesthesia consisting of an abrupt curtailment of the oxygen in the inhaled mixture to produce deep anesthesia, with oxygen given afterwards to correct overdosage and relax muscles.

secondary sensory nucleus *n.* See **terminal nucleus**.

secondary sex character *n.* Any of various characteristics specific to females or males but not directly concerned with reproduction.

secondary spermatocyte *n.* The spermatocyte derived from a primary spermatocyte by the first meiotic division and giving rise by the second meiotic division to two spermatids.

second cranial nerve *n.* See **optic nerve**.

second-degree burn *n.* A burn that blisters the skin and is more severe than a first-degree burn.

sec·ond·hand smoke (sĕk′ənd-hănd′) *n.* Cigarette, cigar, or pipe smoke that is inhaled unintentionally by nonsmokers and may be injurious to their health if inhaled regularly or continuously over a long period.

second heart sound *n.* The heart sound that signifies the beginning of diastole and is caused by closure of the semilunar valves.

second molar *n.* The seventh permanent or fifth deciduous tooth in the upper and lower jaw on either side.

second tooth *n.* See **permanent tooth**.

se·cre·ta (sĭ-krē′tə) *n.* Substances secreted by a cell, a tissue, or an organ.

se·crete (sĭ-krēt′) *tr.v.* **-cret·ed, -cret·ing, -cretes.** To generate and separate a substance from cells or bodily fluids.

se·cre·tin (sĭ-krēt′n) *n.* A polypeptide hormone produced in the duodenum, especially on contact with acid, that stimulates secretion of pancreatic juice.

se·cre·tion (sĭ-krē′shən) *n.* **1.** The process of secreting a substance from a cell or gland. **2.** A substance, such as saliva, mucus, tears, bile, or a hormone, that is secreted.

se·cre·tor (sĭ-krē′tər) *n.* **1.** A cell, a tissue, or an organ that produces a secretion. **2.** A person whose

saliva and other body fluids contain ABO antigens.

se·cre·to·ry (sĭ-krē′tə-rē) *adj.* Relating to or performing secretion.

secretory duct *n.* See **salivary duct**.

secretory nerve *n.* A nerve conveying impulses that excite functional activity in a gland.

sec·tion (sĕk′shən) *n.* **1.** A cut or division. **2.** The act or process of separating or cutting, especially the surgical cutting or dividing of tissue. **3.** A thin slice, as of tissue, suitable for microscopic examination. — *v.* **-tioned, -tion·ing, -tions. 1.** To separate or divide into parts. **2.** To cut or divide tissue surgically.

sec·tor·a·no·pi·a (sĕk′tər-ə-nō′pē-ə) *n.* Loss of vision in a sector of the visual field.

se·cun·di·grav·i·da (sĭ-kŭn′dĭ-grăv′ĭ-də) *n.* A woman in her second pregnancy.

se·cun·dines (sē-kŭn′dīnz′, sĕk′ən-dīnz′) *pl.n.* See **afterbirth**.

se·cun·dip·a·ra (sĕk′ən-dĭp′ər-ə) *n.* A woman who has given birth twice.

se·date (sĭ-dāt′) *tr.v.* **-dat·ed, -dat·ing, -dates.** To administer a sedative to; calm or relieve by means of a sedative drug.

se·da·tion (sĭ-dā′shən) *n.* **1.** Reduction of anxiety, stress, irritability, or excitement by administration of a sedative agent or drug. **2.** The state or condition induced by a sedative.

sed·a·tive (sĕd′ə-tĭv) *adj.* Having a soothing, calming, or tranquilizing effect; reducing or relieving anxiety, stress, irritability, or excitement. — *n.* An agent or a drug having a soothing, calming, or tranquilizing effect.

sed·i·ment (sĕd′ə-mənt) *n.* Insoluble material that sinks to the bottom of a liquid.

sed·i·men·ta·tion (sĕd′ə-mən-tā′shən, -mĕn-) *n.* The act or process of depositing or forming a sediment.

sedimentation rate *n.* The degree of rapidity with which red blood cells sink in a specimen of drawn blood.

sedimentation test *n.* A radiographic procedure for viewing the stomach, in which a mixture of a contrast salt, such as barium or bismuth, in water is used to coat the stomach wall, thus allowing visualization of the shape and movement of the organ as well as lesions on the walls.

sed·i·men·tom·e·ter (sĕd′ə-mən-tŏm′ĭ-tər) *n.* A photographic apparatus for the automatic recording of the blood sedimentation rate.

seg·ment (sĕg′mənt) *n.* **1.** A clearly differentiated subdivision of an organism or part. **2.** A part of an organ having independent function, supply, or drainage. **3.** See **zona** (sense 1).

seg·men·tal anesthesia (sĕg-mĕn′tl) *n.* Loss of sensation limited to an area supplied by one or more spinal nerve roots.

seg·men·ta·tion cavity (sĕg′mən-tā′shən, -mĕn-) *n.* See **blastocoel**.

seg·men·tec·to·my (sĕg′mən-tĕk′tə-mē, -mĕn-) *n.* Excision of a segment of an organ or a gland.

seg·ment·ed cell (sĕg′mĕn′tĭd, sĕg-mĕn′-) *n.* A

cell having a nucleus that is divided into lobes connected by a fine filament.

seg·re·ga·tion (sĕg'rĭ-gā'shən) *n.* **1.** The removal of certain parts or segments from a whole or mass. **2.** The separation of paired alleles especially during meiosis, so that the members of each pair of alleles appear in different gametes.

seg·re·ga·tor (sĕg'rĭ-gā'tər) *n.* An apparatus for obtaining urine from each kidney separately.

sei·zure (sē'zhər) *n.* A sudden attack, spasm, or convulsion, as in epilepsy.

se·lec·tion (sĭ-lĕk'shən) *n.* A natural or artificial process that favors or induces survival and perpetuation of one kind of organism over others that die or fail to produce offspring.

se·lec·tive inhibition (sĭ-lĕk'tĭv) *n.* See **competitive inhibition.**

se·le·ni·um (sĭ-lē'nē-əm) *n.* A nonmetallic element with atomic number 34 that is an essential mineral and believed to be closely associated with vitamin E in its functions.

self (sĕlf) *n., pl.* **selves. 1.** The total, essential, or particular being of a person; the individual. **2.** One's consciousness of one's own being or identity; the ego.

self-a·buse (sĕlf'ə-byōos') *n.* **1.** Abuse of oneself or one's abilities. **2.** Masturbation.

self-a·nal·y·sis (sĕlf'ə-năl'ĭ-sĭs) *n.* An independent methodical attempt by one to study and comprehend one's own personality or emotions.

self-a·ware·ness (sĕlf'ə-wâr'nĭs) *n.* Realization of oneself as an individual entity or personality.

self-care (sĕlf'kâr') *n.* The care of oneself without medical, professional, or other assistance or oversight.

self-con·cept (sĕlf'kŏn'sĕpt) *n.* A person's assessment of his or her status on a single trait or on many human dimensions using societal or personal norms as criteria.

self-con·trol (sĕlf'kən-trōl') *n.* Control of one's emotions, desires, or actions by one's own will.

self-di·ag·no·sis (sĕlf'dī'əg-nō'sĭs) *n.* Diagnosis of one's own illness or disease without professional medical consultation.

self-ex·am·i·na·tion (sĕlf'ĭg-zăm'ə-nā'shən) *n.* Examination of one's own body for medical reasons.

self-i·den·ti·ty (sĕlf'ī-dĕn'tĭ-tē) *n.* Awareness of and identification with oneself as a separate individual.

self-im·age (sĕlf'ĭm'ĭj) *n.* The conception that one has of oneself, including an assessment of qualities and personal worth.

self-lim·it·ed (sĕlf-lĭm'ĭ-tĭd) *adj.* Running a definite course within a specific period; little modified by treatment. Used of a disease.

self-love (sĕlf'lŭv') *n.* The instinct or desire to promote one's own well-being.

self-med·i·ca·tion (sĕlf'mĕd'ĭ-kā'shən) *n.* Medication of oneself without professional supervision to alleviate an illness or condition, as by using an over-the-counter drug or preparation.

self-re·tain·ing catheter (sĕlf'rĭ-tā'nĭng) *n.* A catheter constructed to be retained in the urethra and bladder.

self-treat·ment (sĕlf'trēt'mənt) *n.* Treatment of oneself without professional supervision to alleviate an illness or condition.

Sel·lick's maneuver (sĕl'ĭks) *n.* A method of preventing regurgitation of an anesthetized patient during endotracheal intubation by applying pressure to the cricoid cartilage.

se·men (sē'mən) *n.* A viscous whitish secretion of the male reproductive organs, containing spermatozoa and consisting of secretions of the testes, seminal vesicles, prostate, and bulbourethral glands.

se·me·nu·ri·a (sē'mə-nŏŏr'ē-ə, -nyŏŏr'-) *n.* Excretion of urine containing semen.

sem·i·ca·nal (sĕm'ē-kə-năl', sĕm'ī-) *n.* A deep groove on the edge of a bone that forms a complete canal when united with a similar groove or part of an adjoining bone; a half canal.

sem·i·cir·cu·lar canal (sĕm'ī-sûr'kyə-lər) *n.* Any of three bony tubes in the labyrinth of the ear within which the membranous semicircular ducts are located.

semicircular duct *n.* Any of three small membranous tubes that lie within the bony labyrinth of the inner ear, form loops in planes at right angles to one another, and open into the vestibule.

sem·i·closed anesthesia (sĕm'ē-klōzd', sĕm'ī-) *n.* Inhalation anesthesia using a circuit in which a portion of the exhaled air is exhausted from the circuit and a portion is rebreathed following removal of carbon dioxide.

sem·i·co·ma (sĕm'ē-kō'mə, sĕm'ī-) *n.* A partial or mild comatose state; a coma from which a person may be roused by various stimuli. — **sem'i·co'·ma·tose'** (-kō'mə-tōs', -kŏm'ə-) *adj.*

sem·i·con·scious (sĕm'ē-kŏn'shəs, sĕm'ī-) *adj.* Not completely aware of sensations; partially conscious.

sem·i·flex·ion (sĕm'ē-flĕk'shən, sĕm'ī-) *n.* The position of a limb or muscle halfway between flexion and extension.

sem·i·lunar bone (sĕm'ē-lōō'nər, sĕm'ī-) *n.* See **lunate bone.**

semilunar valve *n.* One of three semilunar segments serving as the cusps of a valve preventing regurgitation, as in the aortic valve and the pulmonary valve.

sem·i·mem·bra·no·sus muscle (sĕm'ē-mĕm'brə-nō'səs, sĕm'ī-) *n.* A muscle with origin from the ischium, with insertion into the tibia and by membrane to the knee joint, the popliteal fascia, and the femur, and whose action flexes the leg, rotates it medially, and makes the capsule of the knee joint tense.

sem·i·nal duct (sĕm'ə-nəl) *n.* Any of the ducts conveying semen outward from the epididymis to the urethra, the vas deferens, the duct of the seminal vesicles, or the ejaculatory duct.

seminal fluid *n.* Semen, especially the fluid part of semen without the spermatozoa.

seminal gland *n.* See **seminal vesicle.**

seminal granule *n.* One of the minute granular bodies present in the spermatic fluid.

seminal vesicle *n.* Either of a pair of pouchlike glands situated on each side of the male urinary bladder that secrete seminal fluid and nourish and promote the movement of spermatozoa through the urethra.

sem·i·na·tion (sĕm′ə-nā′shən) *n.* Insemination.

sem·i·nif·er·ous epithelium (sĕm′ə-nĭf′ər-əs) *n.* Epithelium that lines the seminiferous tubules of the testis.

seminiferous tubule *n.* One of two or three twisted curved tubules in each lobule of the testis in which spermatogenesis occurs.

sem·i·no·ma (sĕm′ə-nō′mə) *n., pl.* **-mas** or **-ma·ta** (-mə-tə). A malignant tumor of the testis arising from sperm-forming tissue.

sem·i·nu·ri·a (sē′mə-nŏŏr′ē-ə, -nyŏŏr′-) *n.* See **semenuria**.

sem·i·o·pen anesthesia (sĕm′ē-ō′pən, sĕm′ī-) *n.* Inhalation anesthesia in which a portion of inhaled gases is derived from an anesthesia circuit while the remainder consists of room air.

sem·i·sys·tem·at·ic name (sĕm′ē-sĭs′tə-măt′ĭk, sĕm′ī-) *n.* A name of a chemical compound that contains both systematic and trivial components, as for many generic names of drugs.

sem·i·ten·di·nous muscle (sĕm′ē-tĕn′də-nəs, sĕm′ī-) *n.* A muscle with origin from the ischium, with insertion into the shaft of the tibia, and whose action extends the thigh, flexes the leg, and rotates it medially.

sen·e·ga (sĕn′ĭ-gə) *n.* The dried roots of the Seneca snakeroot, used medicinally as an expectorant.

se·nes·cence (sĭ-nĕs′əns) *n.* The process of growing old; aging.

Sengs·ta·ken–Blake·more tube (sĕngz′tā′kən-blāk′môr′) *n.* A triple-lumen tube of which one lumen is used to drain the stomach and two lumen are used to inflate attached gastric and esophageal balloons; used for treatment of bleeding esophageal varices.

se·nile (sē′nīl′, sĕn′īl′) *adj.* **1.** Relating to, characteristic of, or resulting from old age. **2.** Exhibiting the symptoms of senility, as impaired memory or the inability to perform certain mental tasks.

senile arteriosclerosis *n.* Arteriosclerosis as a result of advanced age.

senile cataract *n.* A cataract occurring spontaneously in the aged and characterized by the increased opacity of the lens followed by its softening and shrinkage.

senile dementia *n.* A progressive, abnormally accelerated deterioration of mental faculties and emotional stability in old age, occurring especially in Alzheimer's disease.

senile lentigo *n.* See **liver spot**.

senile plaque *n.* A spherical mass of amyloid fibrils surrounded by distorted interwoven neuronal processes, found in the cerebral cortex in Alzheimer's disease.

senile psychosis *n.* A mental disturbance occurring in old age and related to degenerative cerebral processes.

senile tremor *n.* A tremor occurring in the aged.

se·nil·ism (sē′nə-lĭz′əm) *n.* Premature senility.

se·nil·i·ty (sĭ-nĭl′ĭ-tē) *n.* **1.** The state of being senile. **2.** The mental and physical deterioration characteristic of old age.

se·no·pi·a (sĭ-nō′pē-ə) *n.* Improvement of near vision sometimes occurring in the aged because of swelling of the crystalline lens in incipient cataract.

sen·sa·tion (sĕn-sā′shən) *n.* **1.** A perception associated with stimulation of a sense organ or with a specific body condition. **2.** The faculty to feel or perceive; physical sensibility. **3.** An indefinite, generalized body feeling.

sense (sĕns) *n.* **1.** Any of the faculties by which stimuli from outside or inside the body are received and felt, as the faculties of hearing, sight, smell, touch, taste, and equilibrium. **2.** A perception or feeling produced by a stimulus; sensation, as of hunger. — *v.* **sensed, sens·ing, sens·es.** To become aware of; perceive.

sense datum *n.* A basic, unanalyzable sensation, such as color, sound, or smell, experienced upon stimulation of a sense organ or receptor.

sense of equilibrium *n.* The sense that makes it possible to maintain a normal upright posture.

sense organ *n.* A specialized organ or structure, such as the eye, ear, tongue, nose, or skin, where sensory neurons are concentrated and which functions as a receptor.

sen·si·bil·i·ty (sĕn′sə-bĭl′ĭ-tē) *n.* **1.** The ability to perceive stimuli. **2.** Receptiveness to impression, whether pleasant or unpleasant; acuteness of feeling. **3.** The quality of being affected by changes in the environment.

sen·si·ble (sĕn′sə-bəl) *adj.* **1.** Perceptible by the senses or by the mind. **2.** Having the faculty of sensation; able to feel or perceive. **3.** Having a perception of something; cognizant.

sensible perspiration *n.* Perspiration excreted in sufficient quantity to appear as moisture on the skin.

sen·si·tive (sĕn′sĭ-tĭv) *adj.* **1.** Capable of perceiving with a sense or senses. **2.** Responsive to a stimulus. **3.** Easily irritated or inflamed, especially because of previous exposure to an antigen. **4.** Of, relating to, or characterizing a sensitized antigen.

sen·si·tiv·i·ty (sĕn′sĭ-tĭv′ĭ-tē) *n.* **1.** The quality or condition of being sensitive. **2.** The capacity of an organ or organism to respond to a stimulus. **3.** The proportion of individuals in a population that will be correctly identified when administered a test designed to detect the presence of a particular disease.

sensitivity training *n.* Training in small groups in which people learn how to interact by developing an awareness and understanding of themselves and of their relationships with others.

sen·si·ti·za·tion (sĕn′sĭ-tĭ-zā′shən) *n.* The act or

process of inducing an acquired sensitivity or allergy.

sen·si·tize (sĕn′sĭ-tīz′) *v.* **-tized, -tiz·ing, -tiz·es.** To make hypersensitive or reactive to an antigen, such as pollen, especially by a second or repeated exposure.

sen·si·tized antigen (sĕn′sĭ-tīzd′) *n.* The complex formed when antigen combines with specific antibody.

sen·sor (sĕn′sər, -sôr′) *n.* **1.** A device, such as a photoelectric cell, that receives and responds to a signal or stimulus. **2.** See **sense organ.**

sensorimotor area *n.* The precentral and postcentral gyri of the cerebral cortex.

sen·so·ri·um (sĕn-sôr′ē-əm) *n., pl.* **-so·ri·ums** or **-so·ri·a** (-sôr′ē-ə). **1.** The part of the brain that receives and coordinates all the stimuli conveyed to various sensory centers. **2.** The entire sensory system of the body.

sen·so·ry (sĕn′sə-rē) *adj.* **1.** Of or relating to the senses or sensation. **2.** Transmitting impulses from sense organs to nerve centers; afferent.

sensory aphasia *n.* Aphasia in which the ability to comprehend written or spoken words is lost.

sensory cortex *n.* The somatic sensory, auditory, visual, and olfactory regions of the cerebral cortex considered as a group.

sensory deprivation *n.* The reduction or absence of usual external stimuli or perceptual opportunities, commonly resulting in psychological distress and sometimes in unpleasant hallucinations.

sensory ganglion *n.* A cluster of primary sensory neurons forming a swelling in a peripheral nerve or its dorsal root and establishing the sole afferent neural connection between the sensory periphery and the central nervous system.

sensory image *n.* An image based on one or more types of sensation.

sensory neuron *n.* A neuron conveying impulses from sensory receptors or nerve endings for processing by the central nervous system to become part of the organism's perception of itself and of its environment.

sensory paralysis *n.* Loss of sensation.

sensory speech center *n.* See **Wernicke's center.**

sensory urgency *n.* Urgent desire to empty the urinary bladder due to bladder and ureter hypersensitivity.

sen·su·al (sĕn′shōō-əl) *adj.* **1.** Relating to or affecting any of the senses or a sense organ; sensory. **2.** Of, relating to, given to, or providing gratification of the physical and especially the sexual appetites.

sen·tient (sĕn′shənt, -shē-ənt) *adj.* **1.** Having sense perception; conscious. **2.** Experiencing sensation or feeling.

sep·a·ra·tion anxiety (sĕp′ə-rā′shən) *n.* A child's apprehension or fear associated with his or her separation from a parent or other significant person.

sep·sis (sĕp′sĭs) *n., pl.* **-ses** (-sēz). **1.** The presence of pathogenic organisms or their toxins in the blood or tissues. **2.** The poisoned condition resulting from the presence of pathogens or their toxins, as in septicemia.

sep·tate uterus (sĕp′tāt′) *n.* A uterus that is divided into two cavities by an anteroposterior septum.

sep·tec·to·my (sĕp-tĕk′tə-mē) *n.* Surgical excision of a septum or part of a septum, especially the nasal or atrial septum.

sep·tic (sĕp′tĭk) *adj.* **1.** Of, relating to, having the nature of, or affected by sepsis. **2.** Causing sepsis; putrefactive.

septic abortion *n.* Abortion complicated by fever, endometritis, and parametritis, often leading to sepsis.

sep·ti·ce·mi·a (sĕp′tĭ-sē′mē-ə) *n.* A systemic disease caused by the multiplication of microorganisms in the blood. — **sep′ti·ce′mic** (-mĭk) *adj.*

septicemic abscess *n.* See **pyemic abscess.**

septicemic plague *n.* A usually fatal form of bubonic plague in which the bacilli are present in the bloodstream and cause toxemia.

sep·ti·co·py·e·mi·a (sĕp′tĭ-kō-pī-ē′mē-ə) *n.* Pyemia and septicemia occurring together. — **sep′ti·co·py·e′mic** *adj.*

septic shock *n.* **1.** Shock associated with sepsis, usually also associated with abdominal and pelvic infection resulting from trauma or surgery. **2.** Shock associated with septicemia caused by gram-negative bacteria.

septic sore throat *n.* An infection of the throat, often epidemic, caused by hemolytic streptococci and characterized by fever and inflammation of the tonsils.

sep·to·plas·ty (sĕp′tə-plăs′tē) *n.* A surgical operation to correct defects or deformities of the nasal septum, often by altering or partially removing supporting structures.

sep·to·rhi·no·plas·ty (sĕp′tō-rī′nō-plăs′tē, -nə-) *n.* A surgical procedure to repair defects or deformities of both the nasal septum and the external nasal pyramid.

sep·tos·to·my (sĕp-tŏs′tə-mē) *n.* The surgical creation of an opening in a septum.

sep·tot·o·my (sĕp-tŏt′ə-mē) *n.* Surgical incision of the nasal septum.

sep·tu·lum (sĕp′chə-ləm) *n., pl.* **-la** (-lə). A tiny septum.

sep·tum (sĕp′təm) *n., pl.* **-ta** (-tə). **1.** A thin partition or membrane that divides two cavities or soft masses of tissue. **2.** The septum pellucidum.

septum pel·lu·ci·dum (pə-lōō′sĭ-dəm) *n., pl.* **septa pel·lu·ci·da** (-də). A thin membrane of nervous tissue that forms the medial wall of the lateral ventricles in the brain.

se·quel·a (sĭ-kwĕl′ə) *n., pl.* **-quel·ae** (-kwĕl′ē). A pathological condition resulting from a disease.

se·quence (sē′kwəns, -kwĕns′) *n.* **1.** A following of one thing after another; succession. **2.** An order of succession; an arrangement. **3.** The order of constituents in a polymer, especially the order of nucleotides in a nucleic acid or of the amino acids in a protein. — *v.* **-quenced, -quenc·ing, -quenc·es. 1.** To organize or arrange in a sequence. **2.** To determine the order of constituents in a polymer, such as a nucleic acid or protein molecule.

se·ques·tra·tion (sē′kwĭ-strā′shən, sĕk′wĭ-) *n.* **1.** The formation of a sequestrum. **2.** Loss of blood or of its fluid content into spaces within the body, so that the circulating volume diminishes.

se·ques·trec·to·my (sē′kwĭ-strĕk′tə-mē) *n.* Surgical removal of a sequestrum.

se·ques·trum (sĭ-kwĕs′trəm) *n., pl.* **-tra** (-trə). A fragment of dead tissue, usually bone, that has separated from healthy tissue as a result of injury or disease.

se·quoi·o·sis (sĕ′kwoi-ō′sĭs) *n.* Extrinsic allergic alveolitis caused by inhalation of redwood sawdust containing spores of various fungi.

Ser *abbr.* serine

ser·al·bu·min (sĕr′ăl-byōō′mĭn) *n.* A protein fraction of serum involved in maintaining osmotic pressure of the blood and used as a substitute for plasma in the treatment of shock.

Ser·e·vent (sĕr′ə-vĕnt′) A trademark for salmeterol xinafoate.

se·ri·al extraction (sĕr′ē-əl) *n.* Selective extraction of certain teeth during the early years of dental development to encourage autonomous adjustment of moderate to severe crowding of the anterior teeth.

serial radiography *n.* The making of sequential x-ray exposures of a region under study over a period of time.

serial section *n.* One of a number of consecutive histological sections.

se·ries (sĕr′ēz) *n., pl.* **series**. **1.** A number of objects or events arranged or coming one after the other in succession. **2.** A group of objects related by linearly varying successive differences in form or configuration, as in a radioactive decay series.

ser·ine (sĕr′ēn′) *n.* An amino acid that is a common constituent of many proteins.

se·ro·con·ver·sion (sĕr′ō-kən-vûr′zhən, -shən) *n.* Development of antibodies in blood serum as a result of infection or immunization.

se·ro·di·ag·no·sis (sĕr′ō-dī′əg-nō′sĭs) *n., pl.* **-ses** (-sēz). Diagnosis of disease based on reactions in the blood serum.

se·ro·ep·i·de·mi·ol·o·gy (sĕr′ō-ĕp′ĭ-dē′mē-ŏl′ə-jē, -dĕm′ē-) *n.* Epidemiologic study through the use of serological testing to detect infection.

se·rol·o·gy (sĭ-rŏl′ə-jē) *n.* **1.** The science that deals with the properties and reactions of serums, especially blood serum. **2.** The characteristics of a disease or an organism shown by study of blood serums. — **se′ro·log′ic, se′ro·log′i·cal** *adj.*

se·ro·ma (sĭ-rō′mə) *n.* A mass or swelling caused by the localized accumulation of serum within a tissue or organ.

se·ro·mu·cous gland (sĕr′ō-myōō′kəs) *n.* A gland containing both serous and mucous secretory cells.

se·ro·neg·a·tive (sĕr′ō-nĕg′ə-tĭv) *adj.* Having a negative reaction to a serological test for a disease, especially to a test for syphilis or AIDS.

se·ro·pos·i·tive (sĕr′ō-pŏz′ĭ-tĭv) *adj.* Having a positive reaction to a serological test for a disease; exhibiting seroconversion.

se·ro·pus (sĕr′ō-pŭs′) *n.* Pus largely diluted with serum.

se·ro·sa (sĭ-rō′sə, -zə) *n., pl.* **-sas** or **-sae** (-sē, -zē). See **serous membrane**.

se·ro·si·tis (sĕr′ō-sī′tĭs) *n.* Inflammation of a serous membrane.

se·ros·i·ty (sĭ-rŏs′ĭ-tē) *n.* **1.** A serous fluid or a serum. **2.** The condition of being serous. **3.** The serous quality of a liquid.

se·ro·syn·o·vi·tis (sĕr′ō-sĭn′ə-vī′tĭs, -sī′nə-) *n.* Synovitis marked by an increase of serous fluid.

se·ro·ther·a·py (sĕr′ō-thĕr′ə-pē) *n.* Treatment of disease by administration of a serum obtained from an immunized animal.

se·ro·to·nin (sĕr′ə-tō′nĭn, sĕr′-) *n.* A neurotransmitter formed from tryptophan and found especially in the brain, blood serum, and gastric mucous membranes, and active in vasoconstriction, stimulation of the smooth muscles, transmission of impulses between nerve cells, and regulation of cyclic body processes.

se·ro·type (sĕr′ə-tīp′, sĕr′-) *n.* A group of closely related microorganisms distinguished by a characteristic set of antigens. — *v.* **-typed, -typ·ing, -types**. To classify according to serotype; assign to a particular serotype.

se·rous (sĕr′əs) *adj.* Containing, secreting, or resembling serum.

serous cell *n.* A cell, especially of the salivary gland, that secretes a watery albuminlike fluid.

serous fluid *n.* Any of various body fluids resembling serum, especially lymph.

serous gland *n.* A gland secreting a watery substance that may or may not contain an enzyme.

serous inflammation *n.* A form of exudative inflammation in which the exudate is predominantly fluid.

serous ligament *n.* Any of a number of peritoneal folds attaching certain of the viscera to the abdominal wall or to one another.

serous membrane *n.* A thin, two-part membrane that secretes a serous fluid and lines a closed body cavity, covering the organs within that cavity.

serous synovitis *n.* Synovitis with a large effusion of nonpurulent fluid.

se·ro·vac·ci·na·tion (sĕr′ō-văk′sə-nā′shən) *n.* A process for producing mixed immunity by administering an injection of a serum as well as a vaccine of a modified or killed culture.

se·ro·var (sĕr′ō-vär′, -văr′) *n.* See **serotype**.

ser·pi·go (ser- pī′gō) *n.* Any creeping eruption.

ser·ra·tion (sə-rā′shən, sĕ-) *n.* **1.** The state of being serrate. **2.** A series or set of teeth or notches. **3.** A single tooth or notch in a serrate edge.

serre·fine (sâr-fēn′, sĕr-) *n.* A small spring forceps used for approximating the edges of a wound, or for temporarily closing an artery during an operation.

Ser·to·li cell (sər-tō′lē, sĕr′tō-lē) *n.* Any of the elongated striated cells in the seminiferous tubules to which spermatids attach during spermiogenesis.

Sertoli cell-only syndrome *n.* Congenital absence of germinal epithelium from the seminiferous tubules, which contain only Sertoli cells, resulting in sterility due to the absence of living sperm cells in the semen.

Sertoli cell tumor *n.* See **androblastoma**.

ser·tra·line hydrochloride (sǝr′trǝ-lēn) *n.* An oral antidepressant that enhances serotonin activity by inhibiting its uptake by neurons of the central nervous system.

se·rum (sēr′ǝm) *n., pl.* **se·rums** or **se·ra** (sēr′ǝ). **1.** A clear watery fluid, especially that moistening the surface of serous membranes or exuded in inflammation of such membranes. **2.** The clear yellowish fluid obtained upon separating whole blood into its solid and liquid components. **3.** Such fluid from the tissues of immunized animals, containing antibodies and used to transfer immunity to another individual.

serum agglutinin *n.* An antibody that coats Rh-positive red blood cells or bacteria, preventing them from agglutinating when suspended in saline.

serum albumin *n.* See **seralbumin**.

serum globulin *n.* A protein fraction of serum composed chiefly of antibodies.

serum hepatitis *n.* See **hepatitis B**.

serum nephritis *n.* Glomerulonephritis occurring in serum sickness.

serum shock *n.* Anaphylactic or anaphylactoid shock caused by the injection of antitoxic or other foreign serum into a sensitized person.

serum sickness *n.* A hypersensitive reaction to the administration of a foreign serum, characterized by fever, swelling, skin rash, and enlargement of the lymph nodes.

serum therapy *n.* See **serotherapy**.

set (sĕt) *v.* **set, set·ting, sets. 1.** To put into a stable position. **2.** To fix firmly or in an immobile manner. **3.** To become fixed or hardened; coagulate. **4.** To bring the bones of a fracture back into a normal position or alignment. —*n.* **1.** The act or process of setting. **2.** The condition resulting from setting. **3.** A permanent firming or hardening of a substance, as by cooling. **4.** The carriage or bearing of a part of the body. **5.** A particular psychological state, usually that of anticipation or preparedness.

se·ta (sē′tǝ) *n., pl.* **-tae** (-tē). A stiff hair, bristle, or bristlelike process or part.

se·ton (sēt′n) *n.* Material such as thread, wire, or gauze that is passed through subcutaneous tissues or a cyst in order to form a sinus or fistula.

sev·enth cranial nerve (sĕv′ǝnth) *n.* See **facial nerve**.

sex (sĕks) *n.* **1.** The property or quality by which organisms are classified as female or male on the basis of their reproductive organs and functions. **2.** Either of the two divisions, designated female and male, of this classification. **3.** Females or males considered as a group. **4.** The physiolog-

ical, functional, and psychological differences that distinguish the female and the male. **5.** The sexual urge or instinct as it manifests itself in behavior. **6.** Sexual intercourse.

sex cell *n.* See **germ cell**.

sex change *n.* The modification of a person's biological sex characteristics, by surgery and hormone treatment, to approximate those of the opposite sex.

sex chromatin *n.* See **Barr body**.

sex chromosome *n.* Either of a pair of chromosomes, usually designated X or Y, that combine to determine the sex and sex-linked characteristics of an individual, with XX resulting in a female and XY in a male.

sex determination *n.* The determination of the sex of a fetus in utero by identifying sex chromatin in amniotic fluid obtained by amniocentesis.

sex gland *n.* A testis or an ovary; a gonad.

sex hormone *n.* Any of various steroid hormones, such as estrogen and androgen, affecting the growth or function of the reproductive organs and the development of secondary sex characteristics.

sex-influenced inheritance *n.* Inheritance that is autosomal but has a different intensity of expression in the two sexes, as that manifested in male pattern baldness.

sex-limited inheritance *n.* Inheritance in which a trait or phenotype is expressed in one sex only, as in hemophilia A.

sex linkage *n.* The condition in which a gene responsible for a specific trait is located on a sex chromosome, resulting in sexually dependent inheritance of the trait.

sex-linked *adj.* **1.** Carried by a sex chromosome, especially an X-chromosome. Used of genes. **2.** Sexually determined. Used especially of inherited traits.

sex-linked character *n.* An inherited character determined by a sex-linked gene.

sex-linked gene *n.* A gene located on a sex chromosome, usually the X-chromosome.

sex-linked inheritance *n.* Inheritance that may result from a mutant gene located on either the X- or Y-chromosome.

sex reversal *n.* See **sex change**.

sex role *n.* Any of the various attitudinal patterns of daily behavior that are associated with masculinity and femininity in a particular society.

sex test *n.* A method of determining genetic sex by examination of stained smears of buccal mucosal squamous epithelial cells for Barr bodies.

sex·u·al (sĕk′shoo-ǝl) *adj.* **1.** Of, relating to, involving, or characteristic of sex, sexuality, the sexes, or the sex organs and their functions. **2.** Of, relating to, or involving the union of male and female gametes. — **sex′u·al·ly** *adv.*

sexual dimorphism *n.* The physical differences between males and females that arise as a consequence of sexual maturation, including the secondary sex characteristics.

sexual generation *n.* Reproduction through the union of male and female germ cells.

sexual intercourse *n.* **1.** Coitus between humans. **2.** Sexual union between humans involving genital contact other than vaginal penetration by the penis.

sex·u·al·i·ty (sĕk′shoō-ăl′ĭ-tē) *n.* **1.** The condition of being characterized and distinguished by sex. **2.** Concern with or interest in sexual activity. **3.** Sexual character or potency.

sexually transmitted disease *n.* Any of various diseases, including chancroid, chlamydia, gonorrhea, and syphilis, that are usually contracted through sexual intercourse or other intimate sexual contact.

sexual orientation *n.* The direction of one's sexual interest toward members of the same, opposite, or both sexes, especially a direction seen to be dictated by physiologic rather than sociologic forces.

sexual preference *n.* The preference one shows by having a sexual interest in members of the same, opposite, or either sex.

sexual reproduction *n.* Reproduction by the union of male and female gametes to form a zygote.

sexual selection *n.* Selection driven by the competition for mates, considered an adjunct to natural selection.

Sé·za·ry syndrome (sā′zə-rē, sā-zä-rē′) *n.* Exfoliative dermatitis characterized by intense itching and caused by the infiltration of atypical mononuclear cells into the skin and the peripheral blood.

sg *abbr.* specific gravity

SH *abbr.* serum hepatitis

shad·ow test (shăd′ō) *n.* See **retinoscopy.**

shaft (shăft) *n.* **1.** An elongated rodlike structure, such as the midsection of a long bone. **2.** The section of a hair projecting from the surface of the body.

shak·en infant syndrome (shā′kən) *n.* A syndrome affecting infants who have been shaken so violently that the brain is damaged, often resulting in seizures, paralysis, coma, or traumas that lead to blindness or other disabilities.

shal·low breathing (shăl′ō) *n.* Breathing with abnormally low tidal volume.

shank (shăngk) *n.* The part of the leg between the knee and ankle.

shap·ing (shā′pĭng) *n.* A procedure used in operant conditioning in which behavior is modified by stepwise reinforcement of behaviors that produce progressively closer approximations of the desired behavior.

shave biopsy *n.* A biopsy technique performed with a surgical blade or a razor blade and used for lesions that are elevated above the skin level or confined to the epidermis and upper dermis.

sheath (shēth) *n., pl.* **sheaths** (shē*th*z, shēths). An enveloping tubular structure, such as the tissue that encloses a muscle or nerve fiber.

sheath of the eyeball *n.* A condensation of connective tissue on the outer sclera aspect, from which it is separated by a narrow cleftlike space.

sheath of Schwann *n.* See **neurilemma.**

Shee·han's syndrome (shē′ənz) *n.* Hypopituitarism arising from a severe circulatory collapse during the postpartum period, resulting in pituitary necrosis.

shell shock *n.* See **war neurosis.**

shi·at·su (shē-ät′soō) *n.* A form of therapeutic massage in which pressure is applied with the thumbs and palms to those areas of the body used in acupuncture.

shield (shēld) *n.* A protective device or structure, such as a lead sheet to protect one from x-rays.

shift (shĭft) *v.* **shift·ed, shift·ing, shifts.** To alter position or place. —*n.* **1.** A change from one person or configuration to another; a substitution. **2.** A change in position.

Shi·ga–Kruse bacillus (shē′gə-krōōz′, -krōō′zə) *n.* A gram-negative bacterium, *Shigella dysenteriae,* that causes dysentery in humans.

Shi·gel·la (shĭ-gĕl′ə) *n.* A genus of aerobic, gramnegative, nonmotile, rod-shaped bacteria that includes some species that cause dysentery.

shig·el·lo·sis (shĭg′ə-lō′sĭs) *n., pl.* **-ses** (-sēz). Dysentery caused by any of various species of *Shigella,* occurring most frequently in areas where poor sanitation and malnutrition are prevalent and commonly affecting children and infants.

shin (shĭn) *n.* **1.** The front part of the leg below the knee and above the ankle. **2.** The shinbone.

shin·bone (shĭn′bōn′) *n.* See **tibia.**

shin·gles (shĭng′gəlz) *n.* An acute infection caused by a herpesvirus and characterized by inflammation of the sensory ganglia of certain spinal or cranial nerves and the eruption of vesicles along the affected nerve path. It usually strikes only one side of the body and is often accompanied by severe neuralgia.

shin splints or **shinsplints** *n.* A painful condition of the shins caused by inflammation of the surrounding muscles, frequently occurring among runners.

shirt-stud abscess (shûrt′stŭd′) *n.* Two abscesses connected by a narrow channel, usually formed by rupture through an overlying fascia.

shock (shŏk) *n.* **1.** Something that jars the mind or emotions as if with a violent, unexpected blow. **2.** The disturbance of function, equilibrium, or mental faculties caused by a blow; violent agitation. **3.** A generally temporary massive physiological reaction to severe physical or emotional trauma, usually characterized by marked loss of blood pressure and depression of vital processes. **4.** The sensation and muscular spasm caused by an electric current passing through the body or a body part. **5.** The abnormally palpable impact of an accentuated heartbeat felt by a hand on the chest wall. —*v.* **1.** To induce a state of physical shock in a person. **2.** To subject a person to an electric shock.

shock lung *n.* The development of edema, impaired perfusion, and reduction in alveolar space so that the alveoli collapse, occurring during shock.

shock therapy *n.* Any of various treatments for mental disorders, such as major depression or schizophrenia, in which a convulsion or brief coma is induced by administering a drug or passing an electric current through the brain.

shock treatment *n.* See **shock therapy.**

short·sight·ed·ness (shôrt'sī'tĭd-nĭs) *n.* Myopia.

short-term memory *n.* The phase of the memory process in which stimuli that have been recognized and registered are stored briefly.

short·wave diathermy (shôrt'wāv') *n.* The therapeutic elevation of temperature in the tissues by means of an oscillating electric current of extremely high frequency.

shot (shŏt) *n.* **1.** A hypodermic injection. **2.** A small amount given or applied at one time.

shot-silk retina *n.* The appearance of numerous, wavelike, opalescent reflexes that can occur in the retinas of children under the age of 10 and sometimes in teenagers.

shoul·der (shōl'dər) *n.* **1.** The joint connecting the arm with the torso. **2.** The part of the body between the neck and upper arm.

shoulder blade *n.* See **scapula.**

shoulder girdle *n.* The pectoral girdle, especially of a human.

shoulder-girdle syndrome *n.* See **brachial plexus neuropathy.**

shoulder-hand syndrome *n.* See **brachial plexus neuropathy.**

shoulder joint *n.* A ball-and-socket joint between the head of the humerus and the glenoid cavity of the scapula.

shoulder presentation *n.* Presentation during birth in which the fetus lies with its long axis transverse to the long axis of the mother's body and with the shoulder as the presenting part.

show (shō) *n.* **1.** The first discharge of blood in menstruation. **2.** The discharge of bloody mucus from the vagina indicating the start of labor.

shunt (shŭnt) *n.* A passage between two natural body channels, such as blood vessels, especially one created surgically to divert or permit flow from one pathway or region to another; a bypass.

shut-in *n.* A person confined indoors by illness or disability. —*adj.* Confined to a home or hospital, as by illness.

Shy–Dra·ger syndrome (shī'drā'gər) *n.* A progressive disorder of the brain and spinal cord affecting the autonomic nervous system and characterized by low blood pressure, atrophy of the iris, incontinence, the absence of sweating, impotence in males, tremor, and muscle wasting.

si·a·lad·en·i·tis (sī'ə-lăd'n-ī'tĭs) or **si·a·lo·ad·e·ni·tis** (sī'ə-lō-ăd'n-) *n.* Inflammation of a salivary gland.

si·a·lad·e·no·sis (sī'ə-lăd'n-ō'sĭs) *n.* Enlargement of the salivary glands, usually the parotids, often seen in conditions such as alcoholism and malnutrition.

si·a·lem·e·sis (sī'ə-lĕm'ĭ-sĭs) or **si·a·le·me·si·a**

(-lə-mē'zē-ə) *n.* **1.** Vomiting caused by or accompanying an excessive secretion of saliva. **2.** Vomiting of saliva.

si·al·ic acid (sī-ăl'ĭk) *n.* Any of a group of amino carbohydrates that are components of mucoproteins and glycoproteins, especially in tissue and blood cells.

si·a·lo·ad·e·nec·to·my (sī'ə-lō-ăd'n-ĕk'tə-mē) *n.* Surgical excision of a salivary gland.

si·a·lo·ad·e·not·o·my (sī'ə-lō-ăd'n-ŏt'ə-mē) *n.* Surgical incision into a salivary gland.

si·a·lo·an·gi·ec·ta·sis (sī'ə-lō-ăn'jē-ĕk'tə-sĭs) *n.* Dilation of salivary ducts.

si·a·lo·do·cho·plas·ty (sī'ə-lō-dō'kə-plăs'tē) *n.* Surgical repair of a salivary duct.

si·al·o·gram (sī-ăl'ə-grăm') *n.* A radiograph of one or more of the salivary ducts.

si·a·log·ra·phy (sī'ə-lŏg'rə-fē) *n.* Radiographic examination of the salivary glands and ducts after the introduction of a radiopaque material.

si·a·lo·lith (sī'ə-lō-lĭth', sī-ăl'ə-) *n.* A calculus occurring in a salivary gland or duct.

si·a·lo·li·thot·o·my (sī'ə-lō-lĭ-thŏt'ə-mē) *n.* Surgical incision into a salivary duct or gland to remove a calculus.

si·a·lo·met·a·pla·sia (sī'ə-lō-mĕt'ə-plā'zhə, -zhē-ə) *n.* Squamous cell metaplasia in the salivary ducts.

si·a·lo·syr·inx (sī'ə-lō-sēr'ĭngks) *n.* A salivary fistula passing from the salivary gland or duct to the exterior of the body, usually through the skin or oral tissues.

Si·a·mese twin (sī'ə-mēz', -mēs') *n.* Either of a pair of identical twins born with their bodies joined at some point, a result of the incomplete division of the ovum from which the twins developed.

sib (sĭb) *n.* **1.** A blood relation; a relative. **2.** A person's relatives considered as a group; kinfolk. **3.** A brother or sister; a sibling. —*adj.* Related by blood; kindred.

sib·i·lant (sĭb'ə-lənt) *adj.* Of, characterized by, or producing a hissing sound like that of (s) or (sh).

sib·ling (sĭb'lĭng) *n.* One of two or more individuals having one or both parents in common; a brother or sister.

sibling rivalry *n.* **1.** Competition among children, especially for the attention, affection, and approval of their parents. **2.** Such a competition but for recognition or rewards, such as school grades.

sib·ship (sĭb'shĭp') *n.* The children produced by one pair of parents.

sic·ca complex (sĭk'ə) *n.* Dryness of the mucous membranes, as of the eyes and mouth, in the absence of a connective tissue disease such as rheumatoid arthritis.

sic·ca·tive (sĭk'ə-tĭv) *n.* A substance added to some medicines to promote drying; a drier.

sick (sĭk) *adj.* **sick·er, sick·est. 1.** Suffering from or affected with a disease or disorder; ailing. **2.** Of or for sick persons. **3.** Nauseated. **4.** Mentally ill or disturbed. **5.** Constituting an unhealthy environment for those working or residing within, as of a building.

sick·bay (sĭk'bā') *n.* **1.** The hospital and dispensary of a ship. **2.** A place where the sick or injured are treated.

sick·bed (sĭk'bĕd') *n.* A sick person's bed.

sick headache *n.* See **migraine**.

sick·le (sĭk'əl) *v.* **-led, -ling, -les. 1.** To deform a red blood cell into an abnormal crescent shape. **2.** To assume an abnormal crescent shape. Used of red blood cells.

sick leave *n.* Paid absence from work allowed an employee because of sickness.

sick·le cell (sĭk'əl) *n.* An abnormal, crescent-shaped red blood cell that results from a single change in the amino acid sequence of the cell's hemoglobin, which causes the cell to contort, especially under low-oxygen conditions.

sickle cell anemia *n.* A chronic, usually fatal inherited form of anemia marked by crescent-shaped red blood cells, occurring almost exclusively in blacks, and characterized by fever, leg ulcers, jaundice, and episodic pain in the joints.

sickle cell C disease *n.* A hereditary blood disease caused by sickle-shaped red blood cells that contain hemoglobin S and hemoglobin C, characterized by anemia, blocked blood vessels, chronic leg ulcers, and bone deformities.

sickle cell hemoglobin *n.* See **hemoglobin S.**

sickle-cell test *n.* A method of determining the percentage of red blood cells containing hemoglobin S.

sickle cell trait *n.* A hereditary condition, usually harmless and without symptoms, in which a person carries only one gene for sickle cell anemia.

sick·ness (sĭk'nĭs) *n.* **1.** The condition of being sick; illness. **2.** A disease or an illness.

sick·room (sĭk'rōōm', -rŏōm') *n.* A room occupied by a sick person.

side effect *n.* A peripheral or secondary effect, especially an undesirable secondary effect of a drug or therapy.

sid·er·o·blast (sĭd'ər-ə-blăst') *n.* An erythroblast containing granules of ferritin.

sid·er·o·cyte (sĭd'ər-ə-sīt') *n.* A red blood cell containing granules of iron that are not part of the cell's hemoglobin.

sid·er·o·der·ma (sĭd'ə-rō-dûr'mə) *n.* A brownish discoloration of the skin on the legs caused by hemosiderin deposits.

sid·er·o·fi·bro·sis (sĭd'ə-rō-fī-brō'sĭs) *n.* Fibrosis associated with small foci in which iron is deposited.

sid·er·oph·i·lin (sĭd'ə-rŏf'ə-lĭn, -rə-fĭl'ĭn) *n.* See **transferrin.**

sid·er·o·sil·i·co·sis (sĭd'ə-rō-sĭl'ĭ-kō'sĭs) *n.* Silicosis due to inhalation of dust containing iron and silica.

sid·er·o·sis (sĭd'ə-rō'sĭs) *n.* **1.** Chronic inflammation of the lungs caused by excessive inhalation of dust containing iron salts or particles. **2.** Discoloration of an organ or a tissue by an iron pigment. **3.** An excess of iron in the blood.

sid·er·ot·ic (sĭd'ə-rŏt'ĭk) *adj.* **1.** Pigmented by iron. **2.** Containing an excess of iron.

SIDS *abbr.* sudden infant death syndrome

sieve graft (sĭv) *n.* A full-thickness skin graft taken after cutting multiple holes in it with a circular punch, leaving islands of skin to heal the area.

sight (sīt) *n.* **1.** The ability to see. **2.** Field of vision.

sigma factor (sĭg'mə) *n.* A protein component of RNA polymerase that determines the specific site on DNA where transcription begins.

sig·moid (sĭg'moid') or **sig·moi·dal** (sĭg-moid'l) *adj.* **1.** Having the shape of the letter S. **2.** Of or relating to the sigmoid flexure of the colon.

sigmoid colon *n.* See **sigmoid flexure.**

sig·moid·ec·to·my (sĭg'moi-dĕk'tə-mē) *n.* Surgical excision of the sigmoid colon.

sigmoid flexure *n.* The S-shaped section of the colon between the pelvic brim and the third sacral segment, continuous with the rectum.

sig·moid·i·tis (sĭg'moi-dī'tĭs) *n.* Inflammation of the sigmoid colon.

sig·moi·do·pex·y (sĭg-moi'də-pĕk'sē) *n.* Surgical attachment of the sigmoid colon to a firm structure to correct rectal prolapse.

sig·moi·do·proc·tos·to·my (sĭg-moi'dō-prŏk-tŏs'tə-mē) *n.* Establishment of an artificial anus by surgically creating an opening at the junction of the sigmoid colon and the rectum.

sig·moi·do·rec·tos·to·my (sĭg-moi'dō-rĕk-tŏs'tə-mē) *n.* See **sigmoidoproctostomy.**

sig·moi·do·scope (sĭg-moi'də-skōp') *n.* A tubular instrument for visual examination of the sigmoid flexure. — **sig'moid·os'co·py** (sĭg'moi-dŏs'kə-pē) *adj.*

sig·moid·os·to·my (sĭg'moi-dŏs'tə-mē) *n.* Establishment of an artificial anus by surgically creating an opening into the sigmoid colon.

sig·moid·ot·o·my (sĭg'moi-dŏt'ə-mē) *n.* Surgical opening of the sigmoid colon.

sign (sīn) *n.* **1.** See **symptom. 2.** Something that suggests the presence or existence of a fact, condition, or quality. **3.** A trace or vestige, as of disease or life.

sig·net-ring cell (sĭg'nĭt rĭng') *n.* A cell with a large cytoplasmic vacuole containing mucin that compresses the nucleus to one side of the cell.

si·lent (sī'lənt) *adj.* Producing no detectable signs or symptoms.

sil·i·con (sĭl'ĭ-kən, -kŏn') *n.* A nonmetallic element occurring abundantly in Earth's crust and having atomic number 14.

sil·i·cone (sĭl'ĭ-kōn') *n.* Any of a group of silicon compounds in solid, liquid, or gel form, characterized by wide-range thermal stability, high lubricity, extreme water repellence, and physiological inertness and used in many commercial and medical products, including surgical implants and dental impression materials.

sil·i·co·sis (sĭl'ĭ-kō'sĭs) *n.* A disease of the lungs caused by continued inhalation of the dust of siliceous minerals and characterized by progressive fibrosis and a chronic shortness of breath. — **sil'i·cot'ic** (-kŏt'ĭk) *adj.*

sil·i·quose (sĭl′ĭ-kwōs′) *adj.* Resembling a long slender pod. Used of a cataract resulting in shriveling of the lens and calcareous deposits in the capsule.

sil·ver (sĭl′vər) *n.* A lustrous ductile malleable metallic element having the highest thermal and electrical conductivity of the metals and atomic number 47.

silver-fork fracture *n.* A Colles′ fracture of the wrist causing a deformity that, in profile, resembles a fork.

silver iodide *n.* A pale yellow, odorless powder that darkens on exposure to light and is used in medicine, especially as an antiseptic.

silver protein *n.* A colloidal preparation of silver oxide and protein, usually gelatin or albumin, used as an antibacterial agent.

si·meth·i·cone (sĭ-mĕth′ĭ-kōn′) *n.* A mixture of dimethyl polysiloxanes and silica gel, used as an antiflatulent.

sim·i·an virus (sĭm′ē-ən) *n.* Any of a number of viruses of variable taxonomic classification isolated from monkeys and from cultures of monkey cells.

Sim·monds disease (sĭm′əndz) *n.* Extreme and progressive emanciation including loss of body hair and premature aging caused by atrophy or destruction of the anterior lobe of the pituitary.

sim·ple absence (sĭm′pəl) *n.* A brief loss or impairment of consciousness accompanied by the abrupt onset of per 3 per sec spikes and waves on an electroencephalograph.

simple epithelium *n.* Epithelium made up of one layer of cells.

simple fission *n.* Division of the nucleus and then the cell body into two parts.

simple fracture *n.* See **closed fracture.**

simple joint *n.* A joint composed of two bones only.

simple mastectomy *n.* Surgical removal of the breast, including the nipple, areola, and most of the overlying skin.

simple protein *n.* A protein, such as a globulin or histone, that yields only alpha-amino acids upon hydrolysis.

simple squamous epithelium *n.* Epithelium made up of a single layer of flattened scalelike cells.

simple sugar *n.* See **monosaccharide.**

Sims′ position (sĭmz) *n.* A position in which the patient lies on one side with the under arm behind the back and the upper thigh flexed, used to facilitate vaginal examination.

sim·u·la·tion (sĭm′yə-lā′shən) *n.* **1.** Close resemblance or imitation, as of one symptom or disease by another. **2.** Reproduction or representation, as of a potential situation or in experimental testing. — **sim′u·late′** (-lāt′) *v.* — **sim′u·la′tor** (-lā′tər) *n.*

sincipital presentation *n.* Head presentation of the fetus during birth in which the large fontanel is the presenting part.

sin·ci·put (sĭn′sə-pət) *n., pl.* **sin·ci·puts** or **sin·cip·i·ta** (sĭn-sĭp′ĭ-tə). **1.** The upper half of the cranium, especially the anterior portion above and including the forehead. **2.** The forehead. — **sin·cip′i·tal** (-sĭp′ĭ-tl) *adj.*

Sind·bis fever (sĭnd′bĭs) *n.* A febrile illness characterized by arthralgia, rash, and malaise. It is caused by the Sindbis virus and transmitted by culicine mosquitoes.

sin·ew (sĭn′yōō) *n.* **1.** A tendon. **2.** Vigorous strength; muscular power.

sin·gle photon emission computed tomography (sĭng′gəl) *n.* Tomographic imaging of local metabolic and physiological functions in tissues. The image is formed by a computer synthesis of data transmitted by single gamma photons emitted by radionuclides administered in suitable form to the patient.

sin·is·ter (sĭn′ĭ-stər) *adj.* On the left side; left. — **sin′is·ter·ly** *adv.* — **sin′is·ter·ness** *n.*

sin·is·tral·i·ty (sĭn′ĭ-străl′ĭ-tē) *n.* Preference for the left hand in performing manual tasks; left-handedness.

sin·is·tro·tor·sion (sĭn′ĭ-strō-tôr′shən) *n.* A twisting to the left, used especially of the eye.

si·no·a·tri·al (sī′nō-ā′trē-əl) or **si·nu·a·tri·al** (sī′-nōō-ā′trē-əl, -nyōō-, sĭn′yōō-) *adj.* Relating to the venous sinus and the right atrium of the heart.

sinoatrial block *n.* Failure of an impulse to leave the sinoatrial node.

sinoatrial node *n.* A small mass of specialized cardiac muscle fibers located in the posterior wall of the right atrium of the heart that acts as a pacemaker by generating at regular intervals the electric impulses of the heartbeat.

si·no·au·ric·u·lar (sī′nō-ô-rĭk′yə-lər) *adj.* Sinoatrial.

sinoauricular block *n.* See **sinoatrial block.**

sinoauricular node *n.* See **sinoatrial node.**

si·nus (sī′nəs) *n.* **1.** A depression or cavity formed by a bending or curving. **2.** A channel for the passage of blood or lymph that is without the coats of an ordinary vessel, such as the blood passages in the gravid uterus or in the cerebral meninges. **3.** Any of various air-filled cavities in the bones of the skull, especially one communicating with the nostrils. **4.** A fistula or tract leading to a pus-filled cavity.

sinus arrest *n.* A pause or cessation of cardiac sinus pacemaker activity.

sinus histiocytosis with massive lymphadenopathy *n.* A chronic disease occurring in children and characterized by massive painless cervical lymphadenopathy due to distension of the lymphatic sinuses by macrophages containing ingested lymphocytes.

si·nus·i·tis (sī′nə-sī′tĭs) *n.* Inflammation of the mucous membrane of a sinus, especially of the paranasal sinuses.

sinus node *n.* See **sinoatrial node.**

si·nu·soid (sī′nə-soid′, -nyə-) *n.* Any of the venous cavities through which blood passes in various glands and organs, such as the adrenal gland and the liver. — *adj.* Resembling a sinus. — **si′nu·soi′dal** (-soid′l) *adj.*

si·nus·ot·o·my (sī'nə-sŏt'ə-mē, -nyə-) *n.* Surgical incision into a sinus.

sinus rhythm *n.* A normal cardiac rhythm proceeding from the sinoatrial node.

si·phon (sī'fən) *n.* A tube bent into an inverted U shape of unequal lengths, used to remove fluid by means of atmospheric pressure from a cavity or reservoir at one end of the tube over a barrier and out the other end. — *v.* **-phoned, -phon·ing, -phons.** To draw off or convey through a siphon.

si·phon·age (sī'fə-nĭj) *n.* The emptying of a cavity, such as the stomach, by means of a siphon.

Sip·ple's syndrome (sĭp'əlz) *n.* An inherited disorder characterized by pheochromocytoma, medullary thyroid carcinoma, and neural tumors.

sis·o·mi·cin sulfate (sĭs'ə-mī'sĭn) *n.* An antibiotic produced by the actinomycete *Micromonospora inyoensis* that has a spectrum of activity similar to that of gentamicin.

Sis·ter Jo·seph's nodule (sĭs'tər jō'səfs) *n.* A nodule in the umbilical region associated with a malignant metastatic intra-abdominal tumor.

Sister Ken·ny's treatment (kĕn'ēz) *n.* Treatment of poliomyelitis by wrapping affected parts with warm moist cloth, and later passively exercising the paralyzed muscles.

site (sīt) *n.* A place; a location.

si·to·ma·ni·a (sī'tə-mā'nē-ə, -mān'yə) *n.* An abnormal craving for food.

si·to·pho·bi·a (sī'tə-fō'bē-ə) *n.* An abnormal aversion to food.

si·to·tax·is (sī'tə-tăk'sĭs) *n.* See **sitotropism.**

si·to·tox·in (sī'tə-tŏk'sĭn) *n.* A food poison, especially one developing in grain.

si·tot·ro·pism (sī-tŏt'rə-pĭz'əm) *n.* The turning of living cells toward or away from food.

si·tus (sī'təs) *n., pl.* **situs.** Position, especially normal or original position, as of a body organ or part.

situs in·ver·sus (ĭn-vûr'səs) *n.* A congenital condition in which the organs of the viscera are transposed through the sagittal plane so that the heart, for example, is on the right side of the body.

sitz bath (sĭts, zĭts) *n.* **1.** A device shaped like a chair in which one bathes in a sitting position, immersing only the hips and buttocks. **2.** A bath taken in such a device especially for therapeutic reasons.

sixth cranial nerve *n.* See **abducent nerve.**

sixth disease *n.* See **exanthema subitum.**

sixth-year molar *n.* The first permanent molar tooth.

Sjö·gren's syndrome (shœ'grĕnz) *n.* A syndrome occurring in menopausal women, characterized by keratoconjunctivitis sicca, dryness of mucous membranes, telangiectasias or purpuric spots on the face, and bilateral parotid enlargement; it is often associated with rheumatoid arthritis, Raynaud's phenomenon, and dental caries.

skat·ole (skăt'ōl, -ôl) *n.* A white crystalline organic compound formed in the intestine by the bacterial decomposition of tryptophan and having a strong fecal odor, present in feces.

ska·tox·yl (skă-tŏk'sĭl) *n.* An oxidation product of skatole formed in the intestine and excreted in the urine in cases of intestinal disease.

skel·e·tal extension (skĕl'ĭ-tl) *n.* See **skeletal traction.**

skeletal muscle *n.* A muscle that connects at either or both extremities with a bone and consists of elongated, multinucleated, transversely striated, skeletal muscle fibers, together with connective tissues, blood vessels, and nerves.

skeletal traction *n.* Traction on a bone structure by means of a pin or wire surgically inserted into the bone.

skel·e·ton (skĕl'ĭ-tn) *n.* **1.** The internal structure composed of bone and cartilage that protects and supports the soft organs, tissues, and other parts of the body. **2.** All the bones of the body taken collectively.

ski·as·co·py (skī-ăs'kə-pē) *n.* See **retinoscopy.** — **ski'a·scope'** (skī'ə-skōp') *n.*

skin (skĭn) *n.* The membranous tissue forming the external protective covering or integument, especially the epidermis and dermis. — *v.* **skinned, skin·ning, skins.** To bruise, cut, or injure the skin of. — **skin'less** *adj.*

skin dose *n.* The quantity of radiation delivered to the skin surface or absorbed in the skin.

skin tag *n.* An outgrowth of epidermal and dermal fibrovascular tissue.

skin test *n.* A test for detecting an allergy or infectious disease, performed by means of a patch test, a scratch test, or an intracutaneous injection of an allergen or extract of the disease-causing organism.

skin traction *n.* Traction on an extremity by means of adhesive tape or another type of strapping applied to the limb.

skull (skŭl) *n.* The bony or cartilaginous framework of the head, made up of the bones of the braincase and face; cranium.

skull·cap (skŭl'kăp') *n.* See **calvaria.**

SLE *abbr.* systemic lupus erythematosus

sleep (slēp) *n.* A natural periodic state of rest for the mind and body, in which the eyes usually close and consciousness is completely or partially lost, so that there is a decrease in bodily movement and responsiveness to external stimuli. During sleep the brain undergoes a characteristic cycle of brain-wave activity that includes intervals of dreaming. — *v.* **slept** (slĕpt), **sleep·ing, sleeps.** To be in the state of sleep.

sleep apnea *n.* Apnea caused by upper airway obstruction during sleep, associated with frequent awakening and often with daytime sleepiness.

sleep-in·duced apnea (slēp'ĭn-dōōst', -dyōōst') *n.* Apnea resulting from failure of the respiratory center to stimulate adequate respiration during sleep.

sleeping sickness *n.* See **encephalitis lethargica.**

sleep paralysis *n.* A condition in which, upon waking, a person is aware of the surroundings but is unable to move.

sleep·walk·ing (slēp'wô'kĭng) *n.* The act of walking or performing another activity associated with wakefulness while asleep or in a sleeplike state. — **sleep′walk′** v. — **sleep′walk′er** n.

slid·ing flap (slī′dĭng) n. A rectangular flap raised in an elastic area with its free end adjacent to a defect, the defect being covered by stretching the flap longitudinally until the end comes over it.

sling (slĭng) n. A supporting bandage or suspensory device, especially a loop suspended from the neck and supporting the flexed forearm.

slipped disk (slĭpd) n. Protrusion of a part of an intervertebral disk through the fibrocartilage, occurring usually in the lower lumbar region and often causing back pain or sciatica.

slip·ping rib (slĭp′ĭng) n. A subluxation of a rib cartilage with costochondral separation.

slit·lamp (slĭt′lămp′) n. See **biomicroscope**.

slow infection n. An infection having a long incubation period, as that caused by a slow virus or by a prion.

slow-reacting factor of anaphylaxis n. See **slow-reacting substance of anaphylaxis**.

slow-reacting substance of anaphylaxis n. A substance released in anaphylactic shock that produces slower and more prolonged contraction of muscle than does histamine.

slow virus n. Any of a group of animal viruses that cause diseases having an unusually slow progressive course, as Creutzfeldt–Jakob disease.

slow virus disease n. A disease caused by a slow virus.

small intestine n. The narrow, winding, upper part of the intestine where digestion is completed and nutrients are absorbed by the blood. It extends from the pylorus to the cecum and consists of the duodenum, the jejunum, and the ileum.

small·pox (smôl′pŏks′) n. An acute, highly infectious, often fatal disease caused by a poxvirus and characterized by high fever and aches with subsequent widespread eruption of papules that blister, produce pus, and form scabs that leave permanent pockmarks.

smallpox vaccine n. A vaccine containing vaccinia virus suspensions prepared from cutaneous vaccinial lesions of calves, inoculated subcutaneously to immunize against smallpox.

smallpox virus n. See **variola virus**.

smear (smēr) n. A sample, as of blood or bacterial cells, spread thinly on a slide and usually stained for microscopic examination or applied to the surface of a culture medium.

smear test n. See **Pap test**.

smeg·ma (smĕg′ma) n. A sebaceous secretion, especially the whitish cheesy secretion that collects under the prepuce of the penis or around the clitoris.

smell (smĕl) v. **smelled** or **smelt** (smĕlt), **smell·ing**, **smells**. To perceive the scent of something by means of the olfactory nerves. — n. The sense by which odors are perceived; the olfactory sense.

smelling salts pl.n. Any of various preparations of ammonium carbonate and perfume, sniffed as a restorative or stimulant especially to relieve faintness and headache.

Smith′s fracture (smĭths) n. A bone fracture of the radius of the wrist in which the lower fragment is displaced forward.

Smith′s operation n. A surgical technique for removing a cataract within its capsule.

smok·er′s cough (smō′karz) n. A rough, dry cough caused by excessive smoking of tobacco.

smooth diet n. A diet containing little roughage.

smooth muscle n. Muscle tissue that contracts without voluntary control, having fine myofibrils but lacking transverse striations and found in the walls of internal organs, blood vessels, and hair follicles.

snap (snăp) n. A short sharp sound; a click. Used especially of cardiac sounds.

snare (snâr) n. A surgical instrument with a wire loop controlled by a mechanism in the handle, used to remove growths, such as polyps.

sneeze (snēz) v. **sneezed, sneez·ing, sneez·es**. To expel air forcibly through the mouth and nose in an explosive, spasmodic involuntary action resulting chiefly from irritation of the nasal mucous membrane. — n. The act or an instance of sneezing.

Snel·len chart (snĕl′an) n. A chart for testing visual acuity, usually consisting of letters, numbers, or pictures printed in lines of decreasing size which a patient is asked to read or identify at a fixed distance.

Snel·len′s test types (snĕl′anz) pl.n. Letters used in testing the acuity of distant vision; the letters vary in size so that each subtends a visual angle of 5 minutes at a particular distance.

Snellen test n. A test for visual acuity using a Snellen chart.

snore (snôr) v. **snored, snor·ing, snores**. To breathe during sleep with harsh, snorting noises caused by vibration of the soft palate.

snot (snŏt) n. Nasal mucus; phlegm.

snout reflex n. Pouting or pursing of the lips caused by light tapping of the closed lips near the midline, seen in defective pyramidal innervation of facial musculature.

snow blindness (snō) n. A usually temporary loss of vision and inflammation of the conjunctiva and cornea caused by exposure to bright sunlight and ultraviolet rays reflected from snow or ice. — **snow′-blind′, snow′-blind′ed** adj.

snow·shoe hare virus (snō′shoo′) n. An arbovirus that is most commonly found in North America and that causes fever, severe headache, and nausea in humans.

snuff (snŭf) v. **snuffed, snuff·ing, snuff** something audibly through the A medicated powder inh into the nose.

snuf·fle (snŭf′al) noisily, as throu act of snuffling. piration, especiall times due to conge

soap (sōp) n. A cleans

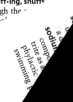

ture of the sodium salts of various fatty acids of natural oils and fats. — **soap** v.

Soa·ve operation (swä'vä, -vě) n. Endorectal pull-through for treatment of congenital megacolon.

so·cial disease (sō'shəl) n. A sexually transmitted disease; a venereal disease.

so·cial·i·za·tion (sō'shə-lĭ-zā'shən) n. The process of learning interpersonal and interactional skills that are in conformity with the values of one's society. — **so'cial·ize** (-shə-līz') v.

so·cial·ized medicine (sō'shə-līzd') n. A system for providing medical care for all at a nominal cost by means of government regulation of health services and subsidies derived from taxation.

so·ci·o·path (sō'sē-ə-păth', -shē-) n. A person affected with a personality disorder marked by aggressive, antisocial behavior. — **so'ci·o·path'ic** adj.

so·ci·op·a·thy (sō'sē-ŏp'ə-thē, -shē-) n. The behavioral pattern exhibited by persons with an antisocial personality disorder.

sock·et (sŏk'ĭt) n. **1.** The concave part of a joint that receives the articular end of a bone. **2.** A hollow or concavity into which a part, such as the eye or a tooth, fits.

so·di·um (sō'dē-əm) n. A soft, light, highly reactive metallic element with atomic number 11 that is naturally abundant in combined forms, especially in common salt. Sodium is an important positive ion in extracellular body fluids and is widely used in medical preparations.

sodium bicarbonate n. A white crystalline compound used therapeutically, usually as an antacid.

sodium borate n. A crystalline compound that is the sodium salt of boric acid and is used as a mild astringent in lotions, gargles, and mouthwashes.

sodium chloride n. Common or table salt, used as a food preservative and seasoning.

sodium cyclamate n. An artificially prepared salt of cyclamic acid, formerly used as a low-calorie sweetener but now banned because of the possible carcinogenic effects of its metabolic products.

sodium fluoride n. A colorless crystalline salt used in fluoridation of water, in treatment of tooth decay, and as an insecticide and a disinfectant.

sodium nitrite n. A white crystalline compound used to lower systemic blood pressure, to relieve local vasomotor spasms, to relax bronchial and intestinal spasms, and as an antidote for cyanide poisoning.

sodium ni·tro·prus·side (nī'trō-prŭs'īd') n. A reddish brown powder or crystalline agent administered intravenously as a treatment for acute hypertension.

sodium peroxide n. A yellowish-white powder used medically as a germicide, an antiseptic, and a disinfectant.

sodium thiosulfate n. A translucent crystalline compound used in conjunction with sodium nitrite as an antidote in cyanide poisoning, as a prophylactic agent against ringworm infections in pools and baths, and as a means to

measure the body's extracellular fluid volume.

sod·o·my (sŏd'ə-mē) n. **1.** Anal copulation of one male with another. **2.** Anal or oral copulation with a member of the opposite sex. **3.** Copulation with an animal. — **sod'o·mize'** (-mīz') v.

soft diet n. A normal diet limited to soft, easily digestible foods.

soft palate n. The movable fold, consisting of muscular fibers enclosed in mucous membrane, that is suspended from the rear of the hard palate and closes off the nasal cavity from the oral cavity during swallowing or sucking.

soft spot n. See **fontanel.**

soft tubercle n. A tubercle with caseous necrosis.

soft wart n. See **skin tag.**

sol (sŏl, sōl) n. A colloidal dispersion of a solid in a liquid.

so·lar cheilitis (sō'lər) n. Mucosal atrophy, crusting, and fissuring of the vermilion border of the lips in older persons, resulting from chronic exposure to sunlight.

solar plexus n. See **celiac plexus** (sense 1).

sol·a·tion (sô-lā'shən,) n. Transformation of a gel into a sol, as by melting gelatin.

sole (sōl) n. The underside of the foot.

so·le·us muscle (sō'lē-əs) n. A muscle with origin from the posterior surface of the head and shaft of the fibula, the medial margin of the tibia, and the tendinous arch passing over the popliteal vessels, with insertion into the tuberosity of the calcaneus, and whose action causes plantar flexion of the foot.

sol·id (sŏl'ĭd) adj. **1.** Of definite shape and volume; not liquid or gaseous. **2.** Firm or compact in substance. **3.** Having no internal cavity or hollow. — n. **1.** A solid substance, body, or tissue. **2.** Food that is relatively firm in substance or that must be chewed before swallowing.

sol·i·tar·y follicle (sŏl'ĭ-tĕr'ē) n. Any of the minute collections of lymphoid tissue in the mucosa of the small and large intestines, especially numerous in the cecum and in the appendix.

sol·u·bil·i·ty test (sŏl'yə-bĭl'ĭ-tē) n. A screening test for sickle-cell hemoglobin.

sol·u·bi·lize (sŏl'yə-bə-līz') v. **-lized, -liz·ing, -liz·es.** To make substances such as fats and lipids soluble in water, as by the action of a detergent.

sol·u·ble (sŏl'yə-bəl) adj. Capable of being dissolved, especially easily dissolved.

sol·ute (sŏl'yōot, sō'lōot) n. A substance dissolved in another substance, usually the component of a solution present in the lesser amount.

so·lu·tion (sə-lōo'shən) n. **1.** A homogeneous mixture of two or more substances, which may be solids, liquids, gases, or a combination of these. **2.** The state of being dissolved. **3.** In pharmacology, a liquid preparation containing a dissolved substance, especially an aqueous solution of a nonvolatile substance. **4.** Termination of a disease by a crisis. **5.** A break, cut, or laceration of the solid tissues.

sol·vent (sŏl'vənt) adj. Capable of dissolving another substance. — n. **1.** A substance in which another substance is dissolved, forming a solution. **2.** A substance, usually a liquid, capable of dissolving another substance.

so·ma (sō′mə) *n., pl.* **-mas** or **-ma·ta** (-mə-tə). **1.** The entire body of an organism, exclusive of the germ cells. **2.** The axial part of a body. **3.** The body of a person as contrasted with the mind or psyche. **4.** See **cell body.**

so·ma·tal·gi·a (sō′mə-tăl′jē-ə, -jə) *n.* Pain in the body due to organic causes.

so·ma·tas·the·ni·a (sō′mə-tăs-thē′nē-ə) or **so·mas·the·ni·a** (sō′măs-) *n.* A condition of chronic physical weakness and fatigue.

so·ma·tes·the·sia (sō′mə-tĕs-thē′zhə) or **so·mes·the·sia** (sō′mĭs-) *n.* Consciousness of one's body; awareness of body sensation. — **so′ma·tes·thet′ic** (-thĕt′ĭk) *adj.*

so·mat·ic (sō-măt′ĭk) *adj.* **1.** Of, relating to, or affecting the body, especially as distinguished from a body part, the mind, or the environment; corporeal or physical. **2.** Of or relating to the wall of the body cavity, especially as distinguished from the head, limbs, or viscera. **3.** Relating to the vegetative, as distinguished from the generative, functions. **4.** Of or relating to a somatic cell or the somatoplasm. — **so·mat′i·cal·ly** *adv.*

somatic antigen *n.* An antigen located in the body of a bacterium.

somatic cell *n.* Any cell other than a germ cell.

somatic death *n.* Death of the entire body.

somatic delusion *n.* A delusion that a part of one's body has been injured or altered in some way.

somatic motor neuron *n.* A motor neuron forming a direct synapse with striated muscle fibers via a motor endplate.

somatic mutation *n.* Mutation occurring in the somatic cells as opposed to the germ cells.

somatic mutation theory of cancer *n.* The theory that cancer is caused by a mutation or mutations in the body cells, rather than germ cells, especially by nonlethal mutations associated with increased proliferation of the mutant cells.

somatic nerve *n.* Any of the nerves of sensation or motion.

somatic swallow *n.* An adult or mature swallowing pattern, marked by muscular contractions that appear to be under control at a subconscious level.

so·ma·ti·za·tion (sō′mə-tĭ-zā′shən) *n.* In psychiatry, the conversion of anxiety into physical symptoms.

somatization disorder *n.* A disorder characterized by an individual's seeking help for and acquiring a complicated medical history of multiple physical symptoms and complaints, but having no detectable organic disorder or injury.

so·mat·o·chrome (sō-măt′ə-krōm′, sō′mə-tə-) *n.* A nerve cell in which there is an abundance of cytoplasm completely surrounding the nucleus.

so·mat·o·form disorder (sō-măt′ə-fôrm′, sō′mə-tə-) *n.* Any of a group of disorders characterized by physical symptoms representing specific disorders for which there is no organic basis or known

physiological cause, but for which there is presumed to be a psychological basis.

so·mat·o·mam·mo·tro·pin (sō-măt′ə-măm′ə-trō′pĭn, sō′mə-tə-) *n.* A peptide hormone closely related to growth hormone in its biological properties but produced by the normal placenta and by certain neoplasms.

so·ma·top·a·thy (sō′mə-tŏp′ə-thē) *n.* Disease of the body.

so·mat·o·plasm (sō-măt′ə-plăz′əm, sō′mə-tə-) *n.* **1.** The entirety of specialized protoplasm, other than germ plasm, constituting the body. **2.** The protoplasm of a somatic cell. — **so′ma·to·plas′tic** (sō′mə-tə-plăs′tĭk) *adj.*

so·mat·o·pleure (sō-măt′ə-plŏŏr′, sō′mə-tə-) *n.* A complex sheet of embryonic cells formed by association of part of the mesoderm with the ectoderm and developing as the internal body wall. — **so·mat′o·pleu′ral** (-plŏŏr′əl), **so·mat′o·pleu′ric** (-plŏŏr′ĭk) *adj.*

so·mat·o·psy·cho·sis (sō-măt′ə-sī-kō′sĭs, sō′mə-tə-) *n.* An emotional disorder associated with an organic disease.

so·mat·o·stat·in (sō-măt′ə-stăt′n, sō′mə-tə-) *n.* A hormone produced in the hypothalamus that inhibits the release of somatotropin by the pituitary gland.

so·mat·o·stat·i·no·ma (sō-măt′ə-stăt′n-ō′mə, sō′mə-tə-) *n.* A somatostatin-secreting tumor of the pancreatic islets.

so·mat·o·ther·a·py (sō-măt′ə-thĕr′ə-pē, sō′mə-tə-) *n.* **1.** Therapy directed at bodily or physical disorders. **2.** Therapy employing chemical or physical methods, especially the treatment of mental illness by such means as drugs, shock therapy, and lobotomy.

so·ma·tot·o·py (sō′mə-tŏt′ə-pē) *n.* The correspondence of receptors in regions or parts of the body via respective nerve fibers to specific functional areas of the cerebral cortex. — **so·mat′o·top′ic** (sə-măt′ə-tŏp′ĭk, -trō′pĭk, sō′mə-tə-) *adj.*

so·mat·o·troph (sō-măt′ə-trŏf′, -trōf′, sō′mə-tə-) *n.* A cell of the anterior lobe of the pituitary gland that produces somatotropin.

so·mat·o·tro·pin (sə-măt′ə-trō′pĭn, sō′mə-tə-) or **so·mat·o·tro·phin** (-trō′fĭn) *n.* A polypeptide hormone secreted by the anterior lobe of the pituitary gland that promotes growth of the body and that influences the metabolism of proteins, carbohydrates, and lipids.

so·mat·o·type (sō-măt′ə-tīp′, sō′mə-tə-) *n.* The structure or build of a person, especially to the extent to which it exhibits the characteristics of an ectomorph, an endomorph, or a mesomorph. — **so·mat′o·typ′ic** (-tĭp′ĭk) *adj.*

so·mite (sō′mīt′) *n.* A segmental mass of mesoderm in the vertebrate embryo, occurring in pairs along the notochord and developing into muscles and vertebrae.

som·nam·bu·lism (sŏm-năm′byə-lĭz′əm) *n.* See **sleepwalking.** — **som·nam′bu·list** *n.* — **som·nam′bu·lis′tic** *adj.*

som·ni·fa·cient (sŏm′nə-fā′shənt) *adj.* Tending to

produce sleep; soporific. — som·ni·fa'cient n.

som·nil·o·quy (sŏm-nĭl'ə-kwē) or som·nil·o·quism (-kwĭz'əm) n. The act or habit of talking in one's sleep. — som·nil'o·quist n.

som·nip·a·thy (sŏm-nĭp'ə-thē) n. A disorder of sleep.

som·no·lence (sŏm'nə-ləns) n. 1. A state of drowsiness; sleepiness. 2. A condition of semiconsciousness approaching coma.

som·no·lent (sŏm'nə-lənt) adj. 1. Drowsy; sleepy. 2. Inducing or tending to induce sleep. 3. In a condition of incomplete sleep; semicomatose.

So·mo·gyi effect or So·mo·gyi phenomenon (sō'mō-jē) n. In diabetes, reactive hyperglycemia following hypoglycemia.

Somogyi unit n. A measure of the level of activity of amylase in blood serum.

son·co·gene (sŏn'kə-jēn, sŏng'-) n. One of a number of genes on specific chromosomes that can suppress the action of oncogenes.

son·i·ca·tion (sŏn'ĭ-kā'shən) n. The process of dispersing, disrupting, or inactivating biological materials, such as viruses, by sound-wave energy.

Son·ne bacillus (sŏn'ə) n. A gram-negative bacterium Shigella sonnei that causes a mild form of dysentery in adults and children.

son·o·gram (sŏn'ə-grăm', sō'nə-) n. An image, as of an unborn fetus or an internal body organ, produced by ultrasonography.

son·o·graph (sŏn'ə-grăf', sō'nə-) n. 1. See ultrasonograph. 2. See sonogram. — so·nog'ra·pher (sə-nŏg'rə-fər) n. — son'o·graph'ic adj.

so·nog·ra·phy (sə-nŏg'rə-fē) n. See ultrasonography.

so·por (sō'pər, -pôr') n. A deep, lethargic, or unnatural sleep.

sop·o·rif·ic (sŏp'ə-rĭf'ĭk, sō'pə-) adj. 1. Inducing or tending to induce sleep. 2. Sleepy; drowsy.

sor·bi·tol (sôr'bĭ-tôl', -tōl') n. A white, sweetish, crystalline alcohol found in berries and fruits or prepared synthetically, used as a flavoring agent, a sugar substitute, and a moisturizer.

sore (sôr) n. An open skin lesion, wound, or ulcer. — adj. Painful to the touch. — sore'ness n.

sore throat n. Any of various inflammations of the tonsils, pharynx, or larynx characterized by pain in swallowing.

s.o.s. abbr. Latin. si opus sit (if needed)

souf·fle (sōō'fəl, sōō'flə) n. A soft blowing sound heard on auscultation.

sound[1] (sound) n. 1. Vibrations transmitted through an elastic material or a solid, liquid, or gas, capable of being detected by the human ear. 2. Transmitted vibrations of any frequency. 3. A distinctive noise. — v. sound·ed, sound·ing, sounds. To auscultate.

sound[2] adj. 1. Free from defect, decay, or damage; in good condition. 2. Free from disease or injury.

sound[3] n. An instrument used to examine or explore body cavities, as for foreign bodies or other abnormalities, or to dilate strictures in them. — v. sound·ed, sound·ing, sounds. To probe a body cavity with a sound.

source amnesia (sôrs, sōrs) n. Memory loss that makes it impossible to recall the origin of the memory of a given event.

South African tick-bite fever n. A typhuslike fever of South Africa caused by Rickettsia rickettsii, and usually characterized by primary eschar and regional adenitis, stiffness, and maculopapular rash on the fifth day, often with severe symptoms of the central nervous system.

South American trypanosomiasis n. A form of trypanosomiasis caused by Trypanosoma cruzi and transmitted by certain species of assassin bugs. In its acute form it causes swelling of the skin at the site of entry with regional lymph node enlargement; in its chronic form it causes various conditions, commonly cardiomyopathy.

South·ern blot analysis (sŭth'ərn) n. An electrophoretic procedure used to separate and identify DNA sequences.

space (spās) n. A particular area, extent, or cavity of the body.

space medicine n. The medical science that is concerned with the biological, physiological, and psychological effects of space flight on humans.

space sickness n. Motion sickness caused by sustained weightlessness during space flight, usually accompanied by disturbance of the inner ear. — space'sick' (spās'sĭk') adj.

spar·ga·no·ma (spär'gə-nō'mə) n. A localized mass resulting from sparganosis.

spar·ga·no·sis (spär'gə-nō'sĭs) n., pl. -ses (-sēz). Infection with the plerocercoid of certain tapeworms, usually in a dermal sore resulting from direct contact with the flesh of an infected host.

spar·ing action (spâr'ĭng) n. The manner in which the presence of a nonessential nutritive component in the diet lowers the requirement for an essential component.

spasm (spăz'əm) n. 1. A sudden involuntary contraction of a muscle or group of muscles. 2. A muscle spasm.

spas·mod·ic (spăz-mŏd'ĭk) adj. 1. Relating to, affected by, or having the character of a spasm; convulsive. 2. Happening intermittently; fitful. — spas·mod'i·cal·ly adv.

spas·tic (spăs'tĭk) adj. 1. Relating to or affected by spasm. 2. Relating to spastic paralysis. — spas'ti·cal·ly adv.

spastic abasia n. Abasia due to spastic contraction of the leg muscles.

spastic gait n. A gait characterized by stiffness of legs, feet, and toes.

spas·tic·i·ty (spă-stĭs'ĭ-tē) n. 1. A spastic state or condition. 2. Spastic paralysis.

spay (spā) v. spayed, spay·ing, spays. To surgically remove the ovaries of an animal.

spe·cial·ist (spĕsh'ə-lĭst) n. A physician whose practice is limited to a particular branch of medicine or surgery, especially one who is certified by a board of physicians.

spe·cial·i·za·tion (spĕsh'ə-lĭ-zā'shən) n. 1. The act of specializing. 2. A specialty. 3. Adaptation, as of an organ or organism, to a specific function or environment. **4.** See **differentiation** (sense 1).

spe·cial·ize (spĕsh′ə-līz′) v. **-ized, -iz·ing, -iz·es. 1.** To limit one's professional attention to a particular specialty or subject area. **2.** To adapt to a particular function or environment.

spe·cial sense (spĕsh′əl) n. Any of the five senses related to the organs of sight, hearing, smell, taste, and touch.

spe·cial·ty (spĕsh′əl-tē) n. A branch of medicine or surgery in which a physician specializes; the field or practice of a specialist.

spe·ci·a·tion (spē′shē-ā′shən, -sē-) n. The evolutionary formation of new biological species, usually by the division of a single species into two or more genetically distinct ones.

spe·cif·ic dynamic action (spĭ-sĭf′ĭk) n. An increase in the production of heat caused by the ingestion of food, especially proteins.

specific gravity n. The ratio of the mass of a solid or liquid to the mass of an equal volume of distilled water at 4°C or of a gas to an equal volume of air or hydrogen under prescribed conditions of temperature and pressure.

specific immunity n. Immunity against a specific antigen or disease.

specific opsonin n. Opsonin formed in response to stimulation by a specific antigen.

specific reaction n. A phenomenon produced by an agent identical with or immunologically related to an agent that has altered the capacity of a certain tissue to react.

spec·i·men (spĕs′ə-mən) n. A sample, as of tissue, blood, or urine, used for analysis and diagnosis.

SPECT abbr. single photon emission computed tomography

spec·ta·cles (spĕk′tə-kəlz) n. A pair of lenses mounted in a frame and used to correct refractive errors of the eyes or to protect the eyes; glasses.

spec·ti·no·my·cin (spĕk′tə-nō-mī′sĭn) n. A broad-spectrum antibiotic obtained from a species of gram-negative bacteria (Streptomyces spectabilis) or produced synthetically, used especially in the treatment of penicillin-resistant gonorrhea.

spec·trin (spĕk′trĭn) n. A contractile protein of high molecular weight that is a component of a network in the membrane of red blood cells, giving the cells flexibility.

spec·trum (spĕk′trəm) n., pl. **-trums** or **-tra** (-trə). **1.** The group of pathogenic organisms against which an antibiotic or other antibacterial agent is effective. **2.** The distribution of a characteristic of a physical system or phenomenon, especially the distribution of energy emitted by a radiant source arranged in order of wavelengths.

spec·u·lum (spĕk′yə-ləm) n., pl. **-lums** or **-la** (-lə). **1.** A mirror or polished metal plate used as a reflector in optical instruments. **2.** An instrument for dilating the opening of a body cavity.

speculum forceps n. A type of tubular forceps for use through a speculum.

speech (spēch) n. **1.** The faculty or act of expressing thoughts, feelings, or perceptions by the artic-

ulation of words. **2.** Vocal communication.

speech bulb n. A prosthetic speech aid used to close a cleft or other opening in the hard or soft palate, or to replace absent tissue necessary for the production of good speech.

speech pathology n. The science concerned with the diagnosis and treatment of functional and organic speech defects and disorders.

speech therapy n. Treatment of speech defects and disorders, especially through use of exercises and audio-visual aids that develop new speech habits.
— **speech therapist** n.

sperm (spûrm) n., pl. **sperm** or **sperms. 1.** A male gamete or reproductive cell; a spermatozoon. **2.** Semen.

sper·ma·cyt·ic seminoma (spûr′mə-sĭt′ĭk) n. A relatively slow-growing, locally invasive type of testicular seminoma that does not metastasize.

sper·mat·ic (spər-măt′ĭk) adj. **1.** Of, relating to, or resembling sperm. **2.** Containing, conveying, or producing sperm.

spermatic cord n. A cordlike structure, consisting of the vas deferens and its accompanying arteries, veins, nerves, and lymphatic vessels, that passes from the abdominal cavity into the scrotum and to the back of the testicle.

spermatic duct n. See **vas deferens.**

sper·ma·tid (spûr′mə-tĭd) n. Any of the four haploid cells formed by meiosis that develop into spermatozoa without further division.

sper·mat·o·blast (spər-măt′ə-blăst′, spûr′mə-tə-) n. See **spermatogonium.**

sper·mat·o·cele (spər-măt′ə-sēl′, spûr′mə-tə-) n. A cystic lesion of the epididymus or rete testis, resulting from obstruction and containing secretions from the testis.

sper·mat·o·cyte (spər-măt′ə-sīt′, spûr′mə-tə-) n. A diploid cell that undergoes meiosis to form four spermatids. A primary spermatocyte divides into two secondary spermatocytes, which divide to form the spermatids.

sper·mat·o·cy·to·gen·e·sis (spər-măt′ə-sī′tə-jĕn′ĭ-sĭs, spûr′mə-tə-) n. See **spermatogenesis.**

sper·mat·o·gen·e·sis (spər-măt′ə-jĕn′ĭ-sĭs, spûr′-mə-tə-) n. Formation and development of spermatozoa by meiosis and spermiogenesis. — **sper·mat′o·ge·net′ic** (-jə-nĕt′ĭk), **sper·mat·o·gen′ic** (-jĕn′ĭk) adj.

sper·mat·o·go·ni·um (spər-măt′ə-gō′nē-əm, spûr′-mə-tə-) n., pl. **-ni·a.** Any of the male germ cells that are the progenitors of spermatocytes.

sper·mat·o·zo·on (spər-măt′ə-zō′ŏn′, -ən, spûr′-mə-tə-) n., pl. **-zo·a** (-zō′ə). The mature male gamete or sex cell that consists of a cylindrical nucleated cell with a short neck and a thin motile tail; sperm.

sper·ma·tu·ri·a (spûr′mə-tŏŏr′ē-ə, -tyŏŏr′-) n. See **semenuria.**

sper·mi·cide (spûr′mĭ-sīd′) n. An agent that kills spermatozoa, especially one used as a contraceptive. — **sper′mi·cid′al** (-sīd′l) adj.

sper·mi·dine (spûr′mĭ-dēn′) n. A polyamine compound found in ribosomes and living tissues and having various metabolic functions. It was originally isolated from semen.

sper·mi·duct (spûr′mĭ-dŭkt′) *n.* **1.** See vas deferens. **2.** See ejaculatory duct.

sper·mi·o·gen·e·sis (spûr′mē-ō-jĕn′ĭ-sĭs) *n.* The stage of spermatogenesis during which spermatids are transformed into spermatozoa.

SPF *abbr.* sun protection factor

S phase *n.* The phase of the mitotic cycle during which DNA synthesis occurs.

sphe·noid (sfē′noid′) *n.* The sphenoid bone. — *adj.* **1.** Of or relating to the sphenoid bone. **2.** Wedge-shaped. — **sphe·noi′dal** (-noid′l) *adj.*

sphenoidal spine *n.* A rearward and downward projection from the greater wing of the sphenoid bone on either side.

sphenoid bone *n.* A compound bone with winglike processes, situated at the base of the skull.

sphenoid crest *n.* A vertical ridge in the midline of the anterior surface of the sphenoid bone that articulates with the perpendicular plate of the ethmoid bone.

sphe·noid·i·tis (sfē′noi-dī′tĭs) *n.* **1.** Inflammation of the sphenoidal sinus. **2.** Necrosis of the sphenoid bone.

sphe·noid·ot·o·my (sfē′noi-dŏt′ə-mē) *n.* Surgical creation of an opening in the anterior wall of the sphenoidal sinus.

sphere (sfēr) *n.* A ball-shaped or globular body. — **spher′al** (sfēr′əl) *adj.*

spher·i·cal (sfēr′ĭ-kəl, sfĕr′-) *adj.* Having the shape of or approximating a sphere; globular. — **spher′i·cal·ness** *n.*

spherical aberration *n.* A blurred image that occurs when light from the margin of a lens or mirror with a spherical surface comes to a shorter focus than light from the central portion.

spherical lens *n.* A lens in which all refracting surfaces are spherical.

spher·o·cyte (sfēr′ə-sīt′, sfĕr′-) *n.* A small spherical red blood cell, characteristic of hereditary spherocytosis and of certain hemolytic anemias. — **spher′o·cyt′ic** (-sĭt′ĭk) *adj.*

spher·o·cy·to·sis (sfēr′ō-sī-tō′sĭs, sfĕr′-) *n.* The presence of spherocytes in the blood.

spher·oid (sfēr′oid′, sfĕr′-) or **sphe·roi·dal** (sfĭ-roid′l) *adj.* Having a generally spherical shape. — **spher′oid′** *n.*

spheroid joint *n.* See ball-and-socket joint.

sphinc·ter (sfĭngk′tər) *n.* A ringlike muscle that normally maintains constriction of a body passage or orifice and that relaxes as required by normal physiological functioning. — **sphinc′ter·al, sphinc·ter′ic** (-tĕr′ĭk) *adj.*

sphinc·ter·ec·to·my (sfĭngk′tə-rĕk′tə-mē) *n.* **1.** Surgical excision of part of the pupillary border of the iris. **2.** Excision of a sphincter muscle.

sphinc·ter·i·tis (sfĭngk′tə-rī′tĭs) *n.* Inflammation of a sphincter.

sphinc·ter·ol·y·sis (sfĭngk′tə-rŏl′ĭ-sĭs) *n.* An operation for freeing the iris from the cornea in an anterior adhesion.

sphinc·ter·o·plas·ty (sfĭngk′tə-rə-plăs′tē) *n.* Reparative or plastic surgery of a sphincter muscle.

sphinc·ter·ot·o·my (sfĭngk′tə-rŏt′ə-mē) *n.* Surgical incision into a sphincter muscle.

sphin·go·lip·id (sfĭng′gō-lĭp′ĭd, -lī′pĭd) *n.* Any of a group of lipids, such as sphingomyelins or cerebrosides, that yield sphingosine or its derivatives upon hydrolysis.

sphin·go·lip·i·do·sis (sfĭng′gō-lĭp′ĭ-dō′sĭs) *n.* Any of various diseases, such as gangliosidosis or Gaucher's disease, characterized by abnormal sphingolipid metabolism.

sphin·go·my·e·lin (sfĭng′gō-mī′ə-lĭn) *n.* Any of a group of phospholipids that are found especially in nerve tissue such as the brain and spinal cord and yield sphingosine, choline, a fatty acid, and phosphoric acid upon hydrolysis.

sphin·go·sine (sfĭng′gə-sēn′) *n.* A basic, long-chain, unsaturated amino alcohol, found combined with lipids in the brain and in nerve tissue.

sphyg·mo·gram (sfĭg′mə-grăm′) *n.* The record or tracing produced by a sphygmograph.

sphyg·mo·graph (sfĭg′mə-grăf′) *n.* An instrument for tracing the form, strength, and variations of the arterial pulse. — **sphyg′mo·graph′ic** *adj.* — **sphyg·mog′ra·phy** (-mŏg′rə-fē) *n.*

sphyg·mo·ma·nom·e·ter (sfĭg′mō-mă-nŏm′ĭ-tər) or **sphyg·mom·e·ter** (sfĭg-mŏm′ĭ-tər) *n.* An instrument for measuring blood pressure in the arteries, especially one consisting of a pressure gauge and a rubber cuff that wraps around the upper arm and inflates to constrict the arteries. — **sphyg′mo·man′o·met′ric** (-măn′ə-mĕt′rĭk) *adj.* — **sphyg′mo·ma·nom′e·try** *n.*

sphyg·mos·co·py (sfĭg-mŏs′kə-pē) *n.* Examination of the pulse.

sphy·rec·to·my (sfī-rĕk′tə-mē) *n.* Surgical removal of the malleus.

sphy·rot·o·my (sfī-rŏt′ə-mē) *n.* Surgical section of a part of the malleus.

spi·ca bandage (spī′kə) *n.* Successive strips of material applied to the body and the first part of a limb, or to the hand and a finger, that overlap slightly so as to resemble an ear of wheat.

spic·ule (spĭk′yōōl) or **spic·u·la** (-yə-lə) *n., pl.* **-ules** or **-u·lae** (-yə-lē). A needlelike structure or part.

spi·der-burst (spī′dər) *n.* Radiating dull-red capillary lines on the skin of the leg, usually without any visible or palpable varicose veins, due to deep-seated venous dilation.

spider nevus *n.* See arterial spider.

Spiel·mey·er–Vogt disease (shpēl′mī′ər-) *n.* The late juvenile type of cerebral sphingolipidosis.

spike (spīk) *n.* A brief electrical event of 3 to 25 milliseconds that gives the appearance in the electroencephalogram of a rising and falling vertical line.

spike potential *n.* The main wave in the action potential of a nerve, followed by negative and positive afterpotentials.

spi·na (spī′nə) *n., pl.* **-nae** (-nē). A spine-shaped or sharp thornlike anatomical process.

spina bif·i·da (bĭf′ĭ-də) *n.* A congenital defect in which the spinal column is imperfectly closed so that part of the meninges or spinal cord may protrude, often resulting in hydrocephalus and other neurological disorders.

spi·nal (spī′nəl) *adj*. **1.** Relating to or situated near the vertebral column or spinal cord. **2.** Relating to any spine or spinous process.

spinal analgesia *n.* The deactivation of sensory nerves by injecting a local anesthetic into the subarachnoid space of the spine.

spinal anesthesia *n.* **1.** Anesthesia produced by injection of a local anesthetic solution into the spinal subarachnoid space. **2.** Loss of sensation produced by disease of the spinal cord.

spinal block *n.* Pathological obstruction of the flow of cerebrospinal fluid in the spinal subarachnoid space.

spinal canal *n.* See **vertebral canal.**

spinal column *n.* The series of articulated vertebrae, separated by intervertebral disks and held together by muscles and tendons, that extends from the cranium to the coccyx, encasing the spinal cord and forming the supporting axis of the body; the spine.

spinal concussion *n.* Sudden transient loss of function of the spinal cord due to trauma.

spinal cord *n.* The thick, whitish cord of nerve tissue that extends from the medulla oblongata down through the spinal column and from which the spinal nerves branch to various body parts.

spinal curvature *n.* Any of several deformities characterized by abnormal curvature of the spine, such as kyphosis or scoliosis.

spinal decompression *n.* The relief of pressure upon the spinal cord as caused by a tumor, cyst, hematoma, or bone, through surgery.

spinal fusion *n.* A surgical procedure in which two or more vertebrae are joined.

spinal ganglion *n.* The ganglion of the posterior root of each spinal segmental nerve, containing the cell bodies of the unipolar primary sensory neurons.

spinal meningitis *n.* Inflammation of the membranes enclosing the spinal cord, especially a usually fatal form that affects infants and young children and is caused by a strain of gram-negative bacteria *(Hemophilus influenzae)* formerly thought to cause influenza.

spinal nerve *n.* Any of 31 pairs of nerves emerging from the spinal cord, each attached to the cord by two roots, anterior or ventral and posterior or dorsal, the latter provided with a spinal ganglion. The two roots unite in the intervertebral foramen, and the nerve almost immediately divides again into ventral and dorsal rami, the former supplying the foreparts of the body and limbs, the latter the muscles and skin of the back.

spinal paralysis *n.* Loss of motor power due to a lesion of the spinal cord.

spinal puncture *n.* See **lumbar puncture.**

spinal reflex *n.* A reflex arc involving the spinal cord.

spinal root *n.* Any of the roots of the accessory nerve that arise from the ventrolateral part of the first five segments of the spinal cord.

spinal tap *n.* See **lumbar puncture.**

spin·dle (spĭn′dl) *n.* **1.** A fusiform structure, usually composed of microtubules. **2.** Mitotic spindle.

spindle cell *n.* A spindle-shaped cell characteristic of certain tumors.

spindle cell lipoma *n.* A microscopically distinctive form of lipoma in which adipose tissue is infiltrated by fibroblasts and collagen.

spindle fiber *n.* One of a network of achromatic filaments that extend inward from the poles of a dividing cell, forming a spindle-shaped figure.

spine (spīn) *n.* **1.** See **spinal cord. 2.** Any of various short pointed projections, processes, or appendages of bone.

spinn·bar·keit (spĭn′bär′kīt, shpĭn′-) *n.* The stringy, elastic character of cervical mucus during the ovulatory period.

spinous process *n.* The dorsal projection from the center of a vertebral arch.

spi·rad·e·no·ma (spī-răd′n-ō′mə) *n.* A benign tumor of the sweat glands.

spi·ral bandage (spī′rəl) *n.* A bandage encircling a limb, with successive turns overlapping the preceding ones.

spiral canal of the cochlea *n.* The winding tube of the bony labyrinth of the ear.

spiral canal of the modiolus *n.* The space in the modiolus in which the spiral ganglion of the cochlear nerve lies.

spiral fracture *n.* A fracture in which the bone has been twisted apart and the line of break is helical.

spiral organ *n.* A specialized structure located on the inner surface of the basilar membrane of the cochlea containing hair cells that transmit sound vibrations to the nerve fibers.

spi·ril·lum (spī-rĭl′əm) *n.*, *pl.* **-ril·la** (-rĭl′ə). **1.** Any of a genus *(Spirillum)* of large, aerobic, gram-negative bacteria having an elongated spiral form and a tuft of flagella. **2.** Any of various other spiral-shaped microorganisms.

spi·ro·chete (spī′rə-kēt′) *n.* Any of various slender, spiral, motile bacteria of the order Spirochaetales, many of which are pathogenic, causing syphilis, relapsing fever, yaws, and other diseases.

spi·ro·che·te·mi·a (spī′rə-kē-tē′mē-ə) *n.* The presence of spirochetes in the blood.

spi·ro·che·to·sis (spī′rə-kē-tō′sĭs) *n.*, *pl.* **-ses** (-sēz). Any of various diseases, such as syphilis, caused by infection with spirochetes.

spi·ro·gram (spī′rə-grăm′) *n.* The tracing made by a spirograph.

spi·ro·graph (spī′rə-grăf′) *n.* An instrument for registering the depth and rapidity of respiratory movements. — **spi·ro·graph′ic** *adj.* — **spi·rog′ra·phy** (spī-rŏg′rə-fē) *n.*

spi·rom·e·ter (spī-rŏm′ĭ-tər) *n.* An instrument for measuring the volume of air entering and leaving the lungs. — **spi′ro·met′ric** (-rə-mĕt′rĭk) *adj.* — **spi·rom′e·try** *n.*

spit·tle (spĭt′l) *n.* Spit; saliva.

splanch·nes·the·sia (splăngk'nĭs-thē'zhə) *n.* See **visceral sense.**

splanch·nes·thet·ic sensibility (splăngk'nĭs-thĕt'ĭk) *n.* See **visceral sense.**

splanch·nic (splăngk'nĭk) *adj.* Of or relating to the viscera; visceral.

splanchnic anesthesia *n.* Loss of sensation in areas of the visceral peritoneum innervated by the splanchnic nerves.

splanch·ni·cec·to·my (splăngk'nĭ-sĕk'tə-mē) *n.* Surgical resection of the splanchnic nerves and usually of the celiac ganglion.

splanch·ni·cot·o·my (splăngk'nĭ-kŏt'ə-mē) *n.* Surgical section of a splanchnic nerve or nerves.

splanch·nop·a·thy (splăngk-nŏp'ə-thē) *n.* Disease of the abdominal viscera.

splanch·no·tribe (splăngk'nə-trīb') *n.* An instrument used for occluding the intestine temporarily prior to resection.

spleen (splēn) *n.* A large, highly vascular lymphoid organ, lying to the left of the stomach below the diaphragm, serving to store blood, disintegrate old blood cells, filter foreign substances from the blood, and produce lymphocytes.

sple·nal·gi·a (splĭ-năl'jē-ə, -jə) *n.* Pain in the spleen.

sple·nec·to·my (splĭ-nĕk'tə-mē) *n.* Surgical removal of the spleen.

splen·ic (splĕn'ĭk) *adj.* Of, in, near, or relating to the spleen.

splenic pulp *n.* The soft, reddish brown substance that fills the sinuses of the spleen.

sple·ni·tis (splĭ-nī'tĭs) *n.* Inflammation of the spleen.

sple·ni·um (splē'nē-əm) *n., pl.* **-ni·a** (-nē-ə). **1.** A compress or bandage. **2.** An anatomical structure resembling a bandaged part.

sple·no·cele (splē'nə-sēl') *n.* A splenic hernia.

sple·nog·ra·phy (splĭ-nŏg'rə-fē) *n.* Radiographic examination of the spleen after injection of contrast material.

sple·no·he·pa·to·meg·a·ly (splē'nō-hĕp'ə-tə-mĕg'ə-lē, -hĭ-păt'ə-) *n.* Enlargement of the spleen and the liver.

sple·no·ma (splĭ-nō'mə) *n.* An enlarged spleen.

sple·no·meg·a·ly (splē'nō-mĕg'ə-lē, splĕn'ō-) *n.* Enlargement of the spleen.

sple·nop·a·thy (splĭ-nŏp'ə-thē) *n.* Disease of the spleen.

sple·no·pex·y (splē'nə-pĕk'sē) *n.* The surgical fixation of an ectopic or floating spleen.

sple·no·por·tog·ra·phy (splē'nō-pôr-tŏg'rə-fē) *n.* X-ray visualization of the portal circulation using a radiopaque material that is introduced into the spleen. — **sple'no·por'to·gram'** (-pôr'tə-grăm') *n.*

sple·no·re·nal shunt (splē'nō-rē'nəl, splĕn'ō-) *n.* Anastomosis of the splenic vein to the left renal vein, usually end-to-side, for control of portal hypertension.

sple·nor·rha·phy (splĭ-nôr'ə-fē) *n.* **1.** Suture of a ruptured spleen. **2.** See **splenopexy.**

sple·not·o·my (splĭ-nŏt'ə-mē) *n.* Surgical incision into the spleen.

sple·no·tox·in (splē'nō-tŏk'sĭn) *n.* A cytotoxin specific for cells of the spleen.

splic·ing (splī'sĭng) *n.* **1.** Gene-splicing. **2.** The removal of introns and the joining of exons from mRNA precursors.

splint (splĭnt) *n.* **1.** A rigid device used to prevent motion of a joint or of the ends of a fractured bone. **2.** A dental appliance put on the teeth to protect them from grinding or from moving out of place. — *v.* **splint·ed, splint·ing, splints.** To support or restrict with a splint.

split (splĭt) *v.* **split, split·ting, splits. 1.** To divide from end to end or as if by a sharp blow; tear. **2.** To break, burst, or rip apart with force; rend. **3.** To separate. **4.** To break apart or divide a chemical compound into simpler constituents.

split personality *n.* See **multiple personality.**

split renal-function test *n.* See **differential ureteralcatheterization test.**

split-skin graft *n.* See **split-thickness graft.**

split-thickness flap *n.* A surgical flap that consists of part of the mucosa and submucosa but does not include periosteum.

split-thickness graft *n.* A skin graft of the epidermis and part of the dermis.

spon·dee (spŏn'dē') *n.* A word or metrical foot having two equally stressed syllables; such words are used in the testing of speech and hearing.

spon·dy·lal·gia (spŏn'dl-ăl'jē-ə, -jə) *n.* Pain in the spine.

spon·dyl·ar·thri·tis (spŏn'dl-är-thrī'tĭs) *n.* Inflammation of the intervertebral articulations.

spon·dy·li·tis (spŏn'dl-ī'tĭs) *n.* Inflammation of one or more of the vertebrae. — **spon'dy·lyt'ic** (-ĭt'ĭk) *adj.*

spon·dy·lop·a·thy (spŏn'dl-ŏp'ə-thē) *n.* Disease of the vertebrae or of the spinal column.

spon·dy·lo·py·o·sis (spŏn'dl-ō-pī-ō'sĭs) *n.* Suppurative inflammation of one or more of the vertebral bodies.

spon·dy·los·chi·sis (spŏn'dl-ŏs'kĭ-sĭs) *n.* Congenital fissure of one or more of the vertebral arches.

spon·dy·lo·sis (spŏn'dl-ō'sĭs) *n.* **1.** Ankylosis of the vertebral bones. **2.** A degenerative disease of the spinal column, especially one leading to fusion and immobilization of the vertebral bones.

spon·dy·lo·syn·de·sis (spŏn'dl-ō-sĭn-dē'sĭs) *n.* See **spinal fusion.**

sponge (spŭnj) *n.* **1.** A piece of absorbent porous material, such as cellulose, plastic, or rubber, used especially for washing and cleaning. **2.** A gauze pad used to absorb blood and other fluids, as in surgery or in dressing a wound. **3.** A contraceptive sponge. — *v.* **sponged, spong·ing, spong·es.** To wash, moisten, or absorb with a sponge.

sponge bath *n.* A bath in which a wet sponge or washcloth is used without immersing the body in water.

spon·gi·o·blast (spŭn'jē-ə-blăst') *n.* Any of the embryonic epithelial cells that give rise to the neuroglia.

spon·gi·o·blas·to·ma (spŭn′jē-ō-blă-stō′mə) *n.* A glioma derived from spongioblasts.

spon·gi·o·cyte (spŭn′jē-ə-sīt′) *n.* **1.** Any of the cells of the neuroglia. **2.** A cell in the zona fasciculata of the adrenal cortex containing many droplets of lipid material that show pronounced vacuolization.

spon·gi·o·sis (spŭn′jē-ō′sĭs) *n.* Intercellular edema of the epidermis.

spon·gi·o·si·tis (spŭn′jē-ə-sī′tĭs) *n.* Inflammation of the corpus spongiosum of the penis.

spong·y (spŭn′jē) *adj.* Resembling a sponge in appearance, elasticity, or porosity; spongelike. — **spong′i·ness** *n.*

spongy bone *n.* **1.** Bone in which the spicules or trabeculae form a latticework, with interstices filled with embryonic connective tissue or bone marrow. **2.** Any of the turbinate bones.

spongy substance *n.* See **spongy bone** (sense 1).

spon·ta·ne·ous abortion (spŏn-tā′nē-əs) *n.* Abortion occurring naturally; miscarriage.

spontaneous amputation *n.* **1.** Congenital amputation. **2.** Amputation resulting from a pathological process rather than from trauma.

spontaneous gangrene of the newborn *n.* Gangrene due to vascular occlusion of unknown cause, usually in marasmic or dehydrated infants.

spontaneous mutation *n.* A mutation arising naturally, not as a result of exposure to mutagens.

spontaneous pneumothorax *n.* A pneumothorax occurring secondary to parenchymal lung disease.

spontaneous version *n.* A turning of the fetus resulting from unaided uterine contraction.

spo·rad·ic (spə-răd′ĭk, spô-) or **spo·rad·i·cal** (-ĭ-kəl) *adj.* **1.** Occurring at irregular intervals. **2.** Occurring singly; not grouped.

spore (spôr) *n.* **1.** A small, usually single-celled asexual or sexual reproductive body that is highly resistant to desiccation and heat and is capable of growing into a new organism, produced especially by certain bacteria, fungi, algae, and nonflowering plants. **2.** A dormant, nonreproductive body formed by certain bacteria in response to adverse environmental conditions.

spo·ro·ag·glu·ti·na·tion (spôr′ō-ə-gloōt′n-ā′-shən) *n.* A method for diagnosing various mycoses based on the presence of specific agglutinins that cause clumping of the fungal spores in the blood serum.

Spo·ro·thrix (spôr′ə-thrĭks′) *n.* A genus of dimorphic imperfect fungi, including the species *S. schenckii*, the causative agent of sporotrichosis.

spo·ro·tri·cho·sis (spôr′ō-trī-kō′sĭs) *n.* A chronic infectious disease of domestic mammals and humans characterized by nodules or ulcers in the lymph nodes and skin and caused by a saprophytic or parasitic fungus of the genus *Sporothrix*, especially *S. schenckii*, commonly found in soil and wood.

Spo·ro·zo·a (spôr′ə-zō′ə) *n.* A large class of parasitic protozoa, most of which reproduce sexually and asexually by means of spores. They are fre-quently transmitted by bloodsucking insects to hosts in which they cause diseases such as malaria and coccidiosis.

spo·ro·zo·an (spôr′ə-zō′ən) *n.* An organism of the class Sporozoa. — **spo′ro·zo′an** *adj.*

sports medicine *n.* The branch of medicine that deals with injuries or illnesses resulting from participation in sports and athletic activities.

spot (spŏt) *n.* **1.** A mark on a surface differing sharply in color from its surroundings. **2.** A stain or blot. — *v.* **spot·ted, spot·ting, spots.** To lose a slight amount of blood through the vagina.

spot·ted fever (spŏt′ĭd) *n.* A tick typhus, such as Rocky Mountain spotted fever, caused by *Rickettsia rickettsii*.

sprain (sprān) *n.* An injury to a ligament when the joint is carried through a range of motion greater than normal but without dislocation or fracture. — *v.* **sprained, sprain·ing, sprains.** To cause a sprain to a joint or ligament.

sprain fracture *n.* An avulsion fracture in which a small portion of bone has been pulled or pushed off, often occurs in the ankle.

sprue (sproō) *n.* A chronic disease characterized by diarrhea, emaciation, and anemia, caused by defective absorption of nutrients from the intestinal tract.

spud (spŭd) *n.* A blunt triangular knife used for removing foreign bodies from the cornea.

spur (spûr) *n.* A spine or projection from a bone.

spu·tum (spyoō′təm) *n., pl.* **-ta** (-tə). Matter coughed up and usually expelled from the mouth, especially mucus or mucopurulent matter expectorated in diseases of the air passages.

SQ *abbr.* subcutaneous

squa·ma (skwā′mə, skwä′-) *n., pl.* **-mae** (-mē′). **1.** A thin platelike mass, as of bone. **2.** A scale or scalelike structure. — **squa′mate′** (-māt′) *adj.*

squa·mous (skwā′məs, skwä′-) or **squa·mose** (-mōs′) *adj.* **1.** Covered with or formed of scales; scaly. **2.** Resembling a scale or scales; thin and flat. **3.** Squamosal. — **squa′mous·ness** *n.*

squamous cell *n.* A flat, scalelike epithelial cell.

squamous cell carcinoma *n.* A carcinoma that arises from squamous epithelium and is the most common form of skin cancer.

squamous epithelium *n.* Epithelium having one or more cell layers, the most superficial of which is composed of flat, scalelike or platelike cells.

squamous odontogenic tumor *n.* A benign epithelial odontogenic tumor that appears radiologically as a lesion closely associated with the tooth root and that is composed of islands of squamous epithelium enclosed by a peripheral layer of flattened cells.

squint (skwĭnt) *n.* See **strabismus**.

stab cell *n.* See **band cell**.

stab drain *n.* A drain passed into the cavity through a puncture made adjacent to a surgical wound to prevent the wound from becoming infected.

sta·bil·i·ty (stə-bĭl′ĭ-tē) *n.* The condition of being stable or resistant to change.

sta·bi·lize (stā′bə-līz′) *v.* **-lized, -liz·ing, -liz·es.** To bring to or reach a stable or steadfast state. — **sta′bi·li·za′tion** (-lĭ-zā′shən) *n.*

sta·ble (stā′bəl) *adj.* **-bler, -blest. 1.** Resistant to change of position or condition. **2.** Not subject to mental illness or irrationality. **3.** Having no known mode of decay; indefinitely long-lived. Used of atomic particles. **4.** Not easily decomposed or otherwise modified chemically.

staff (stăf) *n.* **1.** A specific group of workers. **2.** See **director.** — *v.* **staffed, staff·ing, staffs. 1.** To provide with a staff of workers or assistants. **2.** To serve on the staff of.

staff cell *n.* See **band cell.**

staff of Aes·cu·la·pi·us (ĕs′kyə-lā′pē-əs) *n.* A rod with a single serpent twining around it, used as the symbol of medicine; it is the emblem of the American Medical Association and various other medical organizations.

stage (stāj) *n.* **1.** A period in the course of a disease. **2.** A particular step, phase, or position in a developmental process.

stag-horn calculus *n.* A calculus of the renal pelvis, with branches extending into the infundibula and calices.

stag·ing (stā′jĭng) *n.* The classification of neoplasms according to the extent of the tumor.

stag·nant anoxia (stăg′nənt) *n.* See **ischemic hypoxia.**

stag·na·tion (stăg-nā′shən) *n.* **1.** The retardation or cessation of the flow of blood in the blood vessels, as in passive congestion. **2.** The accumulation of a normally circulating fluid in a part or an organ.

stain (stān) *n.* **1.** A reagent or dye used for staining microscopic specimens. **2.** A procedure in which a dye or a combination of dyes and reagents is used to color the constituents of cells and tissues. — *v.* **stained, stain·ing, stains.** To treat microscopic specimens with a reagent or dye that makes certain structures visible.

stair·case (stâr′kās′) *n.* A series of reactions or responses that follow one another in progressively increasing or decreasing intensity, so that a chart shows a continuous rise or fall.

staircase phenomenon *n.* See **treppe.**

stalk (stôk) *n.* A slender or elongated support or structure, as one that connects or supports an organ.

stam·mer (stăm′ər) *n.* A speech disorder characterized by hesitation and repetition of sounds, or by mispronunciation or transposition of certain consonants, especially *l, r,* and *s.* — *v.* **-mered, -mer·ing, -mers.** To speak with a stammer.

stan·dard (stăn′dərd) *n.* **1.** An acknowledged measure of comparison for quantitative or qualitative value; a criterion. **2.** An object that under specified conditions defines, represents, or records the magnitude of a unit. — *adj.* **1.** Serving as or conforming to a standard of measurement

or value. **2.** Widely recognized as a model of authority or excellence.

stan·dard·ize (stăn′dər-dīz′) *v.* **-ized, -iz·ing, -iz·es. 1.** To cause to conform to a standard. **2.** To evaluate by comparing with a standard.

stand·still (stănd′stĭl′) *n.* Complete cessation of activity or progress.

Stan·ford–Binet intelligence scale (stăn′fərd-) *n.* See **Stanford–Binet test.**

Stanford–Binet test *n.* A standardized intelligence test adapted from the Binet–Simon scale for use in the United States, especially in the assessment of children.

stan·nous fluoride (stăn′əs) *n.* A preparation of stannous tin and fluoride used to fluoridate toothpaste and other dental preparations.

sta·pe·dec·to·my (stā′pĭ-dĕk′tə-mē, -pē-) *n.* Surgical removal of all or part of the stapes of the middle ear and replacement with a prosthesis.

sta·pes (stā′pēz) *n., pl.* **stapes** or **sta·pe·des** (stā′pĭ-dēz′). The smallest of the three auditory ossicles, whose base fits into the oval window and whose head is articulated with the lenticular process of the long limb of the incus.

stapes-mobilization operation *n.* An operation involving the fracture of tissue that has immobilized the stapes; it is performed to restore hearing, especially in patients with otosclerosis.

staph (stăf) *adj.* Staphylococcus. — **staph** *adj.*

staph·y·lec·to·my (stăf′ə-lĕk′tə-mē) *n.* See **uvulectomy.**

staph·yl·e·de·ma (stăf′ə-lĭ-dē′mə) *n.* Edema of the uvula.

staph·y·lo·coc·ce·mi·a (stăf′ə-lō-kŏk-sē′mē-ə) *n.* The presence of staphylococci in the blood.

staph·y·lo·coc·co·sis (stăf′ə-lō-kŏ-kō′sĭs) *n., pl.* **-ses** (-sēz). Infection by a staphylococcus bacterium.

staph·y·lo·coc·cus (stăf′ə-lō-kŏk′əs) *n., pl.* **-coc·ci** (-kŏk′sī, -kŏk′ī). A spherical gram-positive parasitic bacterium of the genus *Staphylococcus,* usually occurring in grapelike clusters and causing boils, septicemia, and other infections. — **staph′·y·lo·coc′cal** (-kŏk′əl), **staph′y·lo·coc·′cic** (-kŏk′-sĭk, -kŏk′ĭk) *adj.*

staph·y·lo·der·ma (stăf′ə-lō-dûr′mə) *n.* Pyoderma due to staphylococci.

staph·y·lo·der·ma·ti·tis (stăf′ə-lō-dûr′mə-tī′tĭs) *n.* Inflammation of the skin due to the action of staphylococci.

staph·y·lo·di·al·y·sis (stăf′ə-lō-dī-ăl′ĭ-sĭs) *n.* See **uvuloptosis.**

staph·y·lo·ki·nase (stăf′ə-lō-kī′nās′, -nāz′, -kĭn′ās′, -āz′) *n.* An enzyme from *Staphylococcus aureus* that catalyzes the conversion of plasminogen to plasmin.

staph·y·lo·ma (stăf′ə-lō′mə) *n.* A bulging of the cornea or sclera due to inflammatory softening.

staph·y·lo·lon·cus (stăf′ə-lŏng′kəs) *n.* A tumor or swelling of the uvula.

staph·y·lo·phar·yn·gor·rha·phy (stăf′ə-lō-făr′-ĭng-gôr′ə-fē) *n.* Surgical repair of defects in the uvula or soft palate and the pharynx.

staph·y·lo·plas·ty (stăf′ə-lō-plăs′tē) *n.* Plastic surgery of the uvula and the soft palate.

staph·y·lop·to·sis (stăf′ə-lŏp-tō′sĭs) *n.* See **uvuloptosis.**

staph·y·lor·rha·phy (stăf′ə-lôr′ə-fē) *n.* See **palatorrhaphy.**

staph·y·los·chi·sis (stăf′ə-lŏs′kĭ-sĭs) *n.* A bifid uvula, with or without cleft of the soft palate.

staph·y·lot·o·my (stăf′ə-lŏt′ə-mē) *n.* **1.** See **uvulotomy. 2.** Surgical division of a staphyloma.

staph·y·lo·tox·in (stăf′ə-lō-tŏk′sĭn) *n.* The toxin produced by a *Staphylococcus* species.

sta·pling (stā′plĭng) *n.* The fastening together of two tissues with a staple or staples.

starch (stärch) *n.* **1.** A naturally abundant nutrient polysaccharide that is the primary storage form of carbohydrates in plants and is found chiefly in seeds, fruits, tubers, roots, and stem pith. **2. starches.** Foods having a high content of starch, such as rice, breads, and potatoes.

star·tle reflex (stär′tl) *n.* **1.** The reflex response of an infant in which the limb and neck muscles contract when the infant is allowed to drop a short distance or is startled by a sudden noise or jolt. **2.** See **cochleopalpebral reflex.**

star·va·tion (stär-vā′shən) *n.* **1.** The act or process of starving. **2.** The condition of being starved.

starve (stärv) *v.* **starved, starv·ing, starves. 1.** To suffer or die from extreme or prolonged lack of food. **2.** To deprive of food.

sta·sis (stā′sĭs, stăs′ĭs) *n., pl.* **sta·ses** (stā′sēz, stăs′-ēz). Stoppage of the normal flow of a body substance, as of blood through an artery or of intestinal contents through the bowels.

stat (stăt) *adv.* With no delay; at once. —*adj.* Immediate.

stat. *abbr. Latin.* statim (immediately)

state (stāt) *n.* A condition or situation; status.

state-dependent learning *n.* Learning associated with a specific state of sleep or wakefulness or with a chemically altered state, such that the learned information cannot be recalled or used unless the subject is restored to the state that existed when learning first occurred.

stat·ic (stăt′ĭk) *adj.* **1.** Of or being at rest; not in motion. **2.** Without force; not dynamic.

static reflex *n.* See **righting reflex.**

stat·in (stăt′ĭn) *n.* Any of a group of drugs used to lower blood cholesterol.

stat·o·ki·net·ic reflex (stăt′ō-kĭ-nĕt′ĭk, kī-) *n.* A reflex that, through stimulation of the receptors in the neck muscles and semicircular canals, brings about movements of the limbs and eyes appropriate to a given movement of the head.

stat·o·ton·ic reflexes (stăt′ə-tŏn′ĭk) *pl.n.* Reflexes that control the tone of the limb muscles to maintain or regain a desired body position.

stat·ure (stăch′ər) *n.* The height of a person.

sta·tus (stā′təs, stăt′əs) *n.* A state or condition.

status ep·i·lep·ti·cus (ĕp′ə-lĕp′tĭ-kəs) *n.* A condition in which one major attack of epilepsy succeeds another with little or no intermission.

status lym·phat·i·cus (lĭm-făt′ĭ-kəs) *n.* See **status thymicolymphaticus.**

status thy·mi·co·lym·phat·i·cus (thī′mĭ-kō-lĭm-făt′ĭ-kəs) *n.* Supposed enlargement of the thymus gland and lymph nodes in infants, formerly believed to be associated with unexplained sudden death.

STD *abbr.* sexually transmitted disease

stead·y state (stĕd′ē) *n.* **1.** A state obtained in moderate muscular exercise when the removal of lactic acid by oxidation keeps pace with its production. If the oxygen supply is adequate, the muscles do not go into debt for oxygen. **2.** A condition in which the formation of substances keeps pace with their destruction so that all volumes, concentrations, pressures, and flows remain constant. **3.** A stable condition that does not change over time or in which change in one direction is continually balanced by change in another.

steal (stēl) *n.* The diversion of blood flow from its normal course.

ste·ap·sin (stē-ăp′sĭn) *n.* A digestive enzyme of pancreatic juice that catalyzes the hydrolysis of fats to fatty acids and glycerol.

ste·ar·ic acid (stē-ăr′ĭk, stēr′ĭk) *n.* A colorless, odorless, waxlike fatty acid occurring naturally in animal and vegetable fats and used in pharmaceutical preparations, ointments, soaps, and suppositories.

Stearns alcoholic amentia (stûrnz) *n.* A temporary mental disorder resulting from alcohol abuse, similar to delirium tremens but longer lasting.

ste·a·ti·tis (stē′ə-tī′tĭs) *n.* Inflammation of adipose tissue.

ste·a·to·cys·to·ma (stē′ə-tō-sĭ-stō′mə) *n.* **1.** A cyst with cells of a sebaceous gland in its wall. **2.** See **sebaceous cyst.**

steatocystoma mul·ti·plex (mŭl′tə-plĕks′) *n.* Widespread, multiple, thin-walled cysts of the skin, lined by squamous epithelium, and including lobules of sebaceous cells.

ste·a·tol·y·sis (stē′ə-tŏl′ĭ-sĭs) *n.* Hydrolysis or emulsion of fat in the digestive process. —**ste′a·to·lyt′ic** (-tə-lĭt′ĭk) *adj.*

ste·a·to·ne·cro·sis (stē′ə-tō-nə-krō′sĭs, -nĕ-) *n.* See **fat necrosis.**

ste·at·o·pyg·i·a (stē-ăt′ə-pĭj′ē-ə, -pī′jē-ə) or **ste·a·to·py·ga** (stē′ə-tō-pī′gə, stē-ăt′ə-) *n.* An excessive accumulation of fat on the buttocks. —**ste′a·to·pyg′ic** (-pĭj′ĭk, -pī′jĭk), **ste′a·to·py′gous** (-pī′gəs) *adj.*

ste·a·tor·rhe·a or **ste·a·tor·rhoe·a** (stē′ə-tə-rē′ə, stē-ăt′ə-) *n.* Excessive discharge of fat in the feces, as occurring in pancreatic disease and in malabsorption syndromes.

ste·a·to·sis (stē′ə-tō′sĭs) *n.* See **fatty degeneration.**

steg·no·sis (stĕg-nō′sĭs) *n.* **1.** A stoppage of any of the secretions or excretions. **2.** A constriction or stenosis.

Stein·berg thumb sign (stīn′bərg) *n.* An indication of Marfan syndrome in which the thumb projects well beyond the ulnar surface of the hand when it is held across the palm of the same hand.

stel·late block (stĕl′āt′) *n.* Injection of local anesthetic solution in the vicinity of the stellate ganglion.

stellate cell *n.* A star-shaped cell, such as an astrocyte, that has many filaments extending radially.

stellate fracture *n.* A bone fracture in which the lines of break radiate from a point, usually from the site of an injury.

stellate ganglion *n.* See **cervicothoracic ganglion**.

Stell·wag's sign (stĕl′wäg′, shtĕl′väks′) *n.* An indication of Graves's disease in which there is infrequent and incomplete blinking of the eye.

stem (stĕm) *n.* A supporting structure resembling the stalk of a plant.

stem cell *n.* An unspecialized cell that gives rise to a specific specialized cell, such as a blood cell.

sten·o·ceph·a·ly (stĕn′ō-sĕf′ə-lē) *n.* Marked narrowness of the head. — **sten′o·ce·phal′ic** (-sə-făl′ĭk), **sten′o·ceph′a·lous** (-sĕf′ə-ləs) *adj.*

sten·o·cho·ri·a (stĕn′ə-kôr′ē-ə) *n.* Abnormal contraction of a canal or orifice, especially of the lacrimal ducts.

ste·no·sal murmur (stə-nō′səl) *n.* An arterial murmur due to a narrowing of the vessel from pressure or organic change.

ste·no·sis (stə-nō′sĭs) *n.*, *pl.* **-ses** (-sēz). A constriction or narrowing of a duct or passage.

sten·o·sto·mi·a (stĕn′ə-stō′mē-ə) *n.* Narrowness of the oral cavity.

sten·o·ther·mal (stĕn′ə-thûr′məl) or **sten·o·ther·mic** (-mĭk) or **sten·o·ther·mous** (-məs) *adj.* Capable of living or growing only within a limited range of temperature. Used of bacteria. — **sten′o·therm′** *n.*

sten·o·tho·rax (stĕn′ō-thôr′ăks′) *n.* A narrow, contracted chest.

stent (stĕnt) *n.* **1.** A device used to maintain a bodily orifice or cavity during skin grafting, or to immobilize a skin graft after placement. **2.** A slender thread, rod, or catheter placed within the lumen of tubular structures to provide support during or after anastomosis.

step·page (stĕp′ĭj) *n.* The peculiar gait seen in neuritis of the peroneal nerve and in tabes dorsalis, characterized by high stepping to allow the drooping foot and toes to clear the ground.

ster·co·bi·lin (stûr′kō-bī′lĭn, -bĭl′ĭn) *n.* A brown degradation product of hemoglobin present in the feces.

ster·co·lith (stûr′kə-lĭth′) *n.* See **coprolith**.

ster·co·ral abscess (stûr′kər-əl) *n.* An abscess containing pus and feces.

stercoral fistula *n.* See **intestinal fistula**.

stercoral ulcer *n.* An ulcer of the colon due to the pressure and irritation caused by retained fecal masses.

ster·cus (stûr′kəs) *n.* See **feces**.

ster·e·o·ar·throl·y·sis (stĕr′ē-ō-är-thrŏl′ĭ-sĭs, stēr′-) *n.* The surgical formation of a new movable joint in cases of bony ankylosis.

ster·e·o·cam·pim·e·ter (stĕr′ē-ō-kăm-pĭm′ĭ-tər, stēr′-) *n.* An apparatus for studying the central visual fields.

ster·e·o·cin·e·fluo·rog·ra·phy (stĕr′ē-ō-sĭn′ē-flŏŏ-rŏg′rə-fē, -flō-) *n.* Motion-picture recording of three-dimensional radiographic images obtained by stereoscopic fluoroscopy.

ster·e·o·e·lec·tro·en·ceph·a·log·ra·phy (stĕr′ē-ō-ĭ-lĕk′trō-ĕn-sĕf′ə-lŏg′rə-fē, stēr′-) *n.* Recording of electrical activity in three planes of the brain by means of surface and depth electrodes.

ster·e·o·en·ceph·a·lom·e·try (stĕr′ē-ō-ĕn-sĕf′ə-lŏm′ĭ-trē, stēr′-) *n.* The localization of brain structures by use of three-dimensional coordinates.

ster·e·o·en·ceph·a·lot·o·my (stĕr′ē-ō-ĕn-sĕf′ə-lŏt′ə-mē, stēr′-) *n.* See **stereotaxis** (sense 1).

ster·e·og·no·sis (stĕr′ē-ŏg-nō′sĭs, stēr′-) *n.* The perception of the form of an object by means of touch. — **ster′e·og·nos′tic** (-nŏs′tĭk) *adj.*

ster·e·o·ra·di·og·ra·phy (stĕr′ē-ō-rā′dē-ŏg′rə-fē, stēr′-) *n.* The taking of radiographs from two slightly different positions so as to obtain a stereoscopic effect.

ster·e·o·scop·ic vision (stĕr′ē-ə-skŏp′ĭk, stēr′-) *n.* The single perception of a slightly different image from each eye, resulting in depth perception.

ster·e·os·co·py (stĕr′ē-ŏs′kə-pē, stēr′-) *n.* An optical technique by which two images of the same object are blended into one, giving a three-dimensional appearance to the single image.

stereotactic instrument *n.* An apparatus attached to the head, used to localize precisely an area in the brain by means of coordinates related to intracerebral structures.

stereotactic surgery *n.* See **stereotaxis** (sense 1).

ster·e·o·tax·is (stĕr′ē-ə-tăk′sĭs, stēr′-) or **ster·e·o·tax·y** (stĕr′ē-ə-tăk′sē, stēr′-) *n.* **1.** A method in neurosurgery and neurological research for precisely locating points within the brain using an external, three-dimensional frame of reference usually based on the Cartesian coordinate system. **2.** Movement of an organism in response to contact with a solid body. — **ster′e·o·tac′tic** (-tăk′tĭk), **ster′e·o·tax′ic** (-tăk′sĭk), **ster′e·o·tac′ti·cal** (-tăk′tĭ-kəl), **ster′e·o·tax′i·cal** (-tăk′sĭ-kəl) *adj.*

ster·e·ot·ro·pism (stĕr′ē-ŏt′rə-pĭz′əm, stēr′-) *n.* See **thigmotropism**. — **ster′e·o·trop′ic** (-ē-ə-trŏp′ĭk) *adj.*

ster·e·o·ty·py (stĕr′ē-ə-tī′pē, stēr′-) *n.* **1.** The maintenance of one attitude for a long period. **2.** The constant repetition of certain meaningless gestures or movements.

ster·ile (stĕr′əl, -īl′) *adj.* **1.** Not producing or incapable of producing offspring. **2.** Free from all living bacteria or microorganisms and their spores. — **ster′ile·ness**, **ste·ril′i·ty** (stə-rĭl′ĭ-tē) *n.*

ster·il·i·za·tion (stĕr′ə-lĭ-zā′shən) *n.* **1.** The act or procedure of sterilizing. **2.** The condition of being sterile or sterilized.

ster·il·ize (stĕr′ə-līz′) *v.* **-ized, -iz·ing, -iz·es. 1.** To make free from live bacteria or other microorganisms. **2.** To deprive of the ability to produce off-spring, as by removing the reproductive organs.

ster·il·iz·er (stĕr′ə-lī′zər) *n.* An apparatus for rendering objects aseptic.

ster·nal (stûr′nəl) *adj.* Of, relating to, or near the sternum.

ster·nal·gi·a (stər-năl′jē-ə, -jə) *n.* Pain in the sternum or in the sternal region.

sternal plane *n.* A plane along the front surface of the sternum.

sternal puncture *n.* Removal of bone marrow from the manubrium of the sternum by means of a needle.

Stern·berg–Reed cell (stûrn′bûrg′-, shtĕrn′bĕrk′-)- *n.* See **Reed–Sternberg cell.**

ster·no·clei·do·mas·toid muscle (stûr′nō-klī′də-mäs′toid) *n.* A muscle with origin by two heads from the anterior surface of the episternum and from the sternal end of the clavicle, with insertion into the mastoid process and the superior nuchal line, and whose action turns the head obliquely to the opposite side and flexes the neck and extends the head when both sides act together.

ster·no·dyn·i·a (stûr′nō-dĭn′ē-ə) *n.* See **sternalgia.**

ster·no·hy·oid muscle (stûr′nō-hī′oid′) *n.* A muscle with origin from the episternum and the first costal cartilage, with insertion into the hyoid bone, and whose action depresses the hyoid bone.

ster·no·mas·toid muscle (stûr′nō-mäs′toid′) *n.* See **sternocleidomastoid muscle.**

ster·no·per·i·car·di·al (stûr′nō-pĕr′ĭ-kär′dē-əl) *adj.* Relating to the sternum and the pericardium.

ster·nos·chi·sis (stər-nŏs′kĭ-sĭs) *n.* Congenital cleft of the sternum.

ster·no·thy·roid muscle (stûr′nō-thī′roid′) *n.* A muscle with origin from the episternum and the first or second costal cartilage, with insertion into the thyroid cartilage, and whose action depresses the larynx.

ster·not·o·my (stər-nŏt′ə-mē) *n.* Incision into or through the sternum.

ster·num (stûr′nəm) *n., pl.* **-nums** or **-na** (-nə). A long flat bone, articulating with the cartilages of the first seven ribs and with the clavicle, forming the middle part of the anterior wall of the thorax, and consisting of the corpus, manubrium, and xiphoid process.

ster·nu·ta·tion (stûr′nyə-tā′shən) *n.* **1.** The act of sneezing. **2.** A sneeze.

ster·oid (stĕr′oid′, stĕr′-) *n.* Any of numerous naturally occurring or synthetic fat-soluble organic compounds, including the sterols and bile acids, adrenocortical and sex hormones, certain natural drugs such as digitalis compounds, and the precursors of certain vitamins. — *adj.* Relating to or characteristic of steroids or steroid hormones. — **ster′oid′, ste·roid′al** (stĭ-roid′l, stĕ-) *adj.*

steroid hormone *n.* See **steroid.**

ste·roid·o·gen·e·sis (stĭ-roi′də-jĕn′ĭ-sĭs, stĕr′oi-, stĕr′-) *n.* The biological synthesis of steroids. — **ste·roid′o·gen′ic** (-jĕn′ĭk) *adj.*

ster·ol (stĕr′ôl′, -ōl′, stĕr′-) *n.* Any of a group of predominantly unsaturated solid alcohols of the steroid group, such as cholesterol and ergosterol, present in the fatty tissues of plants and animals.

ster·tor (stûr′tər) *n.* A heavy snoring inspiratory sound occurring in coma or deep sleep, sometimes due to obstruction of the larynx or upper airways. — **ster′to·rous** *adj.* — **ster′to·rous·ly** *adv.*

ste·thal·gi·a (stĕ-thăl′jē-ə, -jə) *n.* Pain in the chest.

steth·o·go·ni·om·e·ter (stĕth′ə-gō′nē-ŏm′ĭ-tər) *n.* An apparatus for measuring the curvatures of the thorax.

steth·o·scope (stĕth′ə-skōp′) *n.* Any of various instruments used for listening to sounds produced within the body. — **steth′o·scop′ic** (-skōp′ĭk), **steth′o·scop′i·cal** (-ĭ-kəl) *adj.* — **steth′o·scop′i·cal·ly** *adv.* — **ste·thos′co·py** (stĕ-thŏs′kə-pē) *n.*

steth·o·spasm (stĕth′ə-spăz′əm) *n.* A chest spasm.

Ste·vens–John·son syndrome (stē′vənz-jŏn′sən) *n.* A severe inflammatory eruption of the skin and mucous membranes, usually occurring in children and young adults following a respiratory infection or as an allergic reaction to drugs or other substances.

Stew·art–Holmes sign (stōō′ərt-, styōō′-) *n.* A sign occurring in cerebellar deficit in which the person is unable to check a movement when passive resistance is suddenly released.

sthe·ni·a (sthē′nē-ə) *n.* A condition of bodily strength, vigor, or vitality.

stiff-man syndrome *n.* A chronic, progressive but variable disorder of the central nervous system having no known cause and associated with fluctuating muscle spasms and stiffness.

stig·ma (stĭg′mə) *n., pl.* **stig·mas** or **stig·ma·ta** (stĭg-mä′tə, -măt′ə, stĭg′mə-). **1.** Visible evidence of a disease. **2.** A spot or blemish on the skin. **3.** A bleeding spot on the skin considered as a manifestation of conversion disorder. **4.** Follicular stigma.

stig·ma·tism (stĭg′mə-tĭz′əm) *n.* The condition of having stigmas.

stig·ma·ti·za·tion (stĭg′mə-tĭ-zā′shən) *n.* The production of stigmas, especially of hysterical origin.

stil·bene (stĭl′bēn′) *n.* A colorless or yellowish unsaturated crystalline hydrocarbon compound that is the chemical basis for diethylstilbestrol and other synthetic estrogenic compounds.

stil·bes·trol (stĭl-bĕs′trôl′, -trōl′) *n.* DES.

still·birth (stĭl′bûrth′) *n.* **1.** The birth of a dead child or fetus. **2.** A child or fetus dead at birth.

still·born (stĭl′bôrn′) *adj.* Dead at birth.

still layer *n.* The layer of the bloodstream next to the wall in the capillary vessels; it flows slowly and transports the white blood cells.

Still's murmur (stĭlz) *n.* A murmur whose sound resembles the noise produced by a twanging string.

stim·u·lant (stĭm′yə-lənt) *n.* An agent that arouses organic activity, strengthens the action of the heart, increases vitality, and promotes a sense of well-being. — *adj.* Serving as or being a stimulant; stimulating.

stim·u·late (stĭm′yə-lāt′) *v.* **-lat·ed, -lat·ing, -lates.**

To arouse a body or a responsive structure to increased functional activity. — stim′u·lat′er, stim′u·la′tor *n*.

stim·u·la·tion (stĭm′yə-lā′shən) *n*. **1.** Arousal of the body or of individual organs or other parts to increased functional activity. **2.** The condition of being stimulated. **3.** The application of a stimulus to a responsive structure, such as a nerve or muscle, regardless of whether the strength of the stimulus is sufficient to produce excitation.

stim·u·lus (stĭm′yə-ləs) *n., pl.* -li (-lī′). **1.** A stimulant. **2.** That which can elicit or evoke an action or response in a cell, an excitable tissue, or an organism.

stimulus sensitive myoclonus *n*. Myoclonus induced by a variety of stimuli, such as talking, loud noises, or tapping.

sting (stĭng) *v*. stung (stŭng), sting·ing, stings. **1.** To pierce or wound painfully with or as if with a sharp-pointed structure or organ, as that of certain insects. **2.** To introduce venom by stinging. — *n*. **1.** The act of stinging. **2.** The wound or pain caused by or as if by stinging. **3.** The venom apparatus of a stinging organism.

stip·pled epiphysis (stĭp′əld) *n*. A congenital abnormality of the epiphyses characterized by ossification from multiple centers that severely deform the long bone and give it a stippled appearance and a thickened shaft.

stip·pling (stĭp′lĭng) *n*. **1.** A speckling of a blood cell or other structure with fine dots when it is exposed to the action of a basic stain. It is due to the presence of free basophil granules in the cell protoplasm. **2.** The orange-peel appearance of normal gingival tissue.

stir·rup (stûr′əp, stĭr′-) *n*. See stapes.

stitch (stĭch) *n*. **1.** A sudden sharp pain, especially in the side. **2.** A single suture. — *v*. stitched, stitch·ing, stitch·es. To suture.

stitch abscess *n*. An abscess around a stitch or suture.

STM *abbr*. short term memory

stock·ing anesthesia (stŏk′ĭng) *n*. Loss of sensation in an area that would be covered by a stocking.

Stokes–Adams disease (stōks′-) *n*. See Adams–Stokes syndrome.

Stokes–Adams syndrome *n*. See Adams–Stokes syndrome.

sto·ma (stō′mə) *n., pl.* -mas or -ma·ta (-mə-tə). **1.** A minute opening or pore, as in the surface of a membrane. **2.** A surgically constructed opening, especially one in the abdominal wall that permits the passage of waste after a colostomy or an ileostomy. — sto′mal *adj*.

stom·ach (stŭm′ək) *n*. The enlarged saclike portion of the digestive tract located between the esophagus and the small intestine, lying just beneath the diaphragm.

stom·ach·ache (stŭm′ək-āk′) *n*. Pain in the stomach or abdomen.

stomach pump *n*. An apparatus for removing the contents of the stomach by means of suction.

stomach tube *n*. A flexible tube inserted into the stomach through which liquid food is passed.

sto·mal ulcer (stō′məl) *n*. An intestinal ulcer in the jejunal mucosa near the opening between the stomach and the jejunum, occurring after gastrojejunostomy.

sto·ma·tal·gi·a (stō′mə-tăl′jē-ə, -jə) *n*. Pain in the mouth.

sto·ma·ti·tis (stō′mə-tī′tĭs) *n*. Inflammation of the mucous membrane of the mouth.

stomatitis med·i·ca·men·to·sa (mĕd′ĭ-kə-mən-tō′sə) *n*. Allergic inflammatory changes in the oral soft tissues associated with use of drugs or medicines, usually those taken systemically.

sto·ma·to·dyn·i·a (stō′mə-tə-dĭn′ē-ə) *n*. See stomatalgia.

sto·ma·tog·nath·ic system (stō′mə-tŏg-năth′ĭk, -tō-năth′-) *n*. All of the structures involved in speech and in the receiving, chewing, and swallowing of food.

sto·ma·to·ma·la·ci·a (stō′mə-tō-mə-lā′shē-ə, -shə) *n*. Pathological softening of any of the structures of the mouth.

sto·ma·to·my·co·sis (stō′mə-tō-mī-kō′sĭs) *n*. A fungal disease of the mouth.

sto·ma·top·a·thy (stō′mə-tŏp′ə-thē) *n*. A disease of the mouth.

sto·ma·to·plas·ty (stō′mə-tə-plăs′tē) *n*. Reconstructive or plastic surgery of the mouth. — sto′-ma·to·plas′tic (-plăs′tĭk) *adj*.

sto·ma·tor·rha·gi·a (stō′mə-tə-rā′jē-ə, -jə) *n*. Bleeding from any part of the oral cavity.

sto·mo·de·um (stō′mə-dē′əm) *n*. A midline ectodermal depression ventral to the embryonic brain and surrounded by the mandibular arch. It becomes continuous with the foregut and forms the mouth. — sto′mo·de′al *adj*.

stone (stōn) *n*. See calculus (sense 1).

Stook·ey–Scarff operation (stook′ē-skärf′) *n*. See third ventriculostomy (sense 1).

stool (stool) *n*. **1.** A discharging of the bowels. **2.** Evacuated fecal matter.

stor·age (stôr′ĭj) *n*. The second of three stages in the memory process, involving mental processes associated with retention of stimuli that have been registered and modified by encoding.

storage disease *n*. Any of various metabolic disorders usually caused by a congenital enzyme deficiency and characterized by the accumulation of a specific substance, such as a lipid or protein, within tissues.

storm (stôrm) *n*. An exacerbation of symptoms or a crisis in the course of a disease.

stra·bis·mom·e·ter (străb′ĭz-mŏm′ĭ-tər, strā′bĭz-) *n*. A calibrated plate with the upper margin curved to conform with the lower eyelid, used to measure strabismus.

stra·bis·mus (strə-bĭz′məs) *n*. A visual defect in which one eye cannot focus with the other on an objective because of eye muscle imbalance. — stra·bis′mal (-məl), stra·bis′mic (-mĭk) *adj*.

stra·bot·o·my (strə-bŏt′ə-mē) *n*. Surgical division

of one or more of the ocular muscles or their tendons for the correction of strabismus.

strain¹ (strān) *v.* **strained, strain·ing, strains. 1.** To pull, draw, or stretch tight. **2.** To stretch or exert one's muscles or nerves to the utmost. **3.** To injure or impair by overuse or overexertion. **4.** To pass a liquid through a filtering agent. **5.** To draw off or remove by filtration. — *n.* **1.** The act of straining. **2.** The state of being strained. **3.** Extreme or laborious effort, exertion, or work. **4.** A great or excessive pressure, demand, or stress on one's body, mind, or resources. **5.** A wrench, twist, or other physical injury resulting from excessive tension, effort, or use.

strain² (strān) *n.* **1.** Any of the various lines of ancestry united in an individual or a family; ancestry or lineage. **2.** A group of organisms of the same species, having distinctive characteristics but not usually considered a separate breed or variety.

strain fracture *n.* A fracture in which a piece of bone attached to a tendon, ligament, or capsule is torn away by an internal or an external force.

strait (strāt) *n.* A narrow passage, such as the upper or lower opening of the pelvic canal.

strait·jack·et or **straight·jack·et** (strāt′jăk′ĭt) *n.* A long-sleeved jacketlike garment used to bind the arms tightly against the body as a means of restraining a violent person.

stran·gle (străng′gəl) *v.* **-gled, -gling, -gles.** To compress the trachea so as to prevent sufficient passage of air; suffocate.

stran·gu·late (străng′gyə-lāt′) *v.* **-lat·ed, -lat·ing, -lates. 1.** To strangle. **2.** To compress, constrict, or obstruct a body part so as to cut off the flow of blood or other fluid. **3.** To be or become strangled, compressed, constricted, or obstructed.

strangulated hernia *n.* An irreducible hernia in which normal blood supply is arrested.

stran·gu·la·tion (străng′gyə-lā′shən) *n.* **1.** The act of strangling or strangulating. **2.** The state of being strangled or strangulated. **3.** Constriction of a body part so as to cut off the flow of blood or another fluid.

stran·gu·ry (străng′gyə-rē) *n.* Slow, painful urination, with the urine passed drop by drop.

strap (străp) *n.* A strip of adhesive plaster. — *v.* **strapped, strap·ping, straps.** To support or bind a part, especially with overlapping strips of adhesive plaster.

strat·i·fi·ca·tion (străt′ə-fĭ-kā′shən) *n.* An arrangement in layers or strata.

strat·i·fied epithelium (străt′ə-fīd′) *n.* Epithelium made up of a series of layers, the cells of each varying in size and shape.

stra·tig·ra·phy (strə-tĭg′rə-fē) *n.* See **tomography.** — **strat′i·graph′ic** (străt′ĭ-grăf′ĭk) *adj.*

stra·tum (strā′təm, străt′əm) *n., pl.* **-tums** or **-ta** (-tə). **1.** A horizontal layer of material, especially one of several parallel layers arranged one on top of another. **2.** Any of the layers of differentiated tissue forming an anatomical structure. — **stra′tal** (-təl) *adj.*

stratum com·pac·tum (kəm-păk′təm) *n.* The superficial layer of decidual tissue in the pregnant uterus.

stratum cor·ne·um (kôr′nē-əm) *n.* The horny outer layer of the epidermis, consisting of several layers of flat, keratinized, nonnucleated, dead or peeling cells.

stratum func·tion·a·le (fŭngk′shə-nā′lē) *n.* The endometrium except for the basal layer, formerly thought to be lost during menstruation but now considered to be only partially discharged.

stratum spon·gi·o·sum (spŏn′jē-ō′səm) *n.* The middle layer of the endometrium, formed chiefly of dilated glandular structures, and flanked by the stratum compactum on the luminal side and by the basal layer on the myometrial side.

straw·ber·ry mark (strô′bĕr′ē) *n.* A raised, shiny, red nevus or birthmark, occurring usually on the face or scalp and resembling a strawberry.

strawberry tongue *n.* The presence of a whitish coat on the tongue through which the enlarged papillae project as red points, characteristic of scarlet fever.

strep (strĕp) *adj.* Streptococcal. — *n.* Streptococcus.

strep throat *n.* See **septic sore throat.**

strep·ti·ce·mi·a (strĕp′tĭ-sē′mē-ə) *n.* See **streptococcemia.**

Strep·to·ba·cil·lus (strĕp′tō-bə-sĭl′əs) *n.* A genus of gram-negative, rod-shaped, often pathogenic bacteria occurring in chains, especially *S. moniliformis,* which causes a type of rat-bite fever.

strep·to·coc·ce·mi·a (strĕp′tə-kŏk-sē′-mē-ə) *n.* The presence of streptococci in the blood.

strep·to·coc·cus (strĕp′tə-kŏk′əs) *n., pl.* **-coc·ci** (-kŏk′sī, -kŏk′ī). A bacterium of the genus *Streptococcus.* — **strep′to·coc′cal, strep′to·coc′cic** *adj.*

Strep·to·coc·cus (strĕp′tə-kŏk′əs) *n.* A genus of gram-positive, anaerobic, often pathogenic bacteria having an ovoid or spherical appearance and occurring in pairs or chains, including many pathogenic species that cause erysipelas, scarlet fever, and septic sore throat.

streptococcus erythrogenic toxin *n.* A culture filtrate of the endotoxin produced by strains of beta-hemolytic streptococci that produces an erythematous reaction at inoculation sites on the skin of susceptible persons.

strep·tol·y·sin (strĕp-tŏl′ĭ-sĭn, strĕp′tə-lī′sĭn) *n.* A hemolysin produced by streptococci.

strep·to·my·cin or **strep·to·my·cin A** (strĕp′tə-mī′sĭn) *n.* An antibiotic obtained from *Streptomyces griseus* and used against the tubercle bacillus and other bacteria.

strep·to·ni·grin (strĕp′tə-nī′grĭn) *n.* A highly toxic antibiotic produced by an actinomycete (*Streptomyces flocculus*) and active against various types of tumors.

strep·to·sep·ti·ce·mi·a (strĕp′tō-sĕp′tĭ-sē′mē-ə) *n.* See **streptococcemia.**

strep·to·zo·cin (strĕp′tə-zō′sĭn) or **strep·to·zot·o·cin** (-zŏt′ə-sĭn) *n.* An antineoplastic agent produced by an actinomycete *(Streptomyces achromogenes)* and active against tumors but damaging to insulin-producing cells and now regarded as a carcinogen.

stress (strĕs) *n.* **1.** An applied force or system of forces that tends to strain or deform a body. **2.** A physical or psychological stimulus which, when acting upon a person, produces mental tension or physiological reactions that may lead to illness.

stress fracture *n.* A fatigue fracture of bone caused by repeated application of a heavy load, such as the constant pounding on a surface by runners, gymnasts, and dancers.

stress reaction *n.* An acute emotional reaction to physical or psychological stress.

stress shielding *n.* Osteopenia occurring in bone as the result of removal of normal stress from the bone by an implant.

stress test *n.* A graded test to measure one's heart rate and oxygen intake while undergoing strenuous physical exercise, as on a treadmill.

stress ulcers *pl.n.* Acute peptic ulcers occurring in association with other conditions, including burns, intracranial lesions, and surgical operations.

stretch·er (strĕch′ər) *n.* A litter, usually of canvas stretched over a frame, used to transport the sick, wounded, or dead.

stretch mark (strĕch) *n.* A shiny line on the skin of the abdomen, breasts, thighs, or buttocks caused by the prolonged stretching of the skin and weakening of elastic tissues as a result of pregnancy or obesity, for example.

stretch receptor *n.* A sensory receptor in a muscle that responds to the stretching of tissue.

stretch reflex *n.* See myotatic reflex.

stri·a (strī′ə) *n., pl.* **stri·ae** (strī′ē). **1.** A thin, narrow groove or channel. **2.** A thin line or band, especially one of several that are parallel or close together. **3.** A thin line, band, stripe, or streak distinguished from the tissue in which it is found; a striation.

striae a·tro·phi·cae (ə-trŏ′fĭ-kē′, ə-trŏf′ĭ-) *pl.n.* Stretch marks.

striae grav·i·dar·um (grăv′ĭ-dâr′əm) *pl.n.* Stretch marks resulting from pregnancy.

stri·ate (strī′āt′) *v.* **-at·ed, -at·ing, -ates.** To mark with striae or striations. — *adj.* or **stri·at·ed** (-ā′-tĭd) **1.** Marked with striae; striped, grooved, or ridged. **2.** Consisting of a stria or striae.

stri·at·ed border (strī′ā′tĭd) *n.* The free surface of the columnar absorptive cells of the intestine formed by microvilli.

striated muscle *n.* Skeletal, voluntary, and cardiac muscle, distinguished from smooth muscle by transverse striations of the fibers.

stri·a·tion (strī-ā′shən) *n.* **1.** The state of being striated or having striae. **2.** A stria.

stric·ture (strĭk′chər) *n.* A circumscribed narrowing of a hollow structure.

stric·tur·ot·o·my (strĭk′chə-rŏt′ə-mē) *n.* Surgical opening or division of a stricture.

stri·dor (strī′dər, -dôr′) *n.* A high-pitched noisy sound occurring during inhalation or exhalation, a sign of respiratory obstruction.

strip (strĭp) *v.* **stripped, strip·ping, strips. 1.** To press out or drain off by milking. **2.** To make a subcutaneous excision of a vein in its longitudinal axis, usually a leg vein.

stroke (strōk) *n.* **1.** A sudden severe attack, as of paralysis or sunstroke. **2.** A sudden loss of brain function caused by a blockage or rupture of a blood vessel to the brain, characterized by loss of muscular control, diminution or loss of sensation or consciousness, dizziness, slurred speech, or other symptoms that vary with the extent and severity of the damage to the brain.

stroke volume *n.* The volume of blood pumped out of one ventricle of the heart in a single beat.

stro·ma (strō′mə) *n., pl.* **-ma·ta** (-mə-tə). **1.** The connective tissue framework of an organ, a gland, or other structure, as distinguished from the tissues performing the special function of the organ or part. **2.** The spongy, colorless framework of a red blood cell or other cell. — **stro′mal** *adj.* — **stro·mat′ic** (-măt′ĭk) *adj.*

stro·muhr (strō′mŏŏr′) *n.* An instrument for measuring the quantity of blood that flows per unit of time through a blood vessel.

stron·gy·loi·di·a·sis (strŏn′jə-loi-dī′ə-sĭs) or **stron·gy·loi·do·sis** (-dō′sĭs) *n.* Infection with the nematode *Strongyloides stercoralis.*

stron·ti·um (strŏn′chē-əm, -tē-əm, -shəm) *n.* A soft, easily oxidized metallic element with atomic number 38.

struc·tur·al gene (strŭk′chər-əl) *n.* A gene that determines the amino acid sequence of a specific protein or peptide.

struc·ture (strŭk′chər) *n.* **1.** The arrangement or formation of the tissues, organs, or other parts of an organism. **2.** A tissue, an organ, or other formation made up of different but related parts.

stru·ma (strōō′mə) *n., pl.* **-mas** or **-mae** (-mē). **1.** Goiter. **2.** See scrofula. — **stru·mat′ic** (-măt′ĭk), **stru′mose** (-mōs′), **stru′mous** (-məs) *adj.*

struma o·var·i·i (ō-vâr′ē-ī′) *n.* A rare ovarian tumor composed mostly of thyroid tissue.

stru·mec·to·my (strōō-mĕk′tə-mē) *n.* Surgical removal of all or a portion of a goitrous tumor.

stru·mi·tis (strōō-mī′tĭs) *n.* Inflammation of the thyroid gland.

strych·nine (strĭk′nīn′, -nĭn, -nēn′) *n.* An extremely poisonous white crystalline alkaloid, derived from plants of the genus *Strychnos,* used as a poison for rodents and formerly used as a central nervous system stimulant.

Stry·ker frame (strī′kər) *n.* A frame that allows a person to be turned in various planes as a single unit without moving parts of the body separately.

stump (stŭmp) *n.* **1.** The extremity of a limb left after amputation. **2.** The pedicle remaining after removal of the tumor to which it was attached.

stump cancer *n.* A carcinoma of the stomach developing after gastroenterostomy or gastric resection for benign disease.

stu·por (stōō′pər, styōō′-) *n.* A state of impaired

consciousness characterized by a marked diminution in the capacity to react to stimuli.

Sturge–Weber syndrome *n.* A congenital syndrome characterized by a port-wine stain nevus in the distribution of the trigeminal nerve, homolateral meningeal angioma with intracranial calcification and neurologic signs, and angioma of the choroid, often with secondary glaucoma.

stut·ter (stŭt′ər) *n.* A phonatory or articulatory disorder characterized by difficult enunciation of words with frequent halting and repetition of the initial consonant or syllable. — *v.* **-tered, -ter·ing, -ters.** To utter with spasmodic repetition or prolongation of sounds.

sty or **stye** (stī) *n., pl.* **sties** or **styes** (stīz). Inflammation of one or more sebaceous glands of an eyelid.

sty·let (stī-lĕt′, stī′lĭt) *n.* **1.** A fine wire that is run through a catheter, cannula, or hollow needle to keep it stiff or clear of debris. **2.** A slender surgical probe.

sty·loid (stī′loid′) *n.* Of, relating to, or designating any of several slender pointed bone processes, especially the spine that projects from the base of the temporal bone.

sty·loid·i·tis (stī′loi-dī′tĭs) *n.* Inflammation of a styloid process.

stype (stīp) *n.* A tampon.

styp·tic (stĭp′tĭk) *adj.* **1.** Contracting the tissues or blood vessels; astringent. **2.** Tending to check bleeding by contracting the tissues or blood vessels; hemostatic. — *n.* A styptic drug or substance. — **styp·tic′i·ty** (-tĭs′ĭ-tē) *n.*

styptic pencil *n.* A short medicated stick, often of alum, applied to a cut to check bleeding.

sub·a·cute (sŭb′ə-kyōot′) *adj.* Between acute and chronic. — **sub′a·cute′ly** *adv.*

sub·a·or·tic stenosis (sŭb′ā-ôr′tĭk) *n.* Narrowing of the outflow tract of the left ventricle caused by an obstruction shortly below the aortic valve.

sub·ap·i·cal (sŭb-ăp′ĭ-kəl, -ā′pĭ-) *adj.* Located below the apex of a part. — **sub·ap′i·cal·ly** *adv.*

sub·a·rach·noid space (sŭb′ə-răk′noid′) *n.* The space between the arachnoid membrane and pia mater; it contains the large blood vessels supplying the brain and spinal cord.

sub·cho·ri·al lake (sŭb-kôr′ē-əl) *n.* See **subchorial space.**

subchorial space *n.* The part of the placenta adjacent to and beneath the chorion.

sub·cla·vi·an artery (sŭb-klā′vē-ən) *n.* An artery originating on the left from the aortic arch and on the right from the brachiocephalic artery with branches to the brain, neck, thorax, and shoulder.

subclavian steal *n.* Obstruction of the subclavian artery proximal to its origin at the vertebral artery. Blood flow through the vertebral artery is reversed, causing symptoms of cerebrovascular insufficiency.

subclavian vein *n.* A continuation of the axillary vein at the lateral border of the first rib, joining

the internal jugular vein and forming the brachiocephalic vein on each side.

sub·clin·i·cal (sŭb-klĭn′ĭ-kəl) *adj.* Not manifesting characteristic clinical symptoms. Used of a disease or condition.

subclinical absence *n.* Transient impairment of thinking without overt manifestations, demonstrable only by psychological testing, and accompanied by an outburst of 3 per second spike and wave complexes on an electroencephalograph.

sub·con·scious (sŭb-kŏn′shəs) *adj.* Not wholly conscious; partially or imperfectly conscious. — *n.* The part of the mind below the level of conscious perception. — **sub·con′scious·ly** *adv.*

sub·con·scious·ness (sŭb-kŏn′shəs-nĭs) *n.* The state in which mental processes take place without one's conscious perception.

sub·cor·tex (sŭb-kôr′tĕks) *n., pl.* **-ti·ces** (-tĭ-sēz′). The portion of the brain immediately below the cerebral cortex. — **sub·cor′ti·cal** (-tĭ-kəl) *adj.* — **sub·cor′ti·cal·ly** *adv.*

sub·cu·ta·ne·ous (sŭb′kyōo-tā′nē-əs) *adj.* Located, found, or placed just beneath the skin; hypodermic. — **sub′cu·ta′ne·ous·ly** *adv.*

subcutaneous emphysema *n.* The presence of air or gas in subcutaneous tissues.

subcutaneous fat necrosis of the newborn *n.* See **sclerema neonatorum.**

subcutaneous flap *n.* A pedicle flap in which the pedicle is denuded of epithelium and buried in the subcutaneous tissue of the recipient area.

subcutaneous mastectomy *n.* Surgical removal of the breast tissues, with preservation of the skin, nipple, and areola, usually followed by the implantation of a prosthesis.

subcutaneous operation *n.* An operation, as for the division of a tendon, performed without incising the skin beyond a minute opening.

subcutaneous tenotomy *n.* Division of a tendon by means of a small pointed knife introduced through skin and subcutaneous tissue without an incision.

subcutaneous tissue *n.* A layer of loose, irregular connective tissue immediately beneath the skin; it contains fat cells except in the auricles, eyelids, penis, and scrotum.

sub·dur·al (sŭb-dŏor′əl, -dyŏor′-) *adj.* Located or occurring beneath the dura mater.

subdural hematoma *n.* See **subdural hemorrhage.**

subdural hemorrhage *n.* Extravasation of blood between the dural and arachnoidal membranes.

subdural space *n.* The narrow space between the dura mater and the arachnoid membrane.

sub·fer·til·i·ty (sŭb′fər-tĭl′ĭ-tē) *n.* A less than normal capacity for reproduction.

sub·gin·gi·val curettage (sŭb-jĭn′jə-vəl, -jĭn-jī′-) *n.* The removal of subgingival calculus or ulcerated epithelial and granulomatous tissues from periodontal pockets with a curette.

sub·grun·da·tion (sŭb′grŭn-dā′shən) *n.* Depression of one fragment of a broken cranial bone below the other.

sub·in·fec·tion (sŭb′ĭn-fĕk′shən) *n.* A secondary

infection occurring in a person exposed to and successfully resisting another infectious disease.

sub·in·vo·lu·tion (sŭb'ĭn-və-lōō'shən) n. Failure of the uterus to return to its normal size following childbirth.

sub·ja·cent (sŭb-jā'sənt) adj. Below or beneath another part. — **sub·ja'cen·cy** n.

sub·jec·tive (səb-jĕk'tĭv) adj. 1. Of, relating to, or designating a symptom or condition perceived by the patient and not by the examiner. 2. Existing only in the mind; illusory. — **sub·jec'tive·ly** adv.

subjective sensation n. A sensation whose cause cannot be readily linked to a verifiable external stimulus.

subjective symptom n. A symptom apparent to the person afflicted but not observable by others.

sub·la·tion (sŭb-lā'shən) n. The detachment, elevation, or removal of a part.

sub·le·thal (sŭb-lē'thəl) adj. Not sufficient to cause death. — **sub·le'thal·ly** adv.

sub·li·mate (sŭb'lə-māt') v. **-mat·ed, -mat·ing, -mates.** To modify the natural expression of an instinctual impulse, especially a sexual one in a socially acceptable manner.

sub·li·ma·tion (sŭb'lə-mā'shən) n. 1. The act or process of sublimating. 2. An unconscious defense mechanism in which unacceptable instinctual drives and wishes are modified into more personally and socially acceptable channels.

sub·lim·i·nal (sŭb-lĭm'ə-nəl) adj. 1. Below the threshold of conscious perception. Used of stimuli. 2. Inadequate to produce conscious awareness but able to evoke a response. — **sub·lim'i·nal·ly** adv.

sub·lin·gual (sŭb-lĭng'gwəl) adj. Below or beneath the tongue; hypoglossal.

sublingual gland n. Either of two salivary glands situated in the mucus membrane on the floor of the mouth beneath the tongue.

sub·lux·a·tion (sŭb'lŭk-sā'shən) n. Incomplete or partial dislocation, as of a bone in a joint.

sub·man·dib·u·lar gland (sŭb'măn-dĭb'yə-lər) n. Either of two major salivary glands situated in the neck near the lower edge of each side of the mandible and emptying into the submandibular duct.

sub·max·il·la (sŭb'măk-sĭl'ə) n. See **mandible.**

sub·max·il·lar·i·tis (sŭb'măk-sĭl'ə-rī'tĭs) n. Inflammation of the submandibular salivary gland, usually due to the mumps virus.

sub·max·il·lar·y (sŭb-măk'sə-lĕr'ē) adj. 1. Of or relating to the lower jaw; mandibular. 2. Situated beneath the maxilla. — n. An anatomical part, such as a gland or nerve, situated beneath the maxilla.

submaxillary gland n. See **submandibular gland.**

sub·mu·co·sa (sŭb'myōō-kō'sə) n. A layer of loose connective tissue beneath a mucous membrane.

sub·nu·cle·us (sŭb'nōō'klē-əs, -nyōō'-) n. A secondary nucleus into which a large nerve nucleus may be divided.

sub·si·dence (səb-sīd'ns, sŭb'sĭ-dns) n. Sinking or

settling in a bone, as of a prosthetic component of a total joint implant.

sub·sid·i·ar·y atrial pacemaker (səb-sĭd'ē-ĕr'ē) n. A secondary source for rhythmic control of the heart, available for controlling cardiac activity if the sinoatrial pacemaker fails. It is located near the inferior vena cava.

sub·stance (sŭb'stəns) n. A material of a particular kind or constitution.

substance abuse n. Excessive use of a potentially addictive substance, especially one that may modify body functions, such as tobacco, alcohol, and drugs. — **substance abuser** n.

substance abuse disorder n. Any of a category of disorders in which pathological behavioral changes are associated with the regular use of substances that affect the central nervous system.

substance P n. A short-chain polypeptide that functions as a neurotransmitter especially in the transmission of pain impulses from peripheral receptors to the central nervous system.

sub·stan·ti·a al·ba (sŭb-stăn'shē-ə ăl'bə) n. See **white matter.**

substantia gris·e·a (grĭs'ē-ə, grĭz'-) n. See **gray matter.**

substantia ni·gra (nī'grə, nĭg'rə) n. A layer of large pigmented nerve cells in the mesencephalon that produce dopamine and whose destruction is associated with Parkinson's disease.

sub·sti·tu·tion (sŭb'stĭ-tōō'shən, -tyōō'-) n. An unconscious defense mechanism by which the unacceptable or unattainable is replaced by something more acceptable or attainable.

substitution therapy n. Replacement therapy in which a substitute substance is used.

substitution transfusion n. See **exchange transfusion.**

sub·strate (sŭb'strāt') n. 1. The material or substance on which an enzyme acts. 2. A surface on which an organism grows or is attached.

sub·struc·ture (sŭb'strŭk'chər) n. A tissue or structure wholly or partly beneath the surface. — **sub·struc'tur·al** adj.

sub·thresh·old stimulus (sŭb-thrĕsh'ōld', -hōld') n. See **inadequate stimulus.**

sub·to·tal hysterectomy (sŭb-tōt'l) n. See **supracervical hysterectomy.**

sub·vo·cal speech (sŭb-vō'kəl) n. Slight movements of the speech muscles, related to thinking but producing no sound.

sub·vo·lu·tion (sŭb'və-lōō'shən) n. The surgical reversal of a flap of mucous membrane to prevent adhesion, as in the operation for pterygium.

suc·cor·rhe·a (sŭk'ə-rē'ə) n. An abnormal increase in the secretion of a digestive fluid.

suck·ing reflex (sŭk'ĭng) n. Sucking movements of an infant's lips elicited by touching them or the adjacent skin.

sucking wound n. See **open pneumothorax.**

su·cral·fate (sōō-krăl'fāt') n. A polysaccharide used to treat duodenal ulcers.

su·crose (sōō'krōs') n. A nonreducing crystalline disaccharide made up of glucose and fructose, found in many plants but extracted as ordinary sugar mainly from sugar cane and sugar beets, and widely used as a sweetener or preservative.

su·cro·se·mi·a (sōō'krō-sē'mē-ə) *n.* The presence of sucrose in the blood.

sucrose pol·y·es·ter (pŏl'ē-ĕs'tər, pōl'ē-ĕs'tər) *n.* A complex synthetic compound of sucrose and fatty acids that the body is unable to digest or absorb, produced commerically as a partial substitute for fats in cooking oils, shortening, butter, and other high-calorie or high-cholesterol foods.

su·cro·su·ria (sōō'krō-sŏŏr'ē-ə) *n.* Excretion of sucrose in the urine.

suc·tion drainage (sŭk'shən) *n.* The closed drainage of a cavity using a suction apparatus attached to a drainage tube.

su·da·men (sōō-dā'mən) *n., pl.* **-dam·i·na** (-dăm'ə-nə). A small vesicle caused by retention of fluid in a sweat follicle or in the epidermis.

su·da·tion (sōō-dā'shən) *n.* Perspiration.

sud·den infant death syndrome (sŭd'n) *n.* A fatal syndrome that affects apparently healthy sleeping infants under a year old, characterized by a sudden cessation of breathing and thought to be caused by a defect in the central nervous system.

su·dor (sōō'dər, -dôr') *n.* Sweat.

su·do·re·sis (sōō'də-rē'sĭs) *n.* Profuse sweating.

su·do·rif·er·ous (sōō'də-rĭf'ər-əs) *adj.* Carrying or producing sweat.

sudoriferous gland *n.* See **sweat gland.**

suf·fo·cate (sŭf'ə-kāt') *v.* **-cat·ed, -cat·ing, -cates.** **1.** To impair the respiration of. **2.** To suffer from lack of oxygen; to be unable to breathe. — **suf'fo·ca'tion** *n.* — **suf'fo·ca'tive** *adj.*

suf·fu·sion (sə-fyōō'zhən) *n.* **1.** The act of pouring a fluid over the body. **2.** A spreading out of a body fluid from a vessel into the surrounding tissues. **3.** The reddening of a surface. — **suf·fuse'** (-fyōōz') *v.*

sug·ar (shŏŏg'ər) *n.* **1.** A sweet crystalline or powdered substance consisting of sucrose and used in many foods, drinks, and medicines to improve their taste. **2.** Any of a class of water-soluble crystalline carbohydrates, including sucrose and lactose, having a characteristically sweet taste and classified as monosaccharides, disaccharides, and trisaccharides.

sugar diabetes *n.* Insulin-dependent diabetes; diabetes mellitus.

sug·gest·i·bil·i·ty (səg-jĕs'tə-bĭl'ĭ-tē, sə-jĕs'-) *n.* Responsiveness or susceptibility to suggestion.

sug·gil·la·tion (sŭg'jə-lā'shən, sŭj'ə-) *n.* **1.** A black-and-blue mark. **2.** See **livedo.**

su·i·cid·al (sōō'ĭ-sīd'l) *adj.* **1.** Of or relating to suicide. **2.** Likely to attempt suicide. — **su'i·cid'al·ly** *adv.*

su·i·cide (sōō'ĭ-sīd') *n.* **1.** The act or an instance of intentionally killing oneself. **2.** One who commits suicide.

sul·cus (sŭl'kəs) *n., pl.* **-ci** (-kī, -sī). **1.** Any of the grooves or furrows on the surface of the brain, bounding the convolutions or gyri; a fissure. **2.** A

long narrow groove, furrow, or slight depression, as in an organ or a tissue. — **sul'cal** *adj.*

sul·fa·cy·tine (sŭl'fə-sī'tēn) *n.* A sulfonamide used as an oral antibiotic in the treatment of urinary tract infections.

sul·fa·di·a·zine (sŭl'fə-dī'ə-zēn) *n.* A sulfa drug used in the treatment of meningitis and other infections.

sul·fa drug (sŭl'fə) *n.* Any of a group of synthetic organic compounds, derived chiefly from sulfanilamide, chemically similar to PABA and capable of inhibiting bacterial growth and activity by interfering with the metabolic processes in bacteria that require PABA.

sul·fa·nil·a·mide (sŭl'fə-nĭl'ə-mīd', -mĭd) *n.* A white, odorless crystalline sulfonamide used in the treatment of various bacterial infections.

sul·fa·ti·date (sŭl'fə-tī'dāt') or **sul·fa·tide** (sŭl'fə-tīd') *n.* Any of the cerebroside sulfuric esters containing sulfate groups in the sugar portion of the molecule.

sulf·he·mo·glo·bi·ne·mi·a (sŭlf-hē'mə-glō'bə-nē'mē-ə) *n.* The presence of sulfmethemoglobin in the blood.

sul·fin·pyr·a·zone (sŭl'fĭn-pĭr'ə-zōn') *n.* A drug that is related to phenylbutazone, promotes urinary excretion of uric acid, and is used in the treatment of gout.

sulf·met·he·mo·glo·bin (sŭlf'mĕt-hē'mə-glō'bĭn) or **sulf·he·mo·glo·bin** (sŭlf-hē'mə-) *n.* The complex formed by the reaction of a sulfide and hemoglobin in the presence of oxygen.

sul·fon·meth·ane (sŭl'fŏn-mĕth'ān', -fŏn-) *n.* A colorless crystalline or powdered compound used medicinally as a hypnotic.

sul·fo·sal·i·cyl·ic acid turbidity test (sŭl'fō-săl'ĭ-sĭl'ĭk) *n.* A test for measuring protein in urine.

sul·fur or **sul·phur** (sŭl'fər) *n.* A yellow nonmetallic element with atomic number 16, occurring widely in nature and used in the manufacture of pharmaceuticals and many sulfur compounds.

su·lin·dac (sə-lĭn'dăk) *n.* A nonsteroidal anti-inflammatory agent with analgesic and antipyretic actions.

sum·ma·tion (sə-mā'shən) *n.* The process by which multiple or repeated stimuli can produce a response in a nerve, muscle, or other part that one stimulus alone cannot produce.

summation gallop *n.* A heart gallop rhythm in which there is superimposition of abnormal third and fourth heart sounds, usually indicative of myocardial disease.

sum·mer diarrhea (sŭm'ər) *n.* Diarrhea affecting infants or young children in hot weather, usually caused by acute gastroenteritis due to infection with *Shigella* or *Salmonella.*

sump drain *n.* A drain consisting of a smaller tube within a larger tube through which fluid passes as a result of suction.

sun block *n.* A preparation, as of PABA, that prevents sunburn by filtering out the sun's ultraviolet rays, usually offering more protection than a sunscreen.

sun·burn (sŭn′bûrn′) *n.* Inflammation and erythema of the skin, often with blistering, caused by overexposure to the ultraviolet rays of direct sunlight. — **sun′burn′** *v.*

sun protection factor *n.* The ratio of the minimal ultraviolet dose required to produce erythema with and without a sunscreen; a measure of the degree to which a sunscreen protects the skin from ultraviolet radiation, the higher the number the greater degree of protection.

sun·screen (sŭn′skrēn′) *n.* A preparation, often in the form of a cream or lotion, used to protect the skin from damaging ultraviolet radiation.

sun·stroke or **sun stroke** (sŭn′strōk′) *n.* A form of heatstroke resulting from undue exposure to the sun's rays; symptoms are similar to those of heatstroke, often without fever, but with prostration and collapse.

su·per·al·i·men·ta·tion (sōō′pər-ăl′ə-měn-tā′-shən) *n.* See **hyperalimentation** (sense 1).

su·per·bug (sōō′pər-bŭg′) *n.* Any of various disease-causing bacteria that develop a resistance to drugs normally used to control or eradicate them.

su·per·cil·i·um (sōō′pər-sĭl′ē-əm) *n.*, *pl.* -i·a (-ē-ə). **1.** The eyebrow. **2.** An individual hair of the eyebrow.

su·per·duct (sōō′pər-dŭkt′) *v.* -duct·ed, -duct·ing, -ducts. To elevate or draw upward.

su·per·e·go (sōō′pər-ē′gō, -ĕg′ō) *n.*, *pl.* -gos. In psychoanalytic theory, the division of the psyche that censors and restrains the ego and has identified itself unconsciously with important persons from early life.

su·per·ex·ci·ta·tion (sōō′pər-ĕk′sī-tā′shən) *n.* **1.** The act of exciting or stimulating unduly. **2.** A condition of extreme excitement or overstimulation.

su·per·fi·cial (sōō′pər-fĭsh′əl) *adj.* **1.** Of, affecting, or being on or near the surface. **2.** Cursory; not thorough.

superficial reflex *n.* A reflex elicited by stimulation of the skin.

su·per·in·duce (sōō′pər-ĭn-dōōs′, -dyōōs′) *v.* -duced, -duc·ing, -duc·es. To introduce as an addition to something already existing.

su·per·in·fect (sōō′pər-ĭn-fĕkt′) *v.* -fect·ed, -fect·ing, -fects. To cause to be further infected with a microorganism; infect a second time or more.

su·per·in·fec·tion (sōō′pər-ĭn-fĕk′shən) *n.* **1.** The act or process of superinfecting a cell or an organism. **2.** An infection following a previous infection, especially when caused by microorganisms that have become resistant to the antibiotics used earlier.

su·pe·ri·or (sōō-pēr′ē-ər) *adj.* **1.** Situated above or directed upward. **2.** Situated nearer the top of the head. — **su·pe′ri·or′i·ty** (-ôr′ĭ-tē) *n.* — **su·pe′ri·or·ly** *adv.*

su·pe·ri·or·i·ty complex (sōō-pēr′ē-ôr′ĭ-tē) *n.* A psychological defense mechanism in which feelings of superiority counter or conceal feelings of inferiority.

superior limb *n.* See **upper extremity**.

superior vena cava *n.* A large vein that receives blood from the head, neck, upper limbs, and chest, and empties into the right atrium of the heart.

su·per·mo·til·i·ty (sōō′pər-mō-tĭl′ĭ-tē) *n.* Excessive motility.

su·per·nu·mer·ar·y (sōō′pər-nōō′mə-rĕr′ē, -nyōō′-) *adj.* Exceeding the normal or usual number; extra.

su·per·o·vu·late (sōō′pər-ō′vyə-lāt′, -ŏv′yə-) *v.* -lat·ed, -lat·ing, -lates. **1.** To produce mature ova at an accelerated rate or in a large number at one time. **2.** To cause to superovulate. — **su′per·o·vu·la′tion** *n.*

su·per·son·ic (sōō′pər-sŏn′ĭk) *adj.* Of or relating to sound waves beyond human audibility. — **su′·per·son′i·cal·ly** *adv.*

su·per·struc·ture (sōō′pər-strŭk′chər) *n.* A structure above the surface.

su·pi·nate (sōō′pə-nāt′) *v.* -nat·ed, -nat·ing, -nates. To assume, or to be placed in, a supine position. — **su′pi·na′tion** *n.*

su·pi·na·tor muscle (sōō′pə-nā′tər) *n.* A muscle with origin from the humerus and the ulna, with insertion into the radius, and whose action supinates the forearm.

su·pine (sōō-pīn′, sōō′pīn′) *adj.* **1.** Lying on the back; having the face upward. **2.** Having the palm of the hand or sole of the foot upward.

support *v.* -port·ed, -port·ing, -ports. **1.** To bear the weight of, especially from below. **2.** To hold in position so as to keep from falling, sinking, or slipping. **3.** To be capable of bearing; withstand. **4.** To keep from weakening or failing; strengthen. **5.** To provide for or maintain. **6.** To endure; tolerate. — *n.* **1.** The act of supporting. **2.** The state of being supported. **3.** One that supports.

sup·pos·i·to·ry (sə-pŏz′ĭ-tôr′ē) *n.* A small plug of medication designed to melt at body temperature within a body cavity other than the mouth, especially the rectum or vagina.

sup·press (sə-prĕs′) *v.* -pressed, -press·ing, -press·es. **1.** To curtail or inhibit the activity of something, such as the immune system. **2.** To deliberately exclude unacceptable desires or thoughts from the mind. **3.** To reduce the incidence or severity of a condition or symptom.

sup·pres·sion (sə-prĕsh′ən) *n.* **1.** The act of suppressing or the state of being suppressed. **2.** Conscious exclusion of unacceptable desires, thoughts, or memories from the mind. **3.** The sudden arrest of the secretion of a fluid, such as urine or bile. **4.** The checking or curtailing of an abnormal flow or discharge. **5.** The effect of a second genetic mutation that reverses a phenotypic change caused by a previous mutation at a different location on the chromosome.

sup·pres·sor mutation (sə-prĕs′ər) *n.* A mutation that alters the anticodon in a tRNA so that it is complementary to a termination codon, thus suppressing termination of the amino acid chain.

sup·pres·sor T cell (sə-prĕs′ər) *n.* A T cell that reduces or suppresses the immune response of B cells or of other T cells to an antigen.

sup·pu·rate (sŭp′yə-rāt′) *v.* **-rat·ed, -rat·ing, -rates.** To form or discharge pus.

sup·pu·ra·tion (sŭp′yə-rā′shən) *n.* The formation or discharge of pus. — **sup′pu·ra′tive** *adj.*

suppurative gingivitis *n.* Gingivitis in which the gums exude pus.

su·pra·cer·vi·cal hysterectomy (sōō′prə-sûr′vĭ-kəl) *n.* Surgical removal of the fundus of the uterus, leaving the cervix in place.

su·pra·duc·tion (sōō′prə-dŭk′shən) *n.* The moving upward of one eye independently of the other.

su·pra·max·il·la (sōō′prə-măk-sĭl′ə) *n., pl.* **-max·il·lae** (-măk-sĭl′ē). The upper jaw or jawbone.

su·pra·nu·cle·ar paralysis (sōō′prə-nōō′klē-ər, -nyōō′-) *n.* Paralysis due to lesions above the primary motor neurons.

su·pra·pu·bic cystotomy (sōō′prə-pyōō′bĭk) *n.* Surgical incision above the pubic symphysis and into the bladder.

su·pra·re·nal·ec·to·my (sōō′prə-rē′nə-lĕk′tə-mē) *n.* See **adrenalectomy.**

su·pra·re·nal gland (sōō′prə-rē′nəl) *n.* See **adrenal gland.**

su·pra·spi·nous muscle (sōō′prə-spī′nəs) *n.* A muscle with origin from the scapula, with insertion into the humerus, and whose action abducts the arm.

su·pra·val·var stenosis (sōō′prə-văl′vər) *n.* Narrowing of the aorta above the aortic valve, usually by a constricting ring.

su·pra·ver·gence (sōō′prə-vûr′jəns) *n.* The upward rotation of one eye while the other eye remains stationary.

su·pra·ver·sion (sōō′prə-vûr′zhən) *n.* **1.** The act or an instance of turning upward. **2.** Sursumversion.

su·pro·fen (sōō-prō′fən) *n.* A nonsteroidal antiinflammatory agent with antipyretic and analgesic properties.

sur·face (sûr′fəs) *n.* The outer or topmost part of a solid structure.

surface analgesia *n.* See **topical anesthesia.**

surface epithelium *n.* Epithelium covering the embryonic genital ridges and the gonads that develop from them.

surface tension *n.* **1.** A property of liquids arising from unbalanced molecular cohesive forces at or near the surface, as a result of which the surface tends to contract and has properties resembling those of a stretched elastic membrane. **2.** A measure of this property.

sur·fac·tant (sər-făk′tənt, sûr′făk′-) *n.* A substance composed of lipoprotein that is secreted by the alveolar cells of the lung and serves to maintain the stability of pulmonary tissue by reducing the surface tension of fluids coating the lung.

surf·er's knobs (sûr′fərz) *pl.n.* Tumorlike skin nodules just below the knees, on the tops of the feet, and often on the toes, common among surfers who paddle in a kneeling position.

sur·geon (sûr′jən) *n.* A physician specializing in surgery.

Surgeon General *n., pl* **Surgeons General. 1.** The chief general officer in the medical departments of the U.S. Army, Navy, or Air Force. **2.** The chief medical officer in the U.S. Public Health Service or in a state public health service.

sur·geon's knot (sûr′jənz) *n., pl.* **surgeons' knots.** Any of several knots, especially one similar to a square knot, used in surgery for tying ligatures or stitching incisions.

sur·ger·y (sûr′jə-rē) *n.* **1.** The branch of medicine dealing with the diagnosis and treatment of injury, deformity, and disease by manual and instrumental means. **2.** A surgical operation or procedure, especially one involving removal or replacement of a diseased organ or tissue. **3.** An operating room or a laboratory of a surgeon or of a hospital's surgical staff. **4.** The work of a surgeon.

sur·gi·cal (sûr′jĭ-kəl) *adj.* **1.** Of, relating to, or characteristic of surgeons or surgery. **2.** Used in surgery. **3.** Resulting from or occurring after surgery.

surgical abdomen *n.* See **acute abdomen.**

surgical anesthesia *n.* **1.** Anesthesia administered so that a surgical procedure can be performed. **2.** Loss of sensation with muscle relaxation adequate for surgery.

surgical diathermy *n.* The use of a high frequency electrocautery for electrocoagulation or cauterization, as for sealing a blood vessel, resulting in local tissue destruction.

surgical microscope *n.* A binocular microscope used to visualize fine structures within the area of a surgical procedure.

surgical pathology *n.* A field in pathology concerned with examination of tissue specimens from living patients to diagnose disease and guide patients' care.

surgical prosthesis *n.* An appliance serving as an aid to or as a part of a surgical procedure, such as a heart valve or cranial plate.

sur·gi·cen·ter (sûr′jĭ-sĕn′tər) *n.* A surgical facility for operations that do not require hospitalization.

sur·ro·gate (sûr′ə-gĭt, -gāt′, sûr′-) *n.* **1.** One that takes the place of another. **2.** A figure of authority who takes the place of the father or mother in a person's unconscious or emotional life. **3.** A surrogate mother.

surrogate mother *n.* A woman who agrees to bear a child for another woman, either through artificial insemination by the other woman's husband or partner or by carrying until birth the other woman's surgically implanted fertilized egg. — **surrogate motherhood** *n.*

sur·sum·duc·tion (sûr′səm-dŭk′shən) *n.* See **supraduction.**

sur·sum·ver·gence (sûr′səm-vûr′jəns) *n.* See **supravergence.**

sur·sum·ver·sion (sûr′səm-vûr′zhən) *n.* The act of moving the eyes upward together.

sur·veil·lance (sər-vā′ləns) *n.* A type of observational study that involves continuous monitoring of disease occurrence within a population.

sus·cep·ti·ble (sə-sĕp′tə-bəl) *adj.* Likely to be affected with a disease, infection, or condition. — **sus·cep′ti·bil′i·ty** (sə-sĕp′tə-bĭl′ĭ-tē) *n.*

sus·pend·ed animation (sə-spĕn′dĭd) *n.* A temporary interruption of the vital functions resembling death.

sus·pen·sion (sə-spĕn′shən) *n.* **1.** A noncolloidal dispersion of solid particles in a liquid, often used for pharmaceutical preparations. **2.** The fixation of an organ to other tissue for support, as the uterus. **3.** The hanging of a part from a support, such as a plaster-encased limb.

sus·pen·so·ry (sə-spĕn′sə-rē) *adj.* Of or relating to a ligament, muscle, or other structure that supports or suspends an organ or another part. — *n.* **1.** A support or truss. **2.** An athletic supporter.

suspensory bandage *n.* An expandable bag used to support the scrotum and its contents.

sus·tained-ac·tion tablet (sə-stānd′ăk′shən) or **sus·tained-re·lease tablet** (-rĭ-lēs′) *n.* A tablet that releases its active ingredient in specified doses at timed intervals.

sus·ten·tac·u·lar cell (sŭs′tən-tăk′yə-lər, -tĕn-) *n.* One of the supporting cells of an epithelial membrane or tissue.

sus·ten·tac·u·lum (sŭs′tən-tăk′yə-ləm, -tĕn-) *n.*, *pl.* **-la** (-lə). An anatomical structure that supports another anatomical structure.

su·ture (sōō′chər) *n.* **1.** The line of junction or an immovable joint between two bones, especially of the skull. **2.** The process of joining two surfaces or edges together along a line by or as if by sewing. **3.** The surgical method used to close a wound or join tissues. **4.** The fine thread or other material used surgically to close a wound or join tissues. **5.** The line so formed. — *v.* **-tured, -tur·ing, -tures.** To join by means of sutures or a suture. — **su′tur·al** *adj.* — **su′tur·al·ly** *adv.*

su·tur·ec·to·my (sōō′chə-rĕk′tə-mē) *n.* The surgical removal of a cranial suture.

SV40 (ĕs′vē-fôr′tē) *n.* A virus that causes cancers in monkeys and that is used widely in genetic and medical research.

swab (swŏb) *n.* **1.** A small piece of absorbent material attached to the end of a stick or wire and used for cleansing or applying medicine. **2.** A specimen of mucus or other material removed with a swab.

swal·low (swŏl′ō) *v.* **-lowed, -low·ing, -lows.** To pass something, as food or drink, through the mouth and throat into the stomach.

swallowing reflex *n.* Swallowing caused by stimulation of the palate, fauces, or posterior pharyngeal wall.

swamp fever *n.* See **malaria.**

Swan–Ganz catheter (swŏn′gănz′) *n.* A soft catheter with an expandable balloon tip that is used for measuring blood pressure in the pulmonary artery.

S wave *n.* A negative deflection of the QRS complex in an electrocardiogram following an R wave.

sweat (swĕt) *v.* **sweat·ed** or **sweat, sweat·ing, sweats.** To excrete perspiration through the pores in the skin; perspire. — *n.* **1.** The colorless saline moisture excreted by the sweat glands; perspiration. **2.** The process of sweating.

sweat gland *n.* Any of the numerous small, tubular glands that are found nearly everywhere in the skin of humans, that secrete perspiration externally through pores, and that comprise the apocrine sweat and eccrine glands.

Swed·ish massage (swē′dĭsh) *n.* A system of therapeutic massage and exercise for the muscles and joints, developed in Sweden in the 19th century.

swell·ing (swĕl′ĭng) *n.* **1.** Something swollen, especially an abnormally swollen body part or area. **2.** A primordial elevation that develops into a fold, ridge, or process.

swim·mer's itch (swĭm′ərz) *n.* See **schistosome dermatitis.**

swine influenza *n.* A highly contagious form of human influenza caused by a filterable virus identical or related to a virus formerly isolated from infected swine.

Swy·er–James syndrome (swī′ər-) *n.* Decrease in size of one lung due to obliterating bronchiolitis, a congenital abnormality, or some other disorder and resulting in compensatory overinflation of the normal lung.

sy·co·ma (sī-kō′mə) *n.* A pendulous figlike growth or wart.

sy·co·sis (sī-kō′sĭs) *n.* A chronic inflammation of the hair follicles, especially of the beard, characterized by the eruption of pimples and nodules.

Syd·en·ham's chorea (sĭd′n-əmz) *n.* An acute toxic or infective disorder of the nervous system, usually associated with acute rheumatic fever, occurring in young persons and characterized by involuntary, irregular, jerky movement of the muscles of the face, neck, and limbs.

sym·bal·lo·phone (sĭm-băl′ə-fōn′) *n.* A stethoscope fitted with two chest pieces, allowing a lateral comparison of sounds.

sym·bi·o·sis (sĭm′bē-ō′sĭs, -bī-) *n.*, *pl.* **-ses** (-sēz). **1.** A close, prolonged association between two or more different organisms of different species that may, but does not necessarily, benefit each member. **2.** A relationship of mutual benefit or dependence.

sym·bleph·a·ron (sĭm-blĕf′ə-rŏn′) *n.* The adhesion of one or both eyelids to the eyeball.

sym·bleph·a·ro·pte·ryg·i·um (sĭm-blĕf′ə-rō-tə-rĭj′ē-əm) *n.* The union of the eyelid to the eyeball by a cicatricial band of membrane similar to a pterygium.

sym·bol (sĭm′bəl) *n.* **1.** Something that represents something else by association, resemblance, or convention, especially a material object used to represent something invisible. **2.** A printed or written sign used to represent an operation, an element, a quantity, or a relation, as in mathematics or chemistry. **3.** A conventional sign.

sym·bol·ism (sĭm′bə-lĭz′əm) n. **1.** A mental state in which everything that happens is regarded by the person as symbolic of his or her own thoughts. **2.** The disguised representation in conscious thought of unconscious or repressed contents or events.

sym·bol·i·za·tion (sĭm′bə-lĭ-zā′shən) n. An unconscious mental mechanism whereby one object or idea is represented by another and is not consciously recognized as such.

sym·brach·y·dac·ty·ly (sĭm-brăk′ē-dăk′tə-lē) n. A condition in which abnormally short fingers or toes are joined or webbed in their proximal portions.

sym·met·ri·cal gangrene (sĭ-mĕt′rĭ-kəl) n. Gangrene affecting the extremities of both sides of the body; seen especially in severe arteriosclerosis and myocardial infarction.

sym·me·try (sĭm′ĭ-trē) n. Exact correspondence of form and constituent configuration on opposite sides of a dividing line or plane or about a center or an axis.

sym·pa·thec·to·my (sĭm′pə-thĕk′tə-mē) or **sym·pa·the·tec·to·my** (sĭm′pə-thē-tĕk′tə-mē) n. Surgical removal of a part of the sympathetic nervous system.

sym·pa·thet·ic (sĭm′pə-thĕt′ĭk) adj. Of, relating to, or acting on the sympathetic nervous system.

sympathetic ganglia n. Any of the ganglia of the autonomic nervous system composed of adrenergic neurons receiving afferent fibers originating from preganglionic visceral motor neurons in the lateral horn of the thoracic and upper lumbar segments of the spinal cord.

sympathetic nerve n. One of the nerves of the sympathetic nervous system.

sympathetic nervous system n. The part of the autonomic nervous system originating in the thoracic and lumbar regions of the spinal cord that in general inhibits or opposes the physiological effects of the parasympathetic nervous system, as in tending to reduce digestive secretions, speeding up the heart, and contracting blood vessels.

sympathetic trunk n. Either of two long ganglionated nerve strands along the vertebral column that are connected to each spinal nerve by gray rami and receive fibers from the spinal cord through white rami connecting with the thoracic and upper lumbar spinal nerves.

sympathetic uveitis n. Inflammation of the uveal tract of the uninjured eye due to a perforating wound of the uveal tract of the other eye.

sym·pa·thet·o·blast (sĭm′pə-thĕt′ə-blăst′) n. See **sympathoblast**.

sym·pa·thet·o·blas·to·ma (sĭm′pə-thĕt′ō-blă-stō′mə) n. See **sympathoblastoma**.

sym·path·i·co·blast (sĭm-păth′ĭ-kō-blăst′) n. See **sympathoblast**.

sym·path·i·co·blas·to·ma (sĭm-păth′ĭ-kō-blă-stō′mə) n. See **sympathoblastoma**.

sym·path·i·co·go·ni·o·ma (sĭm-păth′ĭ-kō-gō′-nē-ō′mə) n. See **sympathoblastoma**.

sym·path·i·co·to·ni·a (sĭm-păth′ĭ-kō-tō′nē-ə) n. A condition in which there is increased tonicity of the sympathetic nervous system, marked by vascular spasm and high blood pressure.

sym·path·i·co·trip·sy (sĭm-păth′ĭ-kō-trĭp′sē) n. Surgical crushing of the sympathetic ganglion.

sym·pa·thin (sĭm′pə-thĭn) n. A substance, such as norepinephrine, that diffuses from the terminals of active sympathetic nerves and serves as a chemical mediator.

sym·pa·tho·blast (sĭm′pə-thō-blăst′) n. A primitive cell derived from neuroglia of the neural crest that develops into a cell of the adrenal medulla.

sym·pa·tho·blas·to·ma (sĭm′pə-thō-blă-stō′mə) n. A completely undifferentiated malignant tumor made up of sympathoblasts and originating from embryonal cells of the sympathetic nervous system.

sym·pa·tho·go·ni·a (sĭm′pə-thō-gō′nē-ə) pl.n. The completely undifferentiated cells that develop into cells of the sympathetic nervous system.

sym·pa·tho·go·ni·o·ma (sĭm′pə-thō-gō′nē-ō′mə) n. See **sympathoblastoma**.

sym·pa·tho·mi·met·ic amine (sĭm′pə-thō-mĭ-mĕt′ĭk, -mī-) n. An agent that elicits physiological responses similar to those produced by adrenergic nerve activity.

sym·pa·thy (sĭm′pə-thē) n. **1.** A relation between parts or organs by which a disease or disorder in one induces an effect in the other. **2.** Mental contagion, as in yawning induced by seeing another person yawn.

sym·phys·i·ot·o·my (sĭm-fĭz′ē-ŏt′ə-mē, sĭm′fə-zē-) n. Surgical division of the pubic symphysis, especially to increase the capacity of a contracted pelvis sufficiently to permit the passage of a fetus during delivery.

sym·phy·sis (sĭm′fĭ-sĭs) n., pl. **-ses** (-sēz′). **1.** A form of cartilaginous joint in which union between two bones is effected by fibrocartilage without a synovial membrane. **2.** A union, meeting point, or commissure of two structures. **3.** A growing together of bones originally separate, as of the two pubic bones or the two halves of the lower jawbone. **4.** A line or junction thus formed. **5.** A pathological adhesion or growing together.

sym·po·di·a (sĭm-pō′dē-ə) n. Fusion of the feet.

symp·tom (sĭm′təm, sĭmp′-) n. An indication of disorder or disease, especially when experienced as a change from normal function, sensation, or appearance.

symp·to·mat·ic (sĭm′tə-măt′ĭk, sĭmp′-) adj. **1.** Of, relating to, or based on symptoms. **2.** Constituting a symptom, as of a disease.

symp·to·ma·tol·o·gy (sĭm′tə-mə-tŏl′ə-jē, sĭmp′-) n. **1.** The medical science of symptoms. **2.** The combined symptoms of a disease.

symptom complex n. A group of symptoms that occur together and are characteristic of a certain disease, disorder, or condition.

symptom formation n. The process of developing

a physical or behavioral substitute for an unconscious impulse or a conflict that causes anxiety, such as avoiding crowds.

symptom substitution *n.* See **symptom formation.**

symp·to·sis (sĭm-tō′sĭs, sĭmp-) *n.* A localized or general wasting of the body.

syn·apse (sĭn′ăps′, sĭ-năps′) *n.* The junction across which a nerve impulse passes from an axon terminal to a neuron, a muscle cell, or a gland cell.

syn·ap·sis (sĭ-năp′sĭs) *n., pl.* **-ses** (-sēz). The side-by-side association of homologous paternal and maternal chromosomes during the early prophase of meiosis.

syn·ap·tic conduction (sĭ-năp′tĭk) *n.* The conduction of a nerve impulse across a synapse.

syn·ap·ti·ne·mal complex (sĭ-năp′tə-nē′məl) *n.* A submicroscopic structure interposed between the homologous chromosome pairs during synapsis.

syn·ar·thro·di·a (sĭn′är-thrō′dē-ə) *n., pl.* **-di·ae** (-dē-ē′). See **immovable joint.**

synarthrodial joint *n.* **1.** See **immovable joint. 2.** See **movable joint** (sense 2).

syn·ar·thro·sis (sĭn′är-thrō′sĭs) *n., pl.* **-ses** (-sēz). **1.** See **immovable joint. 2.** See **movable joint** (senses 1, 2).

syn·can·thus (sĭn-kăn′thəs) *n.* Adhesion of the eyeball to the orbital structures.

syn·ceph·a·lus (sĭn-sĕf′ə-ləs) *n.* Conjoined twins having a single head.

syn·chei·li·a or **syn·chi·li·a** (sĭn-kī′lē-ə) *n.* Congenital adhesion of the lips.

syn·chei·ri·a or **syn·chi·ri·a** (sĭn-kī′rē-ə) *n.* A form of dyscheiria in which a stimulus applied to one side of the body is referred to both sides.

syn·chon·dro·di·al joint (sĭng′kŏn-drō′dē-əl, sĭn′-) *n.* See **synchondrosis.**

syn·chon·dro·se·ot·o·my (sĭn′kŏn-drō′sē-ŏt′ə-mē) *n.* A procedure for cutting through a synchondrosis, especially cutting through the sacroiliac ligaments and closing the arch of the pubes in the treatment of exstrophy of the bladder.

syn·chon·dro·sis (sĭng′kŏn-drō′sĭs, sĭn′-) *n., pl.* **-ses** (-sēz). A rigid union between two bones formed by hyaline cartilage or by fibrocartilage.

syn·chon·drot·o·my (sĭn′kŏn-drŏt′ə-mē) *n.* See **symphysiotomy.**

syn·chro·ni·a (sĭn-krō′nē-ə, sĭng-) *n.* **1.** See **synchronism. 2.** The origination, development, involution, or functioning of tissues or organs at the usual time.

syn·chro·nism (sĭng′krə-nĭz′əm, sĭn′-) *n.* Coincidence in time; simultaneousness.

syn·co·pe (sĭng′kə-pē, sĭn′-) *n.* A brief loss of consciousness caused by a sudden fall of blood pressure or failure of the cardiac systole, resulting in cerebral anemia.

syn·cy·ti·al bud (sĭn-sĭsh′ē-əl) *n.* See **syncytial knot.**

syncytial knot *n.* A localized aggregation of syncytiotrophoblastic nuclei in the villi of the placenta during early pregnancy.

syn·cy·ti·o·tro·pho·blast (sĭn-sĭsh′ē-ō-trō′fə-blă-

st′) *n.* The syncytial outer layer of the trophoblast.

syn·cy·ti·um (sĭn-sĭsh′ē-əm) *n., pl.* **-cy·ti·a** (-sĭsh′-ē-ə). A mass of cytoplasm having many nuclei but no internal cell boundaries.

syn·dac·tyl·i·a (sĭn′dăk-tĭl′ē-ə) *n.* See **syndactyly.**

syn·dac·tyl·ism (sĭn-dăk′tə-lĭz′əm) *n.* See **syndactyly.**

syn·dac·ty·ly (sĭn-dăk′tə-lē) *n.* Webbing or fusion of the fingers or toes, involving soft parts only or including bone structure.

syn·de·sis (sĭn′dĭ-sĭs, sĭn-dē′-) *n.* See **arthrodesis.**

syn·des·mec·to·my (sĭn′dĕz-mĕk′tə-mē, -dĕs-) *n.* The cutting away of a section of a ligament.

syn·des·mec·to·pi·a (sĭn-dĕz′mĕk-tō′pē-ə, -dĕs′-) *n.* Displacement of a ligament.

syn·des·mi·tis (sĭn′dĕz-mī′tĭs, -dĕs-) *n.* Inflammation of a ligament.

syndesmodial joint *n.* See **syndesmosis.**

syn·des·mo·pex·y (sĭn-dĕz′mə-pĕk′sē, -dĕs′-) *n.* The surgical joining of two ligaments or the attachment of a ligament in a new place.

syn·des·mo·phyte (sĭn-dĕz′mə-fīt′, -dĕs′-) *n.* An osseous excrescence attached to a ligament.

syn·des·mo·plas·ty (sĭn-dĕz′mə-plăs′tē, -dĕs′-) *n.* Plastic surgery on a ligament.

syn·des·mor·rha·phy (sĭn′dĕz-môr′ə-fē, -dĕs-) *n.* The suturing or repair of ligaments.

syn·des·mo·sis (sĭn′dĕz-mō′sĭs, -dĕs-) *n., pl.* **-ses** (-sēz). A form of fibrous joint in which opposing surfaces that are relatively far apart are united by ligaments. — **syn′des·mot′ic** (-mŏt′ĭk) *adj.*

syn·des·mot·o·my (sĭn′dĕz-mŏt′ə-mē, -dĕs-) *n.* The surgical division of a ligament.

syn·drome (sĭn′drōm′) *n.* A group of symptoms that collectively indicate or characterize a disease, a psychological disorder, or another abnormal condition.

syn·er·e·sis (sĭ-nĕr′ĭ-sĭs) *n., pl.* **-ses** (-sēz′). The contraction of a gel, as a blood clot, and the exudation of part of its liquid component.

syn·er·gis·tic muscles (sĭn′ər-jĭs′tĭk) *pl.n.* Muscles having similar and mutually helpful functions or actions.

syn·er·gy (sĭn′ər-jē) *n.* The interaction of two or more agents or forces so that their combined effect is greater than the sum of their individual effects.

syn·es·the·sia (sĭn′ĭs-thē′zhə) *n.* **1.** A condition in which one type of stimulation evokes the sensation of another, as when the hearing of a sound produces the visualization of a color. **2.** A sensation felt in one part of the body as a result of stimulus applied to another, as in referred pain. — **syn′es·thet′ic** (-thĕt′ĭk) *adj.*

syn·ga·my (sĭng′gə-mē) *n.* The fusion of two gametes in fertilization. — **syn·gam′ic** (sĭn-găm′ĭk), **syn′ga·mous** (sĭng′gə-məs) *adj.*

syn·ge·ne·ic (sĭn′jə-nē′ĭk) *adj.* Genetically identical or closely related, so as to allow tissue transplant; immunologically compatible.

syngeneic graft *n.* See **syngraft.**

syngeneic homograft *n.* See **syngraft.**

syn·gen·e·sis (sĭn-jĕn′ĭ-sĭs) *n*. See **sexual repro-duction**. — **syn′ge·net′ic** (-jə-nĕt′ĭk) *adj*.

syn·graft (sĭn′grăft′) *n*. A graft of tissue that is obtained from a donor genetically identical to the recipient.

syn·ki·ne·sis (sĭn′kə-nē′sĭs, -kī-, sĭng′-) *n*. Involuntary movement of muscles or limbs accompanying a voluntary movement. — **syn′ki·net′ic** (-nĕt′ĭk) *adj*.

syn·os·te·ot·o·my (sĭn-ŏs′tē-ŏt′ə-mē) *n*. See **arthrotomy**.

syn·o·vec·to·my (sĭn′ō-vĕk′tə-mē) *n*. Excision of part or all of the synovial membrane of a joint.

syn·o·vi·a (sĭ-nō′vē-ə) *n*. A clear, thixotropic lubricating fluid secreted by membranes in joint cavities, tendon sheaths, and bursae. — **syn·o′vi·al** *adj*.

synovial bursa *n*. A sac containing synovial fluid at sites of friction, as between a tendon and a bone over which it moves, or subcutaneously over a bony prominence.

synovial fluid *n*. See **synovia**.

synovial joint *n*. See **movable joint** (sense 1).

synovial ligament *n*. One of the large synovial folds in a joint.

synovial membrane *n*. The connective-tissue membrane that lines the cavity of a synovial joint and produces the synovial fluid.

synovial sheath *n*. The membrane lining the cavity of bone through which a tendon moves.

syn·o·vi·o·ma (sĭ-nō′vē-ō′mə) *n*. A tumor of synovial origin, involving a joint or tendon sheath.

syn·o·vi·tis (sĭn′ə-vī′tĭs, sī′nə-) *n*. Inflammation of a synovial membrane.

synovitis sic·ca (sĭk′ə) *n*. See **dry synovitis**.

syn·o·vi·um (sĭ-nō′vē-əm) *n*. See **synovial membrane**.

syn·the·sis (sĭn′thĭ-sĭs) *n*., *pl*. **-ses** (-sēz′). **1.** The combining of separate elements or substances to form a coherent whole. **2.** Formation of a chemical compound from simpler compounds or elements. **3.** A period in the cell cycle.

syn·the·size (sĭn′thĭ-sīz′) *v*. **-sized, -siz·ing, -siz·es**. **1.** To combine so as to form a new, complex product. **2.** To form or produce by chemical synthesis.

syn·the·tase (sĭn′thĭ-tās′, -tāz′) *n*. See **ligase**.

syn·thet·ic (sĭn-thĕt′ĭk) *adj*. **1.** Relating to or involving synthesis. **2.** Produced by chemical synthesis, especially not of natural origin. — *n*. A synthetic chemical compound or material.

syn·tro·pho·blast (sĭn-trō′fə-blăst′) *n*. See **syncytiotrophoblast**.

syn·tro·py (sĭn′trə-pē) *n*. **1.** The occasional tendency of two diseases to coalesce into one. **2.** The psychological state of wholesome association with others. **3.** A number of similar structures inclined in one general direction, such as the ribs.

syph·i·lid (sĭf′ə-lĭd) *n*. Any of the cutaneous and mucous membrane lesions characteristic of secondary and tertiary syphilis.

syph·i·lis (sĭf′ə-lĭs) *n*. A chronic infectious disease caused by a spirochete (*Treponema pallidum*), either transmitted by direct contact, usually in sexual intercourse, or passed from mother to child in utero, and progressing through three stages characterized respectively by local formation of chancres, ulcerous skin eruptions, and systemic infection leading to general paresis.

Syr·ette (sĭ-rĕt′) A trademark used for a collapsible tube having an attached hypodermic needle containing a single dose of medicine.

syr·ing·ad·e·no·ma (sĭr′ĭng-ăd′n-ō′mə, -găd′-) or **sy·rin·go·ad·e·no·ma** (sə-rĭng′gō-) *n*. A benign sweat gland tumor showing the glandular differentiation typical of secretory cells.

sy·ringe (sə-rĭnj′, sĭr′ĭnj) *n*. **1.** An instrument used to inject fluids into the body or draw them from it. **2.** A hypodermic syringe.

syr·in·gec·to·my (sĭr′ĭn-jĕk′tə-mē) *n*. See **fistulectomy**.

syr·in·gi·tis (sĭr′ĭn-jī′tĭs) *n*. Inflammation of the eustachian tube.

sy·rin·go·car·ci·no·ma (sə-rĭng′gō-kär′sə-nō′mə) *n*. A malignant epithelial tumor that has undergone cystic change.

sy·rin·go·cyst·ad·e·no·ma (sə-rĭng′gō-sĭ-stăd′-n-ō′mə) *n*. A benign cystic tumor of the sweat glands.

syr·in·go·ma (sĭr′ĭng-gō′mə) *n*. A benign, often multiple, tumor of the sweat glands composed of very small round cysts.

sy·rin·go·my·e·li·a (sə-rĭng′gō-mī-ē′lē-ə) *n*. A chronic disease of the spinal cord characterized by the presence of fluid-filled cavities and leading to spasticity and sensory disturbances. — **sy·rin′-go·my·el′ic** (-ĕl′ĭk) *adj*.

sy·rin·go·my·e·lo·cele (sə-rĭng′gō-mī′ə-lə-sēl′) *n*. A form of spina bifida in which the fluid of the syrinx in the spinal cord is increased, expanding the cord tissue into a thin-walled sac that in turn expands through the vertebral defect.

syr·in·got·o·my (sĭr′ĭng-gŏt′ə-mē) *n*. See **fistulotomy**.

syr·up (sĭr′əp, sûr′-) *n*. A concentrated solution of sugar in water, often used as a vehicle for medicine.

sys·tem (sĭs′təm) *n*. **1.** A group of interacting, interrelated, or interdependent elements forming a complex whole. **2.** An organism or body as a whole, especially with regard to its vital processes or functions. **3.** A group of physiologically or anatomically complementary organs or parts.

sys·tem·a·tized delusion (sĭs′tə-mə-tīzd′) *n*. Any of various delusions that are logically founded upon false premises and form part of an organized group of related delusions.

sys·tem·ic (sĭ-stĕm′ĭk) *n*. **1.** Or or relating to a system. **2.** Of, relating to, or affecting the entire body or an entire organism. **3.** Relating to or affecting a particular body system, especially the nervous system. **4.** Relating to systemic circula-

systemic anaphylaxis *n*. See **generalized anaphylaxis**.

systemic circulation *n*. Circulation of blood

throughout the body through the arteries, capillaries, and veins, which carry oxygenated blood from the left ventricle to various tissues and return venous blood to the right atrium.

systemic lupus er·y·the·ma·to·sus (ĕr′ə-thē′mə-tō′səs, -thĕm′ə-) *n.* A chronic multisystemic inflammatory disease with variable features, including fever, fatigability, joint pains or arthritis, skin lesions on the face, neck, or upper extremities, and often affecting the kidneys, spleen, and various other organs.

systemic vascular resistance *n.* An index of arteriolar constriction throughout the body, calculated by dividing the blood pressure by the cardiac output.

sys·to·le (sĭs′tə-lē) *n.* The rhythmic contraction of the heart, especially of the ventricles, by which blood is driven through the aorta and pulmonary artery after each dilation or diastole. — **sys·tol′ic** (sĭ-stŏl′ĭk) *adj.*

systolic gallop *n.* A triple cadence to the heart sounds in which the extra sound occurs during systole, usually in the form of a systolic click.

systolic murmur *n.* A murmur heard during ventricular systole.

systolic pressure *n.* The highest arterial blood pressure reached during any given ventricular cycle.

sys·trem·ma (sĭ-strĕm′ə) *n.* A muscular cramp in the calf of the leg in which the contracted muscles form a hard ball.

~ ~ ~ ~ ~ ~ T ~ ~ ~ ~ ~ ~

t *abbr.* temperature (usually in italics).

T *abbr.* absolute temperature (usually in italics); temperature; tetanus toxoids vaccine; tetanus vaccine; tidal volume (used as a subscript); tocopherol

T4 *abbr.* thyroxine

ta·ba·nid (tə-bā′nĭd, -băn′ĭd) *n.* Any of various bloodsucking dipterous flies of the family Tabanidae, including the horseflies, that are involved in the transmission of several blood-borne parasites.

ta·bes (tā′bēz) *n., pl.* **tabes. 1.** Progressive bodily wasting or emaciation. **2.** Tabes dorsalis. — **ta·bes′cence** (tə-bĕs′əns) *n.* — **ta·bes′cent** *adj.* — **ta·bet′ic** (tə-bĕt′ĭk) *adj.*

tabes dor·sa·lis (dôr-sā′lĭs, -săl′ĭs) *n.* A late form of syphilis marked by hardening of the dorsal columns of the spinal cord, shooting pains, emaciation, loss of muscular coordination, and disturbances of sensation and digestion.

ta·ble·spoon (tā′bəl-spōōn′) *n.* A measure of about 4 fluid drams, ½ fluid ounce, or 15 milliliters.

tab·let (tăb′lĭt) *n.* A small flat pellet of medication to be taken orally.

tache (tăsh, täsh) *n.* A circumscribed discoloration of the skin or mucous membrane, as a freckle.

tache noir (nwär′) *n.* A necrotic area covered with a black crust that characteristically appears at the site of the bite in certain tick-borne diseases.

ta·chis·to·scope (tă-kĭs′tə-skōp′, tə-) *n.* An apparatus that projects a series of images onto a screen at rapid speed to test visual perception, memory, and learning. — **ta·chis′to·scop′ic** (-skŏp′ĭk) *adj.*

tach·y·ar·rhyth·mi·a (tăk′ē-ə-rĭth′mē-ə) *n.* An excessively rapid heartbeat accompanied by arrhythmia.

tach·y·car·di·a (tăk′ĭ-kär′dē-ə) *n.* A rapid heart rate, especially one above 100 beats per minute in an adult.

tach·y·pha·gia (tăk′ə-fā′jə, -jē-ə) *n.* Rapid eating; bolting of food.

tach·yp·ne·a (tăk′ĭp-nē′ə, tăk′ĭ-nē′ə) *n.* Rapid breathing.

tach·y·rhyth·mi·a (tăk′ə-rĭth′mē-ə) *n.* See **tachycardia.**

ta·chys·ter·ol (tə-kĭs′tə-rôl′, -rōl′) *n.* An isomer of ergosterol that forms vitamin D_2 when irradiated with ultraviolet light.

tac·rine (tăk′rēn′) *n.* Drug that halts or reverses memory loss temporarily in some people with Alzheimer's disease, but does not alter the course of the disease.

tac·tile (tăk′təl, -tīl′) *adj.* **1.** Perceptible to the sense of touch; tangible. **2.** Used for feeling. **3.** Of, relating to, or proceeding from the sense of touch.

tactile anesthesia *n.* Loss or impairment of the sense of touch.

tactile corpuscle *n.* Any of numerous minute oval end organs of touch in areas of sensitive skin, such as on the palms, fingertips, and soles of the feet.

tactile fremitus *n.* The vibration felt by a hand placed on a chest during vocal fremitus.

tactile image *n.* An image of an object as perceived by the sense of touch.

tactile papilla *n.* Any of of the papillae of the skin containing a tactile corpuscle.

tac·to·re·cep·tor (tăk′tō-rĭ-sĕp′tər) *n.* A receptor that responds to touch.

tae·ni·a·sis or **te·ni·a·sis** (tē-nī′ə-sĭs) *n.* Infestation with tapeworms.

TAF *abbr.* tumor angiogenic factor

tag (tăg) *n.* A small outgrowth or polyp. — *v.* **tagged, tag·ging, tags.** To incorporate into a compound a more readily detected substance whereby the compound can be detected and its metabolic or chemical history followed.

Tag·a·met (tăg′ə-mĕt′) A trademark used for the therapeutic drug cimetidine.

tail·bone (tāl′bōn′) *n.* See **coccyx.**

tai·lor's muscle (tā′lərz) *n.* See **sartorius muscle.**

Ta·ka·ha·ra's disease (tăk′ə-hăr′əz, tä′kə-hä′rəz) *n.* See **acatalasemia.**

talc (tălk) *n.* A fine-grained white, greenish, or gray mineral, having a soft soapy feel and used in dusting powder.

tal·co·sis (tăl-kō′sĭs) *n., pl.* **-ses** (-sēz) A form of pneumoconiosis caused by the inhalation of talc mixed with silicates.

tal·cum (tăl′kəm) *n.* See **talc.**

tal·i·ped (tăl′ə-pĕd′) *adj.* Having a clubfoot; clubfooted. — *n.* A person with a clubfoot.

tal·i·pes (tăl′ə-pēz′) *n.* See **clubfoot.**

ta·lus (tā′ləs) *n., pl.* **-li** (-lī′). **1.** The bone of the ankle that articulates with the tibia and fibula to form the ankle joint. **2.** The ankle.

tam·bour sound (tăm′bŏŏr′, tăm-bŏŏr′) *n.* A heart sound, usually the aortic- or pulmonic-valve closure sound when it has a booming and ringing quality like that of a drum.

Tamm–Hors·fall mucoprotein (tăm′hôrs′fôl) *n.* A substance derived from the secretion of renal tubular cells, a normal constituent of urine.

ta·mox·i·fen (tə-mŏk′sə-fĭn) *n.* A nonsteroidal estrogen antagonist used in the treatment of advanced breast cancer in women whose tumors are estrogen-dependent.

tam·pon (tăm′pŏn′) *n.* A plug of absorbent material inserted into a body cavity or wound to check a flow of blood or to absorb secretions, especially one designed for insertion into the vagina during menstruation. — *tr.v.* **-poned, -pon·ing, -pons.** To plug or stop with a tampon.

tam·pon·ade (tăm′pə-nād′) or **tam·pon·age** (tăm′pə-nĭj) *n.* The insertion or use of a tampon.

tan·gen·ti·al·i·ty (tăn-jĕn′shē-ăl′ĭ-tē) *n.* A disturbance in the associative thought process in which one tends to digress readily from one topic under discussion to other topics that arise through association.

Tan·gier disease (tăn-jîr′) *n.* An inheritable disorder of lipid metabolism characterized by almost complete absence from plasma of high-density lipoproteins, by storage of cholesterol esters in foam cells, and by enlargement of the liver, spleen, and lymph nodes.

tan·go·re·cep·tor (tăng′gō-rĭ-sĕp′tər) *n.* A cutaneous receptor that responds to touch and pressure.

Tan·ner growth chart (tăn′ər) *n.* A series of charts for measuring different aspects of the physical development of children according to sex, age, and stages of puberty.

tan·ta·lum (tăn′tə-ləm) *n.* A hard heavy metallic element with atomic number 73, used in surgical instruments, sutures, and implants.

T antigen *abbr.* tumor antigen

tan·trum (tăn′trəm) *n.* A fit of bad temper.

tap (tăp) *n.* The removal of fluid from a body cavity. — *tr.v.* **tapped, tap·ping, taps. 1.** To withdraw fluid from a body cavity, as with a trocar and cannula, hollow needle, or catheter. **2.** To strike lightly with the finger or a hammerlike instrument, as in percussion or to elicit a tendon reflex.

tape·worm (tāp′wûrm′) *n.* Any of various ribbonlike, often very long flatworms of the class Cestoda, that lack an alimentary canal and are parasitic in the intestines of vertebrates, including humans.

ta·pote·ment (tə-pōt′mənt, tä-pôt-mäN′) *n.* A striking with the side of the hand, usually with partly flexed fingers, used in massage.

ta·ran·tu·la (tə-răn′chə-lə) *n., pl.* **-las** or **-lae** (-lē′). Any of various large, hairy, chiefly tropical spiders of the family Theraphosidae, capable of inflicting a painful but not seriously poisonous bite.

tar·dive (tär′dĭv) *adj.* Having symptoms that develop slowly or appear long after inception. Used of a disease.

tardive dyskinesia *n.* A chronic disorder of the nervous system characterized by involuntary jerky movements of the face, tongue, jaws, trunk, and limbs, usually developing as a late side effect of prolonged treatment with antipsychotic drugs.

tardive oral dyskinesia *n.* See **tardive dyskinesia.**

target cell *n.* **1.** A red blood cell having a dark center surrounded by a light band that is itself encircled by a darker ring, and occurring in certain anemias and after splenectomy. **2.** A cell selectively affected by a particular agent, such as a virus, drug, or hormone.

target gland *n.* An endocrine gland directly affected by the hormone of another gland.

target organ *n.* A tissue or organ that is affected by a specific hormone.

target response *n.* See **operant.**

tars·ad·e·ni·tis (tär′săd-n-ī′tĭs) *n.* Inflammation of the tarsal borders of the eyelids and meibomian glands.

tar·sal (tär′səl) *adj.* **1.** Of, relating to, or situated near the tarsus of the foot. **2.** Of or relating to the tarsus of the eyelid.

tarsal bone *n.* Any of the seven bones of the tarsus.

tar·sal·gi·a (tär-săl′jē-ə, -jə) *n.* See **podalgia.**

tarsal gland *n.* See **meibomian gland.**

tarsal tunnel syndrome *n.* A syndrome characterized by pain and numbness in the sole of the foot, caused by entrapment neuropathy of the posterior or tibial nerve.

tar·sec·to·my (tär-sĕk′tə-mē) *n.* **1.** Surgical excision of the tarsus of the foot. **2.** Surgical excision of a segment of the tarsus of an eyelid.

tar·si·tis (tär-sī′tĭs) *n.* **1.** Inflammation of the tarsus of the foot. **2.** Inflammation of the tarsal border of an eyelid.

tar·so·chei·lo·plas·ty (tär′sō-kī′lə-plăs′tē) *n.* Plastic surgery on the edge of the eyelid.

tar·soc·la·sis (tär-sŏk′lə-sĭs) or **tar·so·cla·sia** (tär′sō-klā′zhə, -zē-ə) *n.* The surgical fracture of the tarsus as a treatment for clubfoot.

tar·so·ma·la·ci·a (tär′sō-mə-lā′shē-ə, -shə) *n.* Softening of the tarsal cartilages of the eyelids.

tar·so·meg·a·ly (tär′sō-měg′ə-lē) *n.* Congenital maldevelopment and overgrowth of a tarsal bone.

tar·so·phy·ma (tär′sō-fī′mə) *n.* A growth or tumor of the tarsus of the eyelid.

tar·sor·rha·phy (tär-sôr′ə-fē) *n.* Partial or complete suture of the eyelid margins to shorten the palpebral fissure or to protect the cornea.

tar·sot·o·my (tär-sŏt′ə-mē) *n.* **1.** Surgical incision of the tarsal cartilage of an eyelid. **2.** An operation on the tarsus of the foot.

tar·sus (tär′səs) *n., pl.* **-si** (-sī). **1.** The area of articulation between the foot and the leg, comprising the seven bones of the instep: the talus, calcaneus, navicular, three cuneiform, and cuboid bones. **2.** The fibrous plate that supports and shapes the edges of the eyelids.

tar·tar (tär′tər) *n.* A hard, yellowish deposit on the teeth, consisting of organic secretions and food particles deposited in various salts, such as calcium carbonate.

tartar emetic *n.* A poisonous crystalline compound used in medicine as an expectorant and in the treatment of parasitic infections, such as schistosomiasis.

tart cell (tärt) *n.* **1.** A granulocyte that has engulfed the nucleus of another cell, the structure of which is still well preserved. **2.** This type of ingested nucleus, especially as found as an artifact in lupus erythematosus cell preparations.

taste (tāst) *n.* **1.** The sense that distinguishes the sweet, sour, salty, and bitter qualities of dissolved substances in contact with the taste buds on the tongue. **2.** This sense in combination with the senses of smell and touch, which together receive a sensation of a substance in the mouth. **3.** The sensation of sweet, sour, salty, or bitter qualities produced by or as if by a substance placed in the mouth. — *v.* **tast·ed, tast·ing, tastes. 1.** To distinguish flavors in the mouth. **2.** To have a distinct flavor.

taste bud *n.* One of a number of flask-shaped receptor cell nests located in the epithelium of the papillae of the tongue and also in the soft palate, epiglottis, and posterior wall of the pharynx that mediate the sense of taste.

taste cell *n.* A darkly staining neuroepithelial cell in a taste bud that makes synaptic contact with sensory nerve fibers, thus serving as receptors for taste.

TAT *abbr.* Thematic Apperception Test

tat·too (tă-tōo′) *n., pl.* **-toos.** A permanent mark or design made on the skin by a process of pricking and ingraining an indelible pigment or by raising scars. — *v.* **-tooed, -too·ing, -toos. 1.** To mark the skin with a tattoo. **2.** To form a tattoo on the skin.

Taus·sig–Bing syndrome (tou′sĭg-bĭng′) *n.* A rare malformation of the heart characterized by transposition of the aorta, ventricular septal defect, hypertrophy of the right ventricle, and a pulmonary artery that is situated behind the aorta.

tax·is (tăk′sĭs) *n., pl.* **tax·es** (tăk′sēz). **1.** The responsive movement of a free-moving organism or cell toward or away from an external stimulus, such as light. **2.** The moving of a body part by manipulation into normal position, as after a dislocation, fracture, or hernia.

Tax·ol (tăk′sôl′) A trademark used for the therapeutic drug paclitaxel.

tax·on (tăk′sŏn′) *n., pl.* **tax·a** (tăk′sə). A taxonomic category or group, such as a phylum, order, family, genus, or species.

tax·on·o·my (tăk-sŏn′ə-mē) *n.* **1.** The classification of organisms in an ordered system that indicates natural relationships. **2.** The science, laws, or principles of classification; systematics.

Tay–Sachs disease (tā′săks′) *n.* The infantile type of cerebral sphingolipidosis.

TB or **T.B.** *abbr.* tuberculosis

T-bandage *n.* See T-binder.

T-binder *n.* Two strips of cloth positioned at right angles and used for retaining a dressing.

TBV *abbr.* total blood volume

T cell *n.* A principal type of white blood cell that completes maturation in the thymus and that has various roles in the immune system, including the identification of specific foreign antigens in the body and the activation and deactivation of other immune cells.

Td *abbr.* tetanus-diphtheria toxoids vaccine

teach·ing hospital (tē′chĭng) *n.* A hospital closely associated with a medical school and serving as a practical educational site for medical students, interns, residents, and allied health personnel.

tear¹ (târ) *n.* A rip or rent in a tissue or part.

tear² (tēr) *n.* A drop of the clear salty liquid that is secreted by the lacrimal gland of the eye to lubricate the surface between the eyeball and eyelid and to wash away irritants.

tear·drop (tēr′drŏp′) *n.* **1.** A single tear. **2.** An object shaped like a tear.

tear gas (tēr) *n.* A gas, such as acetone, that causes irritation of the eyes and profuse tearing.

tear·ing (tēr′ĭng) *n.* Epiphora.

tear sac *n.* See lacrimal sac.

tear stone (tēr) *n.* See dacryolith.

tease (tēz) *v.* **teased, teas·ing, teas·es.** To separate the structural parts of a tissue, with a needle, in order to prepare it for microscopic examination.

tea·spoon (tē′spōon′) *n.* A measure of about 1 fluid dram or 5 milliliters.

teat (tēt, tĭt) *n.* **1.** See nipple. **2.** The female breast; mamma. **3.** A papilla.

tech·ne·ti·um (těk-nē′shē-əm, -shəm) *n.* A radioactive metallic element with atomic number 43 that was the first synthetically produced element, and is used in tracers and radiotherapeutic procedures.

tech·ni·cian (těk-nĭsh′ən) *n.* One whose occupation requires training in a specific technical process.

tech·nique (těk-nēk′) or **tech·nic** (těk′nĭk) *n.* The skill and procedure with which a surgical operation or experiment, for example, is carried out.

tech·nol·o·gist (tĕk-nŏl′ə-jĭst) *n.* See **technician**.

tec·ton·ic keratoplasty (tĕk-tŏn′ĭk) *n.* The surgical grafting of corneal material in an area where corneal tissue has been lost.

tec·tum (tĕk′təm) *n.*, *pl.* **-ta** (-tə). A rooflike structure of the body, especially the dorsal part of the mesencephalon. — **tec′tal** (-təl) *adj.*

teeth·ing (tē′thĭng) *n.* The eruption or cutting of the teeth.

teeth·ridge (tēth′rĭj′) *n.* The ridge of gum behind the upper front teeth.

teg·men (tĕg′mən) *n.*, *pl.* **-mi·na** (-mə-nə). A covering or an integument of a part.

teg·men·tum (tĕg-mĕn′təm) *n.*, *pl.* **-ta** (-tə). 1. See **tegmen**. 2. The mesencephalic tegmentum. — **teg·men′tal** (-təl) *adj.*

teg·u·ment (tĕg′yə-mənt) *n.* A natural outer covering; an integument.

tei·chop·si·a (tī-kŏp′sē-ə) *n.* A transient visual sensation of bright shimmering colors, as that preceding scintillating scotoma in migraine.

te·la (tē′lə) *n.*, *pl.* **-lae** (-lē). 1. A thin weblike structure. 2. A tissue, especially of delicate formation.

tel·an·gi·ec·ta·sia (tĕl-ăn′jē-ĕk-tā′zhə) or **tel·an·gi·ec·ta·sis** (-ĕk′tə-sĭs) *n.* Chronic dilation of groups of capillaries causing elevated dark red blotches on the skin. — **tel·an′gi·ec·tat′ic** (-tăt′-ĭk) *adj.*

tel·an·gi·o·sis (tĕl-ăn′jē-ō′sĭs) *n.* Disease of the capillaries and terminal arterioles.

tel·e·di·ag·no·sis (tĕl′ĭ-dī′əg-nō′sĭs) *n.* A diagnosis made by a physician who is at a location that is geographically removed from that of patient and is based on the evaluation of data transmitted from patient-monitoring instruments and a transfer link to a diagnostic center.

tel·en·ceph·a·lon (tĕl′ĕn-sĕf′ə-lŏn′, -lən) *n.* The anterior portion of the prosencephalon, constituting the cerebral hemispheres and composing with the diencephalon the prosencephalon. — **tel′en·ce·phal′ic** (-sə-făl′ĭk) *adj.*

tel·e·op·si·a (tĕl′ē-ŏp′sē-ə) *n.* A vision disorder characterized by errors in judging the distance of objects and arising from lesions in the parietal temporal region of the brain.

te·lep·a·thy (tə-lĕp′ə-thē) *n.* Communication by means other than through the normal senses.

tel·e·ra·di·og·ra·phy (tĕl′ə-rā′dē-ŏg′rə-fē) *n.* Radiography performed with the tube held about six feet (two meters) from the body, thereby securing practical parallelism of the rays.

tel·er·gy (tĕl′ər-jē) *n.* See **automatism** (sense 3).

tel·e·roent·gen·og·ra·phy (tĕl′ə-rĕnt′gə-nŏg′-rə-fē, -jə-, -rŭnt′-) *n.* See **teleradiography**.

tel·e·ther·a·py (tĕl′ə-thĕr′ə-pē) *n.* Radiation therapy that is administered at a distance from the body.

tel·lu·ri·um (tĕ-lŏŏr′ē-əm) *n.* A brittle metallic element with atomic number 52.

tel·o·gen (tĕl′ə-jĕn′, tē′lə-) *n.* The resting phase of the follicle in the hair growth cycle.

tel·o·mere (tĕl′ə-mēr′, tē′lə-) *n.* Either end of a chromosome; a terminal chromosome.

tel·o·phase (tĕl′ə-fāz′, tē′lə-) *n.* The final stage of mitosis or meiosis during which the chromosomes of daughter cells are grouped in new nuclei. — **tel′o·phas′ic** *adj.*

te·maz·e·pam (tə-măz′ə-păm′) *n.* A benzodiazepine sedative used primarily to relieve insomnia.

temp. *abbr.* temperature.

tem·per (tĕm′pər) *n.* 1. A state of mind or emotions; mood. 2. A tendency to become easily angry or irritable. 3. An outburst of rage.

tem·per·a·ment (tĕm′prə-mənt, tĕm′pər-ə-) *n.* 1. The manner of thinking, behaving, or reacting characteristic of a specific person. 2. Disposition; temper.

tem·per·ance (tĕm′pər-əns, tĕm′prəns) *n.* 1. Moderation and self-restraint, as in behavior or expression. 2. Restraint in the use of or abstinence from alcoholic liquors.

tem·per·a·ture (tĕm′pər-ə-chŏŏr′, -chər, tĕm′-prə-) *n.* 1. The degree of hotness or coldness of a body or an environment. 2. A specific degree of hotness or coldness as indicated on or referred to a standard scale. 3. The degree of heat in the body of a living organism, usually about 37.0°C (98.6°F) in humans. 4. An abnormally high condition of body heat caused by illness; a fever.

tem·plate or **tem·plet** (tĕm′plĭt) *n.* A molecule, such as DNA, that serves as a pattern for the synthesis of a macromolecule, as of RNA.

tem·ple (tĕm′pəl) *n.* 1. The flat region on either side of the forehead. 2. Either of the sidepieces of a frame for eyeglasses that extends along the temple and over the ear.

tem·po·ral (tĕm′pər-əl, tĕm′prəl) *adj.* Of, relating to, or near the temples of the skull.

temporal artery *n.* 1. An artery with its origin in the superficial temporal artery and with distribution to the temporal fascia and muscle; middle temporal artery. 2. Either of two arteries with their origin in the maxillary artery and with distribution to the temporal muscle; deep temporal artery. 3. An artery with its origin in the external carotid artery and with distribution to the superficial areas of the face and head; superficial temporal artery.

temporal bone *n.* Either of a pair of compound bones forming the sides and base of the skull.

temporal lobe *n.* The lowest of the major subdivisions of the cortical mantle of the brain, containing the sensory center for hearing and forming the rear two-thirds of the ventral surface of the cerebral hemisphere. It is separated from the frontal and parietal lobes above it by the fissure of Sylvius and is arbitrarily delineated from the occipital lobe with which it is continuous posteriorly.

temporal muscle *n.* A muscle with origin from the temporal fossa, with insertion into the mandible, and whose action closes the jaw.

temporal plane *n.* A slightly depressed area on the side of the cranium, formed by the temporal and parietal bones, the greater wing of the sphenoid, and a part of the frontal bone.

temporal process *n.* The posterior projection of the zygomatic bone articulating with the zygomatic process of the temporal bone to form the zygomatic arch.

tem·po·rar·y cartilage (těm′pə-rěr′ē) *n.* Cartilage that normally becomes converted to bone to form a part of the skeleton.

temporary tooth *n.* See **deciduous tooth**.

tem·po·ro·man·dib·u·lar (těm′pə-rō-măn-dĭb′-yə-lər) *adj.* Of, relating to, or formed by the temporal bone and the mandible.

temporomandibular joint *n.* See **mandibular joint**.

temporomandibular joint dysfunction *n.* Impaired functioning of the temporomandibular articulation of the jaw.

temporomandibular joint syndrome *n.* A disorder caused by faulty articulation of the temporomandibular joint and characterized by facial pain, headache, ringing ears, dizziness, and stiffness of the neck.

te·nac·u·lum (tə-năk′yə-ləm) *n., pl.* **-la** (-lə). A long-handled, slender, hooked instrument for lifting and holding parts, such as blood vessels, during surgery.

tenaculum forceps *n.* A forceps with jaws ending in sharp inward-pointing hooks.

te·nal·gi·a (tě-năl′jē-ə, -jə) *n.* Pain in a tendon.

ten·der (těn′dər) *adj.* **-er, -est. 1.** Easily crushed or bruised; fragile. **2.** Easily hurt; sensitive. **3.** Painful; sore.

ten·der·ness (těn′dər-nĭs) *n.* The condition of being tender or sore to the touch.

ten·di·ni·tis or **ten·do·ni·tis** (těn′də-nī′tĭs) *n.* Inflammation of a tendon.

ten·di·no·plas·ty (těn′də-nə-plăs′tē) *n.* See **tenontoplasty**.

ten·di·no·su·ture (těn′də-nō-sōō′chər) *n.* See **tenorrhaphy**.

ten·di·nous synovitis (těn′də-nəs) *n.* See **tenosynovitis**.

ten·dol·y·sis (těn-dŏl′ĭ-sĭs) or **te·nol·y·sis** (tě-nŏl′ĭ-sĭs) *n.* The surgical release of a tendon from adhesions.

ten·don (těn′dən) *n.* A band of tough, inelastic fibrous tissue that connects a muscle with its bony attachment and consists of fascicles of very densely arranged, almost parallel, collagenous fibers; rows of elongated cells; and a minimum of ground substance.

tendon cell *n.* Any of various elongated fibroblastic cells arranged in rows between the collagenous tendon fibers.

tendon reflex *n.* A myotatic or deep reflex in which the muscle stretch receptors are stimulated by percussing the tendon of a muscle.

ten·do·plas·ty (těn′də-plăs′tē) *n.* See **tenontoplasty**.

ten·dot·o·my (těn-dŏt′ə-mē) *n.* See **tenotomy**.

te·nec·to·my (tě-něk′tə-mē) *n.* The surgical resection of part of a tendon.

te·nes·mus (tə-něz′məs) *n.* A painful spasm of the anal sphincter accompanied by an urgent desire to evacuate the bowel or bladder and involuntary straining that results in the passing of little or no matter.

ten·nis elbow (těn′ĭs) *n.* A painful inflammation of the tissue surrounding the elbow, caused by strain from playing tennis and other sports.

tennis thumb *n.* Tendonitis with calcification in the tendon of the long flexor of the thumb, caused by exercise in which the thumb is subject to pressure or strain.

te·nod·e·sis (tə-nŏd′ĭ-sĭs, těn′ə-dē′sĭs) *n.* The surgical anchoring of a tendon, as to a bone.

ten·o·dyn·i·a (těn′ə-dĭn′ē-ə) *n.* See **tenalgia**.

ten·o·my·o·plas·ty (těn′ō-mī′ə-plăs′tē) *n.* See **tenontomyoplasty**.

ten·o·my·ot·o·my (těn′ō-mī-ŏt′ə-mē) *n.* See **myotenotomy**.

ten·o·nec·to·my (těn′ə-něk′tə-mē) *n.* See **tenectomy**.

ten·o·ni·tis (těn′ə-nī′tĭs) *n.* **1.** Inflammation of the sheath of the eyeball or its associated connective tissue. **2.** Tendinitis.

ten·o·nom·e·ter (těn′ə-nŏm′ĭ-tər) *n.* A tonometer.

Te·non's capsule (tē′nənz, tə-nôNz) *n.* See **sheath of the eyeball**.

ten·on·ti·tis (těn′ən-tī′tĭs) *n.* Tendinitis.

te·non·to·dyn·i·a (tə-nŏn′tə-dĭn′ē-ə, těn′ən-tō-) *n.* See **tenalgia**.

te·non·to·my·o·plas·ty (tə-nŏn′tō-mī′ə-plăs′tē) *n.* A surgical procudure used in the radical correction of hernia that combines tenontoplasty and myoplasty.

te·non·to·plas·ty (tə-nŏn′tə-plăs′te′) *n.* Reparative or plastic surgery of the tendons.

ten·o·phyte (těn′ə-fīt′) *n.* A bony or cartilaginous growth in or on a tendon.

ten·o·plas·ty (těn′ə-plăs′tē) *n.* See **tenontoplasty**.

ten·o·re·cep·tor (těn′ō-rĭ-sěp′tər) *n.* A receptor in a tendon, activated by increased tension.

te·nor·rha·phy (tě-nôr′ə-fē) *n.* Suture of the divided ends of a tendon.

ten·os·to·sis (těn′ŏ-stō′sĭs) *n.* Ossification of a tendon.

ten·o·sus·pen·sion (těn′ō-sə-spěn′shən) *n.* The use of a tendon as a suspensory ligament.

ten·o·su·ture (těn′ō-sōō′chər) *n.* See **tenorrhaphy**.

ten·o·syn·o·vec·to·my (těn′ō-sĭn′ō-věk′tə-mē) *n.* Excision of a tendon sheath.

ten·o·syn·o·vi·tis (těn′ō-sĭn′ə-vī′tĭs, -sī′nə-) or **ten·do·sy·no·vi·tis** (těn′dō-) *n.* Inflammation of a tendon and its enveloping sheath.

te·not·o·my (tě-nŏt′ə-mē) *n.* The surgical division of a tendon to correct a deformity caused by congenital or acquired shortening of a muscle, as for the correction of strabismus.

ten·o·vag·i·ni·tis (těn′ō-văj′ə-nī′tĭs) or **ten·do·vag·i·ni·tis** (těn′dō-) *n.* See **tenosynovitis**.

TENS (těnz) *n.* Transcutaneous electrical nerve stimulation; a technique used to relieve pain in an injured or diseased part of the body in which electrodes applied to the skin deliver intermittent stimulation to surface nerves and block the transmission of pain signals.

ten·sion (tĕn′shən) *n*. **1.** The act or process of stretching something tight. **2.** The condition of so being stretched; tautness. **3.** A force tending to stretch or elongate something. **4.** The partial pressure of a gas, especially that of a gas dissolved in a liquid such as blood. **5.** Mental, emotional, or nervous strain.

tension cavity *n*. A cavity in the lung in which the air pressure is greater than that of the atmosphere.

tension curve *n*. A line tracing the direction of the trabeculae in cancellous bone tissue, indicating the direction of tension placed on the bone.

tension headache *n*. A headache associated with nervous tension, anxiety, or stress, often related to chronic contraction of the scalp muscles.

tension suture *n*. See retention suture.

ten·sor (tĕn′sər, -sôr′) *n*. A muscle that stretches or tightens a body part.

tent (tĕnt) *n*. A canopy used in various types of inhalation therapy to control the humidity and oxygen concentration of inspired air.

tent *n*. A small, cylindrical plug of lint or gauze used to keep open or probe a wound or an orifice. — *v*. **tent·ed, tent·int, tents.** To keep a wound or an orifice open with such a plug.

tenth cranial nerve *n*. See vagus nerve.

ten·to·ri·um (tĕn-tôr′ē-əm) *n*., *pl*. **-to·ri·a** (-tôr′-ē-ə). A membranous cover or horizontal partition.

ter·as (tĕr′əs) *n*., *pl*. **ter·a·ta** (tĕr′ə-tə). A malformed fetus with deficient, redundant, misplaced, or grossly misshapen parts.

ter·a·tism (tĕr′ə-tĭz′əm) *n*. A congenital malformation.

ter·a·to·blas·to·ma (tĕr′ə-tō-blă-stō′mə) *n*. See teratoma.

ter·a·to·car·ci·no·ma (tĕr′ə-tō-kär′sə-nō′mə) *n*. **1.** A malignant teratoma occurring most commonly in the testis. **2.** A malignant epithelioma arising in a teratoma.

te·rat·o·gen (tə-răt′ə-jən, tĕr′ə-tə-) *n*. An agent, such as a virus, a drug, or radiation, that causes malformation of an embryo or a fetus.

ter·a·to·gen·e·sis (tĕr′ə-tə-jĕn′ĭ-sĭs) *n*. The production of physical malformations during embryonic development.

ter·a·to·gen·ic (tĕr′ă-tō- jen′ik) or **ter·a·to·ge·net·ic** (-jĕ-net′ik) *adj*. Of, relating to, or causing malformations of an embryo or fetus.

ter·a·tog·e·ny (tĕr′ə-tŏj′ə-nē) *n*. See teratogenesis.

teratoid tumor *n*. See teratoma.

ter·a·tol·o·gy (tĕr′ə-tŏl′ə-jē) *n*. The biological study of malformations that occur during embryonic development.

ter·a·to·ma (tĕr′ə-tō′mə) *n*., *pl*. **-mas** or **-ma·ta** (-mə-tə). A tumor consisting of different types of tissue, as of skin, hair, and muscle, caused by the development of independent germ cells. — **ter′a·to′ma·tous** (-tō′mə-təs) *adj*.

te·ra·zo·sin hydrochloride (tə-rā′zə-sĭn) *n*. A crystalline compound that blocks adrenergic receptors and is used to treat hypertension.

ter·bi·um (tûr′bē-əm) *n*. A soft metallic rare-earth element with atomic number 65.

ter·es major muscle (tĕr′ēz, tĕr′-) *n*. A muscle with origin from the lower border of the scapula, with insertion into the humerus, and whose action adducts and extends the arm and rotates it medially.

teres minor muscle *n*. A muscle with origin from the lateral border of the scapula, with insertion into the humerus, and whose action adducts the arm and rotates it laterally.

ter·fen·a·dine (tər-fĕn′ə-dēn′) *n*. An antihistamine used to treat a variety of allergic symptoms and having less of a sedative effect than other antihistamines.

term (tûrm) *n*. **1.** A limited period of time. **2.** The end of a normal gestation period.

ter·mi·nal (tûr′mə-nəl) *adj*. **1.** Of, relating to, situated at, or forming a limit, a boundary, an extremity, or an end. **2.** Of, relating to, occurring at, or being the end of a section or series; final. **3.** Causing, ending in, or approaching death; fatal.

terminal artery *n*. See end artery.

terminal boutons *pl.n*. See axon terminals.

terminal bronchiole *n*. The last portion of a conducting airway, which subdivides into respiratory bronchioles.

terminal hair *n*. A mature hair.

terminal nucleus *n*. Any of the groups of nerve cells in the rhombencephalon and spinal cord in which the afferent fibers of the spinal and cranial nerves terminate.

term infant *n*. An infant born between the beginning of the 38th week and the end of the 42nd week of gestation.

ter·pene (tûr′pēn′) *n*. Any of various unsaturated hydrocarbons found in essential oils, resins, and balsams, and used in organic syntheses.

ter·race (tĕr′ĭs) *v*. **-raced, -rac·ing, -rac·es.** To suture in several rows, as when closing a wound through a considerable thickness of tissue.

Ter·ra·my·cin (tĕr′ə-mī′sĭn) A trademark used for oxytetracycline.

ter·ri·to·ri·al·i·ty (tĕr′ĭ-tôr′ē-ăl′ĭ-tē) *n*. **1.** A behavior pattern in animals consisting of the occupation and defense of a territory. **2.** A similar behavior pattern in humans consisting of the tendency to defend a particular domain or sphere of influence or interest.

ter·ri·to·ri·al matrix (tĕr′ĭ-tôr′ē-əl) *n*. The basophilic material surrounding groups of cartilage cells derived from the same embryonic tissue.

ter·tian (tûr′shən) *adj*. Recurring every other day or, when considered inclusively, every third day. Used of a fever. — *n*. A tertian fever, such as vivax malaria.

ter·ti·ar·y syphilis (tûr′shē-ĕr′ē) *n*. The final stage of syphilis, marked by the formation of gummas, cellular infiltration, and cardiovascular and central nervous system lesions.

test (tĕst) *n.* **1.** A procedure for critical evaluation; a means of determining the presence, quality, or truth of something; a trial, examination, or experiment. **2.** A physical or chemical change by which a substance may be detected or its properties ascertained. **3.** A reagent used to cause or promote such a change. — *v.* **test·ed, test·ing, tests. 1.** To subject to a test; try. **2.** To determine the presence or properties of a substance. **3.** To administer a test. **4.** To exhibit a given characteristic when subjected to a test.

tes·tal·gi·a (tĕs-tăl′jē-ə, -jə) *n.* See **orchialgia**.

tes·tec·to·my (tĕs-tĕk′tə-mē) *n.* See **orchiectomy**.

tes·ti·cle (tĕs′tĭ-kəl) *n.* A testis, especially one contained within the scrotum.

tes·tic·u·lar (tĕ-stĭk′yə-lər) *adj.* Of or relating to a testicle or testis.

testicular cord *n.* See **spermatic cord**.

tes·tis (tĕs′tĭs) *n., pl.* **-tes** (-tēz). The male reproductive gland, the source of spermatozoa and the androgens, normally occurring paired in an external scrotum.

tes·ti·tis (tĕ-stī′tĭs) *n.* See **orchitis**.

test meal *n.* Bland food, such as toast or crackers, given to stimulate gastric secretion before analysis of gastric contents.

tes·tos·ter·one (tĕs-tŏs′tə-rōn′) *n.* A steroid hormone and the most potent naturally occurring androgen that is formed by the interstitial cells of the testes or made synthetically, and used in the treatment of hypogonadism, cryptorchism, carcinomas, and hypermenorrhea.

test profile *n.* An array of laboratory tests usually conducted using automated methods and equipment and designed to gather biochemical and other information on the organ systems of people admitted to a hospital or clinic.

test tube *n.* A clear, cylindrical glass tube usually open at one end and rounded at the other, used in laboratory experimentation.

test-tube baby *n.* A baby conceived by the process of in vitro fertilization and then implanted in the uterus of the biological mother or a surrogate.

test types *pl.n.* Letters printed in various sizes used to test the acuity of vision.

te·tan·ic (tĕ-tăn′ĭk) *adj.* **1.** Of or causing tetanus or tetany. **2.** Marked by sustained muscular contractions. — *n.* An agent that in poisonous doses produces tonic muscular spasm. — **te·tan′i·cal·ly** *adv.*

tet·a·nize (tĕt′n-īz′) *v.* **-nized, -niz·ing, -niz·es.** To affect with tetanic convulsions; produce or induce tetanus in. — **tet′a·ni·za′tion** (tĕt′n-ĭ-zā′-shən) *n.*

tet·a·node (tĕt′n-ōd′) *n.* The quiet interval between the recurrent tonic spasms in tetanus.

tet·a·no·spas·min (tĕt′n-ō-spăz′mĭn) *n.* The neurotoxin of *Clostridium tetani* that causes the characteristic signs and symptoms of tetanus.

tet·a·nus (tĕt′n-əs) *n.* **1.** An acute, often fatal disease characterized by spasmodic contraction of voluntary muscles, especially those of the neck and jaw, and caused by the toxin of the bacillus *Clostridium tetani*, which typically infects the body through a deep wound. **2.** A state of continuous muscular contraction, especially when induced artificially by rapidly repeated stimuli.

tetanus-diphtheria toxoids vaccine *n.* One of the forms of the diphtheria, tetanus toxoids, and pertussis vaccine, containing tetanus and diphtheria toxoids and used to immunize against tetanus and diphtheria.

tetanus toxin *n.* The neurotropic heat-labile exotoxin of *Clostridium tetani* that causes tetanus.

tetanus toxoids vaccine *n.* One of the forms of the diphtheria, tetanus toxoids, and pertussis vaccine, containing tetanus toxoid and used to immunize against tetanus.

tetanus vaccine *n.* Tetanus toxoids vaccine.

tet·a·ny (tĕt′n-ē) *n.* An abnormal condition characterized by periodic painful muscular spasms and tremors, caused by faulty calcium metabolism and associated with diminished function of the parathyroid glands.

teth·ered cord syndrome (tĕth′ərd) *n.* Sacral retention of the spinal cord by the terminal filum, causing incontinence and progressive motor and sensory impairment in the legs.

tet·ra·chlo·ride (tĕt′rə-klôr′īd′) *n.* A chemical compound containing four chlorine atoms per molecule.

tet·ra·cy·clic antidepressant (tĕt′rə-sī′klĭk, -sĭk′-lĭk) *n.* Any of a class of antidepressants, such as maprotiline, similar to the tricyclic antidepressants.

tet·ra·cy·cline (tĕt′rə-sī′klēn′, -klĭn) *n.* **1.** A yellow crystalline compound synthesized or derived from certain microorganisms of the genus *Streptomyces* and used as a broad-spectrum antibiotic. **2.** An antibiotic, such as chlortetracycline and oxytetracycline, having the same basic structure.

tet·rad (tĕt′răd′) *n.* **1.** A group or set of four. **2.** A group of four chromatids formed from each of a pair of homologous chromosomes that split longitudinally during the prophase of meiosis.

te·tral·o·gy (tĕ-trăl′ə-jē, -trŏl′-) *n.* A complex of four symptoms.

tetralogy of Fallot *n.* See **Fallot's tetralogy**.

tetramer *n.* A polymer consisting of four identical monomers. — **tet′ra·mer′ic** (-mĕr′ĭk) *adj.*

tet·ra·mer·ic (tĕt′răr-mer′ĭk) or **te·tram·er·ous** (tĕ-trăm′ĕr-əs) *n.* having four parts, or parts arranged in groups of four, or capable of existing in four forms.

tet·ra·ploid (tĕt′rə-ploid′) *adj.* Having four times the haploid number of chromosomes in the cell nucleus. — *n.* A tetraploid individual.

te·tro·do·tox·in (tĕ-trō′də-tŏk′sĭn) *n.* A potent neurotoxin, found in many puffer fish and certain newts.

tet·ter (tĕt′ər) *n.* Any of various skin diseases, such as eczema, psoriasis, or herpes, characterized by eruptions and itching.

text blindness *n.* See **alexia**.

tex·ture (tĕks′chər) *n.* The composition or structure of a tissue or organ. — **tex′tured** *adj.*

thal·a·men·ceph·a·lon (thăl′ə-mĕn-sĕf′ə-lŏn′) *n.*

The part of the diencephalon comprising the thalamus and its associated structures.

thal·a·mot·o·my (thăl'ə-mŏt'ə-mē) *n.* Destruction of a portion of the thalamus by stereotaxy for the relief of pain, involuntary movements, epilepsy, or emotional disturbances.

thal·a·mus (thăl'ə-məs) *n., pl.* **-mi** (-mī'). A large ovoid mass of gray matter that forms the larger dorsal subdivision of the diencephalon and is located medial to the internal capsule and to the body and tail of the caudate nucleus. It functions in the relay of sensory impulses to the cerebral cortex. — **tha·lam'ic** (thə-lăm'ĭk) *adj.* — **tha·lam'i·cal·ly** *adv.*

thal·as·se·mi·a (thăl'ə-sē'mē-ə) *n.* Any of a group of inherited forms of anemia occurring chiefly among people of Mediterranean descent, caused by faulty synthesis of part of the hemoglobin molecule.

tha·lid·o·mide (thə-lĭd'ə-mīd') *n.* A sedative and hypnotic drug withdrawn from sale after it was found to cause severe birth defects when taken during pregnancy. It is sometimes prescribed to treat leprosy, and is used investigationally as an angiogenesis inhibitor in the treatment of certain cancers.

thal·li·um (thăl'ē-əm) *n.* A soft, malleable, highly toxic metallic element with atomic number 81.

than·a·tol·o·gy (thăn'ə-tŏl'ə-jē) *n.* The study of death and dying, especially of their psychological and social aspects.

Than·a·tos or **than·a·tos** (thăn'ə-tōs') *n.* See **death instinct.**

THC (tē'ăch-sē') *n.* Tetrahydrocannabinol; a compound obtained from cannabis or made synthetically; it is the primary intoxicant in marijuana and hashish.

the·ca (thē'kə) *n., pl.* **-cae** (-sē', -kē'). A case, covering, or sheath of an anatomical part.

theca-cell tumor *n.* See **thecoma.**

theca fol·lic·u·li (fə-lĭk'yə-lī') *n.* The wall of a vesicular ovarian follicle.

the·ci·tis (thē-sī'tĭs) *n.* Inflammation of a tendon sheath.

the·co·ma (thē-kō'mə) *n.* A tumor derived from ovarian mesenchyme and consisting chiefly of spindle-shaped cells that frequently contain small droplets of fat; it may form considerable quantities of estrogens, causing development of secondary sexual features in prepubertal girls or endometrial hyperplasia in older persons.

the·lar·che (thē-lär'kē) *n.* The beginning of development of the breasts in the female.

the·le·plas·ty (thē'lə-plăs'tē) *n.* See **mammillaplasty.**

the·li·um (thē'lē-əm) *n., pl.* **-li·a** (-lē-ə). **1.** A papilla. **2.** A cellular layer. **3.** See **nipple.**

T-helper cell *n.* See **helper T cell.**

The·mat·ic Apperception Test (thĭ-măt'ĭk) *n.* A psychological test in which the subject is asked to tell a story about a set of standard pictures showing everyday situations, thereby revealing his or her own attitudes and feelings.

the·nar (thē'när', -nər) *n.* The fleshy mass on the palm of the hand at the base of the thumb. — *adj.* Of or relating to the thenar.

the·o·bro·mine (thē'ō-brō'mēn') *n.* A bitter, colorless alkaloid derived from the cacao bean, found in chocolate products and used in medicine as a diuretic, vasodilator, and myocardial stimulant.

the·oph·yl·line (thē-ŏf'ə-lĭn, thē'ō-fĭl'ēn') *n.* A colorless crystalline alkaloid derived from tea leaves or made synthetically, used as a cardiac stimulant and diuretic.

the·o·ry (thē'ə-rē, thêr'ē) *n.* **1.** A systematically organized body of knowledge applicable in a relatively wide variety of circumstances, especially a system of assumptions, accepted principles, and rules of procedure devised to analyze, predict, or otherwise explain the nature or behavior of a specified set of phenomena. **2.** Abstract reasoning; speculation.

thèque (tĕk) *n.* An aggregation of nevus cells or other cells in the epidermis.

ther·a·peu·tic (thĕr'ə-pyōō'tĭk) or **ther·a·peu·ti·cal** (-tĭ-kəl) *adj.* **1.** Having or exhibiting healing powers. **2.** Of or relating to therapeutics.

therapeutic abortion *n.* Abortion induced because of the mother's physical or mental health, or to prevent the birth of a deformed child or of a child conceived as a result of rape or incest.

therapeutic crisis *n.* A turning point in psychiatric treatment leading to positive or negative change.

ther·a·peu·tics (thĕr'ə-pyōō'tĭks) *n.* Medical treatment of disease; the art or science of healing. — **ther'a·peu'tist** *n.*

ther·a·pist (thĕr'ə-pĭst) *n.* One who specializes in the provision of a particular therapy.

ther·a·py (thĕr'ə-pē) *n.* **1.** Treatment of illness or disability. **2.** Psychotherapy. **3.** Healing power or quality.

ther·ma·co·gen·e·sis (thûr'mə-kō-jĕn'ĭ-sĭs) *n.* Elevation of body temperature by the use of a drug.

ther·mal (thûr'məl) *adj.* **1.** Of, relating to, using, producing, or caused by heat. **2.** Intended or designed in such a way as to help retain body heat.

thermal anesthesia or **ther·mic anesthesia** (thûr'mĭk) *n.* See **thermoanesthesia.**

ther·mal·gi·a (thər-măl'jē-ə, -jə) *n.* Burning pain.

therm·an·al·ge·si·a (thûrm'ăn-əl-jē'zē-ə, -zhə) *n.* See **thermoanesthesia.**

therm·es·the·sia (thûrm'ĭs-thē'zhə) *n.* See **thermoesthesia.**

therm·es·the·si·om·e·ter (thûrm'ĭs-thē'zē-ŏm'ĭ-tər) *n.* See **thermoesthesiometer.**

ther·mo·an·es·the·sia (thûr'mō-ăn'ĭs-thē'zhə) *n.* Loss of the ability to distinguish between heat and cold.

ther·mo·cau·ter·y (thûr'mō-kô'tə-rē) *n.* Cauterization using heat, as with a heated wire.

ther·mo·chem·is·try (thûr'mō-kĕm'ĭ-strē) *n.* The chemistry of heat and heat-associated chemical phenomena.

ther·mo·co·ag·u·la·tion (thûr'mō-kō-ăg'yə-lā'shən) *n.* The use of heat produced by high-frequency electric current to bring about local-ized destruction of tissues.

ther·mo·dif·fu·sion (thûr′mō-dĭ-fyōō′zhən) *n.* The diffusion of fluids as influenced by their temperature.

ther·mo·dy·nam·ics (thûr′mō-dī-năm′ĭks) *n.* **1.** Physics that deals with the relationships between heat and other forms of energy. **2.** Thermodynamic phenomena and processes.

ther·mo·es·the·sia (thûr′mō-ĭs-thē′zhə) *n.* Ability to feel hot or cold; sensitivity to variations in temperature.

ther·mo·es·the·si·om·e·ter (thûr′mō-ĭs-thē′zē-ŏm′ĭ-tər) *n.* An instrument for testing sensitivity to variations in temperature.

ther·mo·gen·e·sis (thûr′mō-jĕn′ĭ-sĭs, -mə-) *n.* Generation or production of heat, especially by physiological processes. — **ther′mo·ge·net′ic** (-jə-nĕt′ĭk), **ther′mo·gen′ic** (-jĕn′ĭk) *adj.*

ther·mo·la·bile (thûr′mō-lā′bĭl, -bīl′) *n.* Subject to destruction, decomposition, or great change by moderate heating. Used especially of biochemical substances. — **ther′mo·la·bil′i·ty** (-bĭl′ĭ-tē) *n.*

ther·mol·y·sis (thər-mŏl′ĭ-sĭs) *n.* **1.** Dissipation of heat from the body, as by evaporation. **2.** Dissociation or decomposition of chemical compounds by heat. — **ther′mo·lyt′ic** (thûr′mə-lĭt′ĭk) *adj.*

ther·mo·mas·sage (thûr′mō-mə-säzh′ -säj′) *n.* Physical therapy using a combination of heat and massage.

ther·mom·e·ter (thər-mŏm′ĭ-tər) *n.* An instrument for measuring temperature.

ther·mom·e·try (thər-mŏm′ĭ-trē) *n.* **1.** Measurement of temperature. **2.** The technology of temperature measurement. — **ther′mo·met′ric** (thûr′-mō-mĕt′rĭk) *adj.*

ther·mo·phore (thûr′mə-fôr′) *n.* A device for applying heat to a body part.

ther·mo·plac·en·tog·ra·phy (thûr′mə-plăs′ən-tŏg′rə-fē) *n.* Determination of placental position by infrared detection of blood flowing through the placenta.

ther·mo·re·cep·tor (thûr′mō-rĭ-sĕp′tər) *n.* A sensory receptor that responds to heat and cold.

ther·mo·reg·u·late (thûr′mō-rĕg′yə-lāt′) *v.* **-lat·ed, -lat·ing, -lates.** To regulate body temperature.

ther·mo·reg·u·la·tion (thûr′mō-rĕg′yə-lā′shən) *n.* Maintenance of a constant internal body temperature independent of the environmental temperature. — **ther′mo·reg′u·la·to′ry** (-rĕg′yə-lə-tôr′ē) *adj.*

ther·mo·ste·re·sis (thûr′mō-stə-rē′sĭs) *n.* Deprivation of heat.

ther·mo·tax·is (thûr′mə-tăk′sĭs) *n., pl.* **-tax·es** (-tăk′sēz). **1.** Movement of a living organism in response to changes in temperature. **2.** Normal regulation or adjustment of body temperature. — **ther′mo·tac′tic** (-tăk′tĭk), **ther′mo·tax′ic** (-tăk′-sĭk) *adj.*

ther·mo·ther·a·py (thûr′mō-thĕr′ə-pē) *n.* Medical therapy involving the application of heat.

ther·mot·ro·pism (thər-mŏt′rə-pĭz′əm) *n.* The tendency of plants or other organisms to bend toward or away from heat. — **ther′mo·trop′ic** (thûr′mə-trŏp′ĭk) *adj.*

theta rhythm *n.* See **theta wave.**

theta wave *n.* A brain wave occurring chiefly in the hippocampus of humans when they are awake but relaxed and drowsy.

thi·a·ben·da·zole (thī′ə-bĕn′də-zōl′) *n.* A white compound used medically as an antifungal agent and as an anthelmintic.

thi·al·bar·bi·tal (thī′ăl-bär′bĭ-tôl′, -tăl′) *n.* A crystalline substance administered intravenously in the form of its sodium salt as a general anesthetic.

thi·a·mine (thī′ə-mĭn, -mēn′) or **thi·a·min** (-mĭn) *n.* A vitamin of the vitamin B complex, found in meat, yeast, and the bran coat of grains, and necessary for carbohydrate metabolism and normal neural activity.

thi·am·y·lal sodium (thī-ăm′ə-lôl′, -lăl′) *n.* A barbiturate, prepared as a mixture with sodium bicarbonate and used intravenously to produce short-term anesthesia.

thi·a·zide (thī′ə-zīd′, -zĭd) *n.* See **benzothiadiazide.**

thick *adj.* **thick·er, thick·est. 1.** Relatively great in extent from one surface to the opposite, usually in the smallest solid dimension; not thin. **2.** Heavy in form, build, or stature; thickset. **3.** Having component parts in a close, crowded state or arrangement; dense. **4.** Having or suggesting a heavy or viscous consistency. **5.** Having a great number; abounding. **6.** Impenetrable by the eyes. **7.** Not easy to hear or understand; indistinctly articulated. **8.** Noticeably affecting sound; conspicuous. **9.** Producing indistinctly articulated sounds. — *adv.* **1.** In a close, compact state or arrangement; densely. **2.** In a thick manner; deeply or heavily.

thick·ness (thĭk′nĭs) *n.* **1.** The quality or condition of being thick. **2.** The dimension between two surfaces of an object, usually the dimension of smallest measure. **3.** A layer or stratum.

thi·e·mi·a (thī-ē′mē-ə) *n.* The presence of sulfur in the circulating blood.

thi·eth·yl·per·a·zine ma·le·ate (thī-ĕth′əl-pĕr′ə-zēn′ mā′lē-āt′, mə-lē′ət) *n.* A drug used to control nausea and vomiting.

thigh (thī) *n.* The part of the leg between the hip and the knee.

thigh·bone (thī′bōn′) *n.* See **femur.**

thig·mes·the·sia (thĭg′mĭs-thē′zhə) *n.* Sensibility to touch.

thig·mo·tax·is (thĭg′mə-tăk′sĭs) *n.* See **stereotaxis** (sense 2). — **thig′mo·tac′tic** (-tăk′tĭk) *adj.*

thig·mot·ro·pism (thĭg-mŏt′rə-pĭz′əm) *n.* The turning or bending response of an organism or part of an organism upon direct contact with a solid surface or object. — **thig′mo·trop′ic** (thĭg′-mə-trŏp′ĭk, -trō′pĭk) *adj.*

thi·mer·o·sal (thī-mĕr′ə-săl′) *n.* A cream-colored crystalline powder used as a local antiseptic for abrasions and minor cuts.

think (thĭngk) *v.* **thought** (thôt), **think·ing, thinks. 1.** To exercise the power of reason, as by conceiving ideas, drawing inferences, and using judgment. **2.** To weigh or consider an idea. **3.** To bring a thought to mind by imagination or invention. **4.** To recall a thought or an image to mind.

thinking through *n.* The psychological process of understanding one's own behavior.

thin section *n.* A section of tissue less than 0.1 micrometer in thickness, fixed and embedded in a plastic resin for examination by electron microscope.

thi·o·nine (thī′ə-nēn′, -nǐn) *n.* A dark-green powder that turns water purple when mixed in solution, used as a basic stain in histology for chromatin and mucin because of its metachromatic properties.

thi·o·pen·tal sodium (thī′ō-pěn′tăl′, -tôl′) *n.* A yellowish-white hygroscopic powder injected intravenously as a general anesthetic and used in psychotherapy to induce a relaxed state.

thi·o·rid·a·zine (thī′ə-rǐd′ə-zēn′) *n.* A white or yellow powder, a derivative of phenothiazine, that is used orally as a tranquilizer to treat various psychotic conditions.

thi·o·sul·fu·ric acid (thī′ō-sŭl-fyoŏr′ǐk) *n.* An acid formed by replacement of an oxygen atom by a sulfur atom in sulfuric acid, known only in solution or by its salts and esters.

thi·o·te·pa (thī′ō-tē′pə, -tĕp′ə) *n.* A sulfur-containing compound used to treat certain malignant diseases such as leukemia, lymphoma, and carcinoma.

thi·o·u·ra·cil (thī′ō-yoŏr′ə-sǐl′) *n.* A white crystalline compound that interferes with the synthesis of thyroxine, used to reduce the action of the thyroid gland, especially in the treatment of hyperthyroidism.

third (thûrd) *adj.* **1.** Coming next after second, as in order, rank, or time. **2.** Being the digit that is adjacent to and on the outermost side of the second digit, as on a foot. — **third** *n.*

third cranial nerve *n.* See oculomotor nerve.

third-degree burn *n.* A severe burn in which the skin and underlying tissues are destroyed and nerve endings are exposed.

third heart sound *n.* The heart sound that occurs in early diastole and corresponds with the first phase of rapid ventricular filling.

third molar *n.* The eighth permanent tooth in the upper and lower jaw on either side.

thirst (thûrst) *n.* **1.** A sensation of dryness in the mouth and throat related to a need or desire to drink. **2.** The desire to drink. — *v.* **thirst·ed, thirst·ing, thirsts.** To feel a need to drink.

thirst·y (thûr′stē) *adj.* Desiring to drink.

thix·ot·ro·py (thǐk-sŏt′rə-pē) *n.* The property exhibited by certain gels of becoming fluid when stirred or shaken and returning to the semisolid state upon standing. — **thix′o·trop′ic** (thǐk′sə-trŏp′ǐk) *adj.*

Thom·as splint (tŏm′əs) *n.* A long leg splint extending from a ring at the hip to beyond the foot, allowing traction to a fractured leg, used in emergencies and for transportation.

Thomp·son's test (tŏmp′sənz, tŏm′-) *n.* A test for determining the extent of gonorrhea infection.

tho·ra·cal·gi·a (thôr′ə-kăl′jē-ə, -jə) *n.* Pain in the chest.

tho·ra·cec·to·my (thôr′ə-sĕk′tə-mē) *n.* Surgical resection of a portion of a rib.

tho·ra·cen·te·sis (thôr′ə-sĕn-tē′sĭs) *n.* Paracentesis of the pleural cavity.

tho·rac·ic (thə-răs′ĭk) *adj.* Of, relating to, or situated in or near the thorax.

thoracic artery *n.* **1.** An artery having its origin in the subclavian artery, with distribution along the anterior wall of the thorax; internal thoracic artery. **2.** An artery having its origin in the axillary artery, with distribution to the muscles of the chest and mammary gland; lateral thoracic artery. **3.** An artery having its origin in the axillary artery, with distribution to the muscles and walls of the chest; superior thoracic artery.

thoracic cavity *n.* The space within the walls of the chest, bounded below by the diaphragm and above by the neck, and containing the heart and the lungs.

thoracic duct *n.* The largest lymph vessel in the body, which collects lymph from the left side of the body above the diaphragm and from all parts of the body below the diaphragm.

thoracic limb *n.* See upper extremity.

thoracic nerve *n.* Any of twelve mixed motor and sensory nerves that arise in pairs below each thoracic vertebra and supply the muscles and skin of the thoracic and the abdominal walls.

thoracic outlet syndrome *n.* Compression of the brachial plexus and subclavian artery by attached muscles in the region of the first rib and the clavicle, characterized by pain in the arm, numbness in the fingers, and weakness in the hand muscles.

tho·ra·co·cen·te·sis (thôr′ə-kō-sĕn-tē′sĭs) *n.* See thoracentesis.

tho·ra·co·dyn·i·a (thôr′ə-kō-dǐn′ē-ə) *n.* See thoracalgia.

tho·ra·col·y·sis (thôr′ə-kŏl′ĭ-sĭs) *n.* The loosening of adhesions of the lung to the chest wall.

tho·ra·co·my·o·dyn·i·a (thôr′ə-kō-mī′ō-dǐn′ē-ə) *n.* Pain in the muscles of the chest wall.

tho·ra·cop·a·thy (thôr′ə-kŏp′ə-thē) *n.* A disease of the thoracic organs or tissues.

tho·ra·co·plas·ty (thôr′ə-kō-plăs′tē) *n.* **1.** Reparative or plastic surgery of the thorax. **2.** Surgical removal of part of the ribs to allow inward retraction of the chest wall and collapse of a diseased lung.

tho·ra·co·scope (thə-rā′kə-skōp′, -răk′ə-) *n.* An endoscope for examination of the chest cavity.

tho·ra·cos·co·py (thôr′ə-kŏs′kə-pē) *n.* Endoscopic examination of the chest cavity.

tho·ra·co·ste·no·sis (thôr′ə-kō-stə-nō′sĭs) *n.* Abnormal narrowness of the chest wall.

tho·ra·cos·to·my (thôr′ə-kŏs′tə-mē) *n.* The surgical formation of an opening into the chest cavity, as for drainage.

tho·ra·cot·o·my (thôr′ə-kŏt′ə-mē) *n.* Surgical incision into the chest wall.

tho·rax (thôr′ăks′) *n., pl.* **tho·rax·es** or **tho·ra·ces** (thôr′ə-sēz′). The part of the body between the neck and the diaphragm, partially encased by the ribs and containing the heart and lungs; the chest.

Tho·ra·zine (thôr′ə-zēn′) A trademark used for chlorpromazine.

tho·ri·um (thôr′ē-əm) *n.* A radioactive metallic element with atomic number 90.

thought *n.* **1.** The act or process of thinking; cogitation. **2.** A product of thinking, such as an idea. **3.** The faculty of thinking or reasoning.

Thr *abbr.* threonine

thread·worm (thrĕd′wûrm′) *n.* **1.** A nematode worm that is an intestinal parasite in humans. **2.** See **pinworm**.

thread·y pulse (thrĕd′ē) *n.* A small fine pulse that feels like a small cord or thread under the finger.

three-glass test *n.* A test to determine the location of an infection affecting the urinary system and involving urination into a series of three tubes, the various samples representing urine washing the anterior urethra; the bladder; and the posterior urethra, prostate, and seminal vesicles.

thre·o·nine (thrē′ə-nēn′, -nĭn) *n.* A colorless crystalline amino acid that is derived from the hydrolysis of protein and is an essential component of human nutrition.

thresh·old (thrĕsh′ōld′, -hōld′) *n.* **1.** The lowest point at which a stimulus begins to produce a sensation. **2.** The minimal stimulus that produces excitation of any structure, eliciting a motor response.

threshold stimulus *n.* A stimulus that is just strong enough to evoke a response.

threshold substance *n.* A material excreted in the urine only when its concentration in the plasma exceeds a certain value.

thrill (thrĭl) *n.* The vibration accompanying a cardiac or vascular murmur, detectable on palpation.

thrix (thrĭks) *n.* Hair; a hair.

throat (thrōt) *n.* **1.** The portion of the digestive tract that lies between the rear of the mouth and the esophagus and includes the fauces and the pharynx. **2.** The anterior portion of the neck.

throb (thrŏb) *v.* **throbbed, throb·bing, throbs.** To beat rapidly or perceptibly, as the heart or a constricted blood vessel. — *n.* A strong or rapid beat; a pulsation.

throm·bas·the·ni·a (thrŏm′băs-thē′nē-ə) or **throm·bo·as·the·ni·a** (thrŏm′bō-ăs-) *n.* An abnormality of blood platelets characteristic of Glanzmann's thrombasthenia.

throm·bec·to·my (thrŏm-bĕk′tə-mē) *n.* Surgical excision of a thrombus.

throm·bin (thrŏm′bĭn) *n.* An enzyme in blood plasma formed from prothrombin that facilitates blood clotting by reacting with fibrinogen to form fibrin.

throm·bo·an·gi·i·tis (thrŏm′bō-ăn′jē-ī′tĭs) *n.* Inflammation of the intima of a blood vessel together with thrombosis.

throm·bo·ar·te·ri·tis (thrŏm′bō-är′tə-rī′tĭs) *n.* Arterial inflammation with thrombus formation.

throm·bo·cy·tas·the·ni·a (thrŏm′bō-sī′tăs-thē′-nē-ə) *n.* A group of hemorrhagic disorders in which the number of platelets may be within or only slightly below the normal range but are morphologically abnormal or are lacking in factors that are effective in the coagulation of blood.

throm·bo·cyte (thrŏm′bə-sīt′) *n.* See **platelet**. — **throm′bo·cyt′ic** (-sĭt′ĭk) *adj.*

throm·bo·cy·the·mi·a (thrŏm′bō-sī-thē′mē-ə) *n.* See **thrombocytosis**.

thrombocytic series *n.* The cells in various stages of thrombocytopoietic development in the bone marrow.

throm·bo·cy·top·a·thy (thrŏm′bō-sī-tŏp′ə-thē) *n.* A disorder of the blood coagulating mechanism that results from dysfunction of the platelets.

throm·bo·cy·to·pe·ni·a (thrŏm′bō-sī′tə-pē′nē-ə) *n.* An abnormal decrease in the number of platelets in the circulating blood. — **throm′bo·cy′to·pe′nic** (-pē′nĭk) *adj.*

throm·bo·cy·to·poi·e·sis (thrŏm′bō-sī′tə-poi-ē′-sĭs) *n.* The process of formation of thrombocytes, usually in the bone marrow. — **throm′bo·cy′to·poi·et′ic** (-ĕt′ĭk) *adj.*

throm·bo·cy·to·sis (thrŏm′bō-sī-tō′sĭs) *n.* An increase in the number of platelets in the circulating blood.

throm·bo·em·bo·lism (thrŏm′bō-ĕm′bə-lĭz′əm) *n.* Occlusion of a blood vessel resulting from a thrombus.

throm·bo·end·ar·ter·ec·to·my (thrŏm′bō-ĕn′-där-tə-rĕk′tə-mē) *n.* An operation to remove a thrombus along with the intima and atheromatous material from an occluded artery.

throm·bo·lym·phan·gi·tis (thrŏm′bō-lĭm′făn-jī′tĭs) *n.* Inflammation of a lymphatic vessel with the formation of a thrombus.

throm·bon (thrŏm′bŏn′, -bən) *n.* The total mass of circulating blood platelets and their precursors.

throm·bop·a·thy (thrŏm-bŏp′ə-thē) *n.* A disorder of blood platelets resulting in defective thromboplastin, without obvious change in the appearance or number of platelets.

throm·bo·phil·i·a (thrŏm′bə-fĭl′ē-ə) *n.* A disorder of the hemopoietic system in which there is an increased tendency for thrombosis.

throm·bo·phle·bi·tis (thrŏm′bō-flĭ-bī′tĭs) *n.* Inflammation of a vein caused by or associated with the formation of a blood clot.

throm·bo·plas·tic (thrŏm′bō-plăs′tĭk) *adj.* **1.** Causing or promoting blood clotting. **2.** Of or relating to thromboplastin. — **throm′bo·plas′ti·cal·ly** *adv.*

throm·bo·plas·tid (thrŏm′bō-plăs′tĭd) *n.* A platelet.

throm·bo·plas·tin (thrŏm′bō-plăs′tĭn) *n.* A plasma protein present in tissues, platelets, and white blood cells necessary for blood coagulation and, in the presence of calcium ions, necessary for the conversion of prothrombin to thrombin.

throm·bosed (thrŏm′bōst, -bōzd) *adj.* **1.** Clotted.

2. Of or being a blood vessel that is the site of thrombosis.

throm·bo·sis (thrŏm-bō′sĭs) *n.*, *pl.* **-ses** (-sēz). Formation or presence of a thrombus.

throm·bo·sthe·nin (thrŏm′bō-sthē′nĭn) *n.* A contractile protein in platelets that is active in the formation of blood clots.

throm·bus (thrŏm′bəs) *n.*, *pl.* **-bi** (-bī). A fibrinous clot formed in a blood vessel or in a chamber of the heart.

through drainage *n.* The passage of an openended perforated tube through a cavity to drain or irrigate the cavity.

thrush (thrŭsh) *n.* A contagious disease caused by a fungus, *Candida albicans,* that occurs most often in infants and children, characterized by small whitish eruptions on the mouth, throat, and tongue, and usually accompanied by fever, colic, and diarrhea.

thu·li·um (thōō′lē-əm, thyōō′-) *n.* A rare-earth element with atomic number 69, having an x-ray emitting isotope used in portable x-ray units.

thumb (thŭm) *n.* The short thick digit of the hand, next to the index finger and opposable to each of the other four digits.

thumb forceps *n.* A forceps operated by compression with thumb and forefinger.

thy·mec·to·my (thī-mĕk′tə-mē) *n.* Surgical removal of the thymus gland.

thy·mic (thī′mĭk) *adj.* Of or relating to the thymus.

thymic alymphoplasia *n.* Thymic hypoplasia that includes an absence of thymic corpuscles and a deficiency of lymphocytes in the thymus and usually in the lymph nodes, spleen, and gastrointestinal tract.

thymic corpuscle or **thymus corpuscle** *n.* Any of numerous small spherical bodies found in the medulla of the lobules of the thymus, composed of keratinized, usually squamous epithelial cells arranged concentrically around clusters of degenerating lymphocytes, eosinophils, and macrophages.

thy·mi·dine (thī′mĭ-dēn′) *n.* A nucleoside composed of thymine and deoxyribose.

thymidine tri·phos·phate (-trī-fŏs′fāt′) *n.* The immediate precursor of thymidylic acid in DNA.

thy·mi·dyl·ic acid (thī′mĭ-dĭl′ĭk) *n.* A nucleotide component of DNA that yields thymine, ribose, and phosphoric acid when hydrolyzed.

thy·mine (thī′mēn′) *n.* A pyrimidine base that is an essential constituent of DNA.

thy·mi·tis (thī-mī′tĭs) *n.* Inflammation of the thymus gland.

thy·mo·cyte (thī′mə-sīt′) *n.* A lymphocyte that develops in the thymus and is the precursor of a T cell.

thy·mo·ma (thī-mō′mə) *n.* A usually benign tumor of the thymus, composed of epithelial and lymphoid cells.

thy·mo·sin (thī′mə-sĭn) *n.* A hormone secreted by the thymus that stimulates development of T cells.

thy·mus (thī′məs) *n.*, *pl.* **-mus·es.** A lymphoid organ that is located in the superior mediastinum and lower part of the neck and is necessary in early life for the normal development of immunological function. It reaches its greatest relative weight shortly after birth and its greatest absolute weight at puberty; it then begins to involute, and much of the lymphoid tissue is replaced by fat.

thy·ro·ac·tive (thī′rō-ăk′tĭv) *adj.* Stimulating activity of the thyroid gland.

thy·ro·ad·e·ni·tis (thī′rō-ăd′n-ī′tĭs) *n.* See **thyroiditis.**

thy·ro·a·pla·sia (thī′rō-ə-plā′zhə, -zē-ə) *n.* Defective development of the thyroid gland and deficiency of its secretion.

thy·ro·cele (thī′rə-sēl′) *n.* Enlargement of the thyroid gland.

thy·ro·cri·co·to·my (thī′rō-krī-kŏt′ə-mē) *n.* Surgical division of the cricoid and thyroid membranes.

thy·ro·glob·u·lin (thī′rō-glŏb′yə-lĭn) *n.* **1.** A protein, usually stored in the colloid of the thyroid gland, that has properties similar to the globulins and that yields various amino acids including iodine-containing amino acids when hydrolyzed. **2.** A substance obtained by the fractionation of thyroid glands from the hog and used as a thyroid hormone in the treatment of hypothyroidism.

thy·roid (thī′roid′) *n.* **1.** The thyroid gland. **2.** The thyroid cartilage. **3.** A dried, powdered preparation of the thyroid gland of certain domestic animals, used in the treatment of cretinism and myxedema, in certain cases of obesity, and in skin disorders. — **thy′roid′** *adj.* — **thy·roi′dal** *adj.*

thyroid bruit *n.* A vascular murmur heard over a hyperactive thyroid gland.

thyroid cartilage *n.* The largest cartilage of the larynx, having two broad processes that join anteriorly to form the Adam's apple.

thy·roid·ec·to·my (thī′roi-dĕk′tə-mē) *n.* Surgical removal of the thyroid gland. — **thy′roid·ec′to·mize′** *v.*

thyroid gland *n.* A two-lobed endocrine gland located in front of and on either side of the trachea and producing various hormones, such as calcitonin.

thyroid hormone *n.* A hormone, especially thyroxine or triiodothyronine, produced by the thyroid gland.

thy·roid·i·tis (thī′roi-dī′tĭs) *n.* Inflammation of the thyroid gland.

thyroid-stimulating hormone *n.* See **thyrotropin.**

thyroid-stimulating hormone stimulation test *n.* A test that measures the uptake of ^{131}I in the thyroid gland before and after the administration of thyroid-stimulating hormone, used to distinguish primary hyperthyroidism from secondary or tertiary hyperthyroidism.

thyroid suppression test *n.* A test of thyroid function used to diagnose difficult cases of hyperthyroidism in which triiodothyronine is administered for a period of from 7 to 10 days; the uptake by the thyroid gland is normally reduced to less than half of the initial uptake.

thy·ro·lib·er·in (thī'rō-lĭb'ər-ĭn) *n.* See **thyrotropin-releasing hormone.**

thy·ro·meg·a·ly (thī'rō-mĕg'ə-lē) *n.* Enlargement of the thyroid gland.

thy·ro·nine (thī'rə-nēn', -nĭn) *n.* An amino acid thats occurs in proteins only in the form of iodinated derivatives such as thyroxine.

thy·ro·par·a·thy·roid·ec·to·my (thī'rō-păr'ə-thī'roi-dĕk'tə-mē) *n.* Surgical removal of the thyroid and parathyroid glands.

thy·rot·o·my (thī-rŏt'ə-mē) *n.* **1.** Surgical incision of the thyroid gland. **2.** See **laryngofissure.**

thy·ro·tox·ic crisis (thī'rō-tŏk'sĭk) *n.* A sudden worsening of thyrotoxicosis following shock, injury, or thyroidectomy.

thy·ro·tox·i·co·sis (thī'rō-tŏk'sĭ-kō'sĭs) *n.* A toxic condition resulting from excessive amounts of thyroid hormones in the body, as that occurring in hyperthyroidism.

thy·ro·troph (thī'rə-trŏf', -trōf') *n.* A cell in the anterior lobe of the pituitary gland that produces thyrotropin.

thy·ro·trop·ic hormone (thī'rə-trŏp'ĭk, -trō'pĭk) *n.* See **thyrotropin.**

thy·ro·tro·pin (thī'rə-trō'pĭn, thī-rŏt'rə-) or **thy·ro·tro·phin** (-fĭn) *n.* A glycoprotein hormone secreted by the anterior lobe of the pituitary gland that stimulates and regulates the activity of the thyroid gland.

thyrotropin-releasing hormone *n.* A tripeptide hormone secreted by the hypothalamus that stimulates the release of thyrotropin.

thyrotropin-releasing hormone stimulation test *n.* A test used primarily to distinguish pituitary from hypothalamic causes of thyroid disorders, in which a person receives an injection of thyrotropin-releasing hormone and levels of thyrotropin are measured.

thy·rox·ine (thī-rŏk'sēn', -sĭn) or **thy·rox·in** (-rŏk'sĭn) *n.* An iodine-containing hormone that is produced by the thyroid gland, increases the rate of cell metabolism, regulates growth, and is made synthetically for treatment of thyroid disorders.

TIA *abbr.* transient ischemic attack

tib·i·a (tĭb'ē-ə) *n., pl.* **-i·as** or **-i·ae** (-ē-ē'). The inner and larger of the two bones of the lower leg, extending from the knee to the ankle, and articulating with the femur, fibula, and talus. — **tib'i·al** *adj.*

tibial nerve *n.* One of two major divisions of the sciatic nerve, supplying the hamstring muscles, the muscles of the back of the leg, the muscles of the plantar aspect of the foot, and the skin on the back of the leg and on the sole of the foot.

tibia val·ga (văl'gə) *n.* Knock-knee.

tic (tĭk) *n.* A habitual spasmodic muscular movement or contraction, usually of the face or extremities.

tick (tĭk) *n.* **1.** Any of numerous small bloodsucking parasitic arachnids of the families Ixodidae and Argasidae, many of which transmit febrile diseases, such as Rocky Mountain spotted fever and Lyme disease. **2.** Any of various usually wingless, louselike insects of the family Hippobosciddae that are parasitic on sheep, goats, and other animals.

tick-borne *adj.* Carried or transmitted by ticks, as certain diseases.

tick-borne encephalitis virus *n.* An arbovirus of the genus *Flavivirus* that occurs in two subtypes, Central European and Eastern, causing two forms of encephalitis.

tick fever *n.* Any of various febrile diseases transmitted by ticks, such as Rocky Mountain spotted fever.

tick paralysis *n.* Ascending paralysis caused by the attachment of certain ticks, especially of the genera *Dermacentor* and *Ixodes.* Removal of the tick usually results in rapid recovery.

tick typhus *n.* Any of various tick-borne rickettsial diseases identified by their immunological reactions and, in some cases, by their pathogenicity.

t.i.d. *abbr. Latin.* ter in die (three times a day)

tidal air *n.* See **tidal volume.**

tidal drainage *n.* The use of an apparatus that can be intermittently filled and emptied to drain the urinary bladder.

tidal volume *n.* The volume of air inspired or expired in a single breath during regular breathing.

tide (tīd) *n.* An alternate rise and fall or increase and decrease, as of levels of a substance in the blood or digestive tract.

Tie·tze's syndrome (tē'tsēz) *n.* Inflammation of the cartilage of the rib cage, causing pain in the chest similar to angina pectoris.

tight junction *n.* An intercellular junction between epithelial cells in which the outer layers of the cell membranes fuse and greatly reduce the ability of water and other large molecules to pass between the cells.

time (tīm) *n.* **1.** A duration or relation of events expressed in terms of past, present, and future, and measured in units such as minutes, hours, days, months, or years. **2.** A certain period during which something is done.

timed-release or **time-release** *adj.* Releasing ingredients gradually to produce a sustained effect.

tim·o·thy hay bacillus (tĭm'ə-thē hā') *n.* An aerobic, gram-negative, nonmotile bacterium, *Mycobacterium phlei,* that is found in soil and dust and on plants.

tin (tĭn) *n.* A malleable metallic element with atomic number 50.

tinc·ture (tĭngk'chər) *n.* **1.** A coloring or dyeing substance. **2.** An alcohol solution of a nonvolatile medicine.

tine (tīn) *n.* **1.** The slender pointed end of an instrument. **2.** An instrument usually containing several individual prongs and used to introduce antigen, such as tuberculin, into the skin.

tin·e·a (tĭn'ē-ə) *n.* Any of various fungal skin infections caused chiefly by species of parasitic fungi, such as of the genus *Trichophyton.* — **tin'e·al** *adj.*

tinea cap·i·tis (kăp'ĭ-tĭs) *n.* A fungal infection of

the scalp, characterized by patches of apparent baldness, scaling, black dots, and occasionally erythema and pyoderma.

tinea cor·po·ris (kôr′pər-ĭs) *n.* A fungal infection of the body, characterized by a scaling macular eruption that frequently forms annular lesions on nonhairy parts of the body.

tinea cru·ris (krōŏr′ĭs) *n.* A fungal infection of the skin of the groin, occurring especially in males.

tinea ver·si·col·or (vûr′sĭ-kŭl′ər) *n.* An eruption of tan or brown patches on the skin of the trunk, caused by the fungus *Pityrosporum furfur* and often appearing white in contrast with hyperpigmented skin after exposure to the summer sun.

Ti·nel's sign (tĭ-nĕlz′, tē-) *n.* A sensation of tingling felt in the distal extremity of a limb when percussion is made over the site of an injured nerve, indicating a partial lesion or early regeneration in the nerve.

tine test *n.* A tuberculin test in which the antigen in introduced into the skin by means of tines.

tin·ni·tus (tĭ-nī′təs, tĭn′ĭ-) *n., pl.* **-tus·es.** A sound in one or both ears, such as buzzing, ringing, or whistling, occurring without an external stimulus and usually caused by a specific condition, such as an ear infection, the use of certain drugs, a blocked auditory tube or canal, or a head injury.

tir·ing (tīr′ĭng) *n.* See **cerclage** (sense 1).

tis·sue (tĭsh′ōō) *n.* An aggregation of morphologically similar cells and associated intercellular matter acting together to perform one or more specific functions in the body. There are four basic types of tissue: muscle, nerve, epithelial, and connective.

tissue culture *n.* **1.** The technique or process of keeping tissue alive and growing in a culture medium. **2.** A culture of tissue grown by this technique or process.

tissue lymph *n.* Lymph derived chiefly from fluid in tissue spaces rather than from the blood.

tissue respiration *n.* The interchange of gases between the blood and the tissues.

tis·sue-spe·cif·ic antigen (tĭsh′ōō-spĭ-sĭf′ĭk) *n.* See **organ-specific antigen.**

ti·ta·ni·um (tī-tā′nē-əm, tĭ-) *n.* A strong, low-density, highly corrosion-resistant metallic element with atomic number 22.

ti·ter or **ti·tre** (tī′tər) *n.* **1.** Concentration of a substance in solution or the strength of such a substance determined by titration. **2.** The minimum volume needed to cause a particular result in titration. **3.** The dilution of a serum containing a specific antibody at which the solution retains the minimum level of activity needed to neutralize or precipitate an antigen but loses the activity at a greater dilution.

ti·tra·tion (tī-trā′shən) *n.* The process, operation, or method of determining the concentration of a substance in a solution to which the addition of a reagent having a known concentration is made in carefully measured amounts until a reaction of definite and known proportion is completed, and then calculating the unknown concentration.

T lymphocyte *n.* See **T cell.**

TMJ *abbr.* temporomandibular joint syndrome

T-mycoplasma *n.* See **Ureaplasma.**

TNM staging (tē′ĕn-ĕm′) *n.* A system of evaluation of tumors, based on three variables: primary tumor (T), regional nodes (N), and metastasis (M).

to·bac·co heart (tə-băk′ō) *n.* A rapid, irregular heart rate resulting from excessive use of tobacco.

tobacco mosaic virus *n.* A retrovirus widely used in the study of viruses and viral diseases.

to·ca·nide hydrochloride (tō-kā′nīd′) *n.* An oral antiarrhythmic agent, similar in action to lidocaine, used in the treatment of ventricular arrhythmias.

to·col (tō′kôl) *n.* A colorless viscous oil produced synthetically and used as an antioxidant.

to·col·o·gy or **to·kol·o·gy** (tō-kŏl′ə-jē) *n.* The science of childbirth; midwifery or obstetrics.

to·coph·er·ol (tō-kŏf′ə-rôl′, -rōl′) *n.* Any of a group of closely related, fat-soluble alcohols that behave similarly to vitamin E and are present in milk, lettuce, and wheat germ oil and certain other vegetable oils.

Todd's paralysis (tŏdz) *n.* Temporary paralysis that occurs in the limb or limbs involved in the convulsions of jacksonian epilepsy after the attack is over.

toe (tō) *n.* Any of the digits of the feet.

toe-drop *n.* A drooping of the toes and front part of the foot due to paralysis of the muscles that flex the foot back.

toe·nail (tō′nāl′) *n.* The thin, horny, transparent plate covering the upper surface of the end of a toe.

toe reflex *n.* **1.** A reflex in which strong passive flexion of the great toe excites contraction of the flexor muscles in the leg. **2.** See **Babinski's reflex.**

tol·bu·ta·mide (tŏl-byōō′tə-mīd′) *n.* An orally active hypoglycemic agent used in the treatment of adult-onset diabetes mellitus.

tolbutamide test *n.* A test to detect insulin-producing tumors in which plasma insulin and glucose are measured at intervals after an intravenous dose of tolbutamide.

tol·er·ance (tŏl′ər-əns) *n.* **1.** Decreased responsiveness to a stimulus, especially over a period of continued exposure. **2.** The capacity to absorb a drug continuously or in large doses without adverse effect; diminution in the response to a drug after prolonged use. **3.** Physiological resistance to a poison. **4.** Acceptance of a tissue graft or transplant without immunological rejection. **5.** Unresponsiveness to an antigen that normally produces an immunological reaction. **6.** The ability of an organism to resist or survive infection by a parasitic or pathogenic organism. **— tol′er·ant** *adj.*

to·mo·gram (tō′mə-grăm′) *n.* An x-ray image produced by tomography.

to·mo·graph (tō′mə-grăf′) *n.* The radiographic equipment used in tomography.

to·mog·ra·phy (tō-mŏg′rə-fē) *n.* Any of several techniques for making detailed x-rays of a predetermined plane section of a solid object, such as the body, while blurring out the images of other planes. — to′mo·graph′ic (tō′mə-grăf′ĭk) *adj.*

tone (tōn) *n.* **1.** The quality or character of sound. **2.** The normal state of elastic tension or partial contraction in resting muscles. **3.** Normal firmness of a tissue or an organ. — *v.* **toned, ton·ing, tones.** To give tone or firmness to.

tongue (tŭng) *n.* A mobile mass of muscular tissue that is covered with mucous membrane, occupies much of the cavity of the mouth, forms part of its floor, bears taste buds, and assists in chewing, swallowing, and speech.

tongue crib *n.* An appliance used to control visceral swallowing and tongue thrusting in infants and to encourage the mature or somatic tongue posture and function.

tongue depressor *n.* A thin blade for pressing down the tongue during a medical examination of the mouth and throat.

tongue-swallowing *n.* A slipping back of the tongue against the pharynx, causing choking.

tongue thrust *n.* The infantile pattern of the suckle-swallow movement in which the tongue is placed between the incisor teeth or between the alveolar ridges during the initial stage of swallowing.

ton·ic contraction (tŏn′ĭk) *n.* The sustained contraction of a muscle, as one that is necessary for maintaining posture.

tonic convulsion *n.* A convulsion in which muscle contraction is prolonged.

tonic epilepsy *n.* A convulsive seizure during which the body is rigid.

to·nic·i·ty (tō-nĭs′ĭ-tē) *n.* **1.** Normal firmness or functional readiness in body tissues or organs. **2.** The sustained partial contraction of resting or relaxed muscles. **3.** The osmotic pressure or tension of a solution, usually relative to that of blood.

ton·o·fi·bril (tŏn′ō-fī′brəl, -fĭb′rəl) *n.* One of a system of fibers found in the cytoplasm of epithelial cells.

ton·o·fil·a·ment (tŏn′ō-fĭl′ə-mənt) *n.* A structural cytoplasmic protein, bundles of which together form a tonofibril.

to·nog·ra·phy (tō-nŏg′rə-fē) *n.* Continuous measurement of intraocular pressure to determine the facility of aqueous outflow, used to determine the pressure of glaucoma.

to·nom·e·ter (tō-nŏm′ĭ-tər) *n.* Any of various instruments for measuring pressure or tension, especially one used in tonography.

ton·sil (tŏn′səl) *n.* **1.** A collection of lymphoid tissue. **2.** A small mass of lymphoid tissue, especially either of two such masses embedded in the lateral walls of the opening between the mouth and the pharynx, believed to help protect the body from respiratory infections.

ton·sil·lar (tŏn′sə-lər) or **ton·sil·lar·y** (tŏn′sə-lĕr′ē) *adj.* Of or relating to a tonsil, especially the palatine tonsil.

tonsillar crypt *n.* One of the deep recesses that extend into the palatine and pharyngeal tonsils.

ton·sil·lec·to·my (tŏn′sə-lĕk′tə-mē) *n.* Surgical removal of tonsils or a tonsil.

ton·sil·li·tis (tŏn′sə-lī′tĭs) *n.* Inflammation of a tonsil, especially the palatine tonsil. — **ton′sil·lit′ic** (-lĭt′ĭk) *adj.*

ton·sil·lo·lith (tŏn-sĭl′ə-lĭth′) *n.* A calcareous concretion in a tonsil.

ton·sil·lot·o·my (tŏn′sə-lŏt′ə-mē) *n.* The cutting away of a portion of a hypertrophied palatine tonsil.

to·nus (tō′nəs) *n.* Body or muscular tone; tonicity.

tooth (tōōth) *n., pl.* **teeth** (tēth). One of a set of hard, bonelike structures rooted in sockets in the jaws, typically composed of a core of soft pulp surrounded by a layer of hard dentin that is coated with cement or enamel at the crown and used primarily for biting or chewing food.

tooth·ache (tōōth′āk′) *n.* An aching pain in or near a tooth.

tooth pulp *n.* See **dental pulp.**

to·pal·gi·a (tə-păl′jē-ə, -jə) *n.* Pain localized in one spot without evident organic basis.

to·pec·to·my (tə-pĕk′tə-mē) *n.* Surgical removal of specific areas of the frontal lobe of the cerebral cortex as a treatment for certain mental disorders.

top·es·the·sia (tŏp′ĭs-thē′zhə) *n.* Ability to recognize the location of tactile sensations.

to·phus (tō′fəs) *n., pl.* **-phi** (-fī). **1.** A deposit of uric acid salts in the skin and tissue around a joint or in the external ear, occurring in gout. **2.** Dental calculus; tartar.

top·i·cal (tŏp′ĭ-kəl) *adj.* Of or applied to a definite or localized area of the body. — **top′i·cal·ly** *adv.*

topical anesthesia *n.* Superficial loss of sensation in mucous membranes or skin, produced by direct application of local anesthetic solutions, ointments, or jellies.

to·pog·ra·phy (tə-pŏg′rə-fē) *n.* The description of the regions of the body or of a body part, especially the regions of a definite and limited area of the surface. — **top′o·graph′ic** (-grăf′ĭk), **top′o·graph′i·cal** (-ĭ-kəl) *adj.*

top·o·nar·co·sis (tŏp′ō-när-kō′sĭs) *n.* Localized cutaneous anesthesia.

TORCH syndrome (tôrch) *n.* A group of congenital infections with similar clinical manifestations: toxoplasmosis, other infections, rubella, cytomegalovirus infection, and herpes simplex.

Torn·waldt's abscess (tôrn′välts) *n.* Chronic infection of the pharyngeal bursa.

tor·pid (tôr′pĭd) *adj.* **1.** Deprived of the power of motion or feeling. **2.** Lethargic; apathetic. — **tor·pid′i·ty** *n.*

tor·por (tôr′pər) *n.* **1.** A state of mental or physical inactivity or insensibility. **2.** Lethargy; apathy. — **tor′po·rif′ic** (-pə-rĭf′ĭk) *adj.*

torque (tôrk) *n.* A turning or twisting force. — **torque** *v.*

Tor·re's syndrome (tôr′āz) *n.* A disorder characterized by multiple tumors of the sebaceous glands often accompanied by malignant gastrointestinal tumors.

tor·sion (tôr′shən) *n.* **1.** A twisting or rotation of a part on its long axis. **2.** Twisting of the cut end of an artery to arrest hemorrhage. **3.** Rotation of the eye around its anteroposterior axis. — **tor′sion·al** *adj.*

torsion forceps *n.* A forceps used for applying torsion on an artery to arrest hemorrhage.

torsion fracture *n.* A bone fracture resulting from the twisting of a limb.

tor·so (tôr′sō) *n., pl.* **-sos** or **-si** (-sē). The body excluding the head and limbs; trunk.

tor·ti·col·lis (tôr′tĭ-kŏl′ĭs) *n.* A contracted state of the neck muscles producing an unnatural position of the head. — **tor′ti·col′lar** (-kŏl′ər) *adj.*

tortuosity *n., pl.* **-ties. 1.** The quality or condition of being tortuous; twistedness or crookedness. **2.** A bent or twisted part, passage, or thing.

tor·u·lop·so·sis (tôr′yə-lŏp-sō′sĭs) *n.* An opportunistic infection caused by the yeast *Torulopsis glabrata* and usually seen in patients with severe underlying disease or in those treated with antibiotics, corticosteroids, or immunosuppressive agents.

tor·u·lus (tôr′yə-ləs) *n., pl.* **-li** (-lī). A minute elevation in the skin.

to·rus (tôr′əs) *n., pl.* **to·ri** (tôr′ī). A bulging or rounded projection or swelling, such as is caused by a bone or muscle.

to·tal body hypothermia (tōt′l) *n.* Deliberate reduction of total body temperature to reduce the general metabolism of the tissues.

total joint arthroplasty *n.* Arthroplasty in which both joint surfaces are replaced with artificial materials, usually metal and high-density plastic.

total lung capacity *n.* The volume of gas contained in the lungs at the end of maximal inspiration.

total parenteral nutrition *n.* Nutrition maintained entirely by intravenous injection or by some other nongastrointestinal route.

total transfusion *n.* See **exchange transfusion.**

to·tip·o·ten·cy (tō-tĭp′ə-tən-sē, tō′tĭ-pōt′n-sē) or **to·tip·o·tence** (tō-tĭp′ə-təns, tō′tĭ-pōt′ns) *n.* The ability of a cell, such as an egg, to give rise to unlike cells and thus to develop into or generate a new organism or part. — **to·tip′o·tent** *adj.*

touch (tŭch) *n.* **1.** The physiological sense by which external objects or forces are perceived through contact with the body. **2.** Digital examination. — **touch** *adj.*

Tou·rette′s syndrome (tōō-rĕts′) or **Tou·rette syndrome** (-rĕt′) *n.* A severe neurological disorder marked by multiple facial and other body tics, usually beginning in childhood or adolescence and often accompanied by grunts and compulsive utterances, as of interjections and obscenities.

tour·ni·quet (tōōr′nĭ-kĭt, tûr′-) *n.* A device, typically a tightly encircling bandage, used to check bleeding by temporarily stopping the flow of blood through a large artery in a limb.

To·vell tube (tə-vĕl′) *n.* An endotracheal tube that has a wire spiral embedded in its wall to prevent compression and kinking when the tube is inserted.

tox·e·mi·a (tŏk-sē′mē-ə) *n.* A condition in which the blood contains toxins produced by body cells at a local source of infection or derived from the growth of microorganisms.

tox·e·mic (tŏk-sē′mĭk) *adj.* Of, affected with, or manifesting the features of toxemia.

tox·ic (tŏk′sĭk) *adj.* **1.** Of, relating to, or caused by a toxin or other poison. **2.** Capable of causing injury or death, especially by chemical means; poisonous. — *n.* A toxic chemical or other substance. — **tox′i·cal·ly** *adv.*

toxic epidermal necrolysis *n.* A syndrome in which a large portion of the skin becomes intensely red and peels off in the manner of a second-degree burn; it is often accompanied by blisters.

toxic megacolon *n.* Acute dilation of the colon, seen in ulcerative colitis.

toxic nephrosis *n.* Necrosis due to chemical poisons, septicemia, or bacterial toxemia.

tox·i·col·o·gy (tŏk′sĭ-kŏl′ə-jē) *n.* The study of the nature, effects, and detection of poisons and the treatment of poisoning. — **tox′i·co·log′i·cal** (-kə-lŏj′ĭ-kəl), **tox′i·co·log′ic** (-ĭk) *adj.* — **tox′i·co·log′i·cal·ly** *adv.* — **tox′i·col′o·gist** *n.*

tox·i·co·sis (tŏk′sĭ-kō′sĭs) *n., pl.* **-ses** (-sēz). **1.** Systemic poisoning. **2.** A diseased condition resulting from poisoning.

toxic shock *n.* See **toxic shock syndrome.**

toxic shock syndrome *n.* An acute infection characterized by high fever, a sunburnlike rash, vomiting, and diarrhea, followed in severe cases by shock, that is caused by a toxin-producing strain of the common bacterium *Staphylococcus aureus,* occurring chiefly among young menstruating women who use vaginal tampons.

tox·i·gen·ic (tŏk′sə-jĕn′ĭk) *adj.* Producing a poison. — **tox′i·ge·nic′i·ty** (-jə-nĭs′ĭ-tē) *n.*

tox·in (tŏk′sĭn) *n.* A poisonous substance, especially a protein, that is produced by living cells or organisms and is capable of causing disease when introduced into the body tissues but is often also capable of inducing neutralizing antibodies or antitoxins.

tox·i·path·ic (tŏk′sə-păth′ĭk) *adj.* Relating to a diseased state caused by a poison.

tox·oid (tŏk′soid′) *n.* A substance that has been treated to destroy its toxic properties but that retains the capacity to stimulate production of antitoxins, used in immunization.

tox·o·plas·mo·sis (tŏk′sō-plăz-mō′sĭs) *n., pl.* **-mo·ses** (-mō′sēz). A disease caused by infection with the sporozoan *Toxoplasma gondii.* The congenital form, apparently resulting from parasites in the infected mother being transmitted to the fetus, is characterized by lesions of the central nervous system that can cause blindness and brain damage. The acquired form of the disease is characterized by fever, swollen lymph nodes, and lesions in the liver, heart, lungs, and brain.

TPI test *abbr.* treponema pallidum immobilization test

TPN *abbr.* total parenteral nutrition

tra·bec·u·la (trə-běk′yə-lə) *n., pl.* **-lae** (-lē′). **1.** Any of the supporting strands of connective tissue projecting into an organ and constituting part of the framework of that organ. **2.** Any of the fine needlelike structures that form a network in cancellous bone. — **tra·bec′u·lar** *adj.*

trabecular bone *n.* See **spongy bone** (sense 1).

tra·bec·u·lo·plas·ty (trə-běk′yə-lə-plăs′tē) *n.* Photocoagulation of the trabecular meshwork of the eye by means of a laser. It is used in the treatment of glaucoma.

tra·bec·u·lot·o·my (trə-běk′yə-lŏt′ə-mē) *n.* Surgical opening of the venous sinus of the sclera to treat glaucoma.

trace element *n.* **1.** A chemical element required in minute quantities by an organism to maintain proper physical functioning. **2.** A minute quantity or amount, as of a chemical compound.

trac·er (trā′sər) *n.* **1.** A substance, such as a dye or a radioactive isotope, that is introduced into and followed through a biological or chemical process, by virtue of its radioactive signature, color, or other distinguishing physical property, thus providing information on the course of the process or on the components or events involved. **2.** An instrument used in dissecting out nerves and blood vessels.

tra·che·a (trā′kē-ə) *n., pl.* **-che·as** or **-che·ae** (-kē-ē′). The airway that extends from the larynx into the thorax where it divides into the right and left bronchi. It is composed of thin rings of hyaline cartilage connected by a membrane called the annular ligament. — **tra′che·al** *adj.*

tracheal cartilage *n.* Any of the incomplete rings of hyaline cartilage forming the wall of the trachea.

tracheal muscle *n.* The band of smooth muscular fibers in the fibrous membrane of the trachea, connecting posteriorly the ends of the tracheal rings.

tracheal tube *n.* See **endotracheal tube**.

tracheal tugging *n.* **1.** A downward pull of the trachea symptomatic of aneurysm of the aortic arch. **2.** A jerky type of inspiration seen when the intercostal muscles and the sternocostal parts of the diaphragm are paralyzed by deep general anesthesia or by muscle relaxants.

tra·che·i·tis (trā′kē-ī′tĭs) or **tra·chi·tis** (trə-kī′tĭs) *n.* Inflammation of the trachea.

tra·che·lec·to·my (trā′kə-lěk′tə-mē, trăk′ə-) *n.* See **cervicectomy**.

tra·che·le·ma·to·ma (trā′kə-lē′mə-tō′mə, -lěm′-ə-, trăk′ə-) *n.* A hematoma of the neck.

tra·che·lism (trā′kə-lĭz′əm, trăk′ə-) or **tra·che·lis·mus** (trā′kə-lĭz′məs, trăk′ə-) *n.* A spasmodic bending backward of the neck, as that preceding an epileptic attack.

tra·che·li·tis (trā′kə-lī′tĭs, trăk′ə-) *n.* See **cervicitis**.

tra·che·lo·cys·ti·tis (trā′kə-lō-sĭ-stī′tĭs, trăk′ə-) *n.* Inflammation of the neck of the bladder.

tra·che·lo·dyn·i·a (trā′kə-lō-dĭn′ē-ə, trăk′ə-) *n.* See **cervicodynia**.

tra·che·lo·pex·y (trā′kə-lō-pěk′sē, trăk′ə-) *n.* Surgical fixation of the uterine cervix.

tra·che·lo·plas·ty (trā′kə-lō-plăs′tē, trăk′ə-) *n.* Surgical repair of the uterine cervix.

tra·che·lor·rha·phy (trā′kə-lôr′ə-fē, trăk′ə-) *n.* Suture of a laceration of the uterine cervix.

tra·che·lot·o·my (trā′kə-lŏt′ə-mē, trăk′ə-) *n.* See **cervicotomy**.

tra·che·o·aer·o·cele (trā′kē-ō-âr′ō-sēl′) *n.* An air cyst in the neck, caused by the distention of a tracheocele.

tra·che·o·bron·chi·tis (trā′kē-ō-brŏn-kī′tĭs, -brŏng-) *n.* Inflammation of the mucous membrane of the trachea and bronchi.

tra·che·o·bron·chos·co·py (trā′kē-ō-brŏng-kŏs′kə-pē) *n.* Endoscopic examination of the interior of the trachea and the bronchi.

tra·che·o·cele (trā′kē-ə-sēl′) *n.* A protrusion of the mucous membrane through a defect in the wall of the trachea.

tra·che·o·ma·la·ci·a (trā′kē-ō-mə-lā′shē-ə, -shə) *n.* Degeneration of the elastic and connective tissue of trachea.

tra·che·o·meg·a·ly (trā′kē-ō-měg′ə-lē) *n.* An abnormally dilated trachea, which may result from infection.

tra·che·o·path·i·a (trā′kē-ō-păth′ē-ə) or **tra·che·op·a·thy** (-ŏp′ə-thē) *n.* Disease of the trachea.

tra·che·oph·o·ny (trā′kē-ŏf′ə-nē) *n.* The hollow voice sound heard on auscultation over the trachea.

tra·che·o·plas·ty (trā′kē-ə-plăs′tē) *n.* Reparative or plastic surgery of the trachea.

tra·che·o·py·o·sis (trā′kē-ō-pī-ō′sĭs) *n.* Suppurative inflammation of the trachea.

tra·che·or·rha·gi·a (trā′kē-ə-rā′jē-ə, -jə) *n.* Hemorrhage from the mucous membrane of the trachea.

tra·che·os·chi·sis (trā′kē-ŏs′kĭ-sĭs) *n.* A congenital fissure of the trachea.

tra·che·os·co·py (trā′kē-ŏs′kə-pē) *n.* Examination of the interior of the trachea, as with a laryngoscope. — **tra′che·o·scop′ic** (-ə-skŏp′ĭk) *adj.*

tra·che·o·ste·no·sis (trā′kē-ō-stə-nō′sĭs) *n.* Abnormal narrowing of the lumen of the trachea.

tra·che·os·to·my (trā′kē-ŏs′tə-mē) *n.* **1.** Surgical construction of a respiratory opening in the trachea. **2.** The opening so made. **3.** A tracheotomy performed in order to insert a catheter or tube into the trachea, especially to facilitate breathing.

tra·che·ot·o·my (trā′kē-ŏt′ə-mē) *n.* Incision into the trachea through the neck.

tracheotomy tube *n.* A curved tube used to keep the stoma unobstructed after tracheotomy.

tra·cho·ma (trə-kō′mə) *n.* A contagious disease of the conjunctiva and cornea, caused by the bacterium *Chlamydia trachomatis* and characterized by inflammation, hypertrophy, and formation of granules of adenoid tissue. It is a major cause of blindness in Asia and Africa.

trac·ing (trā′sĭng) *n.* A graphic record of mechanical or electrical events recorded by a pointed instrument.

tract (trăkt) *n.* **1.** An elongated assembly of tissue or organs having a common origin, function, and termination, or a serial arrangement having a common function. **2.** A bundle of nerve fibers having a common origin, termination, and function.

trac·tion (trăk′shən) *n.* **1.** The act of drawing or pulling. **2.** A pulling force. **3.** A sustained pull applied mechanically, especially to the arm, leg, or neck, to correct fractured or dislocated bones, overcome muscle spasms, or relieve pressure.

trac·tot·o·my (trăk-tŏt′ə-mē) *n.* Incision of a nerve tract in the brainstem or spinal cord, usually for the relief of pain.

trait (trāt) *n.* A characteristic, especially one that distinguishes a person from others.

trance (trăns) *n.* An altered state of consciousness as in hypnosis or catalepsy.

tran·ex·am·ic acid (trăn′ĭk-săm′ĭk) *n.* A competitive inhibitor of plasminogen activation and of plasmin. It is used in hemophilia to reduce or to prevent hemorrhage.

tran·quil·ize or **tran·quil·lize** (trăng′kwə-līz′, trăn′-) *v.* **-ized** or **-lized, -iz·ing** or **-liz·ing, -iz·es** or **-liz·es.** **1.** To make tranquil; pacify. **2.** To sedate or relieve of anxiety or tension by the administration of a drug. **3.** To become tranquil; relax. **4.** To have a calming or soothing effect. — **tran′·quil·i·za′tion** (-kwə-lĭ-zā′shən) *n.*

tran·quil·iz·er (trăng′kwə-līz′ər, trăn′-) *n.* A drug that promotes tranquility by calming, soothing, quieting, or pacifying without depressant effects.

trans·ac·tion·al analysis (trăn-săk′shə-nəl, -zăk′-) *n.* A system of psychotherapy that analyzes personal relationships and interactions in terms of conflicting or complementary ego states that correspond to the roles of parent, child, and adult.

trans·cel·lu·lar fluid (trăn-sĕl′yə-lər) *n.* A body fluid that is not inside cells but is separated from plasma and interstitial fluid by cellular barriers.

tran·scrip·tion (trăn-skrĭp′shən) *n.* **1.** The act or process of transcribing. **2.** Something that has been transcribed. **3.** The process by which messenger RNA is synthesized from a DNA template resulting in the transfer of genetic information from the DNA molecule to the messenger RNA. — **tran·scrip′tion·al** *adj.* — **tran·scrip′tion·ist** *n.*

trans·cy·to·sis (trăns′sī-tō′sĭs, trănz′-) *n.* A mechanism for transcellular transport in which a cell encloses extracellular material in an invagination of the cell membrane to form a vesicle, then moves the vesicle across the cell to eject the material through the opposite cell membrane by the reverse process.

trans·der·mal patch (trăns-dûr′məl, trănz-) *n.* A medicated adhesive pad that is placed on the skin to deliver a timed-release dose of medication through the skin into the bloodstream.

trans·duc·er cell (trăns-dōō′sər, -dyōō′-, trănz-) *n.* Any of various cells capable of responding to a

mechanical, thermal, photic, or chemical stimulus by generating an electrical impulse that is synaptically transmitted to a sensory neuron in contact with the cell.

trans·duc·tion (trăns-dŭk′shən, trănz-) *n.* Transfer of genetic material or characteristics from one bacterial cell to another by a bacteriophage or plasmid.

tran·sec·tion (trăn-sĕk′shən) *n.* **1.** A cross section along the long axis of a part. **2.** Division by cutting across.

trans·fer (trăns′fər) *n.* **1.** The conveyance or removal of something from one place to another. **2.** A condition in which learning in one situation influences learning in another situation. It may be positive, as when learning one behavior facilitates the learning of something else, or negative, as when one habit interferes with the acquisition of another. — **trans·fer′** (trăns-fûr′, trăns′fər) *v.*

trans·fer·ence (trăns-fûr′əns, trăns′fər-əns) *n.* In psychoanalysis, the process by which emotions associated with one person, such as a parent, unconsciously shift to another, especially to the analyst.

transference neurosis *n.* In psychoanalytic theory, the release of early traumas and conflicts through transference that allows a person to become aware of the origin of conflict-causing attitudes and behaviors while attempting to learn more appropriate responses.

transfer factor *n.* A substance free of nucleic acid and antibody, that is obtained from the white blood cells of a person with a delayed-type sensitivity and will transfer the specific sensitivity to the recipient after injection into the skin of a nonsensitive person.

trans·fer·rin (trăns-fĕr′ĭn) *n.* A beta globulin in blood serum that combines with and transports iron.

transfer RNA *n.* tRNA.

trans·fix·ion (trăns-fĭk′shən) *n.* In amputation, passing the knife from side to side through tissues close to the bone and dividing muscles from within outward.

transfixion suture *n.* **1.** A crisscross stitch placed so as to control bleeding from a tissue surface or small vessel when it is tied. **2.** A suture used to fix the lower portion of the nasal septum.

trans·for·ma·tion (trăns′fər-mā′shən, -fôr-) *n.* **1.** See **metamorphosis** (sense 1). **2.** The genetic alteration of a bacterial cell by introduction of DNA from another cell or from a virus.

trans·form·ing factor (trăns-fôr′mĭng) *n.* The DNA responsible for bacterial transformation.

trans·fuse (trăns-fyōōz′) *v.* **-fused, -fus·ing, -fus·es.** To administer a transfusion of or to. — **trans·fus′i·ble, trans·fus′a·ble** *adj.* — **trans·fu′sive** (-fyōō′sĭv, -zĭv) *adj.*

trans·fu·sion (trăns-fyōō′zhən) *n.* **1.** The transfer of whole blood or blood products from one person to another. **2.** The intravascular injection of physiological saline solution.

transfusion nephritis *n.* Renal failure and tubular

damage resulting from the transfusion of incompatible blood; the hemoglobin of the hemolyzed red cells is deposited as casts in the renal tubules.

trans·hi·a·tal (trăns'hī-āt'l, trănz') *adj.* Across or through a hiatus.

transhiatal esophagectomy *n.* Resection of the esophagus by blunt dissection from a cervical incision from above and transhiatal approach through an abdominal incision.

tran·sient ischemic attack (trăn'shənt, -zhənt, -zē-ənt) *n.* A temporary blockage of the blood supply to the brain caused by a blood clot and usually lasting ten minutes or less, during which dizziness, blurring of vision, numbness on one side of the body, and other symptoms of a stroke may occur.

tran·si·tion·al denture (trăn-zĭsh'ə-nəl, -sĭsh'-) *n.* A partial denture that serves as a temporary prosthesis and allows for the addition of more teeth as more natural teeth are lost and that will be replaced once the tissue changes that follow the extraction of natural teeth have occurred.

transitional epithelium *n.* Stratified epithelium in which the individual layers are formed by a transformation of the cells from the layer below.

transitional zone *n.* **1.** The region of the lens of the eye where cells from the anterior epithelial capsule become transformed into the fibers that compose the lens substance. **2.** The portion of a scleral contact lens that joins the corneal and scleral sections.

tran·si·tion mutation (trăn-zĭsh'ən, -sĭsh'-) *n.* A point mutation involving substitution of one base pair for another by replacement of one purine by another purine and of one pyrimidine by another pyrimidine but without change in the purine-pyrimidine orientation.

trans·late (trăns-lāt', trănz-, trăns'lāt', trănz'-) *v.* **-lat·ed, -lat·ing, -lates. 1.** To render in another language. **2.** To put into simpler terms; explain or interpret. **3.** To subject messenger RNA to translation. — **trans·lat'a·ble** *adj.*

trans·la·tion (trăns-lā'shən, trănz-) *n.* **1.** The act or process of translating, especially from one language into another. **2.** The state of being translated. **3.** A translated version of a text. **4.** The process by which mRNA, tRNA, and ribosomes effect the production of a protein molecule from amino acids, the specificity of synthesis being controlled by the base sequences of the mRNA. **5.** Movement of a tooth through alveolar bone without change in axial inclination. — **trans·la'tion·al** *adj.*

trans·lo·cate (trăns-lō'kāt', trănz-) *v.* **-cat·ed, -cat·ing, -cates. 1.** To change from one place or position to another; displace. **2.** To transfer a chromosomal segment to a new position; cause to undergo translocation.

trans·lo·ca·tion (trăns'lō-kā'shən, trănz'-) *n.* Transposition of two segments between nonhomologous chromosomes as a result of abnormal breakage and refusion of reciprocal segments.

trans·mi·gra·tion (trăns'mī-grā'shən, trănz'-) *n.*

Movement from one site to another, which may entail the crossing of some usually limiting membrane or barrier, as in diapedesis.

trans·mis·si·ble (trăns-mĭs'ə-bəl, trănz-) *adj.* Capable of being conveyed from one person to another.

trans·mis·sion (trăns-mĭsh'ən, trănz-) *n.* **1.** The conveyance of disease from one person to another. **2.** The passage of a nerve impulse across synapses or at myoneural junctions.

trans·mit (trăns-mĭt', trănz-) *v.* **-mit·ted, -mit·ting, -mits. 1.** To send from one person, thing, or place to another; convey. **2.** To cause (an infection, for example) to spread; pass on. **3.** To impart or convey to others by heredity or inheritance; hand down. — **trans·mit'ta·ble** *adj.*

trans·mu·ta·tion (trăns'myōō-tā'shən, trănz'-) *n.* **1.** A change; transformation. **2.** In physics, the transformation of one element into another by one or a series of nuclear reactions.

tran·spi·ra·tion (trăn'spə-rā'shən) *n.* The passage of watery vapor through the skin or through any membrane.

trans·pla·cen·tal (trăns'plə-sĕn'tl) *adj.* Passing through or occurring across the placenta. — **trans'pla·cen'tal·ly** *adv.*

trans·plant (trăns-plănt') *v.* **-plant·ed, -plant·ing, -plants.** To transfer a tissue or an organ from one body or body part to another. — *n.* (trăns'plănt'). **1.** The act or process of transplanting. **2.** The tissue or organ so used.

trans·plan·ta·tion (trăns'plăn-tā'shən) *n.* The act or process of transplanting a tissue or an organ from one body or body part to another.

trans·port (trăns'pôrt') *n.* The movement or transference of biochemical substances in biological systems.

transport maximum *n.* The maximal rate of secretion or reabsorption of a substance by the renal tubules.

trans·pos·ase (trăns-pō'zās', -zāz') *n.* An enzyme required for transposition of DNA segments.

trans·pose (trăns-pōz') *v.* **-posed, -pos·ing, -pos·es.** To transfer one tissue or organ to the place of another.

trans·po·si·tion (trăns'pə-zĭsh'ən) *n.* **1.** Removal from one place to another. **2.** The state of being transposed or of being on the wrong side of the body. **3.** Transfer of a segment of DNA to a new position on the same or another chromosome, plasmid, or cell.

transposition of the great vessels *n.* A congenital cardiovascular malformation in which the aorta arises from the right ventricle while the pulmonary artery arises from the left ventricle.

trans·po·son (trăns-pō'zŏn) *n.* A segment of DNA having a repeat of an insertion sequence element at each end as well as genes specific to some other activity such as sugar fermentation or resistance to antibiotics; it is capable of migrating to a new position within the same or another chromosome, plasmid, or cell and thereby transferring genetic properties.

trans·sex·u·al (trăns-sĕk′shoō-əl) *n*. **1.** A person with the external genitalia and secondary sexual characteristics of one sex, but whose personal identification and psychosocial configuration is that of the opposite sex. **2.** A person who has undergone a sex change. —*adj*. **1.** Of or relating to such a person. **2.** Relating to medical and surgical procedures designed to alter a patient's external sexual characteristics so that they resemble those of the opposite sex.

trans·sex·u·al·ism (trăns-sĕk′shoō-ə-lĭz′əm) *n*. **1.** The state of being a transsexual. **2.** The desire to change one's anatomic sexual characteristics to conform physically with one's perception of self as a member of the opposite sex.

trans·tho·rac·ic (trăns′thə-răs′ĭk) *adj*. Across or through the thoracic cavity or chest wall. —**trans′tho·rac′i·cal·ly** *adv*.

transthoracic esophagectomy *n*. Resection of the esophagus through a thoracotomy incision.

tran·su·date (trăn-soō′dāt′, -syoō′-, trăn′soō-dāt′, -syoō-) or **tran·su·da·tion** (trăn′soō-dā′-shən, -syoō-) *n*. **1.** A product of the process of passing through a membrane, pore, or interstice. **2.** A substance that transudes.

tran·sude (trăn-soōd′, -syoōd′, -zoōd′, -zyoōd′) *v*. **-sud·ed, -sud·ing, -sudes.** To pass through pores or interstices in the manner of perspiration. —**tran·su′da·to′ry** (trăn-soō′də-tôr′ē, -syoō′-) *adj*.

trans·u·re·ter·o·u·re·ter·os·to·my (trăns′yoō-rē′tə-rō-yoō-rē′tə-rŏs′tə-mē, trănz′-) *n*. The suture of the transected end of one ureter into the intact opposite ureter.

trans·u·re·thral resection (trăns′yoō-rē′thrəl, trănz′-) *n*. Surgical removal of the prostate gland or bladder lesions by means of an endoscope inserted through the urethra, usually for the relief of prostatic obstruction or for treatment of bladder malignancies.

trans·vec·tor (trăns-vĕk′tər, -tôr′, trănz-) *n*. An animal that transmits a toxic substance that it does not produce but that has accumulated in its body from other sources.

trans·verse (trăns-vûrs′, trănz-, trăns′vûrs′, trănz′-) *adj*. Lying across the long axis of the body or of a part.

transverse colon *n*. The part of the colon that lies across the upper part of the abdominal cavity.

trans·ver·sec·to·my (trăns′vər-sĕk′tə-mē, trănz′-) *n*. Surgical excision of the transverse process of a vertebra.

transverse fracture *n*. A fracture in which the line of break forms a right angle with the axis of the bone.

transverse hermaphroditism *n*. Pseudohermaphroditism in which the external genital organs are characteristic of one sex and the gonads are characteristic of the other sex.

transverse plane *n*. See **horizontal plane.**

transverse presentation *n*. An abnormal presentation during birth that is neither head nor breech, in which the fetus is positioned transversely in the uterus across the axis of the birth canal.

transverse process *n*. A process projecting on either side of the arch of a vertebra.

trans·ver·sion (trăns-vûr′zhən, trănz-) *n*. Eruption of a tooth in a position normally occupied by another.

transversion mutation *n*. A point mutation involving base substitution in which the orientation of purine and pyrimidine is reversed.

trans·ves·tism (trăns-vĕs′tĭz′əm, trănz-) or **trans·ves·ti·tism** (-tĭ-tĭz′əm) *n*. Dressing or masquerading in the clothes of the opposite sex.

trans·ves·tite (trăns-vĕs′tīt′, trănz-) *n*. One who practices transvestism.

Tran·tas dot (trăn′təs, trän′täs) *n*. Any of the pale, grayish-red gelatinous nodules occurring on the edge of the conjunctiva in vernal conjunctivitis.

tra·pe·zi·al (trə-pē′zē-əl) *adj*. Relating to a trapezium or to the trapezius muscle.

tra·pe·zi·us muscle (trə-pē′zē-əs) *n*. A large, flat, triangular muscle of the upper back, with origin from the occipital bone, the nuchal ligament, and the spinous processes of the seventh cervical and thoracic vertebrae, with insertion into the posterior surface of the clavicle, the medial side of the acromion, and the upper border of the scapula, and whose action draws the head to one side or backward and rotates the scapula.

trau·ma (trô′mə, trou′-) *n., pl*. **-mas** or **-ma·ta** (-mə-tə). **1.** A serious injury or shock to the body, as from violence or an accident. **2.** An emotional wound or shock that creates substantial, lasting damage to the psychological development of a person, often leading to neurosis. —**trau·mat′ic** (-măt′ĭk) *adj*.

trau·mas·the·ni·a (trô′măs-thē′nē-ə, trou′-) *n*. Nervous exhaustion following an injury.

traumatic amputation *n*. Amputation resulting from an accidental injury.

traumatic anesthesia *n*. Loss of sensation resulting from nerve injury.

traumatic neuroma *n*. A proliferation of Schwann cells and axons that may develop at the proximal end of a severed or injured nerve.

traumatic neurosis *n*. A mental disorder following an accident, injury, or other traumatic event.

trau·ma·tism (trô′mə-tĭz′əm, trou′-) *n*. **1.** The physical or psychological condition produced by a trauma. **2.** A wound or an injury.

trau·ma·tol·o·gy (trou′mə-tŏl′ə-jē, trō′-) *n*. The branch of medicine dealing with the treatment of serious wounds, injuries, and disabilities. —**trau′-ma·to·log′i·cal** *adj*. —**trau′ma·tol′o·gist** *n*.

trau·ma·top·ne·a (trô′mə-tŏp-nē′ə, trou′-) *n*. Passage of air in and out through a wound of the chest wall.

trav·el·ers′ diarrhea or **trav·el·er′s diarrhea** (trăv′əl-ərz, trăv′lərz) *n*. Diarrhea and abdominal cramps occurring among travelers to regions where sanitation is poor, commonly caused by a toxin-producing strain of the bacterium *Escherichia coli*.

treat (trēt) *v.* **treat·ed, treat·ing, treats. 1.** To give medical aid to someone. **2.** To give medical aid to counteract a disease or condition.

treat·ment (trēt′mənt) *n.* Administration or application of remedies to a patient or for a disease or an injury; medicinal or surgical management; therapy.

Trem·a·to·da (trĕm′ə-tō′də) *n.* A class of flatworms that includes species that are both internal and external parasites of humans, that have a thick outer cuticle and one or more suckers or hooks for attaching to host tissue.

trem·a·tode (trĕm′ə-tōd′) *n.* Any of numerous flatworms of the class Trematoda.

trem·a·to·di·a·sis (trĕm′ə-tō-dī′ə-sĭs) *n.* Infestation or infection with trematodes, often caused by ingestion of inadequately cooked food.

trem·or (trĕm′ər) *n.* **1.** An involuntary trembling movement. **2.** Minute ocular movement occurring during fixation on an object.

trem·u·lous (trĕm′yə-ləs) *adj.* Characterized by tremor. — **trem′u·lous·ness** *n.*

trench fever (trĕnch) *n.* An acute infectious disease characterized by chills and fever, caused by the microorganism *Rickettsia quintana,* and transmitted by the louse *Pediculus humanus.*

trench foot *n.* A condition of the foot resembling frostbite, caused by prolonged exposure to cold and dampness.

trench mouth *n.* An acute, sometimes recurrent lesion of the mouth, gums, and throat commonly associated with certain bacilli and spirochetes, characterized by ulceration and necrosis of the gum margin, destruction of the interdental papillae, and foul breath.

Tren·de·len·burg position (trĕn′dl-ən-bûrg′) *n.* A supine position with the patient inclined at an angle of 45° so that the pelvis is higher than the head, used during and after operations in the pelvis or for shock.

Tren·de·len·burg's test (trĕn′dl-ən-bûrgz′) *n.* A test of the valvular competence of the leg veins in which the leg is raised above the level of the heart until the veins are empty and then the leg is rapidly lowered; in cases of varicosity and incompetence of the valves, the veins will at once become distended.

tre·pan (trĭ-păn′) *n.* A trephine. — *v.* **-panned, -pan·ning, -pans.** To trephine.

treph·i·na·tion (trĕf′ə-nā′shən) *n.* Removal of a circular piece of bone, especially of the skull, by a trephine.

tre·phine (trĭ-fīn′) *n.* A cylindrical or crown saw for the removal of a disc of bone, especially from the skull, or of other firm tissue such as that of the cornea. — *v.* **-phined, -phin·ing, -phines.** To operate on with a trephine.

trep·i·da·ti·o cor·dis (trĕp′ĭ-dā′shē-ō kôr′dĭs) *n.* Palpitation of the heart.

trep·i·da·tion (trĕp′ĭ-dā′shən) *n.* **1.** An involuntary trembling or quivering. **2.** A state of anxious fear; apprehension.

Trep·o·ne·ma (trĕp′ə-nē′mə) *n.* A genus of anaerobic spirochetes, including species that cause syphilis, pinta, and yaws.

trep·o·ne·ma·to·sis (trĕp′ə-nē′mə-tō′sĭs) *n., pl.* **-ses.** See treponemiasis.

trep·o·neme (trĕp′ə-nēm′) *n.* A member of the genus *Treponema.*

trep·o·ne·mi·a·sis (trĕp′ə-nē-mī′ə-sĭs) *n.* Infection caused by bacteria of the genus *Treponema.*

trep·pe (trĕp′ə) *n.* The occurrence of a successive increase in amplitude of the first few contractions of cardiac muscle that has received a number of stimuli of the same intensity following a quiescent period.

tret·i·noin (trĕt′ĭ-noin′) *n.* An isomer of retinoic acid, used in the treatment of acne.

TRH *abbr.* thyrotropin-releasing hormone

tri·al denture (trī′əl, trīl) *n.* A setup of artificial teeth made for placement in a patient's mouth before a denture is completed.

trial frame *n.* An adjustable frame that holds trial lenses used during retinoscopy or refraction tests on the eye.

trial lens *n.* Any of a set of cylindrical and spherical lenses used in testing vision.

tri·am·cin·o·lone (trī′ăm-sĭn′ə-lōn′) *n.* A synthetic glucocorticoid used as an anti-inflammatory drug in the treatment of allergic and respiratory disorders.

tri·an·gu·lar bandage (trī-ăng′gyə-lər) *n.* A piece of cloth cut in the shape of a right-angled triangle and used as a sling.

tri·a·zo·lam (trī-ā′zə-lăm) *n.* A benzodiazepine derivative used as a sedative and hypnotic.

tri·bra·chi·a (trī-brā′kē-ə) *n.* A condition seen in conjoined twins when the fusion has merged the adjacent arms to form a single one, so that there are only three arms for the two bodies.

tri·car·box·yl·ic acid cycle (trī′kär-bŏk-sĭl′ĭk) *n.* See Krebs cycle.

tri·ceps (trī′sĕps′) *n., pl.* **-ceps·es** (-sĕp′sĭz) or **tri·ceps. 1.** A three-headed muscle of the upper arm, the long head having origin from the lateral border of the scapula; the lateral head having origin from the lateral and posterior surface of the humerus; and the medial head having origin from the posterior surface of the humerus; with insertion into the olecranon of the ulna, and whose action extends the forearm; the triceps brachii. **2.** The gastrocnemius and soleus muscles of the calf considered as one muscle; the triceps surae.

triceps reflex *n.* A sudden contraction of the triceps muscle caused by a firm tap on its tendon when the forearm hangs loosely at a right angle with the upper arm.

triceps su·rae reflex (sŏŏr′ē) *n.* See Achilles reflex.

tri·chi·a·sis (trĭ-kī′ə-sĭs) *n.* A condition in which the hair adjacent to a natural opening turns inward and causes irritation, as in the inward turning of the eyelashes upon the eye.

trich·i·lem·mo·ma (trĭk′ə-lĕ-mō′mə) *n.* A benign tumor derived from the outer root sheath epithelium of a hair follicle.

tri·chi·na (trĭ-kī′nə) *n., pl.* **-nae** (-nē). A small, slender parasitic nematode worm *(Trichinella spiralis)* that infests the intestines of various mammals and whose larvae move through the bloodstream, becoming encysted in muscles.

Trich·i·nel·la (trĭk′ə-nĕl′ə) *n.* A genus of parasitic nematodes, including the species *Trichinella spiralis,* the pork or trichina worm, which causes trichinosis.

trich·i·no·sis (trĭk′ə-nō′sĭs) *n.* A disease caused by eating undercooked meat, usually pork, that contains trichinae, which develop as adults in the intestines and as larvae in the muscles, causing intestinal disorders, fever, nausea, muscular pain, and edema of the face.

tri·chi·tis (trĭ-kī′tĭs) *n.* Inflammation of the hair bulbs.

tri·chlo·ro·meth·ane (trī-klôr′ō-mĕth′ān′) *n.* Chloroform.

trich·o·dis·co·ma (trĭk′ō-dĭ-skō′mə) *n.* See **haarscheibe tumor**.

trich·o·ep·i·the·li·o·ma (trĭk′ō-ĕp′ə-thē′lē-ō′mə) *n.* One of multiple small, benign nodules, occurring mostly on the skin of the face, derived from basal cells of hair follicles enclosing keratin pearls.

trich·o·lith (trĭk′ə-lĭth′) *n.* A small mass of hair; a hairball.

trich·o·lo·gi·a (trĭk′ə-lō′jē-ə) *n.* A nervous habit of plucking at the hair.

trich·o·meg·a·ly (trĭk′ə-mĕg′ə-lē) *n.* A congenital condition marked by abnormally long eyelashes.

trich·o·mo·nad (trĭk′ə-mō′năd′) *n.* Any of various flagellate protozoans of the genus *Trichomonas.*

Trich·o·mon·as (trĭk′ə-mō′nəs) *n.* A genus of parasitic protozoan flagellates that cause trichomoniasis.

trich·o·mo·ni·a·sis (trĭk′ə-mə-nī′ə-sĭs) *n.*, *pl.* **-ses** (-sēz′). **1.** A vaginal inflammation caused by a trichomonad *(Trichomonas vaginalis)* and resulting in a refractory discharge and itching. **2.** An infection caused by trichomonads, as a disease of cattle that commonly results in infertility or abortion in infected cows.

trichomoniasis vaginitis *n.* Acute or subacute vaginitis or urethritis caused by infection with the protozoan *Trichomonas vaginalis.* Infection is usually venereal but may be transmitted by other forms of contact.

trich·o·my·co·sis (trĭk′ō-mī-kō′sĭs) *n.* **1.** Trichonocardiosis. **2.** Trichomycosis axillaris.

trichomycosis ax·il·lar·is (ăk′sə-lâr′ĭs) *n.* Infection of the axillary and pubic hairs with development of yellow, black, or red concretions around the hair shafts.

trich·o·no·car·di·o·sis (trĭk′ə-nō-kär′dē-ō′sĭs) *n.* An infection of hair shafts, especially of the axillary and pubic regions, with microorganisms of the genus *Nocardia.* Yellow, red, or black concretions develop around the infected hair shafts.

trich·o·no·sis (trĭk′ō-nō′sĭs) *n.* See **trichopathy**.

tri·chop·a·thy (trĭ-kŏp′ə-thē) *n.* Disease of the hair. — **trich′o·path′ic** (trĭk′ə-păth′ĭk) *adj.*

tri·choph·a·gy (trĭ-kŏf′ə-jē) *n.* Habitual biting of the hair.

trich·o·phy·tid (trĭk′ə-fī′tĭd, trī-kŏf′ĭ-) *n.* An eruption caused by an allergic reaction to infection with *Trichophyton.*

trich·o·phy·to·be·zoar (trĭk′ə-fī′tō-bē′zôr′) *n.* An indigestible mass of hair and vegetable fibers found usually in the stomach of ruminant animals or occasionally in the stomach of humans.

Trich·o·phy·ton (trĭk′ə-fī′tŏn′, trī-kŏf′ĭ-) *n.* A genus of pathogenic fungi that cause infections of the skin, hair, and nails.

trich·o·phy·to·sis (trĭk′ə-fī-tō′sĭs) *n.* A superficial fungus infection caused by species of *Trichophyton.*

tri·chop·ti·lo·sis (trĭ-kŏp′tə-lō′sĭs, trĭk′ə-tə-) *n.* A splitting of the shaft of the hair, giving it a feathery appearance.

trich·or·rhex·is (trĭk′ə-rĕk′sĭs) *n.* A condition in which the hairs readily break or split.

tri·chos·chi·sis (trĭ-kŏs′kĭ-sĭs) *n.* See **trichorrhexis**.

tri·cho·sis (trĭ-kō′sĭs) *n.* See **trichopathy**.

Trich·o·spo·ron (trĭk′ə-spôr′ŏn′, trī-kŏs′pə-rŏn′) *n.* A genus of imperfect fungi that are part of the normal flora of the intestinal tract of humans and that includes the causative agent of trichosporosis.

trich·o·spo·ro·sis (trĭk′ə-spə-rō′sĭs, -spô-) *n.* A superficial mycotic infection of the hair in which nodular masses of fungi become attached to the hair shafts.

trich·o·til·lo·ma·ni·a (trĭk′ō-tĭl′ə-mā′nē-ə, -măn′-yə) *n.* A compulsion to pull out one's own hair.

tri·chro·ma·top·si·a (trī′krō-mə-tŏp′sē-ə) *n.* Normal color vision; the ability to perceive the three primary colors.

trich·u·ri·a·sis (trĭk′yə-rī′ə-sĭs) *n.*, *pl.* **-ses** (-sēz). Infection with a species of *Trichuris.* It is usually asymptomatic and not associated with peripheral eosinophilia, but in massive infections it frequently causes diarrhea or rectal prolapse.

Trich·u·ris (trī-kyŏŏr′ĭs) *n.* A genus of nematodes related to the trichina worm and parasitic in the intestines of mammals.

tri·cus·pid atresia (trī-kŭs′pĭd) *n.* The congenital absence of the normal right ventricular opening.

tricuspid murmur *n.* A murmur produced at the tricuspid orifice.

tricuspid orifice *n.* See **right ventricular opening**.

tricuspid stenosis *n.* Pathological narrowing of the orifice of the tricuspid valve.

tricuspid valve *n.* The three-segmented valve of the heart that keeps blood in the right ventricle from flowing back into the right atrium.

tri·cy·clic antidepressant (trī-sī′klĭk, -sĭk′lĭk) *n.* Any of a class of antidepressants, such as amitriptyline, that are structurally related to the phenothiazine antipsychotics.

tri·fo·cal lens (trī-fō′kəl, trī′fō′-) *n.* A lens having one section that corrects for distant vision, a second section that corrects for intermediate vision, and a third that corrects for near vision.

tri·gem·i·nal nerve (trī-jĕm′ə-nəl) *n.* The chief

sensory nerve of the face and the motor nerve of the muscles of chewing. The nuclei of the nerve are in the mesencephalon and in the pons and extend down into the cervical portion of the spinal cord.

trigeminal neuralgia *n.* Paroxysmal shooting pains of the facial area around one or more branches of the trigeminal nerve, of unknown cause, but often precipitated by touching specific areas in or about the mouth.

trigeminal pulse *n.* A pulse in which the beats occur in threes, with a pause after every third beat.

trigeminal rhizotomy *n.* Division or section of a sensory root of the trigeminal nerve.

trigeminal rhythm *n.* A cardiac dysrhythmia in which heartbeats occur in groups of threes, usually composed of a sinus beat followed by two extrasystolic beats.

tri·gem·i·nus (trī-jĕm′ə-nəs) *n.* See **trigeminal nerve.**

tri·gem·i·ny (trī-jĕm′ə-nē) *n.* See **trigeminal rhythm.**

trig·ger area (trĭg′ər) *n.* A point or circumscribed area that when irritated or stimulated will give rise to physiological or pathological change elsewhere.

trig·gered activity (trĭg′ərd) *n.* One or a series of spontaneously generated heartbeats originating from an action potential that produces an afterdepolarization that reaches activation threshold.

trigger point *n.* A specific point on the body at which touch or pressure will elicit pain.

trigger zone *n.* An area that, when stimulated by touch or pressure, excites an attack of neurologic pain.

tri·glyc·er·ide (trī-glĭs′ə-rīd′) *n.* Any of a group of lipids that are esters composed of three fatty acids and one molecule of glycerol, are the chief constituents of adipose tissue, and are found in the blood as lipoproteins.

tri·go·ni·tis (trī′gə-nī′tĭs) *n.* Inflammation of the urinary bladder, localized in the mucous membrane of the inner surface of the bladder near the openings for the ureters and urethra.

trig·o·no·ceph·a·ly (trĭg′ə-nō-sĕf′ə-lē, trī-gŏ′nō-) *n.* A malformation characterized by a triangular configuration of the skull, due in part to premature fusion of the cranial bones with accompanying compression of the cerebral hemispheres. — **trig′o·no·ce·phal′ic** (-sə-făl′ĭk) *adj.*

tri·io·do·thy·ro·nine (trī′ī′-ə-dō-thī′rə-nēn′) *n.* An iodine-containing hormone derived from thyroglobulin and used in the form of its sodium salt in the treatment of hypothyroidism.

tri·labe (trī′lāb′) *n.* A three-pronged forceps for removal of foreign bodies from the bladder.

tril·o·gy of Fallot (trĭl′ə-jē) *n.* An atrial septal defect associated with pulmonic stenosis and right ventricular hypertrophy.

tri·lo·stane (trī′lə-stān′) *n.* An adrenal steroid inhibitor used in the treatment of adrenal hyperfunction in Cushing's syndrome.

tri·mes·ter (trī-mĕs′tər, trī′mĕs′-) *n.* A period of three months.

tri·meth·a·di·one (trī-mĕth′ə-dī′ōn′) *n.* A white crystalline substance used as an anticonvulsant in the treatment of epilepsy.

tri·meth·yl·a·mine (trī-mĕth′ə-lə-mēn′, -lăm′ēn, -mə-thĭl′ə-mēn′) *n.* A degradation product of nitrogenous plant and animal substances.

tri·meth·yl·am·i·nu·ri·a (trī-mĕth′ə-lăm′ə-nŏōr′ē-ə, -nyŏōr′-) *n.* Increased excretion of trimethylamine in urine and sweat, with a characteristic fishy body odor.

tri·me·trex·ate (trī′mī-trĕk′sāt′) *n.* An antineoplastic agent and antiprotozoal orphan drug used in the treatment of pneumonia in AIDS patients caused by *Pneumocystis carinii.*

tri·nu·cle·o·tide (trī-nŏō′klē-ə-tīd′, -nyŏō′-) *n.* A triplet of nucleotides; a codon.

tri·ple·gi·a (trī-plē′jē-ə, -jə) *n.* **1.** Paralysis of an upper and a lower extremity and of the face. **2.** Paralysis of both extremities on one side and one extremity on the opposite side.

tri·ple response (trĭp′əl) *n.* The triphasic response to the firm stroking of the skin characterized by sharply demarcated erythema, a brief blanching of the skin, and release of histamine from the mast cells, followed by arteriolar dilation causing an intense red flare that extends beyond the margins of the line of pressure, and ending with the appearance of a line wheal having the configuration of the original stroking.

trip·let (trĭp′lĭt) *n.* **1.** Any of three children delivered at the same birth. **2.** A unit of three successive nucleotides in a molecule of DNA or RNA that codes for a specific amino acid; a codon or anticodon.

triple vision *n.* See **triplopia.**

trip·loid (trĭp′loid′) *adj.* Having three times the haploid number of chromosomes in the cell nucleus. — *n.* A triploid organism or cell. — **trip′loi·dy** *n.*

trip·lo·pi·a (trĭp-lō′pē-ə) *n.* A visual defect in which three images are seen of the same object.

tri·que·trum (trī-kwē′trəm) *n.* A bone of the wrist in the proximal row of the carpus, articulating with the lunate, pisiform, and hamate bones.

tris·mus (trĭz′məs) *n.* A firm closing of the jaw due to tonic spasm of the muscles of mastication from disease of the motor branch of the trigeminal nerve. It is usually associated with general tetanus.

tri·so·my (trī-sō′mē, trī′sō′-) *n.* The condition of having three copies of a given chromosome in each somatic cell rather than the normal number of two. — **tri·so′mic** *adj.*

trisomy 21 syndrome *n.* See **Down syndrome.**

tri·stich·i·a (trī-stĭk′ē-ə) *n.* The presence of three rows of eyelashes.

tri·ton tumor (trī′tŏn′) *n.* A peripheral-nerve tumor with striated muscle differentiation, often seen in neurofibromatosis.

tRNA (tē′är-ĕn-ā′) *n.* Transfer RNA; one of a class of RNA molecules that transport amino acids to ribosomes for incorporation into a polypeptide undergoing synthesis.

tro·car (trō′kär′) *n.* A sharp-pointed surgical instrument, used with a cannula to puncture a body cavity for fluid aspiration.

tro·chan·ter (trō-kăn′tər) *n.* Any of several bony processes on the upper part of the femur of many vertebrates.

tro·che (trō′kē) *n.* A small, circular medicinal lozenge; a pastille.

troch·le·a (trŏk′lē-ə) *n., pl.* **-le·ae** (-lē-ē′). **1.** An anatomical structure that resembles a pulley, especially the part of the distal end of the humerus that articulates with the ulna. **2.** A fibrous loop in the eye socket near the nasal process of the frontal bone, through which the tendon of the superior oblique muscle of the eye passes.

troch·le·ar nerve (trŏk′lē-ər) *n.* A cranial nerve that originates in the midbrain and supplies an extrinsic eye muscle. It controls movement of the eyeball and eye muscle sense.

tro·choid joint (trō′koid′, trŏk′oid′) *n.* A joint in which a section of a cylinder of one bone fits into a corresponding cavity on the other, as in the proximal articulation between the radius and ulna.

troph·ec·to·derm (trŏf-ĕk′tə-dûrm′, trō-fĕk′-) *n.* The cell layer from which the trophoblast differentiates.

troph·ic (trŏf′ĭk, trō′fĭk) *adj.* Of or relating to nutrition.

trophic ulcer *n.* An ulcer due to impaired nutrition of the part.

tro·pho·blast (trō′fə-blăst′) *n.* The outermost layer of cells of the blastocyst that attaches the fertilized ovum to the uterine wall and serves as a nutritive pathway for the embryo. — **tro′pho·blas′tic** *adj.*

trophoblastic lacuna *n.* One of the spaces in the chorion that becomes an intervillous space after the chorionic villi are formed.

tro·pho·derm (trō′fə-dûrm′) *n.* See **trophoblast**.

tro·pho·tax·is (trō′fō-tăk′sĭs) *n.* See **trophotropism**.

tro·phot·ro·pism (trō-fŏt′rə-pĭz′əm) *n.* Movement of living cells toward or away from nutritive material. — **tro′pho·trop′ic** (trō′fə-trŏp′ĭk) *adj.*

tro·pho·zo·ite (trō′fə-zō′īt′) *n.* A vegetative protozoan, especially a sporozoan during its growing stage.

tro·pi·a (trō′pē-ə) *n.* **1.** Abnormal deviation of the eye. **2.** See **strabismus**.

trop·i·cal abscess (trŏp′ĭ-kəl) *n.* See **amebic abscess**.

tropical diarrhea *n.* See **tropical sprue**.

tropical eosinophilia *n.* Eosinophilia characterized by cough, asthmatic attacks, and enlarged spleen, and believed to be caused by filarial infection; it occurs most frequently in India and southeast Asia.

tropical medicine *n.* The branch of medicine that deals with diseases occurring in tropical countries.

tropical sore *n.* The lesion occurring in cutaneous leishmaniasis.

tropical sprue *n.* Sprue occurring in the tropics, often associated with enteric infection and nutritional deficiency, and frequently complicated by anemia due to folic acid deficiency.

tropical typhus *n.* See **scrub typhus**.

tro·pism (trō′pĭz′əm) *n.* The turning or bending movement of a living organism or part toward or away from an external stimulus, such as light, heat, or gravity. — **tro′pic, tro·pis′tic** *adj.*

tro·po·col·la·gen (trō′pə-kŏl′ə-jən, trŏp′ə-) *n.* The molecular component of a collagen fiber, consisting of three polypeptide chains coiled around each other.

tro·po·my·o·sin (trō′pə-mī′ə-sĭn, trŏp′ə-) *n.* Any of a group of muscle proteins that bind to molecules of actin and troponin to regulate the interaction of actin and myosin.

tro·po·nin (trŏp′pə-nĭn, trōp′ə-) *n.* A calcium-regulated protein in muscle tissue occurring in three subunits with tropomyosin.

Trous·seau's sign (trōō-sōz′) *n.* An indication of latent tetany in which carpal spasm occurs when the upper arm is compressed, as by a tourniquet or a blood pressure cuff.

true hermaphrodite *n.* A person having both ovarian and testicular tissues.

true knot *n.* An intertwining of a segment of umbilical cord, usually without obstructing circulation, usually formed by the fetus slipping through a loop of the cord.

true rib *n.* Any of the seven upper pairs of ribs attached to the sternum by costal cartilage.

trunk (trŭngk) *n.* **1.** The body of a human excluding the head and limbs. **2.** The main stem of a blood vessel or nerve apart from the branches. **3.** A large collecting lymphatic vessel.

truss (trŭs) *n.* A supportive device, usually consisting of a pad with a belt, worn to prevent enlargement of a hernia or the return of a reduced hernia. — *v.* **trussed, truss·ing, truss·es.** To support or brace with a truss.

truth serum *n.* Any of various hypnotic or anesthetic drugs, such as scopolamine or thiopental sodium, used to induce a subject under questioning to talk without inhibition.

Try *abbr.* tryptophan

Try·pan·o·so·ma (trĭ-păn′ə-sō′mə) *n.* A genus of parasitic flagellate protozoans of the family Trypanosomatidae, transmitted to the vertebrate bloodstream, lymph, and spinal fluid by certain insects and often causing diseases such as sleeping sickness.

try·pan·o·some (trĭ-păn′ə-sōm′) *n.* A member of the genus *Trypanosoma* or of the family Trypanosomatidae. — **try·pan′o·so′mal, try·pan′o·som′ic** (-sŏm′ĭk) *adj.*

try·pan·o·so·mi·a·sis (trĭ-păn′ə-sō-mī′ə-sĭs) *n., pl.* **-ses** (-sēz′). A disease or an infection caused by a trypanosome.

tryp·sin (trĭp′sĭn) *n.* An enzyme of pancreatic juice that hydrolyzes proteins to form smaller polypeptide units.

tryp·sin·o·gen (trĭp-sĭn′ə-jən) or **tryp·so·gen** (trĭp′-sə-jən) *n.* The inactive precursor of trypsin, produced by the pancreas and converted to trypsin in the small intestine.

tryp·tic (trĭp′tĭk) *adj.* Relating to or resulting from trypsin.

tryp·to·phan (trĭp′tə-făn′) or **tryp·to·phane** (-făn′) *n.* An essential amino acid formed from proteins during the digestive process by the action of proteolytic enzymes.

tryp·to·pha·nu·ri·a (trĭp′tə-fə-nŏŏr′ē-ə, -nyŏŏr′-) *n.* Increased urinary excretion of tryptophan.

tset·se fly or **tzet·ze fly** (tsĕ′tsē, tsē′tsē) *n.* Any of several two-winged bloodsucking African flies of the genus *Glossina,* often carrying and transmitting pathogenic trypanosomes to humans and livestock.

TSH *abbr.* thyroid-stimulating hormone

TSS *abbr.* toxic shock syndrome

tsu·tsu·ga·mu·shi disease (tsŏŏ′tsə-gə-mŏŏ′shē) *n.* See **scrub typhus.**

tu·bal (tŏŏ′bəl, tyŏŏ′-) *adj.* Of, relating to, or occurring in a tube, such as the fallopian tube or the eustachian tube.

tubal ligation *n.* A method of female sterilization in which the fallopian tubes are surgically tied.

tubal pregnancy *n.* An ectopic pregnancy developing in the fallopian tube.

tube (tŏŏb, tyŏŏb) *n.* **1.** A hollow cylinder, especially one that conveys a fluid or functions as a passage. **2.** An anatomical structure or organ having the shape or function of a tube; a duct.

tu·bec·to·my (tŏŏ-bĕk′tə-mē, tyŏŏ-) *n.* See **salpingectomy.**

tubed flap *n.* A surgical flap in which the sides of the pedicle are sutured together to create a tube, with the entire surface covered by skin.

tu·ber (tŏŏ′bər, tyŏŏ′-) *n., pl.* **tubers** or **-ber·a** (-bər-ə). A localized rounded projection or swelling; a knob, tuberosity, or eminence.

tu·ber·cle (tŏŏ′bər-kəl, tyŏŏ′-) *n.* **1.** An anatomical nodule. **2.** A small elevation on the surface of a tooth. **3.** A nodule or swelling, especially a mass of lymphocytes and epithelioid cells forming the characteristic granulomatous lesion of tuberculosis.

tubercle bacillus *n.* The rod-shaped aerobic gram-negative bacterium *Mycobacterium tuberculosis* that causes tuberculosis.

tubercle of rib *n.* The knob on which a rib articulates with the transverse process of a vertebra.

tu·ber·cu·lar (tŏŏ-bûr′kyə-lər, tyŏŏ-) *adj.* **1.** Of, relating to, or covered with tubercles; tuberculate. **2.** Of, relating to, or affected with tuberculosis. —*n.* A person having tuberculosis.

tu·ber·cu·lid (tŏŏ-bûr′kyə-lĭd, tyŏŏ-) *n.* A lesion of the skin or of mucous membrane resulting from sensitization to the tubercle bacillus.

tu·ber·cu·lin (tŏŏ-bûr′kyə-lĭn, tyŏŏ-) *n.* A sterile liquid culture containing proteins of tubercle ba-

cilli used chiefly in diagnostic tests for tuberculosis.

tuberculin test *n.* Any of various skin tests used to determine infection with *Mycobacterium tuberculosis,* in which tuberculin or its purified protein is introduced into the skin by injection or by means of tines.

tu·ber·cu·li·tis (tŏŏ-bûr′kyə-lī′tĭs, tyŏŏ-) *n.* Inflammation of a tubercle.

tu·ber·cu·lo·cele (tŏŏ-bûr′kyə-lə-sēl′) *n.* Tuberculosis of the testes.

tu·ber·cu·lo·ma (tŏŏ-bûr′kyə-lō′mə, tyŏŏ-) *n.* A rounded non-neoplastic mass, usually in the lungs or brain, caused by a localized tuberculous infection.

tu·ber·cu·lo·sis (tŏŏ-bûr′kyə-lō′sĭs, tyŏŏ-) *n.* **1.** An infectious disease of humans and animals caused by the tubercle bacillus and characterized by the formation of tubercles on the lungs and other tissues of the body, often developing long after the initial infection. **2.** Tuberculosis of the lungs, characterized by the coughing up of mucus and sputum, fever, weight loss, and chest pain.

tuberculosis vaccine *n.* See **Bacillus Calmette–Guérin vaccine.**

tu·ber·cu·lous (tŏŏ-bûr′kyə-ləs, tyŏŏ-) *adj.* **1.** Of, relating to, or having tuberculosis. **2.** Of, affected with, or caused by tubercles.

tuberculous abscess *n.* An abscess caused by the tubercle bacillus.

tu·ber·cu·lum (tŏŏ-bûr′kyə-ləm, tyŏŏ-) *n., pl.* **-la** (-lə). **1.** See **tubercle** (sense 1). **2.** A circumscribed, rounded, solid elevation on the skin, mucous membrane, or surface of an organ. **3.** A slight elevation from the surface of a bone giving attachment to a muscle or ligament.

tu·ber·os·i·ty (tŏŏ′bə-rŏs′ĭ-tē, tyŏŏ′-) *n.* A projection or protuberance, especially one at the end of a bone for the attachment of a muscle or tendon.

tu·ber·ous sclerosis (tŏŏ′bər-əs, tyŏŏ′-) *n.* An inherited disease characterized by hamartomas of the brain, retina, and viscera, as well as epileptic seizures, mental retardation, and skin nodules of the face.

tu·bo·plas·ty (tŏŏ′bō-plăs′tē, tyŏŏ′-) *n.* See **salpingoplasty.**

tu·bo·tor·sion (tŏŏ′bō-tôr′shən, tyŏŏ′-) *n.* The twisting of a tubular structure, such as a fallopian tube.

tu·bu·lar forceps (tŏŏ′byə-lər, tyŏŏ′-) *n.* Long slender forceps intended for use through a cannula or other tubular instrument.

tubular gland *n.* A gland composed of one or more tubules ending in a blind extremity.

tu·bule (tŏŏ′byŏŏl, tyŏŏ′-) *n.* A very small tube or tubular structure; tubulus.

tu·bu·lin (tŏŏ′byə-lĭn, tyŏŏ′-) *n.* A globular protein that is the basic structural constituent of microtubules.

tu·bu·lo·ac·i·nar gland (tŏŏ′byə-lō-ăs′ĭ-nər, -när′-) *n.* A gland having branching tubules each of which ends in a secretory acini.

tubuloalveolar gland *n.* A gland whose secretory

portions end in tubular and alveolar configurations.

tu·bu·lo·in·ter·sti·tial nephritis (tōō'byə-lō-ĭn'-tər-stĭsh'əl, tyōō'-) *n.* Nephritis affecting renal tubules and interstitial tissue, with infiltration by plasma cells and mononuclear cells. It is seen in lupus nephritis, allograft rejection, and methicillin sensitization.

tu·la·re·mi·a (tōō'lə-rē'mē-ə, tyōō'-) *n.* An infectious disease caused by the bacterium *Francisella tularensis* that chiefly affects rodents but can also be transmitted to humans, in whom it causes intermittent fever and swelling of lymph nodes.

tu·me·fac·tion (tōō'mə-făk'shən, tyōō'-) *n.* **1.** The act or process of puffing or swelling. **2.** A swollen condition. **3.** A puffy or swollen part; tumescence.

tu·me·fy (tōō'mə-fī', tyōō'-) *v.* **-fied, -fy·ing, -fies.** To swell or cause to swell.

tu·mes·cence (tōō-mĕs'əns, tyōō-) *n.* **1.** A swelling or an enlarging. **2.** A swollen condition. **3.** A swollen part or organ.

tu·mes·cent (tōō-mĕs'ənt, tyōō-) *adj.* **1.** Somewhat tumid. **2.** Becoming swollen; swelling.

tu·mor (tōō'mər, tyōō'-) *n.* **1.** An abnormal growth of tissue resulting from uncontrolled, progressive multiplication of cells and serving no physiological function; a neoplasm. **2.** A swollen part; a swelling.

tumor angiogenic factor *n.* A substance released by solid tumors that induces formation of new blood vessels to supply the tumor.

tumor antigen *n.* Any of several antigens present in tumors induced by certain types of adenoviruses and papilloma viruses or in cells transformed in vitro by those viruses.

tumor burden *n.* The total mass of tumor tissue carried by a person with cancer.

tu·mor·i·gen·e·sis (tōō'mər-ə-jĕn'ĭ-sĭs, tyōō'-) *n.* Formation or production of tumors.

tumor marker *n.* A substance, released into the circulation by tumor tissue, whose detection in the serum indicates the presence of a specific type of tumor.

tumor necrosis factor *n.* A protein produced by macrophages in the presence of an endotoxin and shown experimentally to be capable of attacking and destroying cancerous tumor cells.

tu·mor·spe·cif·ic transplantation antigen (tōō'-mər-spĭ-sĭf'ĭk, tyōō'-) *n.* Any of several surface antigens of virus-transformed tumor cells, which elicit an immune rejection of the virus-free cells when transplanted into a person who has been immunized against the specific cell-transforming virus.

tumor stage *n.* The extent of the spread of a malignant tumor from its site of origin.

tumor virus *n.* See **oncogenic virus.**

tung·sten (tŭng'stən) *n.* A hard brittle corrosion-resistant metallic element with atomic number 74.

tu·nic (tōō'nĭk, tyōō'-) *n.* A coat or layer enveloping an organ or a part; tunica.

tu·ni·ca (tōō'nĭ-kə, tyōō'-) *n., pl.* **-cae** (-kē', -sē'). An enclosing or enveloping membrane or layer of tissues, as of a blood vessel or other tubular structure.

tunica ad·ven·ti·ti·a (ăd'vĕn-tĭsh'ē-ə) *n.* The outermost fibrous coat of a vessel or of an organ that is derived from the surrounding connective tissue.

tunica ex·ter·na (ĭk-stûr'nə) *n.* The outer of two or more enveloping layers of any structure, especially the outer fibroelastic coat of a blood or lymph vessel.

tunica in·ti·ma (ĭn'tə-mə) *n.* The innermost membrane of a blood or lymph vessel.

tunica me·di·a (mē'dē-ə) *n.* The middle, usually muscular, coat of a blood or lymph vessel.

tunica mus·cu·lar·is (mŭs'kyə-lâr'ĭs) *n.* The muscular, usually middle, layer of a tubular anatomical structure.

tun·nel (tŭn'əl) *n.* A passage through or under a barrier.

tunnel vision *n.* Vision in which the visual field is severely constricted.

tur·bid (tûr'bĭd) *adj.* Having sediment or foreign particles stirred up or suspended; muddy; cloudy. **— tur·bid'i·ty** *n.*

tur·bi·nate bone (tûr'bə-nĭt, -nāt') *n.* A small curved bone that extends horizontally along the lateral wall of the nasal passage.

tur·bi·nec·to·my (tûr'bə-nĕk'tə-mē) *n.* Surgical removal of a turbinate bone.

tur·bi·not·o·my (tûr'bə-nŏt'ə-mē) *n.* Surgical incision into or excision of a turbinate bone.

Tur·cot syndrome (tər-kō') *n.* An inherited syndrome characterized by polyps of the colon and brain tumors.

tur·ges·cence (tûr-jĕs'əns) *n.* **1.** The condition of being swollen; tumescence. **2.** The process of swelling.

tur·gor (tûr'gər, -gôr') *n.* **1.** The state of being turgid. **2.** The normal fullness or tension produced by the fluid content of blood vessels, capillaries, and cells.

tu·ris·ta (tōō-rē'stə) *n.* Diarrhea occurring in travelers as a result of a change in food and water. Not in technical use.

Tur·ner's syndrome (tûr'nərz) *n.* A congenital condition of females associated with a defect in or an absence of an X-chromosome, characterized by short stature, webbed neck, outward-turning elbows, shield-shaped chest, sexual underdevelopment, and amenorrhea.

turn·o·ver flap (tûrn'ō'vər) *n.* A hinged flap that is turned over 180°, usually to receive a second flap.

tus·sis (tŭs'ĭs) *n., pl.* **-ses** (-sēz). A cough.

tus·sive fremitus (tŭs'ĭv) *n.* The vibration felt by a hand placed on the chest of one who is coughing.

T wave *n.* The first deflection in the electrocardiogram following the QRS complex, representing ventricular repolarization.

twelfth cranial nerve *n.* See **hypoglossal nerve.**

twelfth-year molar *n.* The second permanent molar tooth.

twi·light sleep (twī′lĭt′) *n.* An amnesic condition characterized by insensibility to pain without loss of consciousness, induced by an injection of morphine and scopolamine, formerly used to relieve the pain of childbirth.

twilight state *n.* A condition of disordered consciousness during which actions may be performed without conscious volition and without any remembrance afterward.

twin (twĭn) *n.* One of two offspring born at the same birth. — *adj.* **1.** Being two or one of two offspring born at the same birth. **2.** Consisting of two identical or similar parts; double.

twinge (twĭnj) *n.* A sharp, sudden physical pain. — *v.* **twinged, twing·ing, twing·es.** To cause to feel a sharp pain.

twin·ning (twĭn′ĭng) *n.* **1.** The bearing of twins. **2.** A pairing or union of two similar or identical objects.

twin-twin transfusion *n.* Direct vascular anastomosis between the placental circulation of twins.

twitch (twĭch) *v.* **twitched, twitch·ing, twitch·es. 1.** To draw, pull, or move suddenly and sharply; jerk. **2.** To move jerkily or spasmodically. **3.** To ache sharply from time to time; twinge. — *n.* A sudden involuntary or spasmodic muscular movement.

two-glass test *n.* See **Thompson's test.**

two-step exercise test *n.* A test for coronary insufficiency in which a person ascends and descends two steps nine inches high while an electrocardiograph records cardiac activity during the exercise and at intervals afterwards.

two-way catheter *n.* See **double-channel catheter.**

ty·lec·to·my (tī-lĕk′tə-mē) *n.* Surgical removal of a tumor from the breast.

Ty·le·nol (tī′lə-nôl′) A trademark used for a brand of acetaminophen.

ty·lo·ma (tī-lō′mə) *n.* See **callosity.**

ty·lo·sis (tī-lō′-sĭs) *n., pl.* **-ses** (-sēz). **1.** Inflammation of the eyelids, characterized by thickening and hardening of the edges. **2.** A thickening of the horny layer of the skin as a result of chronic pressure or friction.

tym·pa·nec·to·my (tĭm′pə-nĕk′tə-mē) *n.* Surgical excision of the eardrum.

tym·pan·ic (tĭm-păn′ĭk) *adj.* **1.** Relating to or resembling an eardrum. **2.** *Also* **tym·pa·nal** (tĭm′pə-nəl). Of or relating to the middle ear or eardrum. **3.** Resonant.

tympanic canal *n.* A minute canal that passes from the temporal bone to the floor of the tympanic cavity and transmits the tympanic branch of the glossopharyngeal nerve.

tympanic cavity *n.* See **middle ear.**

tympanic membrane *n.* See **eardrum.**

tympanic nerve *n.* A nerve from the inferior ganglion of the glossopharyngeal nerve, passing to the tympanic cavity and forming the tympanic plexus that supplies the mucous membrane of the middle ear, the mastoid cells, and the eustachian tube.

tym·pa·ni·tes (tĭm′pə-nī′tēz) *n.* A distention of the abdomen resulting from the accumulation of gas or air in the intestine or peritoneal cavity. — **tym′pa·nism** *n.*

tym·pa·nit·ic resonance (tĭm′pə-nĭt′ĭk) *n.* A drumlike resonance obtained by percussing over a large space filled with air, such as the stomach, intestine, or large pulmonary cavity.

tym·pa·no·cen·te·sis (tĭm′pə-nō-sĕn-tē′sĭs) *n.* Puncture of the eardrum with a needle to aspirate fluid from the middle ear.

tym·pa·no·mas·toid·i·tis (tĭm′pə-nō-măs′toi-dī′tĭs) *n.* Inflammation of the middle ear and the mastoid cells.

tym·pa·no·plas·ty (tĭm′pə-nə-plăs′tē, -nō-) *n.* Surgical repair or reconstruction of the middle ear.

tym·pa·nos·to·my (tĭm′pə-nŏs′tə-mē) *n.* See **myringotomy.**

tympanostomy tube *n.* A small tube inserted through the eardrum after myringotomy to aerate the middle ear; often used in the treatment of secretory otitis media.

tym·pa·not·o·my (tĭm′pə-nŏt′ə-mē) *n.* See **myringotomy.**

tym·pa·num or **tim·pa·num** (tĭm′pə-nəm) *n.* **-nums** or **-na** (-nə). **1.** See **middle ear. 2.** See **eardrum.**

tym·pa·ny (tĭm′pə-nē) *n.* **1.** A low-pitched, resonant, drumlike note obtained by percussing the surface of a large air-containing space. **2.** See **tympanites.**

type (tīp) *n.* **1.** A number of people or things having in common traits or characteristics that distinguish them as a group or class. **2.** The general character or structure held in common by a number of people or things considered as a group or class. **3.** A person or thing having the features of a group or class. **4.** An example or a model having the ideal features of a group or class. **5.** A taxonomic group, especially a genus or species, chosen as the representative example in characterizing the larger taxonomic group to which it belongs. **6.** The specimen on which the original description and naming of a taxon is based. — *v.* **typed, typ·ing, types.** To determine the antigenic characteristics of a blood or tissue sample.

type I diabetes *n.* See **diabetes mellitus.** (sense 1).

type II diabetes *n.* See **diabetes mellitus.** (sense 2).

type A behavior *n.* A behavior pattern characterized by tenseness, impatience, and aggressiveness, often resulting in stress-related symptoms such as insomnia and indigestion and possibly increasing the risk of heart disease.

type A personality *n.* See **type A behavior.**

type B behavior *n.* A behavior pattern characterized by a relaxed manner, patience, and friendliness that possibly decreases one's risk of heart disease.

type B personality *n.* See **type B behavior.**

typh·lec·to·my (tĭf-lĕk′tə-mē) *n.* See **cecectomy.**

typh·lo·pex·y (tĭf′lə-pĕk′sē) *n.* See **cecopexy.**

typh·lor·rha·phy (tĭf-lôr′ə-fē) *n.* See **cecorrhaphy.**

typh·los·to·my (tĭf-lŏs′tə-mē) *n.* See **cecostomy.**

typh·lot·o·my (tĭf-lŏt′ə-mē) *n.* See **cecotomy**.

ty·phoid (tī′foid′) *n.* Typhoid fever.

typhoid bacillus *n.* An aerobic, gram-negative, rod-shaped bacterium *Salmonella typhi* that causes typhoid fever.

typhoid fever *n.* An acute infectious disease caused by *Salmonella typhi* and characterized by a continued fever, physical and mental depression, an eruption of rose-colored spots on the chest and abdomen, tympanites, and diarrhea.

typhoid vaccine *n.* A vaccine containing a suspension of inactivated *Salmonella typhi*, used to immunize against typhoid fever.

ty·phus (tī′fəs) *n.* Any of several forms of infectious disease caused by species of *Rickettsia*, especially those transmitted by fleas, lice, or mites, and characterized generally by severe headache, sustained high fever, depression, delirium, and the eruption of red rashes on the skin. — **ty′phous** (-fəs) *adj.*

typhus vaccine *n.* A vaccine containing a suspension of inactivated *Rickettsia prowazekii* that has been grown in eggs that differentiate into an embryo, used to immunize against epidemic typhus.

typ·ing (tī′pĭng) *n.* The process of classifying organisms or things according to type.

Tyr *abbr.* tyrosine

ty·ro·ma (tī-rō′mə) *n.* A tumor affected by caseation.

ty·ro·sine (tī′rə-sēn′) *n.* A white crystalline amino acid that is derived from the hydrolysis of proteins such as casein and is a precursor of epinephrine, thyroxine, and melanin.

ty·ro·si·ne·mi·a (tī′rə-sĭ-nē′mē-ə) *n.* An inherited disorder of tyrosine metabolism characterized by an increase in the concentration of tyrosine in the blood, an increase in urinary excretion of tyrosine and related compounds, hepatosplenomegaly, nodular cirrhosis of the liver, multiple renal tubular reabsorptive defects, and vitamin D-resistant rickets.

ty·ro·si·nu·ri·a (tī′rə-sĭ-nŏŏr′ē-ə, -nyŏŏr′-) *n.* Excretion of tyrosine in the urine.

~ ~ ~ ~ ~ ~ **U** ~ ~ ~ ~ ~ ~

u·bi·qui·none (yōō′bĭ-kwĭ-nōn′, -kĭn′ōn) *n.* A quinone compound found in the inner membranes of mitochondria and functioning during oxidative phosphorylation in cellular respiration.

u·biq·ui·tin (yōō-bĭk′kwĭ-tĭn) *n.* A polypeptide that participates in a variety of cellular functions including protein degradation, is found in all eukaryotic cells including plant cells, and has an amino acid structure that has apparently remained largely unchanged throughout evolution.

Uht·hoff sign (ŏot′hŏf) *n.* An indication of multiple sclerosis in which vasodilation from exposure to heat or from exertion may cause transient visual impairment or weakness.

ul·cer (ŭl′sər) *n.* A lesion of the skin or of a mucous membrane such as the one lining the stomach or duodenum that is accompanied by formation of pus and necrosis of surrounding tissue, usually resulting from inflammation or ischemia.

ul·cer·ate (ŭl′sə-rāt′) *v.* **-at·ed, -at·ing, -ates.** To develop an ulcer; become ulcerous. — **ul′cer·a′tive** (-sə-rā′tĭv, -sər-ə-tĭv) *adj.*

ul·cer·a·tion (ŭl′sə-rā′shən) *n.* **1.** Development of an ulcer. **2.** An ulcer or an ulcerous condition.

ulcerative colitis *n.* A chronic disease of unknown cause, characterized by ulceration of the colon and rectum, with bleeding, mucosal crypt abscesses, and inflammatory pseudopolyps; it frequently causes anemia, hypoproteinemia, and electrolyte imbalance.

ulcerative stomatitis *n.* See **canker sore**.

ul·cer·ous (ŭl′sər-əs) *adj.* **1.** Of the nature of ulcers or an ulcer. **2.** Having ulcers or an ulcer. — **ul′cer·ous·ness** *n.*

ul·na (ŭl′nə) *n., pl.* **-nas** or **-nae** (-nē). The medial and larger of the two bones of the forearm, extending from the elbow to the wrist on the side opposite the thumb, and serving as the bony pivot for hand rotation. — **ul′nar** *adj.*

u·lo·der·ma·ti·tis (yōō′lō-dûr′mə-tī′tĭs) *n.* Inflammation of the skin resulting in destruction of tissue and the formation of scars.

u·loid (yōō′loid′) *adj.* Resembling a scar. — *n.* A scarlike lesion due to a degenerative process in deeper layers of skin.

ul·tra·li·ga·tion (ŭl′trə-lĭ-gā′shən) *n.* Ligation of a blood vessel beyond the point where a branch is given off.

ul·tra·mi·cro·scope (ŭl′trə-mī′krə-skōp′) *n.* A microscope with high-intensity illumination used to study very minute objects, such as colloidal particles that scatter the light and appear as bright spots against a dark background.

ul·tra·son·ic (ŭl′trə-sŏn′ĭk) *adj.* **1.** Of or relating to acoustic frequencies above the range audible to the human ear. **2.** Of, relating to, or involving ultrasound. — **ul′tra·son′i·cal·ly** *adv.*

ul·tra·son·ics (ŭl′trə-sŏn′ĭks) *n.* **1.** The acoustics of ultrasonic sound. **2.** The science and technology that deals with the study and application of ultrasound.

ul·tra·son·o·gram (ŭl′trə-sŏn′ə-grăm′, -sō′nə-) *n.* See **sonogram**.

ul·tra·son·o·graph (ŭl′trə-sŏn′ə-grăf′, -sō′nə-) *n.*

An apparatus for producing images obtained by ultrasonography.

ul·tra·so·nog·ra·phy (ŭl′trə-sə-nŏg′rə-fē) *n*. Diagnostic imaging in which ultrasound is used to visualize an internal body structure or a developing fetus. — **ul′tra·so·nog′ra·pher** *n*. — **ul′tra·son′o·graph′ic** (-sŏn′ə-grăf′ĭk, -sō′nə-) *adj*.

ul·tra·sound (ŭl′trə-sound′) *n*. **1.** Ultrasonic sound. **2.** The use of ultrasonic waves for diagnostic or therapeutic purposes, specifically to visualize an internal body structure, monitor a developing fetus, or generate localized deep heat in the tissues.

ultrasound cardiography *n*. See **echocardiography.**

ul·tra·vi·o·let (ŭl′trə-vī′ə-lĭt) *adj*. Of or relating to the range of invisible radiation wavelengths from about 4 nanometers, on the border of the x-ray region, to about 380 nanometers, just beyond the violet in the visible spectrum. — *n*. Ultraviolet light or the ultraviolet part of the spectrum.

ultraviolet lamp *n*. A lamp, especially a mercury-vapor lamp, that produces ultraviolet rays.

ultraviolet microscope *n*. A microscope having quartz and fluorite optics that allow the transmission of light waves shorter than those of the visible spectrum.

ul·tra·vi·rus (ŭl′trə-vī′rəs) *n*. A filterable virus.

um·bil·i·cal (ŭm-bĭl′ĭ-kəl) *adj*. **1.** Of or relating to the navel. **2.** Relating to the umbilical region of the abdomen. — **um·bil′i·cal·ly** *adv*.

umbilical cord *n*. The flexible cordlike structure connecting a fetus at the navel with the placenta and containing two umbilical arteries and one vein that transport nourishment to the fetus and remove its wastes.

umbilical hernia *n*. A hernia of part of the intestine through the abdominal wall under the skin at the navel.

umbilical region *n*. The middle region of the abdomen centered around the navel.

umbilical vesicle *n*. See **yolk sac.**

um·bil·i·ca·tion (ŭm-bĭl′ĭ-kā′shən) *n*. **1.** A pit or navellike depression. **2.** Formation of a depression at the apex of a papule, vesicle, or pustule.

um·bil·i·cus (ŭm-bĭl′ĭ-kəs, ŭm′bə-lī′kəs) *n., pl* **-ci** (-sī′). See **navel.**

um·bo (ŭm′bō) *n., pl.* **um·bos** or **um·bo·nes** (ŭm-bō′nēz). A small anatomical projection on a surface, such as that on the inner surface of the eardrum at the end of the manubrium of the malleus, corresponding to the most elevated point of the eardrum. — **um′bo·nal** (ŭm′bə-nəl, ŭm-bō′nəl), **um·bon′ic** (ŭm-bŏn′ĭk) *adj*.

un·bal·anced translocation (ŭn-băl′ənst) *n*. A condition resulting from fertilization of a gamete containing a translocation chromosome by a normal gamete. The person so affected would have 46 chromosomes, but a segment of the translocation chromosome would be represented three times in each cell and a trisomic state would exist.

un·ci·nate epilepsy (ŭn′sə-nāt′, -nĭt) *n*. A form of psychomotor epilepsy initiated by a dreamy state and hallucinations of smell and taste; usually the result of a lesion of the medial temporal lobe.

un·con·di·tioned reflex (ŭn′kən-dĭsh′ənd) *n*. An instinctive reflex not dependent on previous learning or experience.

unconditioned response *n*. A natural, usually unvarying response evoked by a stimulus in the absence of learning or conditioning.

unconditioned stimulus *n*. A stimulus that elicits an unconditioned response; for example, food is an unconditioned stimulus for a hungry person, and salivation is the unconditioned response.

un·con·scious (ŭn-kŏn′shəs) *adj*. **1.** Of or in a state of unconsciousness; not conscious. **2.** Occurring in the absence of conscious awareness or thought, as an emotion or motive. **3.** Without conscious control; involuntary or unintended. — *n*. In psychoanalytic theory, the division of the mind containing elements of psychic makeup, such as memories or repressed desires, that are not subject to conscious perception or control but that often affect conscious thoughts and behavior. — **un·con′scious·ly** *adv*.

un·con·scious·ness (ŭn-kŏn′shəs-nĭs) *n*. A state of impaired consciousness in which one shows a total lack of responsiveness to environmental stimuli but may respond to deep pain with involuntary movements.

unc·tion (ŭngk′shən) *n*. The action of applying or rubbing with an ointment or oil.

un·der·bite (ŭn′dər-bīt′) *n*. Malocclusion in which the lower teeth overlap the upper teeth.

un·der·de·vel·oped (ŭn′dər-dĭ-vĕl′əpt) *adj*. Not adequately or normally developed; immature.

un·der·shoot (ŭn′dər-shōōt′) *n*. A temporary decrease below the final steady-state value that may occur immediately following the removal of an influence that had been raising that value.

un·der·weight (ŭn′dər-wāt′) *adj*. Weighing less than is normal, healthy, or required. — *n*. Insufficiency of weight.

un·de·scend·ed testicle (ŭn′dĭ-sĕn′dĭd) *n*. An undescended testis.

un·de·scend·ed testis (ŭn′dĭ-sĕn′dĭd) *n*. A testis that has remained in the abdomen or inguinal canal and has not descended into the scrotum.

un·de·ter·mined nitrogen (ŭn′dĭ-tûr′mĭnd) *n*. The concentration of nitrogen in a biological sample, such as blood or urine, but not of urea, uric acid, amino acids, and similar substances, that can be estimated.

un·du·lant fever (ŭn′jə-lənt, ŭn′dyə-, -də-) *n*. See **brucellosis.**

undulating pulse *n*. A pulse in which there is a succession of waves.

ung. *abbr. Latin.* unguentum (unguent; ointment)

un·gual (ŭng′gwəl) *adj*. Of or relating to fingernails or toenails.

un·guent (ŭng′gwənt) *n*. A soothing or medicinal salve. — **un′guen·tar′y** (-tĕr′ē) *adj*.

un·guis (ŭng′gwĭs) *n., pl.* **-gues** (-gwēz). Any of the thin, horny, translucent plates covering the upper surface at the end of each finger and toe, consisting of a visible body and a root concealed under a fold of skin; a fingernail or toenail.

u·ni·ax·i·al joint (yōō′nē-ăk′sē-əl) *n.* A joint that permits movement around one axis only.

u·ni·cel·lu·lar (yōō′nĭ-sĕl′yə-lər) *adj.* Having or consisting of a single cell, as the protozoans; one-celled. — **u′ni·cel′lu·lar′i·ty** (-lăr′ĭ-tē, -lâr′-) *n.*

unicellular gland *n.* A single secretory cell, such as a goblet cell.

u·ni·corn uterus (yōō′nĭ-kôrn′) *n.* A uterus with only one lateral half, the other being undeveloped or absent.

u·ni·lat·er·al (yōō′nə-lăt′ər-əl) *adj.* On, having, or confined to one side. — **u′ni·lat′er·al·ly** *adv.*

unilateral anesthesia *n.* See **hemianesthesia.**

unilateral hermaphroditism *n.* Hermaphroditism in which there is gonadal tissue typical of both sexes on one side of the body and either an ovary or testis on the other.

u·ni·loc·u·lar joint (yōō′nə-lŏk′yə-lər) *n.* A joint having only one cavity.

un·ion (yōōn′yən) *n.* **1.** The joining or amalgamation of two or more bodies. **2.** The structural adhesion of the edges of a wound.

u·ni·po·lar (yōō′nĭ-pō′lər) *adj.* **1.** Having a single fibrous process. Used of a neuron. **2.** Situated at only one extremity of a cell. — **u′ni·po·lar′i·ty** (-pō-lăr′ĭ-tē, -pə-) *n.*

unipolar lead (lēd) *n.* **1.** A lead of an electrocardiograph in which one electrode is placed on the chest in the vicinity of the heart or on one of the limbs, while the other is placed at an area that will not register electrical variation. **2.** A record obtained from such a lead.

unipolar neuron *n.* A neuron whose cell body emits a single axonal process resulting from the fusion of two polar processes during development; the process has one branch serving as a sensory nerve fiber and a second branch that enters into synaptic contact with neurons in the spinal cord or brainstem.

u·ni·port (yōō′nə-pôrt′) *n.* Transport of a molecule or ion through a membrane by a carrier mechanism without known coupling to any other molecule or ion transport.

u·nit membrane (yōō′nĭt) *n.* A trilaminar structure of the cell membrane as seen in cross-sectional study with an electron microscope.

u·ni·ver·sal donor (yōō′nə-vûr′səl) *n.* A person whose red blood cells do not contain agglutinogen A or B and are therefore not agglutinated by plasma containing either of the ordinary isoagglutinins, alpha or beta; a person who has group O blood.

universal recipient *n.* A person who has group AB blood and is therefore able to receive blood from any other group in the ABO system.

unmyelinated fiber *n.* Any of the nerve fibers that lack a fatty myelin sheath but like other nerve fibers are enveloped by a sheath of Schwann cells.

un·san·i·tar·y (ŭn-săn′ĭ-tĕr′ē) *adj.* Not sanitary.

un·sat·u·rat·ed (ŭn-săch′ə-rā′tĭd) *adj.* **1.** Of or relating a solution in which the solvent is capable of dissolving still more of the solute; not saturated. **2.** Of or relating to a chemical compound in which all the affinities are not satisfied, so that still other atoms or radicals may be added to it. **3.** Of or relating chemical compounds containing double and triple bonds.

unsaturated compound *n.* An organic compound containing carbon atoms connected by double or triple bonds.

unsaturated fat *n.* A fat having chains of unsaturated fatty acids.

unsaturated fatty acid *n.* A fatty acid whose carbon chain possesses one or more double or triple bonds and hence can incorporate additional hydrogen atoms.

un·stri·at·ed (ŭn-strī′ā′tĭd) *adj.* Lacking striations; smooth-textured. Used of the smooth or involuntary muscles.

un·sys·tem·a·tized delusion (ŭn-sĭs′tə-mə-tīzd′) *n.* One of a group of apparently discrete, disconnected delusions.

up·per airway (ŭp′ər) *n.* The portion of the respiratory tract that extends from the nostrils or mouth through the larynx.

upper extremity *n.* The shoulder, arm, forearm, wrist, or hand.

upper motor neuron *n.* A motor neuron whose cell body is located in the motor area of the cerebral cortex and whose processes connect with motor nuclei in the brainstem or the anterior horn of the spinal cord.

up·take (ŭp′tāk′) *n.* The absorption by a tissue of a substance, such as a nutrient, and its permanent or temporary retention.

u·ra·cil (yōōr′ə-sĭl) *n.* A pyrimidine base that is an essential constituent of RNA.

u·ra·ni·um (yōō-rā′nē-əm) *n.* An easily oxidized radioactive toxic metallic element with atomic number 92.

u·ra·no·plas·ty (yōōr′ə-nə-plăs′tē) *n.* See **palatoplasty.**

u·ra·nor·rha·phy (yōōr′ə-nôr′ə-fē) *n.* See **palatorrhaphy.**

u·rar·thri·tis (yōōr′är-thrī′tĭs) *n.* Gouty inflammation of a joint.

u·rate (yōōr′āt′) *n.* A salt of uric acid.

u·ra·te·mi·a (yōōr′ə-tē′mē-ə) *n.* Presence of urates, especially sodium urate, in the blood.

u·ra·tu·ri·a (yōōr′ə-tŏŏr′ē-ə, -tyŏŏr′-) *n.* Presence of an increased amount of urates in the urine.

u·re·a (yōō-rē′ə) *n.* A water-soluble compound that is the major nitrogenous end product of protein metabolism and is the chief nitrogenous component of the urine in humans and other mammals.

urea clearance *n.* The volume of plasma or blood that would be completely cleared of urea by one minute's excretion of urine.

urea cycle *n.* The sequence of chemical reactions occurring in the liver that results in the production of urea. The key reaction is the hydrolysis of arginine by arginase to ornithine and urea.

urea frost *n.* Minute flakes of urea sometimes observed on the skin, particularly of the face, in patients with uremia.

u·re·a·gen·e·sis (yŏo-rē'ə-jĕn'ĭ-sĭs) *n.* Formation of urea, especially the metabolism of amino acids to urea.

urea nitrogen *n.* The concentration of nitrogen in a biological sample, such as blood or urine, derived from urea.

U·re·a·plas·ma (yŏo-rē'ə-plăz'mə) *n.* A genus of nonmotile gram-negative bacteria that require urea and cholesterol for growth and are associated with nongonococcal urethritis and prostatitis in males and with genitourinary tract infections and reproductive failure in females.

u·re·a·poi·e·sis (yŏo-rē'ə-poi-ē'sĭs) *n.* See **ure·agenesis**.

u·re·ase (yŏor'ē-ās', -āz') or **u·rase** (yŏor'ās', -āz') *n.* An enzyme that catalyzes the hydrolysis of urea into carbon dioxide and ammonia.

u·re·de·ma (yŏor'ĭ-dē'mə) or **u·ro·e·de·ma** (yŏor'ō-) *n.* Edema due to infiltration of urine into the subcutaneous tissues.

u·re·mi·a or **u·rae·mi·a** (yŏo-rē'mē-ə) *n.* **1.** The accumulation of urinary waste products in the blood, usually due to kidney disease. **2.** A toxic condition caused by uremia. — **u·re'mic** *adj.*

uremic frost *n.* Powdery deposits of urea and uric acid salts on the skin, especially the face, due to the presence of nitrogenous compounds in the sweat, usually the result of severe uremia.

u·re·si·es·the·sia (yŏo-rē'sē-ĕs-thē'zhə) *n.* The normal urge to urinate.

u·re·sis (yŏo-rē'sĭs) *n.* See **urination**.

u·re·ter (yŏo-rē'tər, yŏor'ĭ-tər) *n.* The long, narrow duct that conveys urine from the kidney to the urinary bladder. — **u·re'ter·al, u're·ter·ic** (yŏor'ĭ-tĕr'ĭk) *adj.*

u·re·ter·al·gi·a (yŏo-rē'tə-răl'jē-ə, -jə) *n.* Pain in the ureter.

u·re·ter·cys·to·scope (yŏo-rē'tər-sĭs'tə-skōp', yŏor'ĭ-tər-) or **u·re·ter·o·cys·to·scope** (yŏo-rē'tə-rō-) *n.* A cystoscope with an attachment for catheterization of the ureters.

u·re·ter·ec·ta·sia (yŏo-rē'tə-rĕk-tā'zē-ə, -zhə, -yŏor'ĭ-tə-) *n.* Dilation of a ureter.

u·re·ter·ec·to·my (yŏo-rē'tə-rĕk'tə-mē) *n.* Surgical excision of all or part of a ureter.

u·re·ter·i·tis (yŏo-rē'tə-rī'tĭs, -yŏor'ĭ-tə-) *n.* Inflammation of a ureter.

u·re·ter·o·cele (yŏo-rē'tə-rō-sēl') *n.* Sacculation of the terminal portion of the ureter at the entrance into the urinary bladder, due to a congenital stricture of the ureteral opening into the bladder.

u·re·ter·o·ce·lor·ra·phy (yŏo-rē'tə-rō'sē-lôr'ə-fē, -sĭ-) *n.* Surgical excision and suturing of a ureterocele, performed through an open cystotomy incision.

u·re·ter·o·co·los·to·my (yŏo-rē'tə-rō-kə-lŏs'tə-mē) *n.* Surgical implantation of the ureter into the colon.

u·re·ter·o·cys·tos·to·my (yŏo-rē'tə-rō-sĭ-stŏs'tə-mē) *n.* See **ureteroneocystostomy**.

u·re·ter·o·en·ter·os·to·my (yŏo-rē'tə-rō-ĕn'tə-rŏs'tə-mē) *n.* Surgical formation of an opening between a ureter and the intestine.

u·re·ter·og·ra·phy (yŏo-rē'tə-rŏg'rə-fē) *n.* X-ray examination of the ureter after injection of contrast media.

u·re·ter·o·il·e·o·ne·o·cys·tos·to·my (yŏo-rē'tə-rō-ĭl'ē-ō-nē'ō-sĭ-stŏs'tə-mē) *n.* Surgical restoration of the continuity of the urinary tract by anastomosis of the upper segment of a partially destroyed ureter to a segment of the ileum, the lower end of which is then implanted into the bladder.

u·re·ter·o·il·e·os·to·my (yŏo-rē'tə-rō-ĭl'ē-ŏs'tə-mē) *n.* Surgical implantation of a ureter into an isolated segment of the ileum which drains through an abdominal stoma.

u·re·ter·o·lith (yŏo-rē'tə-rō-lĭth') *n.* A calculus in the ureter.

u·re·ter·o·li·thi·a·sis (yŏo-rē'tə-rō-lĭ-thī'ə-sĭs) *n.* Formation or presence of a calculus or calculi in one or both ureters.

u·re·ter·o·li·thot·o·my (yŏo-rē'tə-rō-lĭ-thŏt'ə-mē) *n.* Surgical removal of a calculus lodged in a ureter.

u·re·ter·ol·y·sis (yŏo-rē'tə-rŏl'ĭ-sĭs) *n.* **1.** Rupture of a ureter. **2.** Paralysis of the ureter. **3.** Surgical freeing of the ureter from surrounding disease or adhesions.

u·re·ter·o·ne·o·cys·tos·to·my (yŏo-rē'tə-rō-nē'ō-sĭ-stŏs'tə-mē) *n.* An operation to implant the upper end of a transected ureter into the bladder.

u·re·ter·o·ne·o·py·e·los·to·my (yŏo-rē'tə-rō-nē'ō-pī'ə-lŏs'tə-mē) *n.* Surgical reimplantation of the ureter into the pelvis of the kidney.

u·re·ter·o·ne·phrec·to·my (yŏo-rē'tə-rō-nə-frĕk'tə-mē) *n.* Surgical removal of a kidney with its ureter.

u·re·ter·op·a·thy (yŏo-rē'tə-rŏp'ə-thē) *n.* Disease of the ureter.

u·re·ter·o·plas·ty (yŏo-rē'tə-rō-plăs'tē) *n.* Reparative or plastic surgery of either or both ureters.

u·re·ter·o·py·e·li·tis (yŏo-rē'tə-rō-pī'ə-lī'tĭs) *n.* Inflammation of the pelvis of a kidney and of its ureter.

u·re·ter·o·py·e·log·ra·phy (yŏo-rē'tə-rō-pī'ə-lŏg'rə-fē) *n.* See **pyelography**.

u·re·ter·o·py·e·lo·ne·os·to·my (yŏo-rē'tə-rō-pī'ə-lō-nē-ŏs'tə-mē) *n.* See **ureteroneopyelostomy**.

u·re·ter·o·py·e·lo·ne·phri·tis (yŏo-rē'tə-rō-pī'ə-lō-nə-frī'tĭs) *n.* See **ureteropyelitis**.

u·re·ter·o·py·e·lo·plas·ty (yŏo-rē'tə-rō-pī'ə-lə-plăs'tē) *n.* Plastic surgery of the ureter and of the pelvis of the kidney.

u·re·ter·o·py·e·los·to·my (yŏo-rē'tə-rō-pī'ə-lŏs'tə-mē) *n.* Surgical formation of a junction between the ureter and the renal pelvis.

u·re·ter·o·py·o·sis (yŏo-rē'tə-rō-pī-ō'sĭs) *n.* Accumulation of pus in a ureter.

u·re·ter·or·rha·gi·a (yŏŏ-rē'tə-rō-rā'jē-ə, -jə) *n.* Hemorrhage from a ureter.

u·re·ter·or·rha·phy (yŏŏ-rē'tə-rôr'ə-fē) *n.* Suture of a ureter.

u·re·ter·o·sig·moid·os·to·my (yŏŏ-rē'tə-rō-sĭg'-moi-dŏs'tə-mē) *n.* Surgical implantation of a ureter into the sigmoid colon.

u·re·ter·os·to·my (yŏŏ-rē'tə-rŏs'tə-mē) *n.* Surgical establishment of an external opening into the ureter.

u·re·ter·ot·o·my (yŏŏ-rē'tə-rŏt'ə-mē) *n.* Surgical incision of a ureter.

u·re·ter·o·u·re·ter·os·to·my (yŏŏ-rē'tə-rō-yŏŏ-rē'tə-rŏs'tə-mē) *n.* The establishment of an anastomosis between the two ureters or between two segments of the same ureter.

u·re·ter·o·ves·i·cos·to·my (yŏŏ-rē'tə-rō-vĕs'ĭ-kŏs'tə-mē) *n.* Surgical joining of a ureter to the bladder.

u·re·thra (yŏŏ-rē'thrə) *n., pl.* **-thras** or **-thrae** (-thrē). The canal through which urine is discharged from the bladder in humans and most other mammals and through which semen is discharged in the male. — **u·re'thral** *adj.*

urethral caruncle *n.* A small, fleshy, sometimes painful growth on the mucous membrane usually occurring at the meatus of the female urethra.

u·re·thral·gi·a (yŏŏr'ĭ-thrăl'jē-ə, -jə) *n.* Pain in the urethra.

u·re·thra·tre·sia (yŏŏ-rē'thrə-trē'zhə, -zhē-ə) *n.* Imperforation or occlusion of the urethra.

u·re·threc·to·my (yŏŏr'ĭ-thrĕk'tə-mē) *n.* Excision of a part or all of the urethra.

u·re·threm·or·rha·gi·a (yŏŏ-rē'thrĕm-ə-rā'jē-ə) *n.* Bleeding from the urethra.

u·re·threm·phrax·is (yŏŏ-rē'thrĕm-frăk'sĭs, yŏŏr'ə-) *n.* Obstruction of the flow of urine through the urethra.

u·re·thrism (yŏŏr'ə-thrĭz'əm) or **u·re·thris·mus** (yŏŏr'ə-thrĭz'məs) *n.* Irritability or spasmodic stricture of the urethra.

u·re·thri·tis (yŏŏr'ĭ-thrī'tĭs) *n.* Inflammation of the urethra.

urethritis pe·trif·i·cans (pə-trĭf'ĭ-kănz') *n.* Urethritis in which there is a deposit of calcareous matter in the wall of the urethra.

u·re·thro·bal·a·no·plas·ty (yŏŏ-rē'thrō-băl'ə-nō-plăs'tē) *n.* Surgical repair of hypospadias and epispadias.

u·re·thro·cele (yŏŏ-rē'thrə-sēl') *n.* A prolapse of the female urethra.

u·re·thro·cys·ti·tis (yŏŏ-rē'thrō-sĭ-stī'tĭs) *n.* Inflammation of the urethra and the bladder.

u·re·thro·cys·tom·e·try (yŏŏ-rē'thrō-sĭ-stŏm'ĭ-trē) *n.* A procedure that simultaneously measures pressures in the urinary bladder and the urethra.

u·re·thro·dyn·i·a (yŏŏ-rē'thrō-dĭn'ē-ə) *n.* See **urethralgia**.

u·re·thro·pex·y (yŏŏ-rē'thrə-pĕk'sē) *n.* Surgical suspension of the urethra from the posterior surface of the pubic symphysis. It is done to correct urinary stress incontinence.

u·re·thro·phrax·is (yŏŏ-rē'thrə-frăk'sĭs) *n.* See **urethremphraxis**.

u·re·thro·phy·ma (yŏŏ-rē'thrə-fī'mə) *n.* A tumor or circumscribed swelling of the urethra.

u·re·thro·plas·ty (yŏŏ-rē'thrə-plăs'tē) *n.* Reparative or plastic surgery of the urethra.

u·re·thror·rha·gi·a (yŏŏ-rē'thrə-rā'jē-ə, -jə) *n.* See **urethremorrhagia**.

u·re·thror·rha·phy (yŏŏr'ə-thrôr'ə-fē) *n.* Suture of the urethra.

u·re·thror·rhe·a (yŏŏ-rē'thrə-rē'ə) *n.* An abnormal discharge from the urethra.

u·re·thro·scope (yŏŏ-rē'thrə-skōp') *n.* An instrument for examining the interior of the urethra. — **u·re'thro·scop'ic** (-skŏp'ĭk) *adj.* — **u're·thros'co·py** (yŏŏr'ə-thrŏs'kə-pē) *n.*

u·re·thro·spasm (yŏŏ-rē'thrə-spăz'əm) *n.* See **urethrism**.

u·re·thro·stax·is (yŏŏ-rē'thrə-stăk'sĭs) *n.* Oozing of blood from the mucous membrane of the urethra.

u·re·thro·ste·no·sis (yŏŏ-rē'thrō-stə-nō'sĭs) *n.* Stricture of the urethra.

u·re·thros·to·my (yŏŏr'ə-thrŏs'tə-mē) *n.* **1.** Surgical construction of an artificial excretory opening from the urethra. **2.** The opening created by such a procedure.

u·re·throt·o·my (yŏŏr'ə-thrŏt'ə-mē) *n.* Surgical incision of a stricture of the urethra.

u·re·thro·vag·i·nal fistula (yŏŏ-rē'thrō-văj'ə-nəl) *n.* A fistula between the urethra and the vagina.

u·re·thro·ves·i·co·pex·y (yŏŏ-rē'thrō-vĕs'ĭ-kə-pĕk'sē) *n.* Surgical suspension of the urethra and the base of the bladder to correct urinary stress incontinence.

urge incontinence (ûrj) *n.* Leakage of urine when the desire to urinate is strong.

ur·gen·cy (ûr'jən-sē) *n.* A strong desire to urinate, accompanied by a fear of leakage.

u·ric (yŏŏr'ĭk) *adj.* Relating to, contained in, or obtained from urine.

uric acid *n.* A semisolid compound that is a nitrogenous end product of protein and purine metabolism and is a nitrogenous component of urine.

u·ri·col·y·sis (yŏŏr'ĭ-kŏl'ĭ-sĭs) *n.* Decomposition of uric acid. — **u'ri·co·lyt'ic** (yŏŏr'ĭ-kō-lĭt'ĭk) *adj.*

u·ri·co·su·ri·a (yŏŏr'ĭ-kə-sŏŏr'ē-ə) *n.* The presence of excessive amounts of uric acid in the urine. — **u'ri·co·su'ric** (-sŏŏr'ĭk) *adj.*

u·ri·dine (yŏŏr'ĭ-dēn') *n.* A white, odorless powder that is the nucleoside of uracil and that plays an important role in carbohydrate metabolism.

uridine diphosphate *n.* A uridine compound that serves as a glycosyl carrier in the synthesis of glycogen and starch.

uridine phosphate *n.* See **uridylic acid**.

uridine tri·phos·phate (trī-fŏs'fāt') *n.* A phosphorylated nucleoside of uridine that participates in the biosynthesis of glycogen.

u·ri·dro·sis (yŏŏr'ĭ-drō'sĭs) or **ur·hi·dro·sis**

(yŏŏr'hī-) n. Excretion of urea or uric acid in the sweat.

u·ri·dyl·ic acid (yŏŏr'ĭ-dĭl'ĭk) n. A nucleoside of uridine formed in the hydrolysis of RNA.

u·ri·nal (yŏŏr'ə-nəl) n. A vessel into which urine is passed.

u·ri·nal·y·sis (yŏŏr'ə-năl'ĭ-sĭs) n., pl. **-ses** (-sēz').
Laboratory analysis of urine, used to aid in the diagnosis of disease or to detect the presence of a specific substance.

u·ri·nar·y (yŏŏr'ə-nĕr'ē) adj. **1.** Relating to urine and its production, function, or excretion. **2.** Of or relating to the organs involved in the formation and excretion of urine.

urinary bladder n. A membranous elastic receptacle situated in the anterior part of the pelvic cavity that distends to serve as the temporary storage place for urine.

urinary calculus n. A hard mass of mineral salts in the urinary tract.

urinary nitrogen n. The nitrogen excreted as urea, amino acids, or uric acid in the urine, used to calculate the metabolism of protein by the body.

urinary sand n. Small hard particles passed in the urine, usually too small to cause symptoms or be identified as calculi.

urinary stress incontinence n. Leakage of urine as a result of coughing, straining, or sudden movement.

urinary stuttering n. Frequent involuntary interruption occurring during the act of urination.

urinary system n. The organs and passages of the urinary tract.

urinary tract n. The passage from the pelvis of the kidney through the ureters, bladder, and urethra to the external urinary opening.

u·ri·nate (yŏŏr'ə-nāt') v. **-nat·ed, -nat·ing, -nates.**
To excrete urine.

u·ri·na·tion (yŏŏr'ə-nā'shən) n. The passing of urine.

u·rine (yŏŏr'ĭn) n. The waste product secreted by the kidneys that in mammals is a yellow to amber-colored, slightly acidic fluid discharged from the body through the urethra.

u·ri·no·ma (yŏŏr'ə-nō'mə) n., pl. **-mas** or **-ma·ta** (-mə-tə). A cyst containing urine.

u·ri·nom·e·ter (yŏŏr'ə-nŏm'ĭ-tər) n. A device for measuring the specific gravity of urine.

u·ri·nom·e·try (yŏŏr'ə-nŏm'ĭ-trē) n. The determination of the specific gravity of urine. — **u'ri·nom'e·ter** (yŏŏr'ə-nŏm'ĭ-tər) n.

u·ri·nos·co·py (yŏŏr'ə-nŏs'kə-pē) n. See **uroscopy.**

u·ro·bi·lin (yŏŏr'ō-bī'lĭn, -bĭl'ĭn) n. A pigment in urine that produces a orange-red color whose intensity varies with its degree of oxidation; it is one of the natural metabolites of hemoglobin.

u·ro·bi·li·ne·mi·a (yŏŏr'ō-bī'lə-nē'mē-ə, -bĭl'ə-) n. The presence of urobilins in the blood.

u·ro·bi·lin·o·gen (yŏŏr'ō-bī'lĭn'ə-jən, -jĕn') n. The precursor of urobilin and a product of the reduction of bilirubin.

u·ro·bi·li·nu·ri·a (yŏŏr'ō-bī'lə-nŏŏr'ē-ə, -nyŏŏr'-)

n. The presence of excess urobilins in the urine.

u·ro·cele (yŏŏr'ə-sēl') n. Extravasation of urine into the scrotal sac.

u·ro·che·si·a (yŏŏr'ə-kē'zē-ə, -zhə) n. Passage of urine from the anus.

u·ro·chrome (yŏŏr'ə-krōm') n. A compound of urobilin and a peptide that is the principal pigment of urine.

u·ro·cys·ti·tis (yŏŏr'ō-sĭ-stī'tĭs) n. Inflammation of the urinary bladder.

u·ro·dyn·i·a (yŏŏr'ə-dĭn'ē-ə) n. Pain on urination.

u·ro·fla·vin (yŏŏr'ə-flā'vĭn) n. A fluorescent product of riboflavin catabolism, found in urine and feces.

u·ro·fol·li·tro·pin (yŏŏr'ō-fŏl'ĭ-trō'pĭn) n. A preparation of gonadotropin used in conjunction with human chorionic gonadotropin to induce ovulation. It is extracted from the urine of postmenopausal women.

u·ro·gas·trone (yŏŏr'ə-găs'trōn') n. A fluorescent pigment extracted from urine that inhibits gastric secretion and motility.

u·ro·gen·i·tal (yŏŏr'ō-jĕn'ĭ-tl) or **u·ri·no·gen·i·tal** (yŏŏr'ə-nō-) adj. Genitourinary.

urogenital canal n. See **urethra.**

urogenital system n. The organs involved in the formation and excretion of urine together with those involved in sexual reproduction.

u·ro·gram (yŏŏr'ə-grăm') n. A radiograph of the urinary tract.

u·rog·ra·phy (yŏŏ-rŏg'rə-fē) n. Radiography of the urinary tract. — **u'ro·graph'ic** (yŏŏr'ə-grăf'-ĭk) adj.

u·ro·ki·nase (yŏŏr'ō-kī'nās, -nāz) n. An enzyme that catalyzes the conversion of plasminogen to plasmin by selectively breaking the bond between arginine and valine; it is produced in the kidney, excreted in the urine, and used to dissolve blood clots.

u·ro·lith·i·a·sis (yŏŏr'ō-lĭ-thī'ə-sĭs) n. A diseased condition resulting from the presence or formation of calculi in the urinary tract.

u·rol·o·gy (yŏŏ-rŏl'ə-jē) n. The medical specialty concerned with the study, diagnosis, and treatment of diseases of the urinary tract in females and of the genitourinary tract in males. — **u·ro·log'ic** (yŏŏr'ə-lŏj'ĭk), **u·ro'log·i·cal** (-ĭ-kəl) adj. — **u·rol'o·gist** n.

u·ron·cus (yŏŏ-rŏng'kəs, -rŏn'-) n. A circumscribed swelling containing extravasated urine.

u·ron·ic acid (yŏŏ-rŏn'ĭk) n. A product of the oxidation of sugar occurring in various polysaccharides and in urine and containing both an aldehyde and a carboxyl group.

u·rop·a·thy (yŏŏ-rŏp'ə-thē) n. A disorder involving the urinary tract.

u·ro·pla·ni·a (yŏŏr'ə-plā'nē-ə) n. Extravasation of urine.

u·ro·poi·e·sis (yŏŏr'ō-poi-ē'sĭs) n. The production and excretion of urine. — **u'ro·poi·et'ic** (-ĕt'ĭk) adj.

u·ro·ra·di·ol·o·gy (yŏŏr'ō-rā'dē-ŏl'ə-jē) n. Examination of the urinary tract by means of a radiological technique.

u·ros·che·o·cele (yŏo-rŏs'kē-ə-sēl') *n.* See **urocele.**

u·ros·che·sis (yŏo-rŏs'kĭ-sĭs) *n.* **1.** The retention of urine. **2.** The suppression of urine.

u·ros·co·py (yŏo-rŏs'kə-pē) *n.* Examination of urine for diagnostic purposes. — **u'ro·scop'ic** (yŏor'ə-skŏp'ĭk) *adj.*

u·ro·sep·sis (yŏor'ō-sĕp'sĭs) *n.* Sepsis resulting from the decomposition of extravasated urine.

u·ros·to·my (yŏo-rŏs'tə-mē) *n.* Surgical construction of an artificial excretory opening from the urinary tract.

u·ro·tho·rax (yŏor'ō-thôr'ăks') *n.* The presence of urine in the thoracic cavity, usually following complex multiple organ trauma.

u·ro·u·re·ter (yŏor'ō-yŏo-rē'tər, -yŏor'ĭ-tər) *n.* See **hydroureter.**

ur·ti·car·i·a (ûr'tĭ-kâr'ē-ə) *n.* A skin condition characterized by intensely itching welts and caused by an allergic reaction to internal or external agents, an infection, or a nervous condition. — **ur'ti·car'i·al** *adj.*

ur·ti·ca·tion (ûr'tĭ-kā'shən) *n.* **1.** The formation or development of urticaria. **2.** The sensation of having been stung by nettles. **3.** A lashing with nettles formerly used to treat a paralyzed part of the body.

u·ru·shi·ol (ŏo-rŏo'shē-ôl', -ōl') *n.* A toxic substance constituting the active allergen of the irritant oil present in poison ivy, poison oak, and poison sumac.

Ush·er's syndrome (ŭsh'ərz) *n.* An inherited syndrome characterized by sensorineural deafness and retinitis pigmentosa.

USPHS *abbr.* United States Public Health Service

ut dict. *abbr. Latin.* ut dictum (as directed)

u·ter·ine (yŏo'tər-ĭn, -tə-rīn') *adj.* Of, relating to, or in the region of the uterus.

uterine cavity *n.* The space within the uterus extending from the cervical canal to the openings of the uterine tubes.

uterine cycle *n.* The menstrual cycle.

uterine placenta *n.* See **maternal placenta.**

uterine souffle *n.* A blowing sound, synchronous with the cardiac systole of the mother, heard on auscultation over the pregnant uterus.

uterine tube *n.* See **fallopian tube.**

u·ter·o·cys·tos·to·my (yŏo'tə-rō-sĭ-stŏs'tə-mē) *n.* Surgical formation of a communication between the uterus and the bladder.

u·ter·o·fix·a·tion (yŏo'tə-rō-fĭk-sā'shən) *n.* See **hysteropexy.**

u·ter·o·lith (yŏo'tər-ə-lĭth') *n.* An abnormal concretion of the uterus, usually a calcified myoma.

u·ter·o·pex·y (yŏo'tər-ə-pĕk'sē) *n.* See **hysteropexy.**

u·ter·o·pla·cen·tal sinus (yŏo'tə-rō-plə-sĕn'təl) *n.* Any of the irregular vascular spaces in the zone of the chorionic attachment to the decidua basalis.

u·ter·o·plas·ty (yŏo'tər-ə-plăs'tē) *n.* Plastic surgery of the uterus.

u·ter·o·sal·pin·gog·ra·phy (yŏo'tə-rō-săl'pĭng-gŏg'rə-fē) *n.* See **hysterosalpingography.**

u·ter·o·scope (yŏo'tər-ə-skŏp') *n.* See **hysteroscope.**

u·ter·os·co·py (yŏo'tə-rŏs'kə-pē) *n.* See **hysteroscopy.**

u·ter·ot·o·my (yŏo'tə-rŏt'ə-mē) *n.* See **hysterotomy.**

u·ter·o·tu·bog·ra·phy (yŏo'tə-rō-tŏo-bŏg'rə-fē, -tyŏo-) *n.* See **hysterosalpingography.**

u·ter·us (yŏo'tər-əs) *n., pl.* **u·ter·us·es** or **u·ter·i** (yŏo'tə-rī'). A hollow muscular organ consisting of a body, fundus, isthmus, and cervix located in the pelvic cavity of female mammals, in which the fertilized egg implants and develops into the fetus.

uterus di·del·phys (dī-dĕl'fĭs) *n.* A double uterus with double cervix and double vagina. It is caused by a failure of the müllerian ducts to unite.

u·tri·cle (yŏo'trĭ-kəl) *n.* **1.** A membranous sac contained within the labyrinth of the inner ear and connected with the semicircular canals. **2.** A minute pouch at the opening of the prostate.

u·tric·u·li·tis (yŏo-trĭk'yə-lī'tĭs) *n.* **1.** Inflammation of the internal ear. **2.** Inflammation of the prostatic utricle.

u·tric·u·lus (yŏo-trĭk'yə-ləs) *n., pl.* **-li** (-lī'). An anatomical sac or pouch, especially the one within the inner ear; utricle.

UV or **U.V.** *abbr.* ultraviolet

u·ve·a (yŏo'vē-ə) *n.* The vascular, pigmentary, middle coat of the eye comprising the choroid, ciliary body, and iris. — **u've·al** *adj.*

u·ve·i·tis (yŏo'vē-ī'tĭs) *n.* Inflammation of the uvea. — **u've·it'ic** (-ĭt'ĭk)

u·ve·o·scle·ri·tis (yŏo'vē-ō-sklə-rī'tĭs) *n.* Inflammation of the sclera due to extension of inflammation from the uvea.

UV index (yŏo'vē') *n.* A zero to ten scale used in estimating the risk for sunburn that an unprotected, fair-skinned person would have if exposed to the ultraviolet radiation in midday sunlight, accounting for conditions such as cloud cover, ozone, and geographic location.

u·vu·la (yŏo'vyə-lə) *n., pl.* **-las** or **-lae** (-lē). A small, conical, pendent fleshy mass of tissue, especially the lobe of the posterior border of the soft portion of the roof of the mouth.

u·vu·lec·to·my (yŏo'vyə-lĕk'tə-mē) *n.* Excision of the uvula.

u·vu·li·tis (yŏo'vyə-lī'tĭs) *n.* Inflammation of the uvula.

u·vu·lop·to·sis (yŏo'vyə-lŏp-tō'sĭs) *n.* Relaxation or elongation of the uvula.

u·vu·lot·o·my (yŏo'vyə-lŏt'ə-mē) *n.* Surgical incision of the uvula.

U wave *n.* A positive wave following the T wave of the electrocardiogram.

V–A *abbr.* ventriculoatrial

vac·ci·nate (văk′sə-nāt′) *v.* **-nat·ed, -nat·ing, -nates.** To inoculate with a vaccine in order to produce immunity to an infectious disease such as diphtheria or typhus. — **vac′ci·na′tor** *n.*

vac·ci·na·tion (văk′sə-nā′shən) *n.* **1.** Inoculation with a vaccine in order to protect against a particular disease. **2.** A scar left on the skin by vaccinating.

vac·cine (văk-sēn′ văk′sēn′) *n.* **1.** A preparation of a weakened or killed pathogen, such as a bacterium or virus, or of a portion of the pathogen's structure that upon administration stimulates antibody production against the pathogen but is incapable of causing severe infection. **2.** A vaccine prepared from the cowpox virus and inoculated against smallpox.

vac·ci·nee (văk′sə-nē′) *n.* One that has been vaccinated.

vaccine lymph *n.* Lymph collected from the vaccinia vesicles of infected calves and used for active immunization against smallpox.

vac·cin·i·a (văk-sĭn′ē-ə) *n.* **1.** See **cowpox. 2.** An infection induced in humans by inoculation with the vaccinia virus in order to confer resistance to smallpox; it is usually limited to the site of inoculation. — **vac·cin′i·al** *adj.*

vaccinia virus *n.* A virus of the genus *Orthopoxvirus* used in the immunization against smallpox.

vac·ci·ni·za·tion (văk′sə-nĭ-zā′shən) *n.* Vaccination repeated at short intervals until the antigen produces no response.

VACTERL syndrome (văk′tərl) *n.* A syndrome seen in embryos and fetuses characterized by abnormalities of vertebrae, anus, cardiovascular tree, trachea, esophagus, renal system, and limb buds; it is associated with the administration of sex hormones during early pregnancy.

vac·u·o·la·tion (văk′yōō-ō-lā′shən) or **vac·u·o·li·za·tion** (-lĭ-zā′shən) *n.* **1.** The formation of vacuoles. **2.** The condition of having vacuoles.

vac·u·ole (văk′yōō-ōl′) *n.* **1.** A small cavity in the cytoplasm of a cell, bound by a single membrane and containing water, food, or metabolic waste. **2.** A small space or cavity in a tissue. — **vac′u·o′lar** (-ō′lər, -lär′) *adj.*

vac·u·tome (văk′yə-tōm′) *n.* An electrically powered dermatome that applies suction to the skin to raise it before an advancing blade, usually for taking a split-thickness skin graft.

vac·u·um (văk′yōō-əm, -yōōm, -yəm) *n., pl.* **-u·ums** or **-u·a** (-yōō-ə). **1.** Absence of matter. **2.** A space empty of matter. **3.** A space relatively empty of matter. **4.** A space in which the pressure is significantly lower than atmospheric pressure.

va·gal attack (vā′gəl) or **va·so·va·gal attack** (vā′-zō-vā′gəl) *n.* A paroxysmal condition characterized by slow pulse, a fall in blood pressure, and sometimes by convulsions, thought to be due to sudden stimulation of the vagus nerve mediated through baroreceptors in the common carotid artery, the aortic arch, or the heart.

va·gi·na (və-jī′nə) *n., pl.* **-nas** or **-nae** (-nē). **1.** The genital canal in the female, leading from the opening of the vulva to the cervix of the uterus. **2.** A sheathlike anatomical structure.

vag·i·nal (văj′ə-nəl) *adj.* **1.** Of or relating to the vagina. **2.** Relating to or resembling a sheath.

vaginal atresia *n.* Imperforation or occlusion of the vagina.

vaginal celiotomy *n.* Incision into the abdomen through the vagina.

vaginal gland *n.* Any of the mucous glands in the mucous membrane of the vagina.

vaginal hysterectomy *n.* Surgical removal of the uterus through the vagina without incising the wall of the abdomen.

vaginal hysterotomy *n.* Surgical incision into the uterus via the vagina.

vaginal opening *n.* The narrowest portion of the vaginal canal, located in the floor of its vestibule, behind the urethral orifice.

vag·i·nec·to·my (văj′ə-něk′tə-mē) *n., pl.* **-mies. 1.** Surgical removal of all or part of the vagina. **2.** Surgical removal of the serous membrane covering the testis and epididymus.

vag·i·nis·mus (văj′ə-nĭz′məs) *n.* A usually prolonged and painful contraction or spasm of the vagina.

vag·i·ni·tis (văj′ə-nī′tĭs) *n.* Inflammation of the vagina.

vag·i·no·cele (văj′ə-nō-sēl′) *n.* See **colpocele** (sense 1).

vag·i·no·dyn·i·a (văj′ə-nō-dĭn′ē-ə) *n.* Vaginal pain.

vag·i·no·fix·a·tion (văj′ə-nō-fĭk-sā′shən) *n.* Suture of a relaxed and prolapsed vagina to the abdominal wall.

vag·i·no·my·co·sis (văj′ə-nō-mī-kō′sĭs) *n.* Inflammation of the vagina due to infection by a fungus.

vag·i·nop·a·thy (văj′ə-nŏp′ə-thē) *n.* Disease of the vagina.

vag·i·no·per·i·ne·o·plas·ty (văj′ə-nō-pĕr′ə-nē′ə-plăs′tē) *n.* Plastic surgery for repair of an injury to the perineum and vagina.

vag·i·no·per·i·ne·or·rha·phy (văj′ə-nō-pĕr′ə-nē-ôr′ə-fē) *n.* Surgical repair of a lacerated vagina and perineum.

vag·i·no·per·i·ne·ot·o·my (văj′ə-nō-pĕr′ə-nē-ŏt′ə-mē) *n.* Surgical division of the outlet of the vagina and of the adjacent portion of the perineum to facilitate childbirth.

vag·i·no·pex·y (văj′ə-nə-pĕk′sē) *n.* See **vaginofixation.**

vag·i·no·plas·ty (văj′ə-nə-plăs′tē) *n.* Plastic surgery of the vagina.

vag·i·nos·co·py (văj′ə-nŏs′kə-pē) *n.* Examination of the vagina, usually by means of an endoscope.

vag·i·no·sis (văj′ə-nō′sĭs) *n.* A disease of the vagina.

vag·i·not·o·my (văj′ə-nŏt′ə-mē) *n.* Surgical incision of the vagina.

va·gi·tus u·ter·i·nus (və-jī′təs yōō′tə-rī′nəs) *n.* Crying of the fetus while still within the uterus, occurring at times when the membranes have been ruptured and air has entered the uterine cavity.

va·gol·y·sis (vā-gŏl′ĭ-sĭs) *n.* Surgical destruction of the vagus nerve.

va·got·o·my (vā-gŏt′ə-mē) *n.* Surgical division of fibers of the vagus nerve, used to diminish acid secretion of the stomach and control a duodenal ulcer.

va·go·to·ni·a (vā′gə-tō′nē-ə) *n.* Overactivity or irritability of the vagus nerve, adversely affecting function of the blood vessels, stomach, and muscles. — **va′go·ton′ic** (-tŏn′ĭk) *adj.*

va·gus (vā′gəs) *n., pl.* **-gi** (-gī, -jī). The vagus nerve.

vagus nerve *n.* A mixed nerve that arises by numerous small roots from the side of the medulla oblongata and supplies the pharynx, larynx, lungs, heart, esophagus, stomach, and most of the abdominal viscera.

vagus pulse *n.* A slow pulse due to the inhibitory action of the vagus nerve on the heart.

Val *abbr.* valine

va·lence (vā′ləns) *or* **va·len·cy** (-lən-sē) *n.* **1.** The combining capacity of an atom or a radical determined by the number of electrons that it will lose, add, or share when it reacts with other atoms. **2.** A positive or negative integer used to represent this capacity. **3.** The number of components of an antigen molecule to which an antibody molecule can bind. **4.** The attraction or aversion that a person feels toward a specific object or event.

Val·en·tine′s position (văl′ən-tīnz′) *n.* A supine position on a table with double inclined plane so as to cause flexion at the hips, used to facilitate urethral irrigation.

val·ine (văl′ēn′, vā′lēn′) *n.* An essential amino acid that is a constituent of proteins, especially fibrous proteins.

Val·i·um (văl′ē-əm) A trademark used for diazepam.

val·pro·ic acid (văl-prō′ĭk) *n.* An anticonvulsive drug used to treat seizure disorders.

Val·sal·va maneuver (văl-săl′və) *n.* **1.** Expiratory effort when the mouth is closed and the nostrils are pinched shut, which forces air into the eustachian tubes and increases pressure on the inside of the eardrum. **2.** Expiratory effort against a closed glottis, which increases pressure within the

thoracic cavity and thereby impedes venous return of blood to the heart.

valve (vălv) *n.* **1.** A membranous structure in a hollow organ or passage, as in an artery or a vein, that folds or closes to prevent the return flow of the body fluid passing through it. **2.** Any of various devices that regulate the flow of gases, liquids, or loose materials through piping or through apertures by opening, closing, or obstructing ports or passageways. **3.** The movable control element of such a device.

val·vo·plas·ty (văl′və-plăs′tē) *n.* See **valvuloplasty.**

val·vot·o·my (văl-vŏt′ə-mē) *n.* **1.** Surgical cutting of a constricted cardiac valve to relieve obstruction. **2.** Incision of a valvular structure.

val·vu·lar (văl′vyə-lər) *adj.* Relating to, having, or operating by means of valves or valvelike parts.

valvular insufficiency *n.* Failure of the cardiac valves to close perfectly, thus allowing regurgitation of blood past the closed valve.

val·vule (văl′vyōōl′) *or* **val·vu·la** (-vyə-lə) *n., pl* **-vules** *or* **-vu·lae** (-vyə-lē′). A small anatomical valve or valvelike structure.

val·vu·li·tis (văl′vyə-lī′tĭs) *n.* Inflammation of a valve, especially a cardiac valve.

val·vu·lo·plas·ty (văl′vyə-lə-plăs′tē) *n.* Plastic surgery to repair a valve, especially a cardiac valve.

val·vu·lot·o·my (văl′vyə-lŏt′ə-mē) *n.* See **valvotomy** (sense 1).

va·na·di·um (və-nā′dē-əm) *n.* A soft ductile metallic element with atomic number 23.

Van Bu·chem′s syndrome (văn bōō′kĕmz) *n.* An inherited skeletal dysplasia characterized by enlargement of the lower jaw and thickening of the long bones and the top of the skull.

van·co·my·cin (văng′kə-mī′sĭn, văn′kə-) *n.* An antibiotic produced by the actinomycete *Streptomyces orientalis,* and effective against staphylococci and spirochetes.

va·nil·lin (və-nĭl′ĭn, văn′ə-lĭn) *n.* A white or yellowish crystalline compound found in the seedpods of vanilla-producing vines and in certain balsams and resins and used in flavorings and pharmaceuticals.

va·nil·lism (və-nĭl′ĭz′əm) *n.* **1.** Irritation of the skin, nasal mucous membrane, and conjunctiva, sometimes seen in people who work with vanilla. **2.** Infestation of the skin by sarcoptic mites found in vanilla-producing seedpods.

van·il·lyl·man·del·ic acid (văn′ə-lĭl′măn-dĕl′ĭk, və-nĭl′əl-) *n.* The major urinary metabolite of adrenal and sympathetic catecholamines.

vanillylmandelic acid test *n.* A test for catecholamine-secreting tumors performed on a 24-hour urine specimen and based on the fact that vanillylmandelic acid is the major urinary metabolite of norepinephrine and epinephrine.

van·ish·ing lung syndrome (văn′ə-shĭng) *n.* A radiologic sign of progressive decrease of the radiologic density of the lung due to a variety of pathophysiologic conditions.

va·por (vā′pər) *n.* **1.** Barely visible or cloudy diffused matter, such as mist, fumes, or smoke, suspended in the air. **2.** The state of a substance that exists below its critical temperature and that may be liquefied by application of sufficient pressure. **3.** The gaseous state of a substance that is liquid or solid under ordinary conditions. **4.** The vaporized form of a medicinal preparation to be administered by inhalation.

va·por·es·cence (vā′pə-rĕs′əns) *n.* Formation of vapor.

va·por·ize (vā′pə-rīz′) *v.* **-ized, -iz·ing, -iz·es.** To convert or be converted into a vapor.

va·por·iz·er (vā′pə-rī′zər) *n.* A device used to vaporize medicine for inhaling.

var·i·a·ble (vâr′ē-ə-bəl, văr′-) *adj.* **1.** Likely to change or vary; subject to variation; changeable. **2.** Tending to deviate, as from a normal or recognized type; aberrant. **3.** Having no fixed quantitative value. — *n.* **1.** Something that varies or is prone to variation. **2.** A quantity capable of assuming any of a set of values. **3.** A symbol representing such a quantity. For example, in the expression $a^2 + b^2 = c^2$, *a, b,* and *c* are variables.

var·i·ant (vâr′ē-ənt, văr′-) *adj.* **1.** Having or exhibiting variation; differing. **2.** Tending or liable to vary; variable. **3.** Deviating from a standard, usually by only a slight difference. — *n.* Something that differs in form only slightly from something else.

var·i·a·tion (vâr′ē-ā′shən, văr′-) *n.* **1.** The act, process, or result of varying. **2.** The state or fact of being varied. **3.** The extent or degree to which something varies. **4.** Something slightly different from another of the same type. **5.** Marked difference or deviation from the normal or recognized form, function, or structure. **6.** An organism exhibiting such difference or deviation. **7.** A function that relates the values of one variable to those of other variables.

var·i·cel·la (văr′ĭ-sĕl′ə) *n.* See **chickenpox.**

varicella-zoster virus *n.* A herpesvirus that causes chickenpox and shingles.

var·i·co·cele (văr′ĭ-kō-sēl′) *n.* A varicose condition of veins of the spermatic cord or the ovaries, forming a soft tumor.

var·i·co·ce·lec·to·my (văr′ĭ-kō-sə-lĕk′tə-mē) *n.* Surgery for the relief of a varicocele by ligature and excision and by ligation of the dilated veins.

var·i·cog·ra·phy (văr′ĭ-kŏg′rə-fē) *n.* Radiography of varicose veins after injection of a radiopaque medium.

var·i·co·phle·bi·tis (văr′ĭ-kō-flĭ-bī′tĭs) *n.* Inflammation of varicose veins.

var·i·cose (văr′ĭ-kōs′) *adj.* Relating to, affected with, or characterized by varices or varicosis.

varicose ulcer *n.* Loss of skin surface in the drainage area of a varicose vein, usually in the leg, resulting from stasis and infection.

varicose vein *n.* **1.** An abnormally dilated or swollen vein. **2.** varicose veins. The condition of having abnormally dilated or swollen veins, especially in the legs.

var·i·co·sis (văr′ĭ-kō′sĭs) *n., pl.* **-ses** (-sēz). **1.** The condition of being varicose. **2.** Formation of a varix or of varices.

var·i·cos·i·ty (văr′ĭ-kŏs′ĭ-tē) *n.* **1.** Varicosis. **2.** A varicose enlargement or swelling.

var·i·cot·o·my (văr′ĭ-kŏt′ə-mē) *n.* Surgical removal of varicose veins.

va·ric·u·la (və-rĭk′yə-lə) *n., pl.* **-lae** (-lē). A varicose condition of the veins of the conjunctiva.

var·i·cule (văr′ĭ-kyōōl′) *n.* A small varicose vein ordinarily seen in the skin.

va·ri·o·la (və-rī′ə-lə, vâr′ē-ō′lə, văr′-) *n.* See **smallpox. — va·ri′o·lar** (-lər), **va·ri′o·lous** (-ləs) *adj.*

variola virus *n.* A virus of the genus *Orthopoxvirus* that causes smallpox.

var·ix (văr′ĭks) *n., pl.* **-i·ces** (-ĭ-sēz′). An abnormally dilated or swollen vein, artery, or lymph vessel.

var·y (vâr′ē, văr′ē) *v.* **-ied** (-ēd), **-y·ing, -ies** (-ēz). **1.** To make or cause changes in the characteristics or attributes of; modify or alter. **2.** To undergo or show change. **3.** To be different; deviate.

vas (văs) *n., pl* **va·sa** (vā′zə). An anatomical duct or canal conveying any liquid, such as blood, lymph, chyle, or semen.

vas·cu·lar (văs′kyə-lər) *adj.* Or, relating to, or containing blood vessels.

vascular hemophilia *n.* See **von Willebrand's disease.**

vas·cu·lar·i·ty (văs′kyə-lăr′ĭ-tē) *n.* The condition of being vascular.

vas·cu·lar·i·za·tion (văs′kyə-lər-ĭ-zā′shən) *n.* **1.** The formation of blood vessels. **2.** An abnormal or pathological formation of blood vessels.

vas·cu·lar·ize (văs′kyə-lə-rīz′) *v.* **-ized, -iz·ing, -iz·es.** To make or become vascular.

vascularized graft *n.* A graft after the recipient vasculature has been connected with the vessels in the graft.

vascular layer *n.* The outer portion of the choroid of the eye, containing the largest blood vessels.

vascular polyp *n.* A bulging or protruding angioma of the nasal mucous membrane.

vascular spider *n.* See **arterial spider.**

vascular system *n.* See **circulatory system.**

vas·cu·la·ture (văs′kyə-lə-chŏŏr′, -chər) *n.* Arrangement of blood vessels in the body or in an organ or a body part.

vas·cu·li·tis (văs′kyə-lī′tĭs) *n.* Inflammation of a blood or lymph vessel.

vas·cu·lo·my·e·li·nop·a·thy (văs′kyə-lō-mī′ə-lə-nŏp′ə-thē) *n.* Vasculopathy of the small cerebral vessels followed by demyelination of the vessels.

vas·cu·lop·a·thy (văs′kyə-lŏp′ə-thē) *n.* Disease of the blood vessels.

vas def·er·ens (văs′ dĕf′ər-ənz, -ə-rĕnz′) *n., pl.* **va·sa def·er·en·ti·a** (vā′zə dĕf′ə-rĕn′shē-ə). The main secretory duct of the testicle, through which semen is carried from the epididymis to the prostatic urethra, where it ends as the ejaculatory duct.

va·sec·to·mize (və-sĕk′tə-mīz′, vā-zĕk′-) *v.* **-mized, -miz·ing, -miz·es.** To perform a vasectomy on.

va·sec·to·my (və-sĕk′tə-mē, vā-zĕk′-) *n*. Surgical removal of all or part of the vas deferens, usually as a means of sterilization.

vas ef·fer·ens (văs′ ĕf′ər-ənz, -ə-rĕnz′) *n*., *pl.* **va·sa ef·fer·en·ti·a** (vā′zə ĕf′ə-rĕn′shē-ə). Any of a number of small ducts that carry semen from the testis to the epididymis.

Vas·e·line (văs′ə-lēn′, văs′ə-lēn′) A trademark used for a brand of petroleum jelly.

vas·i·fac·tion (văs′ə-făk′shən) *n*. See **angiopoiesis**. — **vas′i·fac′tive** *adj*.

va·so·ac·tive (vā′zō-ăk′tĭv) *adj*. Causing constriction or dilation of blood vessels.

vasoactive amine *n*. A substance containing amino groups, such as histamine or serotonin, that acts on the blood vessels to alter permeability or cause vasodilation.

va·so·con·stric·tion (vā′zō-kən-strĭk′shən) *n*. Constriction of a blood vessel, as by a nerve or drug.

va·so·con·stric·tor (vā′zō-kən-strĭk′tər) *n*. Something, such as a nerve or drug, that causes vasoconstriction. — *adj*. Producing vasoconstriction.

va·so·de·pres·sion (vā′zō-dĭ-prĕsh′ən) *n*. Reduction of tone in blood vessels with vasodilation and resulting lowered blood pressure.

va·so·di·la·tion (vā′zō-dī-lā′shən, -dī-) or **va·so·dil·a·ta·tion** (-dĭl′ə-tā′shən, -dī′lə-) *n*. Dilation of a blood vessel, as by the action of a nerve or drug.

va·so·ep·i·did·y·mos·to·my (vā′zō-ĕp′ĭ-dĭd′ə-mŏs′tə-mē) *n*. Surgical creation of a passage between the vas deferens and the epididymis.

va·so·for·ma·tion (vā′zō-fôr-mā′shən) *n*. See **angiopoiesis**. — **va′so·form′a·tive** (-fôr′mə-tĭv) *adj*.

va·so·form·a·tive cell (vā′zō-fôr′mə-tĭv) *n*. See **angioblast** (sense 2).

va·so·gan·gli·on (vā′zō-găng′glē-ən) *n*. A mass of blood vessels.

va·sog·ra·phy (vā-zŏg′rə-fē) *n*. Radiography of blood vessels.

va·so·li·ga·tion (vā′zō-lī-gā′shən) *n*. Surgical ligation of the vas deferens as a means of sterilization. — **va′so·li′gate** (-lī′gāt) *v*.

va·so·mo·tion (vā′zō-mō′shən) *n*. Change in the caliber of a blood vessel.

va·so·mo·tor (vā′zō-mō′tər) *adj*. Causing or regulating dilation or constriction of blood vessels.

vasomotor nerve *n*. A motor nerve effecting dilation (a vasodilator nerve) or contraction (a vasoconstrictor nerve) of the blood vessels.

vasomotor paralysis *n*. See **vasoparesis**.

va·so·neu·rop·a·thy (vā′zō-nŏō-rŏp′ə-thē, -nyŏō-) *n*. A disease involving the nerves and the blood vessels.

va·so·or·chi·dos·to·my (vā′zō-ôr′kĭ-dŏs′tə-mē) *n*. Surgical reestablishment of blocked seminiferous channels by uniting the tubules of the epididymis or of the rete testis to the divided end of the vas deferens.

va·so·pa·ral·y·sis (vā′zō-pə-răl′ĭ-sĭs) *n*. Paralysis or lack of constricting ability in blood vessels.

va·so·pa·re·sis (vā′zō-pə-rē′sĭs, -păr′ĭ-sĭs) *n*. A mild degree of vasoparalysis.

va·so·pres·sin (vā′zō-prĕs′ĭn) *n*. A hormone, related to oxytocin, that is secreted by the posterior lobe of the pituitary gland, constricts blood vessels, raises blood pressure, stimulates intestinal motility, and reduces the excretion of urine.

va·so·punc·ture (vā′zō-pŭngk′chər) *n*. The puncture of a blood vessel with a needle.

va·so·re·flex (vā′zō-rē′flĕks′) *n*. A reflex that increases or decreases the caliber of blood vessels.

va·so·re·lax·a·tion (vā′zō-rē′lăk-sā′shən) *n*. Reduction in tension of the blood vessel walls.

va·so·sec·tion (vā′zō-sĕk′shən) *n*. See **vasotomy**.

va·so·spasm (vā′zō-spăz′əm) *n*. A sudden constriction of a blood vessel, causing a reduction in blood flow. — **va′so·spas′tic** (-spăs′tĭk) *adj*.

va·sos·to·my (vā-zŏs′tə-mē) *n*. Surgical creation of an opening into the vas deferens.

va·sot·o·my (vā-zŏt′ə-mē) *n*. Incision into or division of the vas deferens.

va·so·trip·sy (vā′zə-trĭp′sē) *n*. See **angiotripsy**.

va·so·va·sos·to·my (vā′zō-vā-zŏs′tə-mē) *n*. Surgical creation of a passage connecting the ends of a severed vas deferens to restore fertility in a vasectomized male.

va·so·ve·sic·u·lec·to·my (vā′zō-vĕ-sĭk′yə-lĕk′tə-mē, -və-) *n*. Surgery excision of the vas deferens and seminal vesicles.

vas·tus muscle of the thigh (văs′təs) *n*. The great muscle of the upper leg, composed of three of the divisions of the quadriceps muscle of the thigh.

VD or **V.D.** *abbr.* venereal disease

VDRL test *n*. A flocculation test for syphilis that uses a phospholipid-lecithin-cholesterol antigen as developed by the Venereal Disease Research Laboratory of the United States Public Health Service.

vec·tion (vĕk′shən) *n*. The transference of pathogens from the sick to the healthy by a vector.

vec·tor (vĕk′tər) *n*. **1.** An organism, such as a mosquito, that carries disease-causing microorganisms from one host to another. **2.** A plasmid, bacteriophage, or other agent that transfers genetic material from one location to another. **3.** A quantity, such as velocity, completely specified by a magnitude and a direction.

vec·tor·car·di·o·gram (vĕk′tər-kär′dē-ə-grăm′) *n*. A graphic representation of the magnitude and direction of the electrical currents of the heart's action in the form of a vector loop.

vec·tor·car·di·og·ra·phy (vĕk′tər-kär′dē-ŏg′rə-fē) *n*. **1.** A form of electrocardiography in which the heart's activation currents are represented by vector loops. **2.** The study and interpretation of vectorcardiograms.

veg·e·tal pole or **vitelline pole** (vĕj′ĭ-tl) *n*. The part of an egg, especially one having the yolk concentrated at one end, where the bulk of the yolk is situated.

veg·e·tar·i·an (vĕj′ĭ-târ′ē-ən) *n*. One who practices vegetarianism. — *adj*. **1.** Of or relating to vegetarianism or vegetarians. **2.** Consisting primarily or wholly of vegetables and vegetable products.

veg·e·tar·i·an·ism (vĕj′ĭ-târ′ē-ə-nĭz′əm) *n*. The

practice of subsisting on a diet composed primarily or wholly of vegetables, grains, fruits, nuts, and seeds, with or without eggs and dairy products.

veg·e·ta·tion (věj'ĭ-tā'shən) *n.* **1.** The process of growth in plants. **2.** An abnormal bodily growth or excrescence, especially a clot composed largely of fused blood platelets, fibrin, and sometimes bacteria that is adherent to a diseased heart valve. **3.** A vegetative state of impaired consciousness.

veg·e·ta·tive (věj'ĭ-tā'tĭv) *adj.* **1.** Of, relating to, or capable of growth. **2.** Of or functioning in processes such as growth or nutrition rather than sexual reproduction. **3.** Of or relating to asexual reproduction, such as fission or budding. **4.** Of or relating to the resting stage of a cell or its nucleus. **5.** Of or relating to a pathological vegetation. **6.** Of or being a state of grossly impaired consciousness, as after severe head trauma or brain disease, in which a person is incapable of voluntary or purposeful acts and only responds reflexively to painful stimuli.

ve·hi·cle (vē'ĭ-kəl) *n.* A substance of no therapeutic value used to convey an active medicine for administration.

veil (vāl) *n.* **1.** See **caul. 2.** See **velum** (sense 1).

vein (vān) *n.* **1.** Any of the branching blood vessels carrying blood toward the heart. All veins except the pulmonary vein carry dark unaerated blood. **2.** A blood vessel. — *v.* **veined, vein·ing, veins.** To supply or fill with veins. — **vein'al** *adj.*

ve·la·men (və-lā'mən) *n., pl.* **-lam·i·na** (-lăm'ə-nə). See **velum** (sense 1).

vel·lus (věl'əs) *n.* The fine hair present on the body before puberty.

ve·loc·i·ty (və-lŏs'ĭ-tē) *n.* Rapidity or speed of motion; specifically, the distance traveled per unit time.

Vel·peau bandage (věl-pō') *n.* A bandage used to support and immobilize an arm, with the forearm positioned obliquely across and upward on the front of the chest.

ve·lum (vē'ləm) *n., pl.* **-la** (-lə). **1.** An anatomical structure resembling a veil or curtain. **2.** See **greater omentum. 3.** A serous membrane or membranous envelope or covering.

ve·na (vē'nə) *n., pl.* **-nae** (-nē). A vein.

vena ca·va (kā'və) *n., pl.* **venae ca·vae** (kā'vē). Either of the two venae cavae, the inferior vena cava and superior vena cava.

ve·na·ca·vog·ra·phy (vē'nə-kā-vŏg'rə-fē) *n.* Angiography of a vena cava.

ve·nec·ta·si·a (vē'něk-tā'zē-ə, -zhə) *n.* See **phlebectasia.**

ve·nec·to·my (vē-něk'tə-mē) *n.* See **phlebectomy.**

ve·neer (və-nēr') *n.* A layer of tooth-colored material, usually porcelain or acrylic resin, attached to and covering the surface of a metal crown or natural tooth structure.

ve·nene (və-nēn', věn'ēn) *n.* A preparation of snake venoms used in medicine, especially in the treatment of epilepsy.

ve·ne·re·al (və-nēr'ē-əl) *adj.* **1.** Transmitted by sexual intercourse. **2.** Of or relating to a sexually transmitted disease. **3.** Of or relating to sexual intercourse. **4.** Of or relating to the genitals.

venereal bubo *n.* An enlarged gland in the groin associated with a venereal disease, especially chancroid.

venereal disease *n.* Any of several contagious diseases, such as syphilis and gonorrhea, contracted through sexual intercourse; a sexually transmitted disease.

venereal ulcer *n.* See **chancroid.**

venereal wart *n.* See **genital wart.**

ven·e·sec·tion (věn'ĭ-sěk'shən, vē'nĭ-) *n.* See **phlebotomy.**

ve·ni·punc·ture or **ve·ne·punc·ture** (vē'nĭ-pŭngk'chər, věn'ĭ-) *n.* Puncture of a vein, as for drawing blood, intravenous feeding, or administration of medicine.

ve·no·gram (vē'nə-grăm') *n.* **1.** A radiograph of a vein after injection of a radiopaque substance. **2.** See **phlebogram.**

ve·nog·ra·phy (vĭ-nŏg'rə-fē) *n.* **1.** Radiography of veins or a vein after injection of a radiopaque substance. **2.** See **phlebography.**

ven·om (věn'əm) *n.* **1.** A poisonous secretion of an animal, such as a snake, spider, or scorpion, usually transmitted by a bite or sting. **2.** A poison.

ve·no·per·i·to·ne·os·to·my (vē'nō-pěr'ĭ-tn-ē-ŏs'tə-mē) *n.* Surgical insertion of either of the major superficial veins of the leg into the peritoneal cavity to drain ascitic fluid.

ve·no·scle·ro·sis (vē'nō-sklə-rō'sĭs) *n.* See **phlebosclerosis.**

ve·nos·i·ty (vē-nŏs'ĭ-tē) *n.* **1.** The quality or condition of being venous or venose. **2.** An excess of venous blood.

ve·nos·ta·sis (vē-nŏs'tə-sĭs, vē'nō-stā'sĭs) *n.* See **phlebostasis** (sense 2).

ve·nos·to·my (vē-nŏs'tə-mē) *n.* See **cutdown.**

ve·not·o·my (vē-nŏt'ə-mē) *n.* See **phlebotomy.**

ve·nous (vē'nəs) *adj.* Of, relating to, or contained in the veins.

venous blood *n.* Blood that has passed through the capillaries of various tissues other than the lungs, is found in the veins, in the right chambers of the heart, and in pulmonary arteries, and is usually dark red as a result of a lower content of oxygen.

venous capillary *n.* A blood capillary opening into a venule.

venous hum *n.* A humming sound, usually continuous, heard during auscultation of the veins at the base of the neck, especially in anemia.

venous insufficiency *n.* Inadequate drainage of venous blood from a part, resulting in edema or dermatosis.

venous pulse *n.* The pulsation occurring in the veins, especially in the internal jugular vein.

venous return *n.* The blood returning to the heart via the inferior and superior venae cavae.

venous sinus of the sclera *n.* A vascular structure near the anterior edge of the sclera and encircling the cornea.

venous sphygmograph *n.* See **phlebograph.**

venous star *n.* A small red nodule formed by a dilated vein in the skin. It is caused by increased venous pressure.

ve·no·ve·nos·to·my (vē'nō-vē-nŏs'tə-mē) *n.* The surgical formation of an anastomosis between two veins.

vent (vĕnt) *n.* An opening into a cavity or canal, especially one through which contents are discharged.

ven·ter (vĕn'tər) *n.* **1.** See **abdomen**. **2.** See **belly** (sense 4). **3.** One of the large cavities of the body. **4.** A cavity or hollowed surface, especially of a bone. **5.** The uterus.

ven·ti·la·tion (vĕn'tl-ā'shən) *n.* **1.** The replacement of fresh air or gas for stale or noxious air or gas in a space. **2.** See **respiration** (sense 1). **3.** Aeration or oxygenation, as of blood. **4.** Verbal expression of feelings or emotions in psychotherapy. — **ven'ti·late'** *v.*

ventilation-perfusion scan *n.* A diagnostic test for pulmonary embolism in which an x-ray of the lung records the distribution and perfusion of a radionuclide that is inhaled and a second radionuclide that is administered intravenously.

Ven·to·lin (vĕn'tl-ĭn) A trademark for albuterol.

ven·tral (vĕn'trəl) *adj.* **1.** Relating to or situated on or close to the abdomen; abdominal. **2.** Relating to or situated on or close to the anterior aspect of the body. **3.** Relating to or situated on or close to the lower surface of an animal body.

ventral column of the spinal cord *n.* See **anterior column of the spinal cord**.

ventral horn *n.* See **anterior horn** (senses 1, 2).

ventral root *n.* The motor root of a spinal nerve.

ven·tri·cle (vĕn'trĭ-kəl) *n.* A small cavity or chamber within a body or an organ, especially the right or left ventricle of the heart or any of the interconnecting ventricles of the brain.

ven·tric·u·lar (vĕn-trĭk'yə-lər) *adj.* Of or relating to a ventricle or ventriculus.

ventricular complex *n.* The QRS complex in an electrocardiogram.

ventricular conduction *n.* See **intraventricular conduction**.

ventricular escape *n.* Cardiologic escape in which a ventricular pacemaker sets the heart's beat before the sinoatrial pacemaker.

ventricular extrasystole *n.* A premature contraction of the ventricle.

ventricular fibrillation *n.* An often fatal form of arrhythmia characterized by rapid, irregular fibrillar twitching of the ventricles of the heart in place of normal contractions, resulting in a loss of pulse.

ventricular fusion beat *n.* A fusion beat that occurs when the ventricles are activated partly by the descending sinus or atrioventricular nodal impulse and partly by an ectopic ventricular impulse.

ventricular rhythm *n.* See **idioventricular rhythm**.

ventricular septal defect *n.* A congenital defect in the septum between the cardiac ventricles, usually resulting from failure of the septum to close the interventricular foramen.

ven·tric·u·li·tis (vĕn-trĭk'yə-lī'tĭs) *n.* Inflammation of the ventricles of the brain.

ven·tric·u·lo·a·tri·al (vĕn-trĭk'yə-lō-ā'trē-əl) *adj.* Of or relating to the ventricles and atria of the heart.

ven·tric·u·lo·cis·ter·nos·to·my (vĕn-trĭk'yə-lō-sĭs'tər-nŏs'tə-mē) *n.* The surgical formation of an opening between the ventricles of the brain and the cerebellomedullary cistern.

ven·tric·u·log·ra·phy (vĕn-trĭk'yə-lŏg'rə-fē) *n.* Radiography of the ventricles of the brain by injection of either a contrast medium or a radiopaque agent.

ven·tric·u·lo·mas·toid·os·to·my (vĕn-trĭk'yə-lō-măs'toi-dŏs'tə-mē) *n.* A surgical procedure used in treating hydrocephalus in which a communication is established between the lateral cerebral ventricle and the mastoid antrum.

ven·tric·u·lo·plas·ty (vĕn-trĭk'yə-lə-plăs'tē) *n.* Surgical repair of a defect in one of the ventricles of the heart.

ven·tric·u·lo·punc·ture (vĕn-trĭk'yə-lō-pŭngk'-chər) *n.* The insertion of a needle into a ventricle.

ven·tric·u·los·co·py (vĕn-trĭk'yə-lŏs'kə-pē) *n.* Examination of a ventricle of the brain by means of an endoscope.

ven·tric·u·los·to·my (vĕn-trĭk'yə-lŏs'tə-mē) *n.* A surgical procedure used in treating hydrocephalus in which an opening is established in a ventricle, usually from the third ventricle to the subarachnoid space.

ven·tric·u·lot·o·my (vĕn-trĭk'yə-lŏt'ə-mē) *n.* Incision into a ventricle of the brain or heart.

ven·tric·u·lus (vĕn-trĭk'yə-ləs) *n.* **1.** A ventricle. **2.** The stomach.

ven·tri·duc·tion (vĕn'trĭ-dŭk'shən) *n.* The drawing of a part toward the abdomen or the abdominal wall.

ven·tros·co·py (vĕn-trŏs'kə-pē) *n.* See **peritoneoscopy**.

ven·trot·o·my (vĕn-trŏt'ə-mē) *n.* See **celiotomy**.

ven·ule (vĕn'yōōl, vēn'-) *n.* A small vein, especially one joining capillaries to larger veins. — **ven'u·lar** (-yə-lər) *adj.*

ver·mic·u·lar movement (vər-mĭk'yə-lər) *n.* See **peristalsis**.

vermicular pulse *n.* A small rapid pulse giving a sensation of a moving worm to the finger.

ver·mic·u·la·tion (vər-mĭk'yə-lā'shən) *n.* Motion resembling that of a worm, especially the wavelike contractions of the intestine; peristalsis.

ver·mi·form appendix (vûr'mə-fôrm') *n.* A wormlike intestinal diverticulum starting from the blind end of the cecum in the lower right-hand part of the abdomen and ending in a blind extremity.

ver·mil·ion border (vər-mĭl'yən) *n.* The exposed red margin of the upper or lower lip.

ver·mil·ion·ec·to·my (vər-mĭl'yə-nĕk'tə-mē) *n.* Excision of the vermilion border of the lip.

ver·min (vûr'mĭn) *n.*, *pl.* **vermin**. Various small animals or insects, such as rats or cockroaches, that are destructive, annoying, or injurious to health.

ver·mi·na·tion (vûr'mə-nā'shən) *n.* **1.** The production or breeding of worms or larvae. **2.** Infestation by vermin, especially parasitic vermin.

ver·mis (vûr'mĭs) *n., pl.* **-mes** (-mēz). The narrow middle zone between the two hemispheres of the cerebellum.

ver·nal conjunctivitis (vûr'nəl) *n.* A chronic form of conjunctivitis affecting both eyes, characterized by abnormal sensitivity to light and intense itching that recurs seasonally during warm weather.

Ver·net's syndrome (vĕr-nāz') *n.* A syndrome characterized by paralysis of the glossopharyngeal, vagus, and accessory cranial nerves, causing paralysis of the soft palate, fauces, pharynx, and vocal cords, most commonly as result of a head injury.

ver·nix ca·se·o·sa (vûr'nĭks kā'sē-ō'sə) *n.* The fatty substance consisting of desquamated epithelial cells and sebaceous matter that covers the skin of the fetus.

ver·ru·ca (və-rōō'kə) *n., pl.* **-cae** (-kē). See **wart.**

verruca a·cu·mi·na·ta (ə-kyōō'mə-nā'tə) *n.* See **genital wart.**

verruca pla·na (plā'nə) *n.* See **flat wart.**

verruca plan·tar·is (plăn-târ'ĭs) *n.* See **plantar wart.**

verruca vul·gar·is virus (vŭl-găr'ĭs) *n.* See **human papilloma virus.**

ver·ru·cous nevus (və-rōō'kəs) *n.* A wartlike, often linear, skin lesion appearing at birth or early in childhood and occurring in various sizes, groupings, and locations.

ver·ru·ga (və-rōō'gə) *n.* See **wart.**

ver·sion (vûr'zhən, -shən) *n.* **1.** Deflection of an organ, such as the uterus, from its normal position. **2.** The changing of position of the fetus in the uterus, either spontaneously or as a result of manipulation. **3.** The conjugate rotation of the eyes in the same direction.

ver·te·bra (vûr'tə-brə) *n., pl.* **-bras** or **-brae** (-brā', -brē'). Any of the bones or cartilaginous segments of the spinal column, usually 33 in number: 7 cervical, 12 thoracic, 5 lumbar, 5 fused sacral (the sacrum), and 4 fused coccygeal (the coccyx).

ver·te·bral (vûr'tə-brəl, vər-tē'brəl) *adj.* **1.** Of, relating to, or of the nature of a vertebra. **2.** Having or consisting of vertebrae. **3.** Having a spinal column.

vertebral arch *n.* The posterior projection from the body of a vertebra that encloses the vertebral foramen.

vertebral canal *n.* The canal that contains the spinal cord, spinal meninges, and related structures and is formed by the vertebral foramina of successive vertebrae of the articulated spinal column.

vertebral column *n.* See **spinal column.**

vertebral foramen *n.* The opening formed by the union of the vertebral arch with the vertebra from which it projects.

vertebral nerve *n.* A nerve that arises from the cervicothoracic ganglion, ascends along the vertebral artery to the level of the axis or atlas, and gives branches to the cervical nerves and meninges.

vertebral rib *n.* See **floating rib.**

ver·te·brate (vûr'tə-brĭt, -brāt') *adj.* **1.** Having a backbone or spinal column. **2.** Of or characteristic of vertebrates or a vertebrate. — *n.* A member of the subphylum Vertebrata.

ver·te·brat·ed catheter (vûr'tə-brā'tĭd) *n.* A catheter made of several segments fitted together so as to be flexible.

ver·te·brec·to·my (vûr'tə-brĕk'tə-mē) *n.* Excision of a vertebra.

ver·tex (vûr'tĕks') *n., pl.* **-tex·es** or **-ti·ces** (-tĭ-sēz'). **1.** The highest point; the apex or summit. **2.** The topmost point of the vault of the skull; the crown of the head.

vertex presentation *n.* Head presentation of the fetus during birth in which the upper back part of the fetal head is the presenting part.

ver·ti·cal (vûr'tĭ-kəl) *adj.* **1.** Of or relating to the vertex of the head. **2.** Being or situated at right angles to the horizon; upright.

vertical banded gastroplasty *n.* A gastroplasty for the treatment of morbid obesity in which an upper gastric pouch is formed by a vertical staple line, with a cloth band applied to prevent dilation at the outlet into the main pouch.

vertical transmission *n.* Transmission of a virus by means of the genetic apparatus of a cell in which the viral genome is integrated.

ver·tig·i·nous (vər-tĭj'ə-nəs) *n.* **1.** Affected by vertigo; dizzy. **2.** Tending to produce vertigo.

ver·ti·go (vûr'tĭ-gō') *n., pl.* **-goes** or **-gos.** A sensation of irregular or whirling motion, either of oneself or of external objects.

ves·i·ca·tion (vĕs'ĭ-kā'shən) *n.* See **vesiculation** (sense 1).

ves·i·cle (vĕs'ĭ-kəl) *n.* **1.** A small structure resembling a bladder. **2.** A small circumscribed elevation of the skin containing serum. **3.** A small sac or cyst containing liquid or gas.

ves·i·co·cele (vĕs'ĭ-kō-sēl') *n.* See **cystocele.**

ves·i·coc·ly·sis (vĕs'ĭ-kŏk'lĭ-sĭs) *n.* The washing out of the urinary bladder.

ves·i·co·fix·a·tion (vĕs'ĭ-kō-fĭk-sā'shən) *n.* The surgical fixation or suture of the uterus to the bladder wall.

ves·i·co·rec·tos·to·my (vĕs'ĭ-kō-rĕk-tŏs'tə-mē) *n.* Surgical formation of a passage between the rear of the bladder and the rectum as a means of diverting the urine.

ves·i·co·sig·moid·os·to·my (vĕs'ĭ-kō-sĭg'moi-dŏs'tə-mē) *n.* Surgical formation of a communication between the bladder and the sigmoid colon.

ves·i·cos·to·my (vĕs'ĭ-kŏs'tə-mē) *n.* Surgical creation of a stoma between the anterior bladder wall and the skin of the lower abdomen, for temporary or permanent lower urinary tract diversion.

ves·i·cot·o·my (vĕs'ĭ-kŏt'ə-mē) *n.* See **cystotomy.**

ves·i·co·u·ter·ine fistula (vĕs′ĭ-kō-yōō′tər-ĭn, -tə-rīn′) *n.* A fistula between the bladder and the uterus.

ve·sic·u·lar (vĕ-sĭk′yə-lər, və-) *adj.* **1.** Of or relating to vesicles. **2.** Composed of or containing vesicles. **3.** Having the form of a vesicle. — **ve·sic′u·lar·ly** *adv.*

vesicular murmur *n.* See **vesicular respiration.**

vesicular resonance *n.* The sound obtained by percussing above the normal lungs.

vesicular respiration *n.* The respiratory murmur heard on auscultation of the normal lung.

vesicular transport *n.* See **transcytosis.**

ve·sic·u·la·tion (vĕ-sĭk′yə-lā′shən, və-) *n.* **1.** The formation of vesicles. **2.** The presence of vesicles.

ve·sic·u·lec·to·my (vĕ-sĭk′yə-lĕk′tə-mē, və-) *n.* Surgical resection of part or of all of each seminal vesicle.

ve·sic·u·li·tis (vĕ-sĭk′yə-lī′tĭs, -və-) *n.* Inflammation of a vesicle, especially a seminal vesicle.

ve·sic·u·log·ra·phy (vĕ-sĭk′yə-lŏg′rə-fē, və-) *n.* Radiography of the seminal vesicles.

ve·sic·u·lo·pros·ta·ti·tis (vĕ-sĭk′yə-lō-prŏs′tə-tī′-tĭs, və-) *n.* Inflammation of the bladder and the prostate.

ve·sic·u·lot·o·my (vĕ-sĭk′yə-lŏt′ə-mē, və-) *n.* Surgical division of the seminal vesicles.

ves·sel (vĕs′əl) *n.* A duct, canal, or other tube that contains or conveys a body fluid such as blood or lymph.

ves·tib·u·lar (vĕ-stĭb′yə-lər) *adj.* Of, relating to, or serving as a vestibule, especially of the ear.

vestibular canal *n.* The division of the spiral canal of the cochlea lying above the spiral bone dividing the spiral canal and the vestibular membrane.

vestibular ganglion *n.* A collection of bipolar neurons forming a swelling on the vestibular part of the eighth cranial nerve in the internal acoustic meatus.

vestibular gland *n.* Any of the glands that open into the vestibule of the vagina.

vestibular labyrinth *n.* The portion of the membranous labyrinth located within the semicircular canals and the vestibule of the osseous labyrinth.

vestibular membrane *n.* The membrane separating the cochlear region from the vestibular canal of the ear.

vestibular nerve *n.* The superior portion of the vestibulocochlear nerve, composed of nerve processes that terminate in hair cells of the ampullae of the semicircular ducts and the maculas of the saccule and utricle and the bipolar neurons of the vestibular ganglion.

vestibular organ *n.* The structure composed of the utricle, saccule, and the three semicircular ducts of the membranous labyrinth of the inner ear.

ves·ti·bule (vĕs′tə-byōōl′) *n.* A cavity, chamber, or channel that leads to or is an entrance to another cavity, especially that of the ear.

ves·tib·u·lo·coch·le·ar nerve (vĕ-stĭb′yə-lō-kŏk′lē-ər, -kō′-klē-) *n.* A composite sensory nerve that emerges from the brainstem at the cerebellopontine angle, innervates the receptor cells

of the membranous labyrinth, and consists of two major anatomically and functionally distinct components: the vestibular nerve and the cochlear nerve.

ves·tib·u·lo·plas·ty (vĕ-stĭb′yə-lō-plăs′tē) *n.* A surgical procedure to restore alveolar ridge height by lowering muscles attaching to the buccal, labial, and lingual aspects of the jaws.

ves·tib·u·lo·spi·nal reflex (vĕ-stĭb′yə-lō-spī′nəl) *n.* Any of many reflexes that originate with vestibular stimulation and control body posture.

ves·tib·u·lot·o·my (vĕ-stĭb′yə-lŏt′ə-mē) *n.* Surgical incision of the vestibule of the labyrinth of the ear.

ves·tige (vĕs′tĭj) *n.* A rudimentary or degenerated, usually nonfunctioning, structure that is the remnant of an organ or a part that was fully developed or functioning in a preceding generation or an earlier stage of development.

ves·tig·i·al (vĕ-stĭj′ē-əl, -stĭj′əl) *adj.* Occurring or persisting as a rudimentary or degenerate structure.

vestigial organ *n.* A rudimentary structure in humans corresponding to a functional structure or organ in ancestral animals.

vet·er·i·nar·i·an (vĕt′ər-ə-nâr′ē-ən, vĕt′rə-) *n.* A person who practices veterinary medicine.

vet·er·i·nar·y medicine (vĕt′ər-ə-nĕr′ē, vĕt′rə-) *n.* The branch of medicine that deals with the causes, diagnosis, and treatment of diseases and injuries of animals, especially domestic animals.

VHDL *abbr.* very high density lipoprotein

vi·a·ble (vī′ə-bəl) *adj.* **1.** Capable of living, developing, or germinating under favorable conditions. **2.** Capable of living outside the uterus. Used of a fetus or newborn. — **vi·a·bil′i·ty** *n.*

Vib·ri·o (vĭb′rē-ō) *n.* A genus of gram-negative, motile, S-shaped or comma-shaped bacteria some species of which are saprophytes in salt and fresh water and in soil, while others are parasites or pathogens.

vib·ri·o·sis (vĭb′rē-ō′sĭs) *n., pl.* **-ses** (-sēz). Infection caused by a species of *Vibrio*, especially an infection caused by *V. parahaemolyticus* as a result of eating undercooked seafood from contaminated waters.

vi·bro·car·di·o·gram (vī′brō-kär′dē-ə-grăm′) *n.* A graphic record of chest vibrations produced by hemodynamic events of the cardiac cycle.

vi·car·i·ous (vī-kâr′ē-əs, -kär′-, vĭ-) *adj.* **1.** Felt or undergone as if one were taking part in the experience or feelings of another. **2.** Occurring in or performed by a part of the body not normally associated with a certain function.

vicarious hypertrophy *n.* Hypertropy of an organ following failure of another organ to which it is functionally related.

vicarious menstruation *n.* Bleeding from a surface other than the mucous membrane of the uterine cavity that occurs at the time when normal menstruation should take place.

vi·cious circle (vĭsh′əs) *n.* A condition in which a

disorder or disease gives rise to another that subsequently affects the first.

vi·dar·a·bine (vī-där′ə-bēn′) *n.* A purine nucleoside obtained from a species of *Streptomyces* and used in the treatment of herpes simplex infections.

vig·il·am·bu·lism (vĭj′ə-lăm′byə-lĭz′əm) *n.* A condition of unconsciousness regarding one's surroundings together with automatism of motion.

vil·lo·ma (vĭ-lō′mə) *n.* See **papilloma**.

vil·los·i·ty (vĭ-lŏs′ĭ-tē) *n.* **1.** The condition of being covered with villi. **2.** A formation, surface, or coating that is or appears to be covered with villi. **3.** A villus.

vil·lus (vĭl′əs) *n., pl.* **vil·li** (vĭl′ī). **1.** A minute projection arising from a mucous membrane, especially one of the vascular projections of the small intestine. **2.** Such a projection of the chorion that contributes to the formation of the placenta in mammals.

vil·lus·ec·to·my (vĭl′ə-sĕk′tə-mē) *n.* See **synovectomy**.

vin·blas·tine sulfate (vĭn-blăs′tēn′) *n.* The sulfate salt of an alkaloid obtained from a plant of the genus *Vinca* and used as an antineoplastic agent in the treatment of Hodgkin's disease, choriocarcinoma, acute and chronic leukemias, and other neoplastic diseases.

Vin·cent's angina (vĭn′sənts) *n.* See **trench mouth**.

vin·cris·tine sulfate (vĭn-krĭs′tēn′) *n.* The sulfate salt of an alkaloid obtained from a plant of the genus *Vinca* that exhibits antineoplastic activity similar to that of vinblastine sulfate and is used especially in the treatment of lymphocytic lymphosarcoma and acute leukemia.

vi·o·my·cin (vī′ə-mī′sĭn) *n.* An antibiotic produced by the actinomycete *Streptomyces puniceus,* used in the treatment of tuberculosis.

vi·po·ma (vĭ-pō′mə) *n.* An endocrine tumor, usually originating in the pancreas that produces a vasoactive intestinal polypeptide believed to cause profound cardiovascular and electrolyte changes with vasodilatory hypotension, watery diarrhea, hypokalemia, and dehydration.

vi·ral (vī′rəl) *adj.* Of, relating to, or caused by a virus.

viral antigen *n.* An antigen having multiple antigenicities that is protein in nature, strain-specific, and intimately associated with the virus particle.

viral dysentery *n.* A profuse watery diarrhea believed to be the result of viral infection.

viral envelope *n.* The outer structure that encloses the nuclear capsids of some viruses.

viral hemagglutination *n.* The agglutination of suspended red blood cells by viruses, usually by the virion itself but in some instances by products of viral growth.

viral hepatitis *n.* Any of various forms of hepatitis caused by a virus, including hepatitis A and hepatitis B.

viral hepatitis type A *n.* Hepatitis A.

viral hepatitis type B *n.* Hepatitis B.

viral hepatitis type D *n.* Acute or chronic hepatitis

which may occur simultaneously with hepatitis B or as a superinfection in a hepatitis B carrier.

viral tropism *n.* The specificity of a virus for a particular host tissue, determined in part by the interaction of viral surface structures with host cell-surface receptors.

vi·re·mi·a (vī-rē′mē-ə) *n.* The presence of viruses in the bloodstream.

vir·gin (vûr′jĭn) *n.* A person who has not experienced sexual intercourse. — **vir′gin·al** (-jə-nəl) *adj.*

vir·gin·i·ty (vər-jĭn′ĭ-tē) *n.* The quality or condition of being a virgin.

vi·ri·cide (vī′rĭ-sīd′) or **vi·ru·cide** (vī′rə-) *n.* An agent that inhibits or destroys viruses. — **vi′ri·cid′al** (-sīd′l) *adj.*

vir·ile (vĕr′əl, -īl′) *adj.* **1.** Of, relating to, or having the characteristics of an adult male, especially the ability to perform sexually as a male. **2.** Having or showing masculine spirit, strength, vigor, or power. **3.** Potent.

vir·i·les·cence (vĕr′ə-lĕs′əns) *n.* The assumption of male characteristics by a female.

vir·il·ism (vĕr′ə-lĭz′əm) *n.* The presence of male secondary sexual characteristics in a female.

vi·ril·i·ty (və-rĭl′ĭ-tē) *n.* **1.** The quality or state of being virile; manly character. **2.** Masculine vigor; potency.

vir·il·i·za·tion (vĕr′ə-lĭ-zā′shən) *n.* Development of male secondary sexual characteristics. — **vir′·il·ize′** (-ə-līz′) *v.*

vi·ri·on (vī′rē-ŏn′, vĕr′ē-) *n.* A complete viral particle, consisting of RNA or DNA surrounded by a protein shell and constituting the infective form of a virus.

vi·ro·gene (vī′rə-jēn′) *n.* A gene capable of specifying the synthesis of a virus in a cell.

vi·rol·o·gy (vī-rŏl′ə-jē) *n.* The study of viruses and viral diseases. — **vi′ro·log′i·cal** (vī′rə-lŏj′ĭ-kəl), **vi′ro·log′ic** (-ĭk) *adj.* — **vi·rol′o·gist** *n.*

vir·tu·al cautery (vûr′chŏo-əl) *n.* See **potential cautery**.

vir·u·lence (vĕr′yə-ləns, vĕr′ə-) *n.* **1.** The quality of being poisonous. **2.** The capacity of a microorganism to cause disease.

vir·u·lent (vĕr′yə-lənt, vĕr′ə-) *adj.* **1.** Extremely infectious, malignant, or poisonous. Used of a disease or toxin. **2.** Capable of causing disease by breaking down protective mechanisms of the host. Used of a pathogen. **3.** Intensely irritating, obnoxious, or harsh.

vi·ru·ri·a (vī-rōŏr′ē-ə) *n.* Presence of living viruses in the urine.

vi·rus (vī′rəs) *n., pl.* **-rus·es. 1.** Any of various simple submicroscopic parasites of plants, animals, and bacteria that often cause disease and that consist essentially of a core of RNA or DNA surrounded by a protein coat. Unable to replicate without a host cell, viruses are typically not considered living organisms. **2.** A disease caused by a virus.

virus-transformed cell *n.* A cell that has been genetically changed to a tumor cell and that passes the change to its daughter cells.

vis·cer·a (vĭs′ər-ə) *pl.n.* **1.** The soft internal organs of the body, especially those contained within the abdominal and thoracic cavities. **2.** The intestines.

vis·cer·al (vĭs′ər-əl) *adj.* Relating to, situated in, or affecting the viscera.

visceral anesthesia *n.* See **splanchnic anesthesia.**

visceral cleft *n.* A cleft between two branchial arches in the embryo.

visceral disease virus *n.* See **cytomegalovirus.**

visceral ganglion *n.* See **autonomic ganglion.**

vis·cer·al·gi·a (vĭs′ə-răl′jē-ə, -jə) *n.* Pain in any part of the viscera.

visceral larva migrans *n.* A disease, chiefly of children, caused by ingestion of nematode ova, usually of *Toxocara canis,* such that the larvae hatch in the intestine, penetrate the gut wall, and wander in the viscera, chiefly the liver; it is characterized by high eosinophilia and often liver enlargement, fever, cough, and hyperglobulinemia.

visceral leishmaniasis *n.* A chronic, often fatal disease occurring chiefly in Asia, caused by a protozoan parasite *(Leishmania donovani)* and characterized by irregular fever, enlargement of the spleen and liver, and emaciation.

visceral node *n.* Any of the lymph nodes draining the viscera of the abdomen or the pelvis.

visceral sense *n.* The perception of the presence of the internal organs.

visceral swallow *n.* An immature swallowing pattern, as of infants, marked by a thrust of the tongue and resembling the peristaltic, wavelike, muscular contractions observed in the gut.

vis·cer·o·meg·a·ly (vĭs′ər-ə-mĕg′ə-lē) *n.* Abnormal enlargement of the viscera.

vis·cer·o·skel·e·ton (vĭs′ə-rō-skĕl′ĭ-tn) *n.* **1.** A bony formation in an organ, as in the heart, tongue, or penis. **2.** The part of the skeleton protecting the viscera, such as the rib cage and the pelvic bones. — **vis′cer·o·skel′e·tal** (-skĕl′ĭ-tl) *adj.*

vis·cid (vĭs′ĭd) *adj.* **1.** Thick and adhesive. Used of a fluid. **2.** Covered with a sticky coating. — **vis·cid′i·ty, vis′cid·ness** *n.*

vis·cos·i·ty (vĭ-skŏs′ĭ-tē) *n.* **1.** The condition or property of being viscous. **2.** The degree to which a fluid resists flow under an applied force, measured by the tangential friction force per unit area divided by the velocity gradient under conditions of streamline flow; coefficient of viscosity.

vis·cous (vĭs′kəs) *adj.* **1.** Having relatively high resistance to flow. **2.** Viscid.

vis·i·ble spectrum (vĭz′ə-bəl) *n.* The part of the electromagnetic spectrum visible to the human eye, extending from extreme red, 7606 Å (760.6 nanometers), to extreme violet, 3934 Å (393.4 nanometers).

vi·sion (vĭzh′ən) *n.* **1.** The faculty of sight; eyesight. **2.** The manner in which one sees or conceives of something.

vis·it·ing nurse (vĭz′ĭ-tĭng) *n.* A registered nurse employed by a public health agency or hospital to promote community health and especially to visit and administer treatment to sick people in their homes.

vi·su·al (vĭzh′ōō-əl) *adj.* **1.** Of or relating to the sense of sight. **2.** Seen or able to be seen by the eye; visible. **3.** Optical.

visual acuity *n.* Sharpness of vision, especially as tested with a Snellen chart. Normal visual acuity based on the Snellen chart is 20/20.

visual allesthesia *n.* A condition in which visual images are transposed from one half of the visual field to the other, either vertically or horizontally.

visual angle *n.* The angle formed at the retina by the meeting of lines drawn from the periphery of the viewed object.

visual field *n.* The area simultaneously visible to one eye without movement.

visual pigment *n.* Any of the photopigments in the retinal cones and rods that absorb light and by photochemical processes initiate the phenomenon of vision.

visual purple *n.* See **rhodopsin.**

visual receptor cell *n.* **1.** A rod cell. **2.** A cone cell.

visual violet *n.* See **iodopsin.**

vi·su·og·no·sis (vĭzh′ōō-ŏg-nō′sĭs) *n.* Recognition and understanding of visual impressions.

vi·tal (vīt′l) *adj.* **1.** Of, relating to, or characteristic of life. **2.** Necessary to the continuation of life; life-sustaining. **3.** Used or done on a living cell or tissue, as in staining. **4.** Destructive to life; fatal, as of an injury.

vital capacity *n.* The amount of air that can be forcibly expelled from the lungs after breathing in as deeply as possible.

vi·tal·i·ty (vī-tăl′ĭ-tē) *n.* **1.** The capacity to live, grow, or develop. **2.** Physical or intellectual vigor; energy.

vitality test *n.* Any of a group of thermal and electrical tests used to aid in assessing the health of dental pulp.

vi·ta·lom·e·ter (vī′tə-lŏm′ĭ-tər) *n.* An electrical device for measuring the vitality of tooth pulp.

vital pulp *n.* Living dental pulp that responds to electric and thermal stimulation.

vi·tals (vīt′lz) *pl.n.* **1.** The vital body organs. **2.** The parts essential to continued functioning, as of a system.

vital signs *pl.n.* The pulse rate, temperature, and respiratory rate of a person.

vital statistics *pl.n.* Statistics concerning the important events in human life, such as births, deaths, marriages, and migrations.

vi·ta·mer (vī′tə-mər) *n.* One of two or more related chemical substances that fulfill the same specific vitamin function.

vi·ta·min (vī′tə-mĭn) *n.* Any of various fat-soluble or water-soluble organic substances essential in minute amounts for normal growth and activity of the body and obtained naturally from plant and animal foods.

vitamin A *n.* A fat-soluble vitamin or a mixture of vitamins, especially vitamin A$_1$ or a mixture of vitamins A_1 and A_2, occurring principally in fish-liver oils, milk, and some yellow and dark green vegetables, and functioning in normal cell growth and development with deficiencies causing hardening and roughening of the skin, night blindness, and degeneration of mucous membranes.

vitamin B *n.* **1.** Vitamin B complex. **2.** A member of the vitamin B complex, especially thiamine.

vitamin B₁ *n.* See **thiamine.**

vitamin B₂ *n.* See **riboflavin.**

vitamin B₆ *n.* Pyridoxine and related compounds.

vitamin B₁₂ *n.* A complex compound containing cobalt, found especially in liver and widely used to treat pernicious anemia.

vitamin B_c *n.* See **folic acid.**

vitamin B_x *n.* See **PABA.**

vitamin B complex *n.* A group of water-soluble vitamins including thiamine, riboflavin, niacin, pantothenic acid, biotin, pyridoxine, folic acid, and vitamin B_{12} and occurring chiefly in yeast, liver, eggs, and some vegetables.

vitamin C *n.* See **ascorbic acid.**

vitamin D *n.* A fat-soluble vitamin occurring in several forms, especially vitamin D_2 or vitamin D_3, required for normal growth of teeth and bones, and produced in general by ultraviolet irradiation of sterols found in milk, fish, and eggs.

vitamin D₂ *n.* A white crystalline compound produced by ultraviolet irradiation of ergosterol.

vitamin D₃ *n.* A colorless crystalline compound found in fish-liver oils, irradiated milk, and all irradiated foods. It has essentially the same biological activity as vitamin D_2.

vitamin E *n.* A fat-soluble vitamin found chiefly in plant leaves, wheat germ oil, and milk and used to treat sterility and various abnormalities of the muscles, red blood cells, liver, and brain.

vitamin G *n.* Riboflavin.

vitamin H *n.* Biotin.

vitamin K *n.* Any of several fat-soluble compounds that are found in alfalfa, hog liver, fish meal, and vegetable oils and are essential for the production of normal amounts of prothrombin.

vitamin K₁ *n.* A yellow viscous oil found in leafy green vegetables or made synthetically, used by the body to form prothrombin and in veterinary medicine as an antidote to certain poisons.

vitamin K₂ *n.* Any of various yellowish crystalline compounds isolated from putrefied fish meal or from various intestinal bacteria and used to stop hemorrhaging and in veterinary medicine as an antidote to certain poisons.

vitamin P *n.* A water-soluble vitamin, found as a crystalline substance especially in citrus juices, that acts to promote capillary resistance to hemorrhaging.

vi·tel·line membrane (vĭ-tĕl′ĭn, -ēn′, vī-) *n.* **1.** The membrane enveloping the yolk of an egg. **2.** The pellucid zone of a mammalian ovum.

vit·i·li·go (vĭt′l-ī′gō, -ē′gō) *n.*, *pl.* **-gos** or **vit·i·lig·i·nes** (vĭt′l-ĭj′ə-nēz) See **leukoderma.**

vit·rec·to·my (vĭ-trĕk′tə-mē) *n.* Surgical removal of the vitreous humor from the eyeball.

vit·re·o·den·tin (vĭt′rē-ō-dĕn′tĭn) *n.* A variety of dentin having a particular brittle hardness.

vit·re·ous (vĭt′rē-əs) *adj.* **1.** Of, relating to, resembling, or having the nature of glass; glassy. **2.** Of or relating to the vitreous body. —*n.* The vitreous body.

vitreous body *n.* A transparent jellylike substance enclosing the vitreous humor and filling the interior of the eyeball behind the lens.

vitreous chamber of the eye *n.* The large space between the lens and the retina, filled with the vitreous body.

vitreous humor *n.* **1.** The clear gelatinous substance that fills the eyeball between the retina and the lens. **2.** The vitreous body.

vit·re·um (vĭt′rē-əm) *n.* See **vitreous body.**

vit·ri·fi·ca·tion (vĭt′rə-fĭ-kā′shən) *n.* The process of using heat and fusion to convert dental porcelain to a glassy substance.

vi·vax (vī′văks) *n.* **1.** The protozoan *(Plasmodium vivax)* that causes the most common form of malaria. **2.** Malaria caused by this protozoan, characterized by the occurrence of febrile paroxysms about every 48 hours.

vi·vax malaria (vī′văks′) *n.* Malaria in which the paroxysms recur every third day, counting inclusively, and are induced by the release of merozoites and their invasion of new red blood cells.

viv·i·fi·ca·tion (vĭv′ə-fĭ-kā′shən) *n.* **1.** The process of converting protein from food into the living matter of the cells. **2.** See **revivification.**

vi·vip·a·rous (vī-vĭp′ər-əs, vĭ-) *adj.* Giving birth to living offspring that develop within the mother's body. Most mammals and some other animals are viviparous.

viv·i·sec·tion (vĭv′ĭ-sĕk′shən, vĭv′ĭ-sĕk′-) *n.* The act or practice of cutting into or otherwise injuring living animals, especially for the purpose of scientific research. —**viv′i·sec′tion·ist** *n.*

VLDL (vē′ĕl-dē′ĕl) *n.* A lipoprotein containing a very large proportion of lipids to protein and carrying most cholesterol from the liver to the tissues; very low density lipoprotein.

vo·cal (vō′kəl) *adj.* **1.** Of or relating to the voice. **2.** Having a voice; capable of emitting sound or speech.

vocal cord *n.* The sharp edge of a fold of mucous membrane stretching along either wall of the larynx from the angle between the laminae of the thyroid cartilage to the vocal process of the arytenoid cartilage. Vibrations of these cords are used in voice production.

vocal fremitus *n.* The vibration felt by a hand placed on the chest of a person who is speaking.

vocal resonance *n.* The voice sounds heard on auscultation of the chest of a person who is vocalizing in some manner.

vocal tic *n.* An involuntary, abrupt, and inappropriate grunt, bark, or other exclamation or utterance, occurring especially in Tourette's syndrome.

voice (vois) *n.* The sound made by air passing out

through the larynx and upper respiratory tract and produced by the vibration of the vocal organs.

void (void) *v.* **void·ed, void·ing, voids.** To excrete body wastes. — *adj.* Containing no matter; empty.

voiding cystogram *n.* See **cystourethrogram.**

vol·a·tile (vŏl′ə-tl, -tīl′) *adj.* **1.** Evaporating readily at normal temperatures and pressures. **2.** That can be readily vaporized. **3.** Tending to violence; explosive, as of behavior.

vo·li·tion (və-lĭsh′ən) *n.* **1.** The act or an instance of making a conscious choice or decision. **2.** A conscious choice or decision. **3.** The power or faculty of choosing; the will. — **vo·li′tion·al** *adj.*

volitional tremor *n.* See **intention tremor.**

vol·ley (vŏl′ē) *n.* The bursting forth of many things together, such as a synchronous group of impulses induced simultaneously by artificial stimulation of either nerve fibers or muscle fibers.

vol·ume (vŏl′yōōm, -yəm) *n.* **1.** The amount of space occupied by a three-dimensional object or region of space, expressed in cubic units. **2.** The capacity of such a region or of a specified container, expressed in cubic units.

vol·u·met·ric solution (vŏl′yōō-mĕt′rĭk) *n.* A solution made by mixing specified volumes of the components.

vol·un·tar·y (vŏl′ən-tĕr′ē) *adj.* **1.** Arising from or acting on one's own free will. **2.** Normally controlled by or subject to individual volition, as of respiration. **3.** Capable of making choices; having the faculty of will.

voluntary muscle *n.* A muscle, such as any of the striated muscles except the heart, whose action is normally controlled by individual volition.

vol·vu·lus (vŏl′vyə-ləs) *n.* Abnormal twisting of the intestine causing obstruction.

vo·mer (vō′mər) *n.* A thin flat bone of trapezoidal shape that forms the inferior and posterior portion of the nasal septum and articulates with the sphenoid and ethmoid bones, the two maxillae, and the two palatine bones. — **vo′mer·ine′** (-mə-rīn′) *adj.*

vom·i·ca (vŏm′ĭ-kə) *n.* **1.** Profuse expectoration of putrid matter. **2.** An abnormal pus-containing cavity, usually in a lung, caused by deterioration of tissue. **3.** The pus contained in such a cavity.

vom·it (vŏm′ĭt) *v.* **-it·ed, -it·ing, -its.** To eject part or all of the contents of the stomach through the mouth, usually in a series of involuntary spasmic movements. — *n.* **1.** The act or an instance of ejecting matter from the stomach through the mouth. **2.** Matter ejected from the stomach through the mouth. **3.** An emetic.

vomiting of pregnancy *n.* Vomiting occurring in the early months of pregnancy, as in morning sickness.

vomiting reflex *n.* Contraction of the abdominal muscles with relaxation of the cardiac sphincter

of the stomach and of the muscles of the throat elicited by a variety of stimuli, especially by a stimulus applied to the region of the fauces.

vom·i·to·ry (vŏm′ĭ-tôr′ē) *adj.* Inducing vomiting; vomitive. — *n., pl.* **-ries. 1.** Something that induces vomiting. **2.** An aperture through which matter is discharged.

vom·i·tu·ri·tion (vŏm′ĭ-chə-rĭsh′ən, -ĭ-tōō-) *n.* Forceful attempts at vomiting without bringing up the contents of the stomach; retching.

vom·i·tus (vŏm′ĭ-təs) *n.* Vomited matter.

von Hip·pel–Lindau disease (vŏn hĭp′əl-, fôn) *n.* See **Lindau's disease.**

von Wil·le·brand's disease (vŏn wĭl′ə-brăndz′, fôn vĭl′ə-bränts′) *n.* A hereditary predisposition to hemorrhaging characterized by bleeding from mucous membranes and various abnormalities in the blood components responsible for clotting.

vor·tex (vôr′tĕks′) *n., pl.* **-tex·es** or **-ti·ces** (-tĭ-sēz′-) A spiral motion of fluid within a limited area, especially a whirling mass of water or air that sucks everything near it toward its center.

vox·el (vŏk′səl) *n.* The basic unit of an electronically generated video image of computed tomography reconstruction.

voy·eur (voi-yûr′) *n.* **1.** A person who derives sexual gratification from observing the naked bodies or sexual acts of others, especially from a secret vantage point. **2.** An obsessive observer of sordid or sensational subjects.

voy·eur·ism (voi-yûr′ĭz′əm) *n.* The practice of being a voyeur.

vul·ner·a·ble phase (vŭl′nər-ə-bəl) *n.* A phase in the cardiac cycle during which an ectopic impulse may lead to repetitive activity, such as flutter or fibrillation, of the affected chamber.

vul·sel·lum (vŭl-sĕl′əm) *n., pl* **-la** (-lə). A forceps with a small hook or hooks at the tip of each blade.

vul·va (vŭl′və) *n., pl.* **-vae** (-vē). The external genital organs of the female, including the labia majora, labia minora, clitoris, and vestibule of the vagina. — **vul′val, vul′var** (-vər, -vär′) *adj.*

vul·vec·to·my (vŭl-vĕk′tə-mē) *n.* Surgical removal of the vulva.

vul·vi·tis (vŭl-vī′tĭs) *n.* Inflammation of the vulva.

vul·vo·vag·i·nal gland (vŭl′vō-văj′ə-nəl) *n.* See **greater vestibular gland.**

vul·vo·vag·i·ni·tis (vŭl′vō-văj′ə-nī′tĭs) *n.* Inflammation of the vulva and vagina, or of the vulvovaginal glands.

V wave *n.* A large pressure wave that is visible in electrocardiographic recordings from either the atrium or the incoming veins and is normally produced by venous return.

V–Y-plas·ty (vē′wī′plăs′tē) *n.* A surgical method for lengthening tissues in one direction by cutting in the lines of a V, sliding the two segments apart, and closing in the lines of a Y.

waist (wāst) *n.* The part of the human trunk between the bottom of the rib cage and the pelvis.

wale (wāl) *n.* A mark raised on the skin, as by a whip; a weal or welt. —*v.* **waled, wal·ing, wales.** To raise marks on the skin, as by whipping.

walk (wôk) *v.* **walked, walk·ing, walks.** To move over a surface by taking steps with the feet at a pace slower than a run. —*n.* **1.** The gait of a human in which the feet are lifted alternately with one part of a foot always on the ground. **2.** The characteristic way in which one walks.

walk·er (wô′kər) *n.* **1.** A frame device used to support someone, such as an infant learning to walk or a convalescent learning to walk again. **2.** A shoe specially designed for walking comfortably. Often used in the plural.

wall (wôl) *n.* A part of a structure that encloses a cavity, chamber, or other anatomical unit.

wall·eye (wôl′ī′) *n.* **1.** Absence of color in the iris. **2.** An opacity having a dense white opacity of the cornea. **3.** See **exotropia.**

waltzed flap (wôltst) *n.* See **caterpillar flap.**

wan·der·ing abscess (wŏn′dər-ĭng) *n.* An abscess formed by pus burrowing along fascial planes and occurring at a distance from the primary focus of infection.

wandering cell *n.* See **ameboid cell.**

wandering kidney *n.* See **floating kidney.**

wandering pacemaker *n.* A disturbance of the normal cardiac rhythm in which the site of the controlling pacemaker shifts from beat to beat, usually between the sinoatrial and atrioventricular nodes.

Wan·gen·steen tube (wăng′gən-stēn′) *n.* A modified siphon that maintains constant negative pressure; used in the treatment of gastric and intestinal distention.

ward (wôrd) *n.* **1.** A room in a hospital usually holding six or more patients. **2.** A division in a hospital for the care of a particular group of patients.

warm-blooded *adj.* Maintaining a relatively constant and warm body temperature independent of environmental temperature.

war neurosis *n.* A nervous disorder, usually temporary but sometimes leading to a permanent neurosis, brought on by the exhaustion and stress of combat or similar situations and characterized by deep anxiety, depression, irritability, and other related symptoms.

wart (wôrt) *n.* A hard, rough lump growing on the skin, caused by infection with certain viruses and occurring typically on the hands and feet.

wart·y dyskeratoma (wôr′tē) *n.* A benign solitary tumor of the skin, usually of the scalp, face, or neck, that appears to arise from a hair follicle and includes extensive epithelial downgrowth.

wash (wŏsh) *v.* **washed, wash·ing, wash·es. 1.** To cleanse, using water or another liquid, usually with soap, detergent, or bleach, by immersing, dipping, rubbing, or scrubbing. **2.** To make moist or wet. —*n.* **1.** The act or process of cleansing or washing. **2.** A solution used to cleanse or bathe a part.

Was·ser·mann reaction (wä′sər-mən) *n.* A complement-fixing reaction in the Wassermann test.

Wassermann test *n.* A diagnostic test for syphilis involving the fixation or inactivation of a complement by an antibody in a blood serum sample.

waste (wāst) *v.* **wast·ed, wast·ing, wastes.** To gradually lose energy, strength, or bodily substance, as from disease. —*n.* The undigested residue of food eliminated from the body; excrement.

waste product *n.* Organic waste matter such as urine, feces, or dead cells.

wast·ing (wā′stĭng) *adj.* **1.** Gradually deteriorating; declining. **2.** Sapping the strength or substance of the body, as a disease; emaciating. —*n.* Emaciation.

wa·ter (wô′tər) *n.* **1.** A clear, colorless, odorless, and tasteless liquid, H_2O, essential for most plant and animal life and the most widely used of all solvents. Freezing point 0°C (32°F); boiling point 100°C (212°F); specific gravity (4°C) 1.0000; weight per gallon (15°C) 8.337 pounds (3.772 kilograms). **2.** Any of the liquids present in or passed out of the body, such as urine, perspiration, tears, or saliva. **3.** The fluid surrounding a fetus in the uterus; amniotic fluid.

water bag *n.* The membranous sac filled with amniotic fluid that protects a fetus during a pregnancy.

water balance *n.* See **fluid balance.**

water blister *n.* A blister having watery contents without blood or pus.

wa·ter·fall (wô′tər-fôl′) *n.* Blood flow in vascular beds where lateral pressure greatly exceeds venous pressure and tends to collapse vessels.

water-hammer pulse *n.* A pulse having a forcible impulse immediately followed by collapse, characteristic of aortic incompetency.

Wa·ter·house–Frid·er·ich·sen syndrome (wô′tər-hous′-frĭd′ə-rĭk′sən) *n.* Acute fulminating meningococcal septicemia occurring mainly in children under 10 years old, characterized by vomiting, diarrhea, purpura, cyanosis, convulsions, and circulatory collapse, usually accompanied by meningitis and hemorrhage into the adrenal glands.

water of metabolism *n.* Water that is formed in the body by oxidation of the hydrogen in foods, as in the metabolism of fat.

water on the brain *n.* Hydrocephalus.

water-trap stomach *n.* A stomach that does not empty itself properly due to a relatively high pyloric outlet.

wa·ter·y (wô′tə-rē) *adj.* **-i·er, -i·est. 1.** Filled with, consisting of, or soaked with water; wet or soggy. **2.** Secreting or discharging water or watery fluid, especially as a symptom of disease.

Wat·son–Crick helix (wät′sən-krĭk′) *n.* See **double helix.**

Watson–Crick model *n.* A three-dimensional model of the DNA molecule, consisting of two polynucleotide strands wound in the form of a double helix and joined in a ladderlike fashion by hydrogen bonds between the purine and pyrimidine bases.

wave (wāv) *n.* **1.** A disturbance traveling through a medium by which energy is transferred from one particle of the medium to another without causing permanent displacement of the medium itself. **2.** A graphic representation of the variation of such a disturbance with time. **3.** A single cycle of such a disturbance.

wax (wăks) *n.* **1.** Any of various natural, oily or greasy heat-sensitive substances, consisting of hydrocarbons or esters of fatty acids that are insoluble in water but soluble in most organic solvents. **2.** Cerumen. **3.** A substance secreted by bees, usually a dull yellow solid.

wax·ing (wăk′sĭng) or **wax·ing-up** (wăk′sĭng-ŭp′) *n.* The shaping of the contours of a trial denture or a crown in wax prior to its casting in metal.

WBC *abbr.* white blood cell; white blood count

weal (wēl) *n.* A ridge on the flesh raised by a blow; a welt.

wean (wēn) *v.* **weaned, wean·ing, weans. 1.** To deprive permanently of breast milk and begin to nourish with other food. **2.** To gradually withdraw from a life-support system.

wear-and-tear pigment *n.* Lipofuscin that accumulates in aging or atrophic cells as a residue of lysosomal digestion.

web (wĕb) *n.* An abnormal membrane or fold of skin connecting the toes or fingers.

webbed (wĕbd) *adj.* United by a common sheath of skin.

web·bing (wĕb′ĭng) *n.* A congenital condition apparent when adjacent structures are joined by a broad band of tissue not normally present.

We·ber's paradox (vā′bərz) *n.* The paradox stating that if a muscle is loaded beyond its power to contract, it may elongate.

Web·er's syndrome (wĕb′ərz) *n.* A form of alternating hemiplegia caused by a lesion in the cerebral peduncle and resulting in paralysis of the oculomotor nerve on the side of the lesion and paralysis of the extremities and of the face and tongue on the opposite side.

We·ber's test (vā′bərz) *n.* A test for differentiating conductive hearing impairment from sensorineu-

ral hearing impairment by applying a vibrating tuning fork to the midline of the forehead.

web·foot (wĕb′fŏŏt′) *n.* A foot with webbed toes.

Wechsler adult intelligence scale *n.* A standardized intelligence test for assessing people aged 16 and older.

Wechsler intelligence scale for children *n.* A standardized intelligence test for assessing children from 5 to 15 years old.

Wechsler preschool and primary scale for intelligence *n.* A standardized intelligence test for assessing preschool children.

wedge bone *n.* Either of two of the cuneiform bones, the lateral or the medial.

wedge pressure *n.* The intravascular pressure reading obtained when a fine catheter is advanced until it completely occludes a small blood vessel.

wedge resection *n.* Surgical removal of a wedge-shaped portion of tissue, as of the ovary.

weight (wāt) *n.* **1.** The force with which a body is attracted to Earth or another celestial body, equal to the product of the object's mass and the acceleration of gravity. **2.** The heaviness of an object.

Weil–Fe·lix test (vīl′fā′lĭcks) *n.* A test to determine infection with a rickettsial bacterium, such as the causative agent of typhus.

Weil's disease (wīlz, vīlz) *n.* A severe form of leptospirosis in humans that is characterized by jaundice, fever, muscle pain, and a tendency to hemorrhage.

Well·bu·trin (wĕl′byōō-trĭn) The trademark for bupropion.

well differentiated lymphocytic lymphoma *n.* A disease that is essentially the same as chronic lymphocytic leukemia except that lymphocytes are not increased in the peripheral blood.

well·ness (wĕl′nĭs) *n.* The condition of good physical and mental health, especially when maintained by proper diet, exercise, and habits.

Wells' syndrome (wĕlz) *n.* Recurrent cellulitis followed by an eruption of skin lesions that are usually brawny, filled with fluid, and heavily infiltrated by eosinophils and histiocytes.

welt (wĕlt) *n.* **1.** A ridge or bump on the skin caused by a lash or blow or sometimes by an allergic reaction. **2.** See **wheal.**

Wer·ner's syndrome (vĕr′nərz) *n.* A hereditary disease of young adults characterized by short stature, early graying, cataracts, vascular disorders, and generally premature aging and death.

Wer·nick·e–Korsakoff syndrome (vĕr′nĭ-kē, -kə) *n.* Wernicke's syndrome and Korsakoff's syndrome occurring together.

Wer·nick·e's center (vĕr′nĭ-kēz, -kəz) *n.* A large region of the parietal and temporal lobes of the left cerebral hemisphere, thought to be essential for understanding and formulating speech.

Wernicke's reaction *n.* A reaction seen in hemianopsia in which the pupil reacts to light directed to the normal side of the retina but not to light directed to the blind side of the retina.

Wernicke's sign *n.* See **Wernicke's reaction.**

Wernicke's syndrome *n.* A disease of the nervous system caused by a deficiency of thiamine and characterized by abnormal eye movements, a loss of muscle coordination, tremors, and confusion; it is almost always followed by amnesia and is most often seen in chronic alcoholics.

Wert·heim's operation (vĕrt′hīmz′) *n.* A radical hysterectomy for treatment of uterine cancer, in which as much as possible of the vagina is excised, and there is wide excision of lymph nodes.

Wes·ter·gren method (wĕs′tər-grĕn′, vĕs′-) *n.* A method for estimating the sedimentation rate of red blood cells in whole blood.

West·ern blot analysis (wĕs′tərn) *n.* An electrophoretic procedure for separating proteins.

Western blot test *n.* A serum electrophoretic analysis used to identify proteins.

wet gangrene *n.* Ischemic necrosis of an extremity with bacterial infection.

wet lung *n.* The lung in pulmonary edema.

wet nurse *n.* A woman employed to breast-feed a child that is not her own.

wet pack *n.* A therapeutic pack moistened in hot or cold water.

Wharton's jelly *n.* The mucous connective tissue of the umbilical cord.

wheal (wēl) *n.* A small swelling on the skin, as from an insect bite, that usually itches or burns.

wheal-and-erythema reaction *n.* See **wheal-and-flare reaction.**

wheal-and-flare reaction *n.* The characteristic immediate reaction to an injected allergen in a skin test, in which an irregular blanched wheal appears, surrounded by an area of redness.

wheel·chair or **wheel chair** (hwēl′châr′, wēl′-) *n.* A chair mounted on large wheels for the use of a sick or disabled person.

wheeze (wēz) *v.* **wheezed, wheez·ing, wheez·es.** To breathe with difficulty, producing a hoarse whistling sound. —*n.* A wheezing sound.

whelk (wĕlk) *n.* An inflamed swelling, such as a pimple or pustule.

whip·lash (wĭp′lăsh′) *n.* Whiplash injury.

whiplash injury *n.* A hyperextension-hyperflexion injury to the cervical spine caused by an abrupt jerking motion of the head, either backward or forward.

Whip·ple's operation (wĭp′əlz) *n.* See **pancreatoduodenectomy.**

whip·worm (wĭp′wûrm′) *n.* See **Trichuris.**

white blood cell *n.* Any of the colorless or white cells in the blood that have a nucleus and cytoplasm and help protect the body from infection and disease through specialized neutrophils, lymphocytes, and monocytes.

white corpuscle *n.* See **white blood cell.**

white gangrene *n.* Death of a body part accompanied by the formation of grayish white sloughs.

white·head (wīt′hĕd′) *n.* **1.** A tiny epidermal cyst-like mass with a narrow or obstructed opening on the skin surface, which may rupture, caused by retention of the secretion of a sebaceous gland. **2.** See **milium.**

White·head's operation (wīt′hĕdz′) *n.* Excision of hemorrhoids by two circular incisions above and below involved veins, allowing normal mucosa to be pulled down and sutured to anal skin.

white line *n.* See **linea alba.**

white matter *n.* Whitish nerve tissue, especially of the brain and spinal cord, chiefly composed of myelinated nerve fibers and containing few or no neuronal cell bodies or dendrites.

white plague *n.* Tuberculosis, especially of the lungs.

white pulp *n.* The part of the spleen that consists of lymphatic nodules and other concentrations of lymphatic tissue.

white rat *n.* A domesticated albino variety of the Norway rat, used extensively in laboratory experiments.

white substance *n.* See **white matter.**

whit·low (wĭt′lō′) *n.* See **felon.**

WHO *abbr.* World Health Organization

whole (hōl) *adj.* **1.** Not wounded, injured, or impaired; sound or unhurt. **2.** Having been restored; healed. **3.** Having the same parents. —*n.* An entity or a system made up of interrelated parts.

whole blood *n.* Blood from which no constituent such as plasma or platelets has been removed.

whole-body counter *n.* A device used to measure the total radiation in the body, usually containing a number of sensitive detectors and shielding to block out ambient radiation.

whole body titration curve *n.* A graphic representation of the ionic changes in blood in response to disturbances in its acid-base balance.

whole-cell vaccine *n.* Vaccine made up of suspensions of killed bacterial cells, as opposed to antigenic fragments of bacteria.

whoop (hoōp, hwoōp, woōp) *n.* The paroxysmal gasp characteristic of whooping cough.

whoop·ing cough (hoō′pĭng, hwoō′-, woō′-, hoōp′ĭng) *n.* A highly contagious disease of the respiratory system, usually affecting children, that is caused by the bacterium *Bordetella pertussis* and is characterized in its advanced stage by spasms of coughing interspersed with deep, noisy inspirations.

whooping cough vaccine *n.* See **pertussis vaccine.**

whorl (wôrl, wûrl) *n.* **1.** A form that coils or spirals; a curl or swirl. **2.** A turn of the cochlea or of the ethmoidal crest. **3.** An area of hair growing in a radial manner. **4.** One of the circular ridges or convolutions of a fingerprint.

Wi·dal test (vē-däl′) *n.* A test of blood serum that uses an agglutination reaction to diagnose typhoid fever.

wild type *n.* The typical form of an organism, strain, gene, or characteristic as it occurs in nature, as distinguished from mutant forms that may result from selective breeding.

Wilms tumor (vĭlms) *n.* A malignant renal tumor occurring in young children and composed of small spindle cells and other tissue.

wind·burn (wĭnd′bûrn′) *n.* A reddened irritation

of the skin caused by exposure to the wind.

win·dow (wĭn′dō) *n.* A fenestra.

wind·pipe (wĭnd′pīp′) *n.* See **trachea**.

wing (wĭng) *n.* **1.** Any of various paired movable organs of flight, as that of a bird or insect. **2.** Something that resembles a wing in appearance, function, or position relative to a main body.

winged catheter (wĭngd) *n.* A soft rubber catheter with little flaps at each side of the end that serve to retain it in the bladder.

wink (wĭngk) *v.* **winked, wink·ing, winks. 1.** To close and open the eyelid of one eye deliberately, as to convey a message, signal, or suggestion. **2.** To close and open the eyelids of both eyes; blink. — *n.* A quick closing and opening of the eyelids; a blink.

wink reflex *n.* Reflex closing of eyelids in response to a stimulus.

wir·ing (wīr′ĭng) *n.* The fastening together of the ends of a broken bone with wire sutures.

wiry pulse *n.* A small, fine pulse that cannot be compressed.

wis·dom tooth (wĭz′dəm) *n.* The third molar tooth on both sides of both jaws that erupts from the 17th to the 23rd year.

wish fulfillment *n.* In psychoanalytic theory, the satisfaction of a desire, a need, or an impulse through a dream, a fantasy, or other exercise of the imagination.

Wis·kott–Aldrich syndrome (wĭs′kŏt-, vĭs′kŏt-) *n.* An inherited immunodeficiency disorder occurring in male children, characterized by thrombocytopenia, eczema, melena, and susceptibility to recurrent bacterial infections.

Wiss·ler's syndrome (wĭs′lərz, vĭs′-) *n.* A condition occurring in children and adolescents, characterized by high intermittent fever, irregularly recurring macular and maculo-papular eruption, leukocytosis, joint pain, and occasionally eosinophilia and raised red blood cell sedimentation rate.

witch hazel *n.* **1.** Any of several deciduous shrubs or small trees of the genus *Hamamelis,* especially *H. virginiana,* of eastern North America, having yellow flowers that bloom in late autumn or winter. **2.** An alcoholic solution containing an extract of the bark and leaves of this plant, applied externally as a mild astringent.

witch's milk *n.* Milk resembling colostrum sometimes secreted from the breasts of newborn infants of either sex three to four days after birth and lasting no longer than two weeks, due to endocrine stimulation from the mother before birth.

with·draw·al (wĭth-drô′əl, wĭth-) *n.* **1.** Detachment, as from social or emotional involvement. **2.** Discontinuation of the use of an addictive substance. **3.** The physiological and mental readjustment that accompanies such discontinuation. **4.** A pattern of behavior, observed in schizophrenia and depression, characterized by a pathological retreat from interpersonal contact and social involvement and leading to self-preoccupation.

withdrawal symptom *n.* Any of a group of physical and psychological symptoms occurring in a person deprived of an accustomed dose of an addicting agent.

wob·ble (wŏb′əl) *n.* **1.** A movement or rotation with an uneven or rocking motion or an unsteady motion from side to side. **2.** The ability of one tRNA anticodon to recognize two mRNA codons, especially as occurs in pairing that does not follow base pairing rules. — **wob′bler** *n.*

Wolfe graft (wŏolf) *n.* A full-thickness skin graft without any subcutaneous fat.

Wolfe–Krause graft *n.* See **Wolfe graft.**

Wolff's law (vŏlfs) *n.* The principle that every change in the form and the function of a bone or in the function of the bone alone, leads to changes in its internal architecture and in its external form.

Wol·man's disease (wŏl′mənz) *n.* An inherited disorder of lipid metabolism caused by a deficiency of lysosomal acid lipase and resulting in the widespread accumulation of cholesterol esters and triglycerides in the internal organs.

womb (wŏom) *n.* See **uterus.**

wool·ly-hair nevus (wŏol′ē-hâr′) *n.* A congenital condition in which hair in a circumscribed area of the scalp is kinky or woolly.

wool-sorter's disease *n.* A pulmonary form of anthrax that results from the inhalation of spores of the bacterium *Bacillus anthracis* in the wool of contaminated sheep.

word deafness *n.* A form of aphasia in which the meaning of ordinary spoken words becomes incomprehensible.

word salad *n.* See **schizophasia.**

work·a·hol·ic (wûr′kə-hô′lĭk) *n.* One who has a compulsive and unrelenting need to work.

work·ers' compensation (wûr′kərz) *n.* Payments required by law to be made to an employee who is injured or disabled in connection with work.

work·up (wûrk′ŭp′) *n.* A thorough medical examination for diagnostic purposes.

worm (wûrm) *n.* **1.** Any of various invertebrates, as those of the phyla Annelida, Nematoda, Nemertea, or Platyhelminthes, having a long, flexible, rounded or flattened body, often without obvious appendages. **2.** Any of various crawling insect larvae, such as a grub or a caterpillar, having a soft, elongated body. **3.** Any of various unrelated animals, such as the shipworm or the slowworm, resembling a worm in habit or appearance. **4. worms.** Infestation of the intestines or other parts of the body with worms or wormlike parasites; helminthiasis.

wound (wŏond) *n.* **1.** Injury to a part or tissue of the body, especially one caused by physical trauma and characterized by tearing, cutting, piercing, or breaking of the tissue. **2.** A surgical incision. — **wound** *v.*

wound clip *n.* A clasp for bringing tissue edges together for the suture of skin incisions.

wo·ven bone (wō′vən) *n.* Bony tissue characteristic of the embryonic skeleton in which the collagen fibers of the matrix are arranged irregularly in the form of interlacing networks.

W-plas·ty (dŭb′əl-yo͞o-plăs′tē, -yo͞o-) *n.* A procedure to prevent the contracture of a straight-line scar in which the edges of a wound are trimmed in the shape of a W and closed in a zigzag fashion.

WR *abbr.* Wassermann reaction

Wright's stain (rīts) *n.* A specially prepared mixture used in staining blood smears.

wrist (rĭst) *n.* **1.** The joint between the hand and the forearm. **2.** See **carpus**.

wrist-drop *n.* Paralysis of the extensor muscles of the wrist and fingers causing the hand to hang down at the wrist.

wrist joint *n.* The joint between the distal end of

the radius and its articular disk and the proximal row of carpal bones, except the pisiform bone.

writ·er's cramp (rītərz) *n.* A cramp or spasm of the muscles of the fingers, hand, and forearm during writing.

wry·neck (rī′nĕk′) *n.* See **torticollis**.

Wu·cher·e·ri·a (wo͞o′chə-rēr′ē-ə, vo͞o′kə-) *n.* A genus of filarial nematodes of the family Onchocercidae characterized by adult forms that live chiefly in lymphatic vessels, causing obstruction to lymph flow and producing large numbers of embryos or microfilariae that circulate in the blood.

wu·cher·e·ri·a·sis (wo͞o′chər-ə-rī′ə-sĭs, vo͞o′kər-) *n.* Infestation with worms of the genus *Wuchereria.*

X

xan·the·las·ma (zăn′thə-lăz′mə) *n.* Xanthoma of the eyelid.

xan·the·mi·a (zăn-thē′mē-ə) *n.* See **carotenemia**.

xan·thine (zăn′thēn′, -thĭn) *n.* **1.** A yellowish-white, crystalline purine base that is a precursor of uric acid and is found in blood, urine, and muscle tissue. **2.** Any of several derivatives of this compound.

xan·thi·nu·ri·a (zăn′thə-no͝or′ē-ə, -nyo͝or′-) *n.* **1.** Excretion of abnormally large amounts of xanthine in the urine. **2.** An inherited metabolic disorder resulting from defective synthesis of an enzyme and characterized by urinary excretion of xanthine in place of uric acid.

xan·thism (zăn′thĭz′əm) *n.* A pigmentary anomaly of blacks characterized by red or yellow-red hair color, copper-red skin, and often fading of the pigment of the iris.

xan·tho·chro·mi·a (zăn′thə-krō′mē-ə) *n.* The occurrence of patches of yellow color in the skin resembling xanthoma but without nodules or plates.

xan·tho·der·ma (zăn′thə-dûr′mə) *n.* **1.** A yellow coloration of the skin. **2.** See **xanthochromia**.

xan·tho·gran·u·lo·ma (zăn′thə-grăn′yə-lō′mə) *n.* An infiltration of retroperitoneal tissue by lipid macrophages, usually occurring in women.

xan·tho·ma (zăn-thō′mə) *n., pl.* **-mas** or **-ma·ta** (-mə-tə). A yellowish-orange, lipid-filled nodule or papule in the skin, often on an eyelid or over a joint.

xanthoma dis·sem·i·na·tum (dĭ-sĕm′ə-nā′təm) *n.* See **xanthomatosis**.

xanthoma pal·pe·brar·um (păl′pə-brâr′əm) *n.* The most common type of xanthoma, consisting of a soft yellow-orange plaque that occurs in groups around the eyes.

xan·tho·ma·to·sis (zăn′thō-mə-tō′sĭs) *n.* A metabolic disorder characterized by excessive accu-

mulation of lipids in the body and a resulting spread of xanthomas.

xan·tho·sine (zăn′thə-sēn′, -sĭn) *n.* A nucleoside that hydrolyzes to yield ribose and xanthine.

xan·tho·sis (zăn-thō′sĭs) *n.* A yellowish discoloration of degenerating tissues, especially in malignant neoplasms.

X-chromosome *n.* The sex chromosome associated with female characteristics, occurring paired in the female and singly in the male sex-chromosome pair.

xen·o·bi·ot·ic (zĕn′ə-bī-ŏt′ĭk, zē′nə-) *adj.* Foreign to the body or to living organisms. Used of chemical compounds. — *n.* A xenobiotic chemical, such as a pesticide.

xen·o·ge·ne·ic (zĕn′ə-jə-nē′ĭk, -nā′-, zē′nə-) *adj.* Derived or obtained from an organism of a different species, as a tissue graft.

xen·o·gen·e·sis (zĕn′ə-jĕn′ĭ-sĭs, zē′nə-) *n.* **1.** The supposed production of offspring markedly different from either parent. **2.** See **alternation of generations**.

xen·o·gen·ic (zĕn′ə-jĕn′ĭk, zē′nə-) or **xe·nog·e·nous** (zə-nŏj′ə-nəs) *adj.* **1.** Originating outside the organism or from a foreign substance introduced into the organism. **2.** Xenogeneic.

xen·o·graft (zĕn′ə-grăft′, zē′nə-) *n.* See **heterograft**.

xe·non (zē′nŏn′) *n.* A colorless, odorless, highly unreactive gaseous element with atomic number 54.

xen·o·pho·bi·a (zĕn′ə-fō′bē-ə, zē′nə-) *n.* Fear and contempt of strangers or foreign peoples.

xen·oph·thal·mi·a (zĕn′ŏf-thăl′mē-ə, zē′nŏf-) *n.* Inflammation resulting from the presence of a foreign body in the eye.

xe·ro·chi·li·a (zēr′ə-kī′lē-ə) *n.* Dryness of the lips.

xe·ro·der·ma (zēr′ō-dûr′mə) or **xe·ro·der·mi·a** (-mē-ə) *n.* Excessive or abnormal dryness of the skin, as in ichthyosis.

xeroderma pig·men·to·sum (pĭg'mən-tō'səm, -mĕn-) *n.* A rare hereditary skin disorder caused by a defect in the enzymes that repair DNA damaged by ultraviolet light and resulting in hypersensitivity to the carcinogenic effect of ultraviolet light.

xe·ro·gram (zēr'ə-grăm') *n.* See **xeroradiograph.**

xe·rog·ra·phy (zĭ-rŏg'rə-fē) *n.* See **xeroradiography.**

xe·ro·ma (zĭ-rō'mə) *n.* See **xerophthalmia.**

xe·ro·me·ni·a (zēr'ə-mē'nē-ə) *n.* The occurrence of the usual physical manifestations at the menstrual period but without the show of blood.

xe·roph·thal·mi·a (zēr'ŏf-thăl'mē-ə) *n.* Extreme dryness of the conjunctiva resulting from disease localized in the eye or from a systemic deficiency of vitamin A.

xe·ro·ra·di·o·graph (zēr'ə-rā'dē-ō-grăf') *n.* A radiograph made by xeroradiography.

xe·ro·ra·di·og·ra·phy (zēr'ə-rā'dē-ŏg'rə-fē) *n.* A dry photographic or photocopying process in which a negative image formed by a resinous powder on an electrically charged plate is electrically transferred to and thermally fixed as positive on a paper or other copying surface.

xe·ro·sis (zĭ-rō'sĭs) *n., pl.* **-ses** (-sēz). **1.** Abnormal dryness, especially of the skin, eyes, or mucous membranes. **2.** The normal hardening of aging tissue.

xe·ro·sto·mi·a (zēr'ə-stō'mē-ə) *n.* Dryness of the mouth resulting from diminished or arrested salivary secretion.

X-inactivation *n.* See **Lyonization.**

xiph·i·ster·num (zĭf'ĭ-stûr'nəm) *n.* See **xiphoid process.** — **xiph'i·ster'nal** *adj.*

xiph·oid cartilage (zĭf'oid') *n.* See **xiphoid process.**

xiph·oid·i·tis (zĭf'oi-dī'tĭs) *n.* Inflammation of the xiphoid process.

xiphoid process *n.* The cartilage at the lower end of the sternum that ossifies as a person ages.

X-linked gene *n.* A gene located on an X-chromosome.

X-linked hypogammaglobulinemia or **X-linked infantile hypogammaglobulinemia** *n.* An X-linked primary immunodeficiency characterized by a deficiency of circulating B-lymphocytes with a corresponding decrease in immunoglobulins and associated with increased susceptibility to infection by pyogenic bacteria, especially pneumococci and *Haemophilus influenzae* beginning after the loss of maternal antibodies.

XO syndrome *n.* See **Turner's syndrome.**

x-radiation *n.* **1.** Treatment with or exposure to x-rays. **2.** Radiation composed of x-rays.

x-ray or **X-ray** *n.* or **x ray** or **X ray 1.** A relatively high-energy photon with wavelength in the approximate range from 0.01 to 10 nanometers. **2.** A stream of such photons, used for their penetrating power in radiography, radiology, radiotherapy, and scientific research. Often used in the plural. **3.** A photograph taken with x-rays. — *v.*

x-rayed or **X-rayed, x-ray·ing** or **X-ray·ing, x-rays** or **X-rays. 1.** To irradiate with x-rays. **2.** To photograph with x-rays.

x-ray microscope *n.* An instrument using x-rays to render a highly magnified image.

x-ray therapy *n.* Medical treatment using controlled doses of x-ray radiation.

XXY syndrome (ĕks'ĕks-wī') *n.* See **Klinefelter's syndrome.**

xy·lose (zī'lōs') *n.* A white crystalline sugar used in diabetic diets and as a diagnostic aid when assessing intestinal function.

xy·lu·lose (zī'lə-lōs', zīl'yə-) *n.* A pentose sugar that is a part of carbohydrate metabolism and is found in the urine in pentosuria.

xys·ma (zĭz'mə) *n.* Any of the shreds of membrane occasionally found in feces.

xys·ter (zĭs'tər) *n.* A surgical instrument for scraping bones.

XYY syndrome (ĕks'wī-wī') *n.* A chromosomal anomaly characterized by the presence of one X-chromosome and two Y-chromosomes and thought to be associated with tallness, aggressiveness, and acne.

~ ~ ~ ~ ~ Y ~ ~ ~ ~ ~

yawn (yôn) *v.* **yawned, yawn·ing, yawns.** To open the mouth wide with a deep inhalation, usually involuntarily from drowsiness, fatigue, or boredom. — *n.* The act of yawning.

yaws (yôz) *n.* An infectious tropical disease caused by *Treponema pertenue,* characterized by the development of crusted granulomatous ulcers on the extremities that may cause bone and joint destruction in later stages of the disease.

Y-chromosome *n.* The sex chromosome associated with male characteristics, occurring with one X-chromosome in the pair of male sex chromosomes.

yeast (yēst) *n.* **1.** Any of various unicellular fungi of the genus *Saccharomyces,* especially *S. cerevisiae,* reproducing by budding and capable of fermenting carbohydrates. **2.** Any of various similar fungi. **3.** A commercial preparation in either powdered or compressed form, containing yeast cells and inert material such as meal and used especially as a leavening agent or as a dietary supplement.

yel·low bile (yĕl'ō) *n.* See **choler.**

yellow bone marrow *n.* Bone marrow in which the meshes of the reticular network are filled with fat.

yellow cartilage *n.* See **elastic cartilage**.

yellow fever *n.* An infectious tropical disease caused by an arbovirus transmitted by mosquitoes of the genera *Aedes,* especially *A. aegypti,* and *Haemagogus,* characterized by high fever, jaundice, and dark-colored vomit resulting from gastrointestinal hemorrhaging.

yellow fever vaccine *n.* A vaccine containing a live attenuated strain of yellow fever virus that has been grown in chick embryos, used to immunize against yellow fever.

yellow fever virus *n.* An arbovirus of the genus *Flavivirus* that causes yellow fever and is transmitted by mosquitoes.

yellow hepatization *n.* The final stage of hepatization of lung tissue in pneumonia, in which the exudate is becoming purulent.

yellow spot *n.* See **macula lutea**.

yer·sin·i·a (yər-sĭn′ē-ə) *n.* A member of the genus *Yersinia*.

Yer·sin·i·a (yər-sĭn′ē-ə) *n.* A genus of gram-negative, parasitic bacteria of the family Enterobacteriaceae that cause various diseases in humans and other animals.

Yersinia pes·tis (pĕs′tĭs) *n.* A bacterium that causes plague and is transmitted from rats to humans by the rat flea *Xenopsylla cheopis*.

yer·sin·i·o·sis (yər-sĭn′ē-ō′sĭs) *n.* An infectious disease caused by *Yersinia enterocolitica* and marked by diarrhea, enteritis, ileitis, pseudoappendicitis, erythema nodosum, and sometimes septicemia or acute arthritis.

Y-linked gene *n.* A gene located on a Y-chromosome.

yo·gurt (yō′gərt) A custardlike food with a tart flavor, prepared from milk curdled by bacteria, especially *Lactobacillus bulgaricus* and *Streptococcus thermophilus,* and often sweetened or flavored with fruit.

yoke (yōk) *n.* See **jugum** (sense 1).

yolk (yōk) *n.* The portion of the egg of an animal that consists mainly of protein, lecithin, and cholesterol, and from which the early embryo derives its primary nourishment.

yolk membrane *n.* See **vitelline membrane** (senses 1, 2).

yolk sac *n.* A membranous sac attached to an embryo and enclosing food yolk.

yolk stalk *n.* A narrow ductlike part that connects the yolk sac to the middle of the embryonic digestive tract.

yt·ter·bi·um (ĭ-tûr′bē-əm) *n.* A soft bright allotropic rare-earth element with atomic number 70.

yt·tri·um (ĭt′rē-əm) *n.* A metallic element, not a rare earth but occurring in nearly all rare-earth minerals, with atomic number 39.

~~~~~~ Z ~~~~~~

zal·ci·ta·bine (zăl′sĭ-tə-bĭn′) *n.* See **DDC**.

Z–DNA *n.* A form of DNA in which the double helix twists in a left-hand direction and has a zigzag appearance.

Zeis gland (zīs, tsīs) *n.* Any of the sebaceous glands opening into the follicles of the eyelashes.

Zeit·geist (tsīt′gīst′, zīt′-) *n.* The taste and outlook characteristic of a period or generation; the spirit of the time.

ze·ro (zēr′ō, zē′rō) *n., pl.* **-ros** or **-roes**. **1.** The numerical symbol 0, indicating the absence of quantity or mass. **2.** The temperature indicated by the numeral 0 on a thermometer. — *v.* To adjust an instrument or a device to zero value.

ze·ta·crit (zā′tə-krĭt′) *n.* Vertical centrifugation of blood in capillary tubes allowing controlled compaction and dispersion of the red blood cells.

ze·ta sedimentation ratio (zā′tə, zē′) *n.* The ratio of the zetacrit to the hematocrit, used as an indicator of the red blood cell sedimentation rate.

zi·do·vu·dine (zĭ-dō′vyōo-dēn′) *n.* Azidothymidine; AZT.

Zie·gler's operation (zē′glərz) *n.* A V-shaped iridotomy for the formation of an artificial pupil of the eye.

zinc (zĭngk) *n.* A lustrous metallic element with atomic number 30; it is an essential part of many enzymes and important in cell division and protein synthesis.

zinc ointment *n.* A salve consisting of about 20 percent zinc oxide with wax, such as beeswax or paraffin, and petroleum jelly, used in the treatment of skin disorders.

zinc oxide *n.* An amorphous white or yellowish powder used as a pigment, in compounding rubber, in the manufacture of plastics, and in pharmaceuticals and cosmetics.

zir·co·ni·um (zûr-kō′nē-əm) *n.* A lustrous strong ductile metallic element with atomic number 40.

zit (zĭt) *n.* A pimple.

zo·ac·an·tho·sis (zō′ăk′ən-thō′sĭs) *n.* An eruption caused by piercing of the skin with the hair, bristles, or stingers of an animal.

Zo·la·dex (zō′lä-dĕks′) *n.* The trademark for goserelin.

Zol·lin·ger–El·li·son syndrome (zŏl′ĭn-jər-ĕl′ĭ-sən) *n.* Peptic ulceration with gastric hypersecretion and non-beta cell tumor of the pancreatic islets.

Zo·loft (zō'lôft') A trademark for sertraline hydrochloride.

zo·na (zō'nə) *n., pl.* **-nae** (-nē). **1.** An encircling or beltlike anatomical structure. **2.** See **shingles**.

zona fas·cic·u·la·ta (fə-sĭk'yə-lā'tə) *n.* The layer of radially arranged cells in the cortical portion of the adrenal gland.

zona glo·mer·u·lo·sa (glŏ-mĕr'yə-lō'sə) *n.* The outer layer of the cortex of the adrenal gland, just beneath the capsule.

zona oph·thal·mi·ca (ŏf-thāl'mĭ-kə) *n.* The occurrence and distribution of herpes zoster in the ophthalmic nerve.

zona pel·lu·ci·da (pə-lōō'sĭ-də, pĕl-yōō'-) *n.* The thick, solid, transparent outer membrane of a developed mammalian ovum.

zona re·tic·u·lar·is (rĭ-tĭk'yə-lâr'ĭs) *n.* The inner layer of the cortex of the adrenal gland in which cell cords form a network.

zone (zōn) *n.* **1.** An area or a region distinguished from adjacent parts by a distinctive feature or characteristic. **2.** See **zona** (sense 1). **3.** A segment.

zo·nes·the·sia (zō'nĭs-thē'zhə) *n.* A sensation of constriction as if a cord were being drawn around the body.

zon·ing (zō'nĭng) *n.* An unexpectedly strong immunologic reaction in a small amount of serum, probably the result of high antibody titer.

zon·ule (zōn'yōōl) *n.* A small zone, as of a ligament. — **zo′nu·lar** (zōn'yə-lər) *adj.*

zo·nu·lol·y·sis (zōn'yə-lŏl'ĭ-sĭs) or **zo·nu·ly·sis** (-lĭ'sĭs) *n.* Enzymatic dissolution of the ciliary zonule to facilitate surgical removal of a cataract.

zo·o·e·ras·ti·a (zō'ō-ə-răs'tē-ə) *n.* See **bestiality**.

zo·o·graft (zō'ə-grăft') *n.* A graft in which tissue from a nonhuman animal is transferred to a human.

zo·o·graft·ing (zō'ə-grăf'tĭng) *n.* See **zooplasty**.

zo·oid (zō'oid') *n.* **1.** An organic cell or organized body that has independent movement within a living organism, especially a motile gamete such as a spermatozoon. **2.** An independent animallike organism produced asexually, as by budding or fission. **3.** One of the distinct individuals forming a colonial animal such as a coral.

zo·o·lag·ni·a (zō'ə-lăg'nē-ə) *n.* Sexual attraction to animals.

zo·on·o·sis (zō-ŏn'ə-sĭs, zō'ə-nō'-) *n., pl.* **-ses** (-sēz'). A disease of animals, such as rabies or psittacosis, that can be transmitted to humans. — **zo′o·not′ic** (zō'ə-nŏt'ĭk) *adj.*

zo·o·phil·i·a (zō'ə-fĭl'ē-ə) or **zo·oph·i·lism** (zō-ŏf'ə-lĭz'əm) or **zo·oph·i·ly** (-ə-lē) *n.* Attraction to or affinity for animals.

zo·o·pho·bi·a (zō'ə-fō'bē-ə) *n.* An abnormal fear of animals.

zo·o·plas·ty (zō'ə-plăs'tē) *n.* Surgical transfer of tissue from an animal to a human.

zos·ter (zŏs'tər) *n.* See **shingles**.

zoster immune globulin *n.* A globulin fraction of pooled plasma from donors who have recovered from infection by herpes zoster, used in the prevention and treatment of chickenpox.

Z-plas·ty (zē'plăs'tē) *n.* A surgical procedure to elongate a contracted scar or to rotate tension 90° in which the middle line of the Z-shaped incision is made along the line of greatest tension or contraction, and triangular flaps are raised on opposite sides of the two ends and then transposed.

zy·gal (zī'gəl) *adj.* Having a shape like othe letter H.

zy·go·gen·e·sis (zī'gō-jĕn'ĭ-sĭs) *n.* Reproduction involving the formation of a zygote.

zy·go·ma (zī-gō'mə, zĭ-) *n.* **1.** See **zygomatic arch**. **2.** See **zygomatic bone**.

zy·go·mat·ic (zī'gə-măt'ĭk, zĭg'ə-) *adj.* Of, relating to, or located in the area of the zygoma.

zygomatic arch *n.* The arch formed by the temporal process of the zygomatic bone that joins the zygomatic process of the temporal bone.

zygomatic bone *n.* A quadrilateral bone that forms the prominence of the cheek and articulates with the frontal, sphenoid, temporal, and maxillary bones.

zygomatic nerve *n.* A branch of the maxillary nerve that divides and supplies the skin of the temporal and zygomatic regions.

zygomatic process *n.* **1.** The rough projection from the maxilla that articulates with the zygomatic bone. **2.** Any of three processes that articulate with the zygomatic bone, especially the process from the temporal bone that articulates to form the zygomatic arch.

zygomatic process of the maxilla *n.* The rough projection of the maxilla that articulates with the zygomatic bone.

Zy·go·my·ce·tes (zī'gō-mī-sē'tēz) *n.* A subclass of fungi characterized by sexual reproduction resulting in the formation of a large multinucleate spore formed by the union of similar gametes.

zy·go·my·co·sis (zī'gō-mī-kō'sĭs) *n.* A fungus infection caused by various genera of the class Zygomycetes.

zy·gon (zī'gŏn') *n.* The short crossbar connecting the branches of a zygal fissure.

zy·go·ne·ma (zī'gə-nē'mə) *n.* See **zygotene**.

zy·go·sis (zī-gō'sĭs, zĭ-) *n., pl.* **-ses** (-sēz). The union of gametes to form a zygote; conjugation.

zy·gos·i·ty (zī-gŏs'ĭ-tē) *n.* The genetic condition of a zygote, especially with respect to its being a homozygote or a heterozygote.

zy·gote (zī'gōt') *n.* **1.** The cell formed by the union of two gametes, especially a fertilized ovum before cleavage. **2.** The organism that develops from a zygote. — **zy·got′ic** (-gŏt′ĭk) *adj.*

zy·go·tene (zī'gə-tēn') *n.* The stage of meiotic prophase during which precise point-for-point pairing of homologous chromosomes begins.

zy·mo·deme (zī'mə-dēm') *n.* An isoenzyme pattern, identified electrophoretically.

zy·mo·gen (zī'mə-jən) *n.* See **proenzyme**.

zy·mo·gen·e·sis (zī′mə-jĕn′ĭ-sĭs) *n*. The process by which a proenzyme is transformed into an active enzyme.

zy·mo·gen·ic (zī′mə-jĕn′ĭk) or **zy·mog·e·nous** (zī-mŏj′ə-nəs) *adj*. **1.** Of or relating to a proenzyme. **2.** Capable of causing fermentation. **3.** Enzyme-producing.

zy·mo·gen·ic cell (zī′mə-jĕn′ĭk) *n*. A cell that forms and secretes an enzyme, especially a secretory cell that lines the lumen of the gastric glands of the stomach and a pepsin-secreting acinar cell of the pancreas.

zy·mol·y·sis (zī-mŏl′ĭ-sĭs) *n*. Fermentation.

zy·mo·sis (zī-mō′sĭs) *n*. **1.** Fermentation. **2.** The process of infection. **3.** An infectious disease, especially one caused by a fungus.

Illustrations

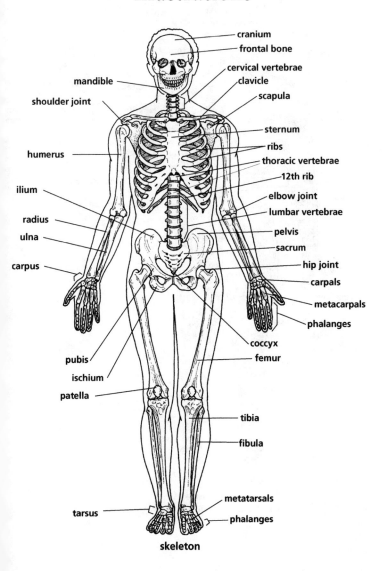

cranium
frontal bone
mandible
cervical vertebrae
clavicle
scapula
shoulder joint
sternum
ribs
thoracic vertebrae
12th rib
humerus
elbow joint
lumbar vertebrae
ilium
pelvis
radius
sacrum
ulna
hip joint
carpus
carpals
metacarpals
phalanges
coccyx
femur
pubis
ischium
patella
tibia
fibula
metatarsals
tarsus
phalanges

skeleton

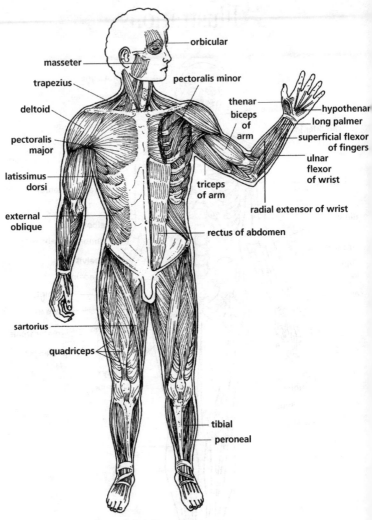

skeletal muscle
Anterior view of skeletal muscles

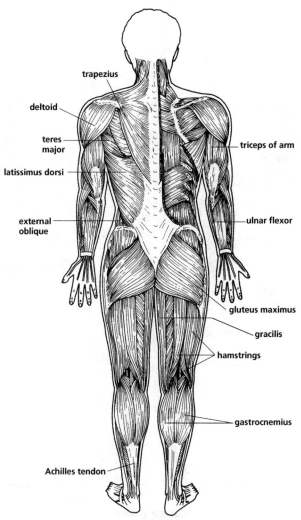

skeletal muscle
Posterior view of skeletal muscles

vascular system

Anterior view with veins shown in black. For veins and arteries that occur on both sides of the body, only one is labeled; eg., the right femoral vein has a matching left femoral vein.

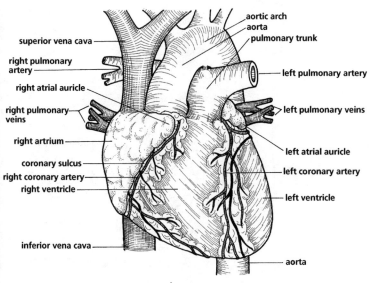

heart
Anterior view

- aortic arch
- aorta
- pulmonary trunk
- superior vena cava
- right pulmonary artery
- right atrial auricle
- right pulmonary veins
- right artrium
- coronary sulcus
- right coronary artery
- right ventricle
- inferior vena cava
- left pulmonary artery
- left pulmonary veins
- left atrial auricle
- left coronary artery
- left ventricle
- aorta

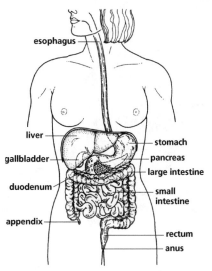

digestive system

- esophagus
- liver
- gallbladder
- duodenum
- appendix
- stomach
- pancreas
- large intestine
- small intestine
- rectum
- anus

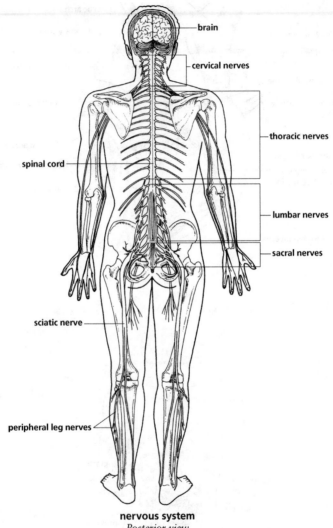

nervous system
Posterior view

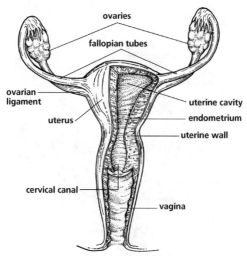

female reproductive system
Posterior view

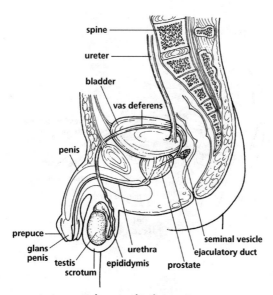

male reproductive system
Sagittal section

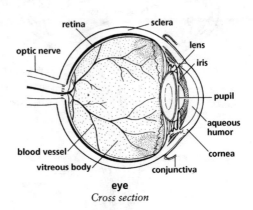

eye
Cross section

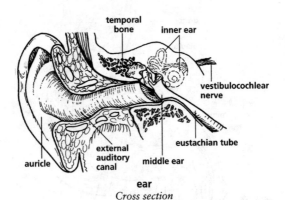

ear
Cross section